The Oxford
Illustrated Companion to

# Medicine

## Dedicated to
## Sir Ronald Bodley Scott (1906–1982)

The son of a general practitioner in Bournemouth, Ronald Bodley Scott was trained at St Bartholomew's Hospital Medical College after obtaining a degree in natural sciences at Brasenose College, Oxford, in 1928. After graduating in medicine in 1931, he joined the family practice in Bournemouth but subsequently was invited to return to St Bartholomew's Hospital as first assistant on the medical professorial unit. His published papers indicate that his interest in hematology began in 1933 and he subsequently published extensively on the reticuloses and hemolytic states, and with A. H. T. Robb-Smith described histiocytic medullary reticulosis in 1939. He distinguished himself in military service in the Middle East in the Second World War, subsequently being elected physician to St Bartholomew's Hospital and developing his research interests in leukemia and lymphoma. He worked ceaselessly towards the integration of laboratory and clinical medicine. He was appointed physician to King George VI in 1949 and to Queen Elizabeth II in 1952, and was knighted in 1964. He delivered the Lettsomian lectures to the Medical Society of London in 1957, and the Langdon-Brown, Croonian, and Harveian Orations to the Royal College of Physicians of London, and was successively counsellor, censor, and vice-president of that College, master of the Society of Apothecaries (1974), and an editor of *Price's Textbook of the Practice of Medicine.* At times appearing somewhat shy and reserved, he nevertheless possessed a rich vein of kindness and humility and an astringent wit, and was a most notable figure in British medicine. With Paul Beeson he conceived the idea of a *Companion,* and the planning of the book was well advanced at the time of his death.

# The Oxford Illustrated Companion to
# Medicine

*Edited by*
Stephen Lock, John M. Last, and George Dunea

*Emeritus editors*
John Walton, Paul B. Beeson, Jeremiah A. Barondess

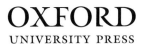

OXFORD
UNIVERSITY PRESS

# OXFORD
UNIVERSITY PRESS

Great Clarendon Street, Oxford OX2 6DP

Oxford University Press is a department of the University of Oxford.
It furthers the University's objective of excellence in research, scholarship,
and education by publishing worldwide in

Oxford New York

Athens Auckland Bangkok Bogotá Buenos Aires Cape Town Chennai
Dar es Salaam Delhi Florence Hong Kong Istanbul Karachi Kolkata
Kuala Lumpur Madrid Melbourne Mexico City Mumbai Nairobi Paris
São Paulo Shanghai Singapore Taipei Tokyo Toronto Warsaw

with associated companies in Berlin Ibadan

Oxford is a registered trade mark of Oxford University Press
in the UK and in certain other countries

Published in the United States
by Oxford University Press Inc., New York

Library of Congress Cataloguing in Publication Data
The Oxford illustrated companion to medicine/edited by Stephen Lock,
John M. Last, and George Dunea; emeritus editors, John Walton,
Paul B. Beeson, Jeremiah A. Barondess.

Rev. ed. of: The Oxford medical companion/edited by John Walton (Lord
Walton of Detchant), Jeremiah A. Barondess, and Stephen Lock.
Includes bibliographical references and indexes.
1. Medicine–Dictionaries 2. Medicine–Biography–Dictionaries I. Lock,
Stephen, 1929– II. Last, John M., 1926– III. Dunea, George. IV. Oxford
medical companion.
[DNLM: 1. Medicine–Dictionary–English. W 13 O976 2001]
R121.O884 2001 610'.3–dc21 2001021799
ISBN 0 19 262950 6 (Hbk.)

10 9 8 7 6 5 4 3 2 1

Typeset in Minion
by Expo Holdings
Printed in Great Britain
on acid-free paper by
Butler & Tanner Ltd, Frome, Somerset

# Acknowledgements

Many authors thank spouses, friends, and colleagues for inspiration and help received with their contributions to this book. The editors also acknowledge with thanks the help they received from family, friends, and colleagues. In particular, we would thank Dr Sanjay Pai and Professor John Pearn for their many comments and suggestions, most of which were instrumental in the shaping of the revised edition.

# How to use this *Companion*

Unlike the two earlier editions, this new *Companion* does not have an entirely alphabetical arrangement. Biographies and other short entries are now often placed near the related main text: for example, Sun Yat-Sen appears within China and the Salerno Medical School within Italy. Such entries are extensively cross-referenced, being shown in the text as small capitals (SALERNO), with the page number in parentheses if they are not in alphabetical order.

References to articles placed in alphabetical order also appear in small capitals in the text. When the treatment is extensive, however, the reference appears at the end of the article (*See also . . .*).

Because of the diversity of the subjects covered, this *Companion* contains no fewer than four indexes. The Topic Index groups articles under broad themes, such as The Arts or Institutions, and its entries overlap those in the other indexes. The List of Individual Conditions and Diseases is confined to the separate medical subjects discussed. The General Index is broader, listing subjects not necessarily covered in the List, but again with some overlap. Finally, the People Index lists non-living persons given a substantial mention or a separate biography (page number in **bold**).

Some articles carried over from the previous editions, and a few new ones, appear without attribution, and the editors take full responsibility for these.

# Preface

A companion is a friend, a guide, and a support in everyday life. This *Companion* is not a dictionary, encyclopedia, or treat-yourself manual. Instead, addressed to the general reader as well as to the professional, it offers explanation and comment in plain English rather than in the technical language that healthcare professionals use among themselves. Such was also the aim of the two previous editions of this work, but here not only have the articles been updated but many new features introduced.

Thus, as well as articles on the history and present-day scope of the principal specialties, there is a greatly increased emphasis on alternative medicine as well as on the other disciplines where medicine impinges: the sciences, fine arts, politics, sociology, and economics, to mention only a few. There are also many more illustrations than before, with color plates interspersed throughout the book for the first time.

We have aimed at choosing expert authors from as wide a variety of countries as possible. The feature on 'Burnout', for example, comes from Finland; that on 'Regulation of the professions' from Australia; and that on 'Serendipity' from India. And the diversity of the earlier editions is continued by separate considerations of medical education and healthcare in countries as different as China and Pakistan, or Russia and Italy.

Another new feature is the highlighting of some killer diseases, whether largely of the past (such as plague and diphtheria) or the present (AIDS or atheroma). Often the margins of these articles now have short biographies of some of the prominent people concerned — a practice used in other articles — so that, together with the extended treatment of some of the greatest names in medicine in the text, there is a strong biographical emphasis.

Self-evidently the wide diversity of subjects is the essence of a Companion that seeks not only to inform but also to entertain, to be for reference but also for browsing. Yet there is a risk that readers might become confused or miss what they seek. We have tackled this problem by providing an index in four parts: one listing all the biographies in the *Companion*; another a Topic Index listing the subjects considered, often in several different articles; and the others a List of Individual Conditions and Diseases and a General Index. In addition, major references to such related topics are cross-indexed in the articles themselves (see the preceding 'How to use this *Companion*').

The authors of the main articles are identified by initials, and the views expressed are their own. In a few instances, such as 'Boxing' and 'the USA', these views are diametrically opposed to those held by one or more of the editors. This may merely reflect the well-known facts that doctors often disagree, and that medical progress is frequently rapid. This is as it should be, for without debate (as this book shows) the course of medicine would have run very differently.

Finally we thank not only all our contributors for sparing the time to write, but also the team at Oxford University Press for their help.

**Stephen Lock** (Aldeburgh, UK), **John M. Last** (Ottawa, Canada), **George Dunea** (Chicago, USA)

# Contents

# List of Color Plates

# List of Contributors

DGA  Douglas G. Altman, University of Oxford, UK

GA  George Alberti, Royal College of Physicians, London, UK

JAA  Johan A. Aarli, University of Bergen, Norway

JKA  J. K. Aronson, University of Oxford, UK

KA  Ken Arnold, Wellcome Trust Centre for the History of Medicine, London, UK

MA  Manzoor Ahmad (Formerly: Medical Services Pakistan Army)

PCA  Peter C. Arnold (Formerly: New South Wales Medical Board, Sydney, Australia)

SA  Stuart Anderson, London School of Hygiene and Tropical Medicine, UK

TA  Tom Arie, University of Nottingham, UK

AGB  Alexander G. Bearn, American Philosophical Society, Philadelphia, USA

AEB  Arnold E. Bender (Deceased) (Formerly: University of London, UK)

CCB  Christopher C. Booth, Wellcome Trust Centre for the History of Medicine, London, UK

DBro  Dorothyanne Brown Last, Public Health Unit, Kingston, Canada

DJB  David J. Bradley, University of London, UK

EEPB  E. E. Peter Barnard (Formerly: Royal Navy, UK)

GB  Glin Bennet (Formerly: University of Bristol, UK)

HB  Harvey Barkun (Formerly: McGill University, Canada)

IB  Ivan Blumenthal, University of Manchester, UK

JABaro  Jeremiah A. Barondess, New York Academy of Medicine, USA

JB  James Barrett, Maudsley Hospital, London, UK

JBai  John Baillie, Duke University Medical Center, North Carolina, USA

JBarr  John Barrett, Cook County Hospital, Chicago, USA

JPBun  John P. Bunker, University of London, UK

LBres  Lester Breslow, UCLA School of Public Health, Los Angeles, USA

LBry  Linda Bryder, University of Auckland, New Zealand

LEB  Lars Erik Böttiger (Formerly: Karolinska Institute, Stockholm, Sweden)

MB  Michael Baum, University of London, UK

OB  O. Blin, Centre Hôpitalo-Universitaire de la Timone, Marseilles, France

PMB  Peter M. Brooks, University of Queensland, Australia

RDHB  Robert D. H. Boyd, University of London, UK

SRB  Solomon R. Benatar, University of Cape Town, South Africa

SBra  Sydney Brandon (Formerly: University of Leicester, UK)

TBB  Thurstan B. Brewin (Deceased) (Formerly: University of Glasgow, UK)

VB  Virginia Berridge, London School of Tropical Medicine and Hygiene, UK

WB  Walter Bodmer, University of Oxford, UK

WFB  William B. Bynum, University of London, UK

WHB  William H. Brock (Formerly: University of Leicester, UK)

AC  Antonio Carreras, Salamanca, Spain

AHCri  Arthur H. Crisp (Formerly: University of London, UK)

ALCrom  A. L. Crombie, University of Newcastle upon Tyne, UK

CC  Charles Clarke, National Hospital for Nervous Diseases, London, UK

DAC  Donald A. Chambers, University of Illinois at Chicago, USA

GC  Geoffrey Chamberlain, Singleton Hospital, Swansea, UK

GCCoo  Gordon C. Cook, Wellcome Trust Centre for the History of Medicine, London, UK

HLC  Helen L. Crimlisk, Maudsley Hospital, London, UK

JC  Jocelyn Chamberlain (Formerly: University of London, UK)

JCoh  Jonathan Cohen, Tufts Medical School, Boston, USA

PBC  Paul B. Cooper, Swiss Re Life and Health Limited, London, UK

RCoo  Roger Cooter, University of East Anglia, UK

RCro  Richard Croxon, Swiss Re Life and Health Limited, London, UK

RLC  Dr Rhonna L. Cohen, University of Illinois, Chicago

RLCru  Richard L. Cruess, McGill University, Montreal, Canada

RYC  Roy Y. Calne, University of Cambridge, UK

| | | | |
|---|---|---|---|
| SC | Suzanne Cherney, UNAIDS, Geneva, Switzerland | SG | Shane Godbolt, British Postgraduate Medical Federation, London, UK |
| SSC | Steven S. Coughlin, Centers for Disease Control and Prevention, Atlanta, USA | TJG | Thomas J. Gamper, University of Virginia, USA |
| TCon | Terence Conway, Cook County Hospital, Chicago, USA | APH | Andrew P. Haines, University of London, UK |
| TGC | Timothy G. Chard, University of London, UK | AHar | Anne Hardy, Wellcome Trust Centre for the History of Medicine, London, UK |
| VKKC | V. K. K. Chatterjee, University of Cambridge, UK | AHol | Arthur Hollman (Formerly: University College Hospital, London, UK) |
| WHC | W.H. Chapman, University of Washington, Seattle, USA | BH | Brian Hurwitz, University of London, UK |
| YC | Yrjö Collan, University of Turku, Finland | BJH | Bruce J. Hillman, University of Virginia, USA |
| AD | Anne Dally, Wellcome Trust Centre for the History of Medicine, London, UK | EJH | Edward J. Huth (Formerly: *Annals of Internal Medicine*, Philadelphia, USA) |
| BMD | Bernard M. Dickens, University of Toronto, Canada | JAH | Jason A. Hannah, McMaster University, Canada |
| EBD | Emery B. Dowell, California Managed Risk Insurance Board, USA | JH | John Havard, British Medical Association, London, UK |
| GD | George Dunea, Cook County Hospital, Chicago, USA | JHaz | Jennifer Hazelgrove, Wellcome Trust Centre for the History of Medicine, London, UK |
| GRD | Gordon R. Dunstan (Formerly: University of London, UK) | JHow | John G. R. Howie, University of Edinburgh, UK |
| J-ARD | Jo-Anne R. Dillon, University of Ottawa, Canada | KH | Keith Hawton, Oxford, UK |
| JMDun | James M. Dunlop, Hull, UK | LAH | Lesley A. Hall, Wellcome Trust Centre for the History of Medicine, London, UK |
| JOD | J. O. Drife, University of Leeds, UK | MH | Mark Harrison, Sheffield Hallam University, UK |
| MD | Michael Donaghy, University of Oxford, UK | MHut | Marten Hutt, Health Services Research Centre, Auckland, NZ |
| RD | Roger Detels, UCLA School of Public Health, Los Angeles, USA | MHyd | Masood Hyder, World Food Programme, New York, USA (this article represents his personal views) |
| TLD | Theo L. Dorpat, University of Washington, Seattle, USA | PH | Patricia Huston, University of Ottawa, Canada |
| AEHE | Alan E. H. Emery, University of Oxford, UK | RH | Robin Higgins (Formerly: Goldsmiths' College, London, UK) |
| BTE | Bryan T. Emmerson, University of Queensland, Brisbane, Australia | RHim | Richard Himsworth, University of Cambridge, UK |
| EE | E. Emanuel, Harvard Medical School, USA | RHof | Raymond Hoffenberg, University of Oxford, UK |
| JGE | John Grimley Evans, University of Oxford, UK | SH | Shigeaki Hinohara, The Life Planning Center, Tokyo, Japan |
| LE | Liz Evans, Human Genome Organization Europe, London, UK | WHec | Winifred Hector (Deceased) (Formerly: St Bartholomew's Hospital, London, UK) |
| MHLE | Marcia H. L. Emery, University of Oxford, UK | WHol | Walter Holland, University of London, UK |
| MTE | Milton T. Edgerton, University of Virginia, USA | WHt | Wimpeter Hart, *Dutch Journal of Medicine*, Amsterdam, The Netherlands |
| AWF | Alfred White Franklin (Deceased) (Formerly: St Bartholomew's Hospital, London, UK) | DJ | Dana Jerome, University of Ottawa, Canada |
| DWF | Derek W. Forrest, Trinity College, Dublin, Republic of Ireland | HJ | Hershel Jick, Boston University Medical Center, USA |
| EF | Erika Frank, Emory University, Atlanta, USA | RKJ | R. K. Jordan, University of Newcastle upon Tyne, UK |
| TGF | Terry G. Feest, University of Bristol, UK | | |
| AMG | Alasdair M. Geddes, University of Birmingham, UK | BJK | Bernard J. Knight (Formerly: University of Wales, UK) |
| CJG | Chris J. Glynn, University of Oxford, UK | | |
| DDG | Denis D. Gibbs (Formerly: The Royal London Hospital, UK) | DK | David N. S. Kerr (Formerly: University of London, UK) |
| GAG | G. Austin Gresham, University of Cambridge, UK | GK | George Kazantzis, University of London, UK |
| JG | John Garfield (Formerly: Wessex Neurological Centre, Southampton, UK) | HiK | Hilda Kalant, British Red Cross, London, UK |
| | | HK | Harold Kalant, University of Toronto, Canada |
| MGG | M. G. Gelder, University of Oxford, UK | KK | Karen Trollope Kumar, McMaster University, Canada |
| MVG | Maria Vittoria Gianelli, University of Genoa, Italy | | |
| PDG | Peter D. Griffith, University of Dundee, UK | BL | Brian Lentle, University of British Columbia, Canada |
| RG | Roy Goulding (Formerly: University of London, UK) | CL | Christopher Lawrence, Wellcome Trust Centre for the History of Medicine, London, UK |

| | |
|---|---|
| DML | Donlin M. Long, Johns Hopkins University, USA |
| EL | Edward Lowbury (Formerly: University of Aston, UK) |
| GL | George Lewith, University of Southampton, UK |
| IL | Irvine Loudon, Wantage, UK |
| JML | John M. Last, University of Ottawa, Canada |
| ML | Maurice Lessof, University of London, UK |
| MLiu | Min Lui, Beijing Union Medical College, China |
| NL | Nicky Leap, Adelaide, Australia |
| PJL | Peter J. Lachmann, University of Cambridge, UK |
| RL | Ray Lewkonia, University of Calgary, Canada |
| RLit | Roland Littlewood, University of London, UK |
| SEL | Susan E. Lederer, Milton S. Hershey Medical Center, USA |
| SLei | Sidney Leibowitz (Deceased) (Formerly: University of London, UK) |
| SPL | Stephen P. Lock (Formerly: *British Medical Journal*, UK) |
| TL | Thomas Lynch, Milford, USA |
| AAFM | Adel A. F. Mahmoud, University Hospitals of Cleveland, USA |
| AAGMor | Andrew A.G. Morrice, Wellcome Trust Centre for the History of Medicine, London, UK |
| AJM | Anthony J. McMichael, University of London, UK |
| AKMay | Alan K. Maynard, University of York, UK |
| FHM | Frank H. Morriss, Jnr, University of Iowa, USA |
| GM | Gordon Macpherson (Formerly: *British Medical Journal*, UK) |
| GMul | Graham Mulley, University of Leeds, UK |
| LMc | Lynn Mcintyre, Dalhousie University, Canada |
| MM | Marshall Marinker, University of London, UK |
| NM | Neil McIntyre, University of London, UK |
| RJRM | Robert J. R. McKendry, University of Ottawa, Canada |
| RM | Robert McNutt, Cook County Hospital, Chicago, USA |
| RMah | R. Mahoney, University of Otago, NZ |
| SGM | S. G. Marketos, University of Athens, Greece |
| TJM | T. Jock Murray, Dalhousie University, Canada |
| WKCM | W. Keith C. Morgan, University of Western Ontario, Canada |
| DN | Derek North, University of Auckland, NZ |
| MNN | M. N. Naylor (Formerly: University of London, UK) |
| ZEN | Zeev E. Neuwirth, New York University School of Medicine, USA |
| AJO | A J. Overbeke, *Dutch Journal of Medicine*, Amsterdam, The Netherlands |
| EO | Eoin O'Brien, University College, Dublin, Republic of Ireland |
| IO | Ian Oswald (Formerly: University of Edinburgh, UK) |
| RKO | R. Kim Oates, University of Sydney, Australia |
| AP | Alex Paton, Chadlington, Oxford, UK |
| APol | Alessandro Polleri, University of Genoa, Italy |
| APor-S | Alberto Portera-Sanchez, Universidad Complutense, Madrid, Spain |
| CP | Christopher Pallis (Formerly: Royal Postgraduate Medical School, London, UK) |
| CPP | C. P. Panaytiotoulos, St Thomas's Hospital, London, UK |
| DPi | Daniel Pick, University of London, UK |
| DPim | David Pimental, Cornell University, USA |
| JHP | John H. Pearn, University of Queensland, Brisbane, Australia |
| KP | Kim Pelis, Armed Forces Institute, Bethesda, USA |
| MCP | Michael C. Petch, Papworth Hospital, Cambridge, UK |
| PP | Peter Piot, UNAIDS, Geneva, Switzerland |
| PPon | Pedro Ponce, Caracas, Venezuela |
| RGP | Robert G. Petersdorf, University of Washington, Seattle, USA |
| RPor | Roy Porter, Wellcome Trust Centre for the History of Medicine, London, UK |
| SAP | Sanjay A. Pai, Bangalore Hospital, India |
| SJP | Stephen J. Proctor, University of Newcastle upon Tyne, UK |
| SKP | Sunil K. Pandya, Jaslok Hospital, Mumbai, India |
| WP-P | William Pryse-Phillips, Memorial University of Newfoundland, Canada |
| AMR | Anne Marie Rafferty, University of London, UK |
| BR | Beverly Raphael, University of Sydney, Australia |
| CGR | Charles G. Roland, McMaster University, Canada |
| GBR | Guenter B. Risse, University of California, San Francisco, USA |
| HJCR | H. J. C. van Rensburg, University of Cape Town, South Africa |
| HRR | Henry R. Rollin (Formerly: Horton Hospital, Epsom, UK) |
| MDR | Michael D. Rawlins, University of Newcastle upon Tyne, UK |
| MIR | Milton I. Roemer (Deceased) (Formerly: University of California, Los Angeles, USA) |
| PJR | P. John Rees, Guy's Hospital, London, UK |
| PRii | Povl Riis, University of Copenhagen, Denmark |
| RR | Ricardo Rangel, Mexico City, Mexico |
| RRic | Ruth Richardson, Wellcome Trust Centre for the History of Medicine, London, UK |
| TJLR | Tessa J. L. Richards, *British Medical Journal*, UK |
| TKRos | Todd K. Rosengart, Cornell University, USA |
| TMRy | T. Michael Ryan (Formerly: University of Wales, UK) |
| VSR | Veena Sona Raleigh, London School of Tropical Medicine and Hygiene, UK |
| ASmi | Tony Smith, *British Medical Journal*, UK |
| ASto | Anthony Storr (Deceased) (Formerly: University of Oxford, UK) |
| CS | Cicely Saunders, St Christopher's Hospice, London, UK |
| CSen | Chendak Sengoopta, Wellcome Trust Centre for the History of Medicine, London, UK |
| CSte | Christine Stevenson, University of Reading, UK |
| DES | Dixie E. Snider, Center for Disease Control and Prevention, Atlanta, USA |
| EDS | E. Dorinda Shelley, Medical College of Ohio, Toledo, USA |

GDS   Gordon D. Schiff, Cook County Hospital, Chicago, USA

GSer  Georges Serratrice, Centre Hôpitalo-Universitaire de la Timone, Marseilles, France

JDS   J. Dean Sandham, University of Calgary, Canada

PNS   Peter N. Sperryn, Brunel University, UK

RAS   Re'ad A. Shakir, Charing Cross Hospital, London, UK

RS    Richard Smith, *British Medical Journal*, UK

RWS   Ralph W. Schaffarzich (Formerly: Blue Shield of California, USA)

US    Udo Schagen, Freie Universität, Berlin, Germany

VWS   Victor W. Sidel, Albert Einstein College of Medicine, New York, USA

WBShe Walter B. Shelley, Medical College of Ohio, Toledo, USA

WES   William E. Seidelman, University of Toronto, Canada

AST   A. Stuart Truswell, University of Sydney, Australia

ET    E. Tapp, Centre for Forensic and Paleopathology, Preston, UK

IT    Ian Tait, Wellcome Trust Centre for the History of Medicine, London, UK

JHT   John H. Tyrer, University of Queensland, Brisbane, Australia

JST   Jeffrey S. Tobias, University College Hospitals, London, UK

PT    Pamela Thompson, Centre for Forensic and Paleopathology, Preston, UK

RBT   R. B. Tattersall, University of Nottingham, UK

TT    Tilly Tansey, Wellcome Trust Centre for the History of Medicine, London, UK

ACU   A. C. Upton, New York University School of Medicine, USA

AV    Adulya Viriyavejakul, Mahidol University, Thailand

BV    Bernard Valman, Northwick Park Hospital, London, UK

IV    Ilkka Vartiovaara, Helsinki, Finland

JPV   Jan P. Vandenbroucke, University of Leiden, The Netherlands

LDV   Leroy D. Vandam, Harvard Medical School, USA

BW    Brian Williams, University of Nottingham, UK

DIWil David Innes Williams (Formerly: University of London, UK)

DW    David Warrell, University of Oxford, UK

DW-T  David Walter-Toews, University of Guelph, Canada

DWea  David Weatherall, University of Oxford, UK

HAW   Anthony W. Waldron, University of London, UK

HNWhi H. N. Whitfield, Institute of Urology, London, UK

HWhi  Harvey White, Royal Marsden Hospital, London, UK

JEAW  John E.A. Wickham (Formerly: Institute of Urology, London, UK)

JLWil John L. Wilkinson (Formerly: University of Wales, UK)

JW    John Walton, University of Oxford, UK

KLW   Kerr L. White (Formerly: The Rockefeller Foundation, New York, USA)

KSW   Kathrine Sorley Walker (Formerly: *The Daily Telegraph*, London UK)

LW    Lise Wilkinson, Wellcome Trust Centre for the History of Medicine, London, UK

LWil  Lori Williamson, Oxford Brookes University, UK

MAW   Michael A. Waugh, Leeds, UK

MWea  Miles Weatherall (Formerly: University of London, UK)

MWor  Michael Worboys, Sheffield Hallam University, UK

NW    Neil Weir, Guildford, UK

PW    Peter Worlock, John Radcliffe Hospital, Oxford, UK

RBW   Richard B. Welbourn (Formerly: University of London, UK)

RGWil Robert G. Will, University of Edinburgh, UK

RWoo  Richard Wootton, Queen's University, Belfast, UK

WFW   William F. Whimster (Deceased) (Formerly: University of London, UK)

YX    Yang Xie, Peking Union Medical College, China

KZ    Kong-lai Zhang, Peking Union Medical College, China

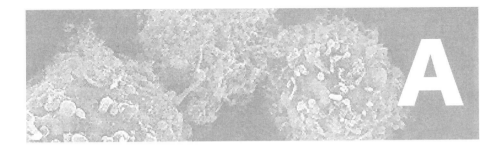

# A

**ABORTION** The loss of an immature embryo or fetus before viability is an abortion. When this happens spontaneously, the softer English word miscarriage is usually used, the word abortion being kept for the intended removal of the fetus from the uterus. Whilst miscarriages are common and are very disappointing to the couple, they are not considered in this entry. The purposeful removal of the embryo from the uterus may be done according to the laws of a country in which the couple reside (legal abortion) or may be performed without the law (illegal abortion).

## Therapeutic abortion

Many countries in the Western world have passed laws that allow pregnancy to be terminated under certain strict conditions. Religious and cultural aspects of termination of pregnancy vary from one country to another and from one religion to another. Termination is unacceptable in many of the world's religions but in fact is performed everywhere regardless of the religious laws or the ethics of the country. Unfortunately, if it is not legal, women will go to untrained and ill-equipped abortionists, with a resulting high rate of illness and death. The WORLD HEALTH ORGANIZATION estimates that world-wide 110 000 women die and six times as many are damaged every year from badly performed illegal abortions.

*Abortion in Britain* Abortion used to be illegal in Britain but gradually by the 1930s it was realized that in certain cases a termination of pregnancy would be medically wise such as pregnancy resulting from rape or for a woman with severe disease who might deteriorate in pregnancy. In 1938 Alec Bourne, a gynecologist, terminated a pregnancy in a 14-year-old girl who had been raped, informing the police that he had done so. This led to a criminal charge and after a long trial Bourne was found not guilty. An *ober dictum* was laid down which became case law for all judges below the Court of Appeal, when the judge said that a doctor may 'terminate a pregnancy if the risk to the mother's health, physical or mental, was greater than the continuation of pregnancy'.

Under such case law, termination of pregnancy was performed in the United Kingdom in the 1940s and 50s but probably never rose above 20 000 per year in the whole country. Towards the end of the 1960s a Liberal member of parliament, David Owen, introduced the Medical Termination of Pregnancy Bill. A free vote in the House of Commons passed the bill and the Abortion Act of 1968 was implemented. It was not until the 1970s that the rate exceeded 100 000 a year and it has plateaued in the last few years. In 1990 the bill was revised to reduce the age of viability from 28 to 24 weeks, in line with pediatric developments, for many babies born at 26 to 27 weeks were saved in neonatal units. A clause was also inserted allowing termination past this time if the baby 'would suffer from such physical or mental abnormalities as to be seriously handicapped'. Neither *substantial risk* nor *seriously handicapped* were defined. The Abortion Act applies to England, Wales, and Scotland but not to Northern Ireland, where political unrest has been shown to arise from religious divides and it was felt that the Abortion Act would cause disruption. Any doctor or nurse in Britain may on grounds of conscience not take part in such procedures.

Most terminations in Britain are performed before the twelfth week of pregnancy and only 2.5% after the twentieth week. Almost 90% of terminations are performed under the clause which states that the risk of injury to the physical or

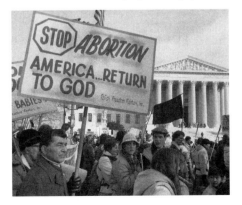

Nearly 70 000 opponents of abortion marched in front of the Supreme Court of the USA in March 1984 to mark the 11th anniversary of the Court's decision to legalize abortion. (© Bettmann/Corbis).

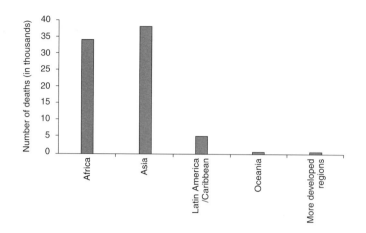

Estimates of deaths from unsafe abortions by continent, late 1980s–early 1990s. (from WHO data.)

mental health of a pregnant women would be greater by continuing the pregnancy than by terminating it. Termination might more commonly be requested by women aged under 20, compared with the distribution of births, which peaks in the late twenties. Any legal termination of pregnancy must be notified to the relevant Department of Health of England, Wales, or Scotland. The figures derived from the notifications are published every quarter and consolidated every year; less good statistics occur in other countries. The penalties for performing a termination of pregnancy outside the Abortion Act are severe. If a doctor or midwife is shown to have performed an illegal termination they are struck off the register and cannot practice; a prison sentence may be involved for those who break this law.

*Methods* A woman considering termination of pregnancy usually goes to her general practitioner. About 80% have made up their minds before arrival there even though the Abortion Act implies that the decision is a medical one and appears to give the woman no choice. If practitioners consider there are reasonable grounds, they sign the certificate and the woman is then referred on to a local gynecological department or private clinic; the second signatory is usually a member of staff of that hospital or clinic. The woman is counselled and the whole procedure discussed beforehand. It is wise to leave time between the decision and the termination, for some women change their minds and should be supported in this decision.

The termination may be performed by either drugs which make the uterus contract to expel the embryo or by instruments which extract the fetus. Both methods require skills and if done incorrectly carry a high risk of death or damage to the mother. Therapeutic termination performed in developed countries has been rendered much more safe because of antiseptics, which

have reduced infection; safer general ANESTHE-SIA; better training of doctors; and the changes in the abortion laws which have encouraged women to seek trained medical advice early. It is much easier to terminate a pregnancy before ten weeks; in later pregnancy it becomes harder and more dangerous. Whether medical or surgical methods are used depends to some extent on the hospital; there are arguments in favor of either method but a medical method does not involve an anesthetic whereas an operation does. However, the woman who has a surgical termination is treated on the spot and may go home usually the same day with the process completed.

The medical methods involve the use of a combination of antiprogesterone hormones (Mifepristone) and prostaglandins. This is used between five and nine weeks after the last menstrual period. It is safe and 95% effective if used before the seventh week (93% after that); two visits to the hospital are required. Commonly surgical abortions are done by vacuum curettage under local or general anesthesia (mostly the latter) and usually between 6 and 13 weeks of pregnancy. It is a day case procedure, taking about ten minutes. The cervix is dilated and the contents of the uterus evacuated through a plastic tube under negative pressure. There are some risks to both the anesthesia and the surgery, but these are minimized with experienced professionals and proper preoperative screening. It is wise to give a prophylactic antibiotic to cover the operation.

Between 13 and 18 weeks the cervix requires even further dilation under anesthesia, the fetus being removed by curettage and extraction; blood loss is heavier than with earlier surgical terminations, and probably involves an overnight stay in hospital. A late medical induction may be done after 13 weeks by producing a mini-labour using Mifepristone and vaginal prostaglandins or injections of prostaglandins and urea straight into the sac surrounding the fetus. This takes some hours of mini-labour and pain relief should be provided, preferably by the epidural route. The placenta may be retained and have to be removed under anesthesia; the risk of infection or damage to the uterus rises with the weeks of pregnancy. Most gynecologists are unhappy with the late terminations of pregnancy not just because of increased operative risks to the mother but because of the psychological effect it has on the women and on the attending health care staff. However, in very few cases a major abnormality is diagnosed after 20 weeks and this leads to the woman's request for a termination of pregnancy. Usually this is performed by injection of prostaglandins and urea into the fetal sac. The latter kills the fetus and delivery follows apace.

The complications of abortion are damage to the uterus, bleeding, or infection. There is a small risk if general anesthesia is given, but this is very small in the western world with properly qualified anesthetists. Afterwards, the woman may have some irregular bleeding, and psychological sequels of distress must be recognized and dealt with. Most well-balanced women who go into a termination of pregnancy wishing it to be done will not be psychologically scarred. If there is any blackmailing or unwillingness of the woman for the procedure, there is a serious risk of depression afterwards.

*Abortion world-wide* In the western world legal abortions have increased in the last 30 years after liberalization of the statutes of most countries, even those of Europe considered to be very Catholic in outlook. Most contain constraints but until 12 weeks of gestation allow abortion, especially if there is danger to life of the mother (95%) or to preserve the physical health of the mother (60%). In few countries now is abortion illegal in all circumstances.

In the USA there are 52 different sets of law — 50 states, the District of Columbia, and New York City all having different interpretations of federal law guidance from the Supreme Court. Since 1990 abortions have declined each year; between 1993 and 1994 there was a 4.7% decrease. Most women were young and white with 88% of terminations before 13 weeks. The debate and the opinions polarize more in the USA than in Britain, with violent and fatal attacks on those who perform terminations by antiabortionists. In Singapore liberal abortion legislation resulted in 35% of all pregnancies being terminated in 1985. This was reduced to 24% by 1993 with the introduction of mandatory counseling. Multiparous women made up 41% of terminations that year, with 95% seeking them for social reasons.

In Eastern Europe abortion was used as a means of contraception as other methods were not available. For example, in Romania at the end of the Ceaucescu government in 1989, repeal of the law banning abortion on demand led to the annual number of terminations rising from about 110 000 to 914 000. This was accompanied by a decline in deaths from unsafe operations from 447 to 142. At present, contraception in Romania is hard to obtain as contraceptives are not produced locally.

## Illegal abortions

In association with the introduction of the Terminations of Pregnancy Act in 1968 there has been a reduction in illegal abortions in the United Kingdom. Now, a procedure that kills almost 20% of women in the world kills none in Britain at all.

In countries where family planning is not easily available for social, religious, or political reasons

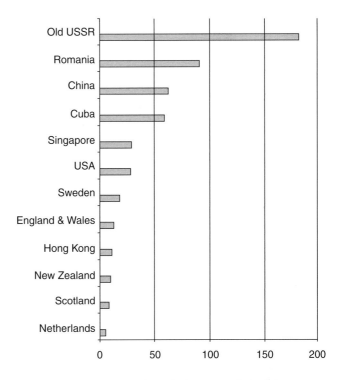

there will be a high incidence of illegal abortion. Further, our current methods of contraception are not fully effective and so women still will seek termination of pregnancy. If they cannot find it medically they will turn to illegal ways. In many societies there are men and women who practice illegal abortions; they become more skilled with time but the methods used are coarse and often damaging. In some regions the abortionist will make a tour arriving in a village at a regular time each week or fortnight. All the women of the area know this and will use the service. Hence a wave of illness and even death follows the abortionist around.

Ineffectual methods used for abortion are legion: jumping off tables, gin, the bark of trees, castor oil, penny royal, quinine, and local potassium permanganate have all been tried with various degrees of ineffectiveness. The production of the antiprogestogen drugs has up to now been carefully controlled and used mostly under medical care. Some illegal abortionists have obtained supplies and are offering them but unless the checks and controls required are maintained, they could prove to be dangerous or ineffectual.

In the developing countries, the abortionist mostly uses physical methods by the introduction of catheters through the cervix often accompanied by an injection of toxic substances. A false air of caution is sought by injecting an antiseptic but these may pass into the body cavities causing

The legal abortion rate per 1000 women aged 15–44 in various countries 1980s–1990s. (from WHO data.)

severe irritation of tissues followed by infection and death. Some try to dilate the cervix with hydroscopic tree bark or seaweed aiming at opening up the neck of the womb and thus allowing expulsion of the fetus. The results are variable.

These methods, particularly the surgical ones, may lead to damage to the woman's genital tract, with sepsis and bleeding. The more fortunate may end up in a local hospital, but in many cases there is no such facility.

## ABSINTHE

Absinthe is a strongly alcoholic drink produced by distillation and flavored by wormwood (*Artemisia absinthium*), prolonged addiction to which notoriously resulted in mental and neurological changes. These may have been related to the presence in it of significant amounts of methanol. The recipe was long associated with the name of Pernod, who in 1797 acquired it from a Frenchman living in Switzerland called Dr Ordinaire. After absinthe became illegal in France and Switzerland (and in the USA), the Pernod firm, of Pontarlier, continued to produce and market an aperitif of the same name but flavored with aniseed rather than absinthium. (Reproduced courtesy of Mary Evans Picture Library.)

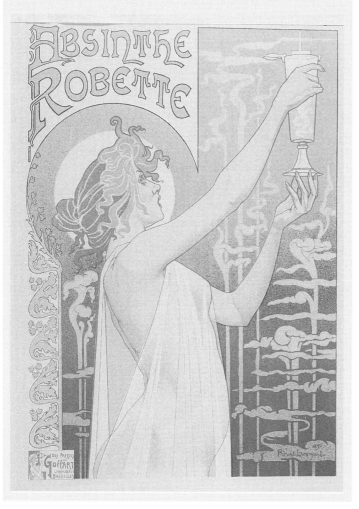

Probably the complications of illegal abortion are the most common reason for admission to gynecological beds in many countries. In developing countries the number of abortions performed will probably increase without regard for the law or religious ideas of the state, for many women have a strong determination not to have a child they did not wish to be conceived.

The wide use of education and easily available contraception should answer this problem. As has been seen in Romania if more effective contraception was provided, the abortion rate may still rise for some years, as traditional abortion practice continues, but hopefully it would eventually level out and reduce.          GC

*See also* OBSTETRICS AND GYNECOLOGY

**ABUSE OF OLD PEOPLE** in public institutions was stimulated as early as 1967 by a British report entitled *Sans everything*, followed by several scandals in such institutions, and later by a paper describing 'granny battering' in families. 'Abuse' was not then a familiar word; but in recent years it has become a widely used term, as abuse — of children, of wives, of old people — has now become a sad commonplace of public scandal. Yet there is no evidence that such abuse is more common than it was. Mistreatment of those who cannot defend themselves has surely always been prevalent. Among recent surveys, 'persistent verbal abuse' was reported as experienced by 5.4% of those interviewed in Britain, which was five times the rate in Boston, USA, and in Canada, and twice that in an Australian survey. By contrast, rates of physical abuse were four times as high in Boston as in Canada. These differences reflect the difficulties of definition and ascertainment, as well as differences in survey method. Most states in the USA have laws for mandatory reporting by relevant professions; their working has been much criticized. How common abuse is we cannot tell; it is clear that it is not rare.

'Elder abuse' has generated many articles, reports, and conferences, and individual media scandals, all of which have helped to 'raise awareness' and, one hopes, in prevention. Abuse may take various forms: physical; psychological; sexual; financial; 'ageist' discriminatory; and humiliating or infantilizing. Of these, the first four are self-explanatory. The most pervasive are the last two. **Discrimination or neglect may occur on grounds of age**, sometimes by individuals, often by covert or even overt 'rationing' — even by deliberate public policies. The last includes **deprivation of privacy, personal possessions, and personal space**, and other such infringements of human rights. A report on a care home by the British Centre for Policy on Ageing wrote: 'The matron does not believe in the basic right of the residents to privacy, in bathing, dressing, and so on. Other individual rights to dignity or choice are positively denied as policy, or withheld as punishments'.

It also includes behavior (often not unkindly meant) such as is indicated in the inspired name of a British radio series on disability: **Does he take sugar?** — talking past people, talking of them in their presence in the third person, assuming that they are 'senile' or deaf, mindlessly addressing old people as 'deary' or 'dad'. Very old people are unlikely to appreciate such imposed familiarity, or jolly fatuities such as 'Have we been a good boy today?' or 'Have we opened our bowels?', which are not confined to the experience of old people.

Physical abuse is probably common, sexual abuse probably much rarer, but it too occurs; women are more often the victims of either or both. An understandable quest to establish specific diagnostic signs of physical abuse has had disappointing results, except in obvious cases; in part this is because very old people often bruise easily, and are more prone to falls, fractures, and other accidents. As with people of other ages, accusations may derive from misunderstanding or malice, or from dementia-related or other confusion. A careful history and careful observation are essential.

Most mistreatment occurs at the hands of family members or carers. Often the latter are 'at the end of their tether': unremitting night and day attendance can break almost anyone's spirit. Sometimes devoted carers let out unkind words or admit to temptation to hit, or to actual hitting, usually with great remorse at the thought, let alone the deed. But much abuse is at the hands of abnormal 'abusive' personalities, or triggered by alcohol. Early identification is crucial, but often difficult. People with dementia are more vulnerable. Often abuse derives from poor past relationships.

### Prevention of abuse

A composite strategy has proved helpful — namely, vigilance, adequate support of carers and of families, better education of staff, and of the public, and appropriate action by the law courts, and publicity. Again, these are probably self-evident. Even devoted carers need both emotional and practical support. This is a challenge which underfunded (and that means most) or ill-planned services do not always meet adequately. An understanding and well-informed family doctor, careful 'assessment', respite admissions, night sitters, day care, help with incontinence, practical advice, and listening (telephone 'Help Lines' are sometimes available), quick availability of practical help when it is needed, and better trained (on the whole they are) staff — all these and other components of good practice and good services are required.

To all these may be added training of carers. There is now much evidence that the coping capacity and the 'morale' of 'informal carers' (family and friends) can be enhanced by specific training programs.

There are many handbooks of good practice in institutional care. There are good texts for the carers of demented people, of which the first is still possibly the best: it is eloquently called *The 36-hour day*. TA

**ACADEMIC MEDICINE** is a term often used but rarely defined because it is felt that most will understand its meaning. The last edition of the *Oxford Companion to Medicine* states that it is 'a term usually taken to imply that part of medicine concerned with teaching and research as well as medical practice, residing largely in universities, academies and other institutions of higher learning. Those engaged in academic medicine may have university titles … and are often full-time university employees'. The reason for the imprecision is that, unlike other formal divisions of medicine, individuals identifying themselves as pursuing careers in academic medicine are found in every branch of medicine. Teaching and the creation of knowledge have undoubtedly existed since healers came to be recognized as physicians. The earliest academics would thus have included HIPPOCRATES (p 382), and his successors would have been those responsible for training apprentices in medicine. The tradition would have continued through the early schools of medicine, and would have begun to change dramatically in the late 18th century as the old medieval order and structure collapsed and new ideas in education and science became dominant. Academic medicine began to achieve greater prominence as a movement towards practical training took place, and as HOSPITALS began to achieve increasing importance in medical education.

The term probably had no real meaning until the early 20th century, when it became possible to contemplate a career in which academic activities rather than practice would predominate. This required both professional and financial rewards for those engaged in academic activities, conditions which did not exist until the turn of the century. The early medical schools in Britain and in North America were a mixture of hospital based institutions, schools located in universities, for-profit enterprises, and loosely structured unaffiliated teaching units offering practical instruction. One element common to them all was the private practitioner, who was responsible for instruction in both clinical medicine and what science was available. Sometimes these instructors were paid by the course, but there was also prestige associated with teaching which would enhance the reputation of the practitioner in the community and hence attract patients.

The concept of the full-time teacher did not exist, and it would not have been possible for one to earn a living as a teacher, much less as an investigator or administrator. This is not to imply that there were not centers or individuals recognized for the quality of their teaching or creativity. The history of medicine in the great Italian cities, Paris, the German centers, and England and Scotland are well documented and their prominence depended on what would today be described as their academic excellence.

Academic medicine developed after the Industrial Revolution as the result of several major changes in society. The Industrial Revolution (itself dependent upon science and technology) provided the resources so that society could pay for both health care and education. The Enlightenment led mankind to have faith in rational thought in science and to an increasing degree, science began to be viewed as forming the basis for modern medicine. Medicine had achieved professional status by the end of the 19th century, and, as a part of its contract with Anglo-American Society, it became responsible for setting and maintaining standards. The General Medical Council in the United Kingdom was given responsibility for the supervision of medical education and licensure, with the Royal Colleges continuing their traditional role in specialty medicine.

### Growth of specialization

The second major influence leading to the establishment of academic medicine was the growth of SPECIALIZATION, which began in the early 20th century and expanded exponentially after World War II. In addition to requiring increasing degrees of complex knowledge on the part of the specialist, this trend required continuous increases in the

## THE GREAT REFORM — THE FLEXNER REPORT

In North America, the responsibility for educational standards originally rested with states and provinces, but without question the emergence of the power of the American Medical Association as spokesperson for the profession had a profound effect on medicine, and its actions greatly facilitated the development of academic medicine. The Council on Medical Education of the American Medical Association had conducted its own internal survey and concluded that many American medical schools failed to meet even minimal standards. It induced the Carnegie Foundation to commission the Flexner Report on the state of medical education in the United States and Canada. Flexner's recommendations, aimed at reforming the medical curriculum, paved the way for the development of a career path for individuals who wished to devote their professional lives to academic endeavors. Flexner recommended that medical schools should be linked to universities, have their own science departments staffed by their own full-time faculty, have firm links with teaching hospitals, and, finally, that clinical departments should be directed and staffed by full-time academics, rather than practicing physicians.

Flexner and Osler (by now at Oxford) testified before the Haldane Commission in 1913, which was examining university education in London. This commission, whose recommendations had an impact beyond London, concurred with Flexner, and recommended that academic clinical units should be established in the major teaching hospitals staffed by full-time university professors. Thus the twin desires of 'professionalizing' teaching and research and of introducing a solid scientific foundation into medical education allowed academic medicine to grow — slowly at first but with increasing impact as the 20th century progressed. Flexner and others were pointing out the frequent problems caused by the private practice of medicine. Practice was viewed as distracting those interested in academic careers from pursuing their academic goals, and many of the proposals were aimed at protecting physicians from this distraction by providing salary support in order to purchase the time required for teaching, research, and, later, for administration.

In retrospect, these recommendations looked forward to the industrial and postindustrial world, where professionalization of tasks, increased specialization, and technology would be major forces. At the time, however, they posed a serious threat to the medical establishment, its structure, and its organization. Leadership roles had traditionally been granted to the most prominent practitioner in the region or to those with powerful connections in the community. There was thus strong opposition to the concept and Johns Hopkins, as the first major university to establish full-time chairs of departments, did so after a very divisive internal debate. Dissenting views were powerfully presented at the Haldane Commission. The controversy centered on two separate but related issues. In the first place many regarded preparation for a career in medicine as 'training', which could be satisfied by a system based on the old apprenticeship model. The medical reformers felt strongly that medical schools should emphasize education. Secondly, there was a linked emphasis on science as the basis of the practice of medicine, and this was opposed by many who observed that science was not of great value in the day-to-day life of the average practitioner. In retrospect the outcome appears to have been predictable, but at the time the issues were very contentious.

There are several reasons why the development of a full-time professoriate was inevitable. The growth of science (and its accompanying technology) and the 'culture of science' which developed in the 20th century, dictated that physicians wishing to contribute to the progress of medicine should take formal and structured training in both science and scientific techniques. This trend started slowly, and in the early 1900s it was still possible to be self-trained and remain competitive. However, by the end of the 20th century a physician would require years of research, and the number of contributions to new knowledge from full-time practitioners was reduced to insignificance. A research career required the commitment of increasing amounts of time to meet the demands of modern research and universities, research institutes, and teaching hospitals were forced to find salary support for this essential activity.

size of full-time faculty of any major medical institution. As long as generalists were present to teach and carry out independent research, the numbers required in any given discipline would be modest. As technology made the generalist extremely rare, universities and their associated teaching hospitals found it necessary to train and recruit increasing numbers of specialists and sub-specialists in order to teach and carry out research in the modern world. This greatly increased the opportunities in academic medicine.

An additional influence has been the growth of the modern teaching hospital, which developed teaching and research in institutions that began with a strong community base and ended with increasing links with the university, and with a value system largely drawn from academe. Both teaching and research changed from activities often based in physicians' offices or clinics to ones that were centered at the bedside or the labora-tory. Thus the practitioner without an academic appointment was largely excluded and those with academic credentials developed into an élite which has come to dominate modern medicine.

The final influence was the shifting economic patterns of the 20th century. Academic medicine developed very slowly until the Second World War, largely because of a lack of financial resources. The Rockefeller FOUNDATION was strongly committed to the directions outlined by Flexner, and made resources available for establishing full-time departmental chairs and research laboratories within medical faculties before World War I, and to an even greater degree in the 1920s. This single organization provided salary support for full-time academic physicians in many countries at a time when university resources were extremely limited. The support continued into the depression years of the early 1930s, when progress would have other-wise been almost impossible to achieve. The other driving forces of science and specialization were creating valid pressures for more full-time appointments.

The economic picture changed dramatically after the Second World War, particularly in North America, which, unlike Europe, had seen its infra-structure largely preserved. The great prosperity of the postwar period provided resources at a time when public faith in science reached an all-time high. Funding of both health care and research in biomedical science expanded, as did the universities with which medical schools were affiliated. Thus academic medicine benefited from the public support of both health and education. Part-time faculty members, while still valued for their very significant contributions to teaching, were largely excluded from this picture. The number of full-time faculty (all of whom would have believed that they were pursuing a career in academic medicine) in the United States increased from about 5000 in 1950 to over 90 000 in 1995. Almost all of this growth occurred in the clinical rather than the basic sciences, occurred because of the prestige of the career choice and because there were substantial financial rewards available.

## Growth in Britain

The growth was much less dramatic in Britain, even though the full-time principle had been accepted and, in fact, endorsed by the Goodenough Commission immediately after the Second World War. It repeated the recommendations of the Haldane Commission and advocated the establish-ment of professorial units in all medical schools in all major disciplines. While the principle of the full-time appointment was largely accepted, the resources available were never as generous as in North America. In addition, the structure of post-graduate training in Britain allowed healthcare to be delivered with a smaller number of university-based personnel and consultants employed by the National Health Service. In many instances the merit award system was used to subsidize the academic activities of consultants, and to serve as a reward for academic prominence.

The profile of the academic physician has changed throughout the century. Before the First World War, specialized training taken by clini-cians would generally have been in a related branch of medicine such as PATHOLOGY or MICROBIOLOGY. Individuals would have been expected to teach, to do research, and to carry out the modest administrative duties required by the academic setting. As science became more tech-nology-driven, and as the problems posed in clin-ical medicine required techniques drawn from the basic sciences, training patterns shifted. More individuals were trained in basic science labora-tories before returning to their clinical discipline to attempt to form a bridge between the basic and clinical sciences. After the Second World War, training requirements became much more rigor-ous and the equivalent of PhD training become more common. While skills in clinical medicine, teaching, and administration were still expected, the emphasis in academic medicine was on science. The value of teaching was without ques-tion diminished by a reward system which favored scientific productivity, and administra-tion was often reserved for the latter stages of a career or for administration in science. These trends were seen throughout the western world.

## Creation of a gulf

The last quarter of the 20th century has seen two trends develop within faculties of medicine. In the first place, reward systems which largely

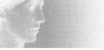

excluded the practitioner have led to a gulf between the academic community and the practitioner. Practitioners have been used extensively by all medical schools to teach clinical medicine, and the resentment caused by the lack of recognition of this essential activity created deep divisions within medical schools. Thus the system itself was challenged, and methods of recognizing teaching as an important activity were devised. This has tended to bring the practitioner closer to medical schools and their full-time personnel, but a gulf still exists. Secondly, specialization reached into the world of the full-time academic, and it became increasingly difficult to maintain true excellence in research, teaching, and administration. This had led to the development of career paths within academic medicine for individuals who wish to be recognized as experts in medical education, and training to prepare for such a career is now available. The administrative complexities which must now be faced if an institution is to function within the modern healthcare system are opening up a third pathway in administration. This also requires either experience or formal training in modern management techniques, and there are structured programs offered to physicians who wish to acquire these skills.

The last two decades of the 20th century have seen great turmoil in the world of healthcare and in the university sector. Since the academic physician must function in both worlds, it is not surprising that these have led to changes. The decrease in university funding and the questioning of university values in the United States have seen a diminution in academic values in North American medical schools. The assault on university funding and on the tenure system in Britain during the Thatcher years had made it more difficult to maintain the structure of academic medicine. In addition, the previous tacit agreement between the National Health Service and the university sector which allowed practitioners considerable time to teach, and permitted full-time university employees time to treat patients is being questioned by cost accountants on both sides. In North America a large portion of the funding of academic departments was derived from the pooled income of clinicians. A part of this money would be recycled to pay the salaries of those engaged in full-time activities. As health maintenance organizations and other third parties used the competitive marketplace to diminish the cost of healthcare, this pooled income was reduced and there was thus less available from what had become a traditional source. Health maintenance organizations do not believe that funding teaching and research is their responsibility, and there has been no ready replacement for the lost income. This has had an impact on the security of the academic career, and it has also led universities and their teaching hospitals to recruit faculty members capable of competing in the entrepreneurial marketplace, thus in part reducing the value system derived from academe.

Looking back to the beginnings of academic medicine, one can see an ebb and flow in terms of the resources available and their sources. It is easy to forget that the principles originally articulated by Flexner and reinforced by Haldane and Goodenough remain dominant. Academic medicine as a career path is firmly established and those devoting significant time to academic activities will continue to be both required and in all likelihood, to dominate both education and research and indeed many aspects of professional life.                                        RLCru

*See also* EDUCATION

**ACADÉMIE DE MÉDECINE, PARIS** The Academy was created by royal ordinance on 20 December 1820. It was charged '*de répondre aux demandes du Gouvernement sur tout ce qui intéresse la santé publique et principalement sur les épidémies, les maladies particuliéres à certains pays, les épizooties, les différents cas de médecine légale, la propagation de la vaccine, l'examen des remédes nouveaux et des remédes tant internes qu'externes, les eaux minérales naturelles ou factices, … .*'

It was intended that the Academy should continue the work of both the Société Royale de Médecine and the Academy of Surgery, which had been suppressed by the Convention in 1793. By doing so, it put an end to the feuding between physicians and surgeons which had characterized French medicine in the 18th century. The authority of the Academy was further strengthened by the inclusion of pharmacists and veterinarians among its membership.

**ACADEMIES** are societies or institutions for the cultivation and promotion of literature, the arts or science, or of some particular branch of science such as medicine, for example, the ACADÉMIE DE MÉDECINE, PARIS; and the National Academy of Sciences, Washington. After 50 years of debate, Britain acquired an academy of medicine in 1998.

**ACUPUNCTURE** literally means 'to puncture with a needle', from the Latin *acus* (needle) and *punctura* (puncture). It is the method of stimulating certain points on the body by inserting special needles, to modify the perception of pain or to normalize physiological functions, to treat or prevent disease. Acupoints may be treated by other techniques such as pressure (shiatsu or acupressure), lasers, and small electrical currents. Ear acupuncture, a particular technique developed mainly in Europe over the last fifty years, owes little to traditional Chinese medicine. The much more widely practiced body acupuncture, however, is part of a complete system of traditional Chinese medicine, which includes herbal medicine, dietary therapy, massage (Tuina), relaxation, and special exercises (Taijiquan, Qigong).

Acupuncture has been practiced in CHINA for several thousand years. The earliest needles were crude tools made of sharpened stone. The oldest known book on acupuncture, The Yellow Emperor's classic of internal medicine, records the basis of traditional Chinese medicine; probably the book is a multi-author text from the Warring States period (475–221 BC). Acupuncture became a specialty during the Sui dynasty (AD 581–618), at which time the Imperial Medical College, with a department of acupuncture, was founded.

The western world first learned of acupuncture in the 17th century from Jesuit missionaries, who also brought western medical practice to China. Acupuncture reached its zenith during the Ming dynasty (AD 1368–1644). It declined during the Qing dynasty (AD 1644–1911) as herbal medicine was emphasized to the extent that in 1822 the authorities ordered the acupuncture-moxibustion department of the Imperial Medical College to be closed. (Moxibustion is burning aromatic herbs, often fixed to acupuncture needles.)

In Europe acupuncture was widely practiced by the medical profession during the first half of the 19th century and good results were reported in the treatment of pain and rheumatism. In 1823 acupuncture was mentioned in the first issue of the *Lancet*, but gradually fell into disrepute as it was not used selectively and discerningly. At present acupuncture is thought to be effective in some painful conditions such as low back pain. In Britain it is widely available in almost all clinics dealing with chronic pain. It is also used in some non-painful conditions such as nausea (early morning sickness, post-anesthetic and chemo-therapeutically-induced nausea). It is believed to work by releasing cerebrospinal fluid endorphins and serum enkephalins, as well as affecting the perception and transmission of pain both peripherally and centrally. Its application in practice remains largely empirical and acupuncture point selection and prescription are frequently based on the information within traditional Chinese medicine.

**Traditional Chinese medicine**

Traditional Chinese medicine involves distinct philosophical concepts which underpin the ancient Chinese view of anatomy, physiology, and pathology treating and preventing illness. Health is defined as a fluctuating balance of two opposing forces; yin (water, cold, and stillness) and yang

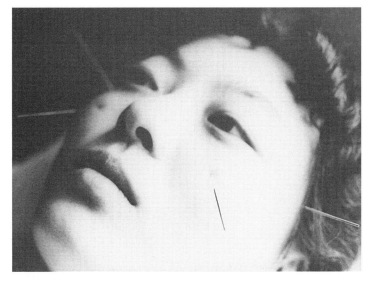

Patient undergoing acupuncture treatment in China. (Reproduced courtesy of the WHO/ National Library of Medicine, Bethesda, MD.)

(fire, heat, and movement). Illness results from a sustained imbalance of these forces. Acupoints cover the body and are grouped into various meridians which represent the energetic balance of each of the main organs. Qi, or vital energy, flows through the meridians and disease is thought to be reflected in an imbalanced flow. The central idea within traditional Chinese medicine is to diagnose the specific reason for this imbalance by taking the patient's history and examination of the tongue and pulse. Acupoints are then selected to correct the imbalance. In traditional Chinese medicine the concept of organ function is similar to conventional western medicine, but each organ has specific attributes. Acupuncture may be carried out by several approaches:

- *Traditional Chinese acupuncture*: the points are selected in accordance with traditional Chinese theories.

- *'Formula' approach ('cookbook' approach)*: a standard formula is used to treat disorders diagnosed on a western medical basis.

- *Trigger point acupuncture*: needling of trigger points in the muscles and the surrounding tissues to treat musculoskeletal pain.

- *'Scientific' acupuncture*: the points are chosen according to modern interpretations of their actions (for example, homeostatic, immune-enhancing, anti-allergy), or according to knowledge of their spinal segments.

Modern acupuncture needles are usually made of stainless steel and are disposable. Patients usually need 4–8 acupuncture treatments to obtain a consistent clinical result, and these may have to be repeated periodically. GL

**ADDICTION** See ALCOHOL; SUBSTANCE ABUSE

**ADVERSE DRUG REACTIONS** The problem of iatrogenic drug-related illness (that is, caused by health professionals) is of broad scientific, political, economic, and public health concern. Medicines with unacceptable toxicity are often discovered in premarketing studies and thus never reach the market. In addition, spontaneous reporting systems have been widely used with some success to identify unacceptable drug toxicity in the first years after marketing. Many medicines, including thalidomide, practolol, and benoxaprofen, have been removed from the market based on spontaneous reports. But some serious toxicity from currently marketed medicines is subtle and can be identified only with formal epidemiologic studies. Such studies often identify important adverse drug effects that were previously unrecognized.

As far back as the early 1970s, congressional hearings in the United States addressed this issue. Testimony was presented that: 'it is now known that billions of wasted dollars, hundreds of thousands of unnecessary hospitalizations for adverse drug reactions, and thousands of lives needlessly lost, are the price society pays for the promotional excesses of the drug industry'. A similarly dramatic statement was made at that time in the *New England Journal of Medicine*: '[the] economic consequences [of drug reactions] are staggering: one-seventh of all hospital days is devoted to the care of drug toxicity, at an estimated yearly cost of US$3 000 000 000'. The documentation for such statements was questionable and there was clearly a need to examine available information to determine their accuracy. Fortunately carefully collected information was available from a large ongoing prospective drug safety research program in the USA which allowed for a reasonably precise quantitative assessment of the extent of iatrogenic drug-caused illness.

Based on information derived from that research program it was possible to estimate, with reasonable confidence, that adverse drug reactions occurred in about 30% of hospitalized medical patients. However, since each patient received on average nine different drugs, the frequency of adverse reactions was only 1 per 20 drugs (5%) received. Reactions which were minor and reversible such as nausea and rash represented over 90% of the adverse effects recorded.

Serious or adverse effects were noted for only 4 out of each 1000 courses of drug treatment. A substantial majority were caused by medicines known to be highly toxic (for example, antitumor agents or anticoagulants) and prescribed to people who were seriously ill. The risk of drug-attributed death was estimated to be about 3 per 10 000 courses of treatment. Again, most patients who died from drug treatment were seriously, often terminally, ill and a few potent medicines accounted for most of the deaths. Based on these findings, it appeared that the above mentioned estimates of the extent of the problem of drug toxicity had been grossly exaggerated.

Since 1974 hundreds of new pharmacologically potent medicines have been marketed in the western world. The use of these drugs is widespread and it is important to reconsider the extent of iatrogenic disease which is caused by them. Based on information derived from over 300 practices which participate in the British-based General Practice Research Database (GPRD), one can estimate that each person in Britain receives, on average, 3.1 drugs per year as an outpatient; persons aged over 50 receive about 4.3. If one adds the number of medicines received in hospital or over the counter, it can be inferred that many hundreds of millions of courses of drug treatment are received each year in Britain. It is in this context that one must consider the problem of iatrogenic drug-caused illness.

Drug safety has been extensively studied for both oral contraceptives and non-steroidal anti-inflammatory drugs; these provide good case studies of the problem of adverse drug reactions and how the risks relate to their benefits.

The major concern about low dose oral contraceptives is the risk of venous thromboembolisms, stroke, and acute myocardial infarction. If the use of oral contraceptives is restricted to healthy women, we can estimate, based on many studies, that the attributable risk for venous thromboembolism is around 2 per 10 000 users per year. Over 90% of cases recover, and deaths from pulmonary embolism occur in about 1 per 100 000 users per year. In view of the almost 100% effectiveness of oral contraceptives together with the documented reduction in the risk for ovarian and endometrial cancer in users, most people would conclude that their benefits far outweigh the risks compared with other forms of birth control. The situation is similar for the risks for stroke and myocardial infarction associated with oral contraceptives in healthy women, particularly those who do not smoke cigarettes.

### Non-steroidal anti-inflammatory drugs

The situation with regard to non-steroidal anti-inflammatory drugs is more complex. Many studies have indicated that these drugs cause about a four-fold increase in the risk for upper gastro-intestinal bleeding and perforation; other serious adverse effects are exceedingly rare. Many millions of people take them each day in Britain and the increased risk for associated gastrointestinal toxicity is primarily present in patients with predisposing gastrointestinal illness, the elderly, and those who use high doses. Given the massive use of non-steroidal anti-inflammatory drugs and their efficacy, the risks from these medicines seem acceptable, particularly if taken by persons at low *a priori* risk for gastrointestinal toxicity.

Similar findings are documented for many medicines currently marketed, which include antibiotics and medicines used to treat cardiovascular illnesses, depression, ulcer disease, pain, and insomnia.

Hence, based on extensive studies of drug safety, despite some alarming gross numbers, most currently available medicines are acceptably safe. At the same time, a need clearly remains to quantitate the toxicity that occurs, to identify populations at highest risk, and to uncover any individual drugs whose toxicity may be unwarranted in relation to the benefit. In addition, careful follow-up of newly marketed medicines to evaluate their safety is essential.

While self-evidently physicians, pharmacists, and patients should be fully informed about the risks for adverse affects caused by medicines, it is also important that they be reassured that extensive research on drug safety indicates that most currently marketed medicines are reasonably safe and effective.    HJ

*See also* PHARMACOLOGY, CLINICAL PHARMACOLOGY, AND THERAPEUTICS

**ADVERTISING** is integral to a modern free market economy. It provides information (and misinformation) about goods and services, and seeks to establish the greatest possible market share for each advertiser's own product. Yet advertising by doctors has been a disciplinary issue, and in Britain effectively 'banned' for most of the 20th century. At one time advertising came under the rubric of medical ethics; today this deals with more serious matters. Similarly the American Medical Association's founding Code of Ethics (1846) instigated a long tradition of professional censure of advertising. Why did doctors decide to swim against the tide of an increasingly commercialized society in this way? This article explores the relationship between advertising and medical professionalism by describing the history of advertising, medical advertising, and the reasons for designating it unprofessional conduct. Unless stated otherwise, all examples are drawn from the history of medicine in Britain.

Medical advertising may be divided into two kinds. Firstly that placed by practitioners, or on their behalf, that simply seeks to draw attention and patients to the individual doctor by whatever means. A handbook for newly qualified doctors issued by the British Medical Association (BMA) in 1926 summed up the ethical injunction against advertising. It advised, 'no medical practitioner should attempt in any way to advertise himself or to gain reputation except by the legitimate means of proficiency in his work and by skill and success in the practice of his profession'. The BMA had in fact been instrumental in inducing the General Medical Council (GMC) to declare, in 1905, that advertising by doctors could warrant erasure from the *Medical Register*, effectively giving disciplinary teeth to the ethical principle of non-advertisement.

A second kind of advertising that concerned medical men deeply at this time was that for medical commodities, appliances, facilities, and drugs, as well as for proprietary medicines used by the public for self-treatment. Some such advertising could also be construed as indirectly advertising a named doctor, and doctors were strongly criticized for allowing their names to appear in such a way, or even for profiting directly from medical trade. By and large this kind of advertising, when undertaken by lay people, was almost always beyond the disciplinary reach of professional organizations. That said, professional bodies managed to severely curtail the claims admissible in such advertising by the 1940s.

Advertising was essentially seen as inimical to the nature of medical professionalism. It was seen to damage the profession's social status, and to run counter to the ideal of disinterested success. Non-advertisement was presented as distinguishing legitimate practitioners from tradesmen and QUACKS, and as an abstention from lying and cheating, but was also closely linked to the desire to prevent doctors competing openly for patients. Objections to advertising, however, were not limited to the medical profession, and have a long history.

The 'free press' and the free market in cures were interdependent from a very early stage. The first news-sheets that appeared in the 17th century made no great distinction between advertisements — information placed for public attention in return for a fee — and the rest of their copy. When Parliament attempted to curtail the activities of the press in the 18th century by placing a flat-rate tax on advertising, many publications were forced to close, and small traders and ordinary readers advertised much less than they had. Nostrum vendors and sick trade showmen, however, continued to advertise in huge numbers.

The Georgian market in healthcare was hurly-burly and practitioners of all shades and types competed openly for patronage and fees. During the early to mid-19th century several proprietary medicine manufacturers, including some med-

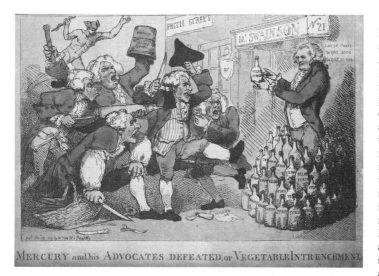

MERCURY and his ADVOCATES DEFEATED, or VEGETABLE INTRENCHMENT

Advertising, 18th-century style: Isaac Swainson promoting his 'Velnos syrup', and facing an onslaught of rival practitioners advocating mercury. Colour etching by T. Rowlandson, 1789. (Reproduced courtesy of the Wellcome Institute Library, London.)

ically qualified men, discovered that systematic advertisement was a reliable route for a fortune. One doctor, James Morison, sold a 'Universal Pill' and supported a large staff of 'Hygeians', presenting his product as a safer more natural alternative to the ghastly depredations of the orthodox doctors with their bloodletting, purging, and mercurial medicines. Thomas Holloway's Pills and Ointment and, later, Beecham's Pills were to sweep the country, earning vast profits on the back of huge advertising campaigns. In addition to these 'big fish' many advertised remedies at this period, and well into the 20th century, were either abortifacients ('Lady Montrose's Miracle Female Tabules') or were presented as cures for venereal disease. Testimonials, which were frequently paid for, were another common feature of such proprietary medicine advertising.

Mid-Victorian businessman, who like doctors preferred to succeed through simple excellence of service and word of mouth recommendation, often felt that advertising was beneath them. This ideal survived far longer among doctors than amongst businessmen. Even after the lifting of various taxes on newspapers in the 1850s, the press continued to rely on advertising and the 'gentlemen of the press' continued to find their association with it embarrassing. By the late 19th century it was not only the advertisements of the 'pox-doctors … and abortionists' but the general ubiquity of advertising, particularly by larger companies, which seemed to be cheapening the whole of national life. Widespread reaction against advertising had set in by the turn of the century. Thomas Carlyle had condemned advertising as against nature, and in the twentieth century writers such as Aldous Huxley and George Orwell were to condemn it as debasing and deceitful.

Advertising men themselves began to put their house in order in response to the criticisms that advertising was debasing and inaccurate. The Advertisers' Protection Society, later renamed the Incorporated Society of British Advertisers, was formed in 1900 and concerned itself with 'ethics', particularly those of 'truthfulness' and 'knocking copy' (running down the opposition). There were also legislative curbs. The 1889 Indecent Advertisements Act banned advertising relating to cures for venereal disease (VD) and the 1917 VD Act made any advertisement for VD cures or for unregistered practitioners offering VD treatment illegal. This 'disease category' model was extended in the 1939 Cancer Act, which banned advertisements claiming cancer cures, and the 1941 Pharmacy and Medicines Act extended the ban to any advertising that claimed to offer a cure for serious chronic complaints such as rheumatoid arthritis, Bright's disease, and tuberculosis.

## 'Secret remedies'

During the 1900s the *British Medical Journal* launched a campaign against 'Secret Remedies' (commercially produced treatments of undisclosed composition) at much the same time that objections to addictive and abortifacient remedies were increasingly put forward by the temperance movement, and publications such as the *Women's Home Journal*. The *BMJ* exposed the worthless or addictive contents of many proprietary medicines, and pressed for legislation to curb the sales and advertising of secret remedies. Not only did many contain high strength alcohol, cocaine, opium, and hemp, but the British Medical Association emphasized that these medications were either worthless, dangerous, or both, and prevented patients from presenting appropriately to their doctor. However, throughout the century the *BMJ*, which like any 'trade journal' relied heavily on advertising revenue, was criticized for the advertising copy it accepted. In 1911 it was challenged by the editor of the *American Medical Journal* to stop advertising a number of secret remedies, and later in the century it was criticized for accepting advertising copy for 'Larson's Swedish Milk'. It is also clear from materials in the BMA's archive that large numbers of doctors not only used, but also endorsed and recommended remedies of undisclosed composition.

## Ethical codes

Advertising by individual doctors rather than commercial advertising was one of the most important disciplinary and ethical issues in the late 19th century and early 20th century. Jukes de Styrap, whose *Code of medical ethics* (editions between 1868 and 1895) was the only British code of medical ethics to appear between 1803 and 1902, condemned it roundly. For him advertising included any communication to those not already bona-fide patients of the practitioner, whether through the press, or by circular, handbill, or calling card. Similarly, publishing signed articles in the press on medical subjects, issuing bulletins on the health of prominent patients, and advertising medical books in the lay press were all unethical practices. Although de Styrap did not use the words mountebank or quack when discussing advertising, these words, which were used interchangeably with 'charlatan', both refer to attempts to attract the attention of the crowd, by climbing on a bench, or by making a noise. The root of the word advertising means 'turning towards' and so the whole linguistic and ethical construct is based on the idea that 'quacks' (those outside the profession, and those of dubious status within it) attempted to attract attention to themselves. The ethical medical man, on the other hand, should rely on reputation alone to attract patients, and even then, scrupulous rules were to be observed in taking over the patients of other doctors to prevent 'poaching'.

Thus late 19th century doctors were enjoined to be conspicuously inconspicuous in the medical marketplace, to distinguish themselves by not distinguishing themselves from their professional brethren. Yet these ideas were pressed into service by a profession that appeared in many areas to be grossly overcrowded. Even medical writers who were at pains to play down the issue of overcrowding had to admit that 'here and there the stress of competition tells, and tells forcibly'. That advertising was linked to competition, and competition to overcrowding is borne out by the fact that complaints of advertising to the GMC ran at a remarkably constant rate in the first half of the 20th century. The exception was during the First World War, when enormous numbers of doctors were transferred to military service, and patients were effectively barred from changing doctors.

Even after 1905, when the GMC's formal 'warning' against advertising came into force, there remained a clear preference to try to explain it as a matter of principle. Indeed, it was frequently used as a rhetorical exposition of medical professionalism and virtues. Robert Saundby's classic *Medical ethics* (1907) stated 'the only advertisement to the public which is now permitted is the doorplate, which should be a modest size'. This plate could state that the practitioner was a surgeon, or physician, but could state no specialty. The window of a building could bear the legend 'surgery' but should on no account display a scale of fees. Saundby explained that the commonplace medical objection to unfair advantage through advertisement was 'superficial'. The matter went deeper than that. He

cited a recent law case in which the proprietors of 'Bile Beans' had sued a rival firm who had also used the term to describe their product. However, in court it emerged that advertising claims to the effect that Bile Beans were the secret elixir of youth for some remote aboriginal tribe were exposed as pure hokum. 'If medical practitioners advertised,' he argued, 'the public would be as little able to discriminate the value of their claims as they are now able to form an opinion as to the real worth of Bile Beans', and if advertising were pursued then the 'scientific worker would be elbowed out'.

## Collegiality

Other writers also enjoined doctors not to see each other as competitors but as 'brethren' and members of a profession. As the century progressed fresh edicts from the GMC and the BMA limited doctors' involvement in newer media such as popular daily papers, radio, and television under the rubric of the designation of advertising and an unethical activity. This was the origin of the now disused, once clichéd newspaper by-line 'a Doctor writes'.

Writers on the medical profession and medical ethics have, however, since the end of the Second World War tended to see the medical ethical ban on advertising as somewhat archaic. In the 1970s several writers characterized older codes of medical ethics that focused on issues such as advertising and the prevention of patient poaching as attempts to control and monopolize the market in healthcare for the profession. At the same time, a new kind of medical ethics based on philosophical principle rather than professional custom and tradition became increasingly influential. The new ethics were concerned largely with matters of experimentation, human rights, and technologies influencing the beginning and ending of human life and in this new agenda a ban on advertising appeared all too self-interested and lacking in ethical rigor. As the critique of medicine launched by writers such as Illich and Szasz began to filter through to a more popular and political level in the 1980s, 'market forces' were also becoming a central political dogma in Britain. Given that the ascendant model of medical ethics (Beauchamp and Childress's 'principalism') emphasized autonomy, a concept easily linked to 'consumer choice' — itself one of the sacred cows of free-market theory — it is not surprising that the medical ban on advertising was to come under attack.

## Against the public interest

In 1989 the GMC was instructed by the Monopolies and Mergers Commission to alter its condemnation of medical advertising in all its forms. The Commission argued that the ban acted against the public interest by limiting access to information about the services doctors offered. Although the GMC still discourages British doctors from advertising as much as it can, advertising itself has ceased to be an activity that warrants removal from the profession. A similar process has occurred in the USA, with the traditional ethical ban on advertising being challenged in 1979 by the Federal Trade Commission. In both countries these moves were resisted by medical organizations. There is little sign in Britain of a resurgence of widespread medical advertising, and less sign of any organized objection to it, and it remains to be seen how advertising will be used and judged by doctors in the 21st century.

The arguments put forward on either side of this debate may be characterized fairly simply. On the one hand, defenders of the older ethical ideal assert that all advertising tends towards deception, omission, and false association, from which the vulnerable sick need defending. On the other hand, their opponents argue that the consumer in the medical marketplace should not be denied information on which choices can be made simply in order to protect doctors from the chill winds of competition and market forces. It would be facile to pretend that there is not some truth in both positions.

Ample evidence exists to show that market forces do not necessarily operate to the benefit of the health of populations or of individuals — the advertising and sponsorship of tobacco products, 'alcohol', or even vitamin and mineral supplementation bear this out. Moreover, most practitioners are aware that determinants of quality and competence are not easily communicated in a form which lends itself to advertising. On the other hand, patients are faced with real dilemmas in choosing medical attendants and treatments, but in a society which embraces 'the market' as its prime organizing factor few alternatives exist that can match the impact of advertising.

The old idea of success through reputation alone rested on word of mouth recommendation, which still remains perhaps the most important reason for choosing a doctor or treatment. In Britain, however, this is limited mainly to the choice of general practitioner (GP). The National Health Service (NHS) has designated GPs a 'gatekeeper' role. In this system access to specialist care is most frequently adjudicated and directed by medically qualified people, for whom word of mouth and personal experience may comprise a more precise set of information and judgements. While an effective professional monopoly, including a ban on advertising, could be argued to favour more objective adjudication of the best practitioners and treatments, it also tends to place most power in the hands of practitioners. Yet in a marketplace that allows heterogeneity of both the methods and quality of medicine, the 'consumer' may have choice, but may have to base that choice on information offered by biased sources, and usually has no chance of returning or trading in any faulty medical 'goods'.

Whilst doctors have almost always sought to make a good living in following their profession, they have also tended to aspire to high standards of practice and to serve their patients' best interest (or have at least recognized the need to behave as if they did). For medical practitioners in the early 20th century banning advertising was one way of ensuring the right balance between these two considerations. It remains to be seen whether tougher regulatory frameworks and increasingly evidence-based practice will achieve this balance better than the older forms of professional self-regulation, and whether they will be sufficient to offset any harmful effects of a rise in medical advertising, should it occur.                               AAGMor

*See also* ASSOCIATIONS; PROFESSIONAL REGULATION

**AFRICA — HISTORY** Some of the earliest evidence of medical practice comes from Africa. The Egyptians were well known, over 5000 years ago, for their advanced knowledge of medicine. Relics from the time of ancient Egypt testify to considerable achievements in medicine. Greek scholars wrote of what they learned from the writings and oral traditions of Africans, with reference particularly to IMHOTEP — an engineer, architect, scribe, priest, and physician (3000 BCE) (p 412) — as the 'historical father of medicine'. He instructed many Greeks in the art of medicine, possibly built the first hospital, and recorded his observations and knowledge about surgery, anatomy, pathology, diagnosis, and experimental scientific observation. An important development in Egyptian medicine was the evolution of physicians into specialists.

Two renowned documents reveal the achievements of early Egyptian medicine: the Code of HAMMURABI — possibly the first codified set of guidelines regarding responsibilities of physicians — and the EBERS PAPYRUS — a type of medical textbook summarizing extant knowledge about several disease categories and offering advice on diagnosis, prognosis, and treatment, including over 800 prescriptions. Medicine and religion were, however, closely intertwined; physicians were also religious leaders. Around 300 BC Alexandria became the center of the intellectual world, where Alexandrian physicians contributed to laying the scientific basis of modern medicine. The Alexandrian school of medicine indeed built on and advanced the ancient theoretical contributions of ARISTOTLE. (p 64)

## Pre-modern Africa

For centuries medicine in Africa was confined to ethnomedicine as offered within the ethno-political contexts of clans, tribes, and later kingdoms and empires. The evolution of these ethnomedical traditions reflected political and other changes in these early societies, and they remain the most common source of healthcare in rural Africa. Because ill-health, disease, and misfortune were amongst natural factors believed to be caused by ancestral spirits, sorcerers, witches, or the violation of taboos, medical practice had a strong magico-religious nature. Activities pertaining to PUBLIC HEALTH included rain-making and rain-control, identification and control of sorcery, control of INFECTIOUS DISEASES, public sanitation services, and health education, with control exerted by the ruling élites (kings, chiefs, and religious leaders). An extensive pharmacopeia of medicinal plant and animal materials was developed, and transfered from generation to generation.

## Missionary medicine and religious influences

Later, medicine in many countries was affected by the spread of Islam, introduced to Africa by the Arabs in the 7th century. The Arabs' intense interest in medicine is reflected in the famous teaching hospitals they built (and the high prestige they bestowed on private physicians), which served as links between Greek medicine and Renaissance medicine. There are many examples of the influence of Islam, resulting in mixed African–Islamic medical systems, and the conversion of magico-religious African medical beliefs and practices to scientific principles fundamental to western medicine. (Even in present-day Islamic Africa there are strong Arabic influences on medicine.)

Although western countries became engaged in Africa long before the arrival of missionaries and colonialists (the Portuguese as early as the mid-15th century), there is little evidence that these early European footholds introduced western medicine to Africa. The exception was 17th century South Africa, where from the beginning the Dutch East India Company deployed ship's doctors, surgeons, and BARBER-SURGEONS (from 1652), and even established hospitals (the first in 1656) to serve mainly sailors but also officials at the Cape refreshment station. As South Africa, Algeria, Kenya, and Zimbabwe were more heavily populated by European settlers than other African countries, Europeans had a more striking influence on medical services there than elsewhere. Early settlers relied heavily on folk medicine and remedies. Western medicine in Africa was predominantly pioneered by Christian missionary societies during the last quarter of the 19th century and early 20th century, mostly well before health services provided by colonial governments.

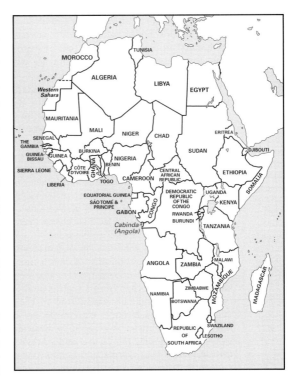

The countries making up the continent of Africa in 1999.

Hundreds of mission hospitals and dispensaries were established and, alongside these, the training of African medical aides. Until 1914, missions in Kenya provided the only western medical services available to the African population.

The religious work of missions was closely linked to medical work. Mission hospitals and mission doctors served as important points of entry of western medicine into African countries, and were the main centers of medical knowledge and practice. The nature of the missions (for example, Protestant or Catholic) and the country of origin of the missionaries (Britain, France, Germany, Switzerland, Belgium, with smaller numbers from Italy, Spain, and Portugal) also influenced the medical practice and the orientation of practitioners. Among these missionaries was Albert SCHWEITZER (p 504), of the Paris Missionary Society, who practiced at Lambaréné, Gabon, during the earlier half of the 20th century. He marked a turning point in missionary thinking that elevated healing to an essential element of the missionary mandate.

Most African countries still rely heavily on missionary hospitals and medical services. Somewhat Africanized church-related health services continue to provide 25–50% of available hospital and health services in most African countries; many, as in colonial times, with grants-in-aid continuing. African populations often prefer church-related healthcare, generally believing it to be superior to that offered by government health departments.

### AFRICAN PIONEERS

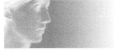

Godfrey Martin **HUGGINS** (1883–1971). British/Rhodesian surgeon and politician. Huggins practiced medicine in London before emigrating to Salisbury, Southern Rhodesia (now Zimbabwe). He practiced surgery there and also took active interest in politics. After his election to the Legislative Council in 1923, he became Prime Minister of Southern Rhodesia 1933–53, when the country became a self-governing colony. He helped bring about the Federation of Rhodesia and Nyasaland and was its first Prime Minister in 1953.

(continued overleaf)

(continued)

Mungo **PARK** (1771–1806). British physician and explorer. Park trained in Edinburgh and in 1791 became a surgeon in the mercantile marine. His first exploration of the Niger was from 1794–7, when he returned to England and published *Travels in the interior districts of Africa* (1799). In 1801 he set up in practice in Peebles, but in 1805 organized another expedition to find the source of the Niger. He was killed with all his companions by natives at Boussa.

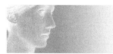

Sir Leander Starr **JAMESON** (1853–1917). British physician and statesman. In 1878 Jameson went out to Kimberley to practice, and there he became a close friend of Cecil Rhodes. In 1889 he was sent to win the concession of Mashonaland from Lobengula, the chief of the Matabele, and succeeded by curing his gout. In 1895 he carried out his ill-conceived raid across the Transvaal border ('the Jameson raid'), was defeated, and taken prisoner. He was in Ladysmith for the siege in 1899. Later he entered the South African parliament and in 1904 became prime minister of Cape Colony.

## Colonial Africa

The European colonization of Africa took place predominantly during the latter 19th and early 20th centuries. State-provided healthcare was restricted during colonial times and only after World War I did colonial governments accept some (usually minimal) responsibility for the medical needs of indigenous populations. Exposure to tropical diseases gave an impetus to medical research and to the spread of western medicine in Africa. Western medical practitioners used modern scientific techniques to support imperial control and protect the interests of the rulers, frequently to the detriment of the ruled. This included the use of western medications — for example, quinine — to facilitate colonial penetration into otherwise inaccessible areas.

Prominent among the factors shaping medicine in Africa were the relationships of domination–exploitation between imperial powers and their colonies. Important characteristics of the mother countries were gradually transferred to their colonies and protectorates. Thus medicine in many African countries was shaped by medicine in Britain, Belgium, the Netherlands, France, Portugal, Italy, and Germany. Simultaneously, colonial influences engrained structural distortions on the emerging public health systems in the colonies. These included racial disparities through reliance on the importation of personnel and the centralized systems of the colonial era featuring strongly in doctor-oriented, hospital-centered, urban-concentrated, and curatively-biased policies and systems. The result was a distribution of medical services favoring upper class and urban citizens. Also recognizable are the crystallization of unequal social relationships and the creation of segregated structures in which 'colonists'/colonizers were geographically separated, more favored, and healthwise more protected than their African counterparts. In most British colonies, the colonial medical system shaped sanitation conditions and stratified healthcare into segregated facilities for Europeans, Asians, and 'Natives' — in that order. In South Africa this 'apartheid in medicine' grew to the fullest extremes of inequality.

## Benefits to medicine

The benefits brought to healthcare in Africa should not be underestimated. Most notable were the introduction of western allopathic medicine to the continent, and the strong tradition of management and administration so typical of the British colonial regimes, which established advanced legislation, administrative structures, and controlling bodies for medicine in several of their colonies. These colonial powers took serious steps to control epidemics, provided the first establishments (hospitals, health posts) of modern western medicine in the colonies, and generously funded and manned several of these.

The liberation of African nations from colonial domination in the mid-20th century set in motion new trends in medicine. Colonial distortions in medicine were countered by radical breaks from the colonial mold. New cadres of health staff emerged, such as village medical helpers, community health workers, clinical nurses, and traditional birth attendants. Progressive Africanization of medicine and professionalization of traditional healing emerged, but the mass emigration of health workers (both state and missionary) from these countries left a great need for trained medical staff. Gradually the vacuum was filled by expatriate doctors from other, especially African, countries, and by graduates from newly established local medical schools, as well as by phasing in less medically or doctor-dependent models of care, such as primary health care and nurse-based health services.

Colonial powers remained varyingly influential in sustaining western medicine in the post-colonial period. In some cases these were largely ousted, and several countries (Tanzania, Angola) leaned towards and drew on the Soviet Union, China, North Korea, and Eastern Bloc countries. Other countries, such as those in the Commonwealth, retained strong ties with the erstwhile European mother countries. Post-colonial and post-independence African governments largely continued to give legitimacy to western medicine; they also reproduced and perpetuated many of its distortions, among others the inherited 'lopsided medical infrastructure'. Post-colonial African rulers also diverged in important ways from colonial patterns, in that they expanded health services to rural areas and accommodated traditional medicine to a larger extent.

Like the rest of the world, Africa has had a long history of disruptive political events — from the 11th century until well into the 20th — which have dislocated masses of people, with devastating effects on health and health systems. The European colonial legacy left serious voids and instabilities which threatened the emerging independent nations in the 1960s. In many cases, conflicts were initiated by withdrawals of colonial powers. In others, independence triggered fierce battles among contending internal factions with a sequence of coups and counter-coups, military regimes, or ensuing undemocratic, authoritarian one-party states. Many of these countries have been dominated by ruinous civil wars, fed by the Cold War, regional rivalries, and internal problems resulting in the establishment of a range of socialist/collectivist political power structures. These have shaped and reformed national health systems towards centralized systems, jeopardizing the already inadequate private healthcare sectors in these countries.

## Effects of instability

Such political instability has disrupted medical training and working conditions of health professionals, many of whom have become exiles. Political disruptions, and resultant dislocation of masses of people, have severely affected the ability of countries to provide medical care. For example, a small country such as Malawi in recent times has absorbed about one million Mozambican refugees. Massive migration and dislocation of millions of people, due to natural disasters, as well as man-made catastrophes have profoundly disrupted both health and the functioning of health systems. In Rwanda, the ethnic massacre in 1994 claimed the lives of one million people within three months.

Since the missionary and colonial eras of Africa's history, African ethnomedicine has been profoundly exposed to western allopathic medicine. As a result, a variegated medical pluralism has evolved. The meeting and mixing of Islam and Christianity with African traditionalism, have also led to new forms of medico-religious practices — syncretic faith healing and prophets within Christian countries, and Islamic divination procedures and other influences in Islamic countries. Another outcome of this contact was the emergence of a relationship between western allopathic and African ethnomedicine best described as one of superiority–inferiority, symbolizing the strengths of imperial and indigenous powers and the official superimposition of western values over African practices. In time, allopathic medicine enjoyed dominant official support over traditional medicine, which was relegated to an officially inferior and often covert position.

Despite these disadvantages traditional healers survived and today, in most African countries, they serve a much larger clientele than western forms of medicine. The two systems exist side by side and when western forms of treatment fail, people return to the more traditional forms. This survival of ethnomedicine may be partly explained by the strength of traditional beliefs, social organization, and customary practices in African societal and tribal life (with particular attention paid to spiritual ailments), but should also be seen in the light of the frequent unavailability and inaccessibility of western medicine in many rural and isolated areas. Here traditional medicine remains the only resort, with success stories playing an important part in its survival. Apart from this, the two systems are based on diverse foundations regarding etiology, diagnosis, and treatment; the magico-religious aura and spiritual nature of traditional medicine are the crux of differences between the two systems.

The relation between the two systems is also not singular; relationships are changing as new policies and legislation emerge. During the colonial period these policies and legislation towards traditional medicine took two forms: herbalists were not forbidden to practice their medicine, but divination, witchcraft, sorcery, ordeals, and oaths were outlawed and prosecuted as criminal offences (the Witchcraft Suppression Acts). In general, colonial governments and early Christian missionaries despised and therefore discouraged or suppressed the use of traditional medicine. Later, this rejection of traditional medicine was carried further by organized professions and councils in the western-scientific mold. In time, however, four broad varieties of relationships crystallized: exclusive (monopolistic) systems, recognizing only scientific medicine; tolerant systems, characterized by *laissez-faire* policies which virtually ignore traditional medicine, yet allow its existence; inclusive (parallel) systems, recognizing traditional health systems alongside scientific medicine; and integrated systems, tending to unite allopathic and traditional medicine in both training and practice. The first type of relationship prevails in the former French and Belgian colonies in Africa; the second was/is typical of the arrangement in former British colonies. Inclusive and integrated systems have not generally been encountered in Africa.

In practice, Africa's large and varied quota of traditional healers is competing with western doctors for scarce resources and a clientele. In most countries the number of African traditional healers far exceeds those of western doctors; in Malawi some 23 000 traditional healers were recently recorded, while in South Africa 150 000 to 200 000 (others suggest nearer to 350 000) are reported practicing. As traditional healers gain more recognition, they increasingly refrain from practicing covertly, and some are now even advertizing their

These traditional healers are still popular, particularly among rural communities in sub-Saharan Africa.

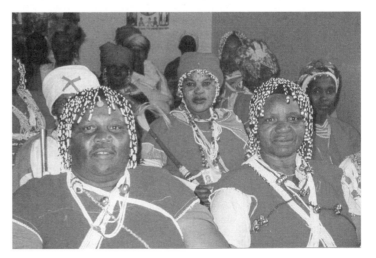

services. The publication of the *South African traditional healers' primary health care handbook*, by the South African Medical Research Council Traditional Medicines' Research Group (1997), reflects the trend towards a growing willingness to integrate diverse systems.                    HCJR, SRB

## AFRICA — PRESENT AND FUTURE

At present Africa comprises 53 independent states: 47 are part of the continent, six are island states. Today Africa has an estimated population of over 600 million. An average annual population growth rate of between 2.2% and 3.3% between 1950 and 1990 resulted in an explosive increase from 170 million to 500 million people. Most of this population is still non-urban. In the mid-1990s life expectancy averaged 53 years in Africa; in only nine African countries is life expectancy over 60 years; in many it is still well below 50 (for example, Zambia, Burundi, Guinea, Malawi, Mali, Niger, Somalia, Uganda) and even lower in Sierra Leone (35 years for women, 32 for men).

Although infant mortality rates have fallen spectacularly during the past century — from levels exceeding 200–300/1000 — they remain high. The highest rates are recorded in Rwanda (145), Mali (156), and Sierra Leone (200), and the lowest in Mauritius (17), Tunisia (41), South Africa, and Algeria (51). Under-5 mortality often exceeds 200/1000, reaching exceptional levels in Mozambique (275), Sierra Leone (284), Angola (292), and Niger (320). In sharp contrast are the low rates in Tunisia (37), Mauritius (23), and Seychelles (20). Only in Botswana, Cape Verde, Mauritius, Namibia, and South Africa, most of the Northern African countries, and possibly Seychelles, are both the infant and under-5 mortality rates below the developing world's averages of 64 and 95/1000, respectively (compared with the developed world's of 14 and 18/1000, respectively). Despite declines in income in the past years, Burkina Faso, Gambia, Senegal, and Zimbabwe have almost halved child mortality between 1980 and 1995. Maternal mortality is of equal concern. In sub-Saharan Africa, at 971/100 000 live births, this is over double the rate of 471/100 000 in the developing world as a whole. For the 1980–90 decade rates were highest in Ghana, Somalia, and Mali: 1000, 1100, and 2000/100 000, respectively.

Africa's burden of disease is high especially in the communicable and preventable categories. In earlier times SMALLPOX, and now TUBERCULOSIS, measles, MALARIA, HIV/AIDS, and many water-borne and other INFECTIOUS DISEASES devastatingly affect health. Tuberculosis is the leading infectious killer in Africa and is increasing, aggravated by the HIV epidemic. Of the world's 30 million people infected with HIV, 21 million live in sub-Saharan Africa, and of 12 million deaths, 83% occurred in Africa. Malaria, another serious problem, is endemic in many countries, with 300–500 million clinical cases (90% of these in Africa) and 1.5–2.7 million deaths each year — mostly in children. The health toll of SCHISTOSOMIASIS also remains high in Egypt and many other parts of Africa. However, the true burden of disease in Africa is difficult to evaluate and may be even greater than estimated.

Understandably such a disease burden profoundly impacts on health, taxing health systems and social services to their limits. However, there have been some limited successes. Of the national tuberculosis control programs in 34 countries, 27 have a central control unit, 11 providing completed short-course treatment for all patients. Regrettably, 19 provide complete treatment for only half of patients. Drug treatment for LEPROSY increased from 7% in 1987 to 27% in 1990 and to 63% in 1993, reducing the prevalence of the disease from 483 000 cases in 1990 to 159 000 in 1993. Vaccination programs have markedly reduced the incidence of neonatal tetanus in 12 African countries, and POLIOMYELITIS is decreasing in several countries. With the recent upsurge in malaria, and the development of widespread resistance to chloroquine, malaria control programs are being given high priority through a World Health Organization global malaria strategy, which includes 17 African countries.

Africa's health status and healthcare needs are conspicuously shaped by poverty, malnutrition, infectious diseases, armed conflict, drought, FAMINE, inadequate access to primary and secondary education, safe water, sanitation, and a range of socio-economic factors propagating inequitable distribution of resources. In turn, these same determinants are the main factors in shaping the nature and status of medicine on the continent.

### Human development and social-economic well-being

On the Human Development Index (measuring human progress [on a 0 to 1 scale] as reflected in longevity, knowledge, and standard of living), African countries fare dismally. On recent gradings, only three African countries (Seychelles, Mauritius, and Libya) rank in the 'high category', and then only in the 52nd, 61st, and 64th positions, respectively. Thirteen African countries are in the 'medium category' (South Africa 90th), while most (35 of them) fall in the 'low category' — with the last 19 positions filled by African countries (the very last being Niger, Rwanda, and Sierra Leone [175th]). Compared with Seychelles' favorable score of 0.845, Sierra Leone has the most unfavorable score (0.176) on the scale — and the 'worst quality of life' and 'poorest health services in the world'. Nevertheless the Human Development Index has improved during 1990–4, from 0.200 to 0.380, though several African countries have recently shown decreases — Rwanda, Botswana, Zambia, Sierra Leone, Guinea, Burundi, Sudan, Zimbabwe, Togo, Congo, Cameroon, Gambia, and Kenya.

## Poverty

Sub-Saharan Africa has the highest proportion of people in — and the fastest growth in — human poverty. The Human Poverty Index, which reflects the combined basic dimensions of poverty, is 40% for the whole of sub-Saharan Africa and exceeds 50% in seven countries in the world. Of these, six (Niger, Sierra Leone, Burkina Faso, Ethiopia, Mali, and Mozambique) are in Africa. Some 220 million people in the region are poor, and by 2000 an estimated half of the people in sub-Saharan Africa will live in such poverty. Women and children, and more so those in rural areas, are disproportionately poor. Economic indicators signal that Africa's annual per capita gross national product in 1996 ranged from a minimum of $80 in Mozambique to a maximum of $6280 in the Seychelles, with a mean of under $500. Africa's economic plight is further aggravated by debt-ridden economies supported by almost valueless currencies; most of the heavily indebted poor countries — 33 of 41 — are in sub-Saharan Africa. Its debt stands at $300 billion, about $370 for every man, woman, and child on the continent. Niger exemplifies Africa's plight: it has a per capita gross national product of $200; 92% of its population lives on $2 a day or less; the debt burden comprises 88% of the gross national product; and three times more money is spent on international debt repayments than on health and education. Rwanda, Burundi, Liberia, the two Congos, Sierra Leone, and Somalia grapple with similar mountainous debts in the aftermath of military conflicts.

National health systems vary in Africa with prevailing political–economic systems. They span the spectrum from predominantly socialist/collectivist (Angola, Mozambique, Tanzania), socialized/ national health service (Kenya), to strongly inclined private/free market dispensations (South Africa). These influence the practice of medicine in Africa — the position of the doctor in society (whether public servants or entrepreneurs); the nature of medical practice (public facilities or private solo or partnership practices); the degree of regulation; and the prevailing financial system (free services or fee-for-service). The health systems of many African countries might, however, be best described as emerging systems — notably unplanned, undifferentiated, uncoordinated, and highly mixed.

Private medicine is generally weakly developed in Africa, although most countries have a private sector of varying size. Many African countries have a weak or progressively dwindling private medical sector, although recent economic reforms have stimulated privatization of medicine. Different models of accommodating the private/ public split also prevail. In Nigeria, for example, public and private doctors function completely separately; public doctors do not run part-time private practices, nor do private doctors use public facilities. By contrast, in Malawi the trend is increasingly to allow public doctors to also run private practices for profit. In a few cases, for example, South Africa, private medicine and private doctors are strongly entrenched and the prevailing pattern. Generally, however, western-style medicine in Africa is provided by the state.

## International health agencies

International influences in African medicine started during colonial times, with three kinds of agencies distributing the bulk of medical care in African countries: governments (through the army, navy, civilian, and development components), missions (particularly for rural Africans); and private companies (for employees and their relatives). Later came international agencies, such as the League of Nations and the International Labor Organization, and even later the United Nations, in particular the multi-lateral World Health Organization, United Nations Children's Fund, and United Nations Development Plan, the European Union, and the Commonwealth. With technical and financial assistance, the World Health Organization has focused on strengthening national healthcare systems, and encouraging integrated healthcare systems that promote services related to medical care, rehabilitation, family health, communicable disease control, environmental health — and with particular emphasis on private health care. Also bilaterals (e.g. Médicin sans Frontières) have played important parts in shaping healthcare and medicine. In addition, the World Bank and the International Monetary Fund have had significant indirect effects on medicine in Africa. Numerous health programs driven by these agencies rescued many African countries, but also created dependency and subscription to their interests and agendas. In the mid 1980s over 70% of Malawi's public sector investment program was donor-funded, and by the 1990s this was over 80%.

Given the part that western medicine should play in Africa, the supply of doctors in African countries is reason for concern. Doctor:population ratios vary greatly: Libya (1:962), Seychelles (1:1064), and South Africa (1:1500) are most favorably supplied, while Malawi (1:50 000), Chad, and Mozambique (both 1:33 333) are the least. Generally the provision in sub-Saharan countries is

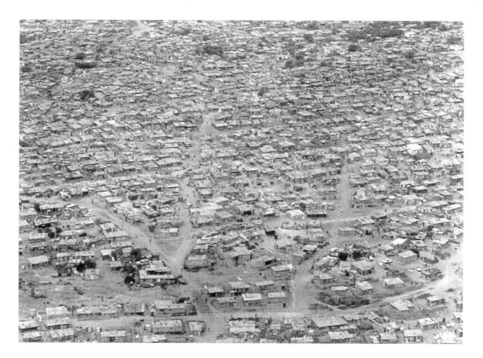

The Crossroads squatter camp near Cape Town in South Africa.

poor to very poor — an average of 1:18 514. Although there have been improvements in the doctor:population ratios in the past years (1970–1988–91) in many African countries (1:97 000 to 1:33 333 in Burkina Faso, 1:86 100 to 1:33 333 in Ethiopia, 1:50 000 to 1: 7692 in Guinea, 1:30 400 to 1:2500 in Lesotho), this ratio has also deteriorated in several African countries. Most notable is the worsening in the doctor:population ratio in Uganda from 1:9200 to 1:25 000; Ghana from 1:14 894 to 1:22 970; Kenya from 1:8000 to 1:20 000; and Mozambique from 1:18 900 to 1:33 333.

### Maldistribution

Featuring prominently in the African context of medicine but not unique to Africa is the regional and rural–urban maldistribution of the medical corps within countries. Sizeable proportions of rural populations have no access to doctor services. Although 85% of Kenya's population live in rural areas, less than 10% of its physicians are located there. African countries have devised various strategies to overcome these shortages and distortions, especially to attract or compel doctors to underserved rural areas or disadvantaged sectors. Many of these were/are to the detriment of the western medical doctor/medical profession in Africa. Among them are the introduction of various less expensive and less qualified medical clinical auxiliary staff categories; compulsory community service in disadvantaged areas by doctors after completion of training; various incentive schemes for doctors to serve in under-

served areas and sectors; and the importation of foreign/expatriate doctors to serve the underserviced areas (Cuban doctors to South Africa being a recent example).

The general shortage of doctors in most African countries has led to the phenomenon of expatriate doctors — the large-scale importation of foreign doctors from abroad and other African countries. In some countries the number of expatriate doctors exceeds that of local doctors (Lesotho and Zambia); in others, the position is just the opposite (Nigeria). Such importation has varying and often detrimental effects on the local medical profession and practitioners.

Henrietta Stockdale, a remarkable person and nurse who started the first training school for nurses in South Africa, achieved professional status for nurses in South Africa in 1891 — the first country where this was achieved. Today nurses outnumber doctors by 10 to 1 in South Africa and play a prominent part in ambulatory and hospital-based healthcare. Together with the rapidly growing community healthcare workers they will increasingly dominate the scene, and will probably work more closely with primary care doctors and members of a transforming traditional healthcare system.

For most of the colonial period the medical profession as a profession scarcely existed in either anglophone or francophone Africa. Doctors were appointed as civil servants and *de facto* members of colonial governments, often under military discipline. Missionary doctors too had a divided allegiance to medicine — it was the appointees of colonial authorities (and not independent professionals) who decided if a doctor's qualifications were acceptable in that colony. Although there were branches of the British Medical Association in the Cape and in Natal in the 1880s, there were too few doctors in most African countries to constitute local autonomous associations, and doctors were too cut off from the mother countries to be included in their professional structure. They were thus not recognized as members of an autonomous organization called a 'medical profession'. By contrast, African medical professionals during the colonial period relied on their professional status to overcome the racial discrimination against them. For them, from early times, professionalization was of paramount importance.

## Professionalization

A self-conscious profession in most of Africa dates back mainly to the 1950s, when African doctors increased in numbers, when private practice outside government or mission hospitals became more common, when university medical schools and teaching hospitals were established — and the whole paraphernalia of a formal profession of medicine was gradually instituted and recognized by the government and the public. Professionalization became part of decolonization; it coincided with the Africanization of staff and curricula; it was to prove, proudly, that the independent states were not content with second best. None the less, the current state of professional medical associations in many African countries is still closely linked to the number of doctors, their employment status, degree of specialization, and the proportions of expatriate and local doctors. In most African countries these associations are still weakly developed. South Africa is an exception, the earliest medical association dating back to 1827 and the current and member-strong Medical Association of South Africa being established in 1926. Despite the weak position of the medical profession in Africa, it nevertheless became dominant as it systematically suppressed and eliminated many of its competitors and subordinated others. The amalgamation of a range of professional medical groups into the South African Medical Association in 1998 opens a new era of potential professional solidarity that might heal some of the wounds that existed between 'conservative' and 'progressive' medical associations in the apartheid era.

## Medical regulating bodies and training

Most English speaking countries have general medical councils responsible for registration, accreditation, ethical standards, and supervision of medical practice. Their policies are more responsive to western European ethical norms and have focused little on social and cultural conditions peculiar to Africa. The factors shaping medical associations also influence the nature of medical councils and controlling bodies in Africa. Many, of quite recent origin (in Malawi since 1987 only), are weak and inefficient. Little attention has been devoted to modern approaches to bioethics and doctors remain paternalistic in their outlook. Fundamental principles such as privacy and confidentiality are generally accepted. The South African Medical Research Council has published guidelines for the ethics of medical research, the latest edition in 1993, and more vigorous teaching programs in medical ethics are being developed in South African medical schools.

## Training and research

Modern medical training started in most African countries only during the 20th century, generally after independence in the 1960s and 1970s. Before the founding of local medical schools, African doctors were mainly trained in former European colonial countries with government or donor grants as well as in non-colonial countries such as Sweden, Canada, or the USA.

There are now about 92 medical schools in Africa, a ratio of 1 per 6 million people (compared with 1 per 2 million in the western world and 1 per 5 million in South Africa). The first medical schools were those of Cape Town (1912), University of the Witswatersrand (1920), and the University of Pretoria (1943). The first medical school in Uganda was founded in 1922, in the Sudan in 1924, in Nigeria in 1948, and in Zimbabwe, Zaire, Kenya, and Zambia only in 1963, 1966, 1967, and 1968, respectively. African countries thus differ greatly in their medical training facilities, self-sufficiency, number of medical schools, and output of doctors. Most smaller countries have one (Malawi, Mozambique, Zambia, Zimbabwe) or none (Botswana, Djibouti, Gabon, Mauritius, Lesotho, and Namibia), while others have several medical schools (South Africa has 8, Sudan 14, and Nigeria 15). The annual output of doctors in Mozambique is about 50; that of Nigerian and South African medical schools approaches 1000.

Many smaller African countries still rely on facilities in Europe, North America, and even Japan and China to train their medical practitioners. Several medical schools (in Nigeria, Kenya, Ghana, South Africa) also train doctors from other African countries, especially those without schools. Many doctors trained overseas do not return to their countries of origin, largely because of unfavorable salaries, conditions of service, and policies regarding medical practice. For many of these same factors a large number of trainees leave their countries of origin — sometimes permanently.

Disease in Africa poses a rich topic for research and has led to renowned campaigns in Africa, such as the French VACCINATION of Senegalese against SMALLPOX in 1887. A laboratory was even established for manufacturing the vaccine. Some missionary doctors made important contributions to the scientific understanding of tropical diseases. During World War II the French conducted an enormous campaign against YELLOW FEVER, vaccinating eleven million Africans. Pioneering research in conquering yellow fever, river blindness, and sleeping sickness are further examples of research break-throughs in Africa. Several medical research institutions in Africa have become known for work in TROPICAL MEDICINE, often under difficult 'frontier' circumstances, and usually with the support of expatriate researchers from previous colonizing countries. The South African Institute for Medical Research in Johannesburg, the Blair Institute in Harare, the Kenyan Medical Research Institute in Nairobi, the Medical Research Council Research Unit in the Gambia and trials on tuberculosis in East Africa, several Pasteur Institutes in Africa, and research units in Makerere (Uganda) are examples. The African Medical and Research Foundation has worked for 40 years with local communities to alleviate the region's health problems and promote research on malaria, hydatid disease, sexual and reproductive health, laboratory services, and health information systems. Most of its research is applied or operational. The *Directory of potential institutions for testing malaria vaccines,* published by the African Malaria Vaccine Testing Network, lists the staffing and activities of infectious disease research institutes in 20 African countries.

Individuals such as Michael Gelfand in Harare, Eldryd Parry and David Warrell in Nigeria, Sir Ian McGregor and others from the Gambia, Anthony Butterworth in Kenya, and indeed many others are well known for their contributions to medical research. Brock's chapter on 'Some highlights of medical research in South Africa' in *A history of scientific endeavour in South Africa,* and a multi-authored book on *South African medical research* provide insights into the extensive research on medical problems in South Africa. The wide range includes infectious and parasitic diseases, nutritional deficiencies, occupational diseases, the porphyrias, iron overload, genetic disorders, organ transplantation (including the first heart transplant in 1967), and cardiovascular and liver diseases. In recent years other major themes and foci such as HIV/AIDS, reproductive health, women's health, mother and child health have started, given the widespread, acute, or devastating nature of these conditions in Africa.

New forms and methods of health research were introduced during the 1980s and 1990s. Essential National Health Research and Health Policy and Health Systems Research are examples. Essential National Health Research aims to establish and strengthen an appropriate health research base in each country; focus research resources on priority health needs; and bridge the research–policy gap. Health Policy and Health Systems Research is steered by the same principles. It focuses primarily on research as supportive in improving health by improving the efficiency of health policy and systems, as well the quality and accessibility of health services. The value of such research has also been shown to be more in line with actual health needs, improve the management of government health facilities, address inefficiencies and inequities, and to reduce waste, all by way of reformative measures resulting from health policy and systems research.

Funding of medical research varies from country to country and is also channelled differently. In South Africa medical research is largely funded by the state (through the Medical Research Council), pharmaceutical industry, and internationally linked non-governmental organizations, such as the Health Systems Trust.

Only a few medical journals in Africa have become widely recognized, arguably the best being the *South African Medical Journal* founded in 1893. The *Central African Journal of Medicine* and the *East Africa Medical Journal* also enjoyed high reputations in the past, but their status has not been sustained. This reflects the extent to which western science and medicine in South Africa have become more deeply entrenched and more successful than elsewhere.

Poverty is one of the most serious problems affecting Africa. Squatter settlement in South Africa.

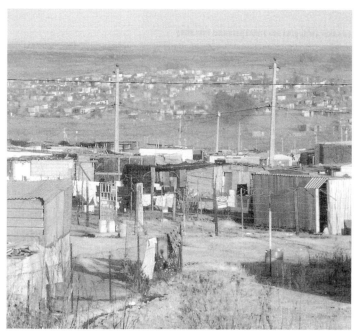

## Transformation of medicine

Amid worsening economic conditions and as part of economic reforms, many African countries have recently embarked on either piecemeal or significant health reforms, particularly in public health and seeking greater efficiency and equity in health. Such reforms are closely linked to current economic structural adjustment programs. These spill over into the health sector as cost-cutting, curbing government expenditure on health, strides towards privatization, the introduction of user-charges and cost-recovery policies, changes in household economies, changes in health and health-seeking behavior. With dwindling economies the emerging healthcare systems are increasingly being directed towards primary healthcare; thus progressively shifting the professional nurse, auxiliary health carers, and semi-professionals to center stage as the main functionaries. Simultaneously the roles of private and solo-practicing doctors and of the medical profession are being reduced. Apart from long-standing shortages of medical doctors, African health systems are becoming less accommodating to and less concerned about advanced medical services and medical specialization.

The shift in emphasis towards primary healthcare, with a de-emphasis on hospitals, poses trends incompatible with the thrust of modern medical services and not sympathetic to the ways doctors approach healthcare. Financially, primary healthcare systems do not stimulate or sustain the high financial demands of private medical practice. Grim economic circumstances and unsatisfactory availability of drugs and medical equipment (mostly to be imported), poor maintenance of buildings, structure and process of care (patient overload, work ethic, neglect, abuse, poor attitudes), and the general decline in the quality of health services do not attract and retain doctors and other health professionals. Rather, these trends are eroding the lean doctor corps in African countries. The result is a dwindling number of medical professionals, with a concomitant shrinking role and declining importance of western medicine in African medical systems. Likewise, medical specialization and medical specialists are making way for general practitioners, generalists, nurses, and community health workers who fit the primary healthcare model better. This trend is also becoming evident in South Africa, where healthcare reform is being based on the primary care approach and the district based system.

What is the future of modern medicine in Africa? Will public medicine increasingly be modeled on the primary healthcare approach, with modern tertiary medical care available only to the wealthy in an exclusive but weakening private sector lacking in the renewal generated through contact with thriving medical schools? Will traditional medicine move towards a more advanced form of herbalism and become incorporated into modern medical practice? What will happen to medical schools in South Africa? The current trend of undermining the tertiary components of those medical schools which offer the prospect of retaining the best of modern medicine within the public sector seems to augur a move towards an almost exclusively primary healthcare approach in the public sector. The role and influence of nurses and other professions allied to medicine will also change. With women making up half or more of medical students in South Africa today the emphasis of healthcare systems may change even more than currently imagined. Clearly the type of modern medical care currently available in the industrialized nations cannot yet become the norm for most Africans. Sensible use of available resources, the development of practical and implementable healthcare policies, attention to more than merely biological aspects of health and disease, and ongoing concern for the care of individuals while instituting policies to improve population health may allow the participation of a wide variety of healthcare professionals and stimulate the development of new and innovative programs.                    SRB, HCJR

**AGE, AGING** See GERIATRIC MEDICINE

**ALCHEMY** The possibility of manipulating matter into substances of commercial value, such as silver and gold on the one hand, or of spiritually uplifting value, such as an elixir of life on the other, led to alchemy. It was, in turn, one of the roots of chemistry and biochemistry as well as chemotherapy. Alchemists derived much of their apparatus and manipulative techniques from the equipment used and developed by artisans, technologists, and pharmacists, whose heating, cooking, subliming, and distillation techniques were grist to the mill of chemists in the 16th century. Alchemy also provided chemistry with the idea of a symbolic language for practitioners of the art. Here, however, the use of a multiplicity of synonyms for the same thing served not merely to obscure matters for the uninitiated but (according to some historians) to increase greatly the degree of symbolic allusion — to the mystification of later readers and interpreters. For example, according to one Greek alchemical lexicon, mercury was 'seed of the dragon', 'talc of the dragon', 'dew', 'milk of the black cow', 'Scythian water', 'water of silver', 'water of the moon', 'river water', and 'divine water'. A Persian source lists over 80 synonyms for the philosopher's stone, a mysterious seed which supposedly precipitated an instant transmutation. Given that the same synonyms were also used for different substances, the resulting poetic mysticism must have been as confusing for alchemical practitioners as it is for the historian. NEWTON (p 544), for example, spent years compiling an *index chemicus* in an attempt to make sense of alchemical allegory.

Historians have delineated three principal traditions underlying alchemical thought and practice: technical, theoretical, and religious (or psychological). Egyptian and Greek dyers, metallurgists, jewelers, and pharmacists are known to have engaged in tincturing and coloring metallic surfaces from at least the 4th century BC onwards. Such procedures, some of whose recipes have come down to us, were not necessarily fraudulent, but were probably equivalent to the modern production of cheaper synthetic products. Needham, the historian of Chinese alchemy, has usefully called this technology aurifiction. Fraud, fakery, and deliberate deceit were only too possible, and much of the rich and entertaining literature of alchemy, such as Ben Jonson's play *The Alchemist* (1610), hinges on trickery, human frailty, and greed.

Faced by such apparently realistic and successful examples of transmutation by artisans, Greek philosophers saw these as aurifactions; that is, as real transformations similar to the change of water into air or an acorn into an oak tree. In the hands of Aristotelian philosophers, transmutation of one metal into another was explained as the transfer of forms and qualities on to a basic, formless, underlying matter. To this esoteric workshop-based aurifiction and aurifaction was added, in the melting-pot of religious and philosophical movements of the 2nd and 1st centuries

BC, a religious and symbolic interpretation of alchemical transmutation. In this esoteric alchemy, the art became a language and ritual concerned more with an individual's quest for spiritual enlightenment and transmutation than with real metallurgy. Indeed, it is by no means clear from the surviving Greek writings whether the chemical experiments described were imaginary or, if carried out, merely a means to a spiritual end.

## Transformations

In most cultures (for alchemy seems to have been a universal technical and spiritual experience) transformations of matter, or of the human condition, were believed to be achieved through the use of a material substance such as 'the philosopher's stone', or elixir, or by combining spiritual practices with revealed knowledge. Whereas Greek alchemy laid stress upon silver and gold as the most perfect metals, or on significant color changes in the search for the stone, Chinese alchemy stressed the role of cinnabar (mercuric sulfide) and potable gold. Needham has also suggested that Chinese alchemists, in developing spiritual and physical exercises for their inner perfection, hit upon ways of preparing sex hormones from human urine (macrobiotics). Modern experimentation has, however, failed to confirm that the Chinese would have been able to prepare sufficient concentrations of steroids to have been of physiological benefit.

On the other hand, Greek, Indian, and Chinese alchemists undoubtedly perfected the art of distillation so much so that, when the practices were passed to the Arabic civilization from the 9th century onwards, they were able to isolate mineral acids such as nitric and hydrochloric acids, as well as alcohol. When knowledge of Greek and Arabic alchemy passed to the Latin West, these new substances were gradually put to use in the preparation of medicinal materials by, among others, John of Rupescissa (*fl.* 1340), whose preparations of 'quintessences' proved useful to PARACELSUS (p 617) and his followers. Paracelsus not only expanded the Arabic doctrine that two principles, sulfur and mercury, were the roots of all things by adding a third principle, salt, but he taught that the universe itself functioned like a chemical laboratory. Indeed, God, the Creator, was a divine alchemist whose macrocosmic drama was mirrored in the microcosmic world of man and earthly creatures. It followed that physiological and pathological processes were chemical in nature and that treatments of diseases were best effected by chemical medicines rather than by the herbal ones of the ancients.

The ramifications of this iatrochemical movement were far-reaching. For the Paracelsians,

A 16th century engraving showing an archetypal alchemist — more magician than scientist, with his black cat and crow, ancient volumes, and wild-eyed dedication. (Reproduced courtesy of the Mary Evans Picture Library.)

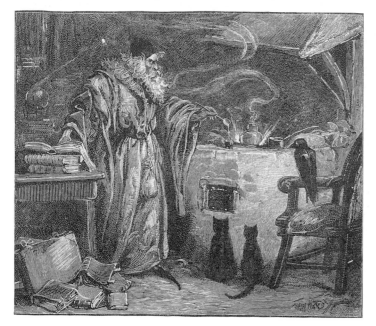

# THE GREAT KILLERS: AIDS

AIDS stands for 'acquired immunodeficiency syndrome' — a syndrome being a cluster of medical conditions. It is caused by the human immunodeficiency virus (HIV), which weakens the body's immune system.

A micro-organism in the family of retroviruses, HIV spreads through sexual intercourse, via blood transfusions, through contaminated needles used for drug-injecting, and from a woman to her child during pregnancy, childbirth, or breast-feeding. Fortunately, the virus is not transmitted via insects, through air or water, or through household contact (for example, eating from the same dish).

HIV is an insidious and slow-acting virus. Most infected people look healthy and feel well for the first five years or so and may not even suspect they have HIV, even though they can unknowingly transmit it to others. An HIV antibody test is the only sure way to find out whether one is seropositive (infected).

Once infected, people are infected for life and will probably succumb to AIDS. As their viral load grows, they come down with conditions such as fatigue, diarrhea, and thrush, and ultimately develop more serious conditions such as opportunistic infections, Kaposi sarcoma, tuberculosis, *Pneumocystis carinii* pneumonia, and meningitis. In the absence of antiretroviral treatment, the life-threatening diseases that characterize AIDS — the end-stage of HIV infection — tend to occur within ten years or so; after this, survival generally does not exceed 3–5 years.

## Care and prevention

While there is no cure for HIV infection, the development of AIDS can now be postponed, survival prolonged, and quality of life improved with therapy involving a mix of protease inhibitors and reverse transcriptase inhibitors — two classes of antiretroviral drugs that work synergistically by attacking HIV at two different points in its cycle of replication. Combination therapy of this kind, using at least three antiretroviral drugs, was introduced in 1995 and became widespread in the industrialized world in 1996, where it has significantly reduced AIDS deaths and changed the image of the epidemic.

Combination drug therapy is not a panacea. It is expensive and difficult to take, and requires an advanced medical infrastructure to monitor patients' side-effects and immune system function. Given that 95% of all people with HIV live in the developing world, where even basic drugs for combating opportunistic infections are often unavailable, antiretroviral therapy is out of practical reach in these countries.

For reducing mother-to-child transmission, research has shown the effectiveness of antiretroviral drugs given to a pregnant seropositive woman. The mother can further reduce her baby's HIV risk by avoiding breast-feeding.

HIV spread through sex and drug use can be reduced by:

- persuading and educating people to avoid unsafe sex and the use of unsterile needles
- tackling social and economic factors that increase behavior (for example, enforced separation from family)
- providing health services and technologies, including education for drug users coupled with harm-reduction measures such as sterile injection equipment; the male condom; the female condom (a polyurethane vaginal sheath that lines the vagina and covers the vaginal opening, thus remaining visible); and prompt antibiotic treatment for sexually transmitted diseases such as chancroid and syphilis which increase 10–300-fold the risk of becoming infected from a single exposure.

Various avenues are being pursued to develop a vaccine that would protect against HIV — a long-term investment but an essential one, for 'behavioral prevention' will never be 100% effective. While a number of candidate vaccines have been shown to be safe and capable of inducing an immune response in human volunteers, just one so far has progressed to the stage of large-scale efficacy trials.

In parallel, research is being conducted to develop a microbicidal cream or foam that a woman could apply vaginally before intercourse, if necessary without her partner's knowledge.

## Scope and shape of the global epidemic

HIV seems to have begun its epidemic spread in the mid-to-late 1970s. By the end of 1999, based on more complete surveillance information than ever before available, the Joint United Nations Programme on HIV/AIDS (UNAIDS) and the World Health Organization (one of the seven UNAIDS co-sponsors) estimated that more than 33 million people were infected with HIV. Around 5.6 million of them — 5 million adults (43% of them women) and close to 600 000 children under age 15 — became infected during 1999. In other words, the epidemic continues to spread at a rate of almost 16 000 new infections a day.

While HIV-infected people in the richer countries are surviving longer, some 75 000 inhabitants of Western Europe and North America became infected during 1999, mainly through drug-injecting or sex between men, although heterosexual transmission gained in importance.

World-wide, over 95% of the new infections in 1999 occurred in the developing world, where poverty, migration, conflicts, and sharp contrasts in wealth and power create fertile soil for the spread of HIV. The country with the single largest infection

(continued overleaf)

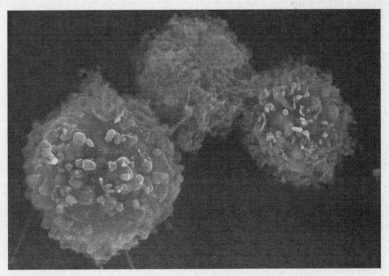

The AIDS virus.

(continued)

burden is India, where an estimated 3–4 million people already have HIV, including drug users, sex workers, and their clients, but also monogamous housewives. In Eastern Europe, where the virus also arrived relatively recently, explosive outbreaks are occurring in the Russian Federation, Ukraine, and elsewhere, largely fueled by drug-injecting.

**A development crisis**

The hardest-hit region of all is still Africa south of the Sahara desert, where over 23 million people are living with HIV. Once concentrated in central and eastern Africa, the epidemic is now spreading fastest in the southern part of the continent, where countries such as Botswana and Zimbabwe, which estimate that up to 26% of all adults aged 15–49 are infected.

This severe and longstanding epidemic poses an urgent threat to development. In the African countries where at least a tenth of the adult population is infected, a child born in 2000–2005 may expect to survive only to age 43, instead of to age 60 had AIDS not been in the picture. By 1996 the direct and indirect costs of AIDS already represented 8% of Namibia's gross domestic product. In Côte d'Ivoire's urban households where the breadwinner has AIDS, family income drops by two-thirds. Because of the epidemic Zimbabwe expected to be burying 350 people a day by the year 2000 and in 2005 to have over 900 000 AIDS orphans.

**What can be done?**

There are no quick fixes, technological or otherwise, to prevent HIV or alleviate the impact of AIDS on families and communities. In the absence of a vaccine, prevention cannot

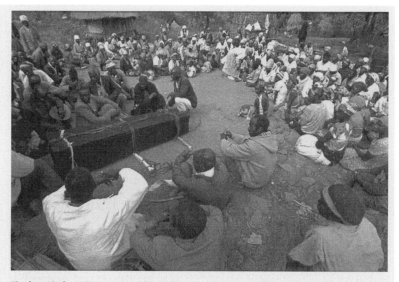

The funeral of an AIDS victim in Africa, where AIDS is now one of the biggest killers.

be imposed on people, only *by* them. But prevention does work, as shown by the documented success of many industrialized countries, Thailand, and Uganda in curbing HIV infection rates. While the industrialized world needs to practice financial solidarity in bringing the global epidemic under control, all countries potentially have an important resource — political courage and leadership. Courage is needed for the hard political choices required for AIDS prevention, including introducing sexual health education in schools (half of all infections today are in young people under 25) and promoting

condoms through the media. Leadership is needed to break through the silence and stigma surrounding AIDS and to extend solidarity and support to people who are already infected or affected by the epidemic. These are the individuals who can speak with authority about AIDS to their friends and neighbors and give the epidemic a human face. So long as HIV remains an unspoken risk, a mere abstraction, ordinary people will not take it seriously and adopt the lifetime changes in their personal, intimate behavior that can protect them and their loved ones from harm. PP, SC

MAJORCAN ALCHEMIST

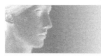

Raymond **LULLY** (1235–1315). Majorcan alchemist. Lully joined the Franciscans and learned Arabic in order to convert North African Moslems to Christianity. He sought the philosopher's stone, which would change base metals into gold, then thought to be a sovereign remedy against most ills. He invented a logic machine, which when fed premises spewed out the appropriate conclusions.

alchemy — or rather chemistry, as it was being called by the 16th century — was to be the handmaiden of medicine. Most notably it meant that chemistry, or at least pharmaceutical chemistry, became part of the European medical curriculum. This was to prove of mutual benefit both for the advancement of medicine and for the emergence of chemistry from the spiritual blanket of esoteric alchemy. Less popular than astrology, the latter continues to inform the doctrines and practices of occultists.                                    WHB

*See also* GREEK MEDICINE; PHILOSOPHER'S STONE

**ALCOHOL**, or ethanol, is a simple organic compound, with the formula $C_2H_5OH$. A colorless liquid, it is produced by using the enzymes in yeast to ferment the sugars and starch found all over nature (from grain to grapes, and vegetables to honey). Pure alcohol is tasteless, but so-called con-

geners give the beverage its characteristic appearance and flavor (and may also be partly responsible for a hangover). Fermentation stops when the alcohol concentration reaches about 13%, because this kills the enzymes, but weaker alcoholic drinks are prepared by stopping fermentation earlier and stronger ones by distillation (heating the liquid to drive off some of the water) or by fortifying wine with spirits. Thus the alcohol concentration in beer is 3–5%, wine 10–12%, sherry and port 15–20%, and spirits 37–60%.

Alcohol is absorbed into the bloodstream from both the stomach and the small intestine. The rate of absorption depends on the strength of the drink (it is maximal with drinks containing 20–30% of alcohol, such as sherry or vermouth) and whether it is part of a meal (starch and sugars in the stomach delay absorption considerably). After absorption, alcohol is distributed widely throughout the body, except in the fatty tissue (which has a poor blood supply). Up to 10% is excreted in the breath and urine, but most is broken down in the liver.

The blood alcohol level reflects many features: how much has been drunk and how quickly; how fast it was absorbed; and body size and gender (since women have relatively more fatty tissue, more alcohol stays in the bloodstream than it does in men).

Even at low blood levels (30–50 mg/100 ml) alcohol affects judgement and performance of skilled tasks: at 80 mg/100 ml the risk of a road accident for a driver is doubled. Given these effects, and the fact that a couple of decades ago drink-driving accidents were rising all over the world, most countries have now introduced legal limits for car driving, though these vary widely — from zero in Sweden through 60 mg/100 ml in many other European Union countries (80 mg/100 ml in Britain) to 100 mg/100 ml in some states in the USA. Such laws have reduced the number of drink-driving accidents and deaths considerably. People in almost all cultures, societies, and nations have used alcohol since before written histories existed. It has been used to soften the harsh realities of an unkind existence, as a sacred ingredient in religious rites and pagan orgies, and to loosen the restraints that inhibit social (and sexual) intercourse. The extent to which alcohol use pervades a nation varies greatly. In orthodox and strict Islamic societies and among RELIGIOUS SECTS in which alcohol consumption is taboo, some furtive drinking takes place regardless. In many nations and communities that have adopted prohibition of alcohol, the law has been widely and often conspicuously flouted, for example, in the USA during PROHIBITION.

Currently doctors are concerned with the harmful effects of alcohol on health and society. In past centuries, however, they relied on it for treating illness (a paradox similar to that with TOBACCO). *Aqua vitae* was popularized at Montpellier by Arnaud de Villeneuve in the 13th century, spirits distilled from grain at Leiden by Francius Sylvius in 1680, and laudanum (an alcoholic tincture of opium) by Thomas SYDENHAM (p 721) in Britain in 1690. In the late 1700s John Brown, another physician, recommended alcohol for all 'asthenic' conditions (those he classified as due to inadequate stimulation). By this time, however, society had become concerned at the evident havoc wrought by cheap spirits; in London alone 11.2 million gallons of spirits were being drunk a year (about 7 gallons per adult). In 1726 the Royal College of Physicians asked one of its fellows to petition Parliament about the evils of excessive spirit drinking, and feeling at large was portrayed by Hogarth in *Gin Lane* some years later. Various Acts of Parliament were passed, and the imposition of a license to dispense spirits was successful eventually in considerably reducing consumption.

Campaigns against alcohol intensified at the turn of the 19th century led by two medical reformers, one American, Benjamin RUSH (p 726), the other British, Thomas Trotter. Both published books, which were to be the foundation of a widespread temperance movement throughout Europe and the USA, lasting throughout the 19th century and persisting into the 20th. The first temperance organizations were formed in the USA in 1808, Ireland in 1829, and Norway and Sweden in 1836 and 1837, and aimed at sanctions against spirits and moderation for other drinks, rather than total abstinence. Their activities waxed and waned for much of this period, though eventually in the 20th century some countries introduced nationwide prohibition, not only in the USA (where several individual states had pioneered such bans), but also in Finland and Sweden. Other countries also came to restrict the availability of alcohol. Given the obvious connection between civil disorder and drinking, Britain (long notorious for its drunkenness) had been the first to do this, introducing licensing laws for ale houses as far back as 1551, but was imitated by few other countries. Nevertheless, again in Britain, concern about its effects on munitions workers during the First World War led to Parliament setting up a liquor control body and passing a Licensing Act drastically limiting the hours when alcohol could be drunk outside the home and could be sold.

**Licensing laws**

Today, though some countries retain licensing laws, few outside the Muslim world have retained a total ban on the sale and consumption of alcohol. Moreover, alcohol is relatively cheaper than in the past and more freely available, as in

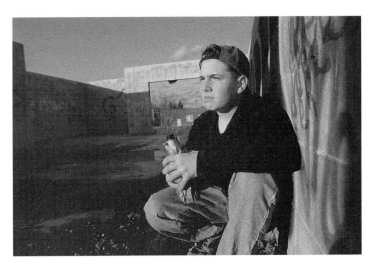

Alcohol abuse is a continuing problem among young people. (© Tony Stone Images.)

## THE CAGE TEST

Do you have difficulty **C**utting down?

Are you **A**ngry because somebody criticized your drinking?

Do you feel **G**uilty about drinking?

Do you take an **E**ye-opener (a morning drink to relieve withdrawal symptoms)?

corner stores and supermarkets, and social drinking has now become even more accepted as part of western social culture. Thus in industrial nations such as the USA, rather more than half the population drinks alcohol daily. Most drinkers consume only modest amounts, one or two alcoholic drinks a day being the mode. Survey data are not consistent, but the evidence suggests that consumption is much higher, and the proportion of heavy drinkers (seven or more drinks a day) is greater in Eastern Europe and Russia than in any other part of the industrialized world. Indeed, in the latter vodka is cited as one of the main factors behind the falling expectation of life since the breakup of the former Soviet Union.

Studies on alcohol consumption have been made easier by the development of an accurate measurement: alcohol units. One unit is 10 g of alcohol, the amount in half a pint (440 ml) of beer, one glass of wine (125 ml), one small glass of sherry, or one measure of spirits. Drinking one unit raises the blood alcohol concentration to 15–20 mg/100 ml — the same amount that can be cleared from the bloodstream in an hour. The current classification gives a recommended limit on the weekly intake of not over 15 units for women and 21 for men (low consumption), defining moderate consumption as 15–35 and 21–50 units, respectively, and high consumption at over 35 and over 50 units. Possibly no level of consumption can be guaranteed as totally safe, but the health risks increase with the amount drunk. Drinkers at the top end of the high range, or over it, will almost certainly have alcohol-related problems, whether due to the excessive use of (abuse) or dependence (addiction) on alcohol — when stopping drinking is associated with serious withdrawal effects.

The damage caused by alcohol includes many different effects: social — accidents, vandalism, wife, husband and baby battering, assault, divorce, and homicide; psychological — alcohol abuse (addiction), depression, and suicide; and physical. These last include effects on:

- the unborn baby (the fetal alcohol syndrome, with deformities of the face and mental retardation)
- digestive system (inflammation of the stomach and pancreas)
- liver (hepatitis, cirrhosis, and cancer)
- heart (hypertension and cardiomyopathy — degeneration of the muscle)
- endocrine system (diabetes, gout, and reduced sexual function in both sexes)
- nervous system (epilepsy, degeneration of nerves and brain substance, Korsakoff syndrome — confusion and incoordination due to the associated deficiency of vitamin B).

The doctor may not suspect that such conditions are linked to alcohol abuse; surveys have shown that only about 1 in 10 heavy drinkers are recognized, but that in Britain an average general practitioner with 2000 adults on his list is likely to have 186 heavy drinkers in this with 37 experiencing problems from abuse and 19 dependent on alcohol. A quarter of hospital patients will be found to be heavy drinkers.

The American Psychiatric Association defines alcohol abuse as a pattern of alcohol use leading to clinically significant impairment or distress, manifested by one or more of the following, over a 12-month period: (a) recurrent alcohol use resulting in failure to fulfil major role obligations at work, school, or home; (b) recurrent alcohol use in situations where it is physically dangerous; (c) recurrent alcohol-related legal problems; (d) continued alcohol use despite a persistent or recurrent social or interpersonal problem caused or exacerbated by the effects of alcohol.

### Alcohol dependency

The Association also defines alcohol dependency as a pattern of alcohol use leading to important distress or impairment as manifested by three or more of the following occurring in the same 12-month period: (a) tolerance; (b) withdrawal effects; (c) alcohol use in greater quantity or for a longer period than intended; (d) persistent desire or unsuccessful efforts to reduce or control alcohol use; (e) a great deal of time spent acquiring, using, or recovering from the effects of alcohol; (f) important social, occupational, or recreational activities given up or reduced because of alcohol use; (g) alcohol use continued despite knowledge of a persistent or recurrent physical or psychological problem caused by using alcohol. With this definition, the one-year prevalence rate of alcohol dependence in the USA is about 3.9%.

Alcohol dependency and alcohol abuse are common among people who have other habits or addictive disorders such as heavy smoking, so tobacco-related diseases tend also to be common. Thus death rates from TUBERCULOSIS, cancer at many sites, stroke and heart disease, pneumonia, and of course accidents, are higher among those who abuse alcohol than in the general population.

In diagnosing alcohol abuse or dependency a doctor has to think of it as the sole or a major cause of a patient's symptoms. Many doctors forget to take a routine drinking history, though four simple questions (the CAGE test) will reveal cause for concern.

The treatment of excessive drinking is more successful than is often acknowledged. Simple recognition of the problem is often sufficient for people to adjust their habits (particularly if they keep a diary of the number of units they are drinking every day). As with stopping smoking, sympathetic but firm advice from a trusted family doctor, or pressure from a spouse or employer, is often the deciding factor in somebody deciding to cut down consumption.

For those who continue to abuse alcohol, the options include taking Antabuse (which sensitizes a person to alcohol), and expert counseling. Notably successful has been Alcoholics Anonymous, a self-help group formed in Akron, Ohio, in 1935 and now with local groups all over the world. With a motto 'One day at a time', its members have to share their problems in group discussions. For those dependent on alcohol expert counseling or detoxification in an institution may be needed, but treatment can sometimes then be continued using Alcoholics Anonymous as a resource.

Against all this it is difficult to quantify the benefits of drinking small amounts of alcohol for the individual. Nevertheless, an unexpected result of recent research has been that one or two glasses of wine a day may be protective against coronary heart disease. Epidemiological studies of risk factors have consistently shown that such light drinkers have lower death rates than either teetotallers or heavier drinkers. Indeed, the all-cause death rates for adult men and women show this same relationship: the lowest death rates are among light or moderate drinkers. The explanation, however, may lie in related behavior patterns rather than in alcohol use by itself — in other words, such people may choose a healthier life-style than most, with particular attention to diet, smoking, and exercise. Another explanation has been that it is the substances present in the skins of the grapes and not the alcohol itself, that have the protective effect on the heart.

Like several other contemporary problems — smoking, obesity, and lack of exercise — excessive alcohol drinking is another self-inflicted problem that may result in preventable but serious illness. Known ways to cut down the problem include restricting the availability and increasing the cost of alcohol. Yet society is unable or unwilling to make such decisions, and to some extent the problem is getting worse, with a rise not only in overall consumption but also in alcohol abuse by professional women. A British survey in 1993 put the health and societal costs of alcohol at £2 billion ($3.5 billion). Against this has to be put the undoubted but unmeasurable pleasure of drinking alcohol, and also the employment it generates (125 000 people in Britain) and the yield in taxes (£7 billion, $11.50 billion). Given the long history of alcohol usage, however, it is unlikely that new solutions will be found to old problems.

SPL, JML

*See also* PATIENTS' ASSOCIATIONS; SUBSTANCE ABUSE

## ALLGEMEINES KRANKENHAUS, VIENNA
See GERMANY, AUSTRIA, AND SWITZERLAND

**ALLERGY** At the time of HIPPOCRATES (p 386) any form of breathing difficulty was 'ASTHMA' and almost any kind of skin disease was 'eczema'. In modern times the use of these Greek terms has been much more restricted. The term asthma now describes the transient wheezing attacks and obstruction to breathing which come and go, while eczema means the slowly developing, weeping, crusting skin reaction which occurs in an allergic subject.

The notion of allergy is itself a modern concept, introduced in 1906 by the Austrian pediatrician Clemens von PIRQUET (p 32) to describe the altered reactions that occur when the body is exposed to specific foreign substances on more than one occasion. The way in which this specific sensitization develops has been worked out as the science of IMMUNOLOGY has developed. What we now recognize as abnormal allergic reactions to harmless inhaled grass pollen (hay fever) or to common foods such as cow's milk were certainly regarded in a different light in earlier centuries.

When MAIMONIDES (p 59) wrote his *Treatise on asthma* in the 12th century, asthma was a difficulty in breathing or a pain in the chest, and the question of an external cause was hardly considered. By the middle of the 16th century, however, reactions to external agents had begun to be noticed and there were several reports of 'rose fever'. A patient of Leonardo Otallo's found that roses made him sneeze, made his nose itch, and gave him headaches. Pietro Mattioli had a patient who was so sensitive to cats that he became ill on entering a room in which a cat was concealed without the man's knowledge. Soon afterwards there was a report of food intolerance in a young count, whose lips swelled up when he ate eggs. Indeed, Pierre Borel, in 1656, confirmed a patient's sensitivity to egg by applying some to his skin and showing that it raised a blister. The use of a skin test to demonstrate altered reactivity thus has a long tradition.

### Bronchial asthma
By 1686, asthma had come to be defined by Salmon as 'difficult respiration, sometimes with and sometimes without fever, sometimes with a noise and sometimes without, arising from an obstruction of the bronchia and cells of the lungs'. Eleven years later, Sir John Floyer observed that exercise and environmental pollution were exacerbating factors, noting that 'Any kind of **smoak** offends the spirits of the asthmatic'. It was left to Bernardino RAMAZZINI (p 583) to emphasize the relevance of specific contact with external agents, when he described the first example of industrial asthma occurring in bakers. The hazards of industrial asthma were not,

## PIONEERS IN ALLERGY

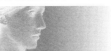

Armand **TROUSSEAU** (1801–67). French physician. Trousseau was the leading French clinician of his day, and became professor of therapy at the Faculté in 1839 and of medicine in 1850, moving from the Hôpital S. Antoine to the Hôtel-Dieu. In 1828 he visited Gibraltar with a commission to report on yellow fever. He was the first to undertake tracheostomy in Paris (1831), published an important monograph on laryngeal tuberculosis (1837), and popularized pleural paracentesis (1843) and intubation (1851). He suggested the eponymic titles of Graves's disease (1860) and Addison's disease (1856), and described the spasm produced by compression of the nerves in latent tetany (Trousseau's sign, 1864). His publication *Clinique médicale de l'Hôtel-Dieu de Paris* (1861) enjoyed immense success.
*(continued on p 32)*

however, fully appreciated until the middle of the 20th century, when the small number of asthma sufferers in agriculture and in the food industry were joined by several workers in the new chemical, plastic, and pharmaceutical industries. In modern Japan, up to 15% of cases of asthma in men are suspected of having an industrial origin.

*Mechanisms* The physiology of asthma begins in the cells of the lungs. Inflammation is now recognized as important, but other triggering agents may contribute, leading to spasm of smooth muscle and reversible airways obstruction, which are both hallmarks of the disease. This kind of 'twitchy lung' may either be part of an allergic reaction (extrinsic asthma) or may occur in people whose bronchial muscle fibers overreact for various other reasons (intrinsic asthma). The factors that can cause this overreaction range from viruses to the inhalation of sulphur dioxide, in industrial air pollution. Exercise and emotion may both cause overbreathing, which makes things worse. The 19th century French physician TROUSSEAU (p 29) was himself an asthmatic and knew that he was sensitive to horses. He could enter his stables without any problems unless, in that enclosed atmosphere, he lost his temper with his coachman and then had an attack of asthma. He had no asthma if he lost his temper in the open air because it needed a combination of allergy and emotion to precipitate an attack.

Wheezing may also occur if the airways are narrowed by retained phlegm or by thickening of the lining of the bronchus and its branches, which both occur in chronic bronchitis. For asthma to be diagnosed, some proof of bronchial irritability or a reversible spasm is therefore needed.

### Hay fever

The 'summer catarrh' which had at first been attributed to roses came to be better understood by the 19th century. In 1831, John Elliotson's lectures in the *London Medical Gazette* laid the blame 'upon the flower of grass, and probably upon the pollen'. Elliotson was also an enthusiastic proponent of MESMERISM and PHRENOLOGY and hence his views were not readily accepted, but a number of his contemporaries certainly debated the grass pollen theory. In 1835, W. P. Kirkman, an asthmatic physician, found some pollinating grass in his hothouse in December, sniffed the pollens, and suffered a severe asthmatic attack.

In the winter of 1871, Charles Blackley came close to repeating Kirkman's experiments when he walked into a previously locked room, disturbed a vase of dried grasses, and gave himself an unseasonal attack of hay fever. He then went further. He scratched pollen into his skin and caused considerable swelling and a vigorous local reaction. The evidence of his sensitivity to pollen was thus confirmed.

Blackley suspected that the transmission of pollen through the atmosphere could occur at a considerable height. He therefore invented a trap with a timed shuttering device, in which he placed a sticky slide with which to collect pollen from the atmosphere. Borne aloft on a tandem series of kites, the sticky slides collected pollen even at a height of 500 m, thus proving Blackley's point. At this stage, he went on to draw some remarkable conclusions. He advised his patients to spend the summer season either on a peninsula or on a yacht. Having shown that tiny amounts of pollen could cause a reaction, he also reviewed his entire approach to the practice of medicine and spent the rest of his career as a homeopathist.

### Skin reactions

The familiar nettle rash occurs when histamine is pricked into the skin by hairs of the nettle. It is similar in appearance to the allergic rash of urticaria (or hives), but it does not follow that every case of urticaria has a similar origin. Nevertheless, urticaria is the most rapidly developing allergic rash — so rapid that the cause, whether it is a food, a drug, a hot bath, or an insect sting, is often recognized by the person who is afflicted. A much more prolonged and insidious skin reaction, with additional inflammatory features, can be present in those who suffer from eczema. Eczema thus presents a far greater challenge, both in diagnosis and treatment.

A house dust mite. (From Davies, R. and Ollier, S. (1989). *Allergy: the facts*, OUP.)

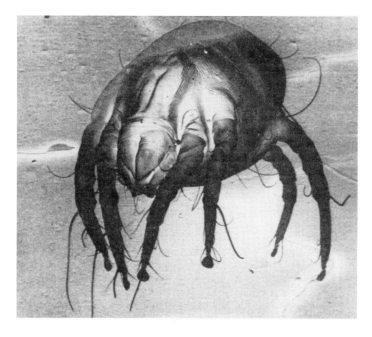

In 1895 in Germany, a dermatologist called Joseph Jadassohn took eczema as his starting point and used patch tests to show the importance of specific sensitivity in the skin. He impregnated lint with his test solutions, attached them to the skin with plaster, and was able to show that areas of inflammation developed in several of those he tested. The method came to be widely adopted and quickly showed that specific sensitivity was not uncommon.

The tendency to develop eczematous skin reactions appears most often in early childhood, when the child may become sensitized to the foreign protein in cow's milk or to the dust mites present in mattress dust and in bedclothes. This type of rash does not only follow direct skin contact but may be provoked when the substance concerned is either inhaled or swallowed. It follows that not all causes of eczema may be easily identified. In childhood, the most common agents involved are cow's milk and sometimes other foods. However, more than one provoking agent can contribute, and the omission of a single food is unlikely to be followed by a complete cure.

## Allergy and anaphylaxis

Von Pirquet based his observations on allergy upon the unpleasant reactions which followed when horse serum was administered during the treatment of diphtheria. It was Charles Richet, however, who discovered extreme form of the same reaction. Richet injected a dog with the venom of a poisonous jellyfish, the Portuguese man-of-war, in the hope that increasing doses of venom could be tolerated when the venom was given a second or third time. Within seconds of giving the next, small dose of venom, the dog became extremely ill and subsequently died. What was intended to be protective *prophylaxis* proved to be the opposite, and in 1903 he called this *anaphylaxis*. Although it would take a further 60 years before the agents which cause this reaction could be identified, several interesting studies were carried out which sought to define the reaction more clearly. Maurice Arthus injected horse serum into rabbits and then found that a further injection could cause intense *local* inflammation. This Arthus reaction, though regarded at first as a local anaphylaxis, helped to show that several different mechanisms contribute to the body's response. These mechanisms may involve not only a variety of specific chemical antidotes which the body can manufacture itself, but also a complex range of cell reactions The chemical antidotes comprise the so-called 'antibody' system, in which proteins are produced with a precise chemical affinity for the provoking substance (antigen or allergen). These proteins belong to five separate classes of immunoglobulin

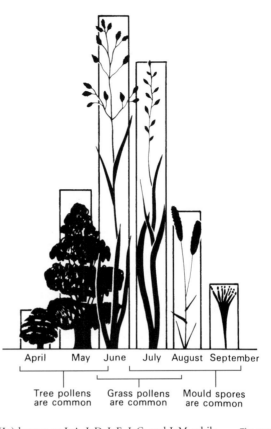

April   May   June   July   August   September

Tree pollens are common   Grass pollens are common   Mould spores are common

The causes of seasonal rhinitis in the UK by month. (From Davies, R. and Ollier, S. (1989). *Allergy: the facts*, OUP.)

(Ig) known as IgA, IgD, IgE, IgG, and IgM, while IgE antibodies have since been shown to be responsible for anaphylaxis and nearly all 'immediate' forms of allergy.

Anaphylaxis is by no means confined to horse serum reactions and can be provoked by insect stings or by food and drugs. An account written in 1765 describes a fatal reaction to a bee sting in a villager who had lost consciousness after two previous stings. On the third occasion he fell to the ground at once and was dead within a few minutes.

There are varying grades of severity of anaphylaxis ranging from flushing of the skin to more severe reactions including asthma, shock, and coma. Reactions to the stings of bees, wasps, or similar insects are now held to account for about four deaths each year in Britain and 10 times that number in the USA. In the latter, also, there may well be over 100 deaths from peanuts and other foods each year.

## Food allergy and intolerance

The most common varieties of food allergy are those that affect infants and young children who vomit or have diarrhea after taking cow's milk, eggs, or fish, or who develop asthma, eczema, hives, or other clear manifestations of an allergic response. As in the USA, there has also been a

(continued)

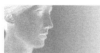

Clemens Freiherr Von **PIRQUET** (1874–1929). Austrian pediatrician of Vienna. Pirquet described a test for tuberculosis in which the surface of the skin is scarified through two drops of old tuberculin, an antigen. A positive result is when after 24–48 hours the site of the scratches shows a red inflamed papule with a central areola. This test confirmed previous tuberculous infection, but did not determine whether the disease was active. Pirquet was one of the founders of the study of allergy.

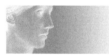

Heinz **KÜSTNER** (1897–1931). German gynecologist and obstetrician. Küstner is remembered for his part in the Prausnitz–Küstner reaction. This is an allergic hypersensitivity response of the skin when the offending substance is injected into the skin of a susceptible subject. Küstner knew that he could not eat cooked fish without experiencing itching, skin weals, coughing, sneezing, and vomiting, the reaction taking about 12 hours to settle down. Prausnitz, in 1912, took some of Küstner's serum and some fish and injected the mixture into his own skin. The area became hot, red, and swollen, and the existence of cutaneous anaphylaxis was established.

striking increase in reports of allergic reactions to peanuts or tree nuts. Whereas most food allergies disappear in later childhood, peanut allergy tends to persist into later life.

The presence of food allergy may certainly be missed, but in recent years it is more often grossly overdiagnosed, even in people who have no allergic symptoms at all. Even in those with undoubted diarrheal or other reactions, allergy is only one cause of food intolerance, most of which are simply solved by avoiding the food concerned.

It now appears that most food intolerance is due to a lack of enzymes or to irritant or toxic substances. It may also occur in association with diseases such as gall bladder disease and gall stones. The mechanism is not always clear, and the occasional relation between certain types of food and the onset of migraine or joint disease is not fully explained either by enzyme defects or by an allergic mechanism.

## Current views

In the early part of the 20th century it was assumed that a special component of blood serum caused allergic reactions, but there was no proof. In a classic experiment, the serum of H. KÜSTNER (this page), who was allergic to fish, was injected into the arm of C. Prausnitz. The next day fish extract was injected into the same site and produced a hypersensitive swelling. Küstner's serum thus contained a 'reagin', a factor which could transfer specific sensitivity to the skin. A. F. Coca, in 1923, suggested that the tendency to produce reagins ran in families, a tendency to which he gave the name of atopy. Forty years later, these reagins were identified for the first time as immunoglobulin E antibodies, shown by the Ishizakas in the USA and Bennich in Sweden to be present in serum in amounts which, although minute, were sufficient to sensitize the skin and the various lining surfaces of the body. The mechanisms of allergy began to be understood.

Another key factor in allergy is the mast cell, together with a rather similar white blood cell, the basophil. Although the mast cell was described by EHRLICH (p 260) in 1877, its function remained a mystery. In the 1940s and 1950s its granules were found to contain heparin and histamine (see below). In fact, the mast cell can synthesize many highly active products which are mediators of inflammation. Since these cells are present below every skin surface and lining membrane of the body, any allergen which penetrates the body surface is likely to come in contact with them. Given the right conditions, this triggers the release of the chemical content of the cells.

The conditions under which this happens are now well understood. Foreign substances to which the body has been exposed provoke the

formation of IgE (immunoglobulin) antibodies tailored to react specifically with them. These antibodies become attached to special receptors on the surface of mast cells, which are thus 'sensitized'. Contact with the same allergen then causes the granules containing histamine to burst through the surface, and other potent mediators and 'cytokines' are produced which attract inflammatory cells to the area. A range of fatty acid derivatives (leukotrienes, prostaglandins, and thromboxanes) increase the local blood flow and have other effects which cause the reaction to build up. If this reaction were to be unrestrained, its crescendo effect would be highly damaging. In fact, powerful switch-off enzymes limit this activity to a level only exceeded in exceptional circumstances.

## Approaches to treatment

In 1901, adrenaline (epinephrine) was discovered, and within two years it had been synthesized. Not only is it the body's main defensive product when anaphylaxis threatens but it has provided a pattern from which anti-allergic drugs can be designed. While interest in adrenaline has therefore continued, the discovery of histamine before the First World War drew attention to another of the body's chemical products, which in this case could trigger the onset of anaphylaxis. In due course chemical engineers designed a large series of antihistamine drugs useful in hay fever and in allergic skin reactions of the nettle rash (urticaria) type. They were, however, strangely ineffective in bronchial asthma. Eventually, with the identification of other mediators, including those derived from arachidonic acid, a whole series of new biologically active agents was found, with molecular patterns which have since been modified to produce designer drugs which can cancel or reinforce the effects of the various chemical mediators.

The administration of anti-asthma drugs by inhalation instead of by tablet or injection has been an example of a further development, of drug 'targeting'. The intention is that the drug should come directly into contact with the cells against which it is directed, in this case the lining cells of the airways. Cortisone and other corticosteroids are used increasingly (but not exclusively) in this way to damp down the inflammation which may contribute to asthmatic attacks. The mast-cell stabilizing cromoglycates are also given by inhalation, and pressurized aerosols and nebulizers can deliver adrenaline-like drugs in this way. As drug delivery systems become more advanced, products are also being developed that are absorbed into the bloodstream and then home directly onto the cells that they are intended to influence.

*Vaccine treatment* In 1911, L. Noon developed a new treatment for hay fever based on the belief that pollen contained a toxin that was responsible for the patient's symptoms. He reasoned, as Richet had before him, that repeated injections of a toxin might accustom the body to its presence and reduce its adverse effects. He used very dilute extracts and his patients claimed to be much improved. He therefore tried to assess his treatment more objectively by instilling different dilutions of pollen under the patient's eyelids both before and after treatment. He was able to show that there was a considerably increased resistance to the allergic effects of pollen after the vaccine treatment.

Subsequently Noon's empirical method was applied to other types of allergy. For example, insect sting allergy came to be treated by injecting extracts of the bodies of bees or wasps, a treatment which Larry Lichtenstein and his colleagues then compared with injections of the venom itself. The venom was effective but — though they had been used for several years — body extracts were not. The use of selected vaccines against allergy, although not without some risk, has thus been shown to provide clinical benefit. It is now known that the pattern of antibody production and cytokine release can be modified by such injections, but the main reasons for the success of the method remain uncertain.

### Unconventional concepts and doubtful tests

The notion that all adverse reactions are allergic is clearly an oversimplification. However, ecologists and environmentalists who are concerned to prevent the contamination of food and the pollution of the atmosphere have often used the term 'allergy' in an undefined sense, to be applied whenever people are adversely affected by a smoky atmosphere or by food. In 1982, there emerged a concept of 'total allergy' which proved to be neither allergic nor total but nevertheless became the subject of much public interest and debate. This centered on the question of whether food allergy and other immune reactions might be so extreme that a specially ventilated atmosphere and specially prepared uncontaminated food had to be used to protect the affected person. Although severe allergies may exist, there was no evidence that allergy was responsible for most of these problems, which were nevertheless much publicized by the press and television.

The separation of fact and fiction deserves some attention. The main thrust of the 'total allergy' claims concerned food allergy, which has indeed come to be accepted as an important allergic disorder, with effects that are not necessarily confined to the bowel itself.

In many cases, the person who is affected by a variety of symptoms insists on blaming food for

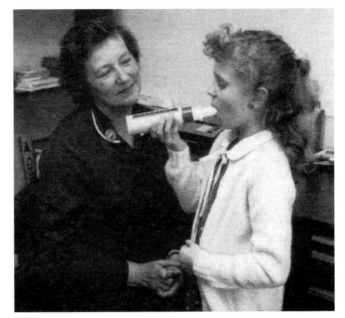

A child using a peak flow meter Mini-Wright. (From Davies, R. and Ollier, S. (1989). *Allergy: the facts,* OUP.)

what is in fact a psychological illness or a food fad, sometimes made worse by an unconscious habit of overbreathing, which may not only cause wheezing episodes but also giddiness, tingling, and malaise.

The public is understandably less concerned with precise definitions than with the relief of their symptoms or, at least, the time to discuss problems. When conventional medicine fails to fulfill these requirements, unorthodox practitioners may offer to fill the gap, sometimes by offering to identify 'allergies' from the radionic examination of a sample of hair, cytotoxic, or immunoglobulin (IgG) tests of the blood, or other unsubstantiated methods. On the results, advice may be given on foods to avoid, the administration of drops under the tongue, or several other treatments that have no evidence of efficacy. In many cases, however, false hopes are raised, nutritionally inadequate diets given, or potentially treatable diseases left undiagnosed until a late stage.

The follow-through from basic science to clinical benefit has been slow and, in spite of advances, there appears to be a rising trend in allergy and asthma world-wide. Better anti-histamines have been developed, topical corticosteroids and other pharmacologic approaches have improved the treatment of asthma, and, for a few conditions, hyposensitizing injections have given more promising results. New methods of diagnosis and treatment are to be welcomed, provided they are evaluated critically before being widely recommended.

33

When John Elliotson, in 1831, identified 'the flower of grass' as the cause of hay fever, he proved to be right. When he espoused mesmerism he proved to be wrong. Charles Blackley, whose method for diagnosing allergy is still in use 100 years later, turned to homeopathy in his later years on a totally false premise. It is well over a century since these highly analytical people jumped to wrong conclusions, but mistakes are as prevalent now as in their time. A critical assessment of new methods of diagnosis and treatment is as necessary now as it was then.      ML

**ALLIED HEALTH PROFESSIONS** (or greater health profession, a term first used by Sir Theodore Fox, editor of the *Lancet*) constitutes a variety of disciplines that make up most of the healthcare workforce and thus form a vital part of the primary, secondary, and tertiary healthcare system infrastructure. The services they provide include prevention, identification, monitoring, and evaluation of diseases and disabilities; health promotion; rehabilitation; health systems management; and dietary and nutritional services. The American Medical Association's Committee on Allied Health Education and Accreditation defines allied health professionals as 'A large cluster of healthcare related professions and personnel whose functions include assisting, facilitating, or complementing the work of physicians and other specialists in the healthcare system, and who choose to be identified as allied health personnel'. Although there is still some debate about who should be counted among the allied health profession, membership is generally defined by a specific educational pathway, a unique scope of practice, common knowledge, self-regulation, accreditation, and licensure.

Most of the health professions, with some exceptions such as PHARMACY, NURSING, and MIDWIFERY, developed from medicine in the first part of the 20th century. Their development was primarily in response to rapid technological and population expansions which included the effects of the First and Second World Wars, and the Industrial Revolution. Before then, health service providers had limited knowledge of the causes of diseases and their treatment. As science and technology progressed, however, physicians and nurses embraced new clinical methods of management (for example, radiography). And as ground breaking technological advancements in medicine became increasingly common, physicians and nurses were replaced by other health care workers, who could specialize in operating medical technology safely and appropriately. This transfer of duties allowed physicians and nurses to practice their professions without becoming overwhelmed with training in new technologies.

With the acquisition of new information and technologies, members of the allied health profession along with their medical counterparts began to conduct research on the effectiveness of new clinical interventions, a feature which continues today.

In 1960, the Professions Supplementary to Medicine Act in the United Kingdom included such occupations as chiropody, dietetics, medical laboratory technology, occupational therapy, physical therapy, radiography, remedial gymnastics, and orthopedics. Today, many more occupations are considered among the allied health profession.

Occupational therapy, physical therapy, and speech-language pathology exemplify how health professions have taken shape over the last century. Other allied health professions generally follow the same patterns.

### Occupational therapy

The roots of occupational therapy go back at least 200 years when the French physician Philippe PINEL (p 77) found that the condition of patients with mental illness who were given menial tasks improved faster than in patients who were idle. The discipline has since evolved into a profession of therapists, who direct their patients in activities designed to help them learn the skills necessary for daily tasks, to diminish or correct pathology, and to promote and maintain health. Occupational therapists use such activities as macramé projects to gain strength or endurance in fine motor hand movements; sorting activities to improve visual discrimination, as well as other games, toys, arts, crafts, music, and dance that lead to functional improvement.

Although a few physicians carried out occupational therapy at the turn of the 19th century, it was during World War I that occupational therapy grew into an established health profession. In 1917, the National Society for the Promotion of Occupational Therapy was established. Three years later, it became what is now known as the American Occupational Therapy Association. In 1923, a major development occurred when the Federal Industrial Rehabilitation Act in the United States required hospitals that treated patients with industrial accidents to provide occupational therapy.

Currently, there are two educational levels for practitioners: technical and professional, and occupational therapists may specialize in gerontology, developmental disabilities, training in activities for daily living, prosthetics training and construction of splints, and rehabilitation for spinal cord injuries and neurological disorders. Accreditation has been granted to standardized educational programs, and licensure is also required for practitioners.

In the past, patients were referred by physicians for occupational therapy. Now, however, many jurisdictions permit direct access to these services for clients (occupational therapists prefer to call patients 'clients'). Occupational therapy is evolving into a profession that enables individuals to perform daily occupations beyond work. Many occupational therapists work in industry, in consulting services, in prisons and schools, and with communities rather than individual clients. In Canada, occupational therapy has been named one of the top two growth professions in healthcare.

### Physical therapy

Physical therapy, also called physiotherapy, has as its primary purpose the promotion of optimal human health and function through the application of scientific principles to prevent, identify, assess, correct, or alleviate acute or prolonged movement dysfunction.

Physical therapy developed during World War I in direct response to the need to rehabilitate large numbers of wounded soldiers. After the war, physical therapists continued to work with hospitalized veterans as well as civilians. 1920 brought the formation of the American Women's Physical Therapeutic Association and subsequently, the American Physical Therapy Association. World War II brought again a sudden increase in demand for physical therapists, which was met by the formation of federally funded university programs to train physical therapists. Although many certificate programs were discontinued after the war, physical therapists were still in demand because of the poliomyelitis epidemics of the 1940s and '50s. During these two decades, physical therapy received massive donations from the private sector; for example, from the National Foundation for Infantile Paralysis for the employment of therapists and the expansion of educational pathways for greater enrollment.

Today, physical therapists have more autonomy than many other health professions. Many practitioners have private practices, and more and more districts allow direct patient access without physician referral. Physical therapists may specialize, for example, in: pulmonary therapy for critically ill patients in intensive care units; developmental assessment of high-risk newborn infants; home care for elderly stroke and arthritis patients; and industrial consulting to reduce back injuries. Currently, all physical therapists in the USA and Canada are required to be licensed, with an accredited degree from a recognized educational institution.

### Speech-language pathology

Speech-language pathologists possess knowledge relevant to speech and language disorders, are skilled in applying this knowledge to solving clinical problems, and have an overriding concern to help patients understand and manage their speech or language problems.

Unlike occupational and physical therapy, speech-language pathology evolved from education, rather than medicine. In the early part of the 20th century, teachers introduced speech correction services into state-funded schools and formed the National Association of Teachers of Speech. As the discipline began to develop, and a professional outlook was defined, a group of speech correctionists formed the American Academy of Speech Correction in 1925 to raise existing standards of practice as well as public recognition of speech correction as an organized profession. As professionalization increased, many practitioners felt their positions were better served among the medical community than the National Association. Today, the Academy is known as the American Speech-Language-Hearing Association, and has been separated completely from the teachers' association. Nevertheless, over 40% of the 45 000 speech-language pathologists working in the USA work in primary and secondary schools. Other work sites include hospitals, nursing homes, speech-language and hearing centers, and private medical clinics.

As with many other health professions, speech-language pathologists are becoming increasingly autonomous, and are expanding their scope of practice. Newer aspects for speech-language pathology now include those with swallowing disorders, and alternative augmentative communication for those who cannot vocalize at all.

### Emerging issues and trends

The diversity of specialized disciplines among the health professions has made it difficult to create a common understanding of the allied health profession. Each profession has a specific and distinct educational environment, professional code of ethics, and body of research that informs its practice. Consequently, practitioners are challenged to foster a sense of identity and belong to a community of the allied health profession. Yet community building is necessary in an era of downsizing and healthcare restructuring resulting from budgetary constraints. For example, one impact of cost-containment is the reduction of the number of employees in hospitals. For allied health professionals, this translates into role-expansion, greater standardization, and multi-skilling. Multi-skilling, or cross-training of professionals to provide more than one function, has been used not only to decrease the cost of healthcare, but to permit administrators to respond with flexibility to changes in patient mix. Quality concerns arise, however, when technical skills are employed without a sound professional grounding in their use.

## PROFESSIONAL-IZATION

The general route by which a health profession comes into existence today may be summarized as follows:

- A technological or clinical intervention is discovered
- experience and knowledge of the indications, precautions, and hazards associated with the new technology/intervention is acquired through continued use
- recognition of adverse clinical effects leads to the realization that more time is needed to master the technology/intervention, thus increasing pressure on the existing workforce. This pressure leads to the creation of a specialized position for the technology/intervention
- initially new specialists are trained on site. Later, however, the demands for consistency in the amount of education, types of training, and certification of competencies leads to formal education in the specialized disciplines
- the need for competency assurance is met through licensing and giving credentials.

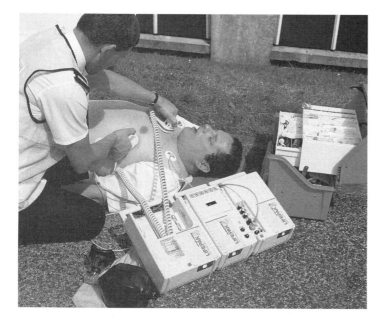

Ambulanceman (paramedic) using a portable defibrillator in an attempt to revive a man who has suffered a heart attack. (Reproduced courtesy of Adam Hart-Davis/ Science Photo Library.)

One major obstacle of role expansion is the protection of turf — encroachment on scope of practice — felt by other professions. Physicians and nurses, who possess the broadest scopes of practice, may feel threatened that the allied health professions are impinging on roles and responsibilities that have traditionally been assigned to them. Turf protection often conflicts with economic constraints, which suggest that if health professionals can provide similar services to nurses and doctors at a lower cost, then role expansion serves its economic purpose. Multiskilling among the allied health professions, such as physical therapy and occupational therapy, may create further interprofessional tensions.

In response to the decrease of hospital positions for allied health professionals, many practitioners have moved into the community. Service delivery is increasingly toward home- and community-based ambulatory care, primary care, and long-term care. Some professionals, traditionally thought of as working under physicians' supervision and receiving patients solely through physician referrals, are moving into more autonomous practice. In striving for autonomy, many health disciplines seek to achieve greater professionalization through upgrading entry-level credential, accreditation, and licensure.

Other trends that are redefining the roles of the allied health profession include encouraging diversity of gender, race, and ethnicity in the professional community; forming strategic alliances with other professions to pursue common goals; expanding links with professional communities in other countries; intensifying internal quality

management; and preparing for less control over work domain boundaries in the workplace.

Although allied health professionals are diverse in terms of the services they provide, in the amount of education they require, the level of autonomy they have achieved apart from the medical establishment, and the regulation that controls their practice, they possess many similarities. Most of the professions share parallel histories and have emerged through similar evolutionary pathways. In addition, the allied health profession works both independently, and cooperatively, to provide the best possible healthcare to the public. However, most occupations among the allied health profession do not strongly identify as allied or among greater health professionals. This lack of identity presents a challenge for these practitioners, if they are to maintain quality care as their priority in an era of budgetary constraint and further technological change. LMc

*See also* GENERAL PRACTICE; LANGUAGE; POLIOMYELITIS; PROFESSIONAL REGULATION

**ALTERNATIVE MEDICINE** See COMPLEMENTARY AND ALTERNATIVE MEDICINE

**ALTITUDE SICKNESS** (or mountain sickness) occurs in humans who ascend to 3000 m or more, unless they do so in commercial aircraft, which are pressurized to the equivalent of 2500 m or less. Symptoms vary according to speed of ascent, age, fitness, exertion, previous acclimatization, and individual susceptibility, but their physiological basis is a reduced blood oxygen level leading to overbreathing and reduced carbon dioxide levels in the blood. They include mental impairment (which may be unnoticed by the person), headache, breathlessness, nausea, vomiting, diarrhea, abdominal pain, and insomnia. Loss of consciousness is usual in unacclimatized persons after several hours at 5500 m. In certain cases altitude sickness is complicated by cerebral or pulmonary edema.

*See also* EXTREME ENVIRONMENTS; MOUNTAINEERING

**ANATOMY — HISTORY** is the scientific study of the structural organization of the body. ARISTOTLE (p 64), one of the earliest students of the subject, gave the science its name, *anatome*, some 2400 years ago. Literally this term means cutting up, and, while Aristotle probably studied animals rather than man, dissection has remained the essential method for the study of human anatomy through the ages.

For centuries, anatomy meant gross anatomy, the structure of the body as seen by the naked eye, but in the last 300 years the boundaries of the subject have widened. Some aspects of studies in physical anthropology are still closely associated with gross anatomy; but, through the use of the microscope, anatomy has come to include micro-anatomy, or histology, and the study of development before birth, or embryology. With the use of radiant energy for diagnosis and treatment, radio-logical anatomy was included, and some new sub-specialties, such as neuroanatomy, have emerged. Just as gross anatomy is recognized as the basic science of surgery, so histology grew up closely related to histopathology, the study of the micro-scopic changes in cells and tissues in disease.

Advances in histology studies depended not only on improved microscopes, but on mechanical means for obtaining thin sections, techniques for the fixation of tissues so that they retained orderly structure, albeit changed from that when living, and of stains to enable components of tissues to be differentiated. Later developments included the development of histo- and cyto-chemistry, the demonstration of chemical compounds, including enzymes, within tissues and cells, and the growing of cells and tissues outside the animal body, in culture. The development of the electron micro-scope, in which use of a beam of electrons instead of light tremendously increased the resolving power, and hence the useful magnifications poss-ible, gave rise to cytology.

Present understanding of the normal structure (and function) of the human body derives from the work of many, but the contribution of the Flemish anatomist Andreas VESALIUS (p 846) must be considered seminal so that, in retrospect, it is possible to see the history of anatomy as divided into a pre- and post-Vesalian period.

## History: before Vesalius

Religious feelings, customary disposal of the dead by burial, cremation, or other ritual means, the belief that corpses were unclean and contact with them defiled, have all inhibited anatomical study, and the systematic practice of human dissection remained condemned until the 20th century.

The ancient civilizations of Greece and Rome were opposed to dissection and, although medi-cine was taught in China as early as about the 4th century BC, the effective study of systematic human anatomy dates from about the year 300 BC. For at least 2000 years the Egyptians practiced the techniques of embalming the dead. Such preservation was religious in its motivations, but the embalmer needed some familiarity with the anatomical basis of his work. It was against this Egyptian background of centuries of familiarity with human cadavers that, with the approval and support of Ptolemy I, the study of human gross anatomy by dissection of corpses of criminals began at Alexandria.

Paradoxically the role of anatomy in medicine apparently diminished over this period.

Dissection of cadavers came to be regarded as unnecessary and degrading in Alexandria, as it was elsewhere. Moreover, dissection was held to give false information, a view ascribed to the 'Empiricists', a group of physicians who allowed that only chance anatomical observations, such as those made on wounded men, were permissible. The study of anatomy was also opposed by another sect, the 'Methodists', whose members were fiercely anti-scientific. This opposition con-tributed to the decline in anatomical studies and, following the withdrawal of royal patronage, the scholars were finally driven out of Alexandria.

GALEN (p 324) studied anatomy for more than 10 years, first at Pergamon under Satyros (an anatomist from Smyrna), then in Smyrna itself, and in Corinth and Alexandria.

Although skeletons were available for study in Galen's time, human dissection was still not poss-ible in Greek cities, although corpses of enemy soldiers killed in battle, of executed criminals, and of stillborn or exposed children might have been subject to some kind of examination. Anatomical writings from the Alexandrian school were avail-able, however, and Galen himself 'condensed' a treatise by Marinus from 20 books to four.

Since studies of practical anatomy based on human dissections were not possible during most of this time, Galen's errors were not recognized, in part from ignorance, but also from adherence to Galen's view that the parts of the body could not be improved upon, and thus further study was not necessary. Thus both his knowledge and his faults were perpetuated. Later teachers encountered, in addition, the problems and com-plications associated with the handing down of Galen's texts over the centuries. Nevertheless Galenic works, errors and all, exerted a great influence on the development of medicine in western Europe well into the 17th century.

During the Early Middle Ages, there was a regression rather than any advance in anatomical and medical knowledge generally. The religious creed of the Muhammadans forbade dissection of human subjects, and little, if any, dissection was carried out in Europe.

Outside the Arab world, the earliest medical school was that founded at SALERNO (p 448), probably as early as the 9th century. From the 13th century universities began to be established throughout western Europe, and in many of these, faculties of medicine were developed. In 1240 the importance of anatomy was recognized when Emperor Frederick II pronounced that sur-geons, before being allowed to practice, had to show knowledge of the anatomy of the human body; but the teaching of anatomy continued to be based on established texts and any anatomical dissection carried out was generally in private.

## FOUNDER OF HISTOLOGY

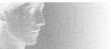

Marcello **MALPIGHI** (1628–94). Italian physician. Malpighi served as professor at Pisa and Messina before being recalled to Bologna in 1668. In 1691 he was sum-moned to Rome as physician to Pope Innocent XII. Malpighi was one of the first microscopists and the founder of histology. In *De pulmonibus observationes anatomicae* (1661) he described the vesicular structure and the capillaries of the lungs. He noted that the blood was composed of a 'host of red atoms' (1661). He described the glomerular tufts in the kidneys (1666) and the Malpighian bodies in the spleen (1666). In *Des viscerum structura* (1666) he records probable examples of Hodgkin's disease. In *De formatio pulli in ova* (1673) he established his place in embryology.

## TWO NOTORIOUS IN ANATOMY

William **HARE** (*fl.* 1827). Hare was the Irish lodging-house keeper in Edinburgh who cooperated with William Burke in murdering his lodgers to provide anatomical specimens. He turned King's evidence and was freed in 1829.

(*continued on p 39*)

# ALZHEIMER'S DISEASE (AND OTHER DEMENTIAS OF THE ELDERLY)

The Latin word *dementia* means 'being out of one's mind'; in this sense it has a long history in literature and common usage. In medicine, it denotes brain diseases in which acquired permanent memory impairment is the most striking feature. Until the 1970s, Alzheimer's disease was the name given to a 'pre-senile' (onset under 65 years) dementia of unknown cause in which plaques and tangles were a microscopic feature. Cases with later onset were called 'senile dementia'. Since the pathological changes at all ages seemed similar, Alzheimer's disease came to be the name for all those later life — mostly very late life — brain diseases in which memory loss is the main, but by no means the only, feature; where there is a typical deteriorating course; and where 'plaque and tangle' pathology is found or inferred. It must be distinguished from the common mild, generally 'benign', forgetfulness of aging, in which recalling names is often the main difficulty.

After Alzheimer's disease the next most common dementia in old age is vascular (or 'arteriosclerotic' or 'multi-infarct') in which death of brain tissue ('infarction') is the result of blockage of blood vessels, and small strokes are common. Quite common too is 'Lewy body' dementia, associated with Parkinson's disease. Often 'Alzheimer' and 'vascular' dementia co-exist. Dementia may also be due to brain injury, to infections, and alcohol abuse, and to many other causes, but in old age about two-thirds of dementias are Alzheimer's. There is no clinical test for Alzheimer's disease.

In Alzheimer's disease all aspects of mind and of personality are disrupted to varying degrees, not just memory, but also thinking, judgement, insight, emotion, language, and skills (including, importantly, self-care skills). Behavior deteriorates, often with incontinence, wandering, constant repetitiveness, nocturnal disturbance, and other taxing features. Eventually the ability to walk, even to stand upright, is lost. Commonly death from 'other causes' intervenes before the last stages.

From the first signs (often recognized only in retrospect) to death may be many years — ten or more is common. There is great variability in the degree to which different features predominate, and in the course in different individuals. No doubt what is known as Alzheimer's disease is a congeries of different entities, of which the process of sorting has only lately begun.

Dementia affects some 3–5% of persons over the age of 65. The rates are similar throughout the world. It is rare in the 'young–old', but about 20% of over-80s suffer from it in moderate or severe degree. Because of the rapidly rising number of the very old in industrial societies the number of sufferers has greatly increased. By its scale and nature (sufferers generally need an eye kept on them around-the-clock, and mostly much more care) it is the most care-consuming condition apart from childhood. The costs — financial, social and emotional pressure on carers, and suffering — are colossal. It is the most common reason for admission to long-stay care.

## Important issues

Legal and ethical issues arise with growing insistence. Reform of the law of incapacity is under discussion. The capacity to drive a car is an important practical and legal issue. Questions are actively debated of how zealously one should strive to preserve life. Standards of long-stay care and its funding are major issues. Other questions derive from now available genetic tests in earlier life which can give estimates of probability of a late life onset of Alzheimer's disease.

Better and more appropriate services, and the new specialty of old age psychiatry, are among the public responses; voluntary and self-help organizations are effective as advocates, and above all as sources of information and support, and none more so than the world-wide Alzheimer Society movement. Alzheimer's has become a household word in many societies.

Twenty years ago there was little research (in 1977 the British Medical Research Council was actively soliciting research proposals). Today research flourishes on all fronts. So far no simple causation or means of prevention have been established. Risk factors (apart from age itself, and Down's disease, in which Alzheimer brain changes are invariable in late middle age) are not well established, and such as there are (for example, past head injury) seem to interact with other predisposing factors, rather than to be causal in themselves.

With the growth of molecular biology, tissue factors (such as the origins of plaques and tangles and of more recently identified changes) are becoming clearer and some gene anomalies have been identified. New brain imaging techniques have advanced research and diagnosis. Understanding deficits of brain 'neurotransmitters' (chemicals involved in nervous messages) has led to the beginnings of rational pharmacological treatment. Some of these substances have lately been licensed for use in various countries but benefits are temporary and unpredictable. Symptomatic tranquillizing treatment has a place. Good, informed, well-supported care is the best bet for maintaining function and minimizing behavioral disturbance.

Genetic testing now makes it possible to identify some people at a higher risk of developing Alzheimer's disease in late life. But other factors influence the expression of genes; and one may die of other causes long before one develops Alzheimer's disease. As in other diseases in which testing for genetic probability has become possible, new questions arise for society.                     TA

*See also* ABUSE OF OLD PEOPLE; PSYCHIATRY

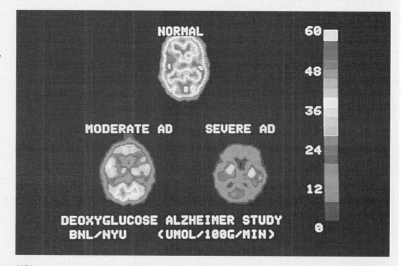

MRI scans comparing a normal brain with those displaying moderate and severe Alzheimer's disease.

BOLOGNA (p 447) occupies a notable place as far as the history of anatomy is concerned. In 1306 Mondino de Luzzi (Mundinus) was appointed to the teaching staff of the university, and, despite opposition from the Church, carried out some human dissection in public during the next few years. He dissected in person, not teaching *ex cathedra* with a demonstrator pointing out the structures revealed in the cadaver by the menial dissector. Mondino wrote a practical text, the *Anathomia*, which appeared in 1316. This contained basic, but often inaccurate, descriptions of organs, but has been regarded as inaugurating a new phase in the study of human anatomy. Another work of equal importance, originating at about the same time, was that of Henri de Mondeville, who lived *c.* 1270–1320. He was a Norman, a contemporary of Mondino, and also studied at Bologna before lecturing at MONTPELLIER (p 319) in the early years of the 14th century. In his lectures he used full-length anatomical pictures and illustrations showing separate organs.

Gradually, albeit with some reluctance on the part of Church and State, however, the proscription was relaxed. In 1377, public dissections were authorized by decree at Montpellier, and similar recognition followed at PADUA (p 447) in 1429 and at Paris in 1478. Pope Sixtus IV, who held office from 1471 to 1484, permitted dissection provided that permission of the Church authorities was obtained.

The corpses made available for public dissection were those of executed criminals, a practice which continued into the 19th century in western Europe. Even when opposition of the Church to the practice had weakened, general distaste and even revulsion hindered anatomical progress. There were also other major problems: first, the number of cadavers officially made available to anatomists was limited, sometimes to one per year or less. Secondly, since there was no means of preserving the cadavers, decomposition was rapid, particularly in the warmer countries of the Mediterranean. Dissections had to be carried out rapidly, perhaps without ceasing over several days, and the most perishable organs, such as the abdominal viscera, were demonstrated first. Midwinter was commonly the season for dissections since at that time decomposition would proceed more slowly than at other times. The public 'anatomies' were generally directed towards the demonstration of the truth of Galenic texts, and little was done to discover and correct their errors.

There seems to have been a considerable stirring of interest in human anatomy at the very end of the 15th century. An increase and wider dissemination of anatomical knowledge resulted from the development of printing and of techniques for the reproduction of illustrations. 'Anatomies' with illustrations began to be available to students.

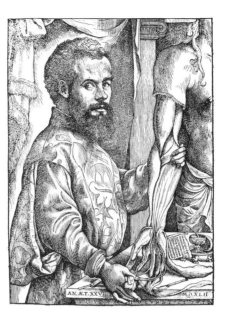

Andreas Vesalius at the age of 28, from *De humani corporis fabrica*, 1543. (Reproduced by permission of the Francis D. Countway Library of Medicine, Boston.)

Nevertheless, the topic was not a major concern of all medical scholars. A 'Humanist' school flourished about this period, whose members held texts to be more valuable than dissections. Books of anatomy based on early writings contained virtually nothing new gained by observation, nor were the texts amended. The early 16th century was thus a time of historically-based anatomical scholarship; but contemporaneously, in some centers of learning, awareness of the importance of practical studies was developing.

In 1514, one of the outstanding figures in the history of anatomy, Andreas Vesalius, was born in Brussels. His most famous work appeared in 1543: this was the *De humani corporis fabrica*, which proved to be one of the most important and significant anatomical texts ever published. The seven books of the *Fabrica* contain large and splendid plates, one series showing progressive stages of dissection from the exposure of superficial structures by removal of skin and underlying connective tissue, through the layers of muscles down to the ligaments and bones. Vessels are shown displayed systematically, suggesting that injected preparations had been made. The drawings were published with terminology in Greek, Latin, Hebrew, and Arabic, in an attempt to reduce the confusion which had resulted from centuries of translation and re-translation of early texts. The *Fabrica* was intended to be an integral work of text and illustrations, both to be appreciated together. He also published, again in 1543, the *Epitome*,

(continued)

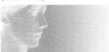

Robert **KNOX** (1791–1862). British anatomist. Knox was appointed an assistant surgeon in the army in 1815 and served at Waterloo and in South Africa. Returning to Edinburgh in 1820, he was appointed Conservator of the Royal College of Surgeons of Edinburgh Museum in 1825. The following year he took over Barclay's school of anatomy and rapidly became the leading teacher of anatomy in the city. Within a year or two the Burke and HARE (p 37) 'resurrectionist' scandals involved him in such obloquy that his school was ruined. He left for London and became pathologist to the Cancer Hospital in Fulham in 1856.

**EPONYMOUS PSYCHIATRIST**

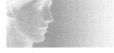

Alois **ALZHEIMER** (1864–1915) In 1907 Alois Alzheimer, working in Munich, published the case of a woman in her early 50s who had died after four years' illness. She had suffered from increasing loss of memory, along with psychotic symptoms and physical deterioration. Under the microscope her much shrunken brain showed 'plaques' and 'tangles' which are characteristic of, though not specific to, what we now call Alzheimer's disease. It was by present usage not a 'typical' case of 'Alzheimer's' — both because the patient was 'young' and because, among other features, arteriosclerotic changes were as prominent as the plaques and tangles.

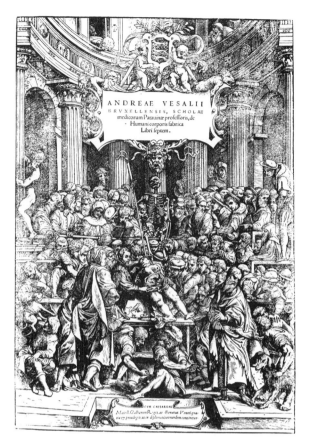

The title page of *De humani corporis fabrica*, 1543. (Reproduced by permission of the Francis D. Countway Library of Medicine, Boston.)

**EARLY ANATOMIST**

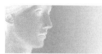

**LEONARDO** Da Vinci (1452–1519). Italian artist and anatomist. Leonardo's distinction as an anatomist has only recently been appreciated with the study of his anatomical notebooks now in the Royal Library at Windsor Castle. The anatomical drawings date from 1487, but from 1506 he dissected as an anatomist. He was a friend of Marcantonio della Tore (1473–1511) professor of anatomy in Pisa and later in PADUA (p 447).

intended to form a guide for students, with little actual description of the plates; this, probably because it was cheaper and simpler, became more popular than the *Fabrica*. The changes in anatomical ideas which followed the publication of the *Tabulae sex*, the *Fabrica*, and the *Epitome* were to transform the subject.

### History: after Vesalius

The great changes in outlook which eventually followed publication of the Vesalian texts were neither immediate nor universal. The *Fabrica* was ill-received in Louvain, and in Paris his former teacher Sylvius took it as an affront. In the schools of Padua, Bologna, and Pisa, however, the work was greeted with approval and Vesalius was invited to conduct anatomies in these places.

The outstanding contribution made by Vesalius to human anatomy lay not only in his texts, but in the size, extensive annotation, and outstanding quality of his illustrations, which were far ahead of anything that had previously appeared, and in the integration of the text and the figures. Subsequently, as anatomical knowledge increased and texts multiplied, so the quality of the illustrations improved. Practicing artists were commonly involved. Indeed, it is generally held that the bulk

of the illustrations for the *Fabrica* were executed in Titian's studio. This work marked the beginning of a long and close association between ART and anatomy. Besides the illustration of anatomical texts, a number of Renaissance artists studied human anatomy and are known to have dissected, among them Raphael, Michelangelo, and Albrecht Dürer. LEONARDO da Vinci (this page) left ample evidence of his knowledge of comparative and human anatomy in his notebooks and drawings, often emphasizing the mechanical principles of anatomical features rather than their pure morphology.

During the 14th century, legal permission to dissect cadavers had been granted to a number of schools in Italy. However, the practical teaching of anatomy developed more slowly in other countries. Public dissections took place in Paris from 1478, and by the end of the 16th century in Basel and the Netherlands. In England, the universities of Oxford and Cambridge were established early and for a long time were the main centers of medical education. David Edwards, who is said to have made the first dissection in England in 1531, was also the first English author of an anatomical text.

### Teaching in Britain

Among the notable teachers concerned in early medical teaching in England was John CAIUS (p 135), master of Gonville College, Cambridge. Caius, who studied with Vesalius in Padua, obtained a grant from the Crown for the dissection of one body each year at Gonville. Meanwhile a Royal Commission examined the system of education at Oxford and formulated revised regulations under which a student of medicine during his six years was to attend two dissections, two disputations, and an examination before being awarded a Bachelor's degree. Further attendance at dissections was required before proceeding to a Doctorate.

During the first half of the 17th century the teaching of anatomy in the two universities fell into neglect, and in 1646 the Senate of the University of Cambridge passed a Grace (a formal decree) to remedy this situation. At the time of the Commonwealth in the mid-17th century, great interest developed in science at Oxford, and in anatomy in particular. Christopher Wren was one who studied the subject, and in 1664 there appeared Thomas Willis's *Cerebri anatome*, with Wren's plates.

In the early 14th century the practice of, and training in, surgery in the City of London were in the hands of two groups, the Company of Barbers and the Fellowship of Surgeons. In 1540 the two groups united. The united company undertook the provision of lectures and demonstrations in anatomy, and was entitled to the corpses of four malefactors each year for dissection. The 'anatomies' and anatomical lectures were held in Barber-Surgeons Hall. Dissections were public and attendance by surgical freemen and by apprentices was compulsory. As the practice of surgery increased over the years and the demand for instruction grew, private schools flourished, and with them came increased competition for the limited number of subjects available for dissection. The Company of BARBER-SURGEONS encountered difficulties in obtaining the bodies to which it was legally entitled, as legal officers often found it more profitable to sell the bodies for private study.

In Edinburgh, instruction in anatomy before the foundation of the medical faculty in 1726 was the responsibility of the surgeons and the Town Council. In Aberdeen two foundations, Marischal College and St Mary's, later King's College, taught medicine, including anatomy, from an early date, but there is no record of human dissection until 1636. In Glasgow a chair of anatomy was established in 1720, and, in Ireland, the teaching of anatomy was taking place in Dublin at about the same time.

Since the centuries-old tradition was that students themselves did not dissect, and their instruction depended on a clear view of the proceedings, many schools built custom-designed anatomical theaters. A permanent anatomical theater was built at Padua in 1594, and a successor, opened in 1783, still exists. Edinburgh had an anatomical theater founded by the Guild of Surgeons in 1697 and in London the Surgeons Hall was built for the teaching of anatomy.

Gradually it was accepted that there was a need for practical anatomical study, at any rate for those training to practice surgical procedures, and the proscription or severe restriction of human dissection was eased. However, the number of corpses granted was small: often only one per year was available. Officially approved occasions for anatomical dissection were thus few, and this constituted a great hindrance to detailed study and teaching. The shortage of legally provided subjects for dissection led to anatomists taking into their own hands the acquisition of additional material for their needs, either by bribing the Sheriff and hangman to provide corpses which should legally have gone to the surgeons and official schools, or ultimately by grave-robbing.

Grave-robbing occurred widely in the British Isles, from Aberdeen to London, and also in Ireland. The practice was prevalent in the USA where it was initially reported in the first decade of American independence. With the exception of Massachusetts, America was slow to legislate for the provision of the considerable number of cadavers needed for teaching, and grave-robbing continued much later than in Britain, where introduction of the Anatomy Act of 1832 curbed the practice.

The fresher the corpse, the more saleable, and the higher the price; and this led a few body-snatchers to murder. The most widely known series of incidents, set in Edinburgh, is that associated with Burke and HARE (p 37) in 1827. Sixteen victims were killed in 10 months, and supplied to the Edinburgh anatomist Robert KNOX (p 39). After the Edinburgh murders, the already strong feeling against both grave-robbers and their clients increased, and led to Parliament passing the Anatomy Act. It empowered the Secretary of State to grant licenses to teachers of anatomy and allowed such persons to receive any dead body for anatomical examination in suitable licensed premises.

Gradually over the early decades of the 20th century individuals began to bequeath their bodies for anatomical purposes after death. This, coupled with modern techniques of preservation, essentially relieved the shortage of subjects for dissection. If dissection is now disappearing from medical curricula, it is not for want of cadavers, but because of fundamental revisions in medical education.                                                RKJ

**ANATOMY** Although anatomy is still occasionally studied as a discipline in its own right, it remains essentially a vocational subject for students of medicine and dentistry. World-wide, medical education is undergoing a major reorientation. With the exponential growth of medical scientific knowledge, older subject disciplines, such as anatomy and physiology, have become increasingly complex and new ones have been recognized in their own right. Consequently the undergraduate curriculum has become overburdened, and it is recognized that there is a pressing need to re-define the core knowledge, skills, and attitudes required of tomorrow's doctors.

There is a move away from separate discipline-based courses of study in favor of some form of integrated multidisciplinary teaching in which groups of teachers deal with various aspects of the structure, function, PATHOLOGY, dysfunction, and treatment relating to a particular system or topic. Such an approach was introduced first at Western Reserve Medical School, USA, in the 1960s, and similar approaches have been introduced subsequently in other centers. The impact of this new approach on the study of teaching of anatomy has been considerable. Indeed, in those schools that have introduced fully integrated curricula, anatomy as a distinct, separately taught subject has virtually disappeared. In most others, the disproportionate time previously allotted in total to the subject, including not only gross anatomy, but the associated topics of neuroanatomy, histology, cytology, and embryology, has been reduced significantly.

Anders Adolf **RETZIUS** (1796–1860). Swedish anatomist. Retzius became professor of comparative anatomy in the veterinary school in the Swedish capital, and later held the chair of anatomy and physiology at the Carolinian Institute. He described the space in front of the urinary bladder which allows it to expand and contract freely, and this space is now known as the cave of Retzius. Certain gyri in the brain were named after him, as has been a ligament of the ankle joint; he discovered the canals in the cornea of the eye, which were later named after Schlemm.

One consequence of this reduction in allotted time is that in most schools students are no longer expected to dissect. Instead they study prosections prepared by demonstrators, often trainee surgeons. Some authorities claim that losing the chance to dissect, and thereby the opportunity for unhurried exploration of the complexity of the human body, diminishes the educational experience. Others hold that the lost opportunity has no effect, as dissection itself does little to enhance students' core knowledge and understanding of clinical anatomy. Indeed, there can be little doubt that in today's medical curriculum there is a need to concentrate anatomical learning upon the principles and concepts essential to the practice of modern medicine and to reduce the teaching of irrelevant and unnecessary detail.

Because of its long and distinguished history, anatomy and its practitioners have recently attracted a reputation for conservatism and resistance to change that is not entirely justified. While the gross structure of the human body and its variations have been well understood since the 19th century (the standard reference Gray's *Anatomy* was first published in 1858), anatomists have been quick to embrace new educational technologies, for example, multimedia applications of information technology and exploit new approaches to learning, for example, problem-based learning. Anatomy has always been taught in relation to clinical medicine and surgery, and its practitioners have responded rapidly to the changing requirements of clinical practice. One recent example of this is the development in a number of schools of clinical and surgical skills laboratories, based upon the use of anatomical models and simulators. Another is the re-introduction of cross-sectional anatomy to meet the needs of modern medical IMAGING techniques such as computerized axial tomography and nuclear magnetic resonance.

## Research

As for anatomical research, there are few boundaries between this and other biological investigations. Like medical education, much of current medical research is multidisciplinary. Anatomical science still has its place, and, while the scalpel is seldom used now, dissection, in the literal sense of 'cutting up', remains the essential reductionist approach to the elucidation of structure. With the advent of new technologies, morphological research has embraced successive levels of structure from the macroscopic to the molecular, and the study of structure has become inextricably associated with the exploration of function. Moreover, anatomical science, now experimentally based, has spawned more new disciplines than any other. Embryology, that branch of anatomy dealing with the study of development before birth, is a good example of this.

Neuroanatomy is one topic where pure structural studies still have a contribution to make. Although the gross topography of the brain and spinal cord were accurately described many years ago, elucidating the fine structure function of the brain remain one of biology's greatest challenges.

Today, human anatomy still forms an essential part of the scientific basis of medicine and allied skills. Those whose concern is the promotion of health and the prevention and treatment of disease must surely continue to work from knowledge of the normal structure and, inseparable from this, the normal function of the human body.           RKJ

**ANEMIA** See HEMATOLOGY

**ANESTHESIA** means loss of feeling, and analgesia, loss of painful sensation; this article deals with the specialty of surgical anesthesia. Humans and all warm-blooded creatures perceive the sensation of PAIN, whether caused by disease, injury, or surgical treatment. Before describing the development of methods to ease surgical pain, it is necessary to explain the phenomenon of PAIN.

Everyone has experienced pain, which is a purely subjective matter, for no one can comprehend the pain experienced by another. As there is no universally identifiable stimulus for pain, in contrast to the other senses — seeing, hearing, touch, taste, and smell — pain is usually described according to prior experiences: burning, stabbing, cutting, aching, throbbing, pricking, and the like. Surely the perception and reaction to pain are colored by one's emotional state and ethnic origins. A confusing factor is that intensification of the classic sensations results in pain: bright light, loud sound, hot and cold, strong tastes, and heavy pressure. Pain is disagreeable and often intolerable: although it is meant to protect against injury, when chronic it can ultimately destroy the sufferer.

Specific receptors for pain exist in the form of naked nerve endings throughout the body, which are dense on the surface and sparse internally; this is why superficial pain is described and located so much more accurately than internal pain. A potentially destructive stimulus is transduced into electrical energy, travelling over a spectrum of specific nerve fibers to the central nervous system, there being decoded and eliciting an appropriate response. According to this schema, pain can be prevented or alleviated peripherally with medications, as in the use of aspirin for treatment of arthritis, or a locally injected anesthetic to dull the effects of the surgeon's scalpel. Centrally acting drugs can alter the perception and significance of pain, as occurs when morphine or other opioids are given. It is just one step further to induce insensibility with a general anesthetic.

Surgical operations were performed far back in antiquity by sorcerers, religious adherents, and itinerant technicians, but always for superficial illness; a fractured bone; limb amputation; trephining the skull to relieve intracranial pressure; to dislodge an ocular lens cataract; or to crush or extract a urinary bladder stone. Other ailments not visible to the eye were assumed, according to galenical concepts (see GALEN (p 324)), to result from an internal imbalance among four HUMORS: blood, phlegm, yellow bile, and black bile. Accordingly, treatments to restore the balance comprised bloodletting or leeching, purging, use of enemas, induction of emesis, and application of heat or cold. Although those practitioners were largely inattentive to the suffering wreaked by surgery, efforts were made to relieve pain through incantation, HYPNOSIS, ACUPUNCTURE, heavy intoxication with alcohol, or inhaling from or sucking upon sponges saturated with extracts of the poppy, henbane, and mandragora root.

### Antecedents of anesthesia

The established route for medication was the gastrointestinal tract, even *c.* 1540, when PARACELSUS (p 617) of Switzerland sweetened the feed of fowl with sweet oil of vitriol, a compound later called ether by Frobenius. The vapor of this liquid was to be inhaled by many a patient over the 130 years following the eventual introduction of surgical anesthesia.

Two centuries later the introduction of anesthesia was prepared for by an emerging comprehension of the physiology of respiration and the circulation to the lungs. HARVEY (p 363), during his observations on the circulation, noticed the change in color — from dark to florid — when blood traversed the lungs. In 1672 Robert BOYLE (p 125), in exhausting air from a vessel containing both a lighted taper and a living bird, succeeded in extinguishing the life of both, thus corroborating the vital nature of a substance in air. Joseph Priestley, in 1774, while heating mercuric oxide, liberated oxygen, which sustained life to a remarkable degree. Incidentally, Priestley also obtained nitrous oxide from nitric oxide. Antoine LAVOISIER (p 321) observed that exhaled air caused a precipitate in lime water, and so must consist in part of chalky-air, or carbon dioxide. Thence it was but a step to conclude that the main purpose of respiration was not only to sustain life with oxygen, but also, to change that element into carbon dioxide.

Eventually, the recognition of these gases and vapors led to the practice of pneumatic medicine and, for the first time, utilization of the lungs as an avenue of therapy, a forerunner of inhalation anesthesia. Around 1794, a group of physicians and scientists established the Pneumatic Institution at Clifton, Bristol, and chose as superintendent of the Institution a youthful chemist and physicist, Humphry Davy. While breathing nitrous oxide, Davy found that a headache associated with indigestion and the pain of an erupting wisdom tooth were considerably diminished. Simultaneously, he experienced a 'thrilling' and an uneasiness swallowed up in pleasure. He was led to write, 'As nitrous oxide in its extensive operation appears capable of destroying pain, it may probably be used with advantage during surgical operations.' Davy's remarks went unheeded, with perhaps one exception. Henry Hill Hickman, general practitioner and surgeon of Shifnal in Shropshire, performed a number of experiments on animals, using carbon dioxide in an asphyxial manner but not for so long that they failed to survive. No matter to whom the glory is accorded, Hickman must be credited with the concept of surgical anesthesia, unfortunately employing the wrong agent.

### Introduction

A fortuitous outcome of Davy's suggestion, plus his repeated demonstration to friends of the exhilarating effects of nitrous oxide, was the public indulgence in frolics, inhaling ether as well. Crawford W. Long participated in such revels and while in practice in Jefferson, Georgia, introduced that wild party to friends, so that one of them, James Venable, underwent excision of a tumor from the nape of the neck in 1842, while under the influence of ether. After the initial publicity it became known that William E. Clarke, a student at the Vermont Medical College, had also employed ether in January 1842.

Another sequence of events took place on 10 December 1844 in Hartford, Connecticut, where Gardner Quincy Colton took a travelling medicine show to allow one and all to experience the effects of inhaling nitrous oxide. The fact that one of the volunteers, Samuel A. Cooley, hurt his leg without noticing it while in the excitement phase of nitrous oxide intoxication intrigued a dentist, Horace Wells, in the audience. On the very next day, while inhaling Colton's nitrous oxide, Wells had one of his own carious teeth painlessly removed by a fellow dentist. Through the mediation of his former dental pupil. William Thomas Green Morton, then practicing in Boston, Wells was accorded the opportunity of demonstrating the benefits of nitrous oxide before a group of Harvard University medical students. But the event, in January 1845, proved to be a shattering defeat for Wells, for the volunteer student cried out in pain as a tooth was extracted, though later claiming no awareness or experience of pain. Undoubtedly, in this case anesthesia failed to progress beyond the excitement phase. This stage of delirium explains why, under less threatening circumstances, nitrous oxide is called laughing gas.

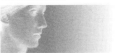

**INTRODUCER OF CHLOROFORM**

Sir James Young **SIMPSON** (1811–70). British obstetrician. He introduced chloroform as an anesthetic in 1847, inhaling it experimentally with his assistants Matthews Duncan and George Keith. He was the leading obstetrician of his day and one of the founders of gynecology. He invented the uterine sound.

W. T. G. Morton, a keen witness to Wells's demonstration, was enrolled at that time in a course of Harvard medical school lectures and had become an expert on dental prosthetics, devising a plate that could be applied to the gums only after the rotted tooth roots had been removed, which was far too painful a venture for all but the most hardy. He accepted the suggestion of Charles T. Jackson, eccentric geologist and chemist, that ether, applied to the gums, would supply, through evaporation, a degree of cold analgesia.

Following experiments on ether inhalation in several animals, in September 1847 Morton, in his Boston office, painlessly extracted an abscessed tooth from the jaw of Eben H. Frost, a merchant of that city. The event, reported in a newspaper on the next day, caught the eye of Henry Jacob Bigelow, an attending surgeon at the Massachusetts General Hospital, who then arranged for a trial at the hospital. The surgeon would be the renowned John Collins Warren, then aged 68, the patient Edward Gilbert Abbott, a young printer with a congenital tumor below the angle of the jaw. On Friday 16 October 1846 the blood vessels leading to the tumor were ligated, with Morton employing a hastily devised glass inhaler containing a sea sponge saturated with ether. On termination of the usual rapid operation, Warren was led to exclaim to the gallery, 'Gentlemen, this is no humbug'.

Although surgical anesthesia was now publicly launched, an interminable period of rancorous controversy ensued over who should be given credit for the discovery. When requested to name the phenomenon, Oliver Wendell Holmes suggested *anesthesia*, from the Greek connoting lack of feeling.

News of the discovery soon reached England so that within 64 days the first operations were being performed with the aid of ether anesthesia. John SNOW (p 48), general practitioner, clinical investigator, and epidemiologist, became the first of a long line of English physician-anesthetists, indeed the first anywhere. Using ether primarily, with a refined apparatus, he was able within several months to report on his experience in a text concerning *The inhalation of the vapour of ether*. Towards the end of 1847, James Young SIMPSON (p 43) abandoned ether as a means of relieving the pain of childbirth, in favor of chloroform. As chloroform was more pleasant to inhale than ether, and more potent with a consequent rapid induction and emergence, it became the more popular anesthetic in England.

After the introduction of anesthesia, surgery made little progress in either the USA or Britain, because the prevailing humoral theory of disease had to be modified to embrace the possibility that medical ailments might be cured by surgical treatment. This attitude changed with the development of pathological anatomy and performance of postmortem examinations. Next, as the concept of the bacterial origin of infection was unknown, postsurgical sepsis was rife after operation. This situation was altered towards the end of the century with acceptance of LISTER's (p 473) technique of antisepsis followed by asepsis, as practiced today. Many deaths due to chloroform were reported early on, as was extensive destruction of the liver. The question was whether sudden, intraoperative death might be related to respiratory standstill or heart failure. Fibrillation of the heart, resulting in circulatory arrest, was later recognized as the cause of death, rather than respiratory failure.

## Local anesthesia

Another approach to anesthesia arose in Vienna in 1884, where Karl Koller and Sigmund FREUD (p 321) were experimenting with agents for the treatment of morphine addiction. Koller applied cocaine, one of the drugs under investigation, to a frog's eye, and noticed that insensitivity to pain resulted. Cocaine, an alkaloid of the coca plant, had been chewed by Peruvians for centuries in the course of their labors, numbing the tongue and causing stimulation and exhilaration. Thus the stage was set for the development of local anesthesia, in contrast to the general method. Within the year, Leonard J. Corning, neurologist of New York City, injected a solution of cocaine into the vicinity of the spinal cord of a man suffering from seminal

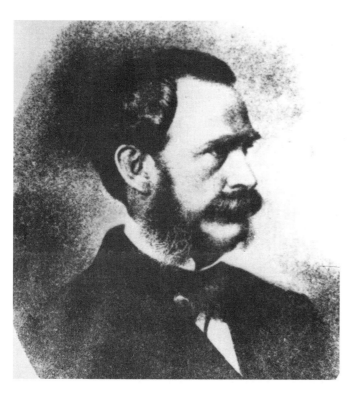

William Thomas Green Morton, anesthetist at the first public demonstration of ether anesthesia.
(Reproduced with permission from the collection of the Boston Medical Library in the Francis A. Countway Library of Medicine.)

incontinence, and anesthesia of the lower half of the body developed. Harvey CUSHING (p 537) later extended the technique to other areas of the body, and coined the term 'regional anesthesia', in contrast to general anesthesia. In 1898, August Bier had spinal anesthesia with cocaine administered to himself by an assistant: a severe lumbar puncture headache developed as a result of extensive cerebrospinal fluid leakage. All manner of regional anesthetic techniques were then devised in the first decade of the 20th century, ranging from mere subcutaneous infiltration of solutions of cocaine, to injection into the major nerves supplying the head, torso, and extremities, and into the large nerve plexuses of the arm and leg. Adrenaline, newly synthesized, was added to the anesthetic mixture to constrict the blood vessels, to afford a bloodless surgical field, and to prolong nerve block.

However, the cocaine molecule was unstable, the solution was not easily sterilized, and it soon became well known for its central exhilarating and stimulating properties that led to addiction. William S. HALSTED (p 746), America's leading surgeon, who became an addict during self-experimentation with the drug, spent much of his career trying to break the habit. Apparently a substitute for cocaine was needed and this came with Alfred Einhorn's synthesis of novocaine, a short-acting anesthetic lacking topical activity. A series of amides: lidocaine, mepivacaine, lignocaine, bupivacaine, and etidocaine followed. The advantages of regional anesthesia lie in its local effect on specific body areas, in contrast to the possible untoward effects on brain, heart, lungs, liver, and kidneys of general anesthesia. Thus, with local anesthesia, fewer systemic sequels are apt to develop.

From the beginning, scientists had pondered on how anesthetics might act on the brain to produce narcosis. Claude BERNARD (p 102), in about 1870, reasoned that narcosis represented a reversible semicoagulation of the substance of the cell, which returned to its original normal state upon elimination of the anesthetic. The potent anesthetics are highly lipid-soluble, and Meyer and Overton, around the turn of the century, independently proposed the lipid solubility theory of narcosis, which postulated physical effects of anesthetics on lipid-containing cell membranes. A strong correspondence exists between lipid solubility and anesthetic potency. Perhaps this physical alteration affects synaptic transmission between nerve cells in the brain, so that clinical anesthesia results. Local anesthetics are also highly soluble in the lipid-containing membranes of nerves.

## Newer anesthetics and techniques

During the first half of the 20th century, as chloroform waned in popularity, a number of new anesthetics were introduced into practice. Ether then shared the same fate as chloroform, so that, of the original agents, only nitrous oxide remained. New halogenated hydrocarbons appeared on the scene; these were distantly related to chloroform but with the incorporation of the fluorine molecule rendering the agent more potent, more stable, and practically non-flammable.

Nowadays, anesthetic practice does not consist in the mere giving of a single inhalation agent, as was originally the case, but in the use of several agents, each ingredient offering one of the desiderata of anesthesia (a unitary term which is no longer an accurate description of the phenomenon): analgesia; lack of awareness and unconsciousness; muscle relaxation; and obtundation of reflex responses to surgical stimuli.

The practice of employing multiple agents began, perhaps, with Claude Bernard's experiments, showing that morphine injected into the dog lessened the amount of chloroform subsequently needed for anesthesia. This experiment antedated the use of preanesthetic medications, which utilized not only opioids but sometimes atropine or scopolamine, both of which reduce respiratory tract secretions.

When regional anesthesia was combined with general anesthesia and with preanesthetic medication, a balanced technique resulted. Synthesis of the short-acting thiobarbiturates resulted in the use of sodium thiopental for intravenous induction of anesthesia, leading to rapid loss of consciousness. In 1942, the use by Griffith and Johnson of intravenous curare (the South American paralysing arrow-poison) for the first time provided still another essential ingredient. In purified form this came to be used frequently during general anesthesia, to avoid excessive depth

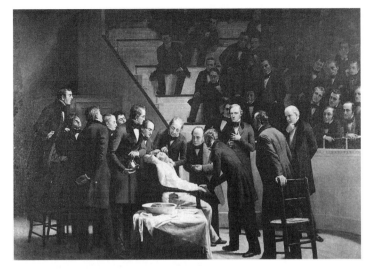

*The first operation with ether*, painted retrospectively by Robert Hinckley over the years 1882–93, begun in Paris and finished in Washington DC, USA. (Reproduced with permission from the collection of the Boston Medical Library in the Francis A. Countway Library of Medicine.)

of narcosis, while giving the patient the muscle relaxation necessary for operation. As the abdominal muscles were paralysed, so were those of respiration — the diaphragm and intercostals. The apnoeic patient therefore required assistance or control of respiration via a mechanical respirator. Better and safer control was afforded by insertion of a tracheal tube attached to the breathing circuit.

Other intravenous agents increased the dimensions of balanced anesthesia. Some were used as preanesthetic medicaments, to supplement regional anesthesia or to prevent awareness during operation in the paralyzed patient. Newer opioids, such as fentanyl, were much more potent and offered fewer adverse effects than the traditional morphine derivatives.

Anesthetists have been responsible for the development of multidisciplinary pain therapy clinics. However, this class of medical specialist is still largely concerned with the overall care of surgical patients even though, of necessity, special expertise is needed in cardiac surgery, pulmonary operations, neuroanesthesia, obstetrics, pediatrics, orthopedics, and ambulatory (outpatient) surgical clinics. Finally, the benefits of training in anesthesia are evident in CRITICAL (intensive) CARE medicine, resuscitation, and neonatology.                LDV

*See also* SURGERY, GENERAL – HISTORY

## ANIMALS AS CARRIERS OF DISEASE

Animals mostly live in harmony with humans, often mutually supporting one another. Interactions among humans and animals are generally more beneficial than harmful, but animals harbor many disease agents that may affect humans. Domesticated animals — pets, livestock, poultry, and fish — and wild species, some of which we regard as pests, are all implicated.

Some diseases are caused by poisons. Ciguatera poisoning is due to a small protozoon (dinoflagellate) that accumulates up the food chain, so it is most potent in large reef fish. Scombrid poisoning is due to histamine and occurs through bacterial spoilage of certain fish such as tuna and shellfish; it also occurs in cheese. A few diseases are allergic, for example, cats' dandruff may precipitate attacks of ASTHMA. Most of the diseases considered here are caused by infectious agents ranging in size and complexity from prions and ultramicroscopic viruses to tapeworms up to a few meters long.

Several categories of carriage may be distinguished. Some infections are transmitted from animals to humans by contact or droplet. Several important epidemic diseases, including some of the zoonoses, are transmitted by insect parasites of animals. Bubonic PLAGUE, TYPHUS, and Rocky Mountain spotted fever are examples, carried from animals to humans respectively by fleas, lice, and ticks. Other categories include many more zoonoses, worms with complex life cycles involving humans and other hosts; vector-borne diseases; and diseases in which animals are passive carriers, that is, the disease agent is a 'passenger' transported from one human host to another by the animal (such as certain kinds of salmonella infection, a potentially serious diarrheal disease that can be carried by houseflies, chickens, ducks, wild birds, and reptiles such as pet tortoises). The animal that carries the disease may be sick, too, or unaffected, whereas humans may be struck down by a serious, even lethal infection.

Some human diseases may be transmitted to domestic animals and pets, and a few disease agents can move in either direction. The endless interrelationship of humans, animals, and disease agents that may move from an animal to a human host and/or vice versa provide many illustrations of the relevance of natural history to epidemic investigation. Plague and typhus were investigated by naturalists, including entomologists, zoologists, and bacteriologists, as well as physicians and epidemiologists. The long, unhappy relationship among humans, rats, lice, and Rickettsia was eloquently described in one of the modern medical

John Snow. (Reproduced with permission from Duncan, B. M. (1947). *Development of inhalation anesthesia*, London.)

classics, Zinsser's *Rats, lice, and history*, as well as in many other works before and since. The similar story of rats, fleas, and the bacillus of plague is celebrated in folklore, myth, and modern parables such as Camus's *La peste* (The plague). Several varieties of virus encephalitis are endemic in wild birds, deer, or horses. They are transmitted by mosquitoes, so transmission is seasonal. Epidemics of viral encephalitis in humans tend to occur in a wet season, perhaps when floods bring mosquitoes and the animal or avian host of the virus closer to where people live or work. The mosquitoes then get their

Animals as carriers: types of animals, disease agents, and diseases

|  | Animal | Agent | Diseases/Infestations |
|---|---|---|---|
| **Domestic animals** | Dogs, cats | Virus | Rabies |
|  |  | Bacteria | Leptospirosis, Salmonellosis, Catscratch fever |
|  |  | Protozoa | Leishmaniasis (kala azar), Toxoplasmosis |
|  |  | Fungus | Ringworm |
|  |  | Helminth (worm) | Hydatids, Hookworm, Toxocara, Trichinella |
|  | Birds (e.g. parrots) | Virus | Encephalitis |
|  |  | Chlamydia | Psittacosis |
|  |  | Bacteria | Campylobacter infection |
|  |  | Fungus | Histoplasmosis |
|  | Reptiles | Bacteria | Salmonellosis |
|  | Cattle, horses | Prion | Spongiform encephalopathy |
|  |  | Virus | Encephalitis |
|  |  | Bacteria | Tuberculosis, Anthrax, Glanders, Tetanus |
|  |  | Rickettsia | Q fever |
|  |  | Fungus | Ringworm |
|  |  | Protozoa | Crytosporidiosis, Sleeping sickness |
|  |  | Helminth (worm) | Tapeworms |
|  | Sheep, goats | Prion | Spongiform encephalopathy |
|  |  | Virus | Orf |
|  |  | Rickettsia | Q fever |
|  |  | Bacteria | Anthrax, Brucellosis, Tularemia, Yersiniosis |
|  |  | Flukes, worms | Clonorchiasis, Tapeworms, Fasciolopsiasis, Hydatids |
|  | Pigs, swine | Virus | Encephalitis, Influenza |
|  |  | Bacteria | Anthrax, Brucellosis, Tularemia, Leptospirosis, Salmonellosis, Yersiniosis |
|  |  | Helminths | Schistosomiasis, Trichinosis, Tapeworms |
|  | Poultry | Virus | Encephalitis, Influenza |
|  |  | Bacteria | Campylobacter infection, Salmonellosis |
| **Pest species** | Rats, mice | Virus | Hemorrhagic fevers, Lassa fever (?), Hantavirus pulmonary syndrome, Meningitis |
|  |  | Rickettsia | Typhus |
|  |  | Bacteria | Plague, Leptospirosis, Ratbite fever, Relapsing fever, Salmonellosis |
|  |  | Protozoa | Babesiosis, Leishmaniasis |
|  |  | Worms | Eosinophilic meningitis, Clonorchiasis, Trichinosis, Tapeworms |
|  | Pigeons | Fungus | Cryptococcus infection, Histoplasmosis |
| **Wild animals** | Deer, etc. | Virus | Orf |
|  |  | Prion | Spongiform encephalopathy |
|  |  | Rickettsia | Rocky Mountain spotted fever (RMSF) |
|  |  | Bacteria | Lyme disease |
|  | Rodents, etc. | Virus | Hemorrhagic fevers, Rabies, Hantavirus pulmonary syndrome |
|  |  | Rickettsia | Typhus, RMSF |
|  |  | Bacteria | Plague, Tularemia, Relapsing fever, Leptospirosis |
|  |  | Protozoa | Giardiasis, Leishmaniasis |
|  | Bears | Helminths | Trichinosis |
|  | Birds | Virus | Arbovirus encephalitis |
|  |  | Fungus | Cryptococcosis |
|  |  | Helminths | Capillariasis |
|  | Fish | Helminths | Schistosomiasis, Tapeworms, Roundworms |
| **Miscellaneous** | Snails, amphibia | Nematode worm | Eosinophil meningitis |

Some vector-borne diseases of public health importance involving animals

| Disease (and agent) | Vector | Control measures |
|---|---|---|
| Malaria (protozoa) | Anopheline mosquito | Ecological measures (drain swamps, etc.) Kill mosquito larvae Nets Antimalarial drugs Human malaria is an exclusively human disease, but other varieties of malaria affect other vertebrates |
| Yellow fever (virus) | Culecine mosquito | Same ecological measures as for malaria Monkeys are alternative hosts Vaccine |
| Schistosomiasis (trematode worm) | Freshwater snail | Ecological measures Molluscicides Protection of exposed skin Chemotherapy not much use Water buffalo is alternative host |
| Leishmaniasis (protozoa) | Sandfly | Dogs, etc., alternative hosts Destroy sandfly habitat Control animal hosts Chemotherapy |
| Trypanosomiasis (sleeping sickness) | Tsetse fly | Destroy fly habitat Domestic and wild animals are alternative hosts |
| Typhus (rickettsia) | Lice | Rats are alternative host Chemotherapy |
| Bubonic plague (bacteria) | Fleas | Rats are principal host Chemotherapy |

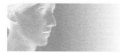

John **SNOW** (1813–58). London doctor, anesthetist, and founder of modern epidemiology. He administered chloroform to Queen Victoria to assist at the births of her two youngest children. His work on CHOLERA included a logical analysis of facts demonstrating that cholera must be transmissible. He did two epoch-making epidemiological investigations. In 1848 he studied a localized epidemic in Soho, demonstrating that the cause was polluted water from a pump in Broad Street. In 1854 cholera returned to London. Snow analyzed the information about cases and their sources of drinking-water, showing beyond doubt that the cause was polluted water — a remarkable feat, completed 30 years before Robert Koch identified the cholera bacillus.

blood meal from humans, and infect them. This seasonal variation is observed with Murray Valley and St Louis encephalitis and some other vector-borne virus infections. Others, such as Ebola virus infection, a frequently fatal hemorrhagic fever, remain a mystery, but those who are studying this disease believe that an animal or other host must be implicated; where else could the Ebola virus go between human outbreaks, if not to some other living creature?

### Zoonoses

These are diseases of vertebrates and humans, who may be accidental hosts, 'caught in the cross-fire', so to speak. Alternatively, zoonoses may be defined as human diseases whose agents are shared in nature with other vertebrate species. Many lethal and dangerous diseases are zoonoses; they include rabies, bubonic plague, anthrax, psittacosis, and several parasitic worm infections. Frequently zoonoses are transmitted by a vector, and some, such as rabies, affect certain species much more severely than others. Rabies appears not to be universally fatal in bats; indeed, in some bat colonies it may be benign.

There are several varieties of zoonoses. Direct zoonoses may be perpetuated in nature by a single species, as with anthrax or leptospirosis. Other zoonoses require two (or more) vertebrate

species; this happens with some parasitic worms, for example, hydatids and some tapeworms. Meta-zoonoses require both vertebrates and invertebrates such as ticks or mosquitoes to complete their life cycle; examples include American trypanosomiasis (Chagas's disease) and LEISHMANIASIS (kala azar). Finally saprozoonoses depend on inanimate reservoirs or development sites such as soil, water, or plants as well as vertebrate hosts; examples include toxoplasmosis and mycotic infections. Some of the spongiform encephalopathies (diseases of the brain, which has a spongy appearance) appear also to be zoonotic infections, although the epidemiological details remain uncertain.

### Helminths

Several parasitic worms have complex life cycles, passing part of their development in human hosts and part in other species, domesticated or wild animals, fish, crustacea, or molluscs such as snails. These complex life cycles are a tantalizing conundrum in evolutionary biology. How did the delicate little worm, the schistosome parasite that lives in and destroys the bladder of Egyptian peasants along the Nile, become mutually dependent on humans and water snails? How did hydatid worms become dependent upon a parasitic existence that requires them to breed in the intestines of carnivorous dogs, foxes, and wolves and an encysted phase in the lungs, or brain of another animal that the canine species might eat? Presumably it is a survival mechanism, for the cysts may survive long after the canine host of the adult worms has died — but how did it evolve? Humans are an accidental intermediate 'dead end' host for hydatid disease because humans are almost never eaten by dogs; but hydatid cysts may gravely damage the human liver and lungs, or wreak awful havoc in a human brain, so that hydatid disease has been a serious problem in countries where people, sheep, and dogs live together, as in Australia and New Zealand (from both of which hydatid disease has been virtually if not entirely eradicated).

### Rats

Rats are champions in the carriage trade. Very hardy, they can live in a wide variety of harsh environmental conditions, almost always close to humans, characteristically in filthy conditions. They carry a diverse array of dangerous diseases, the agents ranging in size and complexity from viruses to large worms, often without apparent harm to themselves.

### Vector-borne diseases

A vector is a living creature — for instance, insect, mollusc, bird — that carries a disease agent which can infect humans. Sometimes the disease agent passes an essential part of its life cycle in the vector, as the malaria parasite does in the mosquito and the schistosome parasite does in freshwater snails. Other vectors are merely passive carriers of infectious agents that are carried rather as passengers might be on a bus; this happens with house flies and perhaps cockroaches (which, despite their unfavorable image, have never been confirmed as carriers of any disease agent). The INSECT vectors of disease are discussed elsewhere. Vector-borne spread involves travel between humans and animals, and also is dependent upon environmental conditions, such as the presence of water for mosquitoes to lay their eggs and the larvae to develop; and ambient environmental temperatures favorable to the vector's breeding cycle. When considering rodents as vectors, their proliferation in breeding and feeding sites close to where humans live, is fostered by the presence of filth, litter, and refuse.

Hence the relationships among humans and other living creatures are complex. These relationships may be clarified only when there is an effective coalition of scientists in the relevant disciplines: physicians, veterinarians, epidemiologists, microbiologists, zoologists, ornithologists, entomologists, botanists, animal behaviorists, and many more.                                                    JML

*See also* WORMS

**ANOREXIA NERVOSA** See EATING DISORDERS

## ANTIBIOTICS AND ANTI-INFECTIVE DRUGS

Six categories of drugs are used in the treatment of infections, according to the type of organism against which they are active:

- antibacterial drugs
- antiviral drugs
- antiprotozoal drugs
- antihelminthic drugs
- antitrematodal drugs
- antifungal drugs

The main classes of antibacterial drugs are listed in the table, along with some examples of drugs that belong to those classes, and of the infections that they are used to treat. The modes of action of some anti-infective drugs are shown in the following figure.

### Antibacterial drugs

The idea that some organisms might contain compounds that destroyed other micro-organisms (*La vie empêché la vie*) was first propounded by Louis PASTEUR (p 620) in 1877, while studying fermentation on behalf on the French wine industry. Thus, the strict definition of an antibiotic is a substance that is produced by living organisms and that is capable of destroying or inhibiting the growth of micro-organisms. For example, streptomycin was originally found in the fungus *Streptomyces griseus*; it is a true antibiotic. However, many types of chemically synthesized drugs, such as the sulfonamides, trimethoprim, and some antituberculous drugs, are also used in the treatment of bacterial infections. These drugs would be better termed chemotherapeutic agents, but they are usually loosely called antibiotics.

*Sulfonamides* The sulfonamides were the first clinically effective anti-infective drugs. They were introduced by Gerhard DOMAGK (p 50) in 1935, after his experiments with azo dyes and their effects on bacterial growth. The first sulfonamide, Prontosil rubrum, was in fact an inactive compound that was metabolized to an active drug in the liver after being taken by mouth. Later, active sulfonamides were synthesized and were widely used to treat many infections. From the 1940s they were gradually superseded by the penicillins and other antibiotics, and they are now little used, because of the risk of severe skin eruptions and other adverse effects. However, sulfamethoxazole, which in combination with trimethoprim is known as co-trimoxazole, is still used in treating pneumonia due to *Pneumocystis carinii*, an infection that is a serious complication of AIDS.

*Penicillins* The anti-infective actions of certain molds had been described in previous centuries, for example, by John Tyndall in 1876. However, not until Alexander FLEMING's (p 50) observations in 1929 was it appreciated that anti-infective drugs might be isolated from molds, and even then it took several years before practical advances were made. The original penicillin, benzylpenicillin or penicillin G, was isolated from a mold called *Penicillium notatum* by FLOREY (p 52), Chain, and Heatley in Oxford in 1940, and was first used in the treatment of infections in Oxford's Radcliffe Infirmary in 1941. In 1945 Florey and Chain, along with Fleming, were awarded the NOBEL PRIZE for their work on penicillin.

**A ROMANIAN BACTERIOLOGIST**

Victor **BABES** (1854–1926). Having studied medicine in Vienna, Babes went on to work at the Histology Institute in Bucharest. He moved to Germany and then to the Pasteur Institute in Paris, where he studied rabies and co-authored (with Cornil) one of the first bacteriology textbooks. In 1887 he became professor of experimental pathology and bacteriology at the University of Bucharest and director of the Antirabies Institute of Romania. He described metachromatic granules (Babes–Ernst bodies) in 1886 and two years later he first discovered the tick-borne protozoa, Babesia, in the red blood cells of cattle (babesiosis, which is rare in humans unless they have had their spleen removed, when it may cause a fatal disease resembling malaria).

A stylized representation of a bacterium, showing the sites of action of some anti-infective drugs. (From Grahame-Smith, D. G. and Aronson, J. K. (1992). *The Oxford textbook of clinical pharmacology and drug therapy*, 2nd edn, OUP.)

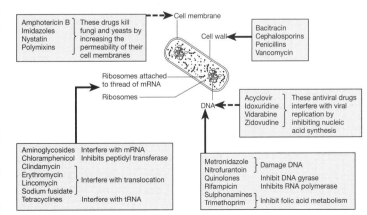

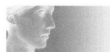
The first development after benzylpenicillin was the synthesis of penicillins that were stable in gastric acid and could therefore be given by mouth (for example, phenoxymethylpenicillin or penicillin V). Next came ampicillin (also effective by mouth and with a slightly broader spectrum of antibacterial activity than penicillin V) and amoxicillin (similar to ampicillin, but better absorbed from the gut). When resistance to the penicillins started to develop among certain organisms, new varieties of penicillins were developed. Flucloxacillin was developed to cope with resistant staphylococci, and piperacillin, ticarcillin, and azlocillin in response to resistance of *Pseudomonas aeruginosa*. The modern phenomenon of methicillin resistance in *Staphylococcus aureus* (so-called MRSA) is causing major problems in the treatment of infections with these organisms, particularly in hospitals.

The penicillins are very safe and can be given in large doses without risk of severe toxicity. However, they cause allergic reactions in about 10% of people, in whom their used is precluded.

*Aminoglycosides* In the 1940s Selman Waksman decided to look for antibiotics in other microorganisms. He had been encouraged by the success of penicillin and stimulated by his colleague and former student René DUBOS (p 247), who had already, in 1939, isolated tyrothricin (actually a mixture of two antibiotics, tyrocidine and gramicidin) from an organism called *Bacillus brevis*. Waksman chose a group of organisms called actinomycetes and isolated the first clinically useful aminoglycoside, streptomycin, from *Streptomyces griseus* in 1943. He invented the word 'antibiotic' and was awarded the NOBEL PRIZE in 1952. The effectiveness of streptomycin in guinea pigs infected with TUBERCULOSIS led to its successful introduction into clinical practice. Since then several other antibiotics of this group have been discovered, including gentamicin, amikacin, netilmicin, and neomycin. These drugs are very toxic after systemic administration. Their main adverse effects are kidney damage and damage to the eighth cranial nerve, which is responsible for hearing and some aspects of balance.

*Tetracyclines* Tetracyclines were first isolated from *Streptomyces aureofaciens* in 1945 by Benjamin Duggar, working at Lederle Laboratories, one of the companies that had been involved in the first commercial production of penicillin when Florey had approached US drug companies in the early 1940s, British companies being too preoccupied with the war in Europe. Their main adverse effects are nausea, vomiting, and diarrhea, and if they lead to dehydration in patients with impaired kidney function they may cause acute kidney failure. They should not be used in children or pregnant women, because they damage growing bones and teeth, in which they are deposited.

*Cephalosporins* Searching for organisms that might produce antibiotics, Giuseppe Brotzu discovered a mold, *Cephalosporium acremonium*, in the sea water near a Sardinian sewer. After his preliminary experiments, cephalosporins were extracted from the mold juice in Oxford in 1949. Numerous derivatives with broader spectra of activity have since been developed. They are generally used as second-line or third-line agents, but are sometimes used as first-line treatment for severe infections in hospitals. The cephalosporins rarely cause adverse effects, except for allergic reactions in about 5% of individuals.

*Macrolides* The most commonly used macrolide, erythromycin, was isolated from *Streptomyces erythreus* by Robert Bunch and James McGuire of Eli Lilly and Company in 1952. They had obtained the organism from a sample of Philippine soil. For many years erythromycin was reserved for treating infections in patients who would have been treated with a penicillin, were it not for allergy. However, it is now also used as the treatment of choice for pneumonia due to unusual organisms, such as *Legionella pneumophila* (Legionnaires' disease) and *Mycoplasma pneumoniae*. Newer compounds are now available, including azithromycin and clarithromycin. Clarithromycin is used in the treatment of peptic ulcers, since it helps to eradicate the bacterium that is associated with them, *Helicobacter pylori*. The main adverse effects of these drugs are liver damage and, more commonly, nausea, vomiting, and loss of appetite.

*Quinolones* The quinolones are synthetic antibacterial drugs and are not therefore true antibiotics. The first of these, nalidixic acid, an analog of a byproduct of chloroquine synthesis, was synthesized by Alexander Surrey of the Sterling-Winthrop Research Institute as part of a search for antimalarial drugs. It was first used in urinary tract infections in 1962. In recent years analogs, such as ciprofloxacin, norfloxacin, and ofloxacin, have been developed and used to treat infections due to a wide range of organisms, although not generally as first choice. The quinolones may cause nausea, vomiting, diarrhea, headache, dizziness, tiredness, and occasionally rashes. They may also worsen epilepsy. They are not given to infants or pregnant women because in tests they damage joints in the fetuses of animals. In patients whose red blood cells are deficient in the enzyme glucose-6-phosphate dehydrogenase they may cause cell breakdown (hemolysis).

*Trimethoprim* The discovery in 1952 that dihydrofolate reductase was a key enzyme in the way in which bacteria use folic acid led to the develop-

Some antibacterial drugs, organisms, and the infections for which they are usually first choice

| | Antibacterial drug | Organisms | Infections |
|---|---|---|---|
| Penicillins | Benzylpenicillin | *Streptococcus pyogenes* | Acute follicular tonsillitis, Cellulitis/erysipelas<br>Acute otitis media (over 5 y; see also co-amoxiclav) |
| | | 'Viridans' streptococci | Endocarditis (+ gentamicin) |
| | | *Streptococcus pneumoniae* | Pneumococcal pneumonia |
| | | *Enterococcus faecalis* | Endocarditis (+ gentamicin) |
| | | *Neisseria gonorrhoeae* | Gonorrhea |
| | | *Neisseria meningitidis* | Meningococcal meningitis |
| | | *Treponema pallidum* | Syphilis |
| | Amoxicillin | *Streptococcus pneumoniae* | Exacerbations of chronic bronchitis, acute bronchitis/pneumonia |
| | | *Streptococcus pyogenes* | Acute otitis media (under 5 y) |
| | | *Streptococcus pneumoniae* | Sinusitis |
| | | *Streptococcus pyogenes* | Sinusitis |
| | | *Listeria monocytogenes* | Listeria septicemia and meningitis |
| | Flucloxacillin | *Staphylococcus aureus* | Wounds, boils, abscesses, septic arthritis, osteomyelitis, pneumonia, endocarditis, impetigo |
| | Piperacillin | *Pseudomonas aeruginosa* | Septicemia (+ gentamicin), urinary tract infection, pneumonia (+ gentamicin), |
| Tetracyclines | (e.g. tetracycline, oxytetracycline, doxycycline) | *Coxiella burnetti*<br>*Rickettsiae*<br>*Chlamydiae* | Q fever, typhus, trachoma, psittacosis, lymphogranuloma venereum, non-specific urethritis |
| Aminoglycosides | (e.g. gentamicin, amikacin, tobramycin) | 'Viridans' streptococci<br>*Enterococcus faecalis* | Endocarditis (+ benzylpencillin)<br>Endocarditis (+ benzylpencillin) |
| | | *Escherichia coli, Klebsiella*<br>*Enterobacter, Proteus* | In severe infections, for example, septicemia, acute pyelonephritis, pneumonia, biliary tract infection |
| | | *Pseudomonas aeruginosa* `<br>(+ azlocillin) | Urinary tract infection |
| Macrolides | (e.g. erythromycin, clarithromycin) | *Legionella pneumophila*<br>*Mycoplasma pneumoniae*<br>*Helicobacter pylori* | Legionnaires' pneumonia<br>Mycoplasma pneumonia<br>In patients with peptic ulcer |
| Trimethoprim | | *Escherichia coli* | Urinary tract infection |
| Chloramphenicol | | *Salmonella typhi*<br>*Haemophilus influenzae* | Typhoid fever<br>Meningitis |
| Metronidazole | | Anaerobic organisms<br>(e.g. *Bacteroides* spp.) | Intra-abdominal infections, e.g. liver abscess, pelvic inflammatory disease, cholangitis, peritonitis, female genital tract infections, Lung abscess, Brain abscess, Endocarditis |
| | | *Clostridium difficile* | Antibiotic-associated diarrhea |
| | | *Helicobacter pylori* | In patients with peptic ulcer |
| Vancomycin | | *Staphylococcus aureus* | Organisms resistant to methicillin |
| | | Coagulase-negative staphylococci | All infections |
| | | *Clostridium difficile* | Antibiotic-associated diarrhea resistant to metronidazole |

ment of a series of reductase inhibitors, of which trimethoprim was found to be antibacterial. For some years it was used in combination with sulfonamides in the treatment of infections of the urinary tract with organisms such as *Escherichia coli* and *Proteus mirabilis*, but it is now used on its own for that purpose. It has few adverse effects.

***Metronidazole*** Metronidazole is one of a group of imidazoles, first synthesized in 1957 at Rhône Poulenc and initially used for the treatment of infections with the protozoan *Trichomonas vaginalis*. However, it is also effective against anaerobic organisms, such as species of *Bacteroides*, for which it is the treatment of first choice. It is also used in the treatment of other protozoan infections, including amebiasis and giardiasis. Other imidazoles (see below) are used in treating fungal infections. Metronidazole rarely causes adverse effects during short-term treatment, but it has a curious interaction with alcohol, whose metabolism it inhibits, causing accumulation of an unpleasant metabolite, acetaldehyde, that makes the patient feel ill.

**Chloramphenicol** Chloramphenicol was isolated from *Streptomyces venezuelae* in 1947 by John Ehrlich and Quentin Bartz of Parke Davis. It was the first so-called broad-spectrum antibiotic, having activity against a very wide range of organisms, and was first used to treat an epidemic of TYPHUS in Bolivia. However, its use was limited because of its severe adverse effects, particularly bone-marrow damage, an idiosyncratic reaction that occurs in about 1 in 250 000 individuals. Nevertheless, it is still the drug of first choice in meningitis due to *Haemophilus influenzae* and in acute typhoid fever. It is also commonly used for local treatment of infections of the eyes.

**Antituberculous drugs** The rifamycins were isolated from *Streptomyces mediterranei* (now called *Nocardia mediterranea*) in 1957 in the Lepetit Research Laboratories in Milan and whimsically named after Jules Dassin's film *Rififi*. They were found to be active against the tubercle bacillus and one of them, rifampicin, has since become one of the mainstays of treatment.

Thiacetazone was developed in the 1940s because of work by Domagk on a group of compounds called thiosemicarbazides. Although it was subsequently replaced by safer drugs, it has recently emerged as a valuable addition to treatment. In 1951 a further derivative, isoniazid, was synthesized from a hydrazine intermediate and proved even more potent; it is still used in the treatment of tuberculosis. Further investigation of these types of compounds led to the development of pyrazinamide, now a first-line drug in developing countries, and ethionamide, a third-line drug (because of its toxicity).

Ethambutol was developed following the discovery that the ethylenediamines had antituberculous activity. It is still used in combination with rifampicin, isoniazid, and pyrazinamide as standard first-line treatment.

The discovery in 1940 that salicylic acid affected oxygen use by the tubercle bacillus led to the development of para-aminosalicylic acid, which was used for many years in the treatment of tuberculosis, but has now been superseded.

The antituberculous drugs have varying adverse effects, but most of them can cause liver damage and have to be used with care in people who have cirrhosis. Other effects include damage to the eyes (ethambutol), peripheral nerves (isoniazid), and hearing (streptomycin).

### Antiviral drugs
A disappointment of the antibiotics was that they are ineffective against viruses. However, some antiviral drugs emerged during the search for anticancer drugs in the 1950s. Modern antiviral drugs are almost all based on the structures of nucleosides, which are important structural components of the nucleic acids, DNA and RNA. The first of these, idoxuridine, was effective against *Herpesvirus* infections, but has been superseded. The nucleoside analogs are themselves inactive, but are activated by intracellular metabolism, generally with greater specificity by viruses than by human cells. This confers therapeutic activity on such agents with minimal toxicity.

Drugs of this kind include acyclovir, used for treating *Herpesvirus* infections; gancyclovir (infection with cytomegalovirus); tribavarin (infection with the respiratory syncytial virus); vidarabine (*Herpesvirus* infections); and zidovudine and didanosine (infection with HIV).

Recently, different approaches have been used in tackling the human immunodeficiency virus (HIV) by attacking specific parts of its structure. For instance, one new group of drugs inhibits a viral enzyme, a protease.

### Antiprotozoal drugs
It has been known since the 17th century that Jesuits' bark, the active ingredient of which is quinine, is effective in the treatment of 'ague', that is, MALARIA. However, it was not until the synthesis of pamaquin in 1925 that the modern series of antimalarial drugs was developed. This group of drugs includes mepacrine, chloroquine, and primaquine, all structurally related to quinine. It is not known how they work, but they seem to bind to components of the DNA of the parasite. Investigations of other structures in the 1940s yielded the unrelated compounds proguanil and pyrimethamine. The antimalarial drugs have few adverse effects, but they may cause hemolysis in people whose red cells are deficient in the enzyme glucose-6-phosphate dehydrogenase. Occasionally there may be allergic reactions. During long-term treatment chloroquine can damage the retina.

One problem in the treatment of malaria is the rapid development of resistance of the malarial parasite, which is currently outstripping the emergence of new effective drugs. New drugs, based on compounds found in *Artemisia* species (for example, artemether), are being increasingly used.

Other important protozoan diseases include amebiasis and giardiasis, for which the imidazoles metronidazole (see above) and tinidazole are effective.

With the discovery in 1906 of the effectiveness of salts of antimony in the treatment of LEISHMANIASIS, various antimonials were developed for treating this protozoan disease. Currently in use are the pentavalent antimony salts (sodium stibogluconate and meglumine antimoniate). An unrelated drug, pentamidine, is also used.

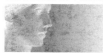

# ANTI-VIVISECTION/ANIMAL RIGHTS MOVEMENTS

Anti-vivisection is a political and moral protest movement which developed in Britain, Europe, and the United States in the 19th century, and which is primarily concerned with protecting animals from harmful experimentation.

At the core of anti-vivisection rationale lies simplistic understanding of right and wrong, of 'respect for all life forms and justice for all species'. Related to these ideas of respect and justice is exploitation of the powerless (animals) by the powerful (humans); this is the key to understanding contemporary and historical issues of animal rights and reasons for 'liberating' animals from oppression. Animal rights advocates assert that exploiting animals involves not only killing them, but also denying them their freedom and causing them fear and pain.

Ideas of pain, exploitation, and the understanding by some individuals of the claims of animals to a pain-free existence were central to the ethical foundations of anti-vivisection sentiment in 19th-century England. A select group of 18th-century animal-loving literati, including Samuel Johnson, Joseph Addison, and Alexander Pope, offered independent criticism of animal experimentation. Animal protection societies, such as the Society for the Prevention of Cruelty to Animals, founded in 1824, were primarily concerned with working-class cruelty to animals in work and sport. However, an organized anti-vivisection movement had to await the mid-19th century, when the public became more aware of experimental work in continental European laboratories, and when English experimentalists began to express a greater willingness to follow the lead of their continental counterparts. In 1875 a Royal Commission was appointed to investigate the extent of animal experimentation in England, and several anti-vivisection societies were established; the policies of each reflected the polarity within the movement as a whole. The restrictionist Society for the Protection of Animals Liable to Vivisection was co-founded by the Anglo-Irish reformer and women's rights advocate, Frances Power Cobbe, and the physician George Hoggan, and George Jesse organized the Society for the Abolition of Vivisection. The abolitionist International Association and the London Anti-Vivisection Society quickly followed. The Society for the Protection of Animals Liable to Vivisection (since 1898 the National Anti-Vivisection Society) figured most prominently in the controversy.

Debate between pro- and anti-vivisectionists escalated throughout the summer of 1876. Petitions poured into Parliament, and in August the first anti-vivisection act, the Cruelty to Animals Act, was passed. This Act introduced a system of licensing and registration for vivisections and of inspection of licensed premises. Fines were to be levied on anyone who had performed vivisections without first having obtained a licence from the Home Secretary — £50 for a first offence and £100 or three months in jail for subsequent offences. Anti-vivisectionists were unimpressed; they believed that the 1876 Act protected physiologists from prosecution, not animals from torture, and anti-vivisection sentiment began to swing in favor of abolition. Several attempts were made by the International Association and the Society for the Protection of Animals Liable to Vivisection to secure Parliamentary support for abolition bills, all of which were unsuccessful. A second Royal Commission into vivisection sat between 1906 and 1912 and a Departmental Enquiry was held in 1965. Not until 1986, however, was the 1876 bill replaced by a more stringent measure, which demanded dual licensing of the person performing the experiment and the experiment being performed.

## First society in USA

The first anti-vivisection society in America was founded in 1883 by Caroline Earle White, who had been encouraged by developments in England. Other organizations followed: the New England Anti-Vivisection Society (1895), the Vivisection Reform Society (1903), and the New York Anti-Vivisection Society (1908). Legislation to regulate animal experimentation in America was introduced first in New York's legislature in 1880, then in the Senate Committee of the District of Columbia in 1896 and 1900. All were unsuccessful and an anti-vivisection act was not passed until 1966 (amended 1970, 1976, 1985).

Issues surrounding animal welfare have become more complex over time. In the 19th century, animals were not considered to have 'rights' per se; as creatures sensitive to pain they had only 'claims' on humans for compassionate treatment. Most anti-vivisectionists agreed with the book of Genesis that man had dominion over animals; few were vegetarian; many were avid hunters. Anti-vivisectionists used both moral and utilitarian arguments to refute the medical claims of their opponents. Vivisection was morally wrong because it involved the torture and destruction of life that God had created; it was scientifically useless because experimentation on an animal said nothing about the human condition. Vivisection destroyed the bodies of animals and the souls of men. Ouida in 1882 referred to vivisection as 'the gigantic system of animal sacrifice' and of laboratories as 'the blood-stained temples of the physiologist'.

Anti-vivisectionists protesting in the late 20th century not only wrestle with physiological research and drug testing, but also cosmetic testing, the illegal monkey trade, and xenotransplantation (organ grafts from animals). These activists do not defend animal welfare on the basis of the claims that animals have, but on their right to enjoy a pain-free existence. Yet there is a lack of agreement about how that existence is to be guaranteed. For example, there is little consistency in vivisection legislation within the European Union. In 1985, a step towards consensus was taken when the Council of Europe adopted a Convention for the Protection of Vertebrate Animals Used for Scientific and Other Purposes.

In the 19th century, the vivisector represented all that was bad with science, and animal experimentation is still interpreted today by the British Union for the Abolition of Vivisection as 'the supreme arrogance of science over humanity'. Protest should not be understood to represent sentiment versus science; members of the medical community are also concerned with the ethical treatment of animals and have formed their own organizations including the Physicians Committee for Responsible Medicine and the Medical Research Modernization Committee. Despite mounting protest, however, animal experimentation is still considered to be vital to medical and scientific research. A recent article in The Guardian, which sets out the clash between the US-based animal rights group, People for the Ethical Treatment of Animals, and individuals supporting medical research, quotes Harold Varmus, director of the National Institutes of Health (an important source of financial support for experimentation in America), as stating that the 'privilege of studying animals is essential to virtually all phases of medical research'. For anti-vivisectionists and animal rights advocates, experimenting upon animals is not a privilege: it is an abuse of power. They see nothing humane in experimental research even if the ultimate goal is to expand knowledge and improve human life.

In 1985, the Council for International Organization of the Medical Sciences, the World Health Organization agency that pronounces on ethical issues, published some international guiding principles for biomedical research involving animals. This document sets out the internationally accepted standards governing ethical justification for animal experiments, varieties of ethically acceptable experiments, standards of care of laboratory animals, and suggests alternatives to animals in biomedical research.                LWil

### Antihelminthic drugs

The imidazoles were first identified as anti-infective drugs when a substance called azomycin was isolated from a species of *Streptomyces* in 1953 in Japan. The nitroimidazole metronidazole was subsequently synthesized in 1957, and since then many related compounds have been synthesized. These include mebendazole, albendazole, and niridazole. Cousins of these compounds, the aminothiazoles, have also been developed; of these levamisole is in current use. These drugs are used in the treatment of infestations with WORMS, including roundworm, whipworm, hookworm, threadworm, and tapeworm.

### Antitrematodal drugs

Older drugs, such as oxamniquine and lucanthone, have been superseded by praziquantel. It is used in the treatment of infections with trematodes, including SCHISTOSOMIASIS; liver fluke infections (for example, opisthorchiasis, clonorchiasis, and fascioliasis); intestinal infections (for example, fasciolopsiasis and echinostomiasis); and lung fluke infections (paragonimiasis).

### Antifungal drugs

In 1950 a substance called nystatin was isolated from *Streptomyces noursci* at the New York State Department of Health (hence the name of the compound). It was followed three years later by the isolation of a similar compound, amphotericin, from *Streptomyces nodosus*. Both of these drugs were found to be effective against fungi.

Several imidazoles, developed since the discovery of metronidazole, are now also used for treating fungal infections. These include clotrimazole, econazole, fluconazole, itraconazole, ketoconazole, miconazole, and tioconazole. They are used to treat infections with *Candida albicans* (thrush) and organisms that infect the skin (dermatophytes), including *Tinea cruris*, *pedis*, *corporis*, *capitis*, and *versicolor*. They are also used in the treatment of systemic fungal infections, including candidiasis, histoplasmosis, coccidioidomycosis, blastomycosis, cryptococcosis, and aspergillosis. Of the antifungal drugs, amphotericin is the most toxic and can cause kidney damage. The imidazoles can cause liver damage.

### Resistance to antibacterial drugs

Ever since anti-infective drugs were used, organisms have developed resistance to them. Profligate use of antibiotics, without careful consideration of their appropriate indications, leads to the emergence of resistant strains. Efforts are currently being made to encourage sensible use of antibiotics in the hope of minimizing this.

The usual way of coping with bacterial resistance is to develop new antibacterial drugs that circumvent the problem. However, in some cases it is possible to enhance the actions of existing drugs. For example, clavulanic acid, although not itself antibacterial, inhibits beta-lactamase and thus combats this form of resistance; it is sometimes used in combination with amoxicillin (the combination being known as co-amoxiclav).

Other drugs prolong the actions of antibacterial drugs in the body by inhibiting their elimination. For example, probenecid inhibits the renal excretion of the penicillins and cilastatin inhibits the inactivation in the kidney of imipenem, a penicillin-like drug.           JKA

*See also* PHYSIOLOGY

**APHASIA** See LANGUAGE

**APOTHECARIES** Throughout medieval Europe, apothecaries were members of trade guilds or associations. Their primary function was to compound and dispense drugs and other medicinal products, although many also engaged in importing and selling other commodities. A few made important contributions to botany and chemistry, the sciences most closely identified with their trade. In Europe, apothecaries eventually became assimilated into the modern profession of PHARMACY, though often with legal rights to advise on health matters and to sell drugs directly to the public which in Britain or the United States would be classified as prescription only. Unusually, in Britain, apothecaries achieved the right of full medical practice and evolved into what by the early 19th century was being called the general practitioner.

For short periods of time apothecaries and spicers in medieval London achieved some autonomy; from 1180 they were associated with the pepperers and grocers. The Grocers Company became one of the wealthiest and most powerful guilds of the 14th century, but apothecaries within the guild had their own identity and from the 16th century tried to secure their independence. After several unsuccessful attempts, the Society of Apothecaries was granted its royal charter by James I, on 6 December 1617, in the face of opposition from the Grocers. Among the Society's founders and early benefactors was Gideon de Laune, who twice served as Master. Thereafter, it was mostly with the Royal College of Physicians that the apothecaries feuded.

The sources of conflict were several. Apothecaries were supposed to compound remedies in accordance with the *Pharmacopoeia Londinensis*, whose compilation was the primary responsibility of the College of Physicians. Apothecaries' shops could be searched by the Physicians in search of faulty or unofficial medicines. The Society objected to a dispensary for the sick poor which the College proposed to establish in 1675; the Physicians protested that many apothecaries were actually practicing medicine. Matters came to a head in 1704, when William Rose, a Liveryman of the Company, was prosecuted by the College for selling medicines directly to a butcher named Seale. The Rose case ultimately went to the House of Lords, where the apothecaries won the legal right to dispense drugs without recourse to a physician's prescription, on the practical grounds that there were not enough physicians to provide healthcare for the whole population.

From the beginning, the Society was based in Black Friars, a precinct which was then outside the jurisdiction of the City of London authorities. The original Apothecaries' Hall was destroyed in the Great Fire of 1666, although many of the Society's records and treasures were saved. Rebuilding started in 1668, and the resulting edifice, with its fine Great Hall, still houses the Society. There were additions in the second half of the 18th century. The 17th-century Society also built and ran a laboratory for producing and selling medicines. It long remained profitable and eventually managed to secure lucrative contracts with the Royal Navy and various hospitals and dispensaries. Its most distinguished superintendent was probably W. T. Brande, who succeeded Sir Humphry Davy as professor of chemistry at the Royal Institution in 1813, and was Master of the Society in 1851–2.

***Botanical garden*** Another 17th-century activity of the Society was the establishment, in 1676, of a botanical garden at Chelsea. The Chelsea Physic Garden (second oldest botanical gardens in England) long remained the responsibility of the Society, during which period it supplied medicinal plants for the laboratories as well as exotic fruits, such as pineapples, for the Society's banquets. Bequests by Sir Hans SLOANE (p 56), Sir Joseph Banks, and others encouraged scientific work, and its 18th-century gardener, Philip Miller, has been described as the greatest botanical horticulturist of his time. As botany became more marginal to medicine, and Society members more actively engaged in routine medical practice, the garden's control passed to a private philanthropy in 1899.

By the end of the 18th century, apothecaries in European countries were closely identified with the professionalization of pharmacy. In France, for instance, the Communauté des Marchands-Apothicaires et Epiciers became the Collège de Pharmacie in 1777, against the opposition of many physicians. Several members of the Collège, such as Antoine Petit and J. J. Virey, contributed to the vigorous scientific life of Revolutionary and Napoleonic France. In Britain, many apothecaries by then considered themselves medical practitioners rather than tradesmen, and the 'surgeon-apothecary' became a common designation for the general practitioner. From the early 19th century,

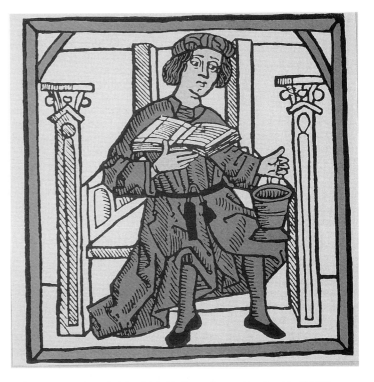

A medieval apothecary. (Reproduced courtesy of the Mary Evans Picture Library.)

various groups attempted to obtain Parliamentary recognition of the apothecary's actual professional status. They included the London Association of Apothecaries, whose president was George Man Burrows, then a surgeon-apothecary, though later to turn to psychiatry (and become a Fellow of the Royal College of Physicians). The Association's agitation for educational reform catalysed the passage of the Apothecaries Act of 1815. Though far from perfect, the Act was important for several reasons. It required anyone who wished henceforth to practice as an apothecary to pursue courses in several medical subjects; to spend six months in attendance at a hospital, infirmary, or dispensary; and to pass the Licentiate examination of the Society (LSA). At one sweep, it extended the Society's jurisdiction from the traditional area of the City of London and six miles around, to the whole country; it turned it from a local livery company into a national medical examining and licensing body.

In many ways, the Society was ill prepared for its new role. Its court of examiners was used to dealing with a handful of apprentices, and, although the apprenticeship was not abolished by the Act, its importance declined as pupils began to spend more of their training years in formal courses. In the first year, 190 candidates (90% from the provinces) presented themselves; by the 1840s, this number had increased to over 400, most of whom also took the Membership Examination of the Royal College of Surgeons

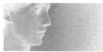

**Sir Hans SLOANE**
(1660–1753). British physician. Sloane trained in medicine in Paris and Montpellier, returning to London in 1684. In 1687 he was appointed physician to the Duke of Albermarle, Governor of the West Indies, and collected many plants and natural curiosities. He attended Queen Anne and in 1716 was the first member of the medical profession to receive a baronetcy. He became physician-general to the Army in 1722 and physician to George II in 1727. He was secretary to the Royal Society from 1693–1712 and president from 1727–41; from 1719–35 he also occupied the position of president of the Royal College of Physicians of London. After his death his collection was bought by the nation for £20 000 and went to form the basis of the British Museum.

(MRCS). Gradually, the traditional oral examinations became written ones, and the whole process was integrated into the Victorian notion of the meritocracy, whereby the examination system was presumed to select those candidates who had best prepared themselves, and were thus most worthy of success. The dual qualification LSA/MRCS became the standard for the general practitioner until 1888, when the Royal Colleges of Physicians and Surgeons joined together to produce their 'conjoint' qualification, LRCP/MRCS.

The exclusion of the Society from the Conjoint examination was a serious blow, although the Society has managed to maintain its status as an independent examining body. Students appreciated that they were eligible to take the Society's examinations before those for the university medical degree, and passing it might be a kind of insurance policy, since the LMSSA (Licentiate in Medicine and Surgery of the Society of Apothecaries, as the LSA became in 1907) was a registrable qualification with the General Medical Council.

While Licentiates of the Society may still call themselves Apothecaries, the term has become largely ceremonial, as the traditional role of the apothecary has been subsumed by that of the pharmacist or general practitioner. WFB

*See also* EDUCATION; HERBAL REMEDIES AND PHYSIC GARDENS; TITLES AND DEGREES

**APPLIANCES** There are over 10 000 appliances and aids for people with disabilities. Aids can be as important for a physically disadvantaged person as drugs are for people with medical conditions. There are as many aids as there are medications in the pharmacopeia. Yet attitudes to aids and drugs differ. There is a huge expenditure on medications, which are carefully designed and thoroughly tested. Drugs are subject to complex clinical trials. Considerable care is taken with dosages, delivery systems, and surveillance of side-effects. Medical students and doctors are taught in depth about PHARMACOLOGY, CLINICAL PHARMACOLOGY, AND THERAPEUTICS.

Enabling equipment has not enjoyed such scientific rigor or medical interest. Many items are developed and marketed without careful evaluation of their shortcomings or dangers. The provision of aids is patchy and uncoordinated and there may be delays in the delivery of important items. Aids are often under-provided, inadequately maintained, inappropriately used, or unused. Most studies of aids have been superficial and unstructured.

### The importance of aids

Physical disabilities may occur at any age but become more common as people get older. Most elderly people are physically independent and do not require any enabling equipment. However, the prevalence of disability increases with age. The population of most countries is aging and there will be large increases in the numbers of old (over 75 years) and very old (over 85) people in the coming decades. Previously, there was a stoical or passive acceptance of impairments and disabilities that may accompany old age: people assumed that deterioration in vision, hearing, and mobility was an inevitable consequence of aging and that little could be done to help them. Now more older people (or their children or other advocates) are beginning to demand better care and rightly expect high standards of rehabilitation.

Traditionally, many disabled older people were cared for in hospitals or care homes. The present trend is away from hospital care (which is increasingly high-technology, intensive, with day care or short-stay treatment) to care 'in the community', usually at home. The emphasis has also been shifting from caring *for* people to helping them to become autonomous. The challenge of enabling people with disabilities to live independently at home (where most of them wish to be) involves detailed assessment, medical treatment, careful goal setting, rehabilitation techniques, advice and support — and the provision of aids and appliances.

Aids may be needed for a short time (after a fracture or a flare-up of arthritis, for example) or over a longer period (for those with amputations, residual weakness after stroke, or with other chronic or progressive disorders). They can be useful in many circumstances (see box).

The main aims of rehabilitation are to restore people with disabling disorders to their optimum level of function and wellbeing. Whereas much medical endeavor has focused on pathology (the underlying disease process) and impairment (the signs and symptoms of disease), more attention is now being given to disability (problems with carrying out everyday activities because of a medical condition), handicap (the social consequences of disability), or quality of life (which includes those things that make life worth living or which give fulfilment).

Aids can help improve function — by allowing people to perform 'basic' activities, such as becoming mobile or self-caring (washing, grooming, dressing, or feeding oneself) or doing other everyday tasks (using public transport, making telephone calls, driving a car). Restoring people's functional abilities will often improve wellbeing: appropriate aids therefore have the capacity to overcome or minimize disability, attenuate handicap, and improve enjoyment of life.

### Aids to allow very disabled people to live in their own homes

These include aids, adaptations, and modifications which allow people to live as normal a life as possible (for example, stair-lifts to help gain access to the upstairs bedroom, toilet, or bathroom); environmental controls, which give people with motor neurone disease and other seriously disabling conditions the ability to open doors to visitors, modulate central heating, operate CD players, videos, and the television); and hoists (to ease the turning, cleaning, and changing of immobile people whilst reducing the risk of back and other injuries to care givers).

### Evolution of mobility aids

Aids can transform people's lives, yet they are not always known about or recommended by health professionals. They may not be provided to those who need them, or they may be rejected or not used by those who do receive them. There are many reasons for this unsatisfactory state of affairs. A consideration of the history and development of common aids to mobility will illustrate some of the problems of development, awareness, provision, and acceptance and indicate how the situation might be improved.

*Walking sticks* Sticks have great historical and symbolic importance. They have long been used as weapons, as a badge of office as well as a means of support and balance. In the Old Testament of the Bible, Moses led his followers with one. In Psalm 23 ('the Lord is my shepherd'), we read 'I fear no evil, for thou art with me; thy rod and thy staff they comfort me'. In ancient Egypt, sticks reflected a person's occupation and status: differ-

ent sticks denoted whether the owner was a shepherd, merchant, or priest.

Ornate sticks have for centuries been a badge of high office — the scepter and mace as a sign of royalty; the bishop's crosier or tau (T-shaped) cross. In Tutankhamun's tomb 132 sticks were found, to help him on his journey into the afterlife. King Henry VIII had bejewelled sticks, and courtiers had rather less ostentatious sticks. Van Dyck's portrait of Charles I shows him with a regal stick. Frederick the Great of Prussia had sticks with ornate jewels and handles. In Regency times, sticks reflected the elegance of the age. They were not only beautifully decorated, they became functional too, concealing blades and firearms as well as money or spirits.

In recent times, sticks have ceased to be fashionable. Many older people will not use them, perceiving them to be a sign of frailty. Some are fearful that the stick may not only identify the user as being disabled, but may be used as a weapon against them. They might instead use umbrellas for support.

Walking sticks can improve balance, ease pain (more effectively if held in the hand opposite to the painful hip or knee), and extend walking distance. They can accommodate a rheumatoid hand (by the provision of Fischer handles). The traditional curved handle, with its echo of a shepherd's crook, is often favored: the more ergonomically-designed straight-handled stick with finger grips not only looks utilitarian, but also cannot be used

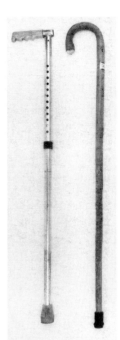

Different types of aids

| Prevention | e.g. hip protectors — to reduce the risk of hip fracture after a fall; low-pressure mattresses or cushions — to help prevent pressure sores; elasticated stockings — to reduce the risk of leg vein thrombosis in immobile or postoperative patients. |
|---|---|
| Therapeutic | walking frames can give stability and confidence to those being restored to full mobility. |
| Comfort | incontinence pads can keep people dry and give them the confidence to resume a more active social life. They should be considered as a first line measure, whilst the cause of the urinary incontinence is being determined and specific treatment arranged. Many people can be treated successfully and can dispense with their pads; others may benefit from longer term use. Bath aids and showers can improve well-being by allowing people to have the pleasure of using these enjoyable aids to hygiene, rather than requiring a strip wash. |
| Prosthetics | devices which replace or compensate for an absent limb or missing part of the body can help psychologically as well as physically. Examples include artificial eyes, breast prostheses for women following removal of a breast, and artificial arms or legs. |
| Orthoses | these aids can help correct the function of a deficient limb or organ. Examples include splints for a rheumatoid hand and ankle-foot orthoses for people who cannot raise their foot when walking (such as those with foot drop or hemiplegia). |
| Aids for impairments | A physical impairment is the malfunctioning of a part of the body as a result of a pathological process. For example, age-related macular degeneration (the most common cause of visual loss in western countries) results in the loss of central vision; artherosclerosis of leg arteries can reduce walking distance by causing claudication (pain in the calves on walking, which is relieved by rest). Aids can mitigate these problems: low visual aids (such as good illumination, large print books, clocks with big numbers, magnifying glasses), and walking sticks (which can increase walking distance in people with painful legs, as well as reducing pain and giving stability) are examples. Others include hearing aids, corsets and collars (to ease the discomfort of arthritis), and trusses (for hernias — though these are better treated surgically wherever possible). |

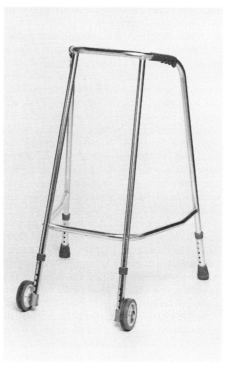

to pick up dropped items, help pull up underpants, or fit neatly over the arm when being carried.

The ideal walking stick should be robust (not too flexible or splintered); comfortable to hold (perhaps with an expanded handle to improve grip by arthritic fingers); and of optimum length (too long, and it will prevent good posture and cause the shoulder to be hitched upwards; too short, and the user will have to lean to one side and bend forwards when walking). It should have a rubber ferrule at the end (ideally with a concentric or studded tip) which has not become worn. If worn ferrules are not replaced, they can slip — particularly on wet surfaces — causing the user to fall. Holding the stick in the opposite, or contralateral, hand (for example, right hand if the left knee is painful) reduces the static forces on the affected joint, and it also allows a more normal reciprocal gait pattern: as the left leg moves forwards, so does the right arm. Holding the stick in the hand at the same side makes for an abnormal, almost amphibian walking pattern.

Sticks can therefore help relieve pain and improve mobility and stability but are not always recommended (perhaps because doctors are more likely to think of analgesics than physical aids), may not be used appropriately, or even used at all. Restoring the fashion status to sticks would help. In China, owning a dragon stick gives the owner kudos. It is cut from a single tree trunk, ornately designed and believed to confer longevity on its owner.

***Walking frames*** We start by walking on all fours, then on two legs. Later, we use three legs (the stick forming the third) and may then use six. The development of the walking frame illustrates some of the problems in recognition, acceptance, and promotion of aids.

In 1924, an American lady fell and broke her hip. She was one of the few in those days to survive, recover, and return home. Mobility was not easy but she found that pushing a chair in front of her gave her stability and confidence. Her 12-year-old nephew had a simple idea. By cutting out the seat from a wooden chair, and using the side arms for support, he developed the fore-runner of the walking frame. The matron of the hospital recognized the usefulness of the device and asked an engineer to fashion modified frames from steel. Years later, the lightweight aluminium frame was developed and the walking frame (often called the zimmer frame, though no one is sure why) became widely used.

Hence a very useful aid is simple — a child designed it. Perhaps because aids were not considered 'scientific', no one in the hospital described the device in a medical journal. Nearly thirty years elapsed between conception and widespread use.

Frames are often transitional aids, and many users graduate to sticks or to independent walking. They produce an unnatural start-stop-start gait pattern. This means that they may be unhelpful in Parkinsonian patients, who have difficulties initiating movements. One way of helping the user to have a smoother progress is to put wheels on the frame. However, this is inadvisable in those Parkinsonian patients with a hurrying gait: with each step, they go progressively more quickly and a wheeled frame would compound this. Aids may therefore be helpful to one person, but hazardous or inhibitory to another. An expert (usually a therapist) should advise on the appropriateness and specifications of an aid, and should instruct the patient and relatives in correct use.

Walking frames are not always used as intended. Sometimes they act as television aerials, often they are a means of drying clothes or supports for plant pots. Aids that are used inappropriately or unused could be retrieved, repaired, serviced, cleaned, and recycled, and this process is beginning to take place in many areas.

***Wheelchairs*** The early wheelchairs were household chairs with wheels attached to the sides, which facilitated indoor mobility. The advent of the railways and the fashion for visiting spas led to the development of chairs that were portable: they were made of lighter woods and could be folded to fit into carriages. Modern wheelchairs are made of metal and have seats which can be compressed but which are not comfortable for sitting in for long periods. They are often used as a seat as well as a means of mobility. They can be a boon: three-quarters of wheelchair users cannot walk at all or can manage only a few steps. Wheelchairs allow them to get around further — visit friends, go shopping, enjoy holidays. Anyone with impaired mobility should therefore be asked if they would benefit from the provision of a wheelchair.

Just as drugs can produce adverse reactions, so too aids and appliances can have untoward effects. Wheelchairs are a cause of pressure sores (indeed, chair sores are now more common than bedsores). If a lap-strap is not provided, the occupant may be tipped forwards and fall out of the chair, and is sometimes even killed. Unless wheelchair tires are kept fully inflated (or lightweight synthetic tire inserts are used instead of pneumatic inner-tubes), the chair will be difficult to propel or steer. The brakes, which work by a metal plate being pushed against the outer rim of the tire, will not work properly and the occupant may fall when getting in or out of the chair. Other wheelchair-related accidents include lacerations, penetrating injuries from exposed bolts, and trapped fingers. Improvements in design are leading to safer chairs, but routine inspection and maintenance are important. It is also helpful for carers to receive written instructions on wheelchair use to complement verbal advice and demonstrations.

## The future

The provision of aids and appliances to people with disabilities is an essential part of promoting independence and well-being. Aids should be considered to be as important as drugs and subject to the same degrees of scrutiny, evaluation, and monitoring of adverse effects. Doctors, nurses, and therapists as well as disabled patients and other care givers should consider aids as important in symptom control, mobility, self care, and an improved quality of life.          GMul

**ARAB MEDICINE** The contribution of Arabic medicine to the evolution of medical knowledge is immense. Arab conquests in the 7th century came at a time when the Greco-Roman civilization was plunging deep into decline and chaos. Europe was entering the Dark Ages and it needed a savior to preserve the classic civilizations of Greece and Rome, which were quickly disappearing. The Arabs, with their new religion, conquered most of the known world within a few decades. Their empire extended from the Ganges across Asia, North Africa, and south-western Europe. They spread their faith into China and as far west as the Pyrenees. During the eight centuries of their empire, medicine flourished, among other scientific and literary endeavors. The new rulers of the empire quickly took to the civilizations they conquered. Greco-Roman, Alexandrian, Byzantine, Persian, Indian, and other cultures were assimilated and cultivated. This was helped by the relative freedom under which Muslims as well as non-Muslim scholars could work. Islam accepted Christianity and Judaism as fellow religions worshipping the same god, and followers of these monolithic faiths could practice their religion in the Muslim state. Islam encouraged scientific and medical endeavors with clear messages in the *Holy Koran:* 'and if any one saved a life, it would be as if he saved the life of all people' (section 5, Surat Al-Maida, verse 32). Medicine was practiced by physicians, who were outside the immediate control of the mosque, in contrast to the view of the Christian Church which prevailed in Europe for several centuries, where medicine was in the hands of the priests, who looked at the human body as a sin, disease as a curse, and suffering a virtue. It is amazing that within a century the Arab nomad conquerors were transformed into benevolent rulers who nurtured and protected the arts and sciences. The libraries, institutions, and universities created in major cities were remarkable.

The initial advances in medicine were quickly established. These involved primarily the translation of Greco-Roman works into Arabic. HIPPOCRATES (p 382) and GALEN (p 324) were thus faithfully translated and preserved. The translations were, by and large, performed by NESTORIAN Christians and Jews. Nestorians were the followers of a Syrian monk, Nestour, who became patriarch of Constantinople in AD 428. He was excommunicated in AD 431 for heresy; his followers were persecuted and fled to Mesopotamia and Persia. They were educated in Greek culture and spoke Syriac, which is a close cousin of Arabic and Hebrew, all being derived from Aramaic. They were the link between the fast-disappearing Greek culture and the newly rising Arab Muslim civilization.

Sedillot (*Histoire des Arabes, Paris, 1854*) said:

> What especially characterized the Baghdad school at its beginning was the truly scientific spirit which presided over all. To go from the known to the unknown, then from effects to causes and only to admit as true what had been demonstrated by experimental work, such were the principles taught by the masters. During the ninth century the Arabs were in possession of this fruitful method which a long time afterward was to be in the hands of modern investigators, the instrument of their finest discoveries.

## EARLY ARABIAN PHYSICIANS

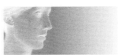

**RHAZES** (Abu Bakr Muhammad ibn Zakariyya) (*c.* 864–925/35). Persian physician. He distinguished smallpox from measles, giving excellent accounts of each. He described the guinea worm (*Dracunculus medinensis*), the recurrent laryngeal nerve, and spina ventosa. He is best known for his Greco-Arabic encyclopedia of medicine, *Kitab al-hawi*, translated into Latin as *Liber continens* in 1279. It was antireligious and critical of GALEN (p 324). The ninth book was the main source of therapeutic knowledge for three centuries.

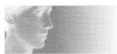

Rabbi Moses Ben Maimon **MAIMONIDES** (Abu Imram Musa ibn Maimum; 'Rambam') (?1135–1204). Hispano-Jewish physician and philosopher. Maimonides was born in Cordoba, where he was a pupil of AVERROES (p 768), moving later to Fez and in 1166 to Egypt. He is buried at Tiberias, where his tomb is still a place of pilgrimage. He codified Talmudic law and wrote on philosophy and theology. His medical writings showed independent and original thought. He was critical of GALEN (p 324) and published a valuable commentary on the aphorisms of HIPPOCRATES (p 382).

*(continued overleaf)*

## Ibn AL-NAFIS (1210–88).

Arabian physician. Living in Damascus, he studied medicine and law and practiced all his life. Regarded by many as second only to Avicenna, (this page) he wrote much, but only his *Compendium medicinae* remains. He concluded that the interventricular septum was solid and that blood passed by the pulmonary artery to the lungs and thence by the pulmonary vein to the left ventricle; he thus precedes Servetus and Colombo in describing the pulmonary circulation.

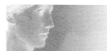

## AVICENNA (Abu Ali al-Hussein Ibn Abdullah Ibn Sina) (980–1037).

Persian physician and philosopher. His tomb is still a place of pilgrimage. Avicenna has been identified, probably erroneously, with the poet Omar Khayyam with whom he shared a taste for wine and minstrelsy. He wrote many philosophical books but his great legacy to medicine was his *Canon of medicine*, a vast encyclopedia in which he attempted to correlate the views of HIPPOCRATES (p 382), GALEN (p 324), and Aristotle (p 64). It was first translated into Latin in the 12th century and was a much consulted textbook of medicine until the 17th century. Avicenna was the first to describe the guinea worm (*Dracunculus medinensis*), and anthrax ('Persian fire'). He is also said to have noted the sweet taste of diabetic urine.

Hunayn Ibn Is 'haq (Johanitius AD 809–873) is considered by many to be the initiator of the renaissance in the East. He was a Christian born in Al-Hira (south-western Iraq). The quality and the breadth of his work make him the principal figure among many scholars who were the custodians of the Greco-Roman culture and its translation into Arabic. His books on medicine alone numbered 84; they included many translations of Galen, Hippocrates, and Plato.

### The sayings of the Prophet

The practice of medicine during the early part of Islam was influenced by the sayings (Hadith) of the Prophet Mohammed (AD 570–632). These have the power of law to Muslims:

> Science is the remedy for the infirmities of ignorance, a comforting beacon in the height of injustice. The study of the sciences has the value of a fast; the teaching of them has the value of prayer; in a noble heart they inspire the highest feelings and they correct and humanize the perverted.

His sayings on medicine were collected in *Al-Tib al-Nabawi* (*Medicine of the prophet*). The practice of medicine evolved quickly. It began early in the 8th century by the establishment of the first hospital in Damascus by the Caliph AI-Walid I in AD 707. The golden age of the Arab civilization was undoubtedly during the reign of Haroon Al-Rashid in Baghdad, AD 787–810. Baghdad was the center of culture and science. During that time the Persian element was added by the Barmakids, who were the wazirs (ministers) of the caliphs. The famous Persian School of Medicine in Jundisapur was gradually transferred to Baghdad.

Medical education and practice were initiated in hospitals, which were built, endowed, and administered by the state. There was regular inspection and certification. Adhudi, Al-Rashid, Al-Muqtadiri in Baghdad, Al-Mansuri, Al-Nasiri, Al-Qashashin in Cairo, Al-Nuri in Damascus were but a few. In the city of Baghdad, on the orders of the caliph, a census of all practicing physicians was made in AD 949. This followed a reported medical mistake leading to a patient's death. There were 860 physicians, excluding those directly working for the government service. They were recertified and licensed. Physicians were licensed to practice their specialty only after an examination. The Arabs were the first to recognize surgery and its practice as part of medicine, which was not the case in Europe with its barber-surgeons even many centuries later.

The practice in hospitals was the backbone of medical learning. Each of the famous doctors was chief physician at a hospital. Al-Razi (RHAZES) (p 59), Ibn Sina (AVICENNA) (this page), and IBN AL NAFIS (this page) were notable in the East; Al-Zahrawi (Abulcassis), and Ibn Zuhr (AVENZOAR)

(p 768) in the West. Several books on hospital organization and management were written, but unfortunately few survived. Al-Razi's book on *Sifat Al-Bimaristan* (*Characteristics of the hospital*) is an excellent example. The word *Bimaristan*, or *Maristan* in Persian, means home for the sick. Al-Razi was chosen to head the old hospital in Baghdad after a careful selection among 100 applicants. The best description of hospitals across the empire is found in the writings of the most famous Arab traveler, Ibn Jubayer, who was born in Valencia and died in Alexandria (AD 1145–1217).

It is difficult to choose the most representative works to cover the many centuries of the Arab Renaissance. Most of the books and manuscripts have been lost. This was mainly due to the massive destruction by the Moguls in the East, when Holagu (AD 1258) plundered and burned Baghdad, and later to the fanatical destruction of the Moorish culture by the later conquerors in south-west

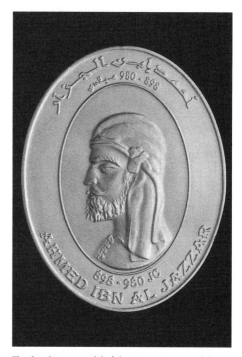

The Ibn al Jazzar medal of the Tunisian Society of the History of Medicine. This medal portrays on the obverse the profile effigy of Dr Ahmed Ibn al Jazzar (898–980 AD) of the Medical School at Kairouan, in Ifriqiya, in present-day Tunisia. Founded c. 820 AD, it was one of the first medical schools in the world. Ibn al Jazzar, a medical polymath, was one of the founders of the disciplines of psychiatry, pediatrics, and travel medicine. The medal was designed by Professor Sleim Ammar, Vice-President of the International Society of the History of Medicine, and was first issued on the occasion of the Society's 36th International Congress, held in Carthage in 1998.

Europe. Andalusia was reported to have had 70 libraries. One of those, the library of Caliph Al-Hakem II in Cordova, had 500 000 books and manuscripts, most of which have disappeared.

Many physicians, translators, and scientists were not ethnic Arabs, or in many cases Muslims, but Nestorians, Christians, Jews, Persians, and other races. The freedom to pursue their endeavors was possible only through the relative tolerance of Islam. With this in mind it is difficult to choose those individuals who contributed most to the progress of medicine during the Arab civilization. This choice is helped by the excellent biographical texts, exemplified by the work of Ibn Usaibiah, *Oyun Al-Anba'a fi Tabaqat Al-Atibba'a* (*Fontes relationum de classibus medicorum; Original news on the classes of doctors*), in which he gave biographies of over 400 physicians. Among other biographers who included many physicians in their works is Ibn Khallikan in his book *Wafiyat Al-Ayan* (*Deaths of notables*), which listed the biographies of 870 distinguished people.

## Four major texts
Perhaps four major texts dominated the period and were the principal medium of transmitting Greco-Roman, Byzantine, Persian, and Indian medical knowledge into Latin. They added an Arabic dimension on clinical observation as well as original surgical, medical, anatomical, therapeutic, and prognostic contributions.

The first was *Al-Hawi* (*Liber continens*) by Abu Baker Mohammed Ibn Zakariya Al-Razi (Rhazes, who was born, as his name implies, in Al-Razy in Persia). He quoted at length from Greek, Persian, and Indian sources. In addition to his encyclopedic work, he produced more specialized succinct monographs such as his masterpiece *Al-Judari wa-Al-Hasbba* (*Smallpox and measles*). This is probably the most concise treatise of Arabic medicine and its last Latin edition was printed in 1866. His clinical abilities were best exemplified in his book *Burr al-Sa'ah* (*Cures in an hour*), in which he described all conditions which a physician can cure in an hour. His other major text, *Al 'Mansuri* (*Liber al-Mansorum*), although smaller than *Liber Continens*, probably had more influence on European medicine, especially the School of SALERNO (p 448). Al-Razi held the view that fever was not a disease but showed that the body was working to bring about a solution to the disease (*Liber continens*, Book XXIII, 347). He was the first to describe the recurrent laryngeal nerve and thought it originated near the trachea.

The second major text was *Kamil al-Sinaah al-Tibbiya*, also known as *Al-Kitab Al-Maliki* (*The complete medical profession;* or *Liber regius*). It was written by Ali Ibn Abbass Al-Majusi, who was a Persian Magian (Zoroastrian). His detailed descriptions of urinary catheterization, tuberculous lymph node excision, and breast cancer removal are a joy to read. The best translation into Latin was by Stephen of Antioch. Other translators were not so scrupulous and some claimed the work for themselves.

### The canon of medicine
The third, and probably best-known, text is *Al-Qanoon fi al-Tibb* (*The canon of medicine*) by Abu Ali Al-Hussain Ibn Abdulla Ibn Sina (Avicenna). Born in Balkh near Bokharra, he practiced all over Persia, and wrote in Arabic not only on medicine but on philosophy, logic, astronomy, music, and mathematics. Perhaps the most noted western Renaissance equivalent figure was LEONARDO da Vinci (p 40). His intellect and early scientific achievements are legendary. Avicenna's eccentricities made him move to many countries and cities. It has to be mentioned that his works were kept and conserved only through the dedicated work of his companion and biographer Abu Ubayid Al-Juzjani, who first met him in AD 1002. *The canon of medicine* was the principal medical text in the Arab world and Europe for around eight centuries. OSLER (p 602) stated that 'The Canon was the Medical Bible for a longer period than any other book'.

The fourth major work was *Al-Taysir fi al-Mudawat wa-al-Tadbir* (*Facilitation, treatment and organization; Facilitatio*) written by Abu Marwan Ibn Malik Abu alAla Ibn Zuhr (Avezoar), who was born in Seville and was a member of a distinguished family of physicians.

Surgery owes much to Abul-Qasim Khalef Ibn Abbass Al-Zahrawi (Abulcassis), who was born in a suburb of Cordova and died in AD 1013. His writings and books are voluminous and highly technical. *Al-Tasrif Lemen Ajeza un Al-Taleaf* (*Practical guide for those who cannot be authors*) was translated into Latin by Gerard of Cremona and influenced medical teaching in medical schools such as those of Salerno and Montpellier. One of his important dictums stated: 'If anatomical knowledge is ignored mistakes will be made and the patient will be killed'. His detailed descriptions of surgical procedures and their contraindications are precise and clear. Although his anatomy and basic surgery were based on Galen and Paul of Aegia, he went much further in describing exact operative detail and illustrations of surgical instruments. He wrote on surgical treatment of liver abscess, goiter, Pott's disease, hydrocephalus, and tracheostomy, as well as on obstetrics and on performing craniotomy when the fetal head was too large.

Other names that should be mentioned include Ibn Nafis, the celebrated physician of the 13th century, who was the dean of the Mansoori Hospital in Cairo and was the first to describe the pulmonary circulation and clearly showed that blood is aerated in the lungs. He disagreed with Avicenna on the blood supply of the heart muscle and suggested the existence of the coronary circulation. Rabbi Musa ibn Maymoon (MAIMONIDES) (p 59) was a Jewish physician born in Cordova who became a physician to Salah al-Din Al-Ayoobi (Saladin) in Egypt. His claim to fame, in addition to his distinguished medical works such as *Fusool Musa* (*Moses' aphorisms*), was his philosophical book on religion, *Dalalat al-Haireen* (*Guide to the perplexed*).

### Pharmacy

PHARMACY as we know it today was started as a separate discipline by the Arabs. The use of chemicals, including sugars and alcohol, to make potions was introduced. The discipline was separated from medicine for the first time and placed under state control and licensing. Ibn-Albitaar (born in Malaga and died in Damascus), a worthy successor of Dioscorides, was the Inspector of Pharmacists in Cairo; he traveled far and wide in search of new plants and remedies. His book, *Al-Jamie le Mufradat Al-Adwia wa Al-Agthia* (*The corpus of simples*), included over 1400 different drugs. This work was translated into French by Leclerc (Paris 1877). Many drugs and medicines were later imported into Europe. This commerce was very large and formed one of the chief sources of income for the Italian maritime republics during the Renaissance.

The Arabic era eventually came to an end and its cultural heritage was transferred to Europe. This happened over centuries, in both the East and the West, but mostly in south-western Europe. Gerbert of Aurillac, who later became Pope Sylvester II (AD 999), traveled to Toledo and brought back Arabic knowledge to medieval Europe. The Crusaders did not really contribute to translation, most of which was carried out in Spain. The School of Translators in Toledo under Archbishop Raymond and Gerard of Cremona was the main venue for transmitting Arabic and Greek writings to Latin. Leclerc (1876) said, 'The Arabs thus repaid unto the Christians of the Western world the services formerly rendered to them by the Christians in the East'.

There were major differences between the eastern Arabic Renaissance, which began in the 8th century, and the western Latin Renaissance six centuries later. In the eastern Renaissance Greek texts were highly valued and sought after and Caliphs searched high and low for Greek masterpieces. In the western Renaissance Arab texts were treated with suspicion and were much less regarded. In the East the schools of translators were organized and well financed, mainly in Baghdad, while in the West they were more individual in different monasteries and universities. Moreover, Arabic was a live and vibrant language which lent itself to development while Latin, into which the works of western Renaissance were translated, was a dead language used only in the Church and in science.

After the demise of the Arab empire in the East, followed by the decline of the Moorish rule in Andalusia, Arab medicine as well as science and literature virtually went into hibernation. During the following eight centuries of Ottoman rule, there was little scientific advancement within the Arab world; on the contrary, the previous achievements declined and practically disappeared.

It was only late in the 19th century that western medicine started to filter back to the Middle East and North Africa. Currently there are two basic schools of medicine in the Arab world. By and large, following colonial influence in the late 19th century, there is an English-speaking school in the East (Egypt, Iraq, Saudi Arabia) and a French-speaking influence in the West (Morocco, Tunisia, Algeria). Medical education is taught in English or in French with one or two exceptions, where it is taught in Arabic.

RAS

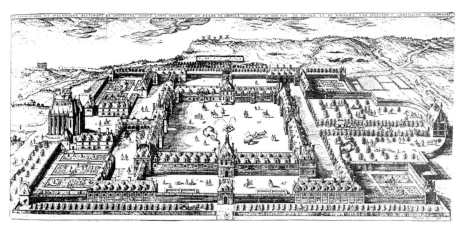

Architecture for controlling infectious diseases. The Plague Hospital at St Louis. (Reproduced courtesy of the Wellcome Institute Library, London.)

**ARCHITECTURE** The healthy built environment promotes neither disease nor injury and may even actively further psychological health. Medicine and architecture, however, have interacted in ways more interesting than this pallid definition might suggest. Such encounters are by no means confined to the hospital, but historically best displayed within that arena.

Hospitals have been the subject of more modern studies than any other kind of building. Such studies emphasize their variety, the number of environments, with different patterns of use and different technical requirements, that must be accommodated. For example, the lighting required in an ophthalmic examination area is different from ward lighting, which must serve both recumbent patients and their upright carers. By the time a new hospital is built, medical techniques, budgets, policies, and patterns of admissions have all changed. This makes hospitals distinctively complex structures with difficult design specifications resulting in the supersession of a prevailing 'machine' model by a more amorphous concept of 'indeterminate' architecture, the ethos of design for change. But does difficulty necessarily follow complexity? Maybe the best that architects can achieve is a robust building shell that can adapt to meet changing needs.

Western medicine's traditional concern with the control of infectious diseases is one precisely, but sometimes inversely, related to enthusiasm for hospitals. In what was for its date an extraordinarily systematic prescription for civic poor relief, *De subventione pauperum* (1526) by Juan Luis Vivès, it was recommended that if a town's existing hospitals (which he assumed would take orphans, travelers, and the handicapped, as well as the sick, as was medieval practice) could not accommodate all the sick poor, then special houses should be set up for them. 'The result will be, as in nature and in shipbuilding, that the foulness will all be restricted to one place, and the rest of the body not infected'. But emanations (variously defined but self-evidently pathogenic) from bowels and bilges can infect the larger body: in 1741, the Governors of the Devon and Exeter Hospital felt obliged to assure the citizens of Exeter that their new hospital was neither a danger to them nor a dangerous place in itself.

During the 18th century, England and Scotland saw the construction of (by one count) 37 purpose-built general hospitals, of which the Devon and Exeter (designed by a local surveyor, John Richards) was one of the first and biggest (160 beds by 1787). By contemporary standards it was also one of the best, simply because its six main wards, superimposed in two wings extended on a line with its center block, had large casement windows on both long sides, admitting light and air. Few

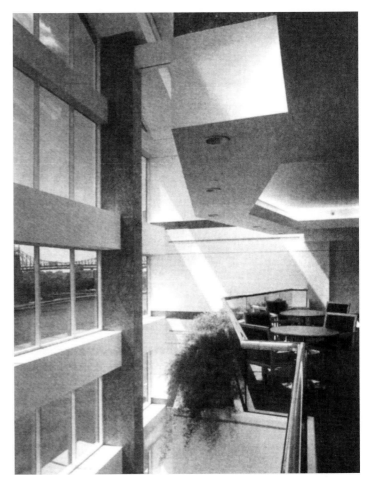

sites permitted such expansiveness, and most hospitals followed U- or H-plans that could throw ward-wings out as similarly permeable units. Long wings make the hospital's 'Structure more complicated, and prevent the Access of free Air', wrote John Foster in 1768, an Edinburgh-trained physician then unique for offering a model hospital plan. Foster envisaged modest rural hospitals for his native Ireland; it was generally assumed that larger establishments would have to be constructed in phases, as money came in and need dictated, and to this procedure the U- and H-plans were very suitable. A modern, computer-assisted study of health centers generated an H-plan in response to the criterion that 'as many rooms as possible should have an exterior wall, permitting daylight and natural ventilation'. The result was judged notably amenable to expansion as required, if extravagant of space. Medical considerations in 18th-century hospital design were of the most common-sensical sort; the best were indeed robust, flexible, and airy shells. Bad ones smelled.

To create a more comforting environment at this world-renowned orthopedics/rheumatology special teaching hospital, the new addition features a dramatic five story atrium that provides daylight and panoramic views of the East River from the patient unit lounges. (Hospital for Special Surgery, Major Modernization Project, New York 1996. Architecture for Health Science and Commerce, PC, architects.)

About an unnamed new London hospital, Florence NIGHTINGALE (p 548) wrote that 'all is complicated, and there is a want of that simplicity of plan which is essential to the free circulation of air'. Complication, as she and Foster suggested, was suspect, and for exactly the same reasons. The word can be interpreted more broadly in the context of an anti-architectural medical rhetoric beginning to develop in the second half of the 18th century. Dr John Aitkin (unfairly) attributed to the architect, who 'considers it his business to manage his room and materials in such a manner, as to accommodate the greatest number of people in the least possible space', all the faults of hospital buildings.

The many plans for rebuilding the Hôtel-Dieu in Paris after a fire in 1772 were not infrequently accompanied by gibes at architects' supposed tendency to what the scientist Jean-Baptiste Le Roy (1720–1800) called the sacrifice of 'principle to props [*l'accessoire*]'; they 'seem to have forgotten that decoration is the least part of such a building'. Today, the generally perceived need for hospitals is to be able to accommodate the unforeseeable results, in publications, in an emphasis on 'principle' that assumes a certain 18th-century flavor. 'Principle' was then associated with 'plan' and especially with ward plans, a focus still apparent in, but less applicable to, studies of modern hospitals, whose wards occupy less and less of their total area. It was a focus given inestimable force by Nightingale's own promotion of the pavilion ward, a promotion with clear 18th-century antecedents, as was her tartness about architects seeking 'external design or appearance' at the expense of the 'good ward'.

Architects are still chided for their supposed neglect of 'principle' at the expense of appearance. They make little use of the numerous publications available to them about hospital design; they spend little time in their own, completed hospitals, or with those hospitals' users; their peers sometimes still judge their work on the basis of glossy photographs or drawings of buildings, often before the building is actually in use. In short, the hostility traditionally directed against architects' supposed enthusiasm for ornamental superfluity endures: but now it comes from psychology and sociology, not medicine.       CSte

**ARISTOTLE** Greek polymath. Son of the court physician to the King of Macedonia, Amyntas II, Aristotle was born in Stagira in Chalcidice and probably learnt his medical knowledge from his father at an early age. After the latter's death, he was sent to Athens in 367BC to study at Plato's Academy and on Plato's death in 347BC he left Athens for Assus, where he set up a school in which he taught for the next three years. He then went on to Lesbos, where he studied natural history and marine

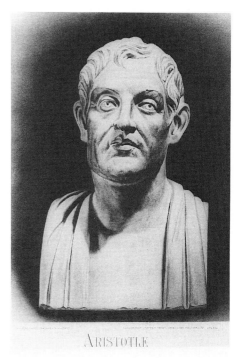

Bust of Aristotle (384–322 BCE). (Reproduced courtesy of the National Library of Medicine, Bethesda, MD.)

biology. In 342BC he was invited by Philip II of Macedonia to become tutor to the prince — later Alexander the Great. On Alexander's accession to the throne in 336BC, Aristotle returned to Athens and established his school, the Lyceum, with its zoo and library. On the death of Alexander in 323BC, Aristotle was accused of impiety by the anti-Macedonian party and he escaped to Chalcis, where he died the following year.

Aristotle has had a profound effect and lasting influence on scientific thought. He was the first to study the observable facts of nature, analyzing and recording them precisely and in scrupulous detail. Once data were assembled and classified, he tried to find an explanation that would fit them all, and, in deriving the universal from the particular, to construct an intelligible universe. His invention of the science of logic established scientific method. He divided reality into spheres of physics, biology, ethics, politics, and psychology, subjecting each to searching analysis. Aristotle is justifiably regarded as the founder of biology, zoology, comparative anatomy, embryology, and psychology.

Aristotle's writings, which survive only in later edited versions, covered most aspects of contemporary thought. They fall into three broad categories: literary essays intended for publication such as the dialogs; set works in literary form written in his later years, such as the *Constitution of Athens*; and treatises written in connection with his courses of lectures such as logic (*Organon*), natural science (*Physica*), the classification of animals (*Historia animalium*), the progression of animals (*De incessu animalium*), and cosmology (*De caelo*).

The breadth of his interests and his influence on posterity have been enormous. In the *Organon* he creates the new science of logic, the art of correct thinking, of defining one's terms, of using a set of propositions to reach a conclusion (the syllogism). Decidedly aristocratic in his views, he sees man as a political animal and describes three basic good forms of governance: by the one (monarchy), the few (aristocracy), or the many (timocracy or polity), and their deviation-forms or perversions: tyranny, oligarchy, and (the least bad of the deviations) democracy. In discussing the principles of comedy and tragedy he lays down the rules of unity of time, pace, and action that dominated western drama until the 17th century. He argues in the *Nichomachean ethics* that all men aim at the good but differ in what they think that good is. True happiness comes from pursuing the contemplative life; moneymaking is undertaken under compulsion; and wealth cannot be the true good but is merely useful for the sake of something else. The virtuous man behaves according to a 'golden mean' between two possible extremes. The educated man should look for precision only so far as the nature of the subject admits. Aristotle distinguishes between scientific knowledge, art, practical wisdom, and true wisdom, 'the most finished of the forms of knowledge'. He discusses the meaning of justice, of pleasure, of friendship, whether it is better to have a few or many friends. Many of his scientific observations were confirmed in later centuries, but by relying on deduction rather than on observation, he also concluded that the function of the brain is to cool the blood, that man has only eight ribs on each side and that women have fewer teeth than men. Yet, as the philosopher Bertrand Russell remarked, all he had to do was to ask Mrs Aristotle to open her mouth and count them.

**ART** From earliest times human disease and its treatment have attracted the attention of artists. This may have been because of the supposed mystical significance of certain diseases, but in most cases because the subject itself was intrinsically fascinating. Attitudes to malformations and diseases, however, have not always been the same. For example, dwarfs in Pharaonic Egypt were characterized by normal faces and very short limbs, in Ancient Greece by snub-noses and prominent foreheads, and in Rome they were often depicted with an over-large phallus. More recently, as in many of Velázquez's paintings, dwarfs are shown much

more sympathetically, as well as more realistically. Furthermore, the artist's intention has sometimes been to use allegorical allusions for a very specific purpose in portraying medical matters. This is particularly true in Dutch genre paintings of the 17th century. In more modern times, as art has become less representational, so paintings have increasingly come to reflect the artist's *subjective impression* of disease and its treatment. Nevertheless, artists at the present day do still occasionally portray malformations and defects in art. For example, achondroplasia in the work of Sarah Lucas (b. 1962) and Gillian Wearing (b. 1963), and thalidomide deformity by James Rielly (b. 1956), were all exhibited at the Royal Academy of Arts' *Sensation* exhibition in London in 1997.

### Disorders in the artist

Artists have, not infrequently, suffered from medical conditions themselves, which in some instances have significantly affected their work. This is most obvious in the case of eye disease.

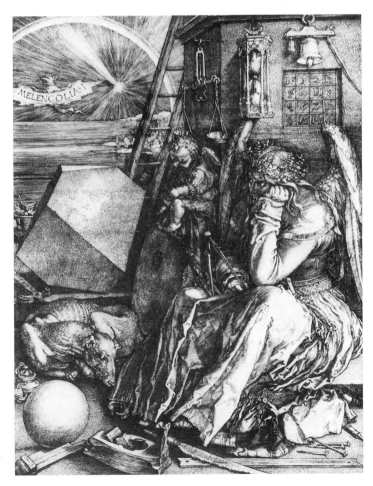

*Melancolia* (1514), Albrecht Dürer. (Photo: Bartsch, A. (1808) *Le Peintre-graveur*, vol VII, Vienna.)

### Henry TONKS

(1862–1937). British surgeon and artist. At the London Hospital he was house surgeon to Sir Henry TREVES (p 261), and later was appointed to the Royal Free Hospital. Increasingly, his painting skills occupied him and in 1894 he was invited by his teacher Frederick Brown, to become his assistant at the Slade School of Art, together with Philip Wilson Steer. Among his early pupils were Augustus John and (Sir) William Orpen. Succeeding Brown as director of the Slade in 1917, retiring in 1930, Tonks became the most influential teacher of his age in Britain. His pictures hang in the Tate, Ashmolean, and other galleries. He produced depictions of war wounds as a war artist in the First World War, when his knowledge of anatomy, surgery, and painting became combined in a unique series of horrific but moving paintings.

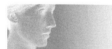

Nicolass TULP (1593–1674). Dutch physician and anatomist. Born Pieterz, he assumed the name of Tulp (= tulip) from sculptures on his house. He practiced in Amsterdam, where he also held civic office and acquired immortality in Rembrandt's painting. *The anatomy lesson of Dr Tulp* (1632). He gave an early account of beriberi (1652) and instituted the first Dutch pharmacopeia.

El Greco's (1541–1614) purported astigmatism is now very much in doubt, but red-green color blindness certainly afflicted Fernand Léger (1881–1955) and Piet Mondrian (1872–1944). It could well be that their particular styles were directly influenced by this. A number of prominent artists have been myopic, for example, Paul Cézanne (1839–1906), Edgar Degas (1834–1917), Georges Braque (1882–1963), and Henri Matisse (1869–1954). It has been suggested that relatively poor central vision may have been a factor in the development of the Impressionist movement. Several artists have suffered from cataracts in later life. A much-quoted example is that of Turner (1775–1851), accounting for the expected predominance of red-brown tints in his later works. But the best authenticated case is that of Claude Monet (1840–1926). After a cataract operation in 1923 his work took on a more bluish tinge. Failing sight leading ultimately to blindness is well documented in Malcolm Drummond (1880–1945) and the Russian painter Mikhail Vrubel (1856–1910), and in the case of Percy Wyndham Lewis (1882–1957) this was due to a pituitary tumor, for which he refused surgery and from which he eventually died. Figure and color distortion in the later stages of increasing blindness would be expected. Pierre Auguste Renoir's (1841–1919) sight also began to fail in later life, but he was by then severely crippled with arthritis, which could have influenced his style of painting.

Paul Klee (1879–1940) was very severely disabled in later years by progressive scleroderma (systemic sclerosis). His anguish is expressed vividly in the painting (self-portrait?) in the year of his death, entitled *Death and fire*, which shows a pale face leering at the observer — the mouth represented by the letter 'T', one eye as 'o' and the other as 'd', thus signifying death.

The influence of mental illness on creativity has been much researched. It is tempting to imagine that madness could, in certain circumstances, lead to heightened artistic creativity. Certainly Richard Dadd's (1819–87) early paintings were attractive but conventional, and it was only after the onset of insanity (which led to his murdering his father and his resultant incarceration in 1844 in BETHLEM and later Broadmoor Hospitals for the rest of his life) that his paintings took on an idiosyncratic strangeness, which has attracted considerable attention ever since. But whether or not his later paintings were actually an improvement and more artistic is debatable. Anthony Storr has argued cogently that in severe bipolar psychosis and schizophrenia, CREATIVITY, rather than being enhanced in some way, is in fact often significantly impaired. Other artists with well-documented mental illness include Carl Frederik Hill (1849–1911), Ernst Josephson (1851–1906), and Edvard Münch (1863–1944). Following a complete break-down the last underwent treatment, including electroconvulsive therapy, and thereafter his work became less anguished and more lyrical and bright. Albrecht Dürer's (1471–1528) engraving *Melencolia* is a graphic representation of profound depression.

### Self-portraits

Self-portraits can sometimes reveal medical disorders in the artist himself. For example, Albrecht Dürer (1471–1528) had a divergent squint, clearly evident in his self-portraits of 1491 and 1498, as well as in several of his other portraits, including his *Mother* (1514), *Caspar Sturm* (1520), and *Laughing peasant woman* (1505).

Henri de Toulouse-Lautrec (1864–1901) frequently portrayed his own deformities in various caricatures as well as in the painting *Au Moulin Rouge* (1892). His deformities have been convincingly attributed to autosomal recessive pyknodysostosis, on the basis of his short stature, bony fractures, and possibly a large fontanelle, prompting him to wear a hat much of the time, and his parents were first cousins.

The Dutch painter Dick Ket (1902–40) probably suffered from Fallot's tetralogy with dextrocardia, and his many self-portraits clearly show finger clubbing, cyanosis, plethora, and possibly some precordial fullness.

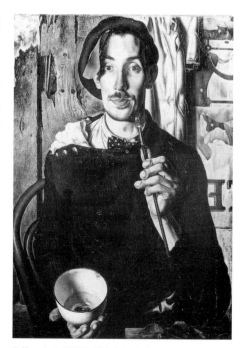

*Self-portrait* (1939), Dick Ket (Reproduced by kind permission of Dr J. R. de Groot, Keeper, Department of Paintings, Gemeentemuseum, Arnhem.)

However, not all artists have been so openly honest. The French painter Jacques-Louis David (1748–1825) had a disfiguring deformity of the left side of his face, which he was very careful to hide in self-portraits, and his pupil, Pierre Langlois, also took care to mask this side of David's face in his portrait of his teacher.

## Portraits of the famous

Detailed and careful portraits of the famous have often revealed evidence of medical disorders, which may not have been fully appreciated or even recognized at the time. For example, the plethoric appearance of King George III in the portrait by Johann Zoffany (1733–1810) may reflect the possibility of the King having ROYAL MADNESS AND PORPHYRIA. More convincing is the portrayal of Prince Alexandre Ypsilante on a Greek stamp commemorating the liberation of Greece. This clearly illustrates his frontal baldness and a somewhat lugubrious expression, associated with his having myotonic dystrophy (see NEUROMUSCULAR DISEASES). But, as in self-portraits, sometimes an artist has consciously hidden a disfigurement, in this case in order to avoid offending a benefactor. The classic example is the portrait (c. 1465) of Federigo da Montefeltro, the Duke of Urbino, by Piero della Francesca (c. 1416–92). Here the artist has portrayed his subject in left profile in order to hide the serious and disfiguring injuries to the right side of his face, including the loss of his right eye, sustained in a jousting match. The Emperor Charles V inherited the so-called 'Hapsburg jaw' with 'gross mandibular prognathism and malocclusion, flat malar areas, and a sloping forehead', but these abnormalities are not at all obvious in the famous portrait by Titian (c. 1487–1576). Thus in portraits, whether of the artist himself or of another, disfigurements, deformities, or disease may, in some cases, have been deliberately obscured.

## Disorders in art

When the manifestations of a disease are clearcut and unmistakable, as in the case of SMALLPOX or crippling arthritis, they can often be identified in paintings from the past. This is also true of certain well-defined congenital malformations and genetic disorders. The most noted examples are those of various dwarfs in the court of King Philip IV of Spain, depicted by Velàzquez (1599–1660). They include achondroplasia in a woman in *Las Meninas* (1656) and in a boy in *El Niño de Vallecas* (1637), and possibly pseudoachondroplasia in *Sebastian de Morra* (c. 1644) and *El Primo* (1644). Van Dyck (1599–1641) depicted an excellent example of a pituitary dwarf in his painting of *Queen Henrietta and her dwarf Sir Jeffrey Hudson* (c. 1633). Other conditions which can be identified in works of art include, for example, digital anomalies, skin diseases, Down's syndrome and various malformations.

However, what may seem obvious on superficial examination may, in fact, prove to be quite different on more careful study. For example, the simplest interpretation of Jusepe de Ribera's (1591–1652) *The clubfooted boy* is that this merely represents talipes equinovarus. But the boy shown also appears to have a right hemiplegia, a suspicion of left facial weakness, and the note he holds in his hand explains that he cannot speak. Thus, he may well have had some form of cerebral palsy.

It is equally possible to dismiss a depicted peculiarity as merely a figment of the artist's imagination, when in fact it represents a true likeness of an unusual condition. An excellent example is L. S. Lowry's (1887–1976) *Woman with a beard*, which the artist actually drew from life. It seems that Lowry was often fascinated by such tragic characters seen in northern industrial towns.

## Diagnosis and treatment

As cultural, economic, and intellectual life in Europe began to flourish in the late Middle Ages, examples are increasingly found of paintings depicting various diagnostic procedures. Pulse-taking and uroscopy were common themes, especially in the 17th and 18th centuries. In more recent times, however, other techniques have been portrayed. For example, there is Théobald Chartran's (1849–1907) painting of René LAËNNEC (p 461) (1781–1826), a French physician credited with having developed the first stethoscope by rolling sheets of paper into a cylinder and later by using a wooden tube. In this painting, Laënnec is seen listening to a patient's heart using the traditional method of putting his ear to the chest. But in his left hand, ready for use, he is holding his cylindrical stethoscope.

Various forms of medical (and surgical) treatment can be seen in illustrations as early as the Middle Kingdom (after 2040 BC) of Ancient Egypt. However, in western art such depictions became most clear by the Middle Ages, for example, Pietro Lorenzetti's (c. 1305–45) *St Humility healing a sick nun*. Miracle treatments have also frequently featured in paintings, for example, in Hogarth's *The Pool of Bethesda* (c. 1735) and *The good Samaritan* (1737), on the staircase of St Bartholomew's Hospital, London. These depict treatment as actually practiced at the time, a tradition that can be traced back not only to the art of Pharaonic Egypt but also to Ancient Greece, and early Arabic texts. The last are often in the form of text ornamentation, but these, and illuminated manuscripts and engravings, have been excluded from the present discussion, where the emphasis is on painting.

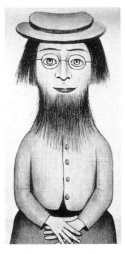

*Woman with a beard* (1957), L. S. Lowry. (Reproduced by kind permission of Mr Martin Bloom.)

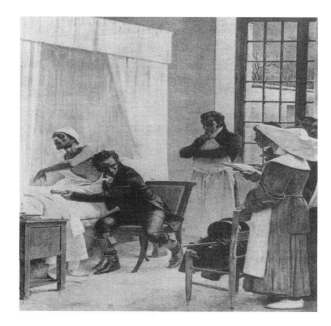

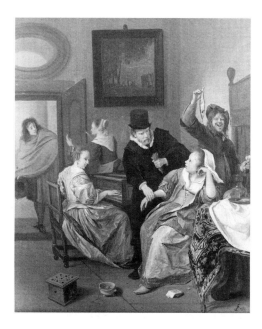

**Above left:**
*The medical examination,*
Godfried Schalken.

**Above right:**
*The doctor's visit* (1663-65),
Jan Steen. (Reproduced by kind
permission of the Philadelphia
Museum of Art: The John G.
Johnson Collection.)

Bloodletting and cupping formed an important part of the physician's armament from Pharaonic times. In Quirijn van Brekelenkam's (*c.* 1620–68) painting *The bloodletting*, an older woman applies a leech to the forearm of a young woman in a quiet domestic interior. This sensitive and sympathetic rendering is in stark contrast to many of the satirical carnival-like scenes of treatments by medical quacks painted by van Brekelenkam's Dutch contemporaries. The latter were often at pains to ridicule the medical profession, whom they viewed as quacks and charlatans, or to make a particular moral point. Thus Dutch genre painters often took the theme of delousing, for example, as having meanings on two levels: outward cleanliness on the one hand and spiritual order and virtue on the other. Furthermore, Dutch genre paintings frequently remind the viewer of patients' gullibility. This is illustrated, for example, in paintings of quacks purporting to treat mental illness.

Some modern artists also appear to view current treatment for mental illness with skepticism, as, for example, in Edvard Münch's *Electric shock treatment.*

### Physician and patient

This was again an important subject of Dutch genre paintings. A particular exponent was Jan Steen (*c.* 1626–79), who painted almost 40 different versions on the theme of 'The doctor's visit', and whose work was much appreciated at the time. His approach was often humorous, but almost always barbed with a warning or moral admonition. The doctor is usually attired in a way that at the time would

clearly have been recognized as antiquated and theatrical. He is often seen assuming a pompous pose. The patient is usually a lovesick maiden, at a time when repressed or unrequited love was believed to cause melancholy. Other elements within the painting often emphasize the theme of lovesickness: a background painting or statue of Cupid or of Venus and Adonis. A ribbon burning in a dish is often included, as nausea induced in the patient in this way was believed to be a test for pregnancy. The doctor is often taking the patient's pulse or inspecting her urine, as these were also believed to be important measures for diagnosing the patient's

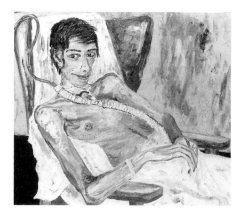

*Boy after a liver transplant* (1989), Sir Roy Calne.
(Reproduced by kind permission of the artist.)

condition. For example, a sudden increase in pulse rate on an unexpected visit from a lover would be considered diagnostic. In one painting, an additional character holds a herring along with two onions (*The doctor's visit*), which clearly also has sexual connotations. In regard to uroscopy and pregnancy, in Godfried Schalcken's (1643–1706) *The medical examination* the painter makes the meaning quite explicit by including a tiny embryo in the flask of urine being examined by the physician. The implication of a fetus in a bottle in the painting *Le foetus* by Gustav-Adolf Mossa (1883–1971) of a gentleman and his courtesan is also quite clear.

In some genre paintings there are clear warnings against licentiousness and unbridled passion. In Steen's *The lovesick girl* (*c.* 1665), in the Metropolitan Museum of Art in New York, the artist included a pair of copulating dogs to emphasize his point, and this offending motif was once painted out by a censorious restorer.

In Victorian times, paintings of physicians attending their patients became very popular and were often dramatic, even bordering on the sentimental, as in *The doctor* by Sir Luke Fildes (1844–1927). Many paintings show the physician in a sympathetic light, bringing comfort and reassurance to his patient.

The artist's interest in portraying medical matters continues to the present day. An excellent example is Sir Roy Calne, professor emeritus of surgery at the University of Cambridge, who helped pioneer liver transplantation and who is himself also a noted artist. One of his early patients was the Scottish painter John Bellany, who subsequently influenced Calne's technique. The latter's painting of a boy with Wilson's disease who had undergone liver transplantation, clearly demonstrates the compassion and understanding the artist felt for his subject (*Boy after a liver transplant*).

Many other aspects of medicine and art could be considered, including the association of art with anatomy, dentistry, surgery, and military medicine. Furthermore, the therapeutic value of art of patients themselves is an important topic in its own right, as is the role of medical illustration and medical photography in current medical practice.

Until comparatively recently, paintings have been essentially representational. But in more recent times, they have increasingly come to reflect the artist's *subjective impression* of disease and its treatment. This is particularly well seen in the work of Frida Kahlo (1907–54), the highly original Mexican painter who was severely injured in her youth and whose subsequent pain, anguish, and frustration are clearly expressed in her paintings, especially her self-portraits.                                          AEHE, MHLE

**ARTHROSCOPY** Examining a cavity in the body through a thin telescope (endoscopy) has been most extensively practiced on the joints — arthroscopy. The concept, initially suggested in 1834, was first applied to the knee in 1934, but was not practicable until 1961, when the technical problems of instrumentation (lighting, lavage) were solved by Watanabe. Since then, diagnostic arthroscopy has become a common procedure. During the last three decades several important technological advances have widened its applicability. They include continuous photographic monitoring that allows subsequent review and study of the findings, and many refinements of the scope (for example, fiberoptics allowing for flexibility). Of greatest importance is the addition of a therapeutic capability to the diagnostic capability. This started in the 1960s as washing out small cartilage fragments representing wear detritus or other contaminants of synovial fluid (such as clots). The instrumentation soon became arthroscopic surgery; for this, instruments were devised to work through the scope, and there were other adjuvants, for example, one could use television for visual control of the surgeon's work, or laser instrumentation to supplement the scalpel. At present, repair of lacerations or incisions are routine, as is excision of pathological tissues.

Arthroscopy has caused rapid advance in understanding lesions of the knee (and their identification and treatment). It now is mandatory for orthopedic surgeons who treat patients with injuries to the knee to be competent in arthroscopy. Many lesions, unknown or not recognized easily before 1961, are now commonly seen and treated. Perhaps the best example would be a partial or complete tear of the anterior cruciate ligament.

Though the knee is still the most common joint for arthroscopic diagnosis and surgery, the techniques are being widely applied to other joints, notably the shoulder and the intervertebral joints of the spine.                                          J Coh

**ARTHRITIS** See RHEUMATOLOGY

*See also* MINIMALLY INVASIVE SURGERY; ORTHOPEDIC SURGERY; SPORTS MEDICINE

**ASSOCIATIONS** National medical associations began to appear in the 19th century when many European countries and the United States were experiencing increases in population and the public health hazards associated with the Industrial Revolution. Although scientific and medical societies had been formed in Britain during the previous century, their meetings (sometimes held at the time of the full moon so that members could find their way home on horseback in the dark) rarely touched on matters affecting medical practice as a whole. The impetus to form national medical associations out of local ones gained added strength with the introduction of insurance for poorly paid workers. Doctors saw the need for a central bargaining body in negotiation with governments, as happened in Germany in 1900, Switzerland in 1911, and in Britain in 1912.

Medical associations, such as the British Medical Association, are often confused with licensing bodies, such as the General Medical Council. Licensing bodies determine and enforce standards for the basic professional education and conduct of physicians and usually have statutory powers of enforcement. Licensing of physicians (or 'registration' in Britain) is mandatory, whereas membership of medical associations is voluntary, except in rare cases where they also act as licensing bodies. Medical associations represent the interests of physicians, particularly in negotiations with government and health service or health insurance authorities which employ them, acting in effect as trade unions. In fact many of them are registered as trade unions, although careful to avoid the more questionable policies of industrial unionism such as the 'closed shop' which are regarded as unethical and inconsistent with the fiercely safeguarded independence of the medical profession.

Medical associations often organize continuing (as opposed to basic) medical education and give priority to developing and issuing guidance on medical ethics, leaving investigation of serious ethical violations to licensing bodies. They involve themselves in public health issues, often promoting legislation on environmental hazards or health education. Thus several Danish health laws explicitly name the Danish Medical Association as an advisory body to official committees and working parties. The larger medical associations provide benefits for their members, mainly insurance, medical defence, employment advisory services, and discount schemes. Many of them publish an official medical journal as well as other publications.

There are a few exceptions to these general differences between medical associations and licensing bodies. For example, membership of the Austrian and Portuguese Medical Associations is compulsory (the former is a trade union, and the latter acts in much the same way as a licensing body).

The foundation and progress of the British Medical Association provide a good illustration of why such organizations arose and why they have prospered. In 1828 Charles Hastings, a leading Worcester physician, started a quarterly journal, in which he drew attention to the large number of patients suitable for study that were available in the provinces of which no use was being made. One main reason for this was the dominance of the profession by the Royal Colleges in London, seen as 'bastions of privilege and nepotism' and said to regard provincial surgeons and physicians as 'beneath their notice'.

Four years later, in 1832, Hastings convened a meeting in Worcester, at which the Provincial Medical and Surgical Association was formed. Four out of its five principal objects were scientific, but the remaining one was 'maintenance of the honor and respectability of the profession generally, in the provinces'. The antipathy of provincial doctors towards London was reflected in its constitution, which restricted the post of president to physicians or surgeons resident in the provinces. Provincial branches of the association were formed in the succeeding period, but a Metropolitan Counties Branch that could include London doctors was not formed until 1853. Three years later, and not

without considerable dissent among its members, the Provincial, Medical, and Surgical Association became the British Medical Association.

At its first anniversary meeting the Provincial Medical and Surgical Association sent a strong recommendation to the Parliamentary committee on parochial registers that reliable statistics should be collected on population and health. This resulted in the introduction in 1836 of births and deaths registration, followed a few years later by death certification. It also set up its own committee on smallpox vaccination, which culminated in the Vaccination Act of 1840. But its most important success was to promote the introduction in 1858 of medical registration which enabled the public to identify properly qualified doctors. During the rest of the century the association's highly influential Parliamentary Bills Committee promoted much important public health legislation. The 20th century has seen the British Medical Association preoccupied with political battles over health services, including the National Health Insurance Act of 1912, and the National Health Service Act of 1948. The adverse publicity attracted by these confrontations with the State invariably failed to mention that both Acts were based on proposals advanced by the British Medical Association itself, whose main concern was that their provisions would allow the profession to provide patients with the best possible service.

The modern British Medical Association is a professional association with well over 100 000 members; a reputation for promoting public health, ethical, and human rights measures; a powerful trade union; and a major international publishing house. The main difference between the British Medical Association and medical associations of many other large countries is that it is more truly national. In other countries there may also be provincial or state medical associations with autonomous or quasi-autonomous powers such as those in Australia, Canada, and USA.

### International medical associations

Almost every medical specialty has its own international association or society, but only a few of them, notably those representing gynecologists and psychiatrists, have had much global impact on specialist practice. The only general and medicopolitical global grouping of medical associations is the World Medical Association, set up by representatives of 33 countries in 1946. The postwar revelation that certain doctors in the Axis countries (particularly Germany, Italy, and Japan) had carried out, or had colluded in, unethical and criminal experiments on detainees was causing much concern at that time and clearly the newly instituted United Nations would need to introduce human rights treaties that would affect medical practice. Initially, therefore, one of the main aims of the World Medical Association was to represent the views of the profession through the United Nations.

The main achievement of the World Medical Association has been to issue a series of important declarations, notably the Declaration of Geneva, which was, in effect, an update of the Hippocratic OATH, and of HELSINKI which, after several revisions, is now accepted as the leading statement on the ethics of medical research.

The British Commonwealth consists of 54 countries with a population of about 1.4 billion, or almost a quarter of the world's population, living mostly in developing countries. Formed in 1962, the Commonwealth Medical Association's main activities have been to advocate improved health services, particularly in reproductive health, and to develop continuing education training modules on adolescent health and on compliance with ethical and human rights standards in healthcare.

The Commonwealth Medical Association now includes in its membership some 40 national medical associations and has held workshops in most of them during the past decade, including 14 in 1997 alone. Its projects are administered through its charitable trust, funded mainly by grants from foundations and from the overseas development agencies of the British and other governments. It has consultative status with the World Health Organization, the United Nations Children's Fund, and the Economic and Social Council of the United Nations, as well as observer status at meetings of Commonwealth Heads of Government and those of their health ministers. JH

*See also* PROFESSIONAL REGULATION

**ASTHMA** The word asthma is derived from the Greek word for panting. The condition has been recognized for over 3000 years and references occur in the works of HIPPOCRATES (p 324), Aretaeus, and GALEN (p 469). John Floyer, a physician with asthma, produced the first English work on the condition in 1698 with a vivid description of nocturnal asthma. The great French physician, LAËNNEC (p 461), described bronchospasm in the early 19th century and appreciated the wheezing through his invention of the stethoscope. The most effective treatments for some time were anticholinergic agents such as stramonium and atropine. Available treatments increased in the second half of the 20th century with the development of beta agonists (drugs that relax smooth muscle and widen air passages) and corticosteroids and the limitation of side effects through the use of inhalers. Work on the pathology and immunology of asthma has expanded in the last

ten years and we have begun to understand the genetics of the condition.

The main feature of asthma is narrowing of the airways, which varies with time and treatment. The importance of inflammation in the wall of the airways in the lung has been recognized in recent years. This inflammation makes the airways irritable so that further inflammation, smooth muscle contraction, and narrowing of the airway occur in response to various stimuli. The inflamed, narrowed airways lead to the shortness of breath, wheeze, and cough that are characteristic of asthma. Modern definitions of asthma include the concept of inflammation and variable obstruction to airflow through the narrowed airways.

White blood cells, such as lymphocytes, eosinophils, neutrophils, and mast cells, are involved in the inflammatory process. A complex system of inflammatory mediators controls the cell movement. The inflamed airway wall is sensitive to further allergic stimuli or to non-specific challenges such as dust, smoke, or drying from the increased respiration during exercise. Continued inflammation with poor control of asthma may result in permanent damage to the airway wall, so that some of the airway narrowing becomes irreversible.

The familial link in asthma and atopic disease has been recognized for many years. Recently there has been a search for specific genes. Links have been found to several different genetic features, including those associated with the tendency to atopic disease and immunoglobulin E

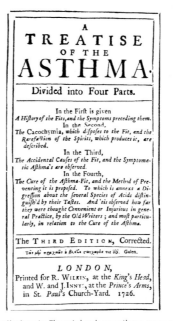

The frontispiece to Floyer's book on asthma. (From Lane, D. L. (1987). *Asthma: the facts*, 2nd edn, OUP.)

those with milder disease, grow out of their asthma during their teenage years, although it may return later. Asthma may develop for the first time in adult life and such cases are often more persistent and difficult to treat.

Some of the increase in prevalence may come from changes in case detection and diagnostic labelling. Various explanations have been suggested for the remainder. Centrally heated homes with warm bedrooms, carpets, and soft furnishings increase the levels of infestation with the house dust mite. Infants with immature immune systems exposed to these allergens may develop sensitivities that emerge later as asthma. Outdoor pollution of various types produces symptoms in asthmatics and may trigger attacks but seems unlikely to explain changes in prevalence. There is a higher prevalence of asthma in first born children. Other children in the home increase the exposure to common viruses in infancy, and these infections help to mature the immune system changing undifferentiated white blood cells (T lymphocytes) away from the type associated with allergy and immunoglobulin E production.

**Effect of smoking**
Maternal smoking during pregnancy and infancy increases the likelihood of a child having asthma and smoking among young women has increased in recent decades. Several studies have shown relationships between asthma and diet related to higher salt intake, or lower intakes of selenium or vitamin C. No one explanation is likely to explain the increases in prevalence seen in different countries.

There are many provoking causes in asthma. Some of these are non-specific causes, such as cold air, exercise, and cigarette smoke. Others are specific allergies, such as the ubiquitous house dust mite, grass pollens, and animal danders. Food sensitivities are less common precipitants. Occupational factors are concerned in around 5% of adults' asthma. Occupational causes include diisocyanates, laboratory animals, platinum salts, and proteolytic enzymes (enzymes that break down proteins); these are recognized compensatable occupational conditions in some countries, including Britain.

There is a variation throughout the day in airway caliber, with the lowest values at 02.00 to 04.00 hours. This typical 'morning dipping' (of measures of airway size) in asthma is often associated with waking at night, with shortness of breath, and with coughing.

The treatment of asthma involves cooperation with the patient to agree on an approach to management. The first important element is avoidance of known precipitating factors so far as possible. Desensitization with small doses of an allergen to which the patient is sensitive is widely used in some

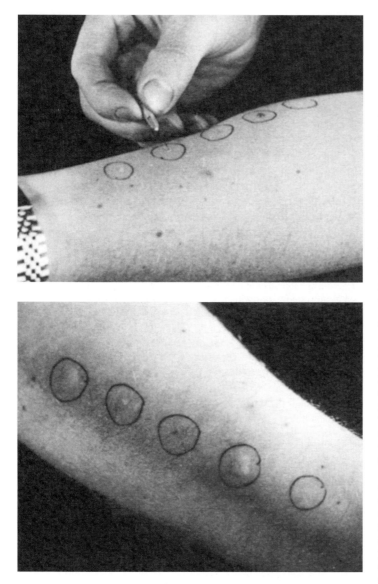

Skin weals produced by skin-prick testing with allergies in an atopic person. (From Lane, D. L. (1987). *Asthma: the facts*, 2nd edn, OUP.)

(an antibody) production. There is no single asthma gene but several genes appear to influence the risk of asthma. The expression of the disease depends on environmental factors interacting with the genetic potential.

The onset of asthma is most often in childhood. Below the age of 18–24 months the diagnosis is difficult and many children who wheeze at this age do not go on to develop asthma. Asthma may develop at any time during life. Studies from many countries show an increase in the prevalence of asthma in the past 20–30 years. In children the prevalence is around 10%, with boys affected more often than girls in a ratio around 1.5: 1. Some of these children, especially boys and

countries. The effects are, in general, less than those achieved by simple safe drug treatment, but improvement in allergens may allow more effective treatment in the future. The variability of asthma and the responses to treatment may be monitored by simple lung function tests. The peak expiratory flow (the maximum speed of breathing out) is measured by cheap, portable peak flow meters. These are particularly useful in a minority of asthmatics who have a poor perception of changes in their airway caliber so that attacks may develop without warning from worsening of symptoms.

Guidelines have been developed for asthma treatment. The two main categories of drugs are bronchodilators, which widen the airways, and anti-inflammatory agents, which reduce the inflammation in the airway wall when used regularly. The guidelines place these treatments in a series of steps. Treatment begins at an appropriate step depending on severity. In mild or moderate chronic asthma the aim is to control asthma, so there are no or minimal symptoms, without adverse effects of treatment. In very mild disease short-acting beta-adrenergic agents (agonists) such as salbutamol or terbutaline are used. If these are needed regularly, an anti-inflammatory agent is added. The most common agent is an inhaled corticosteroid. Corticosteroids by the inhaled route have very few adverse effects at low doses. Alternative drugs at this stage directed at the inflammatory process include sodium cromoglycate and leukotriene receptor antagonists. If these two steps fail to produce good control, higher doses of inhaled steroid or long-acting inhaled beta-agonists are added. Alternative bronchodilators are theophyllines and anticholinergic drugs such as ipratropium bromide.

Acute exacerbations of asthma need to be detected early and treated vigorously. They are often preceded by a period of poorer asthma control identifiable from worsening symptoms or rapidly deteriorating peak flow. Intervention at this point with an increase in regular treatment or a short course of oral steroids may avert the acute attack. Over 1500 deaths from acute asthma occur in Britain every year, and many of these are associated with a lack of appreciation of the severity of the attack by the patient, relative, or doctor.

In chronic asthma that is very difficult to control, it may be necessary to use oral corticosteroids for a prolonged period. Such treatment is likely to be associated with the long-term side-effects of steroids. Studies monitoring treatment show that only around half of prescribed asthma treatment is taken appropriately. Explanation and involvement of the patient in an agreed management plan improves the adherence to appropriate treatment and improves the control of asthma.          PJR

*See also* ALLERGY; SMOKING AND HEALTH

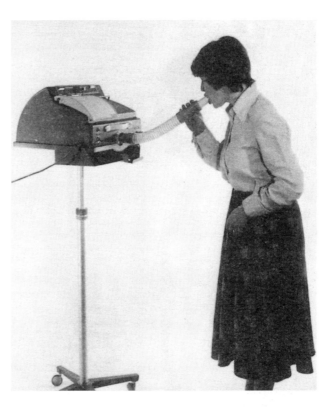

The vitallograph spirometer, used to measure how much air is coming out of the chest during a forced breath. (From Lane, D. L. (1987). *Asthma: the facts*, 2nd edn, OUP.)

**ASYLUMS** The last decades of the 18th century in Britain were illuminated by an increasing awareness of the sufferings of the underprivileged. No better example can be found than those who suffered the double deprivation of poverty and mental disorder, the 'pauper lunatics' as they were opprobriously called. The well-heeled lunatics by comparison were amply cared for in private madhouses, which flourished particularly in the first half of the 19th century.

A further important contemporary event was destined to elevate the status of the mentally ill and the 'mad business' as well as those who traded in it. George III, a popular and much-loved monarch, fell victim to recurrent episodes of mental derangement. The King's physicians were out of their depth. Reluctantly, they sent for the Rev. Dr WILLIS (p 727), known to be of 'peculiar skill and practice in intellectual maladies'. From then on, PSYCHIATRY, having been found to be 'of assistance in the treatment of a great personage', could no longer be ignored and its respectability as a branch of medicine was assured. The King improved, in all probability quite spontaneously. Dr Willis was given the credit and so it could be claimed that lesser mortals suffering from comparable maladies could be expected to benefit.

# ASTROLOGY

Astrology is usually defined as a pseudo-science based upon the supposed influence of the stars and planets on human affairs. Astrologers believed that the situations and different aspects of heavenly bodies might foretell future events. Until the end of the 17th century, there was no demarcation between astrology and what has become orthodox science. This is particularly so in medicine, where most 17th-century medical practitioners either cast horoscopes or accepted that the pattern of human disease was influenced by events in the heavens.

Astrological belief and practice were of two kinds: natural and judicial (so named because judgement and interpretation were involved). The former dealt with astral influences on natural phenomena, such as the weather and agriculture, or with large-scale political, religious, and medical events (such as epidemics); the latter dealt more with predictions concerning individuals. Judicial astrology used nativities (a personal horoscope mapped at birth), or horoscopes based upon the positions of the planets at the time a person first fell ill. Judicial astrology was always faced by the religious problem of free will if human life was predetermined by the stars. The astrologers' defence was that as astral influences descended through the celestial sphere towards the earth they weakened and the human will became stronger; but this did not remove the implication that God's power was predetermined. Broadly speaking, natural astrology has been subsumed into science (weather forecasting is, for example, part of meteorology and deploys mathematics and physical measurements), while judicial astrology has disintegrated into folklore and popular psychology. Both aspects demanded a detailed knowledge of the heavens and therefore contributed to the growth of astronomical observation and theory.

Astrology was first developed as an exact mathematical and astronomical science by the Babylonians and transmitted to the Egyptians, Greeks, and Romans, whence it was transmitted to the Latin west by the Arabs in the 11th and 12th centuries. The most important ancient text on the subject was the *Tetrabiblos* (Four Books) of Ptolemy (c. D 100–170), who also devised, in the complementary *Almagest*, the most precise and complex set of mathematical tables concerning planetary motion known in the ancient world. The *Almagest* enabled readers to predict the positions of the planets, while the *Tetrabiblos* described their influences on terrestrial bodies and events. Since the sun and moon obviously affected terrestrial life, Ptolemy argued, all other heavenly bodies necessarily had physical effects. Ptolemy articulated an influential system which, while not mathematically certain (as he emphasized), would enable the astrologer to make useful predictions, including those concerning health and disease. It was this system that was transmitted to the Islamic world and then to western Europe from the 11th century onwards. With additions and modifications it has remained the basis of all subsequent astrology. It is a mistake to suppose that astrology was disproved when Copernicus showed that our solar system is sun-, and not earth-, centered. Astronomical (and therefore astrological) calculations were and are always made from an earthly base line; moreover, the theory of universal gravitation developed by Newton in 1687 might be said to have confirmed, rather than disproved, solar, lunar, and planetary influences upon the earth. On the other hand, given that the fixed stars forming traditional constellations are widely separated in space, it would be impossible for them to influence our destinies. For example, the bright stars Betelgeux and Rigel in the constellation of Orion are 500 and 900 light years away, respectively, and appear to lie in the same direction only when viewed from the earth.

Astrologers located planetary influences in three principal ways. Signs of the zodiac (the twelve constellations of Aries, Taurus, Gemini, Cancer, Leo, Virgo, Libra, Scorpius, Sagittarius, Capricornus, Aquarius, and Pisces), that each occupy 30° of the ecliptic, controlled temperament and parts of the body (thus, a person born under Aries might be prone to head diseases). Twelve 'houses' based upon the earth's daily rotation with respect to the zodiac revealed aspects of life, for example, fortune, friendship, relationships, health, and marriage, and 'aspects', the degrees of angular separation along the ecliptic between each planet, were also significant. In medical horoscopes, for example, five aspects were held to be important: conjunction (0° separation), sextile (60°), quartile or square 90°), trine (120°), and opposition (180°). The mathematics (trigonometry) was complex until the wide distribution of astronomical tables and almanacs in the 16th century made casting a horoscope relatively simple. Almanacs, combining a calendar with the year's astronomical events and a compilation of prognostications, formed the most popular literature after the Bible before the 1660s.

Interpretation (which might vary from astrologer to astrologer) depended upon sets of arcane symbols drawn from Aristotelian, Platonic, and Paracelsian cosmology. Each planet had unique properties bearing on the dichotomies of masculine/feminine, hot/cold, or dry/moist, or ruled over different parts of the body. Houses might be friendly or hostile to each planet, and provide specific readings, while the signs of the constellations could indicate felicitous or contrary events — for example, the Sun in Aries was good, but in Libra, bad). Finally, planetary aspects might indicate good or bad fortune.

*(continued opposite)*

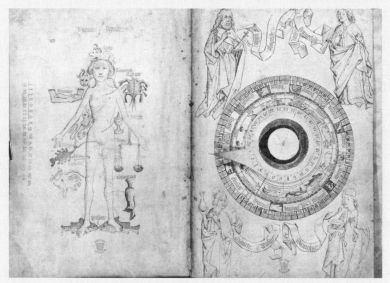

Zodiac man from a 15th-century English manuscript. (The British Library, Egerton MS2572, f.50v–51.)

*(continued)*

All this was put to use by medical astrologers such as Simon Forman (d. 1634) and Nicholas Culpeper, who built up huge general practices. In a competitive healing market aspiring medical men had use for predictive knowledge since prognosis is a source of power and proof of learning. By studying physics, a medical practitioner became a true physician. Clinical signs were not ignored and historians have drawn analogies between the use of horoscopes to aid diagnosis and our contemporary use of blood tests and X-rays to help the doctor focus upon important symptoms.

**Death by success**

Astrology, however, was killed by its own success in Britain, where, despite the existence of royalist practitioners, astrologers tended to be radical in politics and religion. Most historians interpret the discipline's downfall after 1660 to the social, political, and religious changes brought by the Restoration. By the end of the century the relative positions between licensed academic medical practitioners and medical astrologers had radically altered, with the latter losing support among the educated. Astrologers

found themselves excluded from sources of authority and control in church, government, and universities. A similar process occurred throughout Europe. Astrological ideas were redescribed in other scientific ways (for example, comets were explained by Newton's cosmology as regular visitors; menstruation was construed in hormonal terms; human individuality and diversity were explained by genetics; while clinical medicine developed a battery of chemical and physical tests to aid prognosis). Nevertheless, popular astrology continued; the London astro-physician, Francis Moore, started an almanac in 1699 and was soon selling 25 000 copies a year to a laboring and rural population. 'OLD MOORE'S ALMANAC' continues publication. In the 19th century judicial astrology found advocates such as R. J. Morrison, A. J. Pearce, and Richard Garnett (1835–1906), keeper of printed books at the British Museum.

However, the horoscopes that appear in popular newspapers and magazines today have little to do with mathematical astrology. Twentieth-century popular astrology was largely the creation of William Frederick Allen (1860–1917), who, influenced by Madame

Blavatsky's theosophy, transformed astrology into character reading and popular 'self-development' psychology.

There have been many attempts to establish the validity of astrology statistically, notably in the *Traité d'astro-biologie* (1939) of Karl E. Krafft, who, having predicted an assassination attempt on Hitler's life in November 1939, was made Himmler's personal astrologer. Krafft's methods and results were shown to be self-deceiving by the statistician and psychologist, Michel Gauquelin in 1959. Double-blind tests by Shawn Carlson, published in *Nature* in 1985, showed that astrologers' predictions were no better than expected on the basis of pure chance. Despite this, Gauquelin was intrigued by a surprising correlation between personality and an individual's zodiacal sign, as well as positive correlations between the natal charts of distinguished continental sports champions, actors, and scientists. Gauquelin speculated that the explanation had to be sought in the earth's magnetic field, which is certainly affected by fluctuations of solar energy. It remains to be seen whether astrobiology can be made into an exact science.      WHB

---

But, for whatever reason, public asylums were built at the end of the 18th century by voluntary public subscription. Examples are those in Manchester (1766) and York (1777), the latter not to be confused with the Retreat at York, opened in 1796. This, a QUAKER foundation, led the civilized world as an example of 'moral management', which meant in practice the virtual abolition of physical restraint.

However, the distinction for first introducing this humane practice belongs to a Frenchman, Phillipe PINEL (p 77), chief physician in turn of the renowned hospitals in Paris, the Bicétre and the Salpetrière. In so doing, he defied both the French public and the Revolutionary Government by unlocking the chains of his patients and prohibiting other barbaric methods. Instead, he introduced a raft of innovations, all designed to bring a semblance of gentleness and friendliness into their hitherto sordid lives.

However, the grand design of the reformers in England was sadly frustrated by the economic and social upheavals, brought about by increasing industrialization and concomitant urbanization, both aggravated by a dramatic rise in the birthrate. Whatever facilities had been provided for the mentally disordered were swamped. The overspill drifted into the streets as vagrants, or into WORKHOUSES, or into houses of correction, or,

even more tragically, into gaols. The appalling state of affairs occasioned a public scandal and so great was the outcry that in 1815, a Parliamentary Select Committee was set up. It found that: 'If the treatment of those mentally disordered in the middling or in the lower classes of life shut up in hospitals, private madhouses or parish workhouses is looked at, your committee are persuaded that a case cannot be found where remedy is more urgent'.

A condemnation as vehement as this could not be ignored, and in 1815, an Act amending that of 1808 (Wynn's Act) was quickly introduced, which enabled counties to borrow to build asylums. But the counties dragged their feet, and by 1844, the number of such asylums actually built was a mere 15. This was intolerable, and in 1845, the counties were no longer exhorted, but compelled to build asylums. Most of the county asylums that were subsequently built, incidentally, are (or were) the psychiatric hospitals of today.

**Benevolence and optimism**

The county asylums were conceived in an atmosphere of benevolence and therapeutic optimism. The good faith of the planners shone out like a beacon: they earnestly believed, naïvely perhaps, that admission to an asylum would cure insanity *per se*.

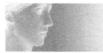

John **DEE** (1527–1608). British mathematician and astrologer. Dee became a fellow of St John's College, Cambridge, in 1545 and the following year a foundation fellow of Trinity College. He incurred considerable unpopularity by dabbling in necromancy, alchemy, and crystal-gazing, but he enjoyed the favor of Elizabeth I, who consulted him when ill.

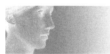

Michael **NOSTRADAMUS** (Michael de Notrèdame) (1503–66). French physician and astrologer, Nostradamus studied medicine at Montpellier and remained in the town during the epidemic of plague, which won him enough popular approval to force an unwilling faculty to accept him. He later practiced at Agen, Aix-en-Provence, and Salon, but, after marrying a rich wife in 1547, turned from orthodox medicine to astrology and casting of horoscopes.

This far-reaching development spread rapidly, overcoming national frontiers, and new asylums were founded all over the civilized world. For example, Jean Esquirol, a successor of Pinel at the Salpetrière, and one of his most ardent disciples, was instrumental in the construction of ten new asylums in France.

But in Britain the ever-increasing proliferation of asylums and the uncontrollable increase in number of beds crammed into them proved to be counter-productive. The rosy optimism of the early planners and the medical staff turned into bitter pessimism as they saw their hospitals choke with the chronically insane, a dire situation which prompted the acid comment, 'a gigantic asylum is a gigantic evil and figuratively speaking a manufactory of chronic insanity'.

During the late 19th and early decades of the 20th centuries, Britain's asylums, like those in Europe and America, languished in the psychiatric doldrums: custodialism took precedence over treatment. However, between the two World Wars, a radical spirit of reform began to creep in, akin to the zeal that motivated the early Victorian reformers such as the 7th Earl of Shaftesbury. In essence, it saw the transformation of the previous quasi-prison/workhouse milieu into one characterized by humanity, active treatment, and rehabilitation.

To crown the vitally important environmental improvements that ensued, the introduction of the era of psychopharmacology in the 1950s gave real hope that rationality and specificity in the treatment of mental illness were on the way. A heart-warming spirit of optimism prevailed: despite some serious inherent structural handicaps and their sheer size, the fame of British mental hospitals — as they were called — reached its zenith.

Nevertheless, it is a bitter irony that at the very time that British mental hospitals basked in their well-deserved fame, plans for their destruction were being laid. Enoch Powell, a brilliant scholar but a sadly flawed politician, was then Minister of Health. In his contentious speech of 1976, based on flawed statistics, he opined, with more eloquence than accuracy, that mental hospitals rather than being 'good objects' were in fact 'bad objects'.

Mr Powell's hospital plan split the psychiatric establishment in two, but in the end he won the day. Mental hospitals were to be destroyed and their patients were to be shared between general hospitals and 'community care' — a most seductive and charismatic slogan. Once begun, the rate of destruction and translocation acquired its own momentum, so fast indeed that the number of beds available had dropped from 150 000 in 1960 to 37 000 in 1998.

But the hospital plan, like its progenitor, was also flawed, a fact that has become increasingly evident as the years have rolled on. Irrespective of political color, the press, for example, has deplored the deteriorating situation. Prominence has been given to the tragic plight of mental patients turned out of mental hospitals into scantily available general hospital beds and, not infrequently, 'community care' which doesn't care. Failing these facilities, the hapless victims of the plan have swollen the number of vagrants, pavement-sleepers, and the petty offenders who choke the penal system. Far more tragic are the 1000 no-hopers who annually commit suicide and the 200 or more who each year commit casual and purposeless murder. Echoes of the same social disorder prompting the outcry leading to the 1815 Parliamentary Select Committee are all too evident.

Public patience and tolerance are fast running out. So intense was the demand for reform that Frank Dobson, the Health Secretary near the end of the 20th century, was compelled to act. In January 1998, he published far-reaching reforms in a Mental Incapacity Bill.

In all fairness, it must be pointed out that Britain was not alone in reaping the bitter harvest of policies both ill considered and too precipitate. In Italy, spear-headed by the late Professor Franco Basaglia, and motivated by Marxist ideology, a law was introduced in 1978 actually forbidding the admission of new patients to mental hospitals, which were to be run down and eventually closed. This has led to a new class of vagrants — the *abbondonnati* — a host of wretched, homeless, mentally sick ex-patients who roam the streets and public places.

America is experiencing the same social upheaval and for virtually the same reasons. Dr Alan Stone, professor of law and psychiatry at Harvard, wrote in 1984, 'Yet madness has not gone out of the world as we hoped, in fact madness is more visible than ever before in this country. One can see chronic mental illness in the streets of every major city in the United States'.

### Impact of Nazism

Psychiatry at the end of the 19th and beginning of the 20th centuries was firmly rooted in Europe, particularly in Germany and Austria. At that time those countries boasted many of the founders of modern psychiatry, such as Alois Alzheimer, A. A. Brill, Emil KRAEPELIN (p 355), Hanz Creutzfeld, Ernst Kretschmer, Otto Binswanger, Josef Breuer, and Baron Richard Von Krafft-Ebing. Of comparable stature in the burgeoning specialty of psychoanalysis, there were Sigmund FREUD (p 321) and his daughter, ANNA (p 676), Alfred ADLER (p 675), Melanie Klein, and her daughter, Melissa Schmiderberg.

The effect on psychiatry, psychiatrists, and the care of the mentally ill of the Second World War was devastating. Nazism was synonymous with anti-semitism, but an anti-semitism of a particularly vile and virulent variety. In Germany, as in Austria, within the ranks of psychiatrists, Jews were substantially over-represented, particularly among the practitioners of psychoanalysis, a subject reviled by the Nazis as 'the despised Jewish science'. The public burning of the works of Freud in 1933 in the quadrangles of German universities was, except symbolically, the least important of the infamies perpetrated by the Nazis; but it was a warning of the shape of things to come. Those Jews who saw the light in time fled, mainly to the USA, and to a lesser extent to Britain. Those who would not, or could not, flee were mercilessly slaughtered or subjected to the unspeakable horrors of the Holocaust. The Aryan psychiatrists left were guilty of condoning the atrocities, or actively promoting them. German psychiatry plunged to its nadir: it was disgraced and discredited.

But Germany and Austria's loss was the gain of whichever country was wise enough to accept the refugees. This was particularly so in America, where psychoanalysis, mainly of the Freudian variety, had taken firm root. The advent of additional skilled Jewish analysts added a decided impetus and popularity, to the point that psychoanalysis was elevated to the status of a cult, or indeed, a religion.

Psychoanalysis aside, America boasted other advantages. It was rich, well-resourced, and had an enviable number of eminent centers for psychiatric research. Important too is that it had not suffered the physical and economic ravages of the most destructive war in history.

Not surprisingly, the cream of Europe's war-weary psychiatrists, underpaid and under-resourced, were tempted to cross the Atlantic in search of a better personal and professional life. And tempted they were. In the 1950s, the brain drain was firmly on its way so much so that, instead of following Europe, as it did in the 19th century, world psychiatry today speaks in English, but with a distinct American accent.

Sadly, in keeping with countries in Europe, particularly in Britain and Italy, certain states in America tried to solve the problem of the 'gigantic asylums' by emptying them and relying on 'community care' to carry the burden of the unfortunate ex-inmates. The result was disastrous in social terms. Nevertheless, the pre-eminence of American psychiatry today is without doubt.

## Psychiatrists versus politicians

Conventional wisdom would have us believe that asylums — or mental hospitals — were designed for the care of the mentally ill. It follows, then, that the overall control of these sick people should lie with doctors, or more precisely, psychiatrists.

In this instance, conventional wisdom is found lacking. Initially, asylums came to be built because of the determined efforts of powerful philanthropists against the will of the politicians. The grand design of the philanthropists was frustrated by their own naïvety and unforeseen social and demographic events, none of which was under the control of the medical staff. The result was the creation of the 'gigantic asylums' and therapeutic stagnation.

And so it remained until the mid-20th century, when, particularly in Britain, a spontaneous movement arose within the psychiatric hierarchy itself to improve the lot of the patients in their care. It was tantamount to a crusade led by the likes of T. P. Rees of Warlingham Hospital, Surrey; T. M. Cuthert of St Luke's, Middlesbrough; Joshua Carse of Graylingwell, Sussex; and Maxwell Jones of Belmont, Surrey. The resultant transformation inspired the term 'therapeutic community', or 'the new moral treatment of the insane'.

The fulsome and universal praise for Britain's humane initiative was, not surprisingly, not echoed in totalitarian countries, where 'psychiatrists' danced to the tune of their political masters, as in Nazi Germany, and in communist Russia, where psychiatric treatment was routinely used, or abused, as an instrument of penal policy.

In the 1960s a new movement emerged to trouble the waters of the psychiatric establishment — anti-psychiatry. The movement, left-wing in politics, sported an international membership including, for example, Ronald Laing and David Cooper in Britain; Thomas Szasz in the USA; and Michel FOUCAULT (p 313) in France, the only one, incidentally, without psychiatric credentials. The gospel according to this zany group was that psychiatry was a form of social repression; that treatment was disguised punishment; and, above all, that mental hospitals must be closed forthwith to avoid further damage to the patients.

The movement for a time enjoyed widespread popularity; but it died because in practice, the results were an unmitigated disaster, as witness David Cooper's venture in Britain in 1962. 'The lunatics have taken over the asylum' was how it was summarized.

And how to epitomize the sorry state of affairs into which politicians have landed us, everywhere? On reflection, there is nothing more apt and succinct than the trenchant comment of a distinguished sociologist, Professor Kathleen Jones, who has experienced at first hand the current situation both in England and in post-Basaglia Italy. She wrote 'Nobody seriously argues

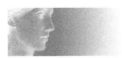

# THE GREAT KILLERS: ATHEROMA

Atheroma or atherosclerosis describes the process by which arteries gradually silt up, becoming narrower and finally blocked. Not all arteries are involved but the most important are the coronary arteries, which supply blood to the heart and which when blocked result in the death of patches of heart muscle and fatal heart attacks. Atheromatous disease of arteries has been present since early times: it is well described in Egyptian MUMMIES; and is occasionally seen in a few old animals such as parrots and monkeys, but in these creatures it is rarely severe enough to cause damage to the heart or other organs. In man, death from coronary disease was not clearly recorded until the beginning of the 20th century; currently it accounts for about half of human deaths in the western world. The word atheroma means a lump of gruel and refers to a mixture of substances such as cholesterol and cells which accumulate on the inside (intima) of arteries.

Arteries are lined by a single layer of thin flattened cells called endothelium. These remarkable cells have many functions. They secrete several substances which control the permeability of the vessel wall and the fluidity of the blood in the artery. Imbalance of endothelial secretions may lead to constriction or relaxation of the muscle of the arterial wall, causing narrowing or widening of the arterial lumen. Imbalance can also lead to blood clotting in the artery or for the tendency of blood constituents, such as lipoproteins, to diffuse into the vessel wall. The earliest stage in the process of atheroma depends on such changes of endothelial cell function.

The early changes of atherosclerosis are still incompletely understood. Early on in life the intima increases in thickness because of the overgrowth of smooth muscle cells; later in childhood spots of yellow intimal thickening appear. They are called fatty streaks or spots and contain cholesterol esters but the overlying intimal endothelial cells appear intact. Later still (in adolescence) the lipid deposits may be covered by a layer of fibrous tissue, the fibrous cap. Complications arise if the fibrous cap splits at the edge of the atheromatous plaque, exposing the contents of the atheroma to the bloodstream; blood may clot on the surface of the plaque, causing more narrowing or even complete blockage of the artery. When this occurs in the coronary arteries it may result in death of part of the heart muscle (myocardial infarction) and acute heart failure. If the full thickness of the wall of the left ventricle dies, the heart may rupture and the pericardial sac around the heart fills with blood, compressing the heart and leading to cardiac arrest.

Other changes occur in the media (muscular wall) of the artery. Muscle cells are destroyed and replaced by fibrous tissue. Pressure of the blood in the artery stretches this fibrous tissue (scar), causing a bulge (aneurysm) in the arterial wall. Aneurysms occur most often in the lower part of the aorta in the abdomen and may rupture with fatal results. Atherosclerotic aneurysms occur in other arteries and produce similar effects.

## Differing incidence

The incidence of atherosclerosis varies greatly in different parts of the world. There is a high prevalence in Scotland but it is much lower in the South of France. In the USA the frequency of atherosclerotic events is falling. The disease is said to be uncommon in other countries such as Africa but this may be because of the lack of diagnostic and reporting facilities. These geographic variations have led to much research into the possible predisposing factors, yet the different incidence between countries is only partly explained. Certain risk factors, however, have been clearly recognized. Atherosclerosis increases with age, is more common in men (though increasing steadily in women), and is more prevalent in the presence of obesity, high blood pressure, cigarette smoking, and diabetes mellitus. Less well defined are the effects of a stressful life and the role of genes. If there is a genetic factor several genes may be involved. The closest association is with raised blood concentrations of fats (lipids), mainly cholesterol and its esters, whereas the association with triglycerides is less well defined.

Cholesterol and its esters are contained within lipids in the blood called lipoproteins. Lipoproteins have a central core of lipids. In addition to cholesterol and its esters there are triglycerides and phospholipids. All these lipids are wrapped in a coat of protein called apolipoprotein. Several apolipoproteins exist and some are more closely related to atherosclerosis than others. Apolipoprotein E is one of the suspects. Various lipoproteins (distinguished by differences in their densities in the ultracentrifuge) may also play a part: the two most important are the low density lipoproteins (LDL), rich in cholesterol and carrying most of the cholesterol present in the blood; and the high density lipoproteins (HDL), rich in phospholipid and involved in the transport of cholesterol to the liver for excretion in the bile. A high HDL blood concentration seems to reduce the risk of atherosclerotic disease; a high LDL is a well-known risk factor for the development of atheroma. Such a raised LDL level may be due to the failure effectively to metabolize

cholesterol, the breakdown of LDL normally being achieved by receptors in the liver that in atheroma may malfunction or be deficient.

Macrophages (a form of white blood cell) can also take up LDL, but this usually occurs when it has been altered, for example, by oxidation. Macrophages become loaded with droplets of lipid and as such may often be seen in the changes of arterial atheroma. Oxidized LDL is toxic and may kill the macrophages that have devoured it. This results in lipid being deposited in the atheroma and may cause damage to the edges of the plaque of atheroma, resulting in its rupture and overlying thrombosis of the artery. Antioxidants such as vitamin E may prevent this process and there is some clinical evidence to support this idea. Many components of the arterial wall may be concerned with the appearance and progress of atheroma. The endothelial lining may be injured by turbulent blood flow, particularly at arterial branches. High blood pressure will create such turbulent blood flow; chemical insults, as found in cigarette smoke, may also damage the endothelium, leading to the adhesion of macrophages and lymphocytes which may, with oxidized LDL, enter the wall of the blood vessel.

These macrophages are white blood cells called monocytes that have phagocytosed materials such as LDL. They produce substances that digest connective tissue and promote smooth muscle cell multiplication in the artery wall. The smooth muscle cells also develop secretory activity and can produce elastin and collagen, which further contributes to the bulk of the atheroma. It has been suggested that the proliferated smooth muscle cells were derived from a single precursor similar to that occurring in new growths such as cancer. This hypothesis raised the possibility that a viral infection or specific chemical injury may be the initiator of atheroma. Other cells that may be involved are T lymphocytes (a type of white blood cell that plays an important part in bodily defences, and is attracted to the diseased area by macrophages and, being able to kill cells, contributes to the atherosclerotic plaque) and blood platelets (adhering to the surface of the plaque and causing thrombosis, and also releasing growth factors that stimulate the proliferation of smooth muscle cells).

Studies using experimental animals have not succeeded in defining the early stages in the development of atherosclerosis. In some animals the role of genetic factors is clear: the white Carneau pigeon breed is prone to develop extensive atheroma of the aorta; the Watanabe rabbit also develops extensive

(continued opposite)

*(continued)*

atheroma spontaneously owing to a deficiency of LDL receptors. The view that a diet rich in saturated fats is an important atherogenic factor has been extensively investigated. Rabbits of many breeds develop lesions rapidly when cholesterol is included in their diet; animals such as primates, rats, and carnivores are much less susceptible to the effects of cholesterol feeding. Soft water was once thought from epidemiological studies to be associated with coronary artery atheroma, and dietary copper has been studied. Copper is a cofactor for the enzyme lysyl oxidase, concerned with the normal synthesis of elastic tissue in the artery wall. The presence of copper in red wine was thought to explain the low incidence of coronary artery disease in parts of France. An increased level of dietary copper did not affect the rupture of atheromatous plaques in the domestic turkey. Clearly there has been no shortage of ideas about atherogenic factors. Vitamin E is the popular agent at present. Doubtless other notions will follow.          GAG

*See also* CARDIOLOGY; DIABETES MELLITUS

for the return of the old mental hospital system; but its abolition has left a chasm between intention and performance. From the 1930s to the 1950s, British mental health policy set a standard for the rest of the world. Only positive action at the highest level can repair the damage of the past three decades'.          HRR

*See also* PSYCHIATRY; 'ROYAL MADNESS' AND PORPHYRIA

**AUDIT** Medical audit is a method of evaluating standards of medical care. It aims at ensuring that practices of known and accepted benefit are given preference over those of more dubious effectiveness and are carried out with maximum efficiency and minimum waste. It was defined by the Department of Health in Britain as 'a systematic analysis of the quality of medical care, including the procedures used for diagnosis and treatment, the use of resources, and the resulting outcome for the patient'.

Audit procedures examine three elements: structure (the quantity and type of resources available – staff, outpatient or operating facilities, number of beds, or radiological or other investigational services); process (an assessment of what is done to the patient, ranging from history taking and physical examination to diagnostic investigations; and treatment, including medication or surgery. This includes input (for instance, financial, administrative) and outcome (the result of clinical intervention).

What really matters is outcome. This depends critically on structure (what resources are available) and process (how these are used). Both of these are relatively easy to evaluate, requiring simply the collection of available numerical or factual information. Outcome may also be easy to assess, provided one keeps to well-defined and measurable indices, such as death rates or length of stay in hospital. It is more problematic when one tries to evaluate less clear-cut end-points such as quality of life after intervention. Many aspects of outcome can be fully assessed only a long time, perhaps years, after intervention, especially where the response is not dramatic or the medical con-

dition being studied is uncommon. In such circumstances there may be no precise or reliable information about outcome. This explains one of the weaknesses of audit procedures: evaluation of the appropriateness of medical care is bound to be arbitrary unless there is exact knowledge of outcome and the extent to which this might be improved by changes in practice.

Because of this lack of an absolute standard for much of medical care, judgements about appropriateness are usually made by consensus view or by comparing the performance of one institution against another. If the outcome for a particular intervention is not as good in one institution as another of comparable size and resources, it needs to be explained. The difference may be due to incompetence or neglect by the doctor or other members of the management team, to a lack of resources, or to the application of inappropriate or ineffective procedures. Once the cause has been identified steps can be taken to remedy it. This notion of feedback is the most important part of audit: analyse performance, identify shortcomings, find the cause and correct it. Without this, the whole process is of little practical value. However, it has an additional and important educational function. By encouraging discussion and analysis of existing practice and exploring ways to eradicate weaknesses and failures, audit educates doctors constantly to be self-critical and to aim at self-improvement.

## Hospital practice

Over the past ten years audit procedures have been introduced into almost all hospitals in Britain and the United States. In the USA since the early 1960s the Professional Activities Study Group of the Commission on Professional and Hospital Activities has conducted routine computerized statistical analyses of all discharges and deaths in most short-stay hospitals. Its primary purpose is audit but the set-up has also generated large data files for analysing the quality of care. Many hospitals have developed their own sets of guidelines for the management of specific conditions, mostly arrived at through a consensus view,

**AUDIT PIONEER**

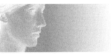

Archibald (Archie) Leman **COCHRANE** (1909–88). British physician and epidemiologist. Between 1946 and 1960 he made major contributions to the aetiology and epidemiology of pneumoconiosis in Wales before becoming director of the MRC Epidemiology Unit in Cardiff, David Davies Professor at the Welsh National School of Medicine, and later, first president of the Faculty of Community Medicine. He is remembered particularly for his application and promotion of randomized CONTROLLED CLINICAL TRIALS.

and therefore not necessarily accepted by other institutions or the profession as a whole.

In recent years the application of audit has been enhanced by the introduction of EVIDENCE-BASED MEDICINE — an attempt to reduce uncertainties by careful studies of outcome to ensure that a particular intervention produces a beneficial result. The concept is not new: in 1971 Archie COCHRANE (p 79) delivered a Rock-Carling lecture under the title '*Effectiveness and efficiency: random reflections on health services*'. He applied the term 'effectiveness' to measurement of the effects of particular medical actions in altering the course of particular diseases for the better, 'efficiency' to the determination of optimal use of personnel and materials (resources). Until recently Cochrane's precepts had produced little change in practice but evidence-based medicine, which demands that all medical interventions are looked at critically in the way Cochrane advocated, has been widely adopted. Special attention is paid to procedures that have been an entrenched part of medical practice for so long that they have become almost sacrosanct. If a procedure can be shown to be effective, it should be retained; if not, it should be abandoned. The development of 'Cochrane centers' simplifies setting appropriate standards and, by audit of local performance against these standards, national and even international comparisons become possible.

Audit has also become an integral part of management. Analysis of structure and process provides managers with the information they need to ensure that resources are being properly used. Perhaps for the first time reliable information exists about such items as the length of waiting lists for each doctor or their prescribing costs, or the number of patients seen or operations carried out per session. Medical care is costly, subsuming from 5 to 15% of national budgets. These vast sums of money can no longer be spent without some accountability. By eliminating ineffective intervention and encouraging the use of tried and tested procedures medical audit should help to control costs without jeopardizing standards of healthcare. Doctors now accept that they owe a duty to provide the highest possible standards of effective care with maximum efficiency and economy.

Yet despite the persuasive arguments in favor of audit, there is a general perception that its introduction has not been an unqualified success. There is some resentment from doctors of the additional work it creates and a lack of conviction that audit really leads to improved clinical care. There is fear that it may be used to force them into action that conflicts with their best clinical judgement. For instance, an insistence on

increased turnover reduces the time spent with the patient, diminishing the opportunity for proper communication, and putting at risk the relationship that is the core of good medical care. Above all, there is suspicion that government and management have seized on audit as a mechanism for driving down costs at the expense of high quality medical care. RHof

**AUSTRALIA** In 1990 the Australian population was 18.53 million, of whom 77.1% were Australian-born. Immigration has been a dramatic feature of the Australian demographic profile since the end of the Second World War; with a relative increase in immigrants of Asian origin since 1980.

There are 238 700 Australians of Aboriginal and Torres Strait Islander descent, or 1.4% of the general population, currently living in Australia (1990 census figures). This group lives primarily in rural or outback communities. Infant mortality rates are higher (up to 25 per 1000 live births) and life expectancy at birth (45 for Aboriginal males) is less for Aboriginal Australians than for those of European origin. Total spending for medical aid to Aboriginal and Torres Strait Islander peoples is $2320 per person, some 8% higher than for other Australians.

In 1990 there were 39 500 doctors in Australia; of these, 23% live outside capital or major cities, as do 41% of the general population.

### Health responsibilities

Three groups provide and control healthcare in Australia — the federal government, the state government, and the private sector. The federal government controls the datum of fees charged by doctors through its scheduled fees list. This is a guide only, as fees are at the discretion of individual medical practitioners. Reimbursement through the federal government's Medicare health scheme is, however, linked to this list of scheduled fees. The federal government also controls the entry of foreign doctors into Australia; and the health standards of immigrants and health aspects of customs and quarantine. The latter is of major importance as Australia, an island continent, is free from rabies, poliomyelitis, cholera, and many of the tropical and subtropical viral encephalitides, and also from many of the great medical and veterinary scourges such as foot-and-mouth disease, swine fever, Newcastle disease, and anthrax. The last case of indigenous malaria occurred in 1962. All incoming air-flights to Australia are fumigated with insecticide.

The federal government provides complete health coverage for members of the armed services but not their dependants; and complete healthcare (including hospital inpatient care) to veterans of the armed services of Australia, through the health division within the Department of Veterans' Affairs. Through the armed services, health and medical care are also provided to some overseas countries in times of crisis or special need (for example, Rwanda in 1994–5; and Papua New Guinea in 1997–9). The federal government also provides healthcare through aid organizations, such as the Australian Development and Assistance Bureau. This aid is targeted particularly to countries in the Indo-Asian-Pacific region. The federal government funds, and by its funding processes controls, undergraduate medical education in Australia.

State governments provide a range of health services, including the provision of government (public) hospitals, throughout the nation. These provide full inpatient and outpatient services, in a hierarchical system of referral and sophistication, with all capital cities having at least two tertiary referral hospitals. Such hospitals also provide the infrastructure for the training of medical students; and provide the infrastructure and control the training and placement of new and graduate doctors in the state (public) hospitals. Medical boards exist in all states and are arms of the state government. They set and control standards of professional competence and practice, establish registers of doctors legally entitled to practice, and supervise professional ethical and disciplinary issues. The legal implications of medical practice are controlled by medical tribunals in each state capital city, these having the status of a court-of-law. State governments also have responsibility for providing integrated medical services, such as psychiatric services, school health services, Aboriginal health services, preventive medicine, and forensic medicine. The current trend is towards district autonomy with public health services broadly based on large tertiary-referral hospitals, but with a 'hospital-without-walls' outreach. These are funded and policy-controlled by state health departments. The eight separate State and Territory departments of health are responsible for all aspects of preventive and public health and for clinical care. All capital cities and regional centers with populations over 500 000 have tertiary referral institutions such as high-dependency neo-natal units, spinal units, burns centers, and specialized surgical units providing, for example, cardiothoracic surgery and neurosurgery.

There are more than 1000 local governments in Australia, and these retain responsibility for local public health issues relating to water supply, sewerage, food safety, water fluoridation, and local environmental safety.

The private sector of health and medicine is very important in Australia. Although Australian political parties champion the concept of socialized medicine, the ethos at the patient level is of privately sought individual medical care. The general practitioner remains pre-eminent in the Australian healthcare system. Many non-governmental institutions have evolved to provide healthcare for geographically or socially disadvantaged groups.

One of the most important of these non-governmental medical institutions is the Royal FLYING DOCTOR Service of Australia, which was established in 1928 in Queensland. It operates with up to 45% federal government funding, up to 45% state government funding, with the balance (in practice, between 10 and 20%) raised by voluntary contributions from the public. It operates from 13 bases in Australia.

The service provides telephone medical consultations to the outback; conducts routine clinics, including immunizations, child health clinics, family planning consultations, and preventive medicine; medical consultations and treatment of all types; and emergency transport and treatment of the sick and injured.

### Payment for healthcare

Historically, much private healthcare was provided by various 'lodge' systems in Australia, and these have evolved into private health-insurance companies. Hundreds of disease-specific voluntary patient advocacy and support groups exist. Private philanthropic funding is important for both healthcare and research. The annual budget of Rotary International (Australia), called Rotary Down Under, now exceeds 10 million Australian dollars specifically targeted to medical research. Similarly, Lions International (Australia) funds medical research and patient-care facilities, targeted particularly to disease-specific aspects such as eye diseases and the preservation of vision; and research into, and help with, the clinical management of patients with chronic renal disease.

Total health expenditure in Australia is $38 770 000 000 (US$24.42 billion, £10.0 billion). Two-thirds of this expenditure is on patients over 60 years of age; and an estimated one-half of the total healthcare expenditure occurs during the last year of life, on average during the eighth decade.

The overall cost of healthcare is shared almost equally among the three contributors to medicine:

- Federal government        35.9%
- State government          33.5%
- Private sector            30.6%

The federal government contributes to healthcare costs through taxation; and, from taxation and

| FLYING DOCTORS | |
| --- | --- |
| Number of flying doctors | 35 |
| Number of nurses | 87 |
| Aircraft | 38 |
| Pilots | 83 |
| Annual patient contacts | 169 500 |

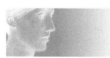
levy revenue, maintains a form of national health service (Medicare). The cost of drugs is covered, in part, to 'public' patients attending general hospitals and to certain disadvantaged members of society, under another federal government scheme called the Pharmaceuticals Benefits Scheme. This currently contributes some 2000 million Australian dollars to subsidies for prescribed pharmaceutical products in Australia.

The federal government controls part-reimbursement of medical costs — consultations, allied health costs, pathology services, and surgery — through a list of scheduled fees. The principles of the Medicare scheme consist of:

- Reimbursement to patients of 85% of the scheduled fee — the patients paying their private medical practitioner in the first instance, and reclaiming costs from the government; or sending their accounts to the Government Medicare Office, which will give to the patient a cheque for 85% of the scheduled fee, which the patient then passes on (with the balance from his or her own purse) to the doctor concerned.

- Doctors are encouraged not to bill patients directly, but to 'bulk bill' directly to the government. This fundamental core of socialized medicine has generally been resisted by the medical profession. Exceptions occur in the case of impecunious or other selected groups of patients, and in a number of instances where entrepreneurial medical services have been set up to take advantage of the system where no 'bad debts' occur. There has been considerable debate in this context about the risks of over-servicing in such a 'bulk bill' socialized system of medicine. Currently, 55% of general practitioners 'bulk bill'.

- Patients are treated free of charge in public hospitals. This point has been the subject of considerable state-to-state variation. In some states (for example, Queensland) public hospital patients are treated free of charge without any means test, but with no Medicare documentation changing hands. In other states (such as New South Wales) patients are subject to a means test before treatment is offered free in public hospitals, and the federal government is billed through the Medicare system.

- Private medical and hospital insurance is not tax-deductible; but expenses for any single medical intervention exceeding $1250 accrue some rebate. From 1997 complex schemes for rebates on premiums for private health insurance, for wage earners with taxable incomes below $35 000 have been introduced. The medical profession generally strongly supports private health and medical insurance, and government measures to promote this.

- The Medicare scheme is funded by a 1.5% levy surcharge on taxable income. When introduced, the Medicare tax levy was 1% on taxable income for tax payers in Australia. With the advances of medicine and increasing costs of delivering the technology and hardware from new medical research, it is anticipated that this Medicare levy will continue to rise inexorably.

The political philosophy of both Labor and Conservative (Liberal–National Party Coalition) federal governments in office in Australia in the past 20 years has been socialized medicine, but with freedom of choice for patients for the selection of both doctor of first contact and for specialist referrals. A Medicare card is issued to everyone aged 16 years or older. A uniform system of scheduled fees operates in all states. Some 2.26% of Australians hold pensioner cards or sickness benefit and healthcare cards. These provide special benefits for pharmaceutical costs; and many doctors voluntarily charge such patients the scheduled fee only.

With the inevitability of increasing costs in medicine, the principle of universal socialized medicine has had to be progressively modified. The Medicare rebate for pathology services has been lowered (85% of the scheduled fee in 1998), private hospital bed subsidies have been abolished for all except aged-care beds, and a strict quota is maintained on these. A patient contribution of $3.20 (US$1.90, £1.19) per item has been introduced for pensioners in the Pharmaceutical Benefits Scheme. Public patients pay up to $20 per pharmaceutical item.

Tension has existed for the past 20 years between the Australian Medical Association (comprising some 70% of the practicing medical profession in Australia) and the federal government-in-office, concerning the broad philosophies of socialized medicine, which the Australian Medical Association does not, in principle, espouse. Hospitals constitute the biggest call (44%) on the Australian healthcare budget.

### Diseases and ill health

The principal international index of a nation's health, the infant mortality rate, is currently 7.0 deaths per 1000 live births and has fallen to this level from a level of 10.5 deaths per 1000 live births over the past two decades. Infant mortality rates measure the combined effect of antenatal care of pregnant women, perinatal care of mother and infant, the incidence of congenital abnormalities, and the sudden infant death syndrome. In Australia, deaths from congenital abnormalities are 1.9 per 1000 live births, and those from the sudden infant death syndrome are 1.0 per 1000 live births. Among the young (up to age 25) violent trauma remains the major cause of death.

Non-melanocytic skin cancers and breast cancer are the most common tumors affecting Australian women. The lifetime risk of an Australian woman developing breast cancer before age 75 is 1 in 11, a risk which has been rising over the past decade. Death rates for breast cancer are 25 per 100 000 women (1999).

Melanoma rates in Australia are the highest in the world, a reflection of high exposure to ultraviolet radiation in a population of which 90% are fair-skinned people. Melanoma currently accounts for 8.7% of all new cancer registrations in men. The rate of new melanoma diagnoses is 49.1 per 100 000 men (1999) annually. Survival rates are relatively high with 5-year survival rates of 86% (men) and 92% (women).

## Medical education

There are eight undergraduate medical schools in Australia; and three graduate medical schools at the Universities of Queensland, Sydney, and Flinders. These range in size from those with an intake of 60 students per year (Flinders University in Adelaide and the University of Tasmania in Hobart) to 230 (the University of Queensland). The criteria for selection to medical schools vary but in all such undergraduate schools most students are selected by the criterion of academic achievement at the competitive matriculation examinations. All schools have subquotas for 'mature age' students, and for 'disadvantaged' and 'refugee' students.

The medical course in all undergraduate Australian universities lasts six years, and four years in the graduate schools. Educational philosophies differ from university to university. Some (for example, Flinders in Adelaide, the Universities of Newcastle in New South Wales, Sydney, and Queensland), adopt a 'problem-oriented' approach from the first year. Currently there is a net annual intake of some 500 medical graduates from overseas into Australia, the equivalent of about the annual output of two large medical schools.

Medical education in Australia which leads to a primary degree in medicine is controlled by the Australian Medical Council, a national audit and policy body which reports to the Department of Health and Family Services. It monitors student course content, curriculum balance, standards, and the numbers of funded places for medical students. The cost of medical education to each student is largely subsidized by federal and state grants; but each medical student pays an annual higher education contribution of $4261.

Postgraduate medical education in Australia is comprehensive and vigorous, and a full and complete postgraduate education to full registration as a specialist is available for all specialties. Such training is provided under the auspices of the various royal colleges, for example, the Royal Australasian College of Surgeons, the Royal Australasian College of Physicians (including the Division of Pediatrics; formerly the Australian College of Pediatrics), and many other similar professional bodies. Training in general practice is conducted by the Royal Australian College of General Practitioners and also by the (federally funded) Family Medicine Programme, a major postgraduate education scheme introduced in 1972.

Future special targeted groups for health in Australia include federal-funded programs targeted to 'at risk' groups of special need. These include the National Aboriginal Health Strategy, the National Women's Health Programme, and the National Campaign against Drug Abuse. This last is currently funded with $40.0 million Australian dollars (US$25.2 million, £15.2 million) of federal money, annually.

The National Better Health Programme aims to achieve a better standard of health for all Australians, with an emphasis on lower socioeconomic groups, and with a strong preventive medicine ethos. This program concentrates on five priority topics — controlling high blood pressure; improving nutrition; the prevention and early detection of malignant diseases; geriatric health; and the prevention of accident injury and trauma. In recent years, this program has had annual funding of 39 million Australian dollars (US$29 million, £19.5 million), from both Commonwealth and state sources. JHP

**AUTHORS — DOCTORS AS** In 1936, Lord Moynihan of Leeds (1865–1936), a famous surgeon, gave a Linacre lecture, published the same year and republished in 1983. He called his lecture: *Truants — the story of some who deserted medicine yet triumphed*. It is fascinating to realize how varied are the achievements of doctors or people who started their careers as doctors. There have been politicians and musicians, philosophers and philanthropists, scientists and botanists, bibliophiles and missionaries, true polymaths, and famous sportsmen. But in no topic are the doctors as many as in LITERATURE.

There are doctor-authors to be found in every country and culture, and that seems always to have been so — Lord Moynihan went as far back as IMHOTEP (p 412), physician to Pharaoh Zoser, more than 2000 years BC, whom he called 'the true father of medicine'.

Why is it that doctors, more than members of any other learned profession, write all sorts of

## CHEKHOV

Many authors have confirmed that their medical training was a great help to them in their work as authors. Anton Chekhov wrote

My study of medicine significantly broadened the scope of my observations and enriched me with knowledge whose value for me as a writer only a doctor can appreciate. It also served as a guiding influence; my intimacy with medicine probably helped me to avoid many mistakes. My familiarity with the natural sciences and scientific methods has always kept me on my guard; I have tried whenever possible to take scientific data into account.

The same testimony has been given to me by several contemporary doctor-authors.

books, fiction and poetry, drama and detective stories, humor and cookery books?

There are obvious similarities between the tasks of a doctor and those of an author. Edmund Pellegrino writes that 'both medicine and literature are ways of looking at man and both are, at heart, moral enterprises'. He continues, 'medicine and literature are linked, too, because they both tell the story of what they see' — all doctors are trained to take and write down the patient's history. Further, 'language, the stuff of literature, is also the means of COMMUNICATION between the patient and the physician. Both medicine and literature probe, although from radically different perspectives, the same subject: the truths that are revealed — and concealed — in man' (E. R. Peschel).

Jean Bernard, famous French doctor-author, member of the French Academy, who started composing poetry when a prisoner of war, divided doctor-authors into three categories, namely:

(1) those who start out as working physicians but, at a specific time, abandon medicine to become full-time authors (such as, T. Smollett, W. Somerset Maugham, A. Conan Doyle)

(2) those who throughout their lives work both as doctors and as writers, but keep the two professions apart (such as, Anton Chekhov, William Carlos Williams)

(3) those whose literary work is filled with, and based entirely upon, their medical experiences.

### British doctor-authors (in alphabetical order)

**Aikin**, John (1747–1822).

**Akenside**, Mark (1721–70). Physician and bibliophile, physician to St Thomas's Hospital, London and to George III's Queen. At the age of 17 he wrote a philosophical poem, *The pleasures of imagination*. Although he continued to write, his later years were more concerned with medicine than poetry. Because of his arrogance he became the target of Tobias Smollett's satire in *Peregrine Pickle*.

**Arbuthnot**, John (1667–1735). Physician to Queen Anne. It has been said that he is remembered only as the recipient of Alexander Pope's *An epistle to Dr Arbuthnot*, but that seems a spiteful and unfair judgement. He wrote *Of the laws of chance* and later, encouraged by Jonathan Swift, a satire, *The history of John Bull*, in which he created John Bull as representing England.

**Beddoes**, Thomas Lovell (1803–49).

**Bell**, Josephine (1897–1987).

**Blackmore**, Sir Richard (?1650–1729).

**Bridges**, Robert (1844–1930). The first and only doctor to be made Poet Laureate, he served in

London hospitals but retired after an attack of pneumonia at the age of 37 to devote himself exclusively to poetry, which he did for more than 45 years. His last work, *The testament of beauty*, is regarded as his most renowned.

**Brown**, John (1810–82).

**Browne**, Sir Thomas (1605–82). He was educated in Oxford, studied medicine at Montpellier, Padua, and Leiden, and returned to Oxford to practice. Later he moved to Halifax and, in 1636, to Norwich, where he stayed until his death in 1682. His *magnum opus, Religio medici*, an elegant and deep work, was first published in a pirate edition in 1642 and only later in a version authorized by the author. It was placed on the *Index expurgatorius* by the Vatican, thus being forbidden reading for Roman Catholics. He also wrote *Pseudodoxia epidemica* (1648), generally called *Vulgar errors*, a great work in seven books, in which he discussed the complete knowledge of the time and, with the help of his own experiments and logic, exposed many of the common superstitions and errors of folklore.

**Campion**, Thomas (1567–1620).

**Chamberlayne**, William (1619–89).

**Cowley**, Abraham (1618–67).

**Crabbe**, George (1754–1832). '… Of all "truants" probably professionally the most incompetent' (Lord Moynihan) — he was ordained as a priest and became curate of Aldeburgh. He was saved from relative obscurity by Benjamin Britten, who based the story of his opera *Peter Grimes* on Crabbe's *The borough*.

**Cronin**, Archibald Joseph (1896–1981). At one time, he was said to be the most read author in the world. He wrote many successful novels from his own experiences as a doctor in the mining districts of Wales: for instance, *Hatter's castle, The stars look down, The citadel*. In later years he wrote an extremely popular series for television, *Dr Finlay's case book*.

**DARWIN**, Erasmus (1731–1802) (see also p 214).

**Deeping**, George Warwick (1877–1950).

**Denton**, William (1605–91).

**Dover**, Thomas (1660–1742).

**Doyle**, Sir Arthur Conan (1859–1930). He practiced for some time in Southsea, but in 1890, when he moved to London, he abandoned medicine and became a full-time author. He created Sherlock Holmes and Dr Watson and their abode in 221b Baker Street. The first Sherlock Holmes story, *A study in scarlet*, appeared in 1887. Doyle also wrote some famous historical novels (*Micah Clarke* and *The white company*) and short stories during his early career (*Doctors — tales from medical life*), and early science fiction — a series of books figuring the eccentric Professor Challenger (see also p 233).

**Freeman**, Robert Austin (1862–1943).

**Garth**, Sir Samuel (1661–1719). During the times of, and after, the plague, he fought against the APOTHECARIES, who wanted to dispense medicines on their own, and supported the Royal College of Physicians, which organized the first DISPENSARY for the poor in 1699. The fight continued, and it was not until Garth had published his famous *The dispensary* that the antagonism between doctors and apothecaries ceased. *The dispensary* is a burlesque poem in Homerian style, ridiculing the disputants who, at the time, could easily be identified.

**Gilbert**, William (1540–1603).

**Gogarty**, Oliver Joseph St John (1870–1957). He was a close friend of James Joyce, who portrayed him as Buck Mulligan in *Ulysses*. A senator in the Irish Parliament; an ear, nose, and throat (ENT) surgeon; and bon vivant, he practiced in London but moved to New York, where he died. He wrote several novels, and his poems, including the moving *Non dolet*, were included by his friend W. B. Yeats in the *Oxford anthology of modern poetry*.

**Goldsmith**, Oliver (1730–74). Perhaps never a qualified doctor? He wrote *The vicar of Wakefield*, of which Lord Moynihan said that 'it will be read as long as the English language exists', and which includes the lines which begin:

When lovely woman stoops to folly
And finds too late that men betray

He also wrote *She stoops to conquer*, a stage comedy in a different vein.

**Grainger**, James (?1721–60).

**Hamilton**, Sir David (1663–1721).

**Harington**, Sir John (1561–1612).

**Harvey**, Gabriel (1545–1630).

**Hoadley**, Benjamin (1706–57).

**Hooker**, Joseph Dalton (1817–1911).

**KEATS**, John (1795–1821). He studied medicine at Guy's Hospital, qualified, and worked a short time as a doctor, but soon abandoned medicine for poetry. He died from tuberculosis at the age of 25. His first volume of poetry was published in 1817; in 1818 came *Endymion* ('A thing of beauty is a joy for ever'), followed by such famous poems as *Hyperion, Ode to a nightingale*, and *Ode on a Grecian urn*. Tennyson regarded Keats as the greatest poet of the 19th century (see also p 659).

**KEYNES**, Sir Geoffrey Langdon (1887–1982) (see also p 119).

**Knowles**, James Sheridan (1784–1862).

**Lever**, Charles James (1806–72).

**Locke**, John (1621–1704).

**Lodge**, Thomas (1558–1625).

**McCrae**, John (1872–1918).

**Maugham**, William Somerset (1874–1965). During his long life he became immensely popular, first as a playwright — in 1908 he had four plays running simultaneously in London — later as an author of novels, and especially short stories. His first novel, *Liza of Lambeth*, is set in the London slum where Maugham, for a short period, worked as an obstetric clerk. He soon abandoned medicine, but later paid his tribute to it when in *The summing up*, he wrote, 'I do not know a better training for a writer than to spend some years in the medical profession.' His most famous novel is *Of human bondage*, an autobiographical story with several similarities to Marcel Proust's *Remembrance of things past*. Other well-known novels are *Cakes and ale, The moon and sixpence*, and the later *The razor's edge*.

**Mayor**, **Osborne** Henry (1888–1951). He studied and practiced medicine, and for a short time was professor of medicine in Glasgow. For the rest of his life he was a very successful playwright and wrote more than 40 plays under the pseudonym James Bridie, the best known being *Tobias and the angel* (1930), *The anatomist* (1931), and *Daphne Laureola* (1949).

**Moir**, David Macbeth (1798–1851).

**Moore**, John (1729–1802).

**ROSS**, Sir Ronald (1857–1932) (see also p 481).

**Smiles**, Samuel (1812–1904).

**Smollett**, Tobias (1721–71). A ship's surgeon and author, he is regarded, together with Richardson, Fielding, and Sterne as an originator of the English novel. He studied in Glasgow and obtained a post as a surgeon's mate during the mismanaged expedition to Cartagena in 1741, later to be described in his first novel. In 1744 he was back in London with a practice in Downing Street and, in 1748, he published his first book, *The adventures of Roderick Random*, based upon his experiences in the navy. He continued in medicine and in 1750 obtained his MD at Aberdeen. The next year saw the appearance of his new novel, *Peregrine Pickle*. He spent some time in Bath and criticized the Bath waters — Bath has an important role in his last novel, *The expedition of Humphrey Clinker* (1771). Before that he had edited the *Critical Review*, and published several other novels, and his *Travels through France and Italy*, regarded as overcritical of all he saw. Smollett's travels appeared in the shadow of Sterne's *A sentimental journey*, in which Sterne ridiculed Smollett as 'Smellfungus'. Smollett also wrote *A complete history of England* (1757–58), which brought him much criticism but also, for the first time, financial security.

The novels that can be read today are *The adventures of Roderick Random* and *The expedition of Humphrey Clinker*. In *Roderick Random*, Smollett was the first novelist 'to draw from the Navy his most notable characters and his liveliest scenes' (H. W. Hodges). We find here the first description of the food and drink on board naval ships:

our provision consisted of putrid salt beef and salt pork, which though neither fish nor flesh, savoured of both; bread, every biscuit whereof, like a piece of clock-work, moved by its own internal impulse, occasioned by the myriads of insects that dwelt within it

and to drink what the sailors styled 'The Necessity'; 'three half-quarters of rum, diluted with a certain quantity of water' — the 'grog', after the admiral 'Old Grog', so named on account of his fondness for a cloak which was made of grogram. *The expedition of Humphrey Clinker* is an epistolary, letters between a traveling gentleman, Mr Bramble, and his physician, a charming story of travels in 18th century England. The very first letter begins, 'Doctor, the pills are good for nothing — I might as well swallow snowballs to cool my veins.' Smollett's reputation sank during the 19th and early 20th centuries but now stands high.

**Stables**, William (Gordon) (1840–1910).

**Stacpole**, Henry de Vere (1863–1951). He is remembered for his romance *The blue lagoon* (1908).

TREVES, Sir Frederick (1853–1923) (see also p 261).

**Vaughan**, Henry (1622–95).

**Warren**, Samuel (1807–77).

WILDE, Sir William (1815–76) (see also p 250).

**Wolcot**, John (1738–1819). Writing under the pseudonym Peter Pindar, he was known for his satirical verse and pamphlets.

**Young**, Francis Brett (1884–1954). He practiced in Devon and served during the First World War in East Africa. He published several novels from the West Midlands and from his African experiences, the best known being *Portrait of Claire* and *My brother Jonathan*.

**Young**, Thomas (1773–1829).

### Non-British doctor-authors

Only a few names are quoted from some of the large language areas, but there are doctor-authors to be found in every country and language.

*Germany/Austria* **Benn**, Gottfried (1886–1956). He is regarded as perhaps the leading poet of 20th-century Germany. He studied medicine in Berlin, in 1912 both graduated and published his first collection of poems, *Morgue*, which made him one of the most important representatives of German expressionism. For a short period he was captured by Nazi ideas, an aberration that cost him dearly, and it was only after the Second World War that he was again accepted in the literary world and could publish his poems. Almost until his death in 1956 he continued a modest practice among the poor and destitute in Berlin. Many of his most famous poems were written during this second active period of his life, poems of solitude and suffering; life only gave emptiness and:

To live is to build bridges
over waters disappearing

**Büchner**, George (1813–37). Author of *Woyzeck*.

**Döblin**, Alfred (1878–1957). A Jewish doctor who himself became an anti-Semite, he lived and worked in the eastern part of Berlin and wrote many novels, the best known being *Berlin Alexanderplatz*, which was made into a famous film by R. W. Fassbinder.

**Hoffmann**, Heinrich (1809–74). A German physician who made important contributions to psychiatry, he wrote the immortal *Struwwelpeter (Schock-Head Peter*, 1847), which, in 1939, when counting stopped, had seen 593 editions and had been translated into most languages.

**Scheffler**, Johannes (Angelus Silesius) (1624–77).

**Schiller**, Johann Christoph Friedrich von (1759–1805).

**Schnitzler**, Arthur (1862–1931).

*France* **Céline**, Louis Ferdinand (1894–1961). He was said to 'crash' into literature with his two novels, *Voyage au bout de la nuit* (1932) and *Mort à crédit* (1936), both with a doctor as the main character and with much autobiographical material. Céline wrote about people at the bottom of society and lived close to them himself, regarding men to be 'disgusting, shocking and absurd!' In his novels, Céline, for the first time, created a modern French written language.

**Duhamel**, Georges (1884–1966).

RABELAIS, François (?1494–1553). He became a Franciscan friar and later got his MD in MONTPELLIER (p 319) in 1530, becoming one of the leading physicians in France. He and his books were several times condemned by the Catholic Church, and Rabelais had to live outside France for long periods. Eventually he was given absolution and could return to France where he ended his days, not as a doctor but as a priest, as vicar of Meudon near Paris.

For many centuries he was thought of only as a jester, but in the 18th century he was rediscovered, and today he is regarded as one of the greatest names in world literature, with an important influence on such authors as Swift, Sterne, and Joyce.

His great work is the story of the giants *Gargantua and Pantagruel*, in five volumes, all with different titles, published between 1532 and 1564. The first tells of the cloister Théleme, with its monastic rule of 'Do as you like', a message which should be seen in context with Rabelais's fight against the rigid ideas of the sophistry of the time. Rabelais is a snorting joker, he snorts from zest for life and happiness, he jokes with everything and everybody. He fills his work with urine and excrements, with anatomy and medicine, with obscenities, with words — he is said to have invented 600 new French words — but his work never gives offence, it leads to laughter (see also p 700).

**Sue**, Eugene (1804–57).

*USA* **Holmes**, Oliver Wendell (1809–94). He was professor of anatomy and physiology at Harvard University and author of novels, poems, and essays. Holmes is famous especially for his *Autocrat at the breakfast-table* (1857–58), essays notable for their kindly humor and width of erudition.

**Percy**, Walker (1916–90). Philosopher, linguist, and author, he published several philosophical works until he realized that nobody read him. He then started writing a series of novels, for example, *The moviegoer*, *The last gentleman*, and *The Thanatos syndrome* (1987), but yet had difficulties in reaching the wide readership he deserves. Percy wrote much of a deep anxiety, of an 'everydayness' which damages life, with people passing each other without meeting.

**Williams**, William Carlos (1883–1963). He was a man in whom medicine and literature had formed a creative symbiosis — he worked his whole life as a practicing physician amongst the poor in New Jersey and wrote whenever he found time. He was primarily a poet — the patients and their lives were his teacher, they inspired him and filled his poems. His fame came late; he was awarded the Pulitzer prize posthumously, at a time when his poetry was published in England for the first time. His most ambitious work was *Paterson*, a long, free verse apotheosis to a suburban industrial city.

*Russia* **Bulgakov**, Mikhail (1891–1940). A Russian prose writer and dramatist, he started his career in medicine, but after the revolution abandoned medicine and became a journalist and author. For long periods he was forbidden to publish, and his plays were banned by the Russian authorities. He tried to emigrate but was never given a passport. His most famous work is *The master and Margarita* (written between 1928 and 1940 but not published until 1966–67); others are *The heart of a dog* and *The white guard*. During his lifetime, when his novels could not be published in Russia, he was famous for his plays, especially *The days of the Turbins*, performed more than 1000 times.

CHEKHOV, Anton (1860–1904) (p 84). When only a schoolboy, he had to take responsibility for his mother and siblings, and he started to write short stories. He studied medicine in Moscow and opened a practice. Later he moved to a country house outside the city, where he practiced medicine among the poor peasants for many years with wide responsibilities: 'my district compasses 25 villages, four factories and a monastery'. He contracted tuberculosis at an early age and by the age of 25 complained of coughing and blood spitting. He denied his tuberculosis for at least

another 12 years, 'I am still far from tuberculosis!', until at the age of 37 he had a major hemorrhage and had to admit that he was ill. He moved to the Crimea but frequently traveled to Moscow, where he married the famous actress Olga Knipper, only a few years before his death in 1904, when only 44 years old.

Chekhov wrote about 700 short stories, many, in fact, with the format of a short novel. During his younger days he wrote small comic pieces; the major short stories were written between 1885 and 1895, and the major plays thereafter. Some of the most famous short stories are *Ward No. 6*, *The steppe*, *The black monk*, and *The lady with the little dog*. The cavalcade of plays began with *The seagull* (1895), the first performance of which, in St Petersburg, was a complete disaster because of the actors' misunderstanding of the play. The new production in 1898 in Moscow started the triumphant, and still ongoing, march over the world's stage of *The seagull*, followed by *Uncle Vanya* (1900), *Three sisters* (1901), and *The cherry orchard* (1904).

Anton Chekhov often paid tribute to his medical studies and training as being important for his authorship, 'There is no doubt in my mind that my study of medicine has had serious impact on my literary activities.' There are, however, remarkably few traces of medicine in his short stories. The opposite could be said of the plays. In all except *The cherry orchard*, doctors, often described as being both incompetent and alcoholic, took important roles with critical comments about what was being enacted on stage.

The principal characteristic in Chekhov's writing lies in his deep understanding of human nature, in his humor, empathy, and compassion. The plays demonstrate that a non-happening may also be genuinely dramatic.

## Why does an author write?

Primo Levi in his book *L'altrui mestière* (*Others' professions*) has given nine answers: because it is necessary, to entertain, to teach, to improve the world, to spread ideas, to get rid of anxiety, to become famous, to get rich, or by habit. Are there other reasons specific for doctors which make them abandon knife and stethoscope for the pen, or, today, for the computer? Many have answered that writing is necessary and that it is great fun. Some say it is escapism, helping them from developing BURN OUT. Jean Bernard wrote to survive. It seems that doctors like to write, although for many it does not come easily. Chekhov once wrote that 'The fire in me burns with an even, lethargic flame; it never flares up or roars!' The US surgeon Richard Selzer says that he writes slowly, only a few pages per day and Oliver Sacks said: 'A deadline might create a dead man!'

In his everyday work the doctor-author lives an exciting story — but there is a danger: if the doctor becomes too artistically sensitive, he might lose the cool objectivity necessary for most doctors' decisions. This is an important reason why some doctor-authors abandon medicine.

In 1735 Alexander Pope, in his famous *An epistle to Dr Arbuthnot*, gave this answer:

> Why did I write? What sin to use unknown
> Dipt me in Ink, my Parent's, or my own?
> As yet a child, nor yet a Fool to Fame,
> I lisp'd in Numbers, for the Numbers came.
> I left no Calling for this idle trade,
> No Duty broke, no Father dis-obey'd.
> The Muse but serv'd to ease some Friend, not Wife
> To help me thro' this long Disease, my life.

LEB

*See also* DANCE; DETECTIVE STORIES; LITERATURE; OPERA; POETRY

**AUTOPSY** — literally to see for oneself — is the dissection and examination of a dead body to determine the cause of death and establish the evolution of a disease. It was coined in 1678, while its synonym 'post-mortem examination' (or post-mortem for short) was first used in 1850 and 'necropsy' in 1856. Although the term 'post-mortem examination' is appropriate etymologically, autopsy is more commonly used. Autopsy forms the cornerstone of PATHOLOGY and has made an important contribution to our current understanding of disease. It has the ability to recognize the mistakes made by doctors and thereby improve their diagnostic skills. At first limited to gross and microscopic anatomy, it may now also make use of specialized techniques such as microbiology, electron microscopy, radiology, toxicology, and chromatography.

## History

The Babylonian phenomenon, 3500 years ago, of 'haruspicy', or examination of animal livers to foretell the future, is probably the earliest known attempt to dissect bodies to gain knowledge of anatomy and pathology. The ancient Greeks and Egyptians did not lay emphasis on anatomic knowledge and dissected the human body (only) for religious or magical reasons. The Alexandrian physician Herophilus performed autopsies to teach normal anatomy, while Erasistratus showed that disease led to changes in anatomy. GALEN (p 324) in the second century AD performed dissections on Barbary apes and extrapolated his findings to man. Since Galenic thought held sway for centuries, this blocked any advances in anatomy, physiology, pathology, and medicine. Sporadic cases of post-mortems, including forensic autopsies in Italy and in China, were recorded in the Middle Ages.

In 1410 Pope Alexander V died suddenly and was autopsied. Towards the end of the 15th century, Pope Sixtus permitted students to dissect human bodies to learn anatomy. One of the earliest autopsies recorded, performed by Bernard Tornius in the 15th century, is that of a child. Antonio Benivienni, a 15th century Florentine physician, correlated his findings with clinical features in 15 cases. The idea that bodies could display clues to diseases that ravaged them began around the 16th century. The impetus given by Andreas VESALIUS (p 846) in 1543 to normal human anatomy dissection led to a change. Theophile Bonet published his *Sepulchretum sive anatomia practica* in 1679; it comprised 3000 autopsies but subscribed to the theory of HUMORS and thus missed the opportunity to recognize the anatomic-pathologic correlation. In 1724 Hermann BOERHAAVE (p 121) documented the first case of esophageal rupture at autopsy. Later Marcello MALPIGHI (p 37) and his students, Albertini and VALSALVA (p 252), showed that anatomy was the seat of all disease. Their student, Giovanni MORGAGNI (p 621), after almost six decades of research in PADUA (p 451), published his *De sedibus et causis morborum per anatomen indagatis* in 1761, in which he described the clinical histories and autopsy findings of over 700 cases. This was the first attempt to show conclusively that there existed a definite correlation between clinical symptoms and the anatomic findings.

At about the same time William (this page) and John HUNTER (p 398) in England and their nephew Matthew Baillie were extraordinary physicians and collectors of specimens. Baillie wrote the first systematic textbook of pathology in 1793. In Paris Corvisart performed autopsies in the Charité hospital, paying specific attention to cardiac pathology and published many volumes on his cases. Marie Francois Xavier Bichat showed that the secrets of health and disease lay within the tissues of the body itself. Not all subscribed to the usefulness of autopsies, though: Thomas SYDENHAM (p 721) decried the procedure.

The golden age of the autopsy was in the mid- and the late 19th century. Karl Rokitansky at the ALLGEMEINES KRANKENHAUS in Vienna (p 352) performed 30 000 autopsies and supervised as many more. He was the first to perform complete autopsies with a definite protocol — the autopsy as we know it today. His approach of performing autopsies without any knowledge of the clinical record had its advantages, but may well have been the beginning of the belief that pathologists live in ivory towers. He restricted himself to gross anatomy for most of his life and it was left to Rudolf VIRCHOW (p 853) of Berlin to introduce microscopy. Virchow singlehandedly changed the face of pathology by introducing the concept of

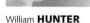

cellular basis of disease. Thus, while Rokitansky was responsible for making autopsy pathology an independent branch of medicine, it was Virchow who made it a scientific and essential aspect of medicine.

Physicians too have had a tremendous influence. Richard BRIGHT (p 522) was the first to show an association between dropsy and renal disease. Much later, Sir William OSLER (p 602) performed 950 autopsies and in Hobart Hare's words went 'into the autopsy room with the joyous demeanor of the youthful Sophocles leading the chorus of victory'. He even left detailed instructions for his own autopsy. That autopsies can detect misdiagnosis was shown by Richard C. CABOT (p 190) of Boston. In his landmark publication in 1912 he showed that there were discrepancies between premortem and post-mortem diagnoses. This, along with the recently published FLEXNER REPORT, which criticized the state of medical education in the USA, was responsible for increasing the rate of autopsies in the USA. In fact, the reputation of an American hospital in the early 20th century was often judged by its autopsy rate.

### Recent history

There has been a world-wide decrease in the autopsy rate since World War II. Attitudes of clinicians, pathologists, and the public contributed to it. In the USA, physicians' belief that clinical and laboratory medicine is infallible and their fear of malpractice lawsuits has resulted in their reluctance to convince patient's relatives to give permission for autopsy. Pathologists avoid autopsies because they take time and the work is unpleasant. The growth of specialties such as surgical and clinical pathology and molecular biology and the fact that autopsy technique has not changed much over two centuries have also contributed to the decrease. Relatives are not enthusiastic because of the mutilation of the body, delay in funeral arrangements, and religious beliefs. The high cost (currently over $2000 per autopsy in the USA) has also been responsible for the decreased number of autopsies.

There is a general belief that the contribution to science is now less dramatic than before, especially in light of new diagnostic facilities available. This fact has been belied by data showing that the incidence of gross error in diagnosis, which contributes to death or illness in patients, has remained roughly the same over decades. This is because of changing patterns of existing disease, emergence of newer diseases, and over-reliance on new technology. Complacence, misinterpretation of tests, and errors of judgement have also been responsible.

### Impact of autopsies

The contribution of autopsy to modern medicine is clear when one realizes that in Cabot's study,

## HAZARDS

Autopsies are not without their hazards. Josef Kolletschka died of sepsis following an infection acquired after sustaining a wound during an autopsy. It was the similarity in his illness and in patients with puerperal fever that led Ignaz Phillip SEMMELWEISS (p 479) to realize that puerperal fever was also caused by infection. Other diseases that pathologists and autopsy attendants are exposed to are TUBERCULOSIS, HIV, and hepatitis B.

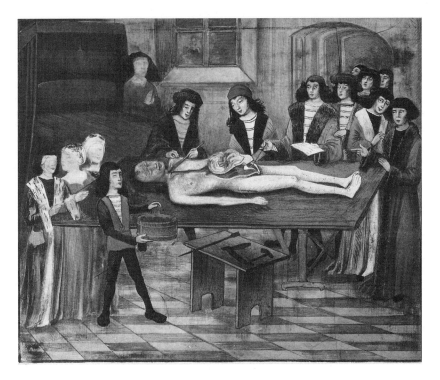

Gouache, after a 15th-century manuscript illustration showing the post-mortem of a woman. (Reproduced courtesy of the Wellcome Institute Library, London.)

clinical misdiagnosis of vertebral tuberculosis, hepatic cirrhosis, and bacterial pneumonias were common — whereas today they are uncommon diagnoses. The autopsy thus acts as a quality control mechanism for clinicians and its capacity to determine a causal relationship with disease is tremendous. Some diseases first detected at autopsy or understood better because of it are Zollinger-Ellison syndrome, veno-occlusive disease of the liver, acute tubular necrosis, secondary hemochromatosis, pancreatic cystic fibrosis; the complications of diabetes mellitus in blood vessels, eye, nerves, and kidney; Creutzfeldt–Jakob disease, subacute sclerosing panencephalitis, Legionnaire's disease, collagen disease, toxic shock syndrome, nosocomial infections, various cancers, AIDS, radiation fibrosis, and appendicitis.

Autopsies can be used to evaluate surgical - procedures, new diagnostic and imaging procedures, as well as drugs and their side-effects. Vital epidemiological statistics may be determined only through autopsy-related data and this may influence the monitoring of public health. Autopsies may assist in genetic counseling and help in the identification of familial disorders. Tissues for transplantation such as bone, corneas, dura, and pituitary glands can be obtained at autopsy. Education of medical students and physicians — including the uncertainty and the limits of medical knowledge — remain an important role for autopsies.

The incidence of autopsies varies world-wide, depending on religious attitudes, nationality, superstition, politics, legislation, and socio-economic factors. For instance, Islam and Judaism do not encourage them, whereas Christian, Hindu, and Buddhist texts and spiritual leaders do not specifically object to them. These religions and their spiritual leaders, in fact, advocate the use of the dead body for organ transplantation, and thus indirectly encourage autopsies. Austria has a very high rate of autopsy even today; Greece has practically no post-mortems; and in India autopsies are restricted to big institutions in large cities such as Bombay, Delhi, and Chandigarth. In western countries autopsies are fairly common; however, the incidence is decreasing.

What does the future hold for the autopsy? Numerous conferences have been held lamenting its decline. Certainly, blindly performing 'routine' autopsies is not the solution. Autopsy reports fill shelves of most pathology departments in the world and contribute little to science and society. Suggestions have been put forward to have only problem-oriented autopsies (to attempt answering specific questions) or limited autopsies. The limitation may denote a restriction in the number of organs studied or in the types of specialized investigations performed. A drawback with this solution would be the lost opportunity to make serendipitous discoveries. It would also restrict the numbers of tissues available for retrospective studies. Autopsies help to eliminate suspicion, provide reassurance to families, and provide facts rather than conjecture by usually giving definitive answers. They may provide better medico-legal defense where required.

The instances in which limited tissue is available from living subjects, such as in neuro-pathology and cardiac pathology, offer the greatest potential for future research. Autopsy material is contributing most to research in neuroscience. In the future, autopsy research could be directed towards shock, neurological disorders, emerging infections, aging, metabolic disorders, environmental poisons, occupational disorders, and changes in disease patterns due to changing socio-economic factors. The proper use of molecular biology techniques in the autopsy is also likely to augment these endeavors.

Thus the words written in the anatomy amphitheatre at the university at Padua and at many autopsy rooms hold true even today 'Hic locus estubi mores gaudet succurrere vitae' — 'This is the place where death delights to help the living'. SAP

**AYURVEDIC MEDICINE** See INDIA; THEORIES OF ILLNESS

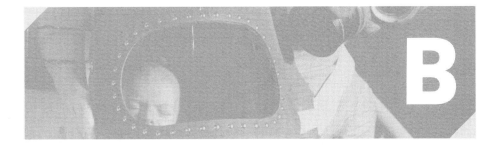

**B**

**BARBER-SURGEONS, COMPANY OF** Granted a Royal Charter by Henry VIII in 1540 at the behest of his personal barber-surgeon Thomas VICARY (this page), the United Company of Barber-Surgeons took the first step in separating the two trades (not complete for another 200 years) and brought together various guilds (such as 'The Mystery and Commonalty of the Barbers and Surgeons of London') which had been scattered and separate. Surgeons were no longer required to be barbers, and barbers were limited to dental surgery. Rules of apprenticeship were laid down, and fines for unlicensed practitioners specified. The Company was empowered to receive the bodies of four executed criminals each year for dissection and anatomical study. The new Company, however, was unable to narrow the gulf between surgeon and physician.

*See also* ANATOMY

**BATTERED BABY SYNDROME** See CHILD ABUSE AND NEGLECT

**BATTLE NEUROSIS** In every conflict in history some servicemen and women have suffered symptoms, inexplicable in terms of physical wounds, which have rendered them incapable of continuing to fight. Some were men whose bravery and endurance had been established in the field, others were newcomers to combat, and yet others were combatants who appeared to have been worn down by the constant demands upon their store of courage. Early Greek, Biblical writings, and Shakespeare include descriptions of such experiences in battle.

Spanish military doctors in the Thirty Years' War (1618–48) used the expression *estar rota* (to be on the point of breakdown) to describe the state of soldiers who could no longer endure battle. Swiss practitioners of this period used the term *nostalgia* to describe a condition of exhaustion, impaired concentration, and loss of appetite among mercenary troops.

Nostalgia associated with longing for a home which was idealized beyond the often harsh reality, with considerable depression and loss of

efficiency, was a major problem during the Napoleonic Wars but did not usually attract much sympathy. Malingering and/or self-inflicted wounds became a matter of concern, and some have claimed that there were nearly as many on disability pensions as those serving in the armed forces. Wellington, like Clausewitz before him, recognized the debilitating effects of battle and wrote: 'Both mind and feelings are exhausted, I am wretched even at the moment of victory, and I always say that next to a battle lost, the greatest misery is a battle gained'.

The American Civil War (1861–5) was the first conflict to approach 'total war', and it was not until the end of the Vietnam War that the combined totals of casualties in all American wars exceeded those of this war. 'Nostalgia or depression' was common and some medical officers recognized that many men died of this condition, despite the fact that a short period of leave from the army might be life-saving. Alcoholism and malingering were also problems. Dr Silas Weir Mitchell, the inventor of the 'rest cure' for neurasthenia, opened a special neurology hospital in Philadelphia in 1863 to detect malingering. George Beard, another Civil War medical officer, afterwards described 'neurasthenia', which was probably based on his war experience but became a fashionable diagnosis among women of leisure.

Da Costa described what has been variously termed as 'soldier's heart', 'irritable heart', or disorderly action of the heart. He noted that many of the soldiers affected had not been involved in combat but had suffered disruption of their normal lives and been obliged to face hardships and unaccustomed physical activity. They suffered breathlessness, fatigue and exhaustion, palpitations and faintness after even modest exercise. The use of artillery with rifling of the barrel ensured more accurate shell fire and 'windage', the precursor of shell shock, was invoked to describe the often bizarre effects of the close passage of shells.

The Crimean War (1853–6) was noted for drunkenness, and many soldiers were unable or unwilling to go into battle without liberal quantities of alcohol. The medical officers were pre-

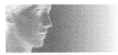

Thomas **VICARY** (d. 1561). British surgeon. Vicary was Master of the Barbers' Company in 1530 and in 1548 was made a governor of St Bartholomew's Hospital in charge of the surgeons. Appointed surgeon to Henry VIII in 1528, he became serjeant-surgeon in 1536 and later to Edward VI, Mary, Philip, and Elizabeth I. He features in Holbein's painting, receiving from Henry VIII in 1541 the Act of Incorporation of the Company of Barber-Surgeons, in the formation of which he was instrumental.

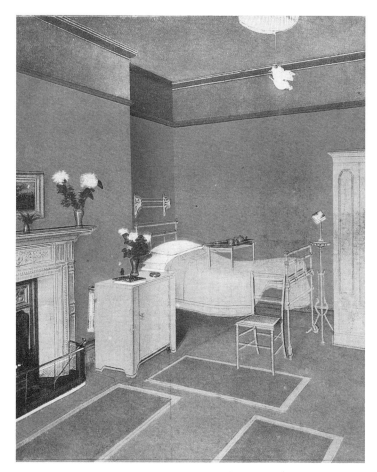

H. Kemp-Prossor's color-cure ward for shell-shock cases.
(Reproduced courtesy of the Mary Evans Picture Library.)

and desolation so familiar from photographs and films of the trenches do little to convey the daily experience of hardship and terror endured by the troops over four years. As the official medical history of the war records, 'during 1914 several men were evacuated from France to England having been "broken" by their experiences in the retreat from Mons'. Within a month, at the base hospitals in France, Lieutenant Colonel Gordon Holmes, an expert on disorders of the nervous system, saw 'frequent examples of gross hysterical conditions which were associated with trivial bullet or shell wounds or even with only slight contusions of the back, arms, or legs'. By the end of the year over 100 000 had been treated for nervous diseases, mainly for what the official history called a 'severe mental disability which rendered the individual, temporarily at any rate, incapable of further service'. By the end of the war 80 000 officers and men had been unable to continue in the trenches, and many had been invalided out of the army altogether for nervous disorders, including what came to be known as 'shell shock'. Sir Thomas LEWIS (p 188) studied 'soldiers' heart' which was 'a chief malady in the war; one such case was numbered for every four cases of wound'. Lewis preferred the term effort syndrome to distinguish it from valvular disease of the heart. By the summer of 1918, 70 000 cases had been classed as cardiovascular disease and of these 44 000 cases of effort syndrome became pensioners. In the last two years of the war it was found that 44% of those diagnosed as effort syndrome had symptoms on enlistment. It was also observed that 53% of effort syndrome cases were teetotal and the more severe cases drank less than those with mild symptoms. Lewis's book *The soldier's heart and the effort syndrome*, first published in 1918, was re-written and published in 1940. The troops received a regular rum ration and quite a number 'went over the top' in a state of inebriation. Some officers believed that this provided Dutch courage and did not impair effectiveness in the heat of battle.

## Shell shock

The asylum doctors of 1914 worked behind closed doors and rarely saw cases of neurosis, for a patient was usually certified insane before they met. Being concerned with the brain, neurologists assumed responsibility for the new discipline of PSYCHIATRY outside the asylums, and were most familiar with Charcot's hysteria. Freudian theory had little impact outside academia, and those medically qualified men who dabbled in it such as W. H. RIVERS (p 93) were usually dubbed psychologists. Academic psychology, on the other hand, was largely theoretical and laboratory based and had little contact with clinical work. The

occupied with malingering and had more than they could cope with in attempting to deal with the rampant infectious diseases. Disease and pestilence accounted for more illness and death than the wounds of war, and continued to do so in future conflicts until exceptionally the Russo-Japanese War (1904–5), when for the first time an army suffered more deaths from enemy action than from disease. This was a tribute to careful medical planning and scrupulous attention to hygiene. The Russians distinguished themselves by establishing forward clearing stations for psychiatric casualties, with good results.

Disorderly action of the heart or effort syndrome became a problem during the Indian Frontier wars, and in the Boer War, when a succession of unimaginative Commissions were inclined to impute the symptoms to unsound harnessing of the soldiers' equipment and to the somewhat rigid forms of drill which then prevailed.

The First World War (1914–18) was expected by the combatants to be over by Christmas but became a war of attrition. The scenes of carnage

various disciplines were thus ill-prepared to take on the task of diagnosing and even less treating those traumatized by the experience of war. C. S. Myers was appointed consulting psychologist to the British Army in 1916 and brought for the first time the recognition that 'shell shock' was a behavioral response to combat and not cowardice or malingering. Lewy reported that 69 394 US soldiers suffered 'neurosis' in World War I and the British Ministry of Pensions reported 120 000 cases of neurosis pensioned by March 1939.

Rivers, a neurophysiologist who practiced psychoanalysis, was brought in to work with the Royal Flying Corps after his success in treating shell-shocked army officers at Craiglockhart Military Hospital. This experience formed the basis for his book *Instinct and the unconscious* (1920), in which he observes 'traumatic neurasthenia, is especially known as the sequel of railway accidents, and since this form of neurosis closely resembles that due to warfare, our knowledge of war neurosis might have advanced more rapidly if this had been taken as a guide'. The War Office Committee of Inquiry into Shellshock (1922) struggled with the dilemma of distinguishing between cowardice and the stress of combat in World War I and failed to reach a satisfactory conclusion. In a scholarly review of soldiers shot for 'cowardice' during the First World War, Judge Anthony Babcock (1983) showed that most of the cases were men who either never should have been accepted for enlistment because of their mental state or were suffering from the effects of combat stress.

The Spanish Civil War (1936–9) was a brutal war in which the Republicans were aided by Russia and the International Brigades, while the 'Nationalist' insurgents were massively aided by the Fascist powers. John Dollard studied 300 survivors of the American Brigade, concluding that fear is a powerful motivating force in training and in battle. Seven out of ten men admitted fear when going into their first action but almost as many believed that fear, which is greatest just before action, diminishes the more times they go into action. Eight out of ten believed that it was better to admit fear and discuss it openly before battle, although they felt that its signs had to be controlled in battle. The most important factors in controlling fear were: devotion to the cause, leadership, training, and matériel. The presence of hunger, thirst, fatigue, ignorance of plans, and idleness increase the danger from fear. Fear may stimulate a soldier to fight harder and better if danger to the self also suggests danger to the unit or cause.

In World War II psychic collapse became known as 'battle fatigue' or 'combat exhaustion', language understandable to front-line troops and an accept-able medical diagnosis. Psychiatrists were attached to Army groups and began to emphasize the value of early, rapid, accessible, and short-term treatment of nervous exhaustion. Troops suffering from battle exhaustion were placed under sedation for 48 hours and removed to a safe situation within the divisional area. They remained soldiers under military discipline and underwent a short period of rehabilitation before being returned to appropriate duties. An estimated 65% of British psychiatric casualties were returned to full combat duty in under two weeks. The principle of PIE (proximity, immediacy, and expectancy) became the accepted policy of military psychiatry.

In the German forces there was no comparable system, and battle exhaustion and other psychiatric disorders received little sympathy. On the Eastern Front the German Army suffered a high incidence of psychiatric illness. In 1942 the German High Command response was to tighten military discipline. All breaches of discipline, regardless of whether these resulted from physical exhaustion, psychiatric breakdown, or unbearable provocation, were treated with the utmost severity. By mid-1944 107 000 German soldiers had been tried for absence without leave, and a further 49 000 for disobedience. Over 7000 were executed for desertion and subversion, compared with only 48 in the First World War. Suicides among German troops also increased appreciably at the end of the war, some 10 000 of them occurring in those with battle neurosis.

## Medical discharges

Over one-third of medical discharges from the allied armed forces were the result, not of physical injury or sickness, but of psychiatric disorders. Over half the psychiatric disorders were 'anxiety cases', stemming directly from combat stress or from many sources, including separation from families and domestic problems. Other reasons for psychiatric discharge were, in descending order of prevalence, 'psychoses', 'mental deficiency', and 'psychopathic personality' — diagnoses rarely declared in senior officers. Deserters were usually dealt with by executive action without taking medical advice, although many were victims of war neurosis.

In World War II the US Army reported only 4000 deserters and the British Army over 100 000. The discrepancy was almost certainly the result of the American Army charging many men with absence without leave rather than desertion, which carried the death penalty. The latter was applied only once, when Private Slovak was executed in 1945 as an example to others. In May 1942 General Auchinleck was so disturbed by the number of deserters during the Desert Campaigns that he recommended the re-introduction

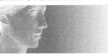

of the death penalty — a request which was denied by the War Office. British and American deserters were almost always infantrymen, mostly very young, and a high percentage of the men were with psychological problems or low intelligence. Many had been poorly adjusted in civilian life before service. After the evacuation from Dunkirk many men were found to be suffering from effort syndrome but most recovered rapidly. Sargent and Slater used a variety of techniques in treatment including drug abreaction (assisted release of repressed emotion). Aubrey Lewis reported a large study showing that 70% manifested anxiety and 50% depression. He diagnosed 18% as psychopaths, 11% as hysterics, and 4% as high grade mental defectives.

After Dunkirk the only offensive action that could be taken in Europe was the bombing campaign. The Royal Air Force was soon involved in nightly bombing raids often over long distances. Even in wartime the Royal Air Force was an entirely volunteer service, but once enlisted in the RAF and accepted for flying training it was not possible to resign. Refusal or inability to continue to fly, in the absence of sufficient medical cause, was regarded as indicative of moral weakness. It was feared that the exhibition of such 'moral' weakness would have a detrimental effect on the morale of others facing danger, and so it became policy to label those who refused to fly as 'Lacking in moral fiber' and they were stripped of rank badges and flying brevets, then LMF was stamped on their paybooks. Officers were reduced to the lowest commissioned rank and required to resign. Most were transferred as privates to the army but any remaining in the Air Force were given menial tasks. Those who went to civilian life were directed to employment at a low level.

What is remarkable is not that some failed to show aggressive spirit but that any could be persuaded to go on raids night after night, despite heavy casualties in their squadron. Since over 8000 British men were killed in accidents while in training, many men started with some fear of flying and more acquired such fears during their training. Some 100 000 men flew with British Bomber Command during the war and 55 573 were killed in action. Overall, between 1939 and 1945, for every 100 aircrew joining a heavy bomber crew in Operational Training Unit only 24 survived unharmed.

The overall figures for removal from flying duties for other than physical causes are:

| Year | Neurosis | Lacking in moral fiber |
|---|---|---|
| 1942–3 | 2503 | 416 |
| 1943–4 | 2989 | 301 |
| 1944–5 | 2910 | 306 |
| Total | 8402 | 1023 |

A third of all cases of lack of moral fiber were disposed of purely by executive action, without involving specialist medical referral. About one-third of neurosis cases came from Bomber Command, one-third from Flying Training Command, and one-third from other commands.

The Royal Navy in World War II was an entirely volunteer service, and it is claimed that their psychiatric casualties were low. In action they served in close communities aboard ship identified closely with their ship and mess, at action stations had clear commitments, and knew their senior ratings and officers — all of which acted as protective factors. More psychiatric breakdown was reported after rather than during action. The loss of a ship was always traumatic and many had to survive in open boats afterwards. There are several accounts of prolonged survival and of the mental states that may result, including collective hallucinations.

**Lessons learnt**
The lessons of every conflict seem to be forgotten before the next. Throughout the command chain there is a reluctance to accept that war neurosis could influence 'our chaps'. Fears are expressed about manpower and morale and the danger that 'loss of the will to fight will spread like wildfire'. People who are adequately trained fight not only for a cause but for their buddies, section, or unit. They identify with their unit, ship, squadron, or army and must have confidence in their leadership. If their cohesion is disrupted by an influx of replacements or they are transferred to other units they become vulnerable. Within these limits, sleep or food deprivation, adverse weather, intensity and duration of exposure to combat, and passive dangers such as mortars, shell fire, or bombing increase the risk of breakdown. In general the more immediate the treatment, the closer to the battle line and the more categorical the expectation of return to duty, the more effective the treatment, with a claimed 60% return rate to duty.                    SBra

*See also* CARDIOLOGY – HISTORY

Henry **BEECHER** (1904–76). American anesthesiologist and ethicist. Apart from wartime service in a field medical unit on the Anzio beachhead, Beecher spent his entire professional life at Harvard, ending up as a professor in his discipline and writing a history of its medical school after he had retired. He carried out important research, including work on the placebo effect and the effect of morphine on pain. His interest on the ethical aspects of research was aroused by reports of the Nuremberg trials, and he gradually became convinced that the ethics of some of the medical research then going on in the 1950s in the USA was debatable, exploring these issues in journal articles and a book *Experimentation in man*. Later, suspecting that the profession was not going to police itself, Beecher wrote an article discussing 22 published studies, where, in particular, informed consent had not been given for work that might entail risk to health or even life. He caused much angry and animated discussion among his colleagues, who reacted as establishments do. Even so, the public reaction led to adoption of the Declaration of Helsinki and the establishment of institutional review boards (called research ethics committees in Britain and elsewhere), where informed scrutiny of proposed research projects is now mandatory.

*See also* BIOETHICS; EXPERIMENTATION IN CHILDREN

**BELLEVUE HOSPITAL** in New York began as a six-bed infirmary in 1736 in a Public Workhouse and House of Correction. From that beginning it has become one of the foremost hospitals of the world, offering a vast range of services, being a public hospital for New York City. In 1811 it moved from the workhouse to its present site on the East River, where there are over 1000 beds, admitting 25 000 patients per annum. It has been a hospital for teaching students in all healthcare disciplines, and it has been an integral part of the New York University School of Medicine since 1968. This arose out of amalgamation of previous medical schools. The University now appoints all the medical staff, numbering about 1300. It is famed for its emergency services, and started the first American hospital-based ambulance service (1809). For the USA it was the first place for many advances, among them anatomy dissection (1750), lying-in wards (1799), a school of nursing (1873), and CESAREAN SECTION (1877). It was there that cardiac catheterization began and this won a NOBEL PRIZE for D. Richards and André Cournand.

**BENEFITS OF CARE** On 12 April 1945 the President of the United States of America Franklin D. Roosevelt died unexpectedly, aged 63. He was suffering from severe HYPERTENSION, for which no treatment was available at that time. As a result of hypertension he also suffered heart failure and kidney damage. The immediate cause of death, and also the direct result of uncontrolled hypertension, was cerebral hemorrhage with rapid loss of consciousness and death shortly afterwards. Writing on the anniversary of his death, Dr Franz Messerli reminded us that 'Today, 50 years later, a powerful therapeutic arsenal to treat all forms of hypertension is at the physician's disposal'.

It is startling to discover how little doctors had to offer during the first half of the 20th century, as a Chicago physician, Dr Theodore Schwartz,

found in reading the third edition of CABOT's (p 190) *Differential diagnosis*, published in 1915. 'Practitioners had available to them a limited number of specific therapies', Schwartz wrote, 'such as arsphenamine for syphilis and thyroid extract for hypothyroidism'. Dr Paul Beeson, Nuffield professor emeritus of clinical medicine at Oxford and an editor of the 1st edition of this *Companion*, compared treatments recommended in the first edition of Cecil's *Textbook of medicine* published in 1927 with its fourteenth edition fifty years later. Many of the recommendations of the first edition were clearly valueless or harmful. Fowler's solution (arsenic trioxide), for example, was recommended for at least forty diseases, including tuberculosis, pellagra, gastroptosis (dropped stomach), and Sydenham's chorea (jerky body movements).

Only 6% of recommended treatments in the 1927 edition were deemed by Beeson to be 'effective and helpful' or 'highly effective'. By 1975, 50% of treatments then recommended were considered effective or highly effective, reflecting how much had been achieved, and, at the same time, how much remains beyond our capacity to treat. As the scientist and author Lewis Thomas reminded us in 1977, 'We have come a long way, indeed, just to have learned enough to be conscious of our ignorance'. Two decades later there have been impressive gains in biomedical knowledge and its application, but the cure for much of human illness remains beyond our grasp.

**First half of the 20th century**
While medicine had few cures to offer in the first half of the 20th century, death rates in America fell from 1700 per 100 000 in 1900 to 840 per 100 000 in 1950 and life expectancy increased from 47.3 to 68.2 years, largely as a result of sanitation, personal hygiene, improved housing, and better nutrition. The first half of the century was one of improved public health and a remarkable reduction of death from infectious disease. Medicine's role in providing immunization against infectious diseases was important, but its contribution to the near doubling of life expectancy was relatively small and remained so until the mid-century 'epidemiologic transition', the shift in illness from one dominated by acute infections to the modern era, in which chronic illness dominates.

Based on the small role of medical care he attributed to the control of acute infections, the epidemiologist Thomas McKeown concluded that medicine as a whole contributes little to health. He based his conclusions mainly on how much of the fall in death rates from individual infections had preceded the introduction of immunization or treatment. His views, summarized in *The role of medicine* and published in 1977, have been

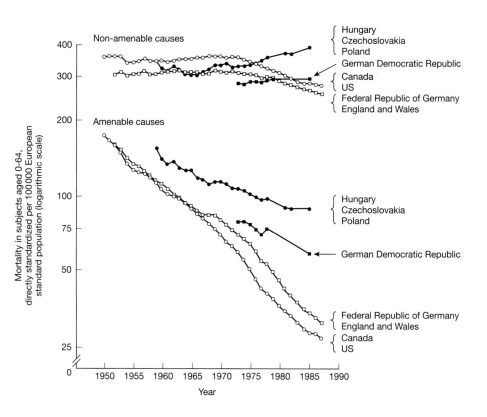

Trends in age-standardized mortality from amenable and non-amenable illness among individuals aged 0–64. The improvements in mortality in the Western democracies were achieved in appreciably different systems of health care. The more modest improvements achieved by Eastern European health systems has been attributed to organization and inefficiency in health services, and not to inadequate numbers of doctors or facilities, since they were comparable to those in the West. (From Boys, J. *et al.* (1991). *Mortality from causes amenable and non-amenable to medical care: the experience of Eastern Europe. British Medical Journal,* with permission.)

widely accepted by social analysts, students of health policy, and many doctors themselves. McKeown attributed the dramatic increase in life expectancy of the previous 100 years to 'provision of food, protection from hazards, and limitation of numbers', that is nutrition, sanitation and other public health measures, and population control; but he conceded that the evidence was no more than circumstantial. He believed that he had shown that medical care had had little effect and concluded that social and environmental factors must therefore have been responsible.

In a second edition McKeown acknowledged that 'it is not possible to estimate with any precision the contribution which therapeutic and other advances have made to the decline of the multiple non-infective causes of death which together were associated with a quarter of the reduction of mortality in this century'. He thus acknowledged the possibility that medical care had made a larger contribution, but as late as 1993 a *British Medical Journal* review of citations of *The role of medicine* concluded that the problem of a 'relatively small impact of clinical medicine on health outcomes [is] still with us'. More recent publications addressing the determinants of health barely mention the contribution of medical care, Ivan Illich and others arguing that it does more harm than good.

McKeown's conclusions did not go unchallenged. Distinguished leaders in medicine argued that medicine does indeed do good. But at that time they were unable to muster epidemiological data with which to mount a rebuttal. Walsh McDermott, emeritus professor of public health at Cornell University, wrote that 'what a doctor does is something that is extraordinarily difficult to analyze and measure'. Professor Beeson expressed disappointment that 'although most clinicians do not doubt that there has been substantial improvement in the treatment of disease during the past few decades, it is difficult to assess the dimensions'.

McKeown has more recently been criticized for his failure to acknowledge the central part played by doctors in the implementation of sanitation and other public health measures; for ignoring the introduction by doctors of hospital isolation that helped to reduce the spread of TUBERCULOSIS early in the 20th century; and for discounting the importance of immunization against SMALLPOX and diphtheria. But McKeown's main conclusion that medical care, narrowly defined as the care of individual patients, had contributed relatively little to the dramatic increase in life expectancy earlier in the century is roughly correct.

McKeown drew his conclusions from public health data for the years before 1971. The quarter century that followed saw an explosion of new treatments, many shown in clinical trials to result in marked improvements in health. Epidemiologic evidence crediting medical care with the extension of life began to appear. The American economist Jack Hadley compared the expenditures of the government's Medicare program for the elderly with regional death rates and calculated that for every 10% increase in expenditure there had been a 1 to 2% fall in mortality. Death rates have continued to fall for all ages and for almost all diseases, but death rates for those diseases considered 'amenable to treatment' were found to fall at much greater rates than death rates for diseases not considered to respond favorably to treatment.

Conflicting data also appeared, however. National age-adjusted death rates were reported to be greater in countries with greater numbers of doctors, and presumably with more medical care. Similarly, death rates for diseases amenable to treatment were found to be greatest in areas with the most medical care resources. Efforts to separate the effects of medical care for an entire population from those of other determinants of health have been fraught with similar difficulties. To overcome these difficulties, my colleagues and I examined the effects of individual medical interventions, one at a time, to create an inventory of their benefits in increasing life expectancy and improving the quality of life.

### Extending the length of life

Life expectancy in America rose by 23 years from 1900 to 1950 and another 7.6 years between 1950 and 1995. (Life expectancy in England and Wales rose by almost the same amount during the same periods.) Falling numbers of deaths from heart disease made by far the greatest contribution to the improvement, accounting for as much as a third of the fall in death rate from all causes since 1950. Even more remarkably, the death rate from cerebrovascular diseases, primarily stroke, fell more than three-fold during the same period.

Based on an analysis of clinical trials, it is estimated that as much as 70% of the decline in cardiac deaths can be attributed to coronary care units, treatment of hypertension, and medical and surgical treatment of coronary artery disease. The diagnosis and treatment of hypertension, by contributing to the dramatic fall in stroke, are also responsible for an important but smaller proportion of the fall in deaths from stroke, equivalent to an increase in life expectancy of 2.5 to 3 months. The treatment of appendicitis, DIABETES, and end-stage renal disease each contributed about a third of a year increase in life expectancy, with lesser contributions from the treatment of several other conditions. Altogether, clinical services, composed of clinical preventive services as well as clinical curative services, can be credited with 5–5$\frac{1}{2}$ of the 30 years' increase in life expectancy since 1900, and roughly half of the 7.6 years of increased life expectancy since 1950.

The 5–5$\frac{1}{2}$ years' increase in life expectancy attributed to medical care is roughly equivalent to a halving of death rates at every age. To put this in perspective, it is roughly equal (and opposite) to the increase in death rate and loss of life expectancy that an individual suffers by smoking a pack of cigarettes a day starting at age 20; and it is roughly equivalent to the difference in life expectancy between the well-off and better educated, on the one hand, and the relatively poor and less well-educated, on the other.

Estimating the contribution of medical care to an improvement in the quality of life requires a somewhat different approach. Complex measurements of quality of life are now in widespread use in clinical research, but only fragmentary data are available by which to estimate the impact of medical care on the quality of life of a population. Ideally, there should be a single index of quality of life comparable with that for life expectancy. One current candidate for this purpose, popular among economists, is the quality-adjusted life year, or QALY. This may be useful as a semi-quantitative basis for resource allocation: it incorporates information on both life expectancy and quality of life, and by providing a single number may give an impression of precision. However, the quality of life component is entirely subjective and may be a poor reflection of what patients actually value.

Whatever its merits in setting priorities for the purchase of medical services, the quality-adjusted life year is of little use to doctors or patients in making clinical decisions. It does not help to answer the patient's question, 'Doctor, will the cataract operation allow me to read again?', nor will it help the doctor to instruct a patient in balancing the risks of stroke or heart attack against the unpleasant side effects of antihypertensive therapy or the pleasures of smoking. To measure these and similar questions more precisely, there are broader, 'multidimensional' indices of quality of life that measure functional status, mental health, and subjective well-being. These are useful in research, but a global index of quality of life would be useful to patients and doctors, and could be used to estimate this important component of medicine's contribution to a population's health.

Global measures of disability-free years and of health-adjusted life years may be estimated for a population, but these present the same problem as do global death rates: there is no way of identifying the effect of disease-specific treatments, let alone how much each contributes. A more useful approach is to estimate the improvement in the quality of life, or more specifically, relief of the poor quality of life associated with individual illnesses.

When medical care is successful in improving the quality of life, or in relieving poor quality of life, it does so in many ways: by relieving pain, shortness of breath, or depression; by restoring function; by improving vision; by preventing stroke; by lessening the likelihood of incurring the debilitating fractures that often occur with osteoporosis. If we want to summarize such disparate conditions, we are faced with a definitional problem. There is, however, a common denominator: severe chronic disease manifests itself in ways that profoundly depress quality of life; these manifestations may be readily measured in months and years and added up, presenting an impressive inventory of the burden of chronic disease. Their prevention or improvement also may be measured to provide an equally impressive index of medicine's contribution to health. On average, based on such an inventory, an individual is spared roughly five years of poor quality life directly as a result of medical care.

Important contributors to the estimated five years of decreased poor quality life include: the diagnosis and treatment of hypertension in decreasing the number of non-fatal, as well as fatal heart attacks and strokes; the diminution of the suffering that peptic ulcer and gall bladder disease cause; the diminution of cough, wheezing, and shortness of breath in ASTHMA. POLIOMYELITIS with paralysis has all but disappeared after the introduction of the Salk and Sabin vaccines. The pain and dysfunction of knee and hip arthritis can be relieved by knee and hip replacement. The widespread and profoundly disabling effects of depression can now be largely controlled with medication. The severe pain of terminal cancer can be almost entirely controlled. The impaired vision of senile cataracts can be corrected surgically. Migraine headaches can be lessened if not prevented.

## Measuring the benefits of visiting the doctor

What happens between the doctor and patient during a medical visit has a profound impact on outcome. Its importance is unquestioned, but it has generally been assumed that it cannot be measured. On close examination, however, there is considerable evidence of benefits. Some can be readily measured: the general practitioner, as primary care doctor, is, by definition, a gate-keeper shielding each patient from the risks of overtreatment, as well as treating or referring for further evaluation and treatment as appropriate. The assessment and recommendation for or against therapeutic intervention have major impacts on outcome, where its magnitude is reflected in two- and three-fold varia-

tions in rates of medical and surgical intervention that patients receive. How the doctor's evaluation is communicated to a patient also has a large impact on outcome. Poor communication about the risks and benefits of therapeutic drugs is probably largely responsible for the failure of a third to half of patients in America to adhere to prescribed drug regimens.

The decision to perform discretionary surgery is similarly affected by the information and advice given to the patient. Variations in surgeons' so-called 'practice-styles', their preferences for one or another therapeutic approach, account for large differences in the number of operations performed and their outcome. When adequately informed, the patient's participation has already resulted in large changes in the number of operations performed for benign prostatic hypertrophy and for early breast cancer.

## Knowledge and belief

Knowledge and belief are also key determinants of a patient's peace of mind. The provision of information can enhance patients' sense of control and, perhaps, optimism, each of which is strongly associated with improved health. Individuals who believe that their health is good live longer than others who manifest similar objective measures of health, but who assess their health as poor. Men recovering from heart attack who comply with prescribed medicine, whether an active drug or a placebo, and who can be assumed to have a more optimistic view of their prospects, die at half the rate of those who fail to take the randomly prescribed medication, whether an active drug or placebo.

The provision of information alone has an important value independent of its use in any medical decision, as physicians at the University of Pennsylvania argue in an article entitled *Knowing for the sake of knowing: the value of prognostic information*. Others have shown that information has monetary value to patients, even if it does not contribute to a medical decision, and that patients provided with the results of diagnostic tests may return to full activity earlier, independent of their clinical usefulness.

## Benefits in context

The importance of medical care in extending life in the first half of the century was surely small, as McKeown claimed in *The role of medicine*. More relevant at the start of a new century is how the current contributions of medicine compare with other factors that affect health.

How we choose to live — that is, whether we smoke, whether we consume alcohol (and how much), whether we are overweight (again by how much), whether we are active or sedentary, and our sexual activity — is important to health. The

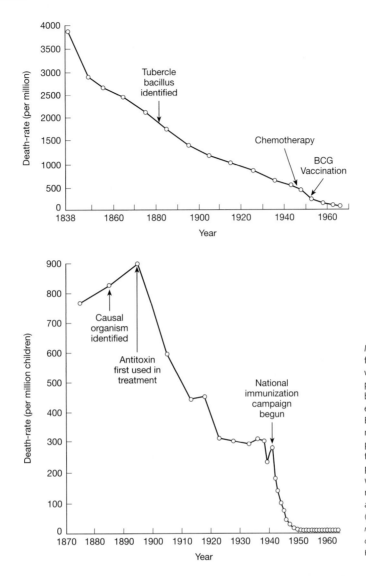

Mortality from tuberculosis fell sharply from the time it was first recorded, a large part of the decline occurring before the introduction of effective treatment in 1947. Equally dramatic declines in mortality and morbidity took place in advance of effective treatment or prevention of poliomyelitis, measles, and whooping cough. Diphtheria represents a major exception, as seen in the lower figure. (From McKeown, T. (1976). *The role of medicine: dream, mirage, or nemesis?* Nuffield Provincial Hospitals Trust, London.)

combined effect of these factors may be responsible for as much as five years' difference in life expectancy: that is, the overweight life-time smoker with a heavy alcohol intake can expect to die, on average, at least five years earlier than an individual who leads a healthier life. He loses about as much in life expectancy as medicine offers gains. Little, if any, of the increase in life expectancy during this half century can be attributed to better health habits. Tobacco-induced lung cancer has increased more than three-fold, and, together with the contribution of tobacco to heart disease, is responsible for a loss of more than a year of the life expectancy of a population consisting of one third to one half of smokers. Smoking by men has begun to fall, and deaths

from lung cancer have begun to drop, but not for women. The drop in smoking by men may have contributed to the fall in cardiac deaths, but not enough to offset the impact of the increase in deaths from lung cancer.

Other life-style risk factors have smaller but important effects on longevity. No credit can be given to them for lengthening life, however, for the proportion of overweight persons in America has increased from 25% in 1960 to 35% in 1994, with similar increases in Britain. There has been a recent small drop in alcohol consumption, any effect of which on life expectancy has been more than offset by the rise in deaths attributed to AIDS (acquired immunodeficiency syndrome).

Health and longevity also vary widely with the quality of the social and physical environment. While bad quality of environmental air can have serious deleterious effects on health, its effects on an entire population have been carefully studied and judged to be small. By contrast, the social environment — that is, the everyday circumstances of our lives — appears to have profound effects. The wealthy and better educated live longer and are healthier than the poor. It is not simply a question of poverty and deprivation, however. Health appears to be strongly related to the social circumstances of our professional lives. A striking example of this is provided by the Whitehall study of British civil servants. This found that administrators are healthier and live longer than senior managers; that senior managers are healthier than those they manage; and that middle managers and technical staff are healthier than those at the bottom of the occupational ladder.

Health is also strongly related to the social circumstances of our personal lives: whether we have strong family and social bonds, and whether we are active in community affairs. In a survey of the residents of Alameda County, California, individuals who were married lived longer than those who were single or widowed, and those who belonged to active social groups (that is, those who are part of a broader 'social network') were the healthiest and lived the longest. Studies in other countries have shown much the same relationship of social and economic circumstances to health and longevity.

## Conclusions

Our health, including how long we live, is the result of an interplay of our inheritance, of the social and physical environment, of the life-style we adopt, and of the benefits of modern medical care. Our inheritance we can do little about. The quality of the physical environment, while often hazardous in the past, has been markedly improved and appears to play only a small part today in observed differences in health among populations. The social environment appears to have a large impact on health, but the mechanism of its effect and how to improve the health of those at risk are unknown. In contrast to the effects of the social environment, however, much is known about the mechanisms by which poor health habits result in poor health, and the benefits of an improved life-style have been well elucidated. Despite this body of knowledge, only a small segment of the population has chosen to adopt healthier habits. In contrast, the potential of medical care can now be clearly demonstrated, and a large measure of the potential has already been realized.

The potential impact of life-style, the social environment, and medical care on health are roughly of the same order of magnitude: medical care can halve death rates; the individual who chooses not to smoke has half the mortality of the smoker; the individual at the bottom of the social/occupational/income ladder has double the mortality of those at the top (and three times or more the mortality if he smokes, is overweight, and is inactive). How much of the potential of each has been realized? What was the contribution of each for the dramatic increase in life expectancy during the 20th century, and more importantly, during the past 50 years? What are their current contributions and their potential for further improvement of the public's health?

Although medical care made an important, but relatively small, contribution to the dramatic increase in life expectancy in the first half of the 20th century, it has made a major impact in the past fifty years, it continues to do so, and there is well-documented potential for further benefit. Apart from smoking, life-style, by contrast, cannot be credited with any past or present improvements in health. Smoking may have had relatively little impact on health at the beginning of the century, for smoking was limited to a smaller segment of the population and deaths from lung cancer were uncommon; while there has been an important recent fall in smoking among men, the century-long negative impact of smoking on health is large. The population has become more sedentary and increasingly overweight over the past few decades and cannot be credited with any of the improvement in health. Likewise, there is no basis for claiming benefits for an improvement in the social environment or for any lessening of inequalities in education and income.

How, then, should society attempt to improve its health? Further efforts to adopt a healthier life-style should certainly be encouraged, but there is little reason for optimism that the public will respond. There are continuing calls for the creation of a more just society, one that is socially more cohesive, and where the distribution of the rewards of an increasingly productive industry is fairer, at the start of the 21st century. However, the discrepancy in wealth and education across the population has widened and continues to grow. The benefits of medical care, by contrast, are large and continue to expand.

If the benefits of medical care are indeed large; if they can be expected to continue to grow; and if they are already greater than we seem willing to pay for, the question society faces is whether they can be afforded. The American economist William Baumol offers an authoritative answer. It is simply a question of how we want to spend the resources and money that an increasingly productive economy makes available. Baumol argues that 'productivity growth in the entire economy means that we can afford more of everything'. If the hours of labor that need to be invested in manufacturing and agriculture continue to fall as they have, more hours of labor are available for medical care, and for other labor-intensive social goods, notably education and the arts. The choice is ours. JPBun

*See also* HYPERTENSION; SKEPTICS; SMOKING AND HEALTH

**BEREAVEMENT** is the term that describes the reaction to loss and includes both the emotional reactions of grief and mourning and the psychological process of relinquishing bonds to the person who has died. The process of resolution of loss may take place over a long time, but for most adults the acute distress of grief lessens progressively in the first few months. This may continue to some degree throughout the first year and with anniversaries or reminders. Losses other than death, for instance, through divorce or separation, injury or illness, or loss of home or country, may also lead to grief and mourning.

The experience of loss is universal and bereavement may occur at any stage of life. It is therefore important to understand the patterns of grief and mourning at different developmental stages and the ways in which loss is adapted to. Different social and cultural influences may also have significance — for instance, role definitions for those bereaved, funeral practice, and the time in which 'recovery' is expected. While these factors may not alter the psychological features of grief, they may define the social behaviors and cultural rituals that ease the aftermath of a loss.

Bereavement is always stressful, involving as it does major life change. Although most people adapt successfully, a few experience untoward health and social consequences. Some circumstances of death and loss are particularly stressful, and may produce greater difficulties of adaptation, for instance, sudden or untimely deaths; deaths of children; violent deaths, such as homicide or suicide; and multiple deaths or losses occurring close together.

Bowlby provided new understandings of grief in his classic description of attachment theory, separation response, and loss. His work has contributed to an understanding of 'normal' and pathological grief, including the phases or stages of grief. However, these stages are not defined entities, but rather dimensions of normal response.

## Normal bereavement

Bereavement has been studied mainly in adults, often following the death of a spouse. Burnett and his colleagues developed a 17-item measure of bereavement phenomena, and used this to study patterns of grief in three non-clinical populations of bereaved adults after the death of a spouse, partner, and child, with more intense grief in the last group. They showed three principal dimensions which diminished incrementally over time: separation, grief, and preoccupation with images of the lost person. A similar pattern was shown by Byrne and Raphael in older widowed men. Items on this scale overlap strongly with those of Jacobs, who described initial numbness or denial, separation distress, and mourning with systematic measures for each dimension.

Bereavement reactions in children are influenced by their development, their relationship to the person who has died, their cognitive understandings of death and its permanency, and the ongoing security and support of their family environment. They too show separation distress and mourning, but these may be intermittent or disguised by behavioral disturbance or withdrawal. It may be difficult for parents and other adults to recognize and respond to a child's grief when their own is overwhelming.

## Pathological bereavement

Bereavement is pathological if it encompasses unusual patterns of grief and mourning, if it is manifest in specific psychiatric disorder (for instance, depression), or if it leads to illness.

The two main forms of pathological grief, reflecting abnormalities in intensity and duration, are chronic grief and absent, inhibited, or delayed grief. Other differing, but overlapping, syndromes include complicated grief disorder and traumatic grief.

All these syndromes show high and continuing levels of intense yearning, longing, preoccupation, and distress about the deceased, of sufficient intensity and duration to disrupt normal functioning. These syndromes are notoriously difficult to treat, the more so because of the bereaved's intense focus on and inability to relinquish ties to the deceased, who is often idealized.

Bereavement has been described and even measured as a model of reactive depression. Questions of whether pathological bereavement is a form of depression have been addressed in several recent reports. There is evidence that, while depressive disorder may be a complication of bereavement, anxiety disorders are also prevalent, and that both are distinct from the phenomenon of bereavement, even when these are intensified to pathological levels.

Clearly if specific disorders supervene, particularly in bereaved people who are vulnerable, those affected should be treated using the best available evidence of effective interventions specifically for the syndromes they present with.

At the same time the issue of grief counseling should be addressed.

Another possible disorder that may overlap with or complicate bereavement is post-traumatic stress disorder. When the circumstances of a death are particularly traumatic — for instance, disaster or violent deaths — then a post-traumatic stress response may appear, locking the person in the traumatic experience, and blocking grieving. A key clinical issue is the identification of such a reaction as separate from bereavement phenomena, and the need for counseling to deal with trauma specifically in addition to grief. This may have to be done in ways that are sensitive to the profound stress involved in such circumstances, and the need to deal with these issues progressively in 'doses' that the bereaved can bear.

Other adverse health outcomes of grief may be an adverse impact on immune functioning and increased mortality. Further research is necessary to clarify the mechanisms of such pathologies of grief when they do occur, but with recognition that most people deal with loss and adapt in their own personal ways to their altered life circumstances.

### Bereavement counseling and other interventions

The distress of those bereaved evokes a natural human response to comfort and console. Recognition that they may not have the social support or personal resources they need to resolve their distress has led to the development of a powerful movement to provide bereavement or grief counseling. There is no evidence that counseling is necessary for those who are grieving normally. However, those at high risk, through either an overly intense reaction, lack of social support, particularly traumatic circumstances of death or particular losses, have been shown to be assisted to better resolution and fewer pathological outcomes. Skilled intervention focusing on grief resolution and enhanced support, intervention by trained volunteer counselors, and self-help have all been shown to be effective for those at high risk after the death of a spouse. A self-help resource kit and support are effective for those at risk after the death of an infant, while family grief intervention is promising for high-risk bereaved families.

Self-help movements for grief also play a part in support, models of recovery, and guidance in social adaptation. There have been systematic studies of psychotherapies showing beneficial outcomes for those with complicated grief. Intervention programs for bereaved children, particularly family counseling, education, and support, have been shown to assist their handling of a loss in the family, even the death of a parent. It is essential, however, that grief is not unduly medicalized; that counseling should be based on the best available evidence of what is likely to be effective; and that it is sensitive to the person's experience, culture, and needs.

### Conclusion

Grief and bereavement are universal human experiences. Learning to grieve and adapt to loss and change are vital personal strengths that should be supported through childhood and adolescence when any loss is faced. Recognition of the normal bereavement response and specific support and counseling for those at risk of bereavement pathology can ease resolution and adaptation for most people. Personal growth also follows loss, with internalization and memories of the lost person and the tribute that grief itself pays to the value of a lost relationship. It has been suggested that the capacity to grieve reinforces essential social bonds, and is a quintessential part of the resilience of the human spirit.                          BR

*See also* DISASTERS; POST-TRAUMATIC STRESS DISORDER

Claude **BERNARD** (1813–78). French physiologist. The son of a vine-grower in the Rhone, after an apprenticeship to a pharmacist and an attempted career as a playwright, Bernard entered the medical school in Paris, qualifying in 1839. He became research assistant to François Magendie at the Collége de France, where he obtained his MD in 1843 with a thesis on the role of gastric juice in the digestion process. He directed his research towards experimental physiology and in 1847 he was appointed lecturer at the Collége de France. In 1852, on the retirement of Magendie, he took on most of the latter's duties, and in 1854 a chair of general physiology in the faculty of sciences at the Sorbonne was created for him. The following year, on Magendie's death, he succeeded him as professor of medicine at the Collége de France. He received numerous honors, including election to the Académie Française and in 1869, he was appointed to the senate by the decree of Emperor Napoleon III. He died in February 1878 of nephritis, receiving a public funeral, the first French scientist to be so honored. One of the greatest physiologists of the 19th century, Bernard was the founder of experimental medicine. His research included the role of the pancreas in the digestion of fat; the function of the liver; the effects of nerves on metabolism; the physiology of fetal tissues and the nutritive role of the placenta; and the suffocating effect of carbon monoxide chemically reacting with hemoglobin. He published widely in the publications of the Academy of Sciences and the *Archives Générales de Médicine* and his treatise *An introduction to the study of*

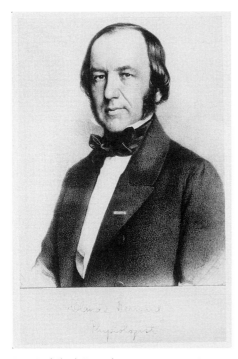

Portrait of Claude Bernard. (Reproduced courtesy of the National Cancer Institute, Bethesda, MD.)

*experimental medicine* was published in 1865. Bernard has two claims to fame: firstly, as an experimenter in his own right, developing new techniques and apparatus and particularly in his insistence on the importance of the milieu intérieur (the consistency of the internal environment); and, secondly, as a teacher, attracting students from all over the world.

**BETHLEM ROYAL HOSPITAL AND THE MAUDSLEY HOSPITAL,** London, have a record of service over several centuries to the mentally ill. The Royal Hospital was founded in 1247 by Simon Fitzmary, alderman of the City of London, and twice sheriff. He gave all his lands in the City to the church of St Mary of Bethlehem to found a priory in London to receive priests of that church when visiting England. The name was contracted to Bethlem, and a corruption of it became bedlam, a new word for the language. There were many early vicissitudes, but by the 14th century it had become a hospice, caring for the sick, wayfarers, and pilgrims. By 1403 it is known that six of the inmates were mentally ill. In 1547 it was incorporated as a royal foundation for the reception of the mentally ill. From then the governance of the hospital was bound up with the other royal hospitals of St Bartholomew's, St Thomas's, Christ's Hospital (an educational foundation), and Bridewell (part house of correction, part prison

for debtors). In 1556 governors were appointed to Christ's and Bethlem, and a year later to Bridewell and Bethlem. This board had a continuous existence until 1948 — the advent of the National Health Service. The old hospital at Bishopsgate in the City was vacated in 1676 for a new building on London Wall. At this time the inmates were exposed to public view for entertainment, and the name of bedlam was applied. However, as public opinion and that of the medical profession changed, the care of the mentally ill became more humane. The hospital was entirely charitable, and at first would not keep patients for over a year, whether they were cured or not. Whatever their state they were then given over to their relatives and friends. This, too, changed over the years and accommodation was provided for the incurable. The fabric of the City hospital decayed rapidly, so in 1815 the hospital was moved to Southwark, to the south and over the river Thames. The site and part of this building remain as the Imperial War Museum. An unusual feature was for the accommodation of Criminal Lunatics, as they were then called. This function of caring for the criminally insane was transferred to Broadmoor in 1863–4. From about this time, gentle humane care began to be practiced, and teaching of students also began. Admissions then also included members of the middle classes as well as paupers. Because of lack of space a unit was built at Witley in Surrey, but this was closed and the hospital finally moved to Beckenham in Kent, on the outskirts of London, when buildings were opened in 1930. In the meantime outpatient departments had been started, and in 1924 the school was admitted as part of the University of London. In 1948 with the start of the NHS the link with Bridewell was broken and the hospital joined with the Maudsley Hospital.

*See also* HOSPITALS; PSYCHIATRY

**BIBLE** It is doubtful if any book in the history of mankind has so decisively affected the developed world as the Bible. It is an incomparable history book and can be used to learn about man's past, including the history of his health. Even so, authors of the books that comprise the Bible record events from their own perspective, which is not necessarily that of the physician today. A good example of this — and the only disease which is fully described in both the *Old* and *New Testaments* — is LEPROSY. The term 'leprosy' has changed its meaning over the centuries. Formerly, it denoted almost any skin condition and as used in the Bible it probably covered scabies, ringworm, psoriasis, and other eruptions. The leprosy of buildings mentioned in *Leviticus* was most likely some kind of fungoid growth such as dry rot.

Pestilence and PLAGUE are frequently mentioned. Modern medical sleuths regularly debate

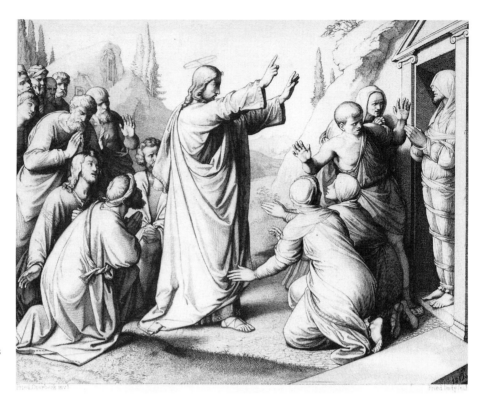

Etching by F. Ludy showing Christ raising Lazarus from his tomb. (Reproduced courtesy of the Wellcome Institute Library, London.)

whether these were accounts of, for example, bubonic or pneumonic plague, TYPHOID, CHOLERA, TYPHUS, SMALLPOX, and INFLUENZA. The primary method of waging war in Biblical times was to encircle the enemy's town, thereby cutting off food supplies to try to force a surrender because of famine. Naturally this took many months and there was ample opportunity for the water supply of both the besiegers and the besieged to become contaminated, particularly from cesspits. This might lead to epidemics of cholera and typhoid, which would spread quickly, as would other diseases such as plague, smallpox, typhus, or influenza, especially amongst the people who were enclosed within the walls of the city.

The Bible gives graphic pen pictures of disease and medical treatment. Did the boy Mephibosheth suffer from poliomyelitis? Was it meningitis which affected the child of the Shunammite woman? Had Jacob a slipped disc after his wrestling match? Did Nabal have a cerebral hemorrhage due to hypertension (he had a history of bad temper perhaps caused by headaches), or did he suffer a coronary thrombosis? Mouth-to-mouth artificial respiration might have caused the revival of the widow's son by Elijah, or even have been used by God to breathe life into Adam. Until modern antibiotics came along, the poultice of

figs used by King Hezekiah would be regarded as the best treatment for a boil. The book of *Daniel* describes the first controlled clinical trial and as a result of its success all prisoners were fed the same diet as Daniel, Shadrach, Meshach, and Abednego.

It has long been recognized that there is a logical medical sequence to the plagues of Egypt; indeed, they might be regarded as celestial biological warfare. Owing to a high level of silt from the Abyssinian mountains after heavy rainfall, the river Nile increased its flow and turned red. The large amount of silt caused the dissolved oxygen level in the water to fall. Because of this, many fish in the Nile died from lack of oxygen and were no longer present to eat frogspawn. The second plague of frogs followed and they spread over the surrounding land during the annual Nile flood. As the increase in silt, flooding, and frogs were all regular happenings the Egyptian 'magicians' could forecast their occurrence. When the floods receded the rotting corpses of the frogs stank and became infested with maggots. This led to the third plague of lice (maggots according to the *New English Bible* translation). The maggots pupated into the fourth plague of flies. The fifth plague was probably a cattle disease spread by ticks called babesiosis. The sixth plague of boils and sores may have occurred because of a lack of water, which meant that dirty clothes chafed the bodies of the Egyptians causing sores. The seventh and later plagues have no obvious medical explanation.

Moses is sometimes described as the first medical officer of health and the books of *Leviticus* and *Numbers* as a PUBLIC HEALTH textbook. In the 14th century, Venice, Ragusa (the modern Dubrovnik), and Marseilles all insisted that travelers spent 40 days in isolation on arrival. This period was inspired by the 40 days passed by Moses on the mountain and other Biblical 40 day periods. The Italian word for 40 is '*quaranta*' and from this our word QUARANTINE is derived.

Job's illness is a conundrum and many diagnostic suggestions have been made. *The book of Job* is most probably a parable and so possibly no diagnosis should be made. Nevertheless, suggestions have included smallpox, anthrax, recurrent staphylococcal abscesses, erythema nodosum, dermatitis herpetiformis, scabies, SYPHILIS, and psoriasis. The three most likely diagnoses are generalized pustular psoriasis, dermatitis herpetiformis, and erythema nodosum.

Saul is an example of a manic depressive. Even in those days it was realized that MUSIC sometimes calms such a person, and so David was introduced to Saul because he was a noted player of the harp.

FREUD (p 321) has interpreted the dreams described in the *Old Testament*, attaching a sexual significance to them — particularly to Joseph's two dreams. Others consider that Joseph's dream that his sheaf stood upright in the field while the sheaves of his brothers bowed before him, and his second dream that the sun, moon, and eleven stars made obeisance to him, simply show Joseph's desire to dominate his brothers.　　JMD

**BILHARZIASIS** See SCHISTOSOMIASIS

**BILLS OF MORTALITY** were weekly official returns of the number of deaths that, from 1592 onwards, were published by the London Company of Parish Clerks for 109 districts in and around London. Although these statistics are inaccurate, they are of value in indicating broad epidemiological trends (see EPIDEMIOLOGY) during the next two centuries, until the first year of death registration in 1837. They illustrate, for example, the gradual rise in SMALLPOX deaths throughout the 17th century, and the subsequent fall, with epidemics in 1681, 1685, and 1694–5.

**BIOETHICS** The word 'bioethics' was coined in the 1960s, and is popularly attributed to Van Rensselaer Potter, a medical researcher at the University of Wisconsin, who combined 'bio', representing biological knowledge or the science of living systems, with 'ethics', representing knowledge of human value systems. The first institutional use of the word was in 1971, when what is now called the Kennedy Institute of Ethics was founded at Georgetown University in Washington, DC, as the Joseph and Rose Kennedy Institute for the Study of Human Reproduction and Bioethics.

The value systems that assess developments in human medicine and biology have ancient roots. They are traceable to ARISTOTLE (p 64) and Plato, and to religious advocates of medical ethics of later centuries. Conscientious care for the sick has long been the inspiration of Christian physicians and nurses, and many hospitals bear the names of Christian SAINTS. Similarly, the 12th century Jewish teacher, physician, and philosopher MAIMONIDES (Moses ben Maimon) (p 59) advanced scholarship based on Jewish law, and a central component of the orthodox Islamic university founded in 972 AD in Cairo associated with the Mosque of El Azhar was its hospital and medical school. Women herbalists and care givers to the sick provided conscientious comfort in pre-Christian Europe, but knowledge of their motivations and *modus operandi* had been lost by the beginning of the 18th century after centuries of their persecution as witches by the Christian Church in Europe and North America.

### Role

Religiously inspired care givers to the sick provide services in accordance with their religious beliefs and sacred teachings, and those inspired by other moral philosophies may invoke their philosophical convictions to justify their conduct towards the sick and suffering. Both tend to be described as bioethicists, but modern bioethics are secular, pluralistic, and multidisciplinary. Some leaders in bioethics come from religious or philosophical traditions, but many others are primarily physicians, nurses, biologists, lawyers, and historians or anthropologists. Bioethicists are interested in working with others outside their disciplines to determine what values should underlie the provision of health care. They make assessments not simply on the basis of religious authority or philosophical claims, but through scientific knowledge and disciplinary interactions.

Bioethics addresses two fundamental questions, namely what should individuals and human communities do, permit, tolerate, or prohibit in biology, particularly affecting existing and future human beings, and how decisions should be made to determine what conduct is mandatory, permissible, tolerable, or prohibited. Bioethics addresses basic issues in the human, institutional, and social management of human birth, sickness, and death, but has come to popular attention through technological developments. These have concerned techniques of human reproduction to overcome infertility, means to limit or remedy undesired conception, mechanical means to replace organ functions, tissue and organ transplantation, or medical means to terminate life.

Bioethicists determine information from a range of scientific and non-scientific disciplines, following the maxim that good bioethics depends on good facts, and propose appropriate conduct in medical care and health services. They often work in hospitals and other healthcare or research institutes, as members or consultants on committees. Governmental and other public or private-sector bodies are increasingly creating ethics committees to make or recommend decisions on bioethical issues.

Bioethics presents language and concepts in which to express ideas about right conduct, and dissent from others' views and preferences. In offering a language of criticism, bioethics also offers a language of explanation and justification. The different orientations, prioritized principles, and levels of bioethical analysis taken together often lead to no self-evident conclusions, but they equip commentators and decision-makers to explain and defend their conclusions, and disagree with others. Concepts of bioethics empower individuals and institutions to react to others in a common language, and to engage in civil discussion about ends and means. Adversaries may recognize each other as following different ethical reasoning rather than as being unethical because their views diverge.

## Bioethical orientations

Several different ethical orientations guide bioethical conclusions. Historical orientations continue in effect today, and reflect the philosophical and religious origins of bioethics.

Duty-based (or deontological) bioethics is attributed to natural reason or natural law, and distinguishes vice from virtue as a matter of the inherent quality of an act or proposal. Natural law, propounded, for instance, by Aristotle, was incorporated into doctrine of the Roman Catholic Church in the 13th century by St Thomas Aquinas to harmonize reason and faith as divine gifts. An exponent of secular duty-based ethics was the late-18th century German philosopher Immanuel Kant, who taught that humans are to be treated as ends in themselves, never only as means towards ends. Duty-based bioethics tends to be absolutist, unaccommodating of ethical relativity and pluralism. The Roman Catholic Church, for instance, once prohibited the reading of Kant's writings.

Duty-based bioethicists believe that good cannot come from evil, and Roman Catholic bioethicists believe that artificial contraception is wrong. They have therefore opposed the distribution of condoms in prisons and schools, intended to contain sexually-transmitted HIV infection. Similarly, Kantians may be troubled by a couple's decision to allow the birth of a child only when prenatal diagnosis proves it to be compatible to donate bone marrow to the couple's existing child who suffers from leukemia and is in need of a transplantation donor, for fear that the new-born child would be regarded only as a means to serve the existing child's ends. In the former case, preventable HIV infection might occur and in the latter, the existing child might die for lack of a donor, but duty-based bioethicists consider that the end does not justify unethical means.

Consequentialist or utilitarian bioethics recognizes moral responsibility for the consequences of individuals' bioethical choices, and judges good or right conduct as that which is useful to promote human well-being or happiness. Ethical conduct serves and maximizes desirable outcomes, and conduct is wrongful if it causes or contributes to harmful or undesirable consequences, judged by communal, democratic, or political assessments of welfare. Consequentialist or utilitarian ethics, unlike duty-based ethics, aspire to be neither universal nor enduring, but are pragmatic responses to varying circumstances.

Under such bioethical orientation, birth control programs would be considered proper to reduce unplanned pregnancies and induced abortion should be lawful to reduce the incidence of back-street abortion resulting in women's death or injury. Similarly, healthcare providers' conscientious objection to such procedures is considered tolerable only when it does not obstruct women's access to early, safe, and convenient abortion services. Further, providers who invoke conscientious objections to their own participation, perhaps because of their religious or other duty-based convictions, should be bound to refer applicants for such services to providers who have no such objections.

Feminist bioethics, sometimes described as the ethics of care or of connectedness, reacts against the exclusion of women from historical sources of moral authority, such as clerical ranks of religions; universities and other learned societies; learned professions such as medicine and law; and legislative assemblies. Exclusion of the relevance of women's voices and experiences, half of the accumulated wisdom of humankind, was often deliberate, but is now considered to discredit the moral authority of exclusionary institutions.

Feminist analysis addresses not only sex, which is biological or genetic, but also gender, which is socially constructed. Not all women are 'feminists', of course, and not all 'feminists' are women, since the focus of this bioethical orientation is on the ethical incorporation of women's social experiences and realities into the value systems of healthcare.

## Contraception and abortion

Much traditional bioethical discussion of contraception and abortion fails to consider the impact of unplanned and undesired pregnancy on women's enjoyment of their lives. Women's inability to influence medical research agendas, and the medical belief that male physiology is 'normal' and women are different only in their reproductive functions, have contributed to inadequate understanding of women's health needs. The role of women as care givers, to their children, parents, and husbands' parents, to the sick or elderly, is often devalued or disregarded, for instance, in discharging patients from medical facilities. It is inadequately recognized that 'home care' and 'community care' mean women's care, and that women are expected to forgo alternative goals and satisfactions to provide it, and condemned if they decline.

Other bioethical orientations exist, such as communitarianism, which seeks to advance human community as a good in itself, but proponents usually acknowledge the seniority of orientations addressed above, and aim to show that their approach is preferable. Casuistry is favored by those who believe that cases should be resolved on their particular merits and not by appeals to universal rules. The orientation of 'principlism', an application of principles of bioethics, is rarely claimed as a virtue by those who follow it, but is the description by which critics condemn the mechanical application or prioritization of a narrow range of perceived principles of bioethics.

## Principles

To escape the contradictions and restrictive orthodoxies of competing bioethical orientations, some analysts have identified a few key principles of bioethical analysis common to different orientations. These appeared as three principles in the Belmont Report (1979) of the US National Commission for the Protection of Human Subjects of Biomedical and Behavioral Research, since the principle of Non-Maleficence (do no harm) was considered implicit in the principle of Beneficence (do good), but the British authority Raanan Gillon considers this principle explicitly separate, and addresses the Four Principles. They are presented here in a conventional sequence, but none has priority over others, and much bioethical controversy concerns which should prevail over others to resolve particular problems.

*Respect for persons* seems a minimal standard for ethical conduct, but its absence often leaves civil bioethical discussion unachievable. The abortion dilemma is insoluble, for instance, when rival proponents characterize the others as child-killers, Nazis, bigots, or zealots.

*Beneficence,* the ethical duty to do good and maximize good, underpins the provision of much medical treatment. The quest for improved therapies and preventive healthcare accords with this principle. It may be limited by patients' autonomy to choose poorly and the choice of individuals who could benefit from care deciding not to seek it. Where poverty limits patients' access to care, charitable aid may assist them. Religiously inspired healthcare providers and service funders enjoy an honorable history of assistance to the poor, under the motivation of beneficence. Laws that permit persons to make posthumous gifts of their own organs or gifts of their deceased family members' organs for TRANSPLANTATION serve this principle. Several countries, particularly in western Europe, have pursued this principle further through laws that make transplantable organs recoverable after death for this purpose without consent, unless the individuals had objected when alive, for instance, because of religious beliefs. However, laws that require individuals to record their religious convictions with public agencies can be oppressive, particularly when the individuals are a minority and fearful of discrimination. The drive towards beneficence may compromise vulnerable persons' interests in protection.

## RESPECT FOR PERSONS

This principle includes:

- Autonomy of capable persons. This principle often seems to transcend all others, particularly in the USA under ascendancy of the so-called 'Me' generation. Patient autonomy requires that patients' consent to treatment be adequately informed and freely given, without undue pressure or inducement. The principle often prevails over Non-Maleficence in that it upholds patients' informed but poor choices, and condemns its compromise as paternalism and as infantilization of patients. The principle is increasingly invoked in support of patients' rights to medically assisted suicide.

- Protection of persons incapable of autonomy. Protection against harm or distress of children is uncontentious, although imposing treatments over children's resistance, such as vaccination against childhood diseases, is often supported because of the highly favorable risk-to-benefit ratio. Female CIRCUMCISION or genital mutilation is often opposed under this principle in countries where it has not customarily been practiced and in some where it has been, and non-religious male circumcision has similarly been questioned. Criteria by which to assess the need for protection can be contentious for adolescents and some adults of low intellect, low income, low social status, or low self-esteem that expose them to personal and social vulnerability and dependency. Normally capable adults may be vulnerable to exploitation, for instance, when physicians on whom they depend for care ask them to participate in risky medical research.

*Non-Maleficence* incorporates the foundational medical ethic *Do no harm*. The principle requires an extended understanding of the senses in which treatment can cause harm. It has been customary for medical investigators to consider a study to pose no risk of harm if it is non-invasive and presents no physical dangers, such as from the withholding of medically indicated treatment. Bioethically, however, harm may also consist in risks of damaged self-esteem or self-confidence — for instance, when participants are presented with soluble problems they fail to solve, or questionnaires that demonstrate to them the disadvantages in life or disabilities they suffer. It is a legitimate function of education to achieve individuals' self-awareness, but the imposition of uninvited self-awareness can cause distress and unhappiness. Similarly, loss of confidentiality or inducing a feeling of having been used, exploited, or treated disrespectfully may be harmful.

Medically induced death is widely condemned in law, but the withdrawal of artificial life supports — such as mechanical ventilators, or intravenous feeding and hydration — results in natural death. This is usually lawful, and in several instances, for the avoidance of doubt, has received prior judicial approval, but it raises bioethical concerns because of the principle of Non-Maleficence. Relief of suffering achievable only by allowing occurrence of natural death may be tolerable and even beneficent, but when a patient is not in pain or mental anguish but is, for instance, in a persistent vegetative state, no relief may be achievable but death may risk harm in foreclosing any prospect of recovery. In life-affirming cultures, toleration of death that could be postponed may appear harmful. By contrast, the utilitarian orientation may argue that using resources to postpone vegetative patients' natural death denies such resources to others whose life would be enhanced by their use.

*Justice* is the ethical principle that the law aims to serve. Bioethics is less concerned with punitive or compensatory justice than with distributive justice. This requires that like cases be treated alike — for instance, in the allocation of scarce resources — and that different cases be treated to show the differences. Bioethical concerns focus on criteria of likeness and difference, since cases that seem alike by some criteria appear different by others. For instance, when transplantation of a single available liver could prolong the life of only one of three persons on the same waiting list — namely, a non-alcoholic patient, a reformed alcoholic patient, and an unreformed alcoholic patient — criteria of allocation among them become a major bioethical concern. A utilitarian criterion of effectiveness would favor the non-alcoholic patient, but if the reformed alcoholic patient has a comparable physiological prognosis and only a minimal risk of relapse, that patient may rank equally with the former. The non-reformed alcoholic patient appears an unpromising candidate since the addiction that damaged the patient's own liver appears to threaten successful functioning of a transplanted liver. By criteria of social justice, however, all three rank equally with each other, so that a non-evaluative criterion is fair, such as who has been on the waiting list longest, or who is closest to death. Disfavoring the non-reformed alcoholic on the ground of addiction may be justified because of moralistic condemnation of drinking, but if addiction is seen as a physical or psychological weakness, treating the patient as ineligible for indicated medical care on the ground of an illness is perverse, contradicting the primary purpose of medical care. Justice requires application of rational, non-discriminatory criteria of allocating resources.

## Levels of analysis

Conventional bioethics has tended to be applied between individuals on the basis of personal conscience, at the so-called *microethical* level. Each person pays each other their ethical due. A physician respects a patient's informed choice whether or not to accept the prepared care and the patient respects the physician's right not to undertake treatment the latter considers countertherapeutic or futile, or to which the physician has a conscientious objection. Classic ethics also considered population groups through analysis conducted at a *macroethical* level. Modern bioethics has not been well developed at this level, but has to consider relations affecting health between rich and poor communities, majority and minority populations, and residents of urban, suburban, and rural regions. It must also address relations between communities and individuals, including community members, outsiders, and immigrants. In public health surveys competing interests of patients in confidentiality of their health records and of communities in determining prevalence rates of diseases and disabilities by review of such records have to be resolved.

Conflicts may concern levels at which issues should be addressed. A feminist approach to abortion has been that it is a microethical issue of choice only between a patient and her doctor, and that political or public intervention should be excluded. However, the same approach to prenatal diagnosis of fetal sex and abortion of female fetuses is that this is macroethical and should be publicly condemned as illegal, because it perpetuates both prejudice against girl children and the devaluation of girls and women in their communities.

Resource allocation by administrative officers or agencies involves *mesoethical* issues, which fall between microethics and macroethics. They implicate principles of beneficence and justice when, for instance, a finite budget bears competing demands from pediatric, geriatric, maternity, emergency, and other services. Authorities allocating resources among primary, secondary, and tertiary healthcare facilities are similarly making mesoethical choices. Transcending regional and national issues are *megaethical* issues. They may affect health through concerns with environmental pollution and the ecological impact of policies, such as the release of wind-borne noxious fumes and chemical effluents that penetrate irrigation and drinking water supplies. At this level, however, bioethics is superseded by ethical concerns that include but go far beyond considerations of human biology.     BMD

*See also* HELSINKI-DECLARATION OF; INFORMED CONSENT; NUREMBERG CODE; RELIGION, PHILOSOPHY, AND MEDICINE

## BIOLOGICAL AND CHEMICAL WARFARE

Chemical and biological weapons are often considered together because they are weapons of mass destruction. Chemical weapons have been used in recent years by nations and terrorist groups but there is no clear evidence that biological weapons have been used since World War II. Use of chemical and biological weapons has been outlawed by international treaties in recent years but stockpiles of these weapons still exist and the threat of their use remains.

### Chemical weapons

Chemical weapons, which have been known since antiquity, are designed to produce direct chemical injury to their victims. They must be differentiated from explosive or incendiary weapons that also involve chemical reactions but produce their injuries by blast or heat.

In the siege of the city of Plataea in 429 BC the Spartans placed enormous cauldrons of pitch, sulfur, and burning charcoal outside the city walls to harass the defenders. Nations signing the 1899 Hague Declaration promised not to use chemical weapons. However, during World War I 125 000 tons were employed, including, in order of use, tear gas, chlorine, phosgene, and mustard gas. They resulted in 1.3 million casualties; one-quarter of all casualties in the American Expeditionary Force in France were caused by them.

In 1925, 28 nations negotiated the Geneva Protocol for the 'prohibition of the use in war of asphyxiating poisonous or other gases and of all analogous liquids, materials or devices and of bacteriological methods of warfare'. The protocol prohibited the use, but not the development, production, testing, or stockpiling of these weapons. Furthermore, many of the nations ratifying the protocol reserved the right to use such weapons in retaliation, and the protocol became in effect a 'no first use' treaty with no verification or enforcement provisions. The United States was one of the initial signers, but the US Senate did not ratify the treaty until 1975.

Despite the protocol, use of chemical weapons continued. Italy used mustard gas during its invasion of Abyssinia (Ethiopia) and Japan used mustard and tear gases in its invasion of China. Germany, with its excellent dye and pesticide industries, developed lethal acetylcholinesterase inhibitors known as nerve gases. The United States and Britain stockpiled chemical weapons during World War II; transportation and storage accidents caused casualties, but there was no direct military use. After World War II, they were used by Egypt in Yemen; mustard and nerve gases were used in the Iran–Iraq war; and Iraq used mustard and nerve gas against Kurdish villages in its own territory. Destruction of the stockpiles and production facilities in Iraq was ordered by the United Nations after the 1991 Persian Gulf War. On 20 March 1995 an apocalyptic religious sect, Aum Shinri-kyo, released nerve gas in the Tokyo subway system. The attack killed eight people outright and injured thousands of others, many of them fatally. The United States and Russia are known to maintain chemical weapons stockpiles and several other countries either have stockpiles or facilities for rapid production.

Troops can be protected against these weapons for limited periods by gas masks and impenetrable garments; however, these reduce the efficiency of troops by as much as half and damage morale, so use or threat of use of chemical weapons may continue to be considered effective against troops. Civilian populations, on the other hand, cannot be adequately protected. Israel, for example, provides every civilian in the country with a gas mask and a self-injectable syringe filled with atropine, a temporary antidote to nerve gas. This limited protection is inadequate against weapons such as mustard gas that attack the skin or against longer-term exposure to nerve gas. Furthermore, poorly trained civilians are likely to injure themselves with equipment such as self-injectable syringes, which caused injuries to hundreds of children in Israel during the Persian Gulf War, even though nerve agents were never used.

In addition to the dangers associated with their actual use, health and environmental risks accompany other chemical weapons-related activities. Their production has been associated with serious accidents to workers and with high levels of pollution in the production sites and nearby coma new international agency, the Organization for the Prohibition of Chemical Weapons, with headquarters in the Hague. Problems with inspections on demand (requiring little prior warning) and other forms of verification, with penalties for noncompliance and with methods for safe disposal of the weapons remain to be solved.

In the 1960s and 1970s the USA used both tear gas and herbicides in Vietnam. Although most nations that are parties to the Geneva Protocol considered tear gas and herbicides used in war to be chemical weapons, and thus prohibited under the provisions of the protocol, the USA until recently rejected that interpretation. Many countries use tear gas on a regular basis to quell civil disorders. For example, police in Korea in 1987 used several hundred thousand canisters of tear gas in a single month for 'riot control', with serious injuries to many people and at least one documented death; Soviet troops in 1990, in quelling a disturbance in Tbilisi, the capital of Soviet Georgia, used what was alleged to be tear gas and produced a large number of casualties. Although the definition of these weapons as chemical weapons is still in dispute, the signatories to the chemical weapons convention have agreed not to use riot control agents or herbicides as weapons of war.

## Biological weapons

Biological weapons depend upon the ability of micro-organisms to infect and multiply in the attacked organism. In this they differ from toxins, which, as biological products used as chemicals, are covered under both chemical and biological weapons treaties. Biological weapons are extremely hard to defend against and are not as controllable or predictable in their use as are chemical weapons.

The effects of biological weapons were officially summarized by a US government agency in 1959: 'Biological warfare is the intentional use of living organisms or their toxic products to cause death, disability, or damage in man, animals, or plants. The target is man, either by causing sickness or death or through limitation of his food supplies or other agricultural resources. Man must wage a continuous fight to maintain and defend himself, his animals, and his plants in competition with insects and micro-organisms. The object of biological warfare is to overcome these efforts by deliberately distributing large numbers of organisms of native and foreign origin, or their toxic products, taking full advantage of the ability to use more effective methods of dissemination and unusual portals of entry. Biological warfare has been aptly described as 'public health in reverse'.

Biological weapons have also been known since antiquity. Persia, Greece, and Rome used diseased corpses to contaminate sources of drinking water.

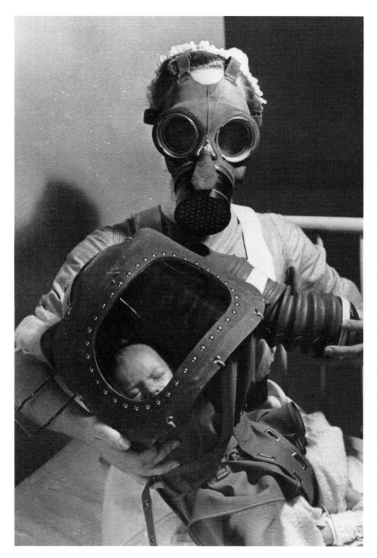

Nurse fitting a baby with its gas mask. (Reproduced courtesy of the Trustees of the Imperial War Museum, London.)

munitions. Tests of mustard gas, nerve agents, and psychochemicals, including lysergic acid diethylamide (LSD), during and after World War II involved thousands of military personnel, many of whom subsequently claimed disabilities from the exposure. Records of participation and of effects are so poor that only a small fraction of those who participated can be identified. Even destruction of the weapons is dangerous, since incineration, one of the preferred methods, can produce toxic ash.

The Chemical Weapons Convention, which prohibits the development, production, storage, and transfer of these weapons and calls for their demilitarization, entered into force in 1997 when it was ratified by the required 65 nations including the United States. The convention establishes

In 1347, Mongols besieging the walled city of Caffa (now called Feodosiya), a seaport on the east coast of the Crimea, began to die of the PLAGUE. The attackers threw their comrades' corpses into the besieged city; the defenders, who were Genoans, fled back to Genoa and carried the plague further into Europe. During the French and Indian Wars, Lord Jeffrey Amherst, commander of the British forces at Fort Pitt, is said to have produced SMALLPOX cases among Native Americans by giving tribal emissaries a gift of blankets in which smallpox victims had slept.

During World War I Germany is alleged to have used the equine disease glanders against the cavalries of eastern European countries. According to testimony at the Nuremberg trials, prisoners in German concentration camps were infected during tests of biological weapons. Great Britain and the United States, fearing the Germans would use biological weapons in World War II, developed anthrax, botulinum toxin, and chemical weapons but did not use them. They tested dispersal of anthrax spores on Gruinard Island, off the coast of Scotland; parts of the island were uninhabitable until recently.

In the 1930s, Japanese troops dropped rice and wheat mixed with plague-carrying fleas from planes, resulting in plague in areas of China that were previously free of it. During World War II, Japanese laboratories conducted extensive experiments on prisoners of war using a variety of organisms selected for possible use as biological weapons, including anthrax, plague, gas gangrene, encephalitis, TYPHUS, TYPHOID, hemorrhagic fever, CHOLERA, smallpox, and tularemia (rabbit fever, deerfly fever). Unlike the Soviet Union, which in 1949 prosecuted twelve of those involved in this work, the United States never prosecuted any of the participants. Instead, US researchers met with Japanese biological warfare experts in Tokyo and urged that the experts be 'spared embarrassment' so that the USA could benefit from their knowledge.

After World War II development of biological weapons continued. None of the numerous allegations of their use has been substantiated (or even fully investigated), but it is known that extensive biological weapons testing has been carried out. In the 1950s and 1960s, for example, the University of Utah conducted secret, large-scale field tests of biological weapons, including tularemia, Rocky Mountain spotted fever, plague, and Q fever, at the US Army Dugway Proving Ground. In 1950 US Navy ships released as simulants (materials believed to be nonpathogenic that mimic the spread of biological weapons) large quantities of bacteria in the San Francisco Bay area to test the efficiency of their dispersal. Some analysts attributed subsequent infections and deaths to one of these organisms. During the 1950s and 1960s, the United States conducted 239 top-secret, open-air disseminations of simulants, involving such areas as the New York City subways and Washington National Airport. The US military developed a large infrastructure of laboratories, test facilities, and production plants related to biological weapons. By the end of the 1960s, the United States had stockpiles of at least ten different biological and toxin weapons. A 1979 outbreak of pulmonary anthrax in the Soviet Union is believed to have been caused by accidental release of anthrax spores from a Soviet biological weapons factory in Sverdlovsk. Recent disclosures by Russian scientists indicate extensive environmental contamination and medical problems in the territories of the former USSR due to weapons production.

In 1969 the Nixon administration, with the concurrence of the Defense Department, which declared that biological weapons lacked 'military usefulness', unconditionally renounced their development, production, and stockpiling, in the USA, and announced that the United States would unilaterally dismantle its biological weapons program. In 1972 the Soviet Union, which had urged a more comprehensive treaty including restrictions on chemical weapons, ended its opposition to a separate biological weapons treaty. The United States, Soviet Union, and other nations negotiated the Convention on the Prohibition of the Development, Prevention, and Stockpiling of Bacteriological (Biological) and Toxin Weapons and on Their Destruction (the Biological Weapons Convention). This Biological Weapons Convention prohibits — except for 'prophylactic, protective, and other peaceful purposes' — the development or acquisition of biological agents or toxins, as well as weapons carrying them and means of their production, stockpiling, transfer, or delivery. The US Senate ratified this Biological Weapons Convention in 1975, the same year it ratified the Geneva Protocol of 1925. By 1987, 110 nations had ratified the Biological Weapons Convention and an additional 25 nations had signed but not yet ratified it.

Invoking the specter of possible new biological weapons and unproven allegations of aggressive biological weapons programs in other countries, the Reagan administration initiated intensive efforts to conduct 'defensive research', permitted under the convention. The budget for the US army biological defense research program, which sponsors programs in a wide variety of academic, commercial, and government laboratories, increased dramatically during the 1980s. Much of this research work is medical in nature, including the development of immunizations and of treatments against organisms that might be used as biological weapons.

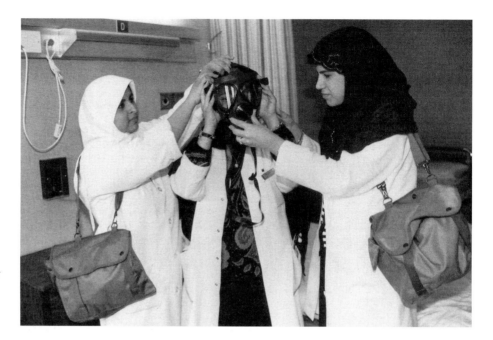

Kuwaiti nurses help a doctor put on a gas mask. (Reproduced courtesy of the Trustees of the Imperial War Museum, London).

While research and development of new biological weapons are outlawed by the convention, possibly these still occur. Novel dangers lie in new genetic technologies, which permit development of genetically altered organisms not known in nature. Stable, tailor-made organisms could travel long distances and still be infectious, rapidly infiltrate a population, cause debilitating effects very quickly, and be resistant to antibiotic treatment.

### Ethical issues for biomedical scientists

Biologists, chemists, biomedical scientists, and physicians have played important parts in chemical and biological weapons research and development. Fritz Haber, awarded the 1918 Nobel prize in chemistry for his synthesis of ammonia, is known as the father of Germany's chemical weapons program of World War I. In his speech accepting the Nobel prize, Haber declared poison gas 'a higher form of killing'. In contrast, during the Crimean War the British government consulted the noted physicist Michael Faraday on the feasibility of developing poison gases; Faraday responded that it was entirely feasible, but that it was inhuman and he would have nothing to do with it.

Many scientists who explicitly recognize the ethical conflicts involved in work on weapons argue that a higher ethical principle — the imperative of defending one's country or of helping to curb what is perceived as evil or destructive — permits or even demands participation in such work. Dr Theodor Rosebury, who worked on bio-

logical weapons during World War II, believed that crisis circumstances, expected to pass in a limited time, required that he should. 'We were fighting a fire, and it seemed necessary to risk getting dirty as well as burnt', he wrote later. Rosebury refused any further participation after the end of the war.

Other scientists resolved their ethical dilemma by arguing that their work on weapons was designed to reduce the devastation of war. For example, Dr Knut Krieger, while working on 'nonlethal' chemical and biological weapons in the 1960s, argued that his research would lead to decreased fatalities: 'if we do indeed succeed in creating incapacitating systems and are able to substitute incapacitation for death it appears to me that, next to stopping war, this would be an important step forward'.

Relevant ethical concerns about 'defensive research' on biological weapons by biomedical scientists include content, safety, context, and locus.

*Content* The Japanese laboratory established in 1933 to develop biological weapons was called the Epidemic Prevention Laboratory. One of its activities was supplying vaccines for troops bound for Manchuria, but its major work was developing and testing biological weapons. Military forces today could conduct research on offensive use of biological weapons under the cover of defensive research. During the parts of the work in which offensive and defensive efforts are parallel, it is possible that new forms of organisms may be found or developed that would be more effective as biological weapons.

**Safety** Research, even if truly defensive in intent, may be dangerous to surrounding communities if toxic materials or virulent infectious organisms are accidentally released.

**Context** Even if truly defensive in intent, research can viewed by a potential military adversary as an attempt to develop protection for a nation's military forces or its noncombatants against weapons the nation itself might wish to use for offensive purposes, thus permitting that nation to protect its own personnel in a first strike. In fact, the military justification for preparing any form of altered organisms is that they are needed for preparation of defenses. It is therefore impossible for adversaries to determine whether a nation's 'defensive' efforts are part of preparation for 'offensive' use of weapons.

**Locus** These fears are usually based on military sponsorship of 'defensive' biological weapons research. Other nations may view with suspicion the intense interest of military forces rather than civilian medical researchers in vaccines or treatment against specific organisms. Such fears can help feed a continuing biological weapons arms race. Just as the US Army supports its requests for appropriation of funds in this area by citing suspicions and possible exaggerations of what others are doing, so the armies of other countries may try to maximize their resources by casting not unreasonable suspicions on what the USA is doing.

More generally, concern has been expressed about the militarization of genetic engineering and of biology in general. Characterization of biological weapons as 'public health in reverse' may therefore have an even broader and more sinister meaning: the entire discipline of biology — and particular aspects of it such as the use of HUMAN GENOME research to design weapons to target specific groups — may be in danger of military subversion to destructive ends. The imprisonment of a chemist by the Russian government and the revocation of his university diploma for publishing an article describing the development of new, highly toxic chemical weapons illustrate the restrictions on scientists engaged in such research.

### Ethical issues for physicians

Is it constructive to view certain ethical responsibilities as peculiar to the physician's social role? Rosebury described the response to physician participation. 'There was much quiet but searching discussion among us regarding the place of doctors in such work ... a certain delicacy con-

centrated most of the physicians into principally or primarily defensive operations'. Rosebury goes on to point out that the modifiers 'principally' and 'primarily' are needed 'because military operations can never be exclusively defensive'. What is seen as the special responsibility of physicians is based largely on an ethical responsibility not to use the power of the physician to do harm (*primum non nocere*). While the Hippocratic OATH as written seems to apply to the relationship of the physician to an individual patient, its meaning has been broadened by many to proscribe physician participation in actions harmful to others in the community.

So far as research on 'offensive' weapons of war is concerned, there seems to be a consensus that physicians participate in such research at their ethical peril, even if their country demands it or they think it useful for 'deterrence' or other 'preventive' purposes. But because of the ambiguity of 'defensive' work the dilemma for the physician is not easily resolved, even for those who believe that 'defensive' efforts are ethically permissible.

Some proponents of defensive research on biological weapons have argued that it is entirely ethical and that responsibility demands that physicians participate. According to this perspective, not only will defenses be needed if such weapons are used but this work may also be useful in developing protection against naturally-occurring diseases. Other analysts take a different position. They believe it unethical for physicians to play a part in military-sponsored research because it has a strong potential for intensifying an arms race and helping to militarize biology, thus increasing the risk of the use of biological weapons and the destructiveness of their effects if they are used.

Where should physicians draw the line? If physicians engage in civilian-sponsored research on disease control that carries an obligation to report all findings in the open literature, even if the research may have implications for biological weapons, such participation, most analysts agree, cannot be ethically faulted. However, if physicians engage in military-sponsored research in which the openness of reporting is equivocal and the purposes ambiguous, it is difficult to distinguish their work ethically from that on the development of weapons.

The responsibility for government-sponsored medical research for prophylactic, protective, and other peaceful purposes in the United States lies largely with the National Institutes of Health and the Centers for Disease Control and Prevention. These might therefore be given the responsibility and the resources for medical research of this type. The US Army may still want to conduct nonmedical defense research and development, such as work on detectors, protective clothing, and other barriers to the spread of organisms. Under this proposed division of effort, such research is less likely to be seen as offensive, less likely to provoke a race, less likely to pervert the science of biology, and less likely to involve physicians.

A different type of ethical issue arose during the Persian Gulf War in 1991. The United States provided protective measures, such as immunization against botulinum toxin and anthrax, for its military forces. Despite the fact that some of these measures were experimental, no informed-consent procedures were used and compliance was often required. Furthermore, these measures were made available to military forces but not to non-combatants in the area.

In addition to the ethical dilemmas involved in these decisions, it may be unethical for physicians simply to ignore the issues. One of the greatest dangers of these weapons may be the apathy of the medical profession toward them. Physicians have specialized knowledge and therefore special responsibility not only to refuse to work on them but also actively to work to reduce the threat of their chemical and biological weapons and therefore their development or use.

### Conclusion

Physicians and biomedical scientists should support methods for international epidemiologic surveillance to detect the use of and to investigate incidents in which use has been alleged after an unexplained disease outbreak and should support the Vaccine for Peace Program for control of 'dual-threat' agents. Support might also be given for measures to strengthen the Biological Weapons Convention by introduction of verification proposals put forth at the regular Review Conferences. With regard to chemical weapons, biomedical scientists and physicians should support effective implementation of the 1993 Chemical Weapons Convention.

More broadly, physicians may wish to explore the connection between biological, chemical, and nuclear weapons. It has been argued that the nuclear powers, by refusing to reduce their vast stockpiles of nuclear weapons substantially and by refusing to agree to verifiable cessation of nuclear-weapons testing and production, provoke non-nuclear powers to contemplate development and production of chemical and biological weapons for 'deterrence' against nuclear weapons. The US Defense Intelligence Agency reported that 'third-world nations view chemical weapons as an attractive and inexpensive alternative to nuclear weapons'. There is much physicians can do, for example, through the International Physicians for the Prevention of Nuclear War (the organization that received the 1985 Nobel Peace Prize) and its

affiliates in many countries, to reduce the provocation and the proliferation of weapons of mass destruction caused by the continuing nuclear-arms race. An advisory opinion by the International Court of Justice (World Court) in 1997 called upon the nations of the world that possess nuclear weapons to move expeditiously toward their elimination.

Individual physicians and scientists can add to the awareness of the dangers of these weapons by signing the pledge, sponsored by the Council for Responsible Genetics, 'not to engage knowingly in research and teaching that will further development of chemical and biological warfare agents'. US physicians also may wish to support legislation to transfer all medical aspects of biological defense from the military to the National Institutes for Health or the Centers for Disease Control and Prevention. Physicians may help awaken the medical profession to the danger of chemical, biological, and nuclear weapons by adding a clause to the oath taken by medical students at graduation from medical school similar to the oath for medical students in the former Soviet Union, requiring them 'to struggle, tirelessly for peace and for the prevention of nuclear war'. The addition might, for example, be worded thus: 'Recognizing that nuclear, chemical and biological arms are weapons of indiscriminate mass destruction and threaten the health of all humanity, I will refuse to play any role that might increase the risk of use of such weapons and will, as part of my professional responsibility, work actively for peace and for the prevention of their use'.                                       VWS

*See also* INFECTIOUS DISEASES

**BLACK BOX (ABRAMS)** A large crowd of doctors gathered on the evening of 16 January 1925 at the Royal Society of Medicine in London to hear a leading medical man, Sir (later Lord) Thomas Horder, communicate the findings of a small committee of experts. They had investigated a diagnostic method which had become fashionable, attracting high profile support from physician Sir James Barr, and Sir Arthur Conan DOYLE (p 233), but which defied orthodox scientific theory and common sense. It is reasonable to assume that most of those gathered there that evening expected to hear Sir Thomas expose the infamous 'Black Box' of Abrams as a complete fraud.

The use of the Black Box had begun in Britain only in the 1920s, but it had been a cause of controversy and heated denunciation in the USA for many years before that. The apparatus was the invention of a wealthy Vienna-trained San Francisco neurologist, who had noticed that the percussion note obtained on patients' abdomens varied according to the point of the compass in which the patient was facing. Abrams went on to conduct more experiments on the phenomenon, and invented a diagnostic method using a device of his own design. Abrams began to manufacture and sell these instruments known as 'ossciloclasts'. The ossciloclast connected a blood or tissue sample, obtained from the patient in question and placed on filter paper, via an 'amplifier' and a pair of variable resistors to the forehead of a patient. No current was supplied to the apparatus. The patient's abdomen was then tapped while the resistors were adjusted to obtain diagnostic information about the patient from whom the sample was taken. Hundreds of practitioners, known as 'electronists', bought a Black Box, undertaking not to open or inspect its contents, and the method rapidly gained notoriety and some popularity.

### USA experiments

Numerous experiments had been made in the USA, without the prior consent or the active participation of 'electronists', and these had demonstrated to Abrams's opponents that the method was a scam, without basis in scientific fact. Horder's team of physicists set out to give the basic underlying assumption of Abrams's technique a fair trial. They wanted 'to ascertain whether the methods concerned ever yielded successful results which could not reasonably be attributed to pure chance, ingenious guess-work, or deception'. They collaborated with a medically qualified homeopath from Glasgow, W. E. Boyd, who had X-rayed his Abrams box to discover its contents, and constructed a novel device of his own. This 'emanometer' still used changes in percussion tone on a subject's abdomen as its 'endpoint'.

Initial trials of Boyd's technique in London failed, but Boyd persuaded the committee that his laboratory in Glasgow, which was fitted with elaborate arrays of copper gauze to exclude interfering 'radiations', was the most suitable place to try the methods. Here they obtained several results indicating a performance well in excess of random chance under conditions that appeared to allow for no deception. The team then devised what they saw as a 'crucial' test. The emanometer was used to distinguish between two visually identical sets of vials containing a homeopathic remedy or lactose powder. Boyd performed spectacularly well in this trial, the chances of his results being due to chance being calculated to be 65 536:1 against. The committee decided to repeat the experiment in the presence of Mr E. J. Dingwall, of the Society for Psychical Research, which was dedicated to exposing fraudulent claims of paranormal phenomena. Similar results were obtained.

Horder told his audience 'that certain substances when placed in proper relation to the emanometer of Boyd produce, beyond reasonable doubt, changes in the abdominal wall of "the subject"… detected by percussion' and concluded that Abrams's technique was probably based on actual phenomena. However, he pointed out that there was no evidence that the method was of diagnostic or therapeutic value, and that 'electronists' had failed to contribute anything to pathology, the 'foundation of medicine'. The meeting was offered a chance to debate the findings, but no interest was expressed by any of those present. Abrams's method slowly disappeared from the stage of fashionable practice during the interwar years, and no further research was carried out into it.

What can we make of the Black Box episode today? First, the method itself appears at first sight to be a form of dowsing, which in the form of water-divining has ancient roots. But Abrams's method was different from 'normal' dowsing, in which the physical changes or reactions are confined to the investigator holding the divining rods or pendulum. The 'Electronic Reaction of Abrams' used a physical response elicited from a third party: the passive patient tapped by the investigator. Dowsing continues to be widely practiced in various forms by unorthodox practitioners, but not using this principle.

The criteria on which treatments and medical methodologies were judged were also relatively unsophisticated, resting on a process of reporting and discussion between researchers using simple statistical methods and relying crucially on the personal integrity of those participating in research work. For Horder's committee, Boyd appeared to be an honorable and honest man, keen to collaborate in research on his methods. The chief objection to 'electronists' were of a social and professional kind. It was the commercialization of such an outlandish method, the refusal of 'electronists' to co-operate in any trial of the method, its apparently beneficial effect on the finances of all who took it up, and its rapid dissemination that most irritated orthodox doctors. Professional ideals insisted that even private medical practice be non-commercial, condemned any secret methods are quackery, and emphasized the importance of sharing knowledge within the profession. It must also be remembered that the state of understanding of radiation and electromagnetic phenomena was not as advanced as today. Radiology and radiotherapy were new disciplines and shaded in many minds imperceptibly into less familiar methods such as ultraviolet light and sunlight therapy.

Perhaps most striking was Horder's courage in presenting such positive findings to a hostile

# THE GREAT KILLERS: BLACK DEATH

Black Death is the popular name given to the most devastating pandemic of plague in history. Occurring between 1348 and 1365, it killed between a third and a half of all Europeans, more in some areas than in others, amounting to 20–25 million in five years. Plague recurred at intervals until the pandemic of 1664–5, the Great Plague, after which it virtually disappeared from northern and western Europe. It probably originated in China, and spread to the rest of Asia and Europe by two main routes: the Silk Road and the pilgrim's way to Mecca. In 1346 some Genoese merchants were besieged by the Tatars in the Crimean city of Kaffa (Feodosiya). An outbreak of plague forced the Tatars to withdraw, but before doing so they catapulted some corpses of plague victims across the walls into the city streets. The Italians were forced to withdraw, but developed plague and brought it back to their home ports — to Messina in 1347 and Genoa the following year, from where it spread to the rest of Europe. In particular, this outbreak, the Black Death, combined three types of plague: bubonic and septicemic (spread by rat fleas) and pneumonic (spread by coughing).

The medical response was to institute quarantine, and also at first to house the victims in former leper houses and then in purpose-built LAZARETTOS (named after St Lazarus). Some Italian cities created health boards, while the Papal proscription of autopsies was temporarily relaxed in the hope of discovering the cause of the disease. The pandemic also led to a search for scapegoats, provoking a wave of antisemitism. In Basle the Jewish population was herded into a wooden building, which was then set on fire. Similar massacres occurred elsewhere, with the result that there was a mass migration of Jews into Poland.

A prominent movement was self-flagellation, of wandering penitents doing penance by scourging themselves, a practice frowned on by the church. Northern and western cultures developed a preoccupation with death in their visual art, and plague became a popular theme in literature. Boccaccio had initiated this for the Black Death itself. His *Decameron* is a series of stories told by fugitives from the plague in Florence, and the theme continued to be used for centuries.

Black Death was the name introduced by the historian Elizabeth Markham in 1823; earlier names included 'Oriental Plague', 'Great Pestilence', and 'Great Mortality'. Although textbooks mostly explain the epithet in terms of cyanosis (blueness of the skin), purpura (small skin hemorrhages), and gangrene, Mrs Markham used 'black' in the sense of disastrous.

SPL

*See also* INSECTS; PLAGUE; QUARANTINE

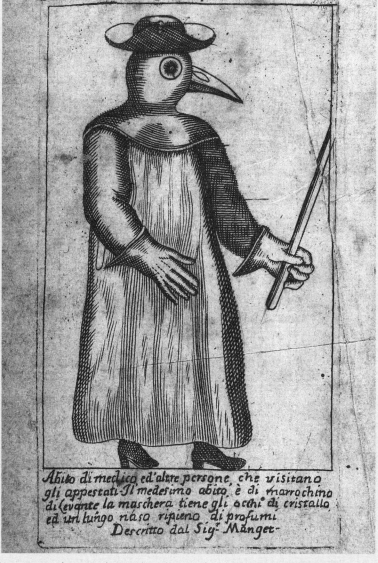

Line engraving showing a physician dressed in protective plague costume. (Reproduced courtesy of the Wellcome Institute Library, London.)

audience. He had sufficient medical and social status to carry this off, and was also keenly interested in bringing diagnostic technologies to the bedside. Having recommended further research at the close of his presentation, he was pressed many years later as to why he did not do any himself. He is reported to have commented that it was not sufficient to show whether or not a method worked. To be truly accepted it was vital to also produce a plausible sounding explanation or proof of how it worked.

AAGMcr

*See also* CULTS AND QUACKERY

Elizabeth **BLACKWELL** (1821–1910). Anglo-American physician. Born in Bristol, she emigrated to New York with her parents in 1832 and after her father's death in 1839 she supported herself by teaching. Her interest in the education of women was thus aroused and she decided to become a doctor. Her attempts to gain entry to a medical school were unavailing until finally she was accepted by the University of Geneva in New York State, from which she graduated MD in 1849. In 1850 she returned to Europe, visiting England and France. In Paris, while attending a school for midwives she acquired a purulent ophthalmia and lost the sight of one eye. In London she attended lectures at St Bartholomew's Hospital with the permission of James PAGET (p 603). Going back to New York she opened a dispensary for women in that city. In 1859, once again in England, she became the first woman to be placed on the British Medical Register. In 1875 she was appointed professor of gynecology and obstetrics at the London School of Medicine for Women. Elizabeth Blackwell was one of the pioneers in the cause of women's education, a subject on which she continued to lecture until an advanced age. She was the first British woman to qualify in medicine.

**BLOOD TRANSFUSION** Across time and cultures, blood has been seen as the harbinger of death and the giver of life. There is, of course, an empirical explanation for these disparate views: we need blood to live; without it, we die. Yet, even today, blood remains at the center of biology, language, and behavior in a manner that underscores its complexity. At one level, blood is a bodily fluid that acts as a specialized connective tissue and is composed of blood cells — red, white, and platelets — floating in plasma. At another, 'blood' is also a metaphor for kinship ('blood brothers'), social division ('blue blood'; 'bad blood'), and solemn truths ('blood oath'). Further, blood has long been the preferred substance of sacrifice and other rituals.

Moved between bodies — by bathing, drinking, or transfusing into veins — blood has been used to rejuvenate failing human bodies and souls. This movement, however, has never been a simple one; instead, it has carried with it the complexities of blood itself. The history of blood's movement between bodies provides myriad examples of blood's ambiguous cultural status. And, while the history of transfusion opens with a clear vision of blood's purer properties, it unfolds — and some have argued, may even end — with an increasing awareness of its more dangerous dimensions.

The more traditional movement of blood between bodies — through drinking or bathing — rested upon blood's multivalent cultural status, frequently crossing the line between purity and

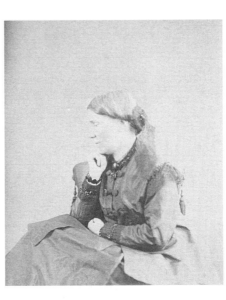

danger. Homer tells of how Odysseus used the blood of goats to substantiate the shades of Hades and force them to speak truthfully to him. In this instance, blood at once reanimates the dead and constrains the nature of their interaction with the living. This latter capacity of blood-as-truth-serum is a recurrent sub-theme in western thought, found in medieval ideas about consuming blood and later continued in connection with transfusion proper. In George Eliot's mid-19th century tale, *The lifted veil*, for example, a woman on the verge of death is temporarily revived by a timely transfusion of blood, only to voice ugly truths that effect the fall of her mistress. Yet it is reanimation itself that is most frequently associated with blood's movement between bodies. In Italy alone, the ancient Romans drank the blood of fallen gladiators to assimilate their vitality; Pope Innocent the VIII was fed the blood of three young boys in a futile effort to prolong his life in 1492; and in 1930, British newspapers announced that Dr Giocondo Protti on the basis of some 2000 experiments had found that blood transfusions from the young rejuvenated the elderly. Outside Italy, in 16th century Hungary, Countess Elizabeth of Bathory bathed in the blood of hundreds of virgins in an effort to maintain her youthful beauty. Moving blood has also been seen to purify its recipient. The Christian Eucharist calls upon believers to drink the blood of Christ to prepare for entry into heaven. The Victorian novelist Bram Stoker juxtaposed good and evil by having the heroes of *Dracula* use transfusion to counteract the deadly and damning effects of vampirically induced anemia. In this same vein, the first actual transfusions were in part an effort to purify fallen humanity.

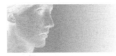

Thomas **WHARTON** (1614–73). British physician. Wharton moved to London during the civil war, where he worked with Cromwell's physician John Bathurst. In 1659 Wharton was appointed physician to St Thomas's Hospital. He remained in the city throughout the plague on condition that he treated the guards and would be appointed physician in ordinary to the King when the position became vacant, but the promise was not fulfilled. As compensation, Wharton was given a coat of arms, but had to pay £10. Having named the thyroid gland, he gave his own to the duct draining the submandibular salivary gland. His friend Izaak Walton mentioned Wharton by name in *The compleat angler*.

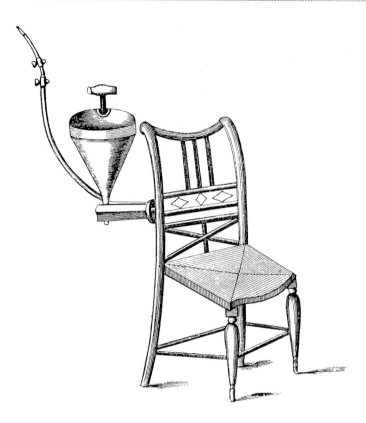

Blundell's Impellor, the first apparatus for giving a blood transfusion. (From *Recherches physiological and pathological*, 1924.)

### First human procedure

The first recorded human blood transfusion was performed in France in 1667 by Jean-Baptiste Denis, at the Académie des Sciences. Denis transfused the blood of a lamb through quills and silver cannulas directly into his patient, who survived the operation. This experiment followed the animal transfusions conducted by the fellows of London's Royal Society from 1665. Certainly, William HARVEY's (p 363) work earlier that century demonstrating that the blood circulated, rather than lapped outward, through the body, was conceptually important to these transfusion experiments. Yet, it has recently been shown that 17th century transfusers were also guided by more traditional, religious concerns: they wanted to effect the moral perfection of their patients. By using the blood of a lamb — which held both temperamental and religious significance — DENYS (p 121) and, in Britain, Richard LOWER (p 119) and Edmund King, hoped to improve the characters of blood recipients, and in this way use science to correct some of the effects of man's fall from grace in the Garden of Eden. The death of one of these recipients (after a transfusion in late 1667), however, swiftly removed the procedure from the realm of acceptable medical practice until the early 19th century.

Transfusion was re-established on a limited but definite scale through the efforts of London obstetrician and physiologist James Blundell. Blundell, who received his MD from Edinburgh University in 1813 and was practicing (and teaching) at Guy's Hospital, began advocating human-to-human transfusion from 1818 — principally to treat women near death from uterine hemorrhage. Donors tended to be husbands or doctors. These donors, however, were far more reticent (at least verbally) than were lambs to have arteries punctured for the sake of direct transfusion — leading Blundell to devise a series of apparatus for the indirect transfusion of blood from donor veins, into a waiting receptacle (at its most simple, a hefty brass syringe/glass container combination), and finally, into patients' veins. He conducted several transfusions over the next 15 years. Those who died were generally thought to have been too near death to be saved; those who lived provided dramatic testimony to blood's reanimating properties. Indeed, it may be argued that belief in blood's powers to rejuvenate — even in small quantities — was an important factor in the operation's re-establishment. This belief, of course, did not disappear in the 18th century; however, in the early 19th, it coincided with increased medical power at the deathbed and a rising fashion of Gothic romances that celebrated the intentional channeling of vital fluids to re-animate the dead (and undead). Though not frequently practiced during the 19th century, transfusion was the subject of animated élite medical debate and became further instrumental evidence in British obstetricians' arguments for superiority over traditional MIDWIVES at the birthing bedside.

There was considerable interest in the physiologic and chemical implications of Blundell's work in Europe. Of particular concern, were questions about blood's coagulability and the effects of mixing blood from different species (heterologous transfusion). In 1821, J. L. Prévost and J. B. A. Dumas confirmed both that blood was far more effective in reanimating the exsanguinated than water and that heterologous transfusion was dangerous. Further, they argued that one could transfuse more simply and effectively by first whipping the blood with a fork, twig, or rod — a process called defibrination. Debates over whether to use defibrinated or unaltered blood, direct or indirect transfusion methods, continued through the 19th century. The 1870s witnessed almost simultaneously a resurgence in the use of animal blood (generally sheep's) for human transfusion, and the production of further physiologic evidence of its danger. The investigations of E. Ponfick (1874) and L. Landois (1875) on the effects of heterologous transfusion helped persuade transfusers to reject non-human blood for human transfusion.

The statistical dimensions of Landois's study gives some idea of transfusion's extension in 19th century European medical practice. Combing the literature, he found accounts of 347 human-to-human transfusions. Twenty-six years earlier, when Britain's C. H. F. Routh had conducted his own statistical study of transfusion's efficacy, he had found evidence of only 48 cases (including the 17th century animal-to-human trials). Indeed, J. Roussel, (simultaneously, but independently, with Britain's J. H. Aveling in 1864) inventor of direct transfusion through india rubber tubes, claimed that his apparatus had been used in the Franco–Prussian War. During the 1870s, surgeons increasingly explored transfusion's applications for treating anemia. Stemming the rising tide of transfusion, however, was a growing belief that infusion of saline solution might replace blood in an equally effective, but far neater, operation. Studies of the relative merits of blood and water, and of the survival of transfused red cells in the patient's body, took a prominent place in the transfusion literature of the 1880s. Classic among these was British physiologist W. Hunter's 1889 piece, which concluded that 'all the advantages to be gained by transfusion may, I believe, be equally well and more readily obtained by infusion of a neutral saline'. Blood transfusion is rarely mentioned in the medical literature of the 1890s and early 1900s.

The American physiological surgeon George Washington Crile is generally credited with reviving interest in blood transfusion. Sceptical whether infused saline could maintain the blood pressure over the long run, he began comparative experiments on shock in 1898. These confirmed his suspicions. However, there remained a difficulty with transfusion's practical application — namely, that blood clotted. When Crile learned of French surgeon Alexis Carrel's new technique for suturing together arteries and veins, he applied it to transfusion, and began experimenting with direct transfusion from donor to patient in 1905. British medical journals received Crile's now-classic 1907 paper advocating transfusion with respectful reserve, the *British Medical Journal* concluding that 'surgeons, we imagine, will find no good reasons given here for abandoning the safe and simple method of saline injection'. With a few exceptions, British practitioners followed this conclusion until midway through the First World War.

In the years before the War, two important discoveries (the one, indeed, more a re-discovery) greatly facilitated transfusion's medical extension. The first was Karl LANDSTEINER's (p 120) discovery of blood groups in 1900–1. 19th-century physi-ologists had appreciated that blood from another species could destroy the cells of transfused patients. Around the turn of the century, serologists noted that a similar reaction — the clumping, or agglutination, of cells — might occur between the blood of individuals of the *same* species. Initially, this was interpreted as a pathological reaction, perhaps brought about by disease. It was Landsteiner who showed that this phenomenon was in fact normal. Human blood naturally occurred in different types (three, he initially thought, though shown to be four by Decastello and Sturli in 1902), and the serum of some types agglutinated the corpuscles of others. Interestingly, though Landsteiner himself pointed to his discovery's applicability to transfusion, blood typing was not systematically used until late in the First World War. Probably Landsteiner's disciplinary distance from medical practice (serology), combined with transfusion's relative obscurity in 1900, effectively marginalized his important discovery. Even into the 1920s, transfusers often pointed to either Jansky's 1907 work, or Moss's 1910 study, as having shown the existence of blood types.

## Anticoagulants

The second important discovery was that sodium citrate could be used as an anticoagulant. During the 19th century, transfusers experimented with various anticoagulants. It was in 1914–15 that three different researchers, working independently in three different countries (A. Hustin, Belgium; R. Lewisohn, USA; L. Agote, Argentina), concluded that sodium citrate, used properly, could delay blood's coagulation without harming the patient. By mixing blood with sodium citrate, doctors could bleed donors into a bottle outside the operating theater — at once creating more space in the theater itself, and simplifying the transfusion operation to the inversion of the bottle and the insertion of a needle into the patient's arm. In 1916, P. ROUS (p 120) and J. R. Turner, of the Rockefeller Institute, devised a procedure that allowed red cells to be preserved and refrigerated for later use. Applied during the War in 1918 by American surgeon O. H. Robertson, this is argued to have been the first blood bank.

The First World War did much to enhance transfusion's favor among surgeons. It was brought to the battlefields of France from 1915 by the North Americans, who, in a classic example of technology transfer, educated British and French army doctors about the operation, and published accounts of their work in British and French medical journals for the consideration of those back home. Moreover, a joint commission on shock, under the auspices of Britain's Medical Research Committee (later Council), brought

**THE TRANSFUSION PIONEERS**

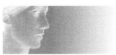

Richard **LOWER** (1631–91). British physician. Lower was assistant to Thomas Willis in Oxford, but later became the most successful physician in London. In 1665 he was the first to undertake direct blood transfusion betweeen two dogs and in 1667 gave the first transfusion of sheep's blood to man in England. He published *Tractatus de corde* (1669).

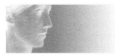

Sir Geoffrey Langdon **KEYNES** (1887–1982). British surgeon. The brother of Maynard (Lord) Keynes, the economist, he became assistant surgeon and later surgeon at St Bartholomew's Hospital. As an army surgeon in the First World War, he became convinced of the importance of blood transfusion for resuscitating wounded soldiers. In the 1920s he wrote a book about this and helped to inaugurate a transfusion service, at first in London and then throughout the country. In the 1930s he pioneered simple removal of the tumor in certain cases of breast cancer ('lumpectomy'), which incurred the wrath of the medical establishment but was shown to give results as good as the more mutilating radical operation usually practiced. In 1942 he performed the first thymectomy for myasthenia gravis in Britain. In close contact with the Bloomsbury Group, he had rushed Virginia Woolf to hospital and had her stomach washed out after she had taken an overdose. (*continued overleaf*)

(continued)

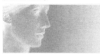

Francis Peyton **ROUS** (1879–1970). American experimental pathologist. After training in pathology at the University of Michigan, Rous joined the staff of the ROCKEFELLER INSTITUTE in 1909, where he remained throughout a long professional career. In 1911 he demonstrated that a sarcoma of chickens could be transmitted by an agent in cell-free sterile filtrates of the tumors, that is, a virus. For this work he received the NOBEL PRIZE 55 years later. During the First World War he conducted studies on the preservation of blood, and showed that by bleeding into a solution of citrate and sugar, blood could be maintained in fluid state, with cells relatively undamaged, for weeks. This finding enabled the later practical development of blood banks.

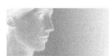

Karl **LANDSTEINER** (1868–1943). Austrian/ American pathologist. He transmitted POLIOMYELITIS from human tissue to monkeys, by intracerebral inoculation. He studied human blood groups, demonstrating the ABO system, thus laying the foundation for safe BLOOD TRANSFUSION. For this work he received the NOBEL PRIZE in 1930. He moved to the USA in 1919 as a member of the ROCKEFELLER INSTITUTE, and continued his immunological research.

(continued opposite)

together the top British and North American surgeons and physiologists, who discussed the means, materials, and applications of the operation. (Indeed, within this group, the specter of the 19th century physiologic debate over whether blood was indeed the best fluid to inject was raised again.) Surgeons tested blood's efficacy initially at evacuation hospitals and later nearer the front, where resuscitation teams transfused soldiers still bleeding and suffering from shock with bottled blood. Donors were never hard to find: the lightly wounded were plentiful and, animated by the spirit of fraternity and the promise of extra time off during their next home leave, eager to donate. Though it is unclear how frequently transfusion was practiced during the Great War, it is clear that the operation won over powerful allies.

Returning home, these converts to the cause of transfusion — principally surgeons — not only practiced the operation, but preached its benefits to the uninitiated. Though some tradition of transfusion existed already in the United States, in Britain, it was essentially introduced into a virgin field. Gradually, it was extended, and was used not only to treat surgical shock and some types of hemorrhage, but also for patients with gas poisoning and various anemias. And, though cold storage and blood substitutes had been explored during war-time, interwar medical practitioners preferred fresh, whole blood. The increasing demand for blood necessitated an increasing demand for blood donors.

In the formation of panels of blood donors, the American lead was again generally followed. Here, individual hospitals — and sometimes surgeons — compiled lists of individuals willing to go to hospital and give blood when a transfusion was needed. Donors tended to be men with type 'O' blood — believed to be 'universal' donors, able to give blood to all types without causing an adverse reaction. (The existence of rhesus positive and negative types was not discovered until 1939–40.) Moreover, these donors were paid, sometimes quite well, for their 'donations'. It was at a small division of the British RED CROSS, however, that a different approach to blood donation was developed and institutionalized. Led by its honorary secretary, Percy Lane Oliver, the Camberwell Division articulated a system that relied exclusively upon unpaid donors of blood. Supported by the élite medical practitioners and administrators of London's voluntary hospitals, and sustained by members of a host of voluntary organizations, the London Blood Transfusion Service grew rapidly, becoming part of the central division of the British Red Cross from 1926. A decade later, in 1936, the Service boasted nearly 2400 donors, who were summoned on roughly

5200 occasions to donate blood to one of the 181 London hospitals served. Already, issues of blood purity were arising in relation to paid and voluntary systems. While in the United States, 'colored' blood was avoided for fear of spreading SYPHILIS, in Britain, Oliver was firmly convinced that voluntarism provided effective protection against contamination: 'Whilst it is not suggested that voluntary donors are immune from such dangers, it may at least be said that the spirit of altruism which induces them to offer their services to unknown sufferers, would be equally effective in causing them to withdraw temporarily or permanently should they chance to contract such a disease'.

### Bleeding cadavers

The 1930s not only witnessed the institutionalization of the voluntary donor, but also introduced new ways of procuring, processing, and delivering blood. In Moscow, doctors bled the cadavers of people who had died suddenly from suicide, accident, or heart attack. This blood was bottled and refrigerated for later use — a process that received attention in Europe and the USA both for its unconventional donors and for its reliance upon cold storage. Perhaps inspired by this latter possibility — neglected since the First World War — F. D. Jorda organized a blood banking system in 1936 to treat casualties of the Spanish Civil War. The next year, Chicago's Cook County Hospital implemented the world's first civilian blood banking program. Although many doctors expressed preference for fresh rather than stored blood, blood banking was firmly established as the favored method of blood delivery during the Second World War.

Blood banking is not the only transfusion-related development to have been encouraged by the war. The use of plasma, particularly in its fresh-frozen form, and of blood-derived biological products — including gamma globulin and serum albumin — received a tremendous boost as a result of war-time needs for efficiency in shipment and distribution. From the 1950s, plastic packs began to be developed and used to replace traditional glass bottles. These now familiar packs offered several advantages: they were sterile, disposable, storable, easily portable, averted the occasional problem of patients reacting to chemicals in the rubber tubing of the glass system (thrombophlebitis), and facilitated the separation of blood into its component parts. They were, however, more expensive; England and Wales's National Blood Transfusion Service did not wholly convert to plastic packs until 1975.

Today, blood transfusion is so fundamental to medical practice that the blood pack is a veritable symbol of medicine itself. At the same time, it has become so routine that it retains little of the romanticized status it had earlier this century. This mundane perception of transfusion is further substantiated by the increasing improbability that any blood donation will go directly to an individual patient: whereas into the 1970s whole blood transfusion was the rule, it is now used for less than 5% of donated blood in England and Wales. A pint of blood is most frequently broken down into its component parts: red cells, platelets, and plasma. Further, a host of blood products may be derived from the blood, from albumin and immunoglobulin to clotting factors. Factor VIII, one such blood product, was licensed in the UK in 1973 and helped increase the life expectancy of individuals suffering from hemophilia from 37 years in 1962 to nearly that of the general population by 1980.

The story of factor VIII is, however, better known for its post-1980 history. Derived from multiple blood donations, this life-extending blood product proved a mortal danger to its recipients in the early years of AIDS, before screening was possible. AIDS, if more dramatic and deadly, is not the first infectious disease to have threatened the purity of the blood supply. MALARIA and syphilis were known dangers to interwar transfusers; hepatitis transmission increasingly concerned those guiding blood donation and using blood in the postwar era. Richard Titmuss, writing in 1970 echoing Oliver's earlier sentiment, argued that voluntary donation dramatically decreased the likelihood of transfusion-related disease transmission. Yet, he did not suggest that blood's potential dangers outweighed its obvious benefits.

Historically, total purity has not been a precondition for transfusion. Indeed, risk has been an integral part of transfusion: from clots and typing errors to hepatitis and AIDS, blood has had the ability to harm or even kill its recipients. Today, while testing for HIV/AIDS has lessened the immediate danger of transfusion, fears that bovine spongiform encephalopathy and therefore variant CREUTZFELDT–JAKOB DISEASE might be transmissible in transfused blood have motivated some to call for the implementation of new procedures to purify the blood supply (such as removing the white blood cells). So expensive are these procedures that, even if they could guarantee 100% purity, they would bankrupt transfusion services — and thereby eliminate transfusion as a medical option.

Why has any risk in transfusion become socially unacceptable? Perhaps it is related to transfusion's success: its routine nature has made it mundane, dislodging it, at least in immediate perception, from its long-standing association with heroism and rejuvenation. Perhaps it is also connected with the increasing technological compartmentalization of a donor's pint of blood — a process that further obscures the tangible meaning of transfusion for the non-medical donating public. Certainly, the devastating effects of AIDS, particularly upon people with hemophilia, galvanized public awareness of blood's danger. At the same time, our current demand for risk-free blood points to the broader fears, needs, and desires of our culture. Titmuss studied transfusion in part because he believed that attitudes towards blood donation both helped illuminate and constitute cultures themselves. In this spirit, one might read our current expectations of risk-free transfusion as a kind of cultural barometer. How best to interpret its readings, I leave to the reader.                                                    KP

Hermann **BOERHAAVE** (1668–1738). Dutch physician, Boerhaave was a scholar of distinction speaking all the European languages as well a being an elegant Latinist. In 1701 he was appointed lecturer in medicine and chemistry at Leiden and rapidly gained a reputation as an outstanding teacher. Promoted professor of medicine and botany in 1709, he added the chair of chemistry in 1718 and his method of bedside teaching drew students from all over Europe. He lectured in Latin and revived the Hippocratic approach to become the founder of the eclectic school. His textbooks, translated into all the European languages, circulated throughout the civilized world. His case report of a man who died from rupture of the esophagus *Atrosis nex descripti prius morbi historia* (1724), was the first to be cast in modern form with history followed by physical examination, diagnosis, course, and autopsy. The modern medical curriculum with its sequence of natural science, anatomy, physiology, and pathology is derived from him. His pupils spread his doctrine throughout Europe; both the Edinburgh and the old Vienna schools owed much to him. His *Aphorismi* (1709) and his *Elementia chemiae* (1732) are perhaps his best-known works. Although he was the most famous man of science in Europe, who raised the status of the medical profession in the eyes of the public and had an immense reputation, he had no enduring influence on medical thought.

**BOLOGNA** See ITALY

**BOOKS AND LIBRARIES** The invention (*c.*1450) of printing from movable type was the most important factor in the development of books and libraries. Scientific and medical printed books soon became available, at first simply reproductions of the works of ancient writers, but soon as an essential factor in the dissemination of developing knowledge. Some

(continued)

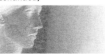

Jean Baptiste **DENYS** (?1640–1704). French physician. He became a member of a scientific group called the 'Montmort Academy' who interested themselves in the work of LOWER (p 119) and others on blood transfusions. Denys, and another, were appointed to study the problem. In 1667 after experiments with dogs and calves he transfused 12 oz (340 g) of lamb's blood into a young man, who improved greatly. Later he had two fatalities, a Swedish traveler, Baron Bunde, and Antoine Mauroy, who was deranged. Denys was accused by Mauroy's wife of murder, although it is possible that she poisoned her husband. In 1668 he was cleared of this charge but the court forbade further transfusions unless sanctioned by the Faculty of Medicine.

books had a profound effect on the medical world. Among these were *De humani corporis fabrica* of Andreas VESALIUS (1543) (p 846), marking the beginning of modern anatomy; the *Oeuvres* of the French military surgeon, Ambroise PARÉ (p 320) (1575), adding greatly to the knowledge of surgery; and William HARVEY's (p 363) *Excertatio anatomica de motu cordis et sanguinis in animabilus* (1628), in which the circulation of the blood was shown conclusively for the first time.

Subsequent prolific writers included SYDENHAM (p 721), LEEUWENHOEK (p 489), MALPIGHI (p 37), BOERHAAVE (p 121), Smellie, and (William) HUNTER (p 88). The importance of publication in books was shown when Edward JENNER's (p 452) paper reporting the successful use of vaccination against smallpox was rejected for publication by the *Philosophical Transactions of the Royal Society*. A referee for that journal had stated that the report was merely anecdotal and the thesis needed more cases to support it, but Jenner was able to disseminate his findings by publishing a pamphlet at his own expense, *An inquiry into the causes and effects of the variolae vaccina*.

The rise of the scientific journal in the 17th century was of great significance. It disseminated news of discoveries more quickly and openly than before, and assured authors enduring identification with their discoveries. Journal publication was fueled by gatherings of the learned in Europe, and later the New World, who met for discussions, conducted experiments, and published their findings. Often these societies developed libraries, comprising books, journals, and archives, whose collections are still of value to scholars today.

At the beginning of the 20th century, an amalgamation of 15 specialist medical societies led to the formation of the Royal Society of Medicine in London, which now houses the largest medical research library in Britain. The Wellcome Library, dating back to 1895, is one of the largest and richest collections of medical and scientific historical literature in the world, also situated in London. In the USA, rich medical collections include the National Library of Medicine, the Francis A. Countway Library in Boston, and the New York Academy of Medicine Library. The libraries of the World Health Organization and those of European nations are important resources.

Two works detail the progress of medical knowledge over the centuries. The first, *Morton's medical bibliography*, records almost 9000 texts, illustrating the history of medicine, which are universal in coverage. The second, *Thornton's Medical books, libraries, and collectors*, is a study of bibliographers and the book trade in relation to the medical sciences from earliest time to the late 20th century. The great medical library collections continue to grow and provide the basis for medical education and a source of medical knowledge.

Today the importance of library services is being increasingly emphasized by the royal colleges and other regulatory bodies. In all countries recognized teaching hospitals and associated centers are expected by the accrediting bodies to provide access to the medical literature for EVIDENCE-BASED practice.

## The National Library of Medicine

Many advances have been pioneered by the world's most important library, the US National Library of Medicine. Founded in 1836, it gained special impetus when the visionary John Shaw Billings took charge in 1864. His monumental achievements included the Index Catalogue of the Library of the Surgeon General's Office and the *Index medicus*, a monthly classified record of the current medical literature. Its major database is MEDLINE, dating from the 1960s, which has been developed to enable doctors and health professionals to have low-cost desk-top access direct from their personal computers.

The National Library of Medicine's home page on the World Wide Web (*http://www.nlm.nih.gov*) links directly to MEDLINE and offers the choice of several user-friendly access systems, Internet Grateful Med and PubMed being the most popular. Both professional and lay readers may follow leads to many sources of information, reflecting the shift which acknowledges the right of the public to have access to the same health information as the professional. A wide range of other sources include AIDSLINE, BIOETHICSLINE, TOXLINE, and health STAR, the healthcare administrative database, and several others. The growing emphasis on consumer health information is reflected in MEDLINEplus, which includes information from many hundreds of links to self-help groups, consumer organizations, clearing houses, health-related organizations, and clinical trials.

## The internet

A major shift, comparable with the invention of printing, is occurring with the changing role of print as a medium for information. The explosion in the use of the World Wide Web now allows doctors, all healthcare professionals, and patients easy access to information down-loaded from the INTERNET. Through developments in information and communication technologies, databases are being established and used globally providing access to words, pictures, sound, and video.

## Medical informatics

Medical informatics, which is the development, use, and evaluation of information technology in health care, is a broad discipline encompassing librarians and information technology specialists working together in new roles around:

- providing literature searching facilities on open access
- providing remote electronic access to the library
- making available electronic books and hypertext learning systems
- receiving and delivering document images
- creating and delivering specialist databases
- offering access to other libraries and information sources
- most important of all, in training and guiding users to appropriate evidence-based sources.

The demand for medical literature is producing new solutions in different parts of the world. Library networks are vital and changing rapidly. Lifelong learning, linked to continuing professional development and potentially to re-accreditation, is becoming a reality for the medical and healthcare professions. Librarians must deliver services and learning opportunities to users in their locality, at work in the hospital or community setting, and at home. They must be able to support all users and to treat those on site equally with those who are distant.

Great changes are taking place in libraries, with increasing emphasis on electronic resources. Librarians are responding by exploiting the potential of networking to enable remote access, training and supporting users, and building centers of evidence. Medical and healthcare libraries of the future may be expected to play an important part in providing and developing information support to practitioners.

Advanced technological systems will continue to develop but can never replace the human element. The real asset of the information age is the expertise of medical and healthcare professionals, including librarians, whose knowledge is accurate, up-to-date, and evidence-based.  SG

## BOVINE SPONGIFORM ENCEPHALOPATHY (BSE) See CREUTZFELD–JAKOB DISEASE (CJD)

**BOXING** The boxer's ambition is to achieve a knockout, an abrupt and temporary loss of consciousness. Normal consciousness embraces a state of alertness, and normal intellectual function. Alertness, which is disrupted in the knockout, depends upon the function of specialized groups of cells located longitudinally and centrally in the brain, extending upwards from the

## EXERCITATIO ANATOMICA DE MOTU CORDIS ET SANGUINIS IN ANIMALIBUS

William HARVEY (p 363) originally communicated his views on the circulation of the blood in the first lecturers he gave as Lumleian Lecturer in Anatomy to the Royal College of Physicians of London, on 16, 17, and 18 April 1616. Twelve years later, aged 50, he published his definitive exposition of the subject in the now classic work, the title of which is usually shortened to *De motu cordis*. In full, it reads in English as follows: *Movement of the heart and blood in animals: an anatomical essay* by William Harvey, Englishman, Physician to the King, and Professor of Anatomy in the College of Physicians of London (Frankfurt: William Fitzer, 1628).

Thus did William Harvey destroy the false Galenic concept of circulation which had held sway for fourteen and a half centuries, and he laid the foundation for all future studies of the cardiovascular system.

Harvey's great work in the original Latin can be studied side by side with an excellent English translation by Kenneth J. Franklin in the volume published in 1957 for the Royal College of Physicians of London by Blackwell Scientific Publications, Oxford, under the title *De motu cordis*.

brainstem to structures between the lower part of the cerebral hemispheres. Such cells and structures are called the 'reticular formation' or 'center-encephalic alerting system'. The effective knockout blow usually lands not on the point of the chin but just to one side, causing a very sudden rotation of the head which may be accompanied by some backward movement. Experiments have shown that acute movement of the brain in relation to the skull, and the momentary distortion of the brain (which has a blancmange-like consistency) follow the acceleration/deceleration and rotation of the skull and the brain. Rotation round a vertical and to some extent horizontal axis will almost certainly selectively impair briefly the function of the neuro-physiological alerting system.

Were the effects of the acute acceleration/deceleration/rotation restricted to the alerting system, the debate about 'punch drunkenness' or 'dementia pugilistica' would be sterile. Unfortunately, the effects, especially if repetitive, may be more diffuse, and produce insidiously neurological and mental sequels. The pathological changes, which may be observed microscopically rather than as gross damage, include: small hemorrhages in relation to very small blood vessels; acute disruption of the extensions (axons) of nerve cells; acute shearing and disruption of the supporting tissues of the brain (glib). The sequels to these acute changes may be areas of scarring (gloss); loss of nerve cells; shrinkage (or atrophy) of the cerebral cortex and deeper structures, upon which depend coordination of movements as well as the higher functions of the brain.

Media attention to boxing gives a misleading impression of the more dramatic types of intracranial pathology, which are very rare. If the acute shearing/rotation is severe, and if there is further severe deceleration of the skull as it hits the

### OSLER'S BIBLIOGRAPHER

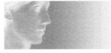

Thomas Archibald **MALLOCH** (1887–1953). American librarian. Upon graduation in medicine from McGill in 1913 'Young Archie', as OSLER (p 602) called him, joined the army and served in France. He spent his leaves with the Oslers at Oxford, and used every opportunity to work in the Bodleian Library on his first book *Finch and Baines, a seventeenth century friendship* (1917). Post-war, Malloch labored at Oxford on the great *Bibliotheca Osleriana* with Dr W. W. Francis and Reginald Hill. Malloch's appointment to the New York Academy of Medicine brought great kudos to its magnificent library. His biographical interests are reflected in his writings on Robin Adair, William Harvey, and John Caius, and also in *Short years*, his biography of John Bruce MacCallum, Osler's most brilliant pupil who died of tuberculosis aged thirty.

canvas, there may be sudden severe, usually irreversible and therefore fatal, swelling of the brain (cerebral edema and vasodilation). Rarely, acute hemorrhage either within the substance of the brain (intracerebral hemorrhage), or over its surface (acute subdural hematoma), may occur immediately or with a short delay. Under those circumstances, transitory recovery from the knockout will be followed by deterioration in level of consciousness. Timely — media dramatic — neurosurgical intervention may occasionally save the boxer's life, but it is very rare for the function of the brain to recover normally. Repeated injuries to eyes or ears may result in serious and permanent disability. The facial skeleton may suffer injuries which produce the deformities that are often caricatured on the stage and screen. It is only when the lovable bruiser speaks that the realities of many past knockouts become apparent.

Inevitably, the final debate centers on 'dementia pugilistica'. The so-called classical features include intellectual impairment, inability to concentrate, fatiguability, impairment of memory, and anxiety. There may also be deterioration of personality or of memory — with disturbance or slurring of speech, tremor, and disturbance of movement similar to that found in Parkinson's disease. Brain scanning, by computerized tomography or magnetic resonance imaging, may show changes in the brain which have been ascribed to repeated knockouts and which may be, but are not commonly, associated with dementia pugilistica.

The great difficulty is to correlate accurately these clinical and radiological features with the severity and frequency of bouts, and knockouts, and with other factors that might be relevant. These include age; pre-existing cerebral function, both intellectual and neurological; and other disorders which may lead to brain atrophy and dementia, either the senile or, particularly, the presenile type. Especially uncertain is any correlation between the speed of apparent recovery from a knockout — or near knockout — and the frequency of microscopic pathological changes in the brain which are believed to lead to dementia pugilistica.

Nevertheless, if the *coup-de-grâce* is to remain a highlight for boxer and spectator, as I believe it should (though almost all doctors argue the opposite), controls can reduce the risk to a boxer of a further knockout within a certain period. Thus the British Boxing Board of Control Ltd has made the medical protection of professional boxers its *raison d'être*. The process includes: licensing of boxers, of whom the vast majority are semi-professional; medical assessment before the bout, with special attention to any psychological, visual, or neurological disorders; and medical assessment at the end of the bout, with a printed card of advice given to every boxer. Furthermore,

a satisfactory report of a magnetic resonance imaging brainscan is required annually, and a report on a magnetic resonance angiogram is required when a boxer first applies for a license.

## The great debate

With all this medical background to the trauma of boxing, it might seem surprising that this sport is allowed to continue in a civilized society. Thus ensues the great boxing debate. The first question is whether boxing is really a noble art, or whether it provides a Roman holiday for a crude populace. Whatever medical, and particularly neurological, disorders may be a consequence of boxing, they will be of little avail to those who wish to curb or control 'the sport', unless the social and immediate physical objectives are examined. Arguably the motorcyclist's desire for the 'ton-up' (driving at 100 miles an hour) has something in common with boxing, and epidemiologically a case could be made for banning motorcycles above a certain engine size. But the motorcyclist and the boxer are as likely to damage themselves as others, so that the element of freedom of choice guides society's view of both activities.

Most of the medical literature on boxing is devoted to the adverse sequels, with little reference to any potential benefits. For this reason, most doctors who have taken an interest in boxing and who have expressed their views publicly, align themselves with its opponents. A balanced view is difficult to find.

Irrespective of the adverse medical effects of boxing, some physical, social, and psychological benefits for the boxer and the spectator deserve attention. Aggressive and physical contact as part of life, and therefore sport, are natural desires for many, especially for young men. There is a strong argument in psychology for not curbing this, and boxing may provide the ideal outlet. Although the proclaimed objective is different, is rugby football so far removed from boxing? The requirements for physical fitness for the boxer are very high and very special; training is medically beneficial. Provided there is reasonable control, the ability to 'take punishment', to 'keep your head', and to retain a certain sporting generosity while being aggressive, is of great benefit. The spectators, now through television in the millions, may be relieved, albeit not physically, of their innate aggression, in a way which does not harm others.

Advocates of boxing, of whom I am one, suggest that all these favorable factors, and especially their prevalence, must be taken into account when drawing conclusions about the risks and benefits of boxing. However, it is very difficult to produce rigorous evidence to support these opinions. It should be remembered that the cases of dementia pugilistica, and of the rare acute intracranial disasters during or immediately after a bout, and which catch the headlines, are often in professional, or semi-professional boxers. But overall most boxing is between amateurs, where there is usually no licensing (for example, by the British Boxing Board of Control) although any recommendations are rightly noted.

Thus in the widest context, the epidemiological evidence shows that the incidence of definite medical injury is very small. A tolerant society should not dismiss the benefits of boxing in the face of pleading by those who have entrenched positions, be they medical or sociological. Thus to restrict, or to abolish, rather than to control, the sport of boxing would diminish the freedom of those who choose to engage in a sport which satisfies natural aggression in a relatively safe way.          JG

*See also* SPORT MEDICINE; VIOLENCE

**Editor's comment**
There is no scientific evidence for any of the alleged benefits of boxing, which are statements of opinion and not facts. Unlike sports in which accidental harm can occur to players, participants in boxing seek deliberately to harm their opponent. Many representative organizations of doctors (e.g. British, American, and Australian Medical Associations, and the American Academy of Pediatrics) have advocated that boxing should either be banned or restricted to adults.          JML

Robert **BOYLE** (1627–91). Anglo-Irish scientist. The seventh son of the first Earl of Cork, he went to Eton College and then travelled with a tutor on the continent of Europe. While living in Oxford his interest in experimental science was stimulated, and he had Robert Hooke as his assistant. Hooke was technically able and a brilliant inventor. Boyle made many contributions to science, the most famous still being known as Boyle's law. More important is the contribution Boyle made to scientific thought, since he helped in the overthrow of the Aristotelian idea of the division of the world into the elements of earth, air, fire, and water. He conceived of the world as made up of particles, with powers of motion and varying organizations. This portended the presently held views of the nature of the world. His outstanding work was *The sceptical chymist* (1661). He was a prominent member of the Royal Society, and a staunch Protestant, thinking that God created the world and set it in motion according to secondary laws which were subject of proper scientific enquiry, without controverting divine law and sinning against it. He never married.

**BRAIN[STEM] DEATH** During the second half of the 20th century significant advances in resuscitation technology began to confront doctors with problems of a new kind. Through the skilled and judicious use of artificial ventilation, of drugs capable of maintaining a collapsing blood pressure, of alimentation via the intravenous route, and of elimination of the waste products of metabolism by dialysis, it became possible to maintain a circulation in bodies whose brains were irreversibly dead. This inevitably led to a profound re-evaluation of what was meant by death. Whether they liked it or not, doctors were forced to confront some basic philosophical issues.

A consensus gradually emerged that human death could be accepted as irreversible loss of the capacity to be conscious, combined with irreversible loss of the capacity to breathe spontaneously, and hence to maintain a spontaneous heart beat. This concept was not really radically new. It was basically a secularized reformulation (in the language of modern neurophysiology) of much older concepts of death. 'Irreversible loss of the capacity for consciousness' was the same as 'departure of the (conscious) soul from the body'. And 'irreversible loss of the capacity to breathe spontaneously' was what many older writers meant by 'loss of the breath of life'.

Most people die because their circulation stops, and doctors can't get it going again. If the circulation resumes within a matter of seconds, the patient will, at worse, have suffered a fainting attack. If the circulation is restored only within 3 or 4 minutes the patient will have suffered severe anoxic brain damage, for anoxia (oxygen deprivation) of this severity not only stops the machine, it wrecks the machinery. The cerebral hemispheres (the part of the brain subserving all perceptive, cognitive, and affective functions) will have been irreversibly damaged, whereas the brainstem (the part of the brain subserving vegetative functions — which is less vulnerable to anoxia) will have been spared. If the heart stops for longer periods, both the cerebral hemispheres and the brainstem will have died, and the patient will be dead according to classic criteria.

Major intracranial catastrophes can also irreversibly destroy the brainstem. When certain parts of the upper brainstem are destroyed, the individual is rendered unconscious, for these parts 'activate' the cerebral hemispheres, generating, as it were, the 'capacity for consciousness'. When the brainstem is destroyed, spontaneous respiration, which is 'driven' by cells in the lower part of the brainstem, will also cease. But if such patients are put on ventilators (and the heart is thereby supplied with oxygenated blood), cardiac function can, for a while, be maintained. This is because the heart beat (unlike breathing) is not 'driven' by the nervous system. Anyone who has seen an isolated frog's heart beating in a jar will be familiar with this phenomenon.

## PRE-CONDITIONS OF BRAINSTEM DEATH

- The patient has to be deeply unconscious, on a ventilator, in an intensive care unit. The diagnosis of brainstem death cannot be made at the roadside, in accident and emergency departments, on patients dying at home, or in the general wards of a hospital.

- The cause of the coma must be known without a shred of doubt. Patients in coma of unknown cause can never be diagnosed as brainstem dead. The cause of the coma must be 'irremediable', 'structural' brain damage. The determination of the 'irremediable' nature of the brain damage is not based on theoretical grounds, but is painstakingly established, after the application of all potentially useful therapeutic measures.

- Conditions such as drug intoxication, hypothermia, or profound metabolic upset (which are capable of causing a reversible disturbance of brainstem function) have to be strictly excluded.

Hence there is only one kind of death (brainstem death), although there are several ways of dying: the brainstem can die because the circulation has ceased for sufficiently long, or it can be destroyed as a result of a primary intracranial catastrophe.

The clinical state which has become known as 'brain death' was first described by two French neurologists in 1958. They called it '*coma dépassé*' (literally a state beyond coma). Affected individuals not only failed to relate to the external environment, they could not even maintain homeostasis (a stable internal environment).

Over the next decade doctors working in intensive care units became increasingly familiar with the condition, and standard criteria for its diagnosis were set up in many countries. It was established that such patients had a 'blocked cerebral circulation'. No blood could enter the head because the intracranial pressure had been lastingly higher than the systolic arterial pressure. Brain death was described by some as 'physiological decapitation'. It was also proved unequivocally that even if ventilation was maintained in such patients, no individual ever regained consciousness. All patients, moreover, developed asystole (cessation of the heart beat) within a relatively short time.

### Diagnosis

The diagnosis of brainstem death is straightforward, despite the very stringent criteria adopted for its identification. Before brainstem death can be diagnosed, certain preconditions have to be fulfilled. If the patient fulfills these preconditions, certain clinical tests are then applied.

Only after the patient has been through these very tight 'filters' is he or she deemed to be a suitable candidate to be tested for irreversible loss of brainstem function.

### Tests

These assess the integrity of the brainstem reflexes and the capacity for spontaneous respiration. The doctors performing the tests have to provide unambiguous answers to several questions:

1. Do the pupils constrict when a bright light is shone into them?

2. Does the patient blink when his/her cornea is touched?

3. Is there grimacing in response to firm supra-orbital pressure or to painful stimuli applied to other parts of the body?

4. Is there any movement of the eyes in response to the irrigation of the eardrums with ice-cold water?

5. Is there any coughing or gagging when a catheter is passed down the airway?

These tests assess function at various levels of the brainstem (in a 'slice by slice' manner), the responses mutually reinforcing one another.

Finally, if all the tests have given negative responses, the doctors then assess whether the individual can breathe spontaneously. After proper preoxygenation, the patient is disconnected from the ventilator. Disconnection is maintained for a period sufficient to allow endogenously produced carbon dioxide to build up to a level of 6.5 kPa (50 mmHg) which would stimulate the respiratory center in the brainstem if it still contained live nerve cells. A failure of inspiratory effort, in response to this concentration of carbon dioxide in the blood, provides the final confirmation that the brainstem has ceased to function.

The tests have to be performed by two doctors of appropriate seniority, who are experienced in the management of such cases. The doctors may be neurologists, neurosurgeons, anesthetists, or intensive care specialists. The relevant tests are always repeated after a short period, to document the fact that the abnormal state has persisted for a period several times longer than nerve cells can survive deprivation of their blood supply.

The diagnosis of brainstem death is made in a systematic and unhurried manner. No haste is involved. The potential recipient of organs may be anxious to receive the organs of a brainstem dead donor. However, the doctors looking after the potential donor remain totally committed to his or her case. Transplant surgeons are not involved in the diagnosis of brainstem death.

The diagnosis of death on neurological (as distinct from cardiological) grounds is now accepted practice in nearly all countries of the world. It has formal legal sanction in many countries. In others it is based on codes elaborated by the highest medical authorities. The British code has been endorsed by the Conference of Medical Royal Colleges and their faculties in Britain, a body which meets periodically to assess national and international developments in this subject.    CP

**BREAST CANCER** awareness campaigns broadcast that one in twelve women will develop breast cancer and then alert women to the importance of breast cancer awareness. The statistic 1 in 12 is true but unhelpful, and an unfortunate side-effect of these campaigns is to generate an atmosphere of anxiety among inappropriate age groups.

There are many ways of describing the incidence of breast cancer and the 1 in 12 ratio applies to women who live to the ripe old age of 85 and have escaped all the competing risks for premature death. Furthermore, the 1 in 12 ratio does not define the number of women who die of breast cancer, which on latest estimates is about 1 in 22.

A much higher proportion of women die of cardiovascular disease, lung cancer if they smoke, or the complications of osteoporosis.

Perhaps a more relevant statistic for women is that breast cancer in women aged under 30 is extremely rare, accounting for about 30 deaths a year in Britain. Therefore health promotion campaigns for this young age group should perhaps be targeted at road traffic accident awareness and tobacco consumption advice. Between the ages of 30 and 50 there is about a 1 per 1000 per year risk of developing breast cancer, on aggregate 2% over this 20 year span. Between the ages of 50 and 69 (the age group most likely to be invited for mammographic screening) the risk goes up to 2 per 1000 per year or 4% over those two decades.

### What does 'relative risk' mean?

When epidemiological studies calculate relative risk for developing breast cancer based on familial or environmental factors, they use a calculation based on the background risk described above. Thus if a study suggests that drinking three glasses of wine a day increases a woman's risk of developing breast cancer twofold, this has to be interpreted as 2 per 1000 per year under the menopause and 4 per 1000 per year after the menopause. Once lay people are equipped to interpret these alarmist statistics, they are better able to make life-style calculations that on balance of probabilities may enhance their length and quality of life.

The table illustrates some of the well-established risk factors for developing breast cancer, but even those with two first degree relatives who may worry about a relative risk of 5.0 for developing breast cancer can put this into perspective when it is translated into a 10% absolute risk of developing the disease before the age of 50, which is certainly of some concern but not sufficient to demand instant intervention.

To clarify the issue of relative risk calculations I will concentrate on the two extremes. What is meant by a relative risk of 1.3 for women using oral contraceptives or hormone replacement therapy, and what is the significance of a risk in a family with a strong likelihood of a genetic predisposition? Recent analyses of all the epidemiological studies on breast cancer risk associated with using oral contraceptives in premenopausal women or hormone replacement therapy in postmenopausal women come up with a figure which is roughly the same — 1.3 on the basis of ever use/never use.

Women in the reproductive years have a risk of 1 per 1000 per year of developing breast cancer over the age of 30, and an almost immeasurable risk under the age of 30. 1.3 times that risk might suggest another 3 cases per 10 000 women over a decade. Furthermore, the cancers that develop under these circumstances tend to be more favorable, and therefore there is no real evidence of an increased death rate from breast cancer. Against this has to be weighed up the convenience of safe and effective contraception and the hazard of illness and death from unwanted pregnancies, which certainly exceeds that of breast cancer. Hence a woman's decision whether or not to take oral contraceptives should not be influenced by the perceived risk of breast cancer.

The same kind of arguments apply to hormone replacement therapy. In the decade 50–60, when women might be considering hormone replacement therapy, the background risk of breast cancer is 2 per 1000 per year — 2% over the decade. A relative risk of 1.3 would suggest an extra 6 cases per 1000 women exposed to hormone replacement therapy, and once again there is no good evidence that this is associated with an excess death rate from breast cancer because the disease that develops seems to be more favorable. Given that hormone replacement therapy protects women from the more common causes of death, through cardiovascular disease and osteoporosis, then the perceived hazard of breast cancer after receiving hormone replacement therapy should not influence a woman's decision on this matter.

### Genetic predisposition

At the other extreme, where the woman's pedigree is strongly suggestive of a genetic predisposition to breast cancer (carrying the genes known as BRCA1 or BRCA2), then the calculations are very different. If there is a germ line mutation passing through the family then any unaffected woman has a 50/50 chance of having inherited the gene. The penetrance of the gene (i.e. the capacity of inducing breast cancer if the woman has the gene) is about 70%, and therefore the absolute risk of developing breast cancer is roughly 35%. Most of this risk is

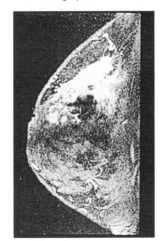

MRI scan showing a cancerous tumor of the breast. (Reproduced courtesy of the National Institute for Cancer, Bethesda, MD.)

Well-established breast cancer risk factors

| Risk factor | Comparison category | Risk category | Relative risk |
|---|---|---|---|
| Age at menarche | 16 years | <12 years | 1.3 |
| Age at menopause | 45–54 years | >55 years | 1.5 |
| Age when first child born alive | <20 years | Nulliparous or >30 years | 1.9 |
| Oral contraceptive | Never use | Ever use | 1.3 |
| Hormone replacement | Never use | Ever use | 1.3 |
| Benign breast disease | No biopsy or fine needle aspiration | Any benign disease | 1.5 |
| | | Proliferative disease | 2.0 |
| | | Atypical hyperplasia | 4.0 |
| Family history | No first-degree relative affected | Mother affected | 1.7 |
| | | Two first-degree relatives affected | 5.0 |

expressed before the women reaches the age of 60. Such women prove an enormous challenge to the medical community because, as yet, there are no clear indications for genetic testing and even interventions such as prophylactic mastectomy are still considered of unproved efficacy.

There is no agreed policy for preventing breast cancer. There is some evidence that regular exercise or a diet rich in phyto-estrogens may be protective if these start early in the reproductive years; in any case these regimens are of value in promoting general health. The most promising drug for the chemoprevention of breast cancer is tamoxifen. Currently clinical trials in Britain, Italy, and the USA are close to their recruitment target and within the next ten years we may know with confidence whether or not taking the drug for five years will have an important effect on breast cancer incidence and breast cancer mortality.

Mammographic screening is not a preventive intervention for breast cancer, but is thought to reduce mortality from breast cancer by detecting the disease at a stage before it has spread and established secondary tumors. There is considerable controversy about the value of mammographic screening among premenopausal women, and in most of Europe and Britain screening programs are considered inappropriate for the premenopausal age group; although, as a result of intense lobbying, such programs are available for the under 50s in the USA. In contrast, reliable data show that mammographic screening for women between the ages of 50 and 69 reduces breast cancer mortality in that population. However, there has to be very tight quality control of the program. The interval between screens should be between two and three years, and ideally each women should have mammograms

that are read by two specialists and involve taking two views of each breast.

If everything goes to plan then this program may result in a 25% reduction in breast cancer death rates in the population screened, or, in other words, a relative risk of 0.75. Women should be given sufficient information to either opt in or opt out of the program. Although screening is of public health value, the chances of an individual woman benefiting may be calculated as follows: between the ages of 50 and 69 about 4 or 5% of the population are likely to develop breast cancer. However, over this same time only about 1 in 4 will die of the disease. Therefore the 0.75 relative risk applies to that 1% — so, in other words, 99.75% of such women are unlikely to benefit. Unfortunately it is impossible to define the women who are winners in the lottery, but sadly it is easy to define those who suffer.

The harm does not come from exposure to radiation but rather from the imperfection of the mammographic test. Even in the best of hands, there is a false reassurance and a false alarm rate. Negative mammograms may be associated with so-called interval cancers, between one screening and the next, and false positives occur when the mammograms are incorrectly interpreted as showing a suspicion of cancer and the woman is subjected to an unnecessary biopsy. Sometimes this biopsy may show a condition known as duct carcinoma in situ (which is the precursor of invasive cancer) but at the same time it has been estimated that only 1 in 5 of such conditions, if left undetected, would proceed to invasive breast cancer (the same applies to screening for prostate cancer in men). For these reasons, women should not be coerced into mammographic screening, but allowed to make an informed choice. At the same time, a successful program will clearly be associated with reducing the burden of breast cancer diagnosis and management on the community as a whole.

## Treatment

So far as treatment is concerned, the news is encouraging. The adoption of breast conserving techniques, using limited surgery followed by radiotherapy, has been confidently demonstrated as equivalent in outcome to the more radical operations of the past, while the use of chemotherapy and tamoxifen after primary surgery (adjuvant systemic therapy) has been associated with a significant improvement in survival. Since the widespread adoption of adjuvant systemic therapy in the mid-1980s, the mortality from breast cancer has fallen throughout the western world.

With a better understanding of risk and risk management, appropriate awareness, and appropriate screening, together with improvements in adjuvant systemic therapy and the exploitation of our new won knowledge on the molecular basis of breast cancer, it is likely that mortality from this disease will continue to fall. Then we shall reach a point where the disease is no longer the dread specter conjured up by the breast cancer awareness campaigns.                    MB

*See also* DIET AND DISEASE; IMAGING; SCREENING

**BRITAIN** As in many western countries, the early medical care of the poor in Britain was provided by the family, neighbors, and priests. The rich were treated in their homes by a mix of 'professionals,' varying from QUACKS to those with a particular skill such as bone setting or cutting for a bladder stone. The few religious or municipal institutions were small, a notable exception being St Leonard's in York, with its 225 beds for the sick and poor, opened in 1278. More usual were the modest HOSPITALS opened, for instance, in Bury St Edmunds in 1150–1260, and later the almshouses, of which there were 500 nationwide by 1400. Even so, such institutions did not treat the usual run of illness, but concentrated on the indigent, the old, pilgrims, and those with leprosy.

Two developments nudged the gradual development of healthcare: the Crusades and the foundation of the universities at Oxford (1167) and Cambridge (1209). Thereafter medicine started to become professionalized, with the foundation of a Fellowship of Surgeons in 1368, a Company of Barbers in 1376, and, rather later, a College of Physicians in 1518 and the Society of APOTHECARIES in 1618. But with the dissolution of the monasteries in the 1530s, healthcare by religious organizations ceased, and most institutions closed. One exception was the City of London,

which bought and staffed the hospitals located there, St Bartholomew's (founded 1123) and St Thomas's (1215), and the more unusual foundation of BETHLEM ROYAL HOSPITAL (1247) (p 103) for the mentally ill.

Elsewhere, however, there were no comparable hospitals for many decades, and the indigent sick had to rely on the Poor Law, introduced in 1601, which compelled parishes to provide impoverished citizens with shelter and work, with the care of the sick as an added function, paid for by local taxes. Hospitals as we know them were largely the creation of the 18th century, with wealthy donors, both aristocrats and merchants, helping to start and fund local enterprises. Infirmaries opened in Edinburgh in 1729, in Winchester in 1736, and subsequently in another 20 of the older cities.

By the end of the century every major town and city had its own hospital, relying on local funding, being managed by boards of local worthies (who could gain admission for their nominees), and often staffed by local practitioners working in voluntary (unpaid) appointments part time. Various religious institutions also continued to provide some residential care. From the middle of the 18th century special hospitals were developed in a few cities, and particularly London, to deal with problems that the new infirmaries would not address — such as incurable illness, SEXUALLY TRANSMITTED DISEASES, fevers, and illegitimate births.

There were several other new types of development. The DISPENSARIES were organizations mostly for outpatient care founded by the doctors themselves from 1770, as were cottage hospitals (the first opening in Cranleigh, Surrey, in 1859), where inpatients could be treated by their own general practitioners — many of whom by then were becoming separate from hospital specialists, though general practitioners did provide some specialist care in the cottage hospitals.

From the 1860s, with the change in the Poor Law, hospitals were built alongside the WORK-HOUSES, where the indigent were now housed. Although the celebrated mental hospital, The Retreat, had opened at York, further development of mental hospitals had to wait until the latter part of the 19th century, when further large ASYLUMS were built often in the countryside miles away from the cities they served. Similar changes occurred in the 20th century when municipal authorities built large SANITARIUMS to treat the myriads of patients with tuberculosis.

NURSING care was an essential part of hospital services and for much of the 19th century it was carried out by poorly educated women, who learnt on the job. The quality was generally poor, but in 1859 Florence NIGHTINGALE (p 548), who had reorganized military nursing during the Crimean

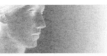
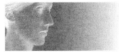

## BEHIND THE BRITISH NATIONAL HEALTH SERVICE

Bertrand Edward **DAWSON** (1864–1945). British physician. Dawson was appointed physician to the London Hospital in 1906. The following year he became physician-extraordinary to Edward VII and later to George V, whose death he hastened by a few hours to save prolonging the final phase. During the First World War he served as consulting physician to the British army. He became president of the Royal College of Physicians of London from 1931–8, of the British Medical Association in 1932 and 1943, and of the Royal Society of Medicine from 1928–30, for which he made important recommendations for the report for the Consultative Council on Medical and Allied Services (the *Dawson Report*). Dawson was a medical statesman and courtier who played an important part in planning the Ministry of Health and the Emergency Medical Service.

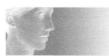

Aneurin **BEVAN** (1897–1960). British politician. Bevan was born in Tredegar, Monmouthshire, the son of a miner. He was returned as Member of Parliament for Ebbw Vale in 1929. In the Labour Government of 1945 he was made Minister of Health and Housing and it became his duty to see the National Health Service Act (1946) on to the statute-book. In his negotiations with the medical profession he proved to be more flexible and possessed of more patience than had been expected, and a successful conclusion was reached in two years. (*continued opposite*)

War, published her influential *Notes on nursing*. A year later she set up a school at St Thomas's Hospital, London, and her teaching initiated a revolution in nursing standards in Britain.

Not surprisingly, haphazard hospital developments resulted in a plethora of voluntary institutions, particularly in London, and the problems of oversupply and shortage of funds continued between the two world wars. The Second World War led to some rationalization of hospital care, with the government setting up the Emergency Medical Service. Even so, at the start of the National Health Service the new authorities were faced by no fewer than 900 hospitals, many of them small, run down, in the wrong place, and staffed by doctors of varying skills.

### Education and registration

Historically, the College of Physicians was responsible for examining, licensing, and monitoring physicians in the City of London and within a 7-mile radius. Elsewhere at first there was no uniform system of medical education and these functions were the responsibility of the local bishop aided by medical and surgical advisers. The physicians were the élite, necessarily members of the Church of England, and almost always graduates of Oxford or Cambridge. Their subordinates, the surgeons and the apothecaries, were usually trained by apprenticeship and regulated by their respective guilds, a situation that was punctuated by a continual series of disputes between them and the physicians for many years.

The 18th century was characterized by the rise of the Edinburgh Medical School, based on the Royal Infirmary with six beds, which opened in 1729. With a strong Leiden connection — five of its founding professors (including the charismatic William Cullen (p 129)) had studied there. Edinburgh had many advantages: tuition was cheap and in English; it imposed no religious requirements on its students; and from 1750 it set up a special clinical ward in which patients were shown at clinical lectures. Nevertheless, London also became a center for medical instruction. Teaching ward rounds started at St Thomas's Hospital in 1718, where there were also four courses of clinical lectures a year. Between 1719 and 1945, no fewer than five new teaching hospitals opened in the capital, including University College Hospital (1836), attached to the non-sectarian University College and the London School of Medicine for Women (1874).

Not surprisingly, standards of medical training had become very variable and the first half of the 19th century was characterized by attempts to tighten them. This started in 1815 with the Apothecaries Act, restricting prescribing to qualified APOTHECARIES. The feeling that provin-

cial doctors were getting a raw deal from the capital came to a head with the formation of several small pressure groups, culminating in the foundation of the Provincial Medical and Surgical Association by Charles Hastings in Worcester in 1832. Subsequently the British Medical Association played an important part in the battle to raise medicine to the status of a profession, eventually resulting in the passing of a Medical Act in 1858, while a General Medical Council, comprising experienced doctors, was formed to oversee standards.

Alongside these developments had been a public health campaign, occasioned by the problems of rapid industrialization and the continual epidemics of the early 19th century, particularly as highlighted by the great CHOLERA outbreaks starting in 1832. Civil registration of births and deaths was introduced into England and Wales with the formation of the Registrar General's Office, and Edwin Chadwick succeeded in having a Public Health Act passed in 1848, with towns being forced to appoint medical officers of health from the 1860s.

### Separation of doctors

The 19th century also saw the increasing separation of general practitioners from hospital specialists. In part, this started because practitioners were asked to tender for the care of paupers in the workhouses, and it was perpetuated in the National Health Insurance Act of 1911, when the liberal statesman David Lloyd George followed the example of Bismarck in introducing a compulsory state insurance scheme. A great advance in its time, the National Health Insurance Act replaced lost wages and paid the cost of general practitioner care for workers, who could choose to be treated by practitioners listed on a local panel. The scheme has been aptly described by the medical historian Roy Porter as helping 'to cement a lasting and valued relationship between the sick and their general practitioners, secured by the authority of the state'. Crucially, however, it did not cover their dependants, members of the middle class, or hospital care, though to some extent such needs were catered for by friendly societies — which offered contributory third party schemes to help people cover the costs of illnesses.

The first, and central, proposal was a universal comprehensive insurance scheme covering the whole population and providing for 'interruption and destruction of earning power and for special expenditure arising at birth, marriage, or death'. Benefits would be paid without test of need in return for contributions made jointly by the insured person, the state, and, where appropriate, the employer. The second and third proposals provided for those whose need was not fully met by social insurance (requiring proof of need), and for flat-rate children's allowances payable irrespective of parental income. Most of these recommendations were implemented by July 1948.

Between the 1911 Act and 1942, when the Beveridge Report appeared, health became a well-established national political issue. In 1913 the Ministry of Health was set up, and the First World War was to show yet again (as in the Crimean and Boer wars) how a substantial proportion of the volunteers was unfit for active service. A report produced by Lord DAWSON (p 130) in 1921 recommended a new pattern of healthcare based on district hospitals and general practitioners working in teams out of purpose-built primary health centers, but it came to nothing because of a financial crisis. Other reports followed, most suggesting some system of nationally organized health care. At the abolition of the Poor Law in 1929 the workhouse hospitals passed to the control of the local authorities, while the voluntary hospitals continued to struggle for survival, being funded mainly by local donations (although some of them were also underwritten by the government for their role as teaching hospitals).

During the Second World War these hospitals were subsidized by the government, which was concerned about the number of air-raid casualties it might be faced with; the Emergency Bed Service was later to facilitate the incorporation of hospitals into the postwar National Health Service. By then, the separation of family and hospital doctors was appreciable: in Britain, at the outbreak of the Second World War, there were 2800 full-time consultants and specialists in the hospitals and 18 000 general practitioners.

In his 1942 government-initiated report, *Social insurance and allied services*, the social scientist and civil servant Sir William BEVERIDGE (this page) proposed setting up the welfare state to slay the 'five giants' — want, disease, ignorance, squalor, and idleness. Though the wartime coalition government had dithered over publishing the report, it became extraordinarily popular both with the fighting forces and with the general population, and there was no going back from implementing its proposals once the war was over. After a series of difficult confrontations between the profession and the new Labour Government (with the ebullient and visionary ANEURIN BEVAN (p 130) as the health minister) a new National Health Service came into being on 1 August 1948, the first free comprehensive medical service in the world.

## Unleashed demand

The experiences with the National Health Service since its beginning have been mixed. A vast demand was suddenly unleashed for elementary necessities such as dentures and spectacles, let alone comfort surgical operations such as hernia repairs and the treatment of varicose veins. The authorities also found run-down plant, not only the hospitals but also general practitioners' premises and public health clinics. Moreover, the plan was started just as Britain (despite its war-ravaged economy) was engaging in a large social program, modernizing education, embarking on large-scale house building and nuclear energy programs as well as on nationalization of the iron and steel industries, the coalmines, and the railways, and assigning independence to former Empire countries, let alone contributing to the Berlin airlift and the Korean War. Specialist excellence was diffused across the country to ensure that the old district hospitals were adequately staffed; however, the first totally new hospital in Britain (at Welwyn) was not opened until 1963, and the subsequent optimism in a dash for economic growth in the late 1960s was extinguished by the international oil crisis in 1973.

The result of all this was to give health a low place in national priorities. The proportion of gross domestic product spent on health was initially 4–5%, compared with up to double that amount spent by Britain's European counterparts, and treble by the USA — proportions that have remained constant despite the increased proportionate spending in all countries. Government officials, regularly embroiled in rows over funding capital investment and staff pay levels, seemed to think that the problems could be addressed by increased efficiency. Certainly, there were isolated instances of extravagance, and a whole series of reforms, such as cutting excess beds, and introducing day-care procedures, showed how much

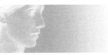

(continued)

William **BEVERIDGE** (Sir, later Lord) (1879–1963). British civil sevant and social reformer. After a brilliant undergraduate career at Oxford he entered the Civil Service. In 1919 he became director of the London School of Economics and in 1937 master of University College, Oxford. Relations with his colleagues were seldom easy; thus when he sought government employment at the oubreak of the Second World War he was relegated to chairmanship of a committee enquiring into the co-ordination of the social services, which was not expected to report until after the war. Within 18 months he had produced the 'BEVERIDGE REPORT' (this page) for a complete social service. It met with a cool reception from government, but in four days 70 000 copies were sold and public acclaim forced its acceptance underpinning a National Health Service.

## DAWSON REPORT, 1920

The interim (and in the event the only) report of the Council on Medical and Administrative Services, set up under the chairmanship of Sir Bertrand DAWSON (later Lord Dawson of Penn) (p 130) shortly after the return to power of Lloyd George's coalition government in 1918. The intention was to make recommendations fulfilling the election promise that a general health service would replace the Poor Laws in medical care. The Council's report in 1920, which was a preliminary document intended for discussion, was revolutionary and farseeing; it introduced the concept of health centers, emphasized the importance of preventive medicine and its integration with therapeutics, and accorded a central role in the reorganized system to the family practitioner. Though generally well received, the work of the Council was overtaken by other urgent matters pressing upon the new Ministry of Health (notably a financial crisis in the voluntary hospitals), and a final report was never published.

## BEVERIDGE REPORT

Basic provision for social security in Britain was influenced by the proposals made by Sir William (later Lord) BEVERIDGE (this page) in 1942. Three systems of benefit were recommended: social insurance payable on a contractual basis; social assistance payable on a test of need; and children's allowances payable to all without contract or test of need.

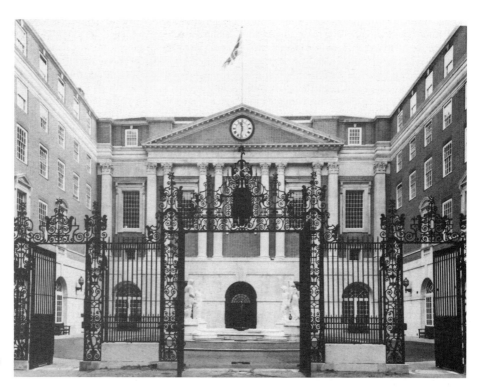

The British Medical Association's headquarters in Tavistock Square, London. (Reproduced courtesy of the British Medical Association.)

## GREAT WINDMILL STREET SCHOOL

The two best-known of the private medical schools of London in the 18th century were located in Great Windmill Street and Leicester Square. Both were associated with John (p 398) and William HUNTER (p 388). William Hunter had bought 16 Great Windmill Street and, after rebuilding it, began a course of lectures there in 1767. Beginning as an anatomy school, it later expanded into chemistry, surgery, and medicine. Other famous doctors connected with it included Matthew Baillie, Sir Charles Bell, and Peter Mark ROGET (p 263). The school, sometimes claimed to be the ancestor of the Middlesex Hospital Medical School, ceased to exist in about 1833. It was the first medical school in London.

could be achieved by increased efficiency. Nevertheless, most studies, including a Royal Commission on the National Health Service in 1979, concluded that money was indeed well spent and that Britain was unlikely to achieve parity with its neighbors unless it spent proportionately more.

One problem has been how to measure value for money: the index often used, the perinatal mortality rate, was lower in Britain than in Germany or the USA, which spent far more on health. Another reason for the population's relative satisfaction was, as Charles Webster (an Oxford historian of the Health Service) suggested, the little-Englandism of the population, who preferred to take refuge in catch-phrases such as 'the envy of the world' rather than looking across the Channel to see what could be achieved without such parsimony. But the result was a series of upsetting reorganizations of the Service, the first in 1973, which achieved little detectable improvement, while boosting the power of the managers at the expense of the hitherto dominant doctors. A downside was that these changes increased the proportion of money spent on administration from a once internationally lean figure of 5% to 12%, and possibly still set to rise. Another defect was that PUBLIC HEALTH suddenly found itself without a well-defined role.

All this was set against a background of media criticism of the Service's failure to cope with

influenza epidemics, a shortage of intensive care facilities, covert rationing of drug treatment or surgical procedures (such as hip or cataract replacements), and waiting lists which may involve patients' waiting for admission to hospital, or even their outpatient appointment to see a specialist, for a year or more. Nevertheless, the National Health Service has always been popular with patients, who endorse the idea that it should be funded by taxes. Moreover, the predicted increase in private medicine has never happened, remaining at a virtually constant 15% for all procedures.

The National Health Service did, however, perhaps create one unique feature that might have been the envy of the world: its general practitioner service. Reforms in the 1960s developed this into a specialist service in its own right, with general practitioners forming groups leading teams of well-trained ancillary workers in purpose-built health centers. Not only was this cost-effective, in that it reinforced the 'gatekeeper' role of GENERAL PRACTICE — in Britain, patients cannot refer themselves to specialists but have to go through a general practitioner — but it was underpinned by a striking intellectual base provided by the Royal College of General Practitioners (founded in 1952), which with its own training programs and higher diploma at last put general practice almost level with some hospital specialties. The result was to

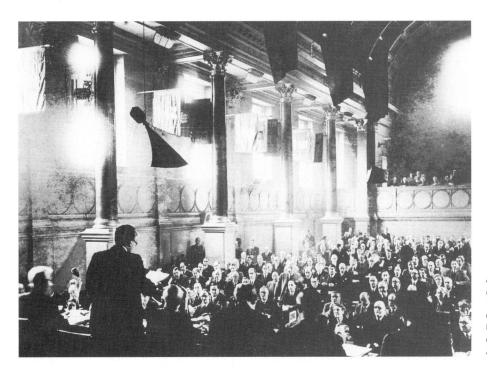

A Special Representative Meeting of the BMA in May 1948 agreed conditional cooperation in the National Health Service. (Reproduced courtesy of the British Medical Association.)

make general practice a popular option with both medical students and newly qualified doctors as well as providing a much-appreciated service for the general population.

The pivotal position of general practice — or primary care, as it is commonly titled — was reinforced in 1991 by the Thatcher government's controversial introduction of an 'internal market' into the National Health Service. This radical reform offered general practitioners an annual budget with which to 'purchase' specialist and community services for their patients from independent healthcare provider trusts. In 1997, however, a change of government led to closure of the National Health Service's managed market before its effectiveness or otherwise could be assessed, leaving primary care facing yet more change.

In 1997 in Britain (excluding Northern Ireland and the 450 public health/community health staff) the National Health Service employed about 24 000 medical and dental consultants supported by around 35 000 trainee staff, many of whom had come temporarily to Britain from either Europe or overseas for employment and training. Juniors had designated training programs leading to higher diplomas in many specialties, administered by various royal college and faculties, and to specialist registration. There was a total of 35 700 doctors working in general practice; in all 102 000 doctors were working in the National Health Service and 8 300 outside it.

There are 25 undergraduate medical schools (7 in London, 13 others in England and Wales, 4 in Scotland, and 1 in Northern Ireland), and numerous specialist institutions which also undertake teaching and research. The latter is funded partly by the Medical Research Council (which was set up as the Medical Research Committee in 1913, mostly to study tuberculosis, and re-formed in 1920) and partly by private foundations, including the WELLCOME FOUNDATION, industry, government, and universities. Many of these aspects are dealt with in much more detail elsewhere in this book.

Meanwhile, as in every country, the pressures on the delivery of healthcare increase. Costly medicines and technology, the greying of the population, rising public expectations (and litigation), ethical dilemmas over rationing, staff shortages, constant media criticism, and uncertain political leadership make its future hard to forecast. Even so, public popularity of the National Health Service endures.               SPL, GM

*See also* ASSOCIATIONS; HEALTHCARE SYSTEMS; HEALTH ECONOMICS; REGULATION OF THE PROFESSIONS

**BULIMIA NERVOSA** See EATING DISORDERS

**BURNOUT SYNDROME** This term was introduced in 1974 by Herbert Freudenberger to describe something common, difficult, and curable. The term was quickly taken up by the media, the medical profession, and the general population, because like stress it stood for something with which many hard working people could identify. Burnout became the syndrome of people who worked long hours and tried to get all their satisfaction in life from work and not from the other aspects of normal living. Burnout also carried the implication that it affected good workers who were victims of organizational deficiencies and eventually developed this syndrome. This idea survives to the present day, perhaps because in part it is true.

Burnout became a fashionable topic during the world-wide economic depression of the 1980s. Many organizations, regardless of size or specialty, set very high goals and had high expectations of their employees. Common wisdom at the time was that people worked very hard. There was also an optimistic feeling in the air: people believed that they could achieve much. With time this unrealistically optimistic view began to erode. Moreover, it did not take into consideration the person's background, their early childhood experiences, genetic make-up, environment, and family support system.

The typical burnout victim, then, would be a good worker who at some point ceased to function well or became chronically depressed. It used to be thought that the reason for this change was an underlying individual flaw, and little was known about the factors that would eventually cause the problems. Indeed, in many work-places the true situation was generally not even recognized.

The symptoms of this many faceted syndrome are those of chronic psychological and emotional exhaustion. Patients feel depressed, tired, and cynical. They experience no good things in life, and see the future as gloomy. Often before reaching this stage they have lived in the fast lane, with work being the most important thing in life. They have thought they could do anything and do it well. They were ready to work many extra hours because they believed that sooner or later they would reach their goal and get their reward. But as time went on and success continued to elude them they began to worry: Why do I not have the energy I had earlier? Why am I so tired all the time? Can this task be accomplished by me or by anyone else? Sleeplessness would follow and the person would wake up after disastrous nights tired and lacking energy. The symptoms are similar to those observed during prolonged stressful situations.

Sometimes burnout represents the final event that follows severe stress. Thus, stress may occur without burnout, but burnout never occurs without stress. There may occur, in addition, a wide selection of psychosomatic disorders. People react to difficulties in various ways, by developing indigestion, diarrhea, headache, aches, and pains, and some have flu-like symptoms all the time and do not sleep well. Medications may be helpful for a while until new symptoms arise. Eventually the patient's entire personality may change becoming cynical, passive, sometimes openly aggressive. This is true at work but also at home. The whole family suffers and may break up; divorce is common.

The burnout patient does not yet understand what is going on, but later, when help is needed, there is nobody there. The partner has had enough, the children have distanced themselves and tried to avoid the parent's problem. When friends are approached, there are none left: the long years at work have destroyed old friendships.

Treatment needs to begin with the patients' understanding that they cannot go on as usual and need help. Some 20% of burnout patients need professional mental health treatment. In addition to a frank discussion of the problems, modern antidepressants and short-acting sleeping pills may be needed, as well as several weeks or months off work. Some 80% of the burnout patients seem to recover spontaneously — largely because they have retained some human friendly contacts to lean on. It is indeed important to have at least one human relationship in which the patient can trust. Such a person does not need to have any special characteristics; it is enough to be reliable, empathetic, and willing to listen.

The outlook is usually favorable. With treatment the patient acquires insight, develops a more optimistic outlook, and eventually begins to function normally again. Interestingly, talk of burnout seems to become less common during economic depressions, when unemployment rates are high. In such times workers are afraid that they would lose their jobs if they complained. As economic times improve, however, people start again to talk about feeling ill, insecure, and depressed. Thus burnout remains a problem, best recognized early so as to prevent its progression to a more severe stage. It is the young and inexperienced who are most prone to develop burnout; older people can provide supportive talk and help. Undoubtedly the best help at the early stage of burnout comes from spouse, friends, co-workers, and other understanding and kind people. IV

John **CAIUS** (1510–73). British physician. Elected a fellow of Gonville Hall, Cambridge, was later enrolled at the University of Padua, where he was a pupil of Montanus, lodged with Vesalius, and lectured on Aristotle with Realdus Columbus. After graduating in 1541 he travelled widely in Europe collating texts of Galen and Celsus which formed the basis of his *Commentaries*. He practiced briefly in Cambridge, Norwich, and Shrewsbury, recording his experiences in *A boke or counsell against the disease commonly called the sweate or sweating sickness* (1552). In 1552 he moved to London and was elected president of the Royal College of Physicians for the years 1555–60, 1562, 1563, and 1571. He presented the president's insignia to the College and strenuously upheld its rights to prevent surgeons from prescribing drugs. At the command of Henry VIII he was the first to teach anatomy publicly at the Barber-Surgeons' Hall. Later he was appointed physician successively to Edward VI, Mary, and Elizabeth I, but was deprived of this office in 1568 because he was a Roman Catholic.

As well as being a scholarly physician and a gifted naturalist, Caius was the most learned classicist of his generation in Europe. In 1557 Philip of Spain and Queen Mary granted Caius letters patent to refound Gonville Hall as Gonville and Caius College. He was a munificent benefactor of his foundation and Master from 1558–73. However, he was unpopular in Cambridge on account of his Catholicism, and in 1573 his lodgings were searched by the vice-chancellor at the instance of the Bishop of London. Much 'popish trumpery' and many books were found and burned in the court of his College. He resigned and died a few months later.

**CANADA**, the second largest country in the world, comprises ten provinces and two territories. Discovered by Jacques Cartier in 1534, legend has it that when he asked the Indians where he was, they gestured towards their settlement and pronounced the word Kanata. In fact, John Cabot, sailing for the King of England, first set foot upon the northern new world when he landed in what is now Newfoundland in 1497. But Newfoundland did not join the Canadian federation until 1949.

The first hospitals were founded in Quebec City in 1637, and in Montreal in 1642. Both were called Hôtel Dieu, and were run by Catholic religious orders. It was not until 1821 that the first secular institution, the Montreal General Hospital, was established, mainly by the Protestant business community in that city. Formal teaching of medicine began concurrently at the site of the Montreal General Hospital when four physicians from Edinburgh were recruited to form the Montreal Medical Institute. During this same period, James McGill, a wealthy local businessman, died and left a will which specified that an institution for higher learning be established on his large estate. By 1829 negotiations were still going on, and, with the specter of the entire estate reverting to McGill's heirs, the Montreal Medical Institute was transferred to the site in question, and became the faculty of medicine, the first faculty of MCGILL UNIVERSITY (p 139).

### Education

Medicine is taught in sixteen faculties of medicine, each of which is part of a university. Each of the ten provinces has at least one faculty of medicine, except for New Brunswick and Prince Edward Island, which contract with other provinces for admission of their residents as medical students. Both health and education are provincial jurisdictions in Canada, and this overriding part of the Canadian constitution highly influences decisions and implementation of all programs in health and education. Concrete examples of such provincial policies in medical education include admission requirements, residency status, and numbers of students admitted to and eventually graduating from medical school. There is financial input for both health and post-secondary education from the federal government, and for health, the federal government has established the national standards governing the healthcare system.

Medicine is taught in English in 12 of the 16 faculties, in French in three faculties, and the

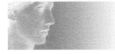

(continued)

Sir Charles **TUPPER**
(1821–1915). Canadian
physician and politician. From
1884 to 1886 he was High
Commissioner for Canada in
London, returning to Canada
as Minister of Finance to be
responsible for floating the
large loan through which the
Canadian Pacific Railway was
completed to the west coast
of Canada. He returned to
London to represent Canada,
but was subsequently
brought back to Ottawa as
Prime Minister of Canada. It
was Tupper's courage and
determination which brought
his native province of Nova
Scotia into the Canadian
confederation. OSLER
(p 602) wrote in his obituary
notice: 'His life is an
illustration of the brilliant
success of the doctor in
politics.'

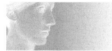

Sir Thomas George
**RODDICK** (1846–1923).
Canadian surgeon. His
greatest work was in forming
the Medical Council of
Canada, after 18 years of
frustrating work through
professional organizations
(he was president of the
Canadian and British Medical
Associations in turn). As a
result, a medical graduate is
able to take examinations
which permit him to practice
anywhere in Canada.

(continued on p 138)

Faculty of Medicine of the University of Ottawa teaches in both English and French. The oldest school is at McGILL UNIVERSITY in Montreal (1821) (p 139); the youngest is at Memorial University of Newfoundland in St John's (1969); the largest is at the University of Toronto, which celebrated its 150th anniversary several years ago, as did l'Université de Montréal. Although there are some differences in admission requirements, in general, students are admitted to medicine after having completed secondary schooling and obtained a university undergraduate degree. The medical course is generally of four years' duration, and, as of 1997, half of Canada's medical schools had adopted curricula based on problem-based learning.

During the fourth and final year, each student must decide whether to become a family physician or a specialist. Beginning with the province of Quebec in 1988, all provinces have decided that licenses to practice, issued by the provincial College of Physicians and Surgeons, will be granted only after full postgraduate training in either family medicine (two years) or a specialty (four to six years depending upon the specialty). Students must make their decisions by February of their final year of studies.

After a lengthy study by health economists in the early 1990s, all provincial ministries of health developed policies to reduce the numbers of students admitted to the study of medicine. As a consequence, the number of graduates has decreased from 1735 in 1990 to 1608 in 1998. At the time of the study, the country had one physician for 530 individuals. Canada's population has increased by over 2 000 000 since then. People are living longer; the elderly, who consume most of the treatment services, comprise a greater percentage of Canada's population; and there is rising concern that by 2003 there will no longer be sufficient physicians to meet the needs.

Formal postgraduate education is required before any license to practice medicine is issued. All such education is under the jurisdiction of universities with faculties of medicine. Medical and surgical residents are recruited, trained, and evaluated on a regular basis by accredited university programs. There are 53 specialty programs accredited by the Royal College of Physicians and Surgeons of Canada, with each faculty of medicine providing training in some or all of these programs. In addition, each faculty has a program in family medicine accredited by the College of Family Physicians of Canada. Final evaluation with the issuing of a licence to practice varies slightly by province, but a common factor is success in the final examinations of the Royal College of Physicians and Surgeons of Canada or the College of Family Physicians.

Currently the requests for residency positions by graduating students are 60% for the specialties and 40% for family medicine. The numbers allotted to each program are fixed by each ministry on a triannual basis after consultation with the medical schools, the medical profession at large, the student and resident unions, and the regional councils of health. (The last bodies have been set up over the past ten years to bring decision-making closer to where the action actually occurs. Their role in the distribution of resident positions by discipline is to reflect need.) Given the longer training period required for specialty training, this results in a practice mode of 50% family physicians and 50% specialists.

## Healthcare system

Canadian physicians practice in a system which provides 'free' medical and hospital care to all Canadian citizens and permanent residents of Canada. The structure, called 'Medicare', has been in place now for over thirty years, and was updated by federal legislation in 1984 entitled the Canada Health Act. The five principles governing the system are as follows:

- Universal: All Canadian citizens and all permanent residents are covered. Landed immigrants become covered as permanent residents three months after their arrival in the country.

- Portable: Benefits are available to all those eligible across the entire country no matter what their province of residence might be. Payment is also made to physicians and hospitals outside Canada, but only at rates paid in the province of origin. Prudent Canadians traveling abroad purchase insurance to cover themselves.

- Comprehensive: All services deemed 'medically necessary' are covered.

- Publically administered: The system is operated by organizations established by the government of each province and territory. Numerous studies have shown the efficiency of the system as compared with structures based on privatization.

- Reasonable access: All efforts must be made to provide quality services at an optimum time, and at a place which is reasonably accessible within that time. This principle is probably the most difficult.

## Finance

In 1991 Canada spent $66.3 billion on healthcare. This represented 9.8% of gross domestic product. 70% of healthcare in Canada is financed through public expenditure. The remaining 30% comes from private insurance premiums and private sources.

## Physician/population ratios

Since the early '90s the population of Canada has continued to increase (current government policy is to admit 200 000 new immigrants annually) while the physician workforce has stabilized. The latter is projected to decrease in the next several years, given the policy decisions to diminish intake into Canadian medical schools. At the same time, foreign trained physicians have little chance of receiving the necessary training for general licensure. However, some provincial licensing authorities recruit fully trained doctors from abroad to provide medical services to mainly rural and underpopulated regions of the country.

The five principles outlined above govern the manner in which medicine is practiced in Canada, and the manner in which the population receives medical services.

The principle of **universality** has provided the entire population of Canada with complete medical and hospital coverage. The system is funded through general and payroll taxation. Services are rendered on presentation of a health card, which is carried by all. Fraudulent use of cards has been a problem from time to time, but **universality** is one of the most appreciated features of the system.

The **comprehensive** aspect of healthcare bases coverage on what is deemed 'medically necessary'. When the system first began some thirty years ago, certain medical acts such as cosmetic surgery were excluded. Over time, new technologies have been added, and some questionable procedures have been removed. Although **comprehensiveness** remains a pillar of the system, the decrease in both federal and provincial funding has contributed to what one may call a 'rationing' of services. For example, a purely elective service, whose effectiveness might be held in question, may have only half its cost covered.

**Public administration** of the system has been one of its most financially attractive features. The provincial bodies set up to administer it have been shown to do so in a most efficient manner, and at a cost well below that of organizations run by private institutions such as insurance companies be they 'for profit' or 'not for profit'. Payment to health professionals is rarely questioned, and is rendered in an acceptable time frame.

**Portability** means that Canadians need only present their health card in any of the ten provinces or two territories in order to receive services. There is never any need to pay initially and wait for reimbursement.

**Reasonable access** has been the most difficult principle to achieve for several reasons. Canada is a vast country with most of its 30 million inhabitants living in urban centers. Urbanization has been increasing and this presents the problem of providing medical services to Canada's rural population. Several programs have been mounted in the attempt to convince graduating physicians to practice in rural Canada, and some have been quite successful. However, the retention rate is not good and small communities may be left without a doctor when a physician leaves to practice in a larger town or city. The two main reasons for such departures are that family does not wish to remain in a rural setting, and that there is no collegial support — physicians burn out after bearing the responsibility for an isolated community, and being on call for most or all of the time.

The accessibility factor has been complicated by the legislated drop in admissions to medical schools; the change in gender make-up of recent medical school classes; and the discrepancy

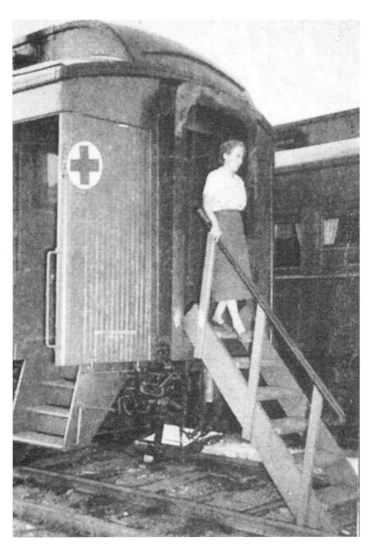

This railroad car was converted into a mobile nursing clinic to be used in northern Manitoba in 1954. (Reproduced courtesy of the National Library of Medicine, Bethesda, MD.)

(continued)

Jonathan Campbell **MEAKINS** (1882–1959). Canadian clinical researcher and medical educator. War-time service led him to work on 'soldier's heart' and on the treatment of gas warfare injuries to the lungs. He served as dean of medicine at McGill, as director general of medical services for Canada's army, and wrote a textbook, *The practice of medicine,* which went through six editions.

Wilder Graves **PENFIELD** (1891–1976). Canadian neurosurgeon. Born in the USA and later naturalized Canadian, Penfield received his surgical training in New York City; he moved to Montreal in 1928 to become surgeon to the Royal Victoria Hospital and first director of the Montreal Neurological Institute. In the course of craniotomies performed under local anesthesia, for treatment of focal epilepsy or for removal of tumors, he was able to add important information to knowledge of areas of cortical function.

between the choice of specialty by graduates, and the need for such specialties. The number of graduates from Canadian medical schools will have gone from a high of 1835 in the mid 1980s to about 1550 at the turn of the century. Women now make up about one half (or slightly more) of first year medical student classes, a trend which began several years ago, and which will probably increase in the future. Repeated surveys have shown that female physicians limit both the number of hours they work, and the specialties in which they train. The result of all of these factors means fewer doctors available to the public.

Some provincial ministries of health have issued directives which increase the number of residency positions in specialties considered 'in need' at the expense of those which are 'over-doctored'. For example, Quebec has increased the number of positions in internal medicine and diagnostic radiology, and limited those in dermatology and plastic surgery. These directives are revised regularly to adjust for changing needs.

Since 1995 there have been funding cuts to health and education in the transfer payments of the federal government to the provinces. The consequence has been a downsizing of the system across the entire country. The number of acute hospital beds has been reduced; hospitals have been obliged to merge; and a number of institutions have closed.

Thus the system does have its problems. The austerity measures which generated them stemmed from the large annual deficits of both the

federal government and the provinces. However, at the end of the 20th century federal government announced a substantial surplus, as did some of the provinces. The remainder were targeting surpluses in the immediate future. There is already discussion concerning increased funding at both the federal and provincial levels. In addition, there has been a marked move to ambulatory care with a pronounced increase in the amount of day surgery and the introduction of new technologies.

The elderly (age over 65) of Canada constituted 12% of the population in 1995, and are projected to make up 20% by 2005. They are becoming ever more autonomous, and much of the emphasis in ambulatory care will be geared to maintaining them in their home setting.

Over the past few years, with the cuts in services, there have been repeated calls for the implementation of a parallel privately funded healthcare system. Repeated polls have shown that Canadians recognize that this might eventually become necessary, but the same polls reveal that Canadians cherish the current system and regard it as the most important of all Canadian social programs. Indeed, it has been said that the system is what distinguishes Canada in the society of nations.

### Research

Canada has a rich tradition of discoveries in the medical sciences. The most well known is the work of BANTING (p 236), BEST (p 236), COLLIP (p 265), and McLeod that led to the discovery and

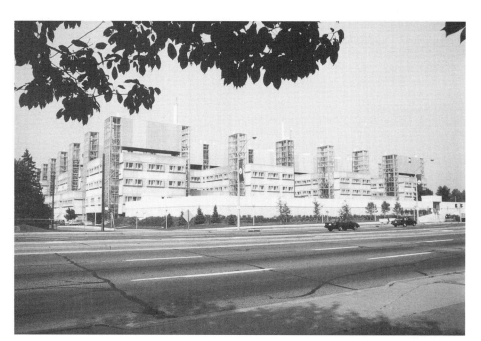

McMaster University, housing one of the largest medical schools in Canada.

development of insulin treatment for diabetes. Internationally renowned original work has been carried out in many other subdisciplines: dermatology, hematology, ophthalmology, neurosciences, and cardiothoracic surgery, to name a few. The work of Wilder PENFIELD (p 138) and others at the Montreal Neurological Institute is almost as well known as the discovery of insulin. Also in Montreal, Hans Selye attracted worldwide attention with his work on the endocrine and neurological basis of stress. At the University of Western Ontario, Charles Drake made important contributions to research and development of techniques for vascular and neurovascular surgery.

Financial support for medical research comes from federal and provincial governments and from foundations and charitable organizations. The Medical Research Council of Canada began as an offshoot of the National Research Council in the mid 1930s. By Act of Parliament it has been an independent agency since 1969. It provides about a quarter of the medical research funds in Canada; in 1996–97 its budget was Cdn$242 million. The Medical Research Council supports basic and clinical medical sciences. Since the late 1980s it has partly supported a National Network of Centers of Excellence initiated by the Canadian Institute for Advanced Research, with support also from provincial governments, foundations, and charities. Research on healthcare organization, the environment, life-styles, and the biology of human populations was given impetus by concepts and recommendations in the Lalonde Report of 1974. It was supported by the National Health Research and Development Program until that program was phased out in the mid-1990s and replaced by new initiatives of the Medical Research Council. These included research on the efficacy and cost-effectiveness of health services, and women's health.

There is also combined federal–provincial support for research on HIV disease and AIDS. At the provincial level, Alberta, British Columbia, Ontario, Quebec, and Saskatchewan have their own health science and medical research funding agencies. Further financial support for research comes from foundations, charities, and increasingly from the corporate and industrial sectors. When mounting federal budget deficits led to deep cuts in Medical Research Council funds in the early 1990s, the pharmaceutical industry began to provide increasing support as compensation to Canadians for the political decision to grant copyright protection for proprietary pharmaceutical preparations for a prolonged period, a decision that means newly developed drugs cost patients more than they would if generic alternatives were allowed on the market. Many independent observers believe that pharmaceutical industry support for medical research comes at a high price: the industry controls at least part of the research agenda, and has not escaped accusations of conflicts of interest.

Two other federal research councils support social sciences and humanities and natural sciences and engineering. There are some overlaps, notably in a combined approach to the ethical problems that may arise in any form of research that involves humans. It is recognized that the boundaries among the three broad categories of federally supported research are often indistinct. Some priority research problems confronting Canada — indeed, the world as a whole — at the beginning of the new century transcend traditional disciplinary boundaries. Moreover, research is increasingly multidisciplinary.

Representatives of the three research councils, the academic sector, the practice sector, and the private sector, have discussed innovative approaches to research in Canada. The Science Advisory Council, a select committee of some 20 prominent Canadians, chaired by Canada's first female astronaut, Dr Roberta Bondar (a physician and research worker in physiology), has begun to explore how to develop effective coalitions of research workers from widely diverse disciplinary backgrounds, as a way to break free of the reductionist approach to science that has been dominant throughout the world for at least the last 150 years. This pathway has already been trodden in research sponsored by the International Development Research Centre. This Canadian development aid agency exists solely to support research and capacity building in developing countries, in health sciences, social sciences, food, nutrition, and agriculture, engineering, and earth sciences. Some of its most successful programs and projects — for example, in provision of safe water supplies to rural communities, and elevation of the status and health of women — have a multidisciplinary makeup that is a template for similar efforts in Canada and other rich industrial nations.                                    HB, JML

*See also* HEALTHCARE SYSTEMS

Girolamo **CARDANO** (1501–76). Italian Renaissance polymath. Cardano's many written works embrace medicine, mathematics, physics, philosophy, religion, music, geology, and the theory of games but his fame now rests chiefly on his contributions to mathematics, especially algebra (for example, 'Cardano's rule' for the solution of third-degree equations), although for many years he was also a successful practicing physician. Born in Pavia the illegitimate son of Pazio Cardano, a distinguished jurist and friend of LEONARDO da Vinci (p 40), Cardano began his university studies

**McGILL UNIVERSITY**

is in Montreal, Canada. Four Edinburgh-trained physicians, working at the Montreal General Hospital, started lectures on medicine in 1822. In 1829 the institution which they founded was accepted as the faculty of medicine by the University which grew out of the original McGill College. William OSLER (p 602) qualified there in 1872 and taught in the faculty from 1874–84. Other hospitals and institutions have been affiliated over the years, one of the more famous being that founded in 1934 by Wilder PENFIELD (p 138) in neurology.

# CANES

The gold-headed cane that originally belonged to Dr John Radcliffe is now a treasured possession of the Royal College of Physicians of London. Its ownership then passed in succession to five generations of

eminent London physicians and Fellows of the College, before it was given in 1825 to the Royal College of Physicians by the widow of Dr Mathew Baillie; the coats of arms of the previous owners are engraved on its gold

head. A book entitled *The gold-headed cane* written by Dr William Macmichael, registrar

(*continued opposite*)

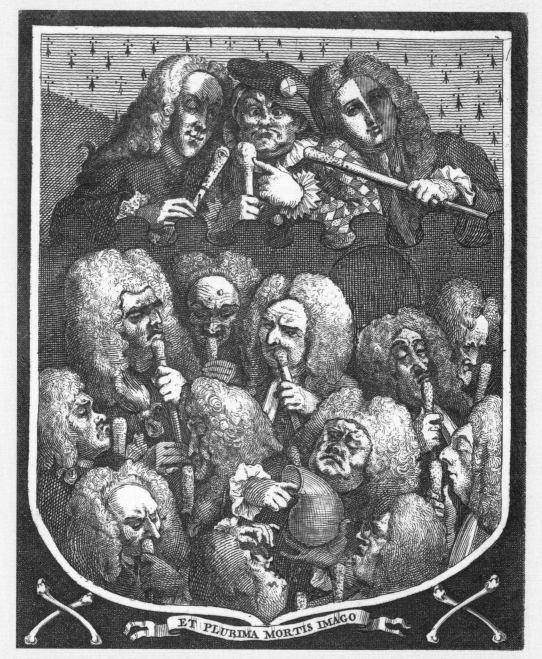

The arms of the Honourable Company of Undertakers by Hogarth shows the company smelling their pomander canes.

(continued)

to the College, was published anonymously in 1827; a second edition was published a year later, and the book has remained in print for most of the time since it first appeared. The third edition, published in 1884, was edited and extended by Dr William Munk. The book belongs to a literary genre, popular at the time, in which an inanimate object tells its story. Thus the gold-headed cane recounted its experiences while in the company of the successive physicians who owned it. As a result, this gold-headed cane became, to some extent, an emblem of physicianly medicine as practiced in the 18th century. Munk's edition continued the story of the gold-headed cane for another fifty years.

**Unusual handle**

In the third edition of *The gold-headed cane* the cane was given the opportunity to explain that its crook or bar-shaped handle was unusual: 'The physician's cane proper has a rounded knob or head, often of gold, sometimes of silver, but in later times generally of ivory. In earlier times this knob was perforated with holes, and it had within, a cavity or chamber, … for aromatic or Marseille vinegar … of sovereign efficacy against all pestilences'. This prophylactic was said 'to have arisen from the confession of four thieves, who during a plague in Marseilles, plundered the dead bodies with perfect security, and who, on being arrested, stated, on condition of their being spared, that the use of aromatic vinegar had preserved them from the influence of the contagion. … The head of the cane was thus a vinaigrette, which the doctor held to his nose when he went into the sick chamber, so that its fumes might protect him from contagion and other noxious exhalations from his patients. You may perhaps remember the lines:

Physic of old, her entry made Beneath th'immense full bottoms shade, While the gilt cane, with solemn pride, To each sagacious nose applied, Seem'd but a necessary prop, To bear the weight of wig at top.'

Dr John Radcliffe's malacca cane with its gold head was functional and decorative, but was not equipped with vinaigrette. In this respect, it was similar to the canes carried by physicians in the 18th century — more in conformity with fashions of dress and accoutrements of the time than for specifically medical purposes. The fashionable physician of the 18th century has been described as 'somewhat of a dandy, with his buckskin breeches and top boots, or stockings and buckled shoes, his velvet or satin coat with gilt-buttons, his wig and three-cornered hat, his gloves and even his muff'. It was also *de rigueur* for such a physician to carry a decorative cane with a gold or silver head and often with a tassle. Though some physicians in the 17th century used vinaigrette canes, they were a small minority. By contrast, ivory-headed pomander canes were widely used by doctors, apothecaries, and quacks in the late 17th century and throughout the 18th century. The perforated heads could be unscrewed so that an olfactorily powerful pomander, relying especially on ambergris, civet, and musk, could be inserted into the hollow top. Such dual-purpose ivory-headed pomander canes proved a gift to caricaturists, who used them to identify not only doctors and apothecaries, but anyone with medical pretensions. In Hogarth's *Company of undertakers*, a motley group of physicians and quacks is portrayed, most of whom are shown sniffing the heads of their pomander canes. The pomander cane was eventually

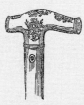

THE

**GOLD-HEADED CANE.**

*SECOND EDITION.*

LONDON:
JOHN MURRAY, ALBEMARLE-STREET.
MDCCCXXVIII.

Title page of *The gold-headed cane,* 2nd edition (1828). John Murray, London.

superseded by the stethoscope as the caricaturist's hallmark for identifying doctors.

At the end of the 18th century John Radcliffe's gold-headed cane remarked: 'I ceased to be considered any longer as a necessary appendage of the profession'. Medical canes were available in the 19th century and were sometimes equipped with gadgets and gimmicks, but such canes are of more interest to present day collectors than representative of cane-carrying by doctors of the time.                    DDG

*See also* EMBLEMS

in his home town and completed them at Padua in 1526. Thereafter he spent six years in medical practice in the nearby small town of Saccolongo, years which he was later to describe as the happiest of his life; they culminated in his marriage to Lucia Bandareni, following cure of the impotence which had afflicted him as a young man. In 1534 he became a teacher of mathematics in Milan but continued to practice medicine to such effect that he became the leading physician in the city, regarded by some as the best medical opinion in Europe next to Vesalius. Among his famous patients was the asthmatic Archbishop of Edinburgh, John Hamilton, whom he treated in Scotland in 1552; other British noblemen came to him as patients and he remained there for most of that year. He had returned to Pavia as professor of medicine in 1543, where he taught until 1560.

Personal and family troubles intervened (the elder of his two sons was executed for poisoning his wife and the younger was dissolute) and in 1562 he removed to the chair of medicine at BOLOGNA (p 457). Eight years later he was imprisoned by the Inquisition for heresy, the accusation being that he had attributed the events of Christ's life to the influence of the stars (astrology was yet another of his manifold interests). After some months in prison, he recanted and on his release went to Rome to try to win the favor of Pope Pius V. This he did, and was granted an annuity until his death in 1576. Overall, his life does not seem to have been a happy one despite his powerful intellect, his encyclopedic learning, and his success in medical practice. Apart from the extraneous troubles which afflicted him (they included controversies over mathematical matters), his personality was unstable and immature, marked by irrational fears and childish credulity. His work, however, has endured. Not only his mathematics, but some of his contributions to hydrodynamics and geology have proved of lasting value.

**CARDIOLOGY — HISTORY** The earliest knowledge of the heart and circulation is found in the EDWIN SMITH PAPYRUS and was possibly written by IMHOTEP (p 412), the first known physician, around 2700 BC. Mummification entailed removal of the viscera and so the anatomy of the heart and vessels was well known to the early Egyptians, who realized that the pulse was due to the action of the heart. However, the progress of knowledge was slow and erratic. HIPPOCRATES (p 382) in the 4th century BC believed that the arteries contained air, although Herophilus in 300 BC described the frequency, rhythm, size, and strength of the pulse and timed it with a water clock. GALEN (p 324) in the 2nd century, suggested that blood went from the right to the left ventricle through invisible pores in the septum and so great was his influence that this and other errors were stoutly upheld for the next 1400 years. The High Renaissance led to excellent work by Italian anatomists such as de Capri, VESALIUS (p 846), Colombo, and Fabricius, who described coronary arteries and the valves in the veins.

### Circulation of the blood

In 1628 came the outstandingly important discovery by William HARVEY (p 363) outlined in his book *De motu cordis*, of the circulation of the blood. By observations in living men showing the direction of blood flow in the veins, on dead animals demonstrating the forward (but not backward) flow in the pulmonary artery, in experiments on living animals, and by calculations of the cardiac output derived from ventricular cavity size, Harvey built up an unchallengeable body of evidence to prove his contention that there was a 'movement, as it were, in a circle'. His experimental work and his reasoning from it were so fine that he has been named the father of physiology and also the father of clinical science. He had to deduce the passage of blood through the lungs and across the systemic circulation because it was not until 1661 that MALPIGHI (p 37) demonstrated capillary anastomoses, an observation that was confirmed by van LEEUWENHOEK (p 489) in 1696 with his invention of the biconvex lens microscope. Harvey's work must have been important to LOWER (p 119), who in 1665 was the first to perform direct transfusion of blood from one animal to another and whose work *Tractatus de corde* contained observations on cardiac tamponade with pericardial effusion. In the next 100 years there was increasing emphasis on

correlating clinical and pathological findings, and MORGAGNI'S (p 621) 1761 five-volume work *De sedibus et causis morborum* was the high point of this development, with many cardiological cases, including rupture of the heart.

Stephen Hales, a clergyman and scientist, was the first to measure directly the arterial blood pressure in 1732. He placed a brass pipe connected to a long glass tube in the crural artery of a mare and noted that the blood had risen to a height of 8 ft 3 in (2.5 m) above the level of the left ventricle.

The next big leap forward was LAËNNEC'S (p 461) discovery of auscultation of the heart by the invention of the monaural stethoscope in 1819. This opened up a completely new chapter in cardiac diagnosis and Laënnec's own pioneer work was soon taken up by James Hope of Edinburgh. Hope's book on the heart published in 1831 described all the murmurs of valve disease. By listening to the exposed heart of stunned donkeys he showed the origin of the second heart sound, and experimentally produced mitral regurgitation by passing a wire through the orifice of the mitral valve between the left atrium and ventricle, while auscultating. The method of clinicopathological correlation which Laënnec used for elucidating auscultatory signs was fruitfully employed by Austin Flint in New Orleans in 1862, when a patient with a mitral presystolic murmur and aortic insufficiency was shown post-mortem to have a normal mitral valve and this murmur was named after him.

The 'opening snap' in mitral stenosis was correctly identified in 1888 by Rouchés, who described it as '*claquement d'ouverture de la mitrale*'. Rouchés's teacher was Potain, who wrote a good account of gallop rhythm in 1885 and who had a particular interest in jugular venous pulsation.

### Instruments

An instrument to record cardiac pulsations had been invented by the physiologist Marey in 1860. It consisted of two tambours which wrote on a smoked drum, and was named the 'polygraph'. James MACKENZIE (p 332) used a modification of both Jacquet's and Dudgeon's sphygmographs when he started his remarkable studies in 1894 on the venous and arterial pulses and cardiac movements when he was a general practitioner in Burnley. The inconvenience of using smoked paper whilst on domiciliary visits led to the invention of the famous Mackenzie ink-writing polygraph. This was excellent for recording abnormal hemodynamics, and was good for arhythmias.

Augustus Waller in 1887 had recorded the electrical activity of the human heart using the capillary electrometer of Lippman, but the records were

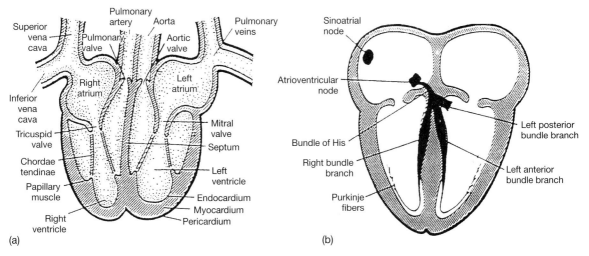

(a)
(b)

Diagram (a) of the heart; (b) of the conduction pathway.

primitive and inaccurate and the invention in 1903 by Willem Einthoven of the string galvanometer revolutionized the electrophysiological study of the heart (electrocardiography). His very precise recordings showed clearly and unequivocally the electrical wave associated with atrial contraction which he labelled P, and those associated with ventricular contraction labelled Q, R, S, T, ($T_1$), and U. He recorded the electromotive force of the heart by recording the electrical current flowing between leads attached respectively to the right and left arms and the left leg and these were called leads I, II, and III. The original Einthoven apparatus occupied two rooms and took five people to operate, so an early redesign was essential. This was first done by Edelmann in Munich and by 1910 a compact machine using continuous paper recording was in daily use at JOHNS HOPKINS Hospital (p 840). The Cambridge Instrument Company produced their own beautifully constructed version which included a twin string carrier for Thomas LEWIS's (p 188) research work. He even used two of these side by side, so that simultaneous four-channel recording was possible by 1913. The inconvenient early practice of placing the limbs in electrode baths was superseded by metal electrode plates in 1920 when the Hindle Company in the USA produced a mobile electrocardiograph. The electrocardiograph (ECG) was especially suitable for arrhythmia analysis and it clarified the nature of the 'irregular irregularity' of the heart which Mackenzie had already shown by auscultation and by polygraph records to be associated with absence of atrial activity. That it was due to atrial fibrillation was convincingly shown by Thomas Lewis in 1910 and Lewis's early mastery of all aspects of clinical and animal work in electrocardiography, and especially the arhythmias, was signaled by his treatise in 1911, *The mechanism of the heart beat*, which

was hailed as the bible of electrocardiography. Good-quality heart-sound records were also obtained, although this phonocardiographic work was not pursued as it should have been at this time and it was much later in 1948 that William Evans followed by Aubrey Leatham reaped this particular harvest in full. After only 20 years or so the analysis of arhythmias was almost complete and progress was being made on evaluating abnormalities of the myocardium. Ventricular hypertrophy, or preponderance as they called it, was also well known, as was congenital dextrocardia (siting of the heart on the right rather than the left side of the chest), while measurement of the heart's electrical axis was in common use. Pardee showed the features of coronary artery occlusion in 1920, but the changes associated with acute pericarditis were still unknown in 1931 and it was after this that the first records of depression of the ST segment in the ECG due to ischemia of the myocardium with angina occurring at rest were obtained. Master described a standardized effort test in 1929 for evaluating cardiac performance and Wood in 1931 was among the first to show ischemic changes in the ECG taken after effort.

The realization in 1931 by Wolferth and Wood, from experimental coronary occlusion in dogs, that clamping the anterior descending artery produced a dramatic visual change in the heart, but none in the limb lead ECG, led them to use an additional electrode attached to the chest wall over the heart (a chest lead), which then revealed the acute changes. At once they applied this clinically and a bipolar chest lead from the precordium to the back, 'lead 4', showed the features of acute anterior infarction, whereas the limb leads did not. Slowly, multiple chest leads came into use, and Wilson's 1934 invention of the central terminal eventually led to universal adoption of this technique with the unipolar leads designated by the letter V. The esophagus is anatomically close to the atria of the heart and Hurst Brown in 1936 showed the value of recording the ECG via an esophageal lead in arhythmia analysis.

### Hemodynamic studies

Electrophysiological work had started in 1855 when von Kölliker showed that an electric current was produced by each beat of a frog's heart and it was marked by equally enthusiastic work in hemodynamics, much of it necessarily done on animals in physiological laboratories. In 1870 Fick introduced the concept of measuring the cardiac output by a dilution method, and this was applied experimentally in horses by Zuntz in 1898 with measurement of the oxygen content from the right heart. An injected indicator for the dilution method in humans was pioneered by Stewart in 1897 using salt solution, while Hamilton introduced the use of blue dye in 1932. The respiratory method was invented by Grollman in 1930 using acetylene gas and he checked his results once in a human against the Fick method by puncture of the right ventricle.

### Heart failure

From von Haller in 1757 to LUDWIG (p 643) in 1855 and Cohnheim in 1877, physiologists in Germany had expressed the view that cardiac ventricular contraction (systole) is less forceful if filling is decreased and stronger if resistance to outflow is increased. In 1881, Martin at Johns Hopkins University devised an isolated mammalian heart preparation. Starling at University College London drew together these endeavors. But Starling's work had no immediate impact on medical practice and the important diagnostic advance in recognizing heart failure was made by Lewis, who emphasized the value of measuring the jugular venous pressure by inspection of the neck veins for early diagnosis. Lewis taught that the heart usually failed as a whole, but the concept of isolated failure of the left side of the heart, which had first been advocated in 1831 by Hope and then rejected by Mackenzie in 1908, gained ground again in the 1920s and was fully established by the work of Evan Bedford in 1939. Advances in treatment of heart failure lagged behind those in diagnosis and, although the mercurial diuretics were an invaluable addition to treatment available in 1920, there remained patients with right-sided heart failure whose severely edematous legs (dropsy) had to be drained mechanically by Southey's tubes or through skin incisions, while those with left heart failure were relieved by venesection.

Digitalis had by now been in use for over 150 years following WITHERING's (p 633) fine deduction in 1785 that the foxglove, *Digitalis purpurea*, must be the active principle in an old Shropshire polypharmacy remedy for dropsy (see HERBAL REMEDIES AND PHYSIC GARDENS). Withering regarded it chiefly as a diuretic, although he did recognize its 'power over the motion of the heart to a degree yet unobserved in any other medicine'. When electrocardiography elucidated the arrhythmias it was shown that digitalis slowed the ventricular rate in atrial fibrillation by acting on the atrioventricular node, and this led to the belief, almost a gospel, that this was its only therapeutic effect and therefore that it had no place in treating cardiac failure when the rhythm was normal. That it could, however, rapidly improve right heart failure without arrhythmia, was shown conclusively by Wood in 1940, but whether it is of long-term benefit to the failing heart in normal rhythm is less certain.

Before the development of modern diuretics which, being effective and available, must not now be withheld from a patient, it would have been ethical to conduct a clinical trial of digitalis alone in chronic heart failure with normal rhythm but unfortunately this was never done.

### Surgery in heart disease

Further examples of how dogma grips men's minds and suppresses enquiry were later supplied by disputes about the management of heart failure due to mitral valve disease. Brunton found in 1902 that the narrowed mitral valve could easily be enlarged at post-mortem examination and he proposed that surgical treatment of mitral stenosis should be considered. In 1925, Souttar attempted finger dilatation of the mitral valve via the left atrium but this brave pioneer attempt failed because the physician had chosen to ignore the patient's mitral systolic murmur (due to valvular incompetence) and there was little stenosis to dilate. There are important historical lessons here. Because innocent systolic murmurs had commonly been misdiagnosed as being due to mitral valve incompetence, thus leading to unjustified cardiac invalidism, there had arisen a virtual embargo on diagnosing mitral incompetence on the basis of systolic murmurs only ('incompetence of the doctor, not the valve') without too much effort being made to separate the one from the other. Cutler in 1923 had also operated upon the mitral valve and, although his technique was wrong, he and Souttar showed that even the diseased heart could readily withstand a direct attack via the atrium or left ventricle. An even worse error was the failure of heart specialists to accept that the narrowed heart valve was directly responsible for the heart failure. In 1933 Paul White wrote 'There are no symptoms of mitral stenosis'. This was a legacy of Mackenzie, to whom failure of the heart in valve disease meant a primary fault in the myocardium. He wrote to Cutler's physician, Levine, 'Dear Sam, What a foolish thing to try to do! The fate of the patient is determined by adaptation of the myocardium.'

But other operations on the heart were not constrained by hypothesis (see also CARDIOTHORACIC SURGERY – HISTORY). In 1820 Napoleon's chief surgeon, LARREY (p 796), incised the pericardium for a traumatic pericardial effusion, and in 1873 Callender removed a needle from the heart. But credit for being the first to operate on the myocardium itself goes to Forina, who sutured a stab wound of the right ventricle in 1896. The thickened pericardium in chronic constrictive pericarditis was an obvious surgical target and the operation of pericardiectomy was first done in 1914 by Rehn.

Attempts to prevent aortic aneurysms from rupturing began in 1864, when Moore and Murchison passed fine wire into the aneurysmal sac hoping that thrombosis would occur and eventually strengthen the wall; amazingly, this rather ineffective treatment was still in use 90 years later. A better approach was that of Matas, whose first account of surgical treatment of aneurysm by 'endo-aneurysmorrhaphy' appeared in 1902.

Pulmonary stenosis was described by William HUNTER (p 88) in 1762 and in 1777 Sandifort wrote of its association with ventricular septal defect — a syndrome that was superbly worked out in 1888 by Fallot, who stated that the cyanosis of this condition was due to venous blood entering the arterial circulation; this is known as Fallot's tetralogy. Another cyanotic congenital heart lesion but with a dilated rather than a stenosed pulmonary artery was named the Eisenmenger complex after its discoverer. Burns, Farre, Bouillaud, and Peacock were among many others who gave good descriptions of congenital heart lesions, but it was the comprehensive collection started in 1908 by Maude ABBOTT (this page) that led to the best understanding of these complex abnormalities, culminating in her *Atlas* of 1935 describing 1000 specimens. Evidence regarding the genetic cause of congenital heart lesions first came from noting the association of certain cardiac defects with other congenital lesions such as Down's syndrome and later by chromosomal analysis, for example, in Turner's syndrome. The very perceptive observation by Gregg in 1940 that congenital cataract follows maternal rubella led to the realization that congenital cardiac anomalies are also caused by this virus infection, and hence may be prevented.

Although the role of other infections in the genesis of heart disease had to await the development of microbiology before they could be fully evaluated, there was, nevertheless, good early evidence of their causative importance. Fernel in 1554 believed that aneurysms were produced by SYPHILIS and in 1863 Wilks demonstrated endarteritis and showed that gumata cause myocardial changes. Wilks also wrote an important paper on infective endocarditis noting its frequent association with chronic valvular heart disease and separating it clearly from rheumatic fever. The importance of blood cultures was shown in 1903 by Lenhartz, who particularly drew attention to an organism he called *Streptococcus parvus* (now *viridans*) as causing a subacute form of bacterial endocarditis (with vegetations containing blood clots and bacteria attached to the heart valves), the clinical features of which, with an account of evanescent subcutaneous nodes, were described by OSLER (p 602) in 1909. That rheumatic fever led to heart disease was recognized by JENNER (p 452) in 1789 and another pre-Laennec report was that of Wells in 1810, but it was Bouillaud in 1836 who showed beyond doubt the etiological association between the two. The unique diastolic murmur of acute rheumatic valvulitis was described in 1907 by Coombs.

## Cardiac ischemia and infarction

Jenner was an early writer on coronary artery disease, which was first described in 1662 by Bellini, and the classic description in 1772 by Heberden of angina pectoris has never been bettered. He recorded nearly 100 patients with severe chest pain accompanied by a 'sense of strangling' coming on with exertion so this 'disorder of the breast' must have been quite common even then. Soon afterwards a man with angina who died suddenly in a fit of anger was shown by FOTHERGILL (p 695) to have severely diseased coronary arteries. This post-mortem was done by the surgeon John HUNTER (p 398), whose distal ligation for arterial aneurysm was celebrated and who died an identical death — which he had anticipated — 'my life is in the hands of any rascal who chooses to annoy me'. The only effective medicine available for treating angina pectoris until 1960 was discovered somewhat by chance by Brunton in 1867 because the patient in whom he showed that amyl nitrite relieved anginal pain had the rare syndrome of nocturnal angina due to aortic regurgitation. Luckily the same effect held good for the angina of coronary disease and the longer-acting glyceryl trinitrate introduced by Murrell in 1879 is still in common use today. But for severe cases it was not enough. In 1932 Blumgart introduced thyroidectomy in order to reduce metabolism and hence lessen cardiac work but the symptoms of myxedema were an unwelcome substitute for angina. Surgical thought naturally turned towards a direct approach to increase myocardial blood flow. Beck tried to do

PEDIATRIC CARDIOLOGIST

Maude Elizabeth Seymour **ABBOTT** (1869–1940). Canadian cardiologist, medical historian. As a woman she was denied admission to McGill University so she trained in the obscure Bishop's University, then spent her professional life almost entirely at McGill, where she became world renowned for her studies of congenital heart disease. She was an authority also on the history of medicine and nursing and became the permanent secretary of the International Association of Medical Museums throughout her lifetime.

this in 1935 by suturing pectoral muscle on to the heart, and in 1936 O'Shaughnessy used a pedicle of omentum. Vineberg extended this idea in 1950 by implanting the internal mammary artery into a myocardial tunnel. Although of little use, these were important early attempts, which helped to catalyze later developments.

The symptom of exertional angina is clear enough, so one might have expected the more dramatic picture of acute myocardial infarction to have been identified sooner than it was, especially as the pathology was noted quite early. In 1749 de Senac described ventricular aneurysm, and in 1761 MORGAGNI (p 621) recorded rupture of the heart. In 1815 Hodgson wrote of a patient with angina who died suddenly and who had softening of the myocardium in the region supplied by a calcified coronary artery, and in 1880 Weigert gave a classic account including microscopy of the changes resulting from sudden coronary occlusion. The first clinical diagnosis with post-mortem control (excepting Hammer's 1878 case with endocarditis) was made by Dock in 1896 and the definitive paper by Herrick followed in 1912. But still the diagnosis was ignored and Herrick later wrote 'The publication aroused no interest. It fell like a dud.' It was the electrocardiographic features pioneered by Herrick, by Pardee in 1920, and by Bedford and Parkinson in 1928 that eventually led to wide recognition of the condition but acceptance had been remarkably slow.

That the pulse could be abnormal in ways other than rate and rhythm was shown by Corrigan in 1832 with the 'water-hammer' or 'collapsing' pulse of aortic incompetence and by Kussmaul in 1873 with the pulsus paradoxus of constrictive pericarditis, but to measure the pressure of the pulse was more difficult. In 1855, von Vierordt compressed the radial artery with weights but this and similar attempts using pneumatic and hydraulic pressure by Marey in 1876 and von Basch in 1887 (*Der Sphygmomanometer ... in der Praxis*) lacked precision. It was Riva-Rocci's invention of the pneumatic cuff in 1896 that enabled the systolic pressure to be measured readily by palpation. Then in 1910 as a result of studying traumatic arterial aneurysms in the Russo-Japanese war KOROTKOFF (p 399) discovered that a partially compressed artery yields a noise with each heart beat and so modern blood-pressure measurement was born; nevertheless, effective treatment for HYPERTENSION had to wait for another 50 years.

### Functional cardiac disorders

During the American Civil War J. M. DaCosta described a syndrome in soldiers who had what were apparently cardiac symptoms such as chest pain and palpitation but who in fact had normal hearts. This condition, often called 'irritable heart' or 'soldiers' heart', caused so much invalidism among British soldiers in World War I that a special heart hospital, directed by Thomas Lewis, had to be set up to deal with it. Lewis re-named it the 'effort syndrome' because the symptoms occurred on exertion and he devised a remedial system of physical exercises which enabled over 35 000 men to be returned to active service. There was no one cause of the syndrome. In some it was undoubtedly due to the terrible strain of trench warfare. But in others, especially in new recruits, it was reasonable to label it neurocirculatory asthenia or cardiac neurasthenia, and to regard it as a form of cardiac neurosis. Hyperventilation was later shown to be a causative factor in some. The condition was well recognized in civilian life even before 1914, so it was not a malady confined to soldiers – with the important exception of those who were totally exhausted by warfare.

The impetus of much new research work in heart disease after 1900 made it essential to have a journal dedicated to that purpose. In 1909 the journal *Heart* was founded and under the editorship of Thomas Lewis it became prestigious. Lewis changed it into *Clinical Science* in 1933 and in 1939 the British Cardiac Society created their own journal, the *British Heart Journal*. In 1996 this journal changed its name to *Heart*.          AHol

*See also* BATTLE NEUROSIS; BLOOD TRANSFUSION; JOURNALS; SPECIALIZATION

## CARDIOLOGY

### Congenital heart disease

About 8 in 1000 babies are born with a recognizable heart defect. A few have very minor defects which are not recognized until later in life, if at all. A few are so severe that life cannot be sustained. For most cases the cause is unknown. The genetic basis for some disorders is beginning to be understood but in others extraneous influences — such as treatment of the mother with warfarin — are causative.

Congenital heart disorders may be classified into those which permit abnormal shunting of blood from the left to the right side of the heart, thus increasing the flow of blood through the lungs; those which obstruct blood flow; and those that are complex, usually because there are several defects. The best known of these is Fallot's tetralogy, which results in reverse shunting of blood from the right to the left side of the heart so that blue (deoxygenated) blood appears in the systemic circuit. This blue discoloration is known as cyanosis.

The most common congenital heart disorder (about 30%) is a ventricular septal defect (a hole between the two ventricles). Many defects can be corrected by surgery so that subsequent life and life-expectancy are both near normal. Techniques using fine catheters, which can be inserted into the circulation from a blood vessel in the arm or leg, often are increasingly successful nowadays and are often the preferred approach.

Congenital heart disease, if severe, causes infants to 'fail to thrive', whereupon urgent treatment is necessary. More commonly the disorder is detected at a routine medical examination by finding a heart murmur. Treatment may then be deferred until the child is older. This has several advantages, both psychological and physical. For example, the larger size makes surgery easier and adult replacement valves can be implanted.

Heart murmurs are noises caused by turbulent blood flow, rather like water gurgling intermittently in a pipe. Murmurs can be heard in normal children and slender adults if the heart is contracting forcefully, as happens if the person is nervous, has recently exercised, or is pregnant. Flow murmurs are also common in old age because the valves are stiffer. The distinction between a 'flow' murmur and a murmur indicating heart disease can usually be made by an experienced doctor. A definite diagnosis is best achieved by echocardiography or ultrasound of the heart. This technique is harmless and painless and has transformed our understanding of cardiac disorders.

Echocardiography involves placing a transducer on the front of the chest, or sometimes, if special views of the back of the heart are required, through a probe in the gullet.

## Coronary heart disease

This is by far the most common form of heart disease. In Britain in 1994 there were 154 842 deaths and 381 083 hospital admissions due to coronary or ischemic heart disease. The disease may present itself in several ways.

A heart attack is a useful term which embraces both sudden cardiac death resulting from a profound disturbance of heart rhythm or the chest pain resulting from dead heart muscle (myocardial infarction) due to a blocked artery. About half of all heart attacks are fatal. If the artery is merely narrowed then the patient may experience chest discomfort on effort which eases with rest; this is known as angina pectoris (literally strangling of the chest). Other manifestations include heart failure, lesser disturbances of cardiac rhythm, and the detection of a silent abnormality at a routine medical or health screening check, when an electrocardiogram is performed, especially after exercise.

The pathology of coronary heart disease is a progressive silting up of the arteries due to an accumulation of fatty substances (ATHEROMA). Fatty streaks can be found in young people; they gradually thicken to form fibrous plaques. Cholesterol and other fats are deposited in the center, and inflammatory cells invade the margins; eventually the plaque may rupture through the inner lining of the arterial wall, provoking a clot to form on the raw surface so that the artery becomes blocked suddenly. The atheromatous process happens very slowly, although not until the narrowing is far advanced does the victim have symptoms.

There is no single cause of coronary heart disease. Five major factors place a person at increased risk: these are age, male sex, smoking habit, raised blood cholesterol concentrations, and high blood pressure. Many other minor risk factors have been described such as mental stress, but none is sufficiently well established to justify advising a change in life-style, with two exceptions: the evidence that regular exercise, and consumption of (in limited quantity) alcohol, such as red wine have a protective effect is well founded.

The long silent incubation period of coronary heart disease and its dramatic presentation make management of the condition difficult. Prevention would clearly be desirable. Health education programs are laudable but have generally been ineffective in changing people's life-styles. Screening for silent coronary disease is bedevilled by false positive clues. The death rate from coronary disease is, however, falling in most developed countries. The most likely explanation for this is that we have better treatments for the disease once it becomes manifest including drugs and surgery. Aspirin, for example, protects against heart attacks. Prompt treatment of an attack with resuscitation and treatment of abnormal rhythms coupled with admission to hospital for the administration of clot-busting drugs (such as streptokinase) and observation in a coronary care unit so that any complications can be dealt with early saves individual lives.

The outcome for patients with coronary disease is governed by the extent of the disease and the damage to the heart muscle. Indirect clues to the extent of the disease can be sought in the history (multiple heart attacks imply extensive damage), physical examination, and the results of investigations, notably electrocardiography. An electrocardiogram is an amplified electrical recording of the signals from the heart. A scar creates an electrical hole, which shows up in the record, thus confirming the diagnosis. Patients with angina usually have a normal electrocardiogram at rest but may develop changes on effort, reflecting the lack of an adequate blood supply. This change may be induced by exercise testing, usually on a treadmill. The time on the treadmill is a reasonable indicator of prognosis, so that this test is widely used in assessing a person's ability to return to work or need for further treatment.

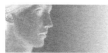
A coronary angiogram involves inserting a catheter into the circulation generally via the groin so that X-ray images of the coronary arteries and left ventricle may be obtained, and a more accurate prognosis given. Precutaneous transluminal coronary angioplasty involves stretching the narrowed segment of artery with a balloon on the end of a catheter. This is immediately successful in over 95% of cases, but recurrent narrowing occurs in up to one third of patients usually within the first three months.

Coronary artery bypass grafting is recommended if there are impassable blockages or more than one or two narrowings. Like angioplasty, a bypass should be undertaken only in patients with continuing angina or a very abnormal exercise test. Unlike angioplasty, coronary artery bypass grafting improves survival, especially in those whose coronary disease is widespread. Veins taken from the legs are the traditional bypasses and these last about 10 years, when angina may recur.

Other investigations and treatments are undertaken less commonly. Nuclear imaging may be used to study the supply of blood through the heart muscle.

### Valve disease

Most valve disease is degenerative, affecting middle-aged and elderly people. The inlet and outlet valves of the left ventricle are chiefly affected. The inlet or mitral valve may become leaky with advancing years as mitral regurgitation or the aortic valve may become narrowed (aortic stenosis), often as a result of imperfect construction and hence increased wear. Both may be detected as murmurs initially and may never

progress. Some valves do deteriorate, however, and this imposes an increasing load on the left ventricle. The ventricle adapts and compensates but ultimately begins to fail. The patient therefore feels nothing until late in the day when shortness of breath is the usual complaint, because the lungs become congested. In aortic stenosis other complaints include lightheadedness or faintness on effort and angina pectoris. Once symptoms develop valve surgery is necessary.

It is sometimes possible to repair a leaking mitral valve but the aortic valve always has to be replaced. The operation carries a risk of death of less than 3%. Complications are rare and most people return home in 7 to 10 days. The replacement valve (prosthesis) is usually mechanical, often a metal frame containing a tilting carbon fiber disc, and since all mechanical prostheses are prone to clotting, blood-thinning treatment with an anticoagulant drug is mandatory.

### Heart failure and cardiomyopathy

In heart failure the heart cannot fully meet the needs of the body. Fatigue and congestion with water logging (edema) of the tissues are the dominant complaints. Congestion of the lungs leads to shortness of breath; of the liver to anorexia; of the ankles to observable swelling; and of other organs to an outpouring of fluid which may embarrass their function, including the heart itself. Any of the foregoing heart diseases may cause failure but the scarred muscle of coronary heart disease is the most common. Various precipitating events may be recognized including a chest infection, change in rhythm, anemia, and pregnancy.

A cardiac pacemaker consists of a battery and associated electronic equipment which generate regular impulses that are transmitted through the attached wires to electrodes implanted in the heart. The device is usually attached under the skin, though sometimes can be worn on the body supported by elastic strapping.

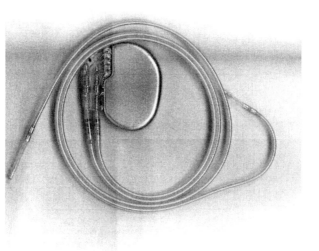

Occasionally the heart muscle fails without obvious reason (congestive or dilated cardiomyopathy). Good and often lasting improvement may be achieved with modern drugs. Those whose condition deteriorates progressively may be recommended for heart transplantation. The results of this operation are very good nowadays, over two thirds of patients surviving five years. The number of operations is limited by the shortage of donors.

Hypertrophic cardiomyopathy is an unusual condition in which there is overgrowth of heart muscle. Some families are affected and sudden death may occur. Screening, however, has uncovered many mild cases who remain free from trouble indefinitely.

### Rhythms and pacemakers

The rhythm of the human heart rarely falters. Missed beats are however a universal phenomenon at some stage in life, although not everyone feels them. The 'miss' is a pause after an early beat called an ectopic or extrasystole. This is not felt because the heart is only half filled but the next beat is over-filled and is detected as a thump after a momentary sinking feeling. They do not matter, although they may be very unsettling. Groups of extrasystoles produce a fast abnormal rhythm known as a tachycardia, which may occur in episodes or paroxysms. Some paroxysmal tachycardias are due to a short-circuit in the electrical pathways of the heart; these have traditionally been treated with drugs. Nowadays the abnormal pathway can be located and abolished by a radiofrequency current, leaving the surrounding tissues unharmed.

Atrial fibrillation is the commonest abnormal rhythm (arrhythmia). Some 2% of the population suffer this at some stage in their lives; the incidence rises with age, so that 5% of people over 65 are affected. This arrhythmia, like those above, usually occurs in an otherwise normal heart and the outlook is excellent. Any of these arrhythmias may also occur in diseased hearts, when the outlook is less certain.

The implantable cardioverter-defibrillator is the latest in a series of implantable devices designed to treat arrhythmias. The principle is the same as external cardioversion, but the devices are expensive. The current implant rates per million population in Britain are 7, in Germany 25, and in the USA 110.

An extremely slow heart rate or bradycardia lies at the other end of the spectrum of rhythm disturbances leading to faintness and blackouts. A pacemaker transforms the victim's life. This can sense the normal heartbeat and if the heart rate falls below a predetermined level, usually 70 beats

Electrocardiogram (ECG). This shows the atria and the ventricles beating independently, secondary to heart block (interruption of several conduction pathways).

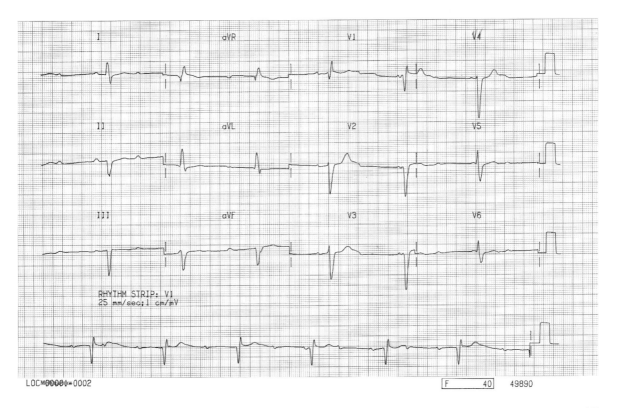

Helen Brooke **TAUSSIG**
(1898–1986). American
pediatric cardiologist. Head of
the first pediatric cardiac
clinic at the JOHNS HOPKINS
Hospital (p 840). With Alfred
Blalock she helped to develop
the Blalock–Taussig operation
for tetralogy of Fallot. She
probably did more towards
the development of pediatric
cardiology than any other
person.

per minute, then the pacemaker cuts in. Most ingenious of all, some contain a small crystal which senses bodily movement and increases the firing rate when the patient takes exercise.     MCP

*See also* IMAGING

## CARDIOTHORACIC SURGERY – HISTORY

Cardiothoracic surgery is a relatively new endeavor in surgery, owing to the technical difficulties of opening the thoracic cavity. The problem of ventilation with a collapsed lung, and the difficulties of working on a beating heart are only two of several such obstacles. Indeed, only some 100 years ago the famous German surgeon BILLROTH (p 518) stated that 'the surgeon who should attempt to suture a wound of the heart would lose the respect of his colleagues'. Nevertheless, in 1897 Rehn successfully repaired a tear of the heart ventricle. In 1913 Doyen unsuccessfully attempted the first internal heart surgery attempting a closed repair of pulmonary valve stenosis. This same operation was successfully developed by Brock and Sellors in London in 1948. Souttar carried out the first successful operation inside the heart, opening a stenotic (narrowed) mitral valve in 1925. Harken and Bailey in the USA completed the first of a series of closed mitral valvotomies in 1948. The first half of the 20th century was marked by other significant milestones in cardiac surgery, including the first resection of a ventricular aneurysm by Sauerbruch in Germany in 1931; the first closure or ligation of a patent ductus arteriosus by Gross at Harvard in 1938; and the first resection of a coarctation (narrowing) of the thoracic aorta by Crafoord in Stockholm in 1945.

The modern era of cardiac surgery was ushered in by two significant advances. The first was the development of the Blalock–Taussig shunt, using the subclavian artery to direct oxygenated arterial blood into the pulmonary circuit via the pulmonary artery. This revolutionized the care of cyanotic ('blue baby') congenital heart disease. The second critical development was the conception and refinement over 20 years of the heart–lung machine by John Gibbon, culminating in 1953 in its use to take over the function of the heart and lungs for the successful repair of an atrial septal defect ('hole in the heart') in 1953. The subsequent 30 years mark the accelerating use of the heart–lung machine to address and correct acquired and congenital heart defects, leading to the current era of cardiothoracic surgery.

The recent history of lung surgery follows a somewhat similar course. Surgery inside the thorax, as indicated above, was limited until the development in 1904 by Sauerbruch and Breslau of positive pressure ventilation that allowed for removal of all or part of the lung without lung collapse. The first

pneumonectomy or removal of a lung using modern techniques was successfully undertaken in 1933 on a child at the JOHNS HOPKINS HOSPITAL (p 840), Baltimore, by Reinhoff. The first successful resection (removal) of the esophagus was completed by Torek in New York in 1913, and Ohsawa and Seou performed the first esophageal resection with the re-establishment of gastroesophageal continuity in 1933.     TKRos

**CARDIOTHORACIC SURGERY** Disease of the heart valves primarily affects the mitral and aortic valves, which, respectively, allow blood to flow in one direction into and out of the left ventricular pumping chamber of the heart. In the modern era of antibiotic therapy, rheumatic heart disease, which typically causes narrowing of the mitral valve, is becoming less common. Today the prevalent forms of valvular heart disease include narrowing of the aortic valve caused by 'wear and tear' in the aging population, and leakage of the mitral valve, occurring primarily in younger patients because of inborn tissue weaknesses.

The surgical correction of valvular disease figured predominantly in the early era of open heart surgery. Replacement of heart valves with mechanical valves was first successfully accomplished in 1961 by Starr in Portland, Oregon, using a ball and cage type device. Subsequently, various forms of tilting disc valves were developed and introduced clinically. Currently, the St Jude tilting disc valve is the most widely used mechanical heart valve in the world, yielding excellent durability and hemodynamic function. The failure rate of this and similar mechanical prostheses is far less than 1% per year. The rate of infection for these prosthetic valves is roughly 0.2% per year. Unfortunately, the prosthetic heart valves do require thinning of the blood, anticoagulation, with oral anticoagulant agents to allow proper function. Despite this precaution, the risk of clotting complications of the valve or embolism of clots from the valve is about 1–2% per year and the complications of bleeding secondary to use of these oral anticoagulants is also 1% per year.

Because of these complications, an alternative substitute after removal of abnormal valves is a bioprosthesis. In general, these valves are harvested from pigs and then sewn onto cloth struts to allow for surgical insertion. These porcine valves are preserved in glutaraldehyde and in general do not require anticoagulant: however, their expected durability is 10–13 years, when patients require reoperation and valve replacement.

More recently, tissue valves engineered from the bovine pericardial lining have been employed. These valves appear to have better hemodynamic performance and enhanced longevity compared with the porcine valves. Ross in London and Barrett-Boyes in Australia have pioneered work in the use of transplanted human cadaveric valves as an alternative, with good results. In what has been called the 'Ross procedure', the homograft valve may be positioned in place of the pulmonary valve, which is then transplanted into the aortic position, with the hope that this 'auto-transplant' will last longer than a foreign, preserved valve in the high pressure aortic valve position.

In recent years, an increasing effort has also been made to repair and not replace diseased valves. This is most applicable to those mitral valves that can be opened by incising between the leaflets. An open operation may be performed, or a ring placed around a leaking valve (annuloplasty), or the torn portions of the mitral valve leaflets repaired (valvuloplasty). Intermediate to long-term results with these procedures are encouraging. In selected cases, the fused leaflets of a narrowed mitral valve (but not the aortic valve), typically occurring through rheumatic heart disease, can also be opened by a balloon introduced through the femoral artery in the leg, thus avoiding an open operation. Significant freedom from the complications associated with valve replacement is a major advantage of this repair procedure.

## Coronary artery grafting bypass (coronary bypass)

Inadequate blood supply to the heart due to atherosclerotic obstruction of the coronary arteries causes chest pressure or pain called angina pectoris, first described in 1768. Another one hundred years passed before the association between coronary artery obstruction and angina was recognized, and still another one hundred years before modern coronary bypass surgery arrived. Saphenous vein bypass grafting (using a long superficial vein taken from the leg) is the current technique for surgical relief of coronary obstruction. It was established in the 1960s by Johnson in Milwaukee and Favaloro at the Cleveland Clinic. The first use of the internal mammary artery (situated just behind the breast bone) in humans dates to the Vineberg procedure, reported in 1946, and the first direct internal mammary artery to coronary graft was performed in 1964 by Kolesov in the Soviet Union and subsequently in the USA.

Trials of medical versus surgical management for coronary artery disease were performed in the early 1970s with the initial growth in expertise in performing coronary bypass surgery. These studies showed that surgery provided superior relief of angina and improvement in functional capacity and a reduction in the incidence of fatal myocardial infarction, but no difference in the frequency of late non-fatal myocardial infarc-

tions. These studies also showed that patients with obstruction of the left main coronary artery or significant obstructions of three major coronary arteries and left ventricular dysfunction enjoyed a significant survival advantage with surgical versus medical treatment.

Current symptomatic indications for coronary bypass surgery include unstable angina that does not respond to standard medical treatment and must be treated with intravenous medications, or that has been increasing in severity, or that occurs at rest. Similarly, severe exertional angina that is unresponsive to medical treatment is also an indication for surgical intervention. Angina that persists after myocardial infarction is a further indication, as is ischemia or hemodynamic instability after an unsuccessful percutaneous angioplasty (blood vessel repair), or after acute myocardial infarction. Cardiogenic shock complicating myocardial infarction, or mechanical complications of a myocardial infarction such as mitral regurgitation or acute ventricular septal defect, may be further indications.

In general, each of these clinical indications needs to be correlated with appropriate anatomic or physiologic abnormalities. These include a greater than 50% blockage of the left main coronary artery, a greater than 50% obstruction of all three major coronary arteries (three vessel disease) with impaired left ventricular function, or three vessel disease with normal left ventricular function but inducible ischemia on physiologic testing. Two vessel disease with significant proximal blockage of the left anterior descending coronary artery, severely depressed left ventricular function with evidence of reversible ischemia, or, less commonly, coronary artery disease associated with life threatening ventricular arhythmias are other surgical indications. Coronary stenoses not normally indicated for surgery may be bypassed concomitant with other indicated procedures such as repair of aortic or mitral valvular disease.

The recent advent of percutaneous transluminal coronary angioplasty and placement of scaffolding devices called 'stents', together with appropriate anti-blood-clotting medications, has generally usurped the role of bypass surgery for single and double vessel disease, but the consensus is that coronary bypass surgery remains the indicated treatment for triple vessel disease. Angioplasty/stenting has an associated 10–30% restenosis rate at six months and roughly a 1–2% acute failure rate. Emergency coronary bypass surgery in the setting of failed angioplasty carries about a 5–10% mortality compared with 1–2% in an elective setting. Therefore, angioplasty should be undertaken with the understanding that an almost 10-fold increase in mortality exists in the event of emergency coronary bypass surgery.

## OBJECTIVES OF BYPASS SURGERY

The potential objectives of coronary bypass surgery include:

- relief of low blood flow to the heart (ischemia)
- relief of anginal symptoms
- prolongation of survival
- prevention of myocardial infarction
- preservation of cardiac function
- improvement in exercise tolerance.

The overall risk of elective coronary bypass surgery is about 1–2% for patients with stable angina, 3% for unstable angina, 5–10% for postinfarction angina or failed angioplasty, and 30% for cardiogenic shock.

Surgery is performed by placing the patient on cardiopulmonary bypass. That requires insertion of a cannula (tube) into the right atrium to carry blood away from the heart into a heart–lung machine which oxygenates the blood and removes carbon dioxide. The blood is then returned to the systemic circulation through a second cannula inserted into the aorta. Access to the heart is obtained by splitting the breast bone (a median sternotomy). After instituting cardiopulmonary bypass, a clamp is placed across the aorta, eliminating blood flow to the heart. Because this creates an ischemic condition, heart function is preserved by using a cold potassium (cardioplegic) solution maintained at 4°C. Such conditions decrease the heart's oxygen consumption by 85% or more, allowing a period of bloodless surgery on a still, non-beating heart.

With these conditions, the coronary arteries can be incised beyond the areas of obstruction and a saphenous vein or internal mammary artery joined ('anastomosed') to the coronary artery. After completing these anastomoses, the cross clamp is removed from the aorta. The blood supply to the heart is restored, and it starts beating again. At this point the proximal portions of the bypass grafts are sewn to the aorta, thus receiving a source of blood flow. During the period of crossclamping the patient is also cooled systemically to about 28°C by a heat exchanger included in the cardiopulmonary bypass circuit. This systemic cooling helps prevent rewarming of the heart from blood flowing around it and allows for maintenance of lower systemic pressures and red blood cell levels.

The results of cardiopulmonary bypass surgery from large studies in the 1970s and more recent data are favorable. For patients with triple vessel disease and ejection fraction between 35 and 50%, the large United States CASS study indicated a significant ten-year survival rate difference of 75% for surgical treatment compared with 58% for medical treatment. Patency of the saphenous veins at ten years is about 50%. The internal mammary artery, on the other hand, enjoys a patency of about 95% at ten years. The long-term occlusion of these vein bypass grafts is due to accelerated atherosclerosis and results in a reoperation rate of roughly 17% at 12 years. Recently, increased use of the internal mammary artery and other arterial grafts, such as the radial artery, have been explored to prevent graft closure.

Valve surgery is performed in an analogous fashion to coronary bypass surgery, except that the heart (left atrium) or aorta is opened to access the mitral or aortic valves, respectively. More recently, 'minimally invasive' procedures have been introduced, whereby the coronary arteries are bypassed either without stopping the heart and lungs ('beating heart' technique), or the heart is approached through smaller sternal splitting incisions or thoracotomy incisions between the ribs.

### Congenital heart disease

Congenital heart disease may most simplistically be classified into two types, cyanotic disease and acyanotic heart disease. Cyanotic patients generally have inadequate pulmonary blood flow and are approached surgically by increasing blood flow to the pulmonary circuit through either the bypass or shunt technique. Acyanotic patients generally have problems of heart failure because excessive blood flow occurs in one portion of the heart through a short-circuiting of the normal flow patterns through a hole in the heart (atrial or ventricular septal defect) or an abnormal or anomalous connection of the major vessels (for example, transposition of the great arteries). Many congenital heart diseases are associated with a combination of these two classes of abnormalities.

Almost all congenital heart defects may now be treated either by complete early correction, with or without cardiopulmonary bypass, or early palliation (for example, by the creation of a temporary shunt to increase blood flow to the lungs) with later definitive treatment. As technical abilities improve, it is increasingly possible to reconstruct the normal anatomy of the heart. Mortality rates for even the most complex of congenital heart operations are now approaching under 5%. Long-term survival data are only recently becoming available since many of these procedures are less than twenty years old, but seem to be favorable.

An early heart operation. (Reproduced courtesy of the WHO/National Library of Medicine, Bethesda, MD.)

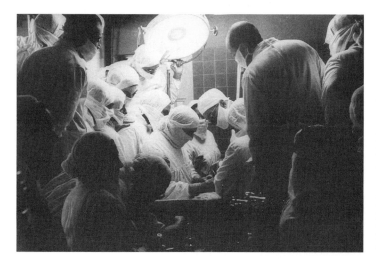

## Pacemakers and automatic implantable cardioverter defibrillator devices

The ability to maintain the normal heartbeat with external electrical stimulation has existed for some thirty years. This requires placement of a wire, or lead, through one of the large veins to the right ventricle of the heart. Occasionally, the lead must be placed through a chest incision directly onto the outside surface of the heart. The lead is connected to the generator unit the size of a woman's compact, which contains a battery and the microcircuitry capable of interpreting and processing the impulses received and transmitted to the lead. The pacemaker generator has a life expectancy of five to ten years, after which it must be replaced. Dual chamber units are available that can sense the patient's own heart rhythm with a second lead placed in the atrium and transmitting this impulse to the ventricle, allowing maintenance of this internal rhythm. The pacemakers available today are capable of external reprogramming and of sensing the patient's motion or activity and increasing the heart rate based upon activity levels.

Until recently, malignant abnormal rhythms originating in the cardiac ventricles, known as ventricular tachycardia and ventricular fibrillation, were commonly associated with sudden death, and were treatable only by medication. The ability to apply an external countershock to reset the electrical rhythm of the heart has, however, existed for many years. The automatic implantable cardioverter defibrillator device, which can sense these abnormal rhythms and internally apply a countershock, has recently gained wide clinical use. These defribrillators may now be routinely implanted using internal lead systems similar to those applied for pacemakers.

## Current advances and future horizons

The last ten years have seen many innovations in cardiac surgery resulting in operations on more seriously ill patients with improved outcomes. The introduction of immunosuppression agents, most notably cyclosporin, has allowed the resurgence of cardiac as well as lung and other organ transplantation. Early and intermediate survival after cardiac transplantation is now about 80%. The introduction of mechanical assist devices — most notably the intraaortic balloon pump — which can bolster the heart's pumping function, has allowed survival of patients with severely compromised heart function. Increasingly accurate monitoring devices, including the transesophageal echocardiogram, allow continuous on-line visualization of the heart and measurement of its pumping function, even with a closed chest. New pharmacologic agents can improve myocardial function and decrease such complications of open heart surgery as bleeding disorders induced by the cardiopulmonary bypass circuit. Finally, much attention is being directed towards biological approaches to myocardial revascularization, including the use of transmyocardial laser revascularization and gene therapy to induce the expression of proteins that cause new blood vessels to grow.

## Thoracic (noncardiac) surgery

Noncardiac thoracic surgery was nearly synonymous with surgery for TUBERCULOSIS in the middle portion of this century. The advent of antituberculosis chemotherapy nearly extinguished the working knowledge of this type of surgery among thoracic surgeons. However, the recent resurgence of tuberculosis, mostly as related to the epidemic of AIDS, has refocused attention on pulmonary surgery for tuberculosis and other infections. The remainder of pulmonary surgery consists primarily of removing the lung or portions of it for lung cancer and other tumors. Advances rely predominantly on changes in chemotherapy and/or radiation therapy and multimodality treatment of these diseases in a synergistic approach to eradicating the tumor, rather than advances in surgical technique. Removal of the esophagus for cancer has been modified in similar ways, although the Japanese have recently advocated wide lymph node dissection for esophageal cancer because of its predilection to spread widely even at an early stage. Perhaps one of the greatest advances in treatment of both of these tumors is the rigorous application of a tumor staging system and advances in staging computerized tomography and ultrasound technology.

The last five years have seen the development of video-assisted thoracic surgery and thoracoscopic surgery. These techniques avoid the significant morbidity of the thoracic incision, which frequently requires excision or division of ribs to allow adequate exposure. Treatment of pleural effusions, pneumothoraces (collapsed lung), open lung biopsies, and even lung resections, lobectomies, and esophageal operations have recently been reported. It is too early to determine whether thoracoscopy will be an appropriate treatment in lung resection for cancer, but this renewed interest in an old technique seems to be revolutionizing thoracic surgery. TKROS

*See also* MINIMALLY INVASIVE SURGERY; TRANSPLANTATION

**CATARACT** See OPHTHALMOLOGY

**CELL AND CELL BIOLOGY** The term 'cell' was first used by the microscopist Hooke in 1665 to describe the structures he saw in thin slices of cork. Although he was not seeing cells but the spaces where cells had been during the life of the tree, in the following years other microscopists made observations that supported his idea of living matter being composed of small structural units. Even so, over 150 years passed before the accumulated observations on cells were brought together into a general 'cell theory', usually attributed to Schleiden and Schwann in 1838. According to this theory, the cell is the smallest component of life that can exist independently. All living organisms are composed of cells and, as concluded by VIRCHOW (p 853) in 1855, cells can arise only from pre-existing cells.

Cells vary enormously in size and shape, which may explain why scientists took so long to recognize their fundamental role in life. The smallest micro-organisms, such as mycoplasmas, are less than one micron ($\mu$m) (less than one-thousandth of a millimeter) in diameter, whereas the ostrich egg has a diameter of several centimeters; skeletal muscle cells are long and thin but red blood cells are biconcave discs; plant cells have rigid thick walls but cells such as the amoeba can change their shape from one moment to the next. Nevertheless, it has been possible to classify living organisms according to the characteristics of the cells of which they are composed and the way in which they are organized.

The first large division is into cells such as bacteria which have no well-defined nucleus (prokaryotes) and organisms composed of cells with nuclei and clearly defined chromosomes (eukaryotes). Eukaryotes may be single-celled or multicellular organisms and most can be classified as either animals or plants; an important difference is that most plants are capable of photosynthesis. Single-celled animals (protozoa) include the MALARIA parasite, trypanosomes, and amoebae; single-celled plants include *Euglena* and yeasts. A few organisms are difficult to classify as animals or plants, and there are also organisms

that can exist during different stages of their life cycles either as single-celled or multicellular organisms. Multicellular organisms develop from one cell (a fertilized egg), which differentiates into many different cell types. The number of cells in a multicellular organism varies greatly from one organism to another; the average human comprises roughly 100 million million cells.

The detailed knowledge we have today about the structure and function of cells is largely due to the development of the electron microscope in the 1940s, and the availability of an increasingly wide range of biochemical and tissue culture techniques.

All cells are surrounded by a thin lipid plasma membrane. This is a very selective barrier, allowing some substances to pass across it and excluding others in order to maintain a relatively constant internal environment. Some of the many different types of proteins embedded in the cell membrane play an active part in transporting substances across the membrane, by acting as pumps or catalysts. Some act as receptors, detecting changes in the external environment and initiating appropriate responses from the cell; others provide a mechanism for cells to interact and communicate. In plant cells the cell membrane is surrounded by a cell wall, a thick, protective cellulose-containing structure which forms the rigid skeleton of the plant.

Little detailed structure may be seen in the cells of prokaryotes, but in eukaryotic cells many different subcellular structures ('organelles') have been identified. Just as the different organs of the human body work together to maintain the body, so the different organelles of a cell each have their own characteristic activities but work together to maintain the cell. What remains inside the cell when the organelles have been removed is the gel-like cytoplasm.

**The nucleus**

The largest organelle in a eukaryotic cell is the nucleus, which is surrounded by a double membrane and contains the genetic material, DEOXYRIBONUCLEIC ACID (DNA). Through the information contained in a coded form within its chemical structure, DNA determines the specific morphological and biochemical characteristics of each type of cell and controls its metabolic activities. Although the same GENETIC information is generally present in each cell of an organism, only some of it is used (expressed) in any given type of cell. Genetic information is expressed in the form of proteins, and the specialized functions of different cell types are to a large extent determined by their protein complement. When a cell divides, the DNA carried in chromosomes in its nucleus is copied and passed on to each daughter cell,

Components of a cell.

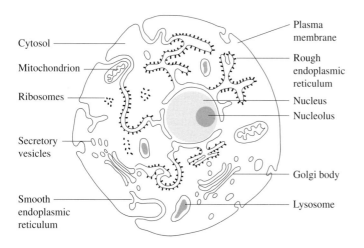

Cytosol

Mitochondrion

Ribosomes

Secretory vesicles

Smooth endoplasmic reticulum

Plasma membrane

Rough endoplasmic reticulum

Nucleus

Nucleolus

Golgi body

Lysosome

thus ensuring that the next generation of cells has all the information needed to function correctly.

Within the nucleus, DNA is combined with histones and other structural proteins to form chromatin, seen under a microscope as a dark, diffuse material. The first visual indication that a cell is about to divide is when the chromatin condenses to form rod-like chromosomes. A constant number of chromosomes is formed in the cells of each species. The somatic cells of humans (that is, not sperm or egg) are described as diploid because they contain two complete sets of chromosomes. There are 23 pairs of chromosomes in each cell, 22 pairs of somatic chromosomes (one of each pair derived from each parent) and one pair of sex chromosomes, either two Xs in the female or an X and Y in the male.

Each nucleus also contains one or more nucleoli. The main function of a nucleolus is to manufacture the precursors of ribosomes. Under the electron microscope ribosomes appear as small, dense particles either free in the cytoplasm or attached to the membranes of the endoplasm (see below). Ribosomes are the sites where protein are synthesized.

The structure of proteins is determined by the 50 000–100 000 or so genes (units of genetic information) contained within the structure of DNA. When a protein is to be synthesized, the information in the corresponding gene is copied into a molecule of messenger RNA (mRNA), which then moves into the cytoplasm, where it associates with ribosomes. Amino acids, the building blocks of proteins, are lined up on the RNA in the correct order and joined together to form the protein. Each amino acid reaches the site of protein synthesis attached to a molecule of transfer RNA (tRNA), which acts like an adapter, ensuring that the sequence of amino acids in the protein is that specified by the genetic instructions passed on from DNA to RNA.

The endoplasm is an intricate system of membranes that spreads throughout the cytoplasm. Part of it is studded with ribosomes and is called rough endoplasm because of its appearance under the electron microscope. Proteins synthesized on these ribosomes move to the smooth endoplasm (areas without ribosomes), the apparatus, and then the cell membrane for secretion. On the way the proteins often have carbohydrates added, turning them into glycoproteins.

The Golgi apparatus consists of a stack of curved, flattened sacs surrounded by many interconnecting tubules and vesicles. Proteins reach one side of the apparatus inside vesicles, which bud off from the surface of the endoplasmic reticulum. Similarly, vesicles bud off from the other side of the Golgi apparatus to carry the proteins to the cell membrane, where the vesicles and membrane fuse and the proteins are secreted into the extracellular fluid.

Running through the cytoplasm is the cytoskeleton, an intricate network of solid fibers and hollow tubes. The cytoskeleton does the same job for the cell as scaffolding on a building site; it determines the basic shape of the cell and provides a framework that allows materials to be moved from one place to another. Unlike the poles and girders of scaffolding, however, the three main components of the cytoskeleton — microtubules, actin filaments, and intermediate filaments — are not permanent static structures. They are themselves assembled from subunits and can be taken apart rapidly and then reassembled in a different way as part of the processes of providing cells with shape and form, moving cells, or moving and organizing things within cells. Microtubules occur as single tubules or as precisely arranged groups of tubules in structures such as cilia (used for moving material past the cell surface), flagella (used for cell locomotion), and the mitotic spindle formed during cell division.

## Organelles

Cells generate energy by oxidizing fuel molecules derived from the diet. Mitochondria (the 'power stations' of the cell) are the main sites of oxidation. Each mitochondrion is a sausage-shaped organelle surrounded by a double membrane, and most of the activities concerned with the energy metabolism of the cell and the synthesis of adenosine triphosphate (ATP) occur on the highly folded inner membrane or in the region within it. Plant cells, but not animal cells, also have chlorophyll-containing organelles called chloroplasts, which can capture light energy and perform the basic reactions of photosynthesis.

Lysosomes are a collection of small vesicles which form the cell's digestive system. The enzymes inside them can degrade any material which the cell needs to digest — whether derived from the cell itself or from its surroundings. In the process of phagocytosis, particulate material is taken into the cell in vacuoles formed by invagination of the cell membrane. The vacuoles fuse with the lysosomes, exposing their contents to the digestive enzymes. The process of pinocytosis, in which fluid is engulfed, is essentially similar.

Another organelle about the same size as the lysosome is the peroxisome. Peroxisomes contain enzymes involved in special oxidation processes, during which peroxides are formed.

The body continually needs to make new cells to grow or to replace cells that have become worn out or lost through the ravages of day-to-day existence. The replacement process occurs in many tissues, but the main sites are those where the cells are in direct contact with the external or internal environment, such as the skin or the lining of the intestine. New cells are formed when existing cells divide, and it is estimated that about 100 000 000 000 ($10^{11}$) cells in the body (about 0.002% of the total) divide each day. During cell division (mitosis) the genetic material in the nucleus, contained within the DNA of the chromosomes, is first duplicated so that identical sets of information are passed onto each of the two daughter cells.

The period between cell divisions is called interphase. The onset of prophase is signaled by the chromatin condensing to form chromosomes. The centromere region of each chromosome then divides, separating the chromosome into two daughter chromatids. During early and late metaphase the membrane of the nucleus is lost and the chromatids attach to the center of a framework of microtubules (the mitotic spindle), which extends across the cell. During anaphase the chromatids move outwards towards the ends of the spindle. Finally, during telophase, they complete their journey, the spindle breaks down, and a nuclear membrane is formed around each new set of chromosomes, which begin to decondense into chromatin. The cytoplasm between the two nuclei then constricts, dividing the parent cell into two.

The daughter cells formed during mitosis have the same total number of chromosomes as the parent cell. In contrast, in meiosis, which occurs during the maturation of the sex cells, the number of chromosomes is halved (as the chromosomes divide once but the cells divide twice) so the gametes — the spermatozoa and ova — are haploid, that is, they have only a single set of chromosomes. During the formation of the gametes, a process of crossing-over (exchange of parts) occurs, ensuring a mixing of the genetic information passed on to the progeny.

The different organs of the body contain different types of cells — nerve cells are typical of the brain, leukocytes and erythrocytes of the blood, and so on. All these cells are derived from a single fertilized egg by mitosis, and most contain exactly the same genetic information. Hence the development of differences among cells (cell differentiation) must require a differential use of the genetic information they contain. The mechanism of cell differentiation is not understood, but it is thought that in early development there are some crucial cell divisions, during each of which at least one of the daughter cells becomes different from its parent. Over many cell divisions divergences accumulate and the process of change becomes irreversible. What has become a liver cell can then no longer regress to a common precursor which could redifferentiate as a nerve cell, for example.

In addition to fully differentiated cells, many tissues of the body contain stem cells, precursor cells which are not fully differentiated. These may divide to produce more stem cells but can also give rise to progeny which can differentiate. Stem cells in the bone marrow, for example, give rise to granulocytes (white blood cells), macrophages, and erythrocytes (red blood cells).

## The growth process

If cell division proceeded unchecked, a single cell would rapidly grow into an unacceptably large mass of tissue, one cell becoming two, two becoming four, and so on. In fact, the growth of tissues is carefully and accurately regulated in response to the specific needs of the body.

The formation of new cells, which accounts for growth, depends on the synthesis of DNA, RNA, and proteins. Many of the molecular mechanisms regulating growth affect the synthesis of these substances during the different phases of the cell's life cycle. The life cycle of a eukaryotic cell has four consecutive phases, designated $G_1$, S, $G_2$, and M. DNA is synthesized during the S phase, RNA and protein during $G_1$, S, and $G_2$. During the M phase (mitosis), RNA synthesis stops and protein synthesis is reduced. Cell division takes place after each full cycle is complete.

Cell growth and differentiation are regulated by growth factors which bind to specific receptors on the cell surface. Chemical signals are generated inside the cell, increasing the production of DNA, RNA, or proteins and leading to an increased rate of mitosis.

## Malignant transformation

If the delicate control of growth breaks down, cells will continue to divide even though there is no need for further cells of that type. Even if the controls in only one cell break down, that cell can multiply to form an unwanted mass of cells (a tumor). The different forms of cancer develop as a result of a series of genetic 'mutations' which increase the rate of growth and independence of cells, and change them from being normal to malignant.

The transformation of normal cells to malignant, cancerous cells may be brought about by mutagenic chemicals, ionizing radiation, or certain viruses. Such transformed cells show several differences from normal ones, with the overall characteristic of growing continuously and chaotically without regard for their neighbors. The abnormal characteristics of transformed cells are passed on to succeeding generations of cells.

Tumor cells synthesize and release large amounts of growth-stimulating factors. Some of these can make normal cells malignant; others stimulate the growth of the cells that produced them, which may be important in establishing and maintaining their malignancy.

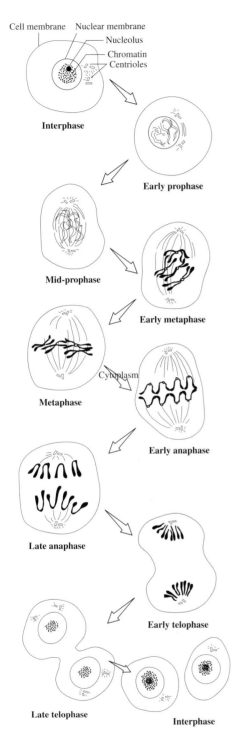

Cell membrane  Nuclear membrane
Nucleolus
Chromatin
Centrioles

**Interphase**

**Early prophase**

**Mid-prophase**

**Early metaphase**

Cytoplasm

**Metaphase**

**Early anaphase**

**Late anaphase**

**Early telophase**

**Late telophase**

**Interphase**

The stages of cell division.

The cancer-forming viruses transform cells by adding cancer-causing genes (oncogenes) to the DNA of the infected cells, or by causing oncogenes that are already present but latent to become active. The oncogenes act by producing proteins that enhance cell proliferation and growth.    LE, WB

*See also* GENETICS, HUMAN

**CHANGING PATTERNS OF DISEASE IN THE 20TH CENTURY** In Britain and other industrial nations at the end of the 20th century, more people than ever survive to old age, and most lead healthier lives than they did at the beginning of the century. Diseases once prevalent and deadly have become uncommon or rare, or even disappeared; but new causes of disability and premature death have emerged. There were greater changes in the incidence, prevalence, severity, and mortality of many diseases and disabilities in the 20th century than in any previous century.

Accounting for these changes were the ascendency of the motor car and labor-saving machinery; increasing affluence; urbanization and suburbanization; changing roles of women; cigarette smoking; expanding technologies, notably new communications media (radio, the cinema, TV) that have helped to transform education and understanding but have also contributed to a sedentary way of life — and raised levels of anxiety — which has had other consequences for health and well-being. Human values have also changed profoundly, notably in relation to sexual behavior. These social and cultural changes have altered the ecology of many diseases, whether caused by infectious pathogens or by other factors such as those we loosely call 'life-style' or 'stress'.

One obvious ecological change is the huge increase of motorized transport. In the late 1990s, traffic injury killed over three quarters of a million people in the world every year and caused permanent disability, much of it due to brain damage, to perhaps 500 000 people every year, many of them adolescents or young adults. The toll of traffic-related premature death and injury is rising rapidly in the industrializing nations of the developing world.

Advances in medical science, leading to understanding of the causes and control of infectious and other diseases, progress in methods of diagnosis and treatment of disease and injury, and above all routine immunization of children against many diseases have played an important part. Since the end of the 19th century infant and child mortality have fallen dramatically. The fall in maternal mortality has been even more dramatic. Having remained at a high level of between 400 and 500 (direct) maternal deaths per 100 000 births from the 19th century up to the mid-1930s,

157

# CESAREAN SECTION

Cesarean section involves incising the abdominal wall and uterus to deliver the baby, at any time during the last three months of pregnancy. A similar but earlier operation to terminate pregnancy before the fetus can survive is called hysterotomy.

Ancient writings in Europe, Egypt, India, and China refer to abdominal delivery, usually (but not always) after the mother's death. In mythology, ASCLEPIUS (p 709) was delivered in this way by his father, APOLLO (p 359), and in Shakespeare's *Macbeth*, Macduff was 'from his mother's womb untimely ripped'. The name was thought to be derived from the birth of Julius Caesar, but this seems unlikely because his mother lived to hear of his invasion of Britain. A more probable derivation is from *caedere* to cut. The Roman law *Lex Caesare* stated that a woman who died in advanced pregnancy should be delivered soon after her death, and if the baby died they should be buried separately.

The first cesarean section of modern times is attributed to a Swiss sow-gelder, Jacob Nufer, who in 1500 gained permission from the local authorities to operate on his wife after she had been in labor for several days. The baby lived for 77 years and the mother subsequently had five successful vaginal deliveries including twins, which leads some to doubt the authenticity of the story.

The operation remained controversial, with a high risk of maternal death. The first cesarean section with survival of the mother was performed in Ireland by a midwife, Mary Donally, in 1738; in England by Dr James Barrow in 1793; and in the USA by Dr John Richmond in 1827. The 'first' in the British Empire was performed in South Africa some time before 1821 by James Miranda BARRY (this page), an Edinburgh graduate who masqueraded successfully as a man from 1809 until her death in 1865. (A grandson of the child she delivered, James Barry Munnik Hertzog, became prime minister of South Africa.) In fact, cesarean sections had been performed in Africa by indigenous healers for many years.

In the 19th century ANESTHESIA was introduced but death rates remained high. To try to reduce infection, cesarean section was combined with hysterectomy but in the 1880s a conservative operation with suturing of the uterus was developed, using antisepsis. In the 1920s the 'classical' operation — a vertical incision in the upper part of the uterus — was replaced by the 'lower segment' operation, which involves a transverse incision low in the uterus behind the bladder and carries less risk of subsequent rupture.

Today 'elective' cesarean section, performed before labor begins, may be for breech presentation, low-lying placenta, or (most commonly) a previous cesarean section — though vaginal delivery is usually possible in a subsequent pregnancy, unless the cesarean section has been for a contracted pelvis. 'Emergency' cesarean section is performed when a complication arises during labor, the most common being slow progress or fetal distress (signs of lack of oxygen in the baby).

Possible complications include infection, which is reduced if antibiotics are given routinely, and venous thrombosis, which is reduced by giving anticoagulants to women at risk. Anesthesia nowadays is safe, most operations being performed under epidural anesthesia. In Britain from 1994 to 1996 over 250 000 cesarean sections were carried out with only one death resulting from anesthesia.

The cesarean section rate is steadily rising in many countries. In Britain it rose from less than 3% in the 1950s to 16% in 1995. In some places, for example, Rio de Janeiro, it is around 90% and some people fear that this is the future for other countries as well. In the USA, however, it reached a peak in the 1980s at around 40% (at least among private patients) before falling to around 25%. Many obstetricians expect the rate in Britain to plateau around 20%, with cesarean section replacing difficult vaginal delivery but not easy labor.

Current debates center on a woman's right to choose her mode of delivery. British courts have ruled that she cannot be compelled to undergo cesarean section in the baby's interests, and some obstetricians believe she has the right to cesarean section on demand. Usually, however, the decision is agreed after discussion among all concerned — the woman, her partner, her midwife, and her doctors.   GC

James Miranda Stewart **BARRY** (1795–1865). Barry masqueraded as a man for her entire adult life. A British Army medical officer, she was appointed Inspector-General of Hospitals for both Upper and Lower Canada in 1857. Barry was thus the first woman to practice medicine in Canada, and carried out the first cesarean section in the British Empire.

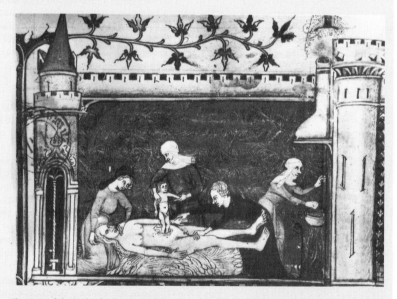

The story of the birth of Julius Caesar by cesarean section (c. 14th century). From Laignel-Lavastin, M. P .M. (1938). *Histoire générale de la médicine*, Michel, A. Paris. (Reproduced courtesy of the Wellcome Institute Library, London.)

it has fallen at almost the same rate every year for the last sixty years to between 6 and 8 (direct and indirect) maternal deaths per 100 000: a reduction by a factor of at least fifty.

At the beginning of the last century, medical care consisted mainly of dealing with brief episodes of acute illness. Chronic disease with age-adjustment was probably at least as prevalent as it is today. Since only slight and ineffective treatments were available, much chronic disease was accepted as part of life and seldom reported to doctors. Since 1900, however, emphasis has switched from acute to chronic disease, which has had effects not expected even fifty years ago, let alone a hundred. For instance, episodes of acute diseases so typical of medical care in the first half of the 20th century, were inexpensive to treat, and short lasting. The management of long-term disease, however, which dominates medical practice at the beginning of the 21st century, involves frequent consultations and is therefore highly demanding in terms of staff and time, and the techniques are often very expensive. In short, medicine gets better at managing chronic disease but requires huge increases in the cost of health services.

## Demographic transition

The demographic transition is another powerful force, especially in relation to chronic disease. The age distribution of the population in most industrial nations has completely changed because of declining birth rates, which have also reduced the average family size from over 7 to less than 4. Less overcrowding reduces the likelihood that infants will be infected by dangerous pathogens. At the same time there is aging of the population, which does not mean that people are living longer, but that higher proportions survive to old age. In Britain the proportion of the population over the age of 75, which was just over 1% in 1901 and 3% in 1951, rose to 7% in 1991. Conversely, as the size of families has decreased, the proportion of the population aged under 25, 52% in 1901, fell to 35% in 1951 and 33% in 1991. It is interesting that the greatest change in the proportion of young people occurred in the first half of the 20th century, and of old people in the second half. Even greater changes in the proportions of young and old have occurred in countries that are further along in the demographic transition; old people suffer and die of quite different diseases from those that afflict infants, children, and young adults.

The two most prominent epidemics of the middle third of the 20th century were coronary heart disease and lung cancer. Many causal and other associated factors of coronary heart disease have been identified, some unequivocally linked to aspects of personal behavior. Cigarette smoking, a diet rich in fats and animal protein, and lack of physical exercise are the most important, all of them identified as aspects of life-style. Recently it has been observed that there is an association between maternal nutrition, birthweight, and the risk of high blood pressure and coronary heart disease among the offspring, especially the males, in middle age. Put simply, a baby which fails to thrive properly in the uterus and is born too small will, even though it 'catches up' in weight and size during early childhood, be more likely to suffer from high blood pressure and coronary heart disease in middle age than babies whose intrauterine life and neonatal period were normal. Much remains to be learnt before this intriguing observation is fully understood, but it suggests that the seeds of disease in middle age can be sown at the very beginning of life.

The epidemic of coronary heart disease began to recede after the 1960s, whether because of altered behavior that followed publicity about presumed causes or for other reasons. By the early 1990s, coronary heart disease incidence and death rates had fallen by over 40% from their peak in the late 1950s and early 1960s in the rich industrial nations, but the epidemic has rapidly gathered momentum in Eastern Europe, the former Soviet Union, and the industrializing nations of Asia.

Cigarette smoking became popular early in the 20th century, and socially acceptable, first among adolescent boys and young men at the time of the Great War (1914–18), then about thirty years later, among girls and young women. Tobacco contains several poisons, and several strong carcinogens. Muller showed the link between cigarettes and cancer in 1939, but it was overlooked in the turmoil of the Second World War. In 1950 Doll and HILL (p 381) in Britain, and Wynder and GRAHAM (p 762) in the USA, published the first of what soon became a torrent of articles that unequivocally revealed cigarette smoking to be the main cause of lung cancer. Later studies have shown that smoking is linked with many cancers, as well as significantly increasing the risk of chronic respiratory and cardiovascular disease, especially coronary heart disease. Attitudes towards smoking as a socially acceptable, even desirable custom, have changed remarkably in the second half of the 20th century. Smoking is no longer socially admired (or even acceptable) in many places. Consequently, lung cancer is beginning to recede as a cause of death among men, though the epidemic is still rising among women, who adopted smoking more recently. The rates therefore will continue to increase for another 25–30 years at least among women.

Another 'lifestyle' factor causing increasing concern is obesity among both adults and children. It seems to be linked to low income families, cheap high-calorie convenience foods, lack of exercise, and the tendency to spend hours in front of television while consuming crisps or candy. League tables have been drawn up, some of which suggest that Germany is said to lead (if 'lead' is the right word) Europe in the tables of excessive obesity. But, as any visitor to the United States will attest, the extreme obesity of many American citizens is particularly striking.

### Nosology

Changing patterns of disease and expanding knowledge are reflected in changes in nosology, the science of the classification and nomenclature of disease. There was no generally agreed classification of disease until the International Classification of Diseases (ICD) was introduced in 1891. It listed 161 causes of death in 14 chapters. Since then, the ICD has gone through successive revisions roughly every decade, with the 10th revision (ICD-10) being published in 1993. Over 1000 diseases and disabilities, arranged in 21 chapters, are identified in ICD-10. Many of the changes have occurred through four processes: description of new or unrecognized diseases; differentiation of a disease into several components; rearrangement and integration of diseases under new rubrics (diagnostic labels); elimination of conditions no longer regarded as diseases, discussed below.

So far as new diseases are concerned, the 1996 Report of the WORLD HEALTH ORGANIZATION listed 30 diseases due to infectious agents that had been identified since 1973. Almost all are serious and several are lethal. HIV/AIDS is the best known. Others include: Legionnaire's disease, Lyme disease, Ebola virus, and several other viral hemorrhagic fevers; several leukemia and lymphoma virus diseases; viruses responsible for several distinct types of hepatitis; the agents responsible for several kinds of transmissible spongiform encephalopathies, including KURU, CREUTZFELDT-JAKOB DISEASE, and 'mad-cow disease'; hantaan virus (causing a lethal hemorrhagic fever); and *Helicobacter pylori*, which causes peptic ulcer disease and possibly some varieties of stomach cancer. Some of these may indeed be new diseases due to micro-organisms that have mutated into forms that can infect humans; others are newly identified infectious agents. Other 'new' diseases are possibly due to environmental factors such as ionizing or non-ionizing radiation, or to ergonomic stressors that have arisen since many of us began to use keyboards and computer screens instead of pen and paper to do our clerical work.

*Splitting, lumping, and bogus diseases* These are three ways in which nosology can change. The process epidemiologists call splitting may be illus-trated by viral hepatitis. This was called catarrhal jaundice in the early 20th century. Epidemics in the 1930s suggested an infectious, presumably viral, origin. Later studies led to differentiation of viral hepatitis into two types: one spread by the fecal–oral route, the other by contaminated blood or serum. Recent studies have differentiated hepatitis C, D, E, F, and perhaps G; some are spread by the fecal–oral route, others by contaminated blood or other body fluids. This is just one example of how, with increasing knowledge, one disease can become many.

The opposite occurs when a rearrangement and integration — a process epidemiologists call lumping — takes place and diseases thought to be distinct entities are found to have the same underlying cause. The best known example is TUBERCULOSIS. Before Robert KOCH (p 455) discovered the tubercle bacillus, phthisis, 'galloping' consumption, scrofula, suppurating lymph nodes, Pott's disease (collapsed spinal vertebrae), and several other conditions were regarded as quite different diseases; however, all are due to Koch's bacillus.

The third way consists of the elimination of diseases, when rigorous scientific investigation allied to healthy skepticism leads to the recognition that what were thought to be diseases are in fact normal healthy variations, and false theories about causes (and treatment) are rejected. This happened in the 20th century to 'focal sepsis' — the theory that infected teeth, tonsils, or the large bowel were the seat of chronic infection, and were treated accordingly by surgeons, who often became richer, though their patients did not. Retroversion of the uterus, a normal variation, was thought to cause dysmenorrhea, backache, infertility, and pain on sexual intercourse, and there are many other examples.

The accompanying graph shows some of the changes in mortality due to different International Classification of Disease (ICD) categories between 1911 and 1991. It shows that deaths from infectious disease declined very steeply during the 20th century, and there was a slighter decline in deaths from respiratory diseases. Deaths from circulatory diseases (diseases of the heart and blood vessels) and deaths from neoplasms (cancer), on the other hand, increased greatly. Interestingly, deaths from 'injuries and poisoning' did not, as one might have expected from the huge rise in the number of motor cars, increase significantly. Such deaths accounted for 3.9% of all deaths in 1911, rose to 4.4% in 1931, and fell to the lowest level of 3.0% in 1991. Each of the many other ICD categories accounted, individually, for less than 5% of deaths throughout 1911–91, and are not included in the graph. The most striking feature of the change illustrated by the graph is this: in 1911 25% of deaths were due to

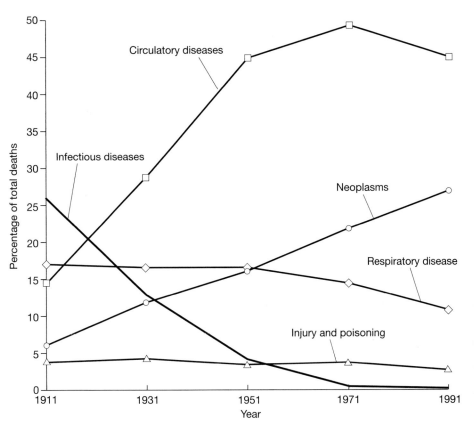

Changes in certain selected ICD categories shown as a percentage of deaths from all causes in England and Wales in 1911, 1931, 1951, 1971, and 1991. (Source: Charlton, J. and Murphy, M. (1997). *The health of adult Britain 1841–1994*, decennial supplement no. 12, HMSO, London.)

infectious disease and 17% to cancer and heart disease combined (neoplasms and circulatory disease). In 1994, however, deaths due to heart disease and cancer had risen to 70% of the total, whereas deaths due to infectious diseases had sunk to 0.6%.                                    IL

*See also* CARDIOTHORACIC SURGERY – HISTORY; DEMOGRAPHY; SMOKING AND HEALTH

**CHARITÉ HOSPITAL, BERLIN** See GERMANY, AUSTRIA, AND SWITZERLAND

**CHARITIES** A charity is a benevolent organization that provides aid or services to those in need. The distinction between a charity and a FOUNDATION is that a foundation has endowments and investments which provide all or most of its income and operating expenses, whereas a charity relies for its financial support mainly on voluntary contributions and donations by the general public to provide the funds for its operating expenses. Some charities generate enough funds to invest and provide an income, but care must be taken to avoid violating taxation law. Most charities rely entirely on donations, sometimes augmented by bequests. A few charities receive direct support from govern-

ment revenues (the number varies, as does the level of support).

To qualify for tax concessions, both for their donors and for the charity, charities in most countries must comply with certain rules. For example, in Britain, a charity must provide something of recognized value to society without benefiting individuals in a way that outweighs its social value. It must not harm anyone. Its aims must be clearly stated. It must be run by an identifiable body of people, who are accountable for its management and control. It must be independent. It must be able to show that any private benefit (such as investment income) is incidental to and a necessary and desirable part of carrying out its charitable aims. It must not pursue partisan political aims.

Many charities support medical or health-related causes. Most have well-defined missions and goals. These include support for medical research; direct service for the victims of specific conditions that are within the mandate or terms of reference of the charity in question; provision of aids of many kinds, such as wheelchairs and prosthetic devices for the handicapped and disabled, or oxygen for sufferers from chronic lung diseases. Some charities, such as Oxfam and Save the Children Fund, focus on the medical and public health problems of people in the poorest countries in the world. At the opposite extreme, some are devoted entirely to support for one aspect of work in a single hospital, for example, the palliative care of cancer patients.

Most of the well-known medical charities target a specific disease or group of conditions such as cancer, lung diseases, heart disease and stroke, arthritis, or multiple sclerosis. Several charities have outlived the diseases for which they were set up. In the first half of the 20th century, prominent charities in Britain, USA, Canada, Australia, and most western European nations were devoted to the care and prevention of TUBERCULOSIS. In the late 1950s this disease began to recede as a cause of premature death and long-term disability; whereupon anti-tuberculosis charities shifted their aims to all chronic disabling diseases of the lungs and respiratory system. The March of Dimes in the USA and its counterparts in other countries raised large amounts of money entirely by voluntary donations, much of it collected in door-to-door campaigns, exclusively to treat and carry out research on the cause and prevention of infantile paralysis (POLIOMYELITIS). This disease had tremendous emotional impact, especially when the president of the United States, Franklin D. Roosevelt, was afflicted. Money from the March of Dimes contributed to support for the research of Jonas SALK (p 664) that led to the development of the first effective vaccine. When the Salk and SABIN (p 664) vaccines led to the virtual disappearance of polio, the March of Dimes could have dissolved itself. Instead, it shifted focus and began to devote its considerable resources to the treatment and research on the prevention of birth defects.

Charities both within and beyond health often compete for support from the same limited pool of voluntary donors to charitable causes. In North America at the beginning of the 21st century, middle-class professional households receive hundreds of begging letters every year; most of these solicit support for charities in medicine and health. Some charities, for example, the Salvation Army, raise at least part of their funds through street collections; one health charity that relies on street solicitation is the Cystic Fibrosis Foundation. Some conduct campaigns by radio or television, and many hold raffles or engage in legalized forms of gambling, with the profits going to the charity in question.                                   JML

**CHEMICAL WARFARE** See BIOLOGICAL AND CHEMICAL WARFARE

**CHEMOTHERAPY** See HEMATOLOGY; ONCOLOGY

**CHEST MEDICINE** Chest medicine, or respirology or pulmonology, as it is known in North America, owes its origin to the treatment of TUBERCULOSIS. With the decline in the incidence and prevalence of tuberculosis, phthisiologists extended their interest to other chest diseases. The advances in understanding pulmonary and cardiac physiology which made possible modern day thoracic and cardiac surgery also stimulated interest in respiratory diseases.

The contemporary chest physician is called on to diagnose and treat many lung and pleural infections; malignant and benign tumors of the lungs; conditions such as emphysema and bronchitis that are induced by cigarette smoking; various fibrotic lung conditions of unknown cause; and occupational and environmental diseases such as asbestosis and silicosis. There are also various conditions related to immunological disorders, and sleep apnea (a condition which is usually associated with obesity), cigarette smoking, and anatomical abnormalities of the nasal and oral air passages.

The prime purpose of the lungs is to maintain the oxygen and carbon dioxide content of the arterial blood within a limited range. This has to be effected despite the fact that oxygen needs and carbon dioxide production are changing constantly with the person's activity and metabolic demands. The lungs fulfill this function by allowing venous blood, from which oxygen has been removed, to come into contact with the inspired air. Such contact takes place over an enormous area, usually referred to as the alveolo-capillary surface. Three essential physiological functions are concerned: (i) ventilation, or the bellows function, moving air in and out of the lungs; (ii) gas transfer or diffusion, the transfer of gas from the alveolus to the capillary (small blood vessels) and vice versa; and (iii) perfusion or blood flow, in which the blood containing oxygen or carbon dioxide is transferred to and from the lungs.

### Infections
*Tuberculosis and related infections* Tuberculosis has been recognized for centuries. HIPPOCRATES (p 382) described a wasting disease known as 'phthisis', which was later referred to as 'the white plague'. He also noted that there was a familial incidence, but the mode of spread was not shown until JA VILLEMIN (p 830) showed in 1865 that it could be transmitted from animal to animal and suggested that the same situation might apply to humans. The tubercle bacillus was isolated by Robert KOCH (p 455) in 1882 and shortly thereafter he isolated an extract from dead bacilli which came to be known as tuberculin. It was subsequently shown that tuberculin could be injected into the skin and if the person had been

# CHERNOBYL

The purpose of the radioactivity in a nuclear power station is to heat water. As in coal-fired power stations, the steam that results drives turbines, which produce electricity. On 20 April 1986, there was a serious accident in the nuclear power station 10 miles from the city of Chernobyl, in the Ukraine, then part of the Soviet Union. Owing to failure to observe safety regulations — and to poor reactor design — the chain reaction in the radioactive core of one of the four reactors was insufficiently controlled. As a result, pressure rose to dangerous levels and there were several steam (not nuclear) explosions and fires that took several hours to put out. But for these fires, immediate evacuation of the reactor site might have been possible and there would then have been few, if any, radiation deaths. Meanwhile, large amounts of radioactive material escaped and were scattered over a wide area and into the atmosphere — later descending in very dilute form as fallout all over the world.

At the reactor, there were two instant deaths from the force of the explosion and 29 later ones from radiation effects — mostly fire fighters who were very close to the escaping radiation for an hour or more. In addition, about 150 others at the reactor site suffered major or minor radiation effects. Contrary to many grossly misleading media reports, there were no deaths or injuries (or any detectable radiation effects) among the 50 000 people living near the power station.

At first it was felt (very reasonably) that the radiation levels to which the local population were exposed were not high enough to justify the disruption and hardship of mass evacuation. But then it was feared that there might be further releases of radioactivity and in view of this — and because of strong public fears — over 100 000 people were finally evacuated and rehoused outside a 30 km exclusion zone. This does not mean that it was actually dangerous (in the sense that most people use the word) to be inside this zone. The three undamaged reactors on the site continued to produce electricity normally and the risk to the workers concerned was very small. In addition, some time later the sensible decision was taken to allow old people to return to their homes in the evacuated zone.

## Radiation effects

In an accident of this kind those very close to the escaping radiation for any appreciable length of time may be in great danger, owing mainly to radiation burns, damage to the lining of the intestines, and impairment of the ability of the bone marrow to maintain a normal supply of blood cells. The precise risk depends on the amount (more correctly, the concentration) of the radiation, the time exposed, and other factors (including the various radioactive substances involved) — all needing expert assessment. Only a short distance away (even just a few hundred meters) the now much less concentrated radiation probably carries for each individual little or no risk of any immediate harm, but each exposed person is slightly more likely to get some kind of cancer in later life than would have been the case had there been no accident.

This cancer risk, which should be neither exaggerated nor minimized, may be put into perspective by comparing it with the risk of smoking cigarettes, both risks having been well studied for many years. The cancer risk from prolonged dilute radiation is considerably less than that of even very modest smoking. Unlike the effect of cigarette smoking, the worst possible effects of the Chernobyl accident will be too small to have any detectable effect on national or international cancer mortality statistics. And the sort of cancers made more common by radiation are

*(continued overleaf)*

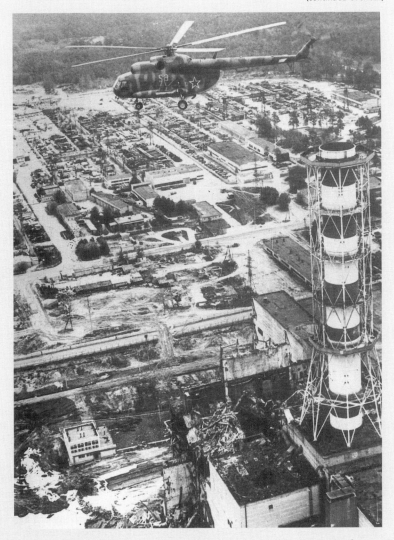

Aerial view of the Chernobyl nuclear power station in the Ukraine taken in May 1986, during the early stages of making the reactor safe. The helicopter is taking radioactivity measurements.
(Reproduced courtesy of Novosti/Science Photo Library.)

(continued)

generally less serious than those caused by smoking.

However, one disturbing effect of the Chernobyl accident did not come to light until several years after the accident. Many children in regions of maximum fallout, especially those in the first year of life at the time of exposure, have since developed cancer of the thyroid gland. This is virtually the only part of the body that needs to concentrate iodine for its proper function and undoubtedly radioactive iodine in the fallout was responsible. Little of this was seen after the nuclear bombing of Japan in 1945. And for many years much higher concentrations of radioactive iodine have been used in treating overactive thyroid glands in adults, without any increase in the incidence of thyroid cancer. So this was quite unexpected, but fortunately thyroid cancer in children is much less aggressive than most other cancers, and so far very few of these children have died.

Another well-known and much feared risk of exposure to radiation is an increase in birth defects. This may occur in two ways. First, there is a theoretical risk due to genetic damage in the testicles of future fathers or in the ovaries of future mothers, but, contrary to widespread belief, this has not been seen as a result of the nuclear bombs dropped on Japan in 1945 or of the Chernobyl accident. A second and separate cause of birth defects is radiation of the unborn child in early pregnancy. This occurred in Japan, but not at all in the Chernobyl region, presumably because of the lower exposure. Media stories and photographs of children in the area with birth defects are irresponsible, since some such cases have always been present in all communities all over the world. No increase has been seen as a result of the accident. As to leukemia, once again, unlike Japan, there has been no increase due to the Chernobyl accident.

As regards the general health of those living near the reactor at the time, not surprisingly many feel that their health has been affected. The fear of any radiation, however dilute, is so strong in communities all over the world — and has been made so much worse by misleading stories in the media — that this was inevitable. But general health comparisons with other communities have not shown any difference.

What can be done to minimize possible harm to exposed populations from such an accident, whether involving a nuclear reactor or a nuclear weapon? The exposure is of three main types: from skin contact, breathing, and eating or drinking. If there is any radioactive material in the air those who don't need to be out of doors can reduce what is probably only a small risk still further by staying indoors as much as possible in the first few days. And if there is radioactive iodine in the fallout, iodine tablets taken as soon as possible will ensure that the thyroid gland will have so much normal iodine that it will not need to absorb the radioactive iodine — which is quickly excreted in the urine. With babies and small children it will then be important in subsequent weeks to avoid any food or drink likely to contain even very small amounts of the radioactive iodine from the fallout.

The effects of mass relocation of populations (to protect them from small risks) and of excessive fear have caused enormous distress and hardship. In such an accident, it is not easy to balance all the conflicting fears and risks. Even in much less serious accidents, such as the Three Mile Island accident in the USA in 1979 — where the amount of escaping radiation exposed local people to less radiation than from the average medical X-ray — there was intense public anxiety. TBB

*See also* DISASTERS; X-RAYS

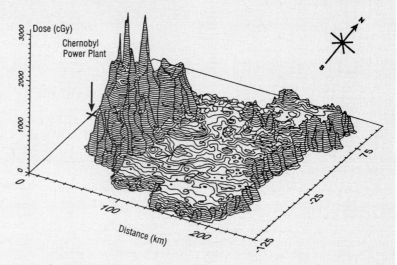

Average distribution of thyroid doses in children born in 1986, Chernlgovskaya region, Ukraine.
(Reproduced with permission from World Health Statistics Quarterly (1996), **49**.)

exposed to tubercle bacilli and these had 'settled' in the body, the skin would respond by producing a red wheal. Tuberculosis is spread mainly by infected people coughing, expelling small droplets containing tubercle bacilli into the air. The moisture evaporates and the bacillus remains in the air. If inhaled it will settle in the lungs.

Before chemotherapy, which became available in the late 1940s and early 1950s, thousands of people were treated for tuberculosis in SANITARIUMS. Over half of these patients were dead within five years, either because of, or despite, the treatment. The latter consisted of bed rest, preferably in cold mountain air, and sundry mutilating operations; the treatment and its bodily and psychological effects are well described in Thomas Mann's *The magic mountain*, or A. E. Ellis's *The rack*. With chemotherapy, patients ceased to be infectious, and it eliminated the need for deforming surgery. Many physicians felt that tuberculosis would disappear rapidly from the world, a viewpoint that subsequently proved optimistic.

The decline of tuberculosis in most western countries was rapid and impressive, but there has been a recent resurgence because of diseases or medications that suppress immune responses. Particularly important are AIDS, the overuse of steroids and other immunosuppressives, and wasting caused by starvation. The inappropriate use of antituberculosis medications, especially in developing countries, has led to the emergence of tubercle bacilli resistant to the standard drugs used.

A recent finding is that some organisms (atypical mycobacteria) look like tubercle bacilli under the microscope, but cause lung disease less frequently. When they do, however, the disease is often more difficult to treat since they may be partially or totally resistant to standard drugs. Moreover, the means or mode of infection differs from that of tubercle bacilli.

*Pyogenic bacterial infections* Numerous bacteria may cause lung infections, ranging from pneumonia to lung abscess. Over the past twenty to thirty years, through the injudicious use of antibiotics, many of the more easily treated infections such as pneumococcal pneumonia (caused by *Streptococcus pneumoniae*) have occurred less frequently but have been replaced by infections with other organisms. Many pyogenic (pus forming) bacteria which used to be suppressed by the commonly used antibiotics such as penicillin, tetracycline, and erythromycin, no longer respond to them. Fortunately the latter have been replaced by new antibiotics (such as the macrolides and fluoroquinolones) but resistance will surely develop unless these newer agents are used with care.

The organism causing most cases of pneumonia — *Streptococcus pneumoniae* — has in certain parts of the world such as Spain and Australia developed a significant resistance to penicillin and the synthetic related drugs. This has arisen as a result of their inappropriate administration to people who did not need them.

*Fungal infections* In North and South America and also in Africa various fungi cause pneumonias. Some of the more common infections include histoplasmosis, blastomycosis, and coccidiodomycosis. The agents responsible for these conditions are seldom found in Europe, but several other fungi, which are much less common, tend to cause lung infections in people whose immune systems are functioning inadequately. This is particularly true of people with AIDS, or who have been taking corticosteroids (cortisone and its derivatives), or chemotherapeutic agents, for malignant disease and those who are malnourished. One common complication of AIDS is a protozoal pneumonia caused by *Pneumocystis carinii*.

### Lung cancer and other malignancies

As tuberculosis has declined, lung cancer has increased, with a counterbalanced increase in the number of deaths. Cigarette smoking causes 95% of lung cancers, either by itself or aided and abetted by other cancer causing agents such as radon daughters (found in uranium mines), asbestos, nickel, arsenic, and other less common agents. Whether passive smoking can cause lung cancer, however, remains uncertain.

While the death rate for lung cancer has decreased in men in the USA, Britain, and some other European countries, that for women has gone up. More women and teenage girls have taken up cigarette smoking and because of the long incubation time the death rate will probably continue to increase for twenty or more years. Cigarette smoking is also associated with an increase in cancer of the larynx, bladder, and kidney.

Surgery is possible in only about 20 to 30% of people with lung cancer, and of them only 20–25% survive for five years. Thus the overall cure rate is around 7–10% of those who develop lung cancer. Chemotherapy as a curative or adjuvant has proved to be much more useful than expected and induces some long remissions.

While giving up cigarette smoking is of benefit and lessens the likelihood of developing cancer, and in addition slows down the rate of decline of lung function in emphysema, a significant risk of lung cancer persists. Thus, while the risk becomes substantially lower after 10 years (with the risk being half that of current smokers), even after 15 to 20 years, the risk persists at about one-tenth of that of a current smoker.

Other malignant tumors of the lung are uncommon and are mostly not related to smoking. Chest physicians have recently seen more of a formerly rare tumor of the pleura known as mesothelioma. Some 80–85% of these result from exposure to asbestos, and in particular to two types known as crocidolite and amosite. The latter are no longer used commercially, but it is likely that mesothelioma will remain a problem for the next one or two decades because the delay between first exposure until the development of the tumor is inordinately long — anything from 25 to 45 years.

### Diseases of the airways

During breathing air is inhaled and first passes through the nose to the nasopharynx and then to the larynx and windpipe (trachea) and its various divisions so that it ultimately reaches the alveoli or distal air spaces where gas exchange occurs. In normal people air is distributed in a uniform fashion to the lungs. The airways contain smooth muscle which can contract and reduce air flow in the conducting airways, that is, the bronchi and bronchioles. Such smooth muscle contraction narrows the airways, which may lead to breathlessness and wheezing. Usually this is precipitated by inflammation in the affected airways, whether induced by viral infections, or numerous other agents. About 5% of ASTHMA is caused by specific agents encountered in the workplace. Bronchial asthma responds to drugs known as beta-agonists, which have an adrenaline-like action

PIONEER CHEST PHYSICIAN

Joseph Leopold
**AUENBRUGGER**
(1722–1809). Austrian physician. He was the son of an inn-keeper and his most noteworthy contribution was to discover the diagnostic value of percussion. Traditionally it was attributed to seeing his father tapping on barrels to determine the levels of wine they contained, but it may be relevant that he was a keen musician and even wrote the libretto for his friend Antonio Salieri's comic opera *Der Rauchfangkehrea (The chimney sweep)*. His book *Inventum novum expercussione thoracis humani ut signo abstrusos interni pectoris morbos detergendi* (1761) made little impact until taken up by Corvisart 50 years later.

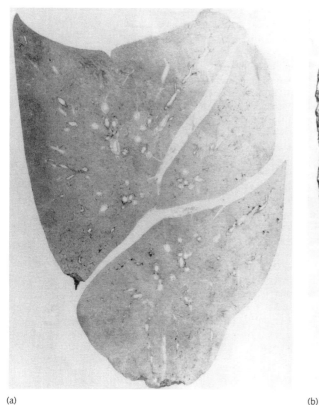

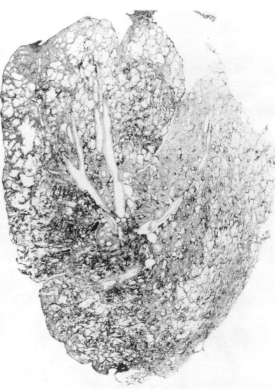

(a)

(b)

(a) Long section of a normal lung; (b) long section of the lung of a person suffering from emphysema.

and widen the bronchi. In many instances the asthmatic attacks recur, and then inhaled steroids are often effective in eliminating or reducing the frequency of asthmatic attacks.

The long continued inhalation of cigarette smoke may lead to several diseases that affect the conducting airways including bronchitis, emphysema, and small airways disease (bronchiolitis).

**Bronchitis** is characterized by cough and sputum in the absence of any destructive lung disease such as tuberculosis or bronchiectasis. Cough and sputum need to be present for at least two months each year for two consecutive years. In bronchitis, the depth and number of the mucous glands found in the walls of the large bronchi (airways) are both increased, and these changes lead to a slight fall in the person's ability to breathe out quickly (the basis of so-called respiratory function tests).

Most people who develop chronic bronchitis do so from cigarette smoking, but the inhalation of dust, or exposure to irritant gases, such as sulfur dioxide, chlorine, and ozone, may also cause it. If such exposure ceases then chronic bronchitis usually regresses within six months.

**Emphysema** is the destruction of the gas exchange surface of the lungs associated with an increase in the amount of air beyond the terminal bronchiole. The terminal bronchiole is the smallest air passage in which no gas exchange occurs.

Emphysema is thought to be due to the presence of various cells in the gas exchanging regions of the lungs (in particular, the respiratory bronchioles). These cells liberate enzymes that dissolve the lung tissue, leading to the formation of dilated spaces and disruption of the alveolar walls. Emphysema is usually associated with airways obstruction and mismatching of ventilation and blood flow from the lungs, thereby reducing the amount of oxygen present in the blood. Stopping smoking has no effect on emphysema and the lung destruction never regresses.

**Small airways disease** Much of the breathlessness and obstruction to airflow associated with smoking is located in the bronchioles — the smaller airways below 0.5 mm in diameter. Cigarette smoking causes an inflammatory response in the bronchioles leading to the development of fibrosis with narrowing and occlusion. Stopping smoking is not associated with improvement in air flow through the small airways.

## Pulmonary fibrosis

This is an excess of scar tissue in the lungs. In one type the fibrotic response is found in nodules throughout the lungs. Examples are the pneumoconioses, such as silicosis and coal workers' pneumoconiosis, and various infections, for example, histoplasmosis. Given that the fibrosis affects a limited area, the alveoli and gas exchanging regions of the lungs are largely spared. The other type, interstitial fibrosis, occurs when the fibrotic agents, for example, asbestos fibers, are deposited in the alveoli and in the respiratory bronchioles. There they induce scar tissue, and if this is extensive enough the lungs become stiff and noncompliant, that is, they do not expand as easily as they should.

Another disease that may result in fibrosis is sarcoidosis, a condition that may affect other organs, including the eyes, kidney, the lymph nodes, the lining layers of the brain and spinal cord, the heart, and the skin.

Early in the disease a good response often results from steroids, but once the lung has become fibrotic these are of little use.

Sarcoidosis most frequently presents in young adults, who develop painful red nodules on the legs (erythema nodosum). On occasion the nodules are accompanied by chest pain. A chest X-ray will usually show enlarged lymph nodes in the area between the two lungs where the great vessels and gullet are located. The presence of erythema nodosum and lymph node enlargement is usually known as Loffgren's syndrome, after the Swedish physician who first described it. Fortunately, Loffgren's syndrome usually disappears without treatment within the year. In other instances, however, sarcoidosis develops in the lungs and spares the mediastinal lymph nodes. Only around half of patients so affected respond to treatment and many are left with reduced lung function. The cause of the disease is unknown.

## Occupational lung diseases

Various diseases may result from occupational exposures. These include the pneumoconioses, such as silicosis, coal workers' pneumoconiosis, asbestosis, and the talcosis and kaolin pneumoconiosis. Pneumoconiosis is defined as the deposition of a mineral dust in the lungs and the tissues' reaction to it. Most pneumoconioses are diagnosed by obtaining a history of exposure and by specific changes in the chest X-ray or on lung function testing.

Other occupational diseases of the lungs include occupational asthma, which may be caused by many agents, ranging from antibiotics and latex, to rat and hamster urine. In the former, those workers manufacturing the antibiotics or using the latex gloves are at risk. It is essential to demonstrate specific sensitization to the agent concerned before a diagnosis of occupational asthma. Pre-existing asthma that becomes worse in a dusty environment or because of irritant odors is not occupational asthma.

A group of inflammatory diseases known as the extrinsic allergic alveolitides is also often related to work exposure. This group of conditions includes farmers' lung, caused by fungal spores found in moist hay. Should the hay be forked or disturbed with the spores allowed to enter the surrounding air, the person may well develop it, especially if he inhales deeply. Four to eight hours later he becomes breathless and develops a fever and an abnormal chest X-ray. Similar extrinsic alveolitides may be caused by other agents, and occur in other groups of workers — those in Scotch whisky distilleries, indoor mushroom growers, sugar cane workers (bagassosis), and pigeon breeders. With a better understanding of occupational lung diseases and more effective industrial hygiene, most of these are becoming less common in North America, Europe, and Australasia, but still occur in the developing countries.

## Collagen vascular diseases

Rheumatoid arthritis and other 'collagen vascular' diseases are often accompanied by chest manifestations. People with rheumatoid arthritis may develop pleurisy with fluid in one of the pleural cavities which surround the lungs. This may be accompanied by inflammation of the outer lining of the heart (pericardium). Small to moderate sized nodules may appear in the lungs. Scleroderma, a condition in which the skin becomes firm and immobile, is often accompanied by similar changes in the gullet or esophagus and by obliteration of the small blood vessels in the lungs.

## Pulmonary embolism

The word embolism was originally used to describe an intercalation or insertion of a day or days into the calendar to correct an error. In medical parlance it has come to mean the insertion of a blood clot into a blood vessel.

Those who have recently undergone surgery have a predisposition for the blood in their veins to clot (thrombose). The propensity to clot is a defence mechanism designed to prevent undue loss of blood. On occasion it oversteps the mark and the blood becomes ultra-'clottable'. Other predisposing factors for venous thrombosis are slowed circulation, such as occurs in heart failure, severe malnutrition, polycythemia (an excessive number of red cells), and sitting still for many hours, for example, on an intercontinental air flight (economy class syndrome). The veins most likely to be affected are those in the calves, thighs, and pelvis.

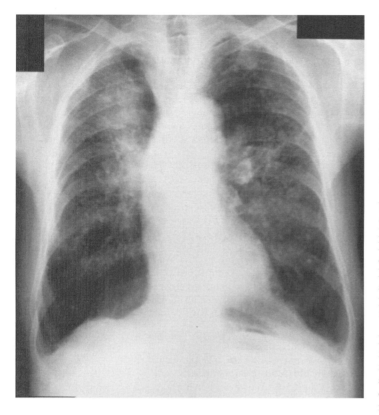

The X-ray of the chest of a man with silicosis. The patient had worked as a driller in a coal mine, setting charges and blasting rock.

the inner aspects of the thoracic cavity, which contains the lungs, heart, and great vessels. The pleura itself is a glistening thin membrane. The small blood vessels (capillaries) supplying the parietal pleura permit fluid to permeate through their walls so that it can enter the pleural cavity. There are always a few milliliters of pleural fluid present in the pleural cavity. This is gradually absorbed by the lymphatics and capillaries underneath the visceral pleura, thereby making its way back into the bloodstream. This leads to homeostasis — the volume of pleural fluid remains relatively constant.

Should the capillaries in the parietal pleura become inflamed or excessively permeable, fluid often accumulates in the pleural cavity since the lymph channels and the capillaries present in the lungs cannot absorb the fluid rapidly enough. The collection of fluid in the pleural cavity is usually known as a pleural effusion. Changes in the pressure of the blood present in the capillaries and parietal pleura will also increase the flow of fluid into the pleural cavity.

Chest injuries such as from car accidents may lead to severe bleeding into the pleural cavity. This is known as hemothorax — a collection of blood in the thoracic cavity. The presence of blood in sufficient quantity in the thoracic cavity requires drainage and the control of bleeding. Pneumonia may also increase the permeability of the capillaries, leading to excess formation of pleural fluid. Bacteria from the lungs in a person who has pneumonia may penetrate the visceral pleura infecting the pleural fluid. The fluid acts as a culture medium in which bacteria flourish, and the pleural fluid may become purulent — in other words, a collection of pus may form in the pleural cavity. When this occurs the patient is said to have developed an empyema. Control of the empyema is best carried out by drainage of the pus and by the administration of suitable antibiotics.

Were smoking to gradually decline and become extinct few common lung diseases would be left for the chest physician to treat. The infectious diseases could be treated by infectious disease specialists and the other conditions could be allocated to other specialties such as rheumatology. Unfortunately cigarette smoking, gluttony, and other bad habits are not likely to decline in the immediate future and the chest physician will be needed for many years.                    WKCM

*See also* ANTIBIOTICS AND ANTI-INFECTIVE DRUGS; CARDIOTHORACIC SURGERY – HISTORY; OCCUPATIONAL HEALTH; SMOKING AND HEALTH; TRAUMA; TUBERCULOSIS

A problem arises when the clots in such veins break off and are carried to the right side of the heart and subsequently to the lungs. If the clot is large enough it is held up in the main pulmonary artery and as a result cuts off most of the blood flow going to the left side of the heart. A large pulmonary embolus which blocks both pulmonary arteries causes sudden death. Smaller clots may be carried to the lungs and if multiple may lead to a strain on the right side of the heart, which in some cases eventually proves to be fatal. Deep venous thrombosis is particularly common after pelvic and orthopedic surgery on the hips and knees.

Much can be done to prevent venous thrombosis. The avoidance of inactivity after surgery or during prolonged journeys can be effected by simple measures. Early physiotherapy should be the accepted standard in the management of abdominal, pelvic, and lower limb orthopedic surgery. The use of anticoagulants such as heparin and coumadin before and immediately after surgery have done much to reduce death rates from pulmonary emboli.

The lungs are separated from the chest wall by the visceral and parietal pleura. The visceral pleura lines the outer surface of the lungs, while the parietal pleura fulfills the same function on

## CHILD ABUSE AND NEGLECT Scarcely a day goes by without public attention being focused on some form of child abuse or neglect.

Newspaper and television reports are common, constantly reminding the public of this problem. Yet the abuse of children is not new. What is new is the awareness of the extent of the problem and the realization of the paradox that children are often in most danger in the places where they should be safest, their own homes.

Child abuse covers a spectrum of physical abuse, sexual abuse, emotional abuse, and neglect. Many abused children experience more than one type of abuse, especially when emotional abuse is included. What started as one form of abuse, such as neglect in infancy, may develop into other forms of abuse, such as physical abuse as a toddler and sexual abuse at school age.

Child abuse and neglect is a complex problem involving attitudes to VIOLENCE and sexual behavior, prior childhood experiences, and learned behavior. As such, it has no simple explanation or treatment.

## Physical abuse

Although there was always awareness that at times children could be seriously injured or killed by adults, there has been considerable denial about the extent of the problem. Medical practitioners who saw children with injuries which could only have been caused by abuse, were reluctant even to consider this diagnosis because of the difficulty in accepting that parents could treat their children in this way. This was despite the fact that abuse was well recognized by child welfare groups. It was not until the 1960s, when pediatricians started to collect and publicize details about children who had suffered serious injury, usually caused by their parents, that the extent and seriousness of the problem were realized.

It is difficult to know the true frequency of physical abuse. Most serious physical abuse occurs to children who are too young to give their account of the injuries and most abusers give a false explanation for the injuries that come to medical attention. All this suggests that the reported incidence of physical abuse is a significant underestimate of the true incidence. In countries which have mandatory reporting laws, the reported incidence of physical abuse is between one and four cases per thousand children, with many experts suggesting that there are at least ten unreported cases for each one that is reported.

Adults may seriously injure children for a number of reasons. It is well accepted that, although serious physical abuse can be caused by strangers, the majority is caused by parents or parent figures. Some authorities suggest that the physical abuse of children is a result of poverty and a society that often condones physical abuse in child rearing. However, poverty is not a sufficient explanation as physical abuse occurs across the entire social spectrum, although it is somewhat more common in families in poorer socio-economic circumstances where lack of access to a supportive network and good quality child care can add to the normal stresses of raising young children. Others believe that abusive behavior in parents is a direct result of the abuse they experienced in their own childhoods and which becomes incorporated into their own adult behavior. This view has led some to predict that abused children will become abusive parents. While this is true in some cases, it is not so for most abused children. Roughly 30% of adults who were abused as children will abuse their own children. It follows that, although there is a strong link between being an abused child and becoming an abusive parent, most abused children do not develop in this way.

It is unclear which features influence whether or not parents will be physically abusive towards their children and it is also difficult to be certain whether a child's injuries are the result of abuse. As the active, exploratory behavior of children may cause them to suffer accidental injuries, and as most severe abuse occurs to pre-verbal children, it is not always easy for the doctor to decide whether or not a child's injury was accidental or due to abuse. Some injuries are very suggestive of abuse. These include fractures in young children, especially in the first year of life. Most children are unable to crawl before eight to ten months and cannot roll until four to five months; thus under these ages infants are unlikely to get into situations where they could injure themselves accidentally. There should be genuine concern when children of this age have poorly explained injuries.

It is sometimes claimed that the injuries occurred when the child fell from a couch or bed. Studies of falls in children have shown that, while it is possible to sustain minor injuries in short distance falls, such as from a bed, it is extremely unlikely that such a fall will cause a serious injury, particularly multiple injuries. Other factors such as the pattern of bruise marks and particular X-ray features will help the experienced medical practitioner to be confident that the child's injuries were inflicted, rather than accidental.

MUNCHAUSEN'S SYNDROME by proxy (factitious disorder by proxy) is a particular form of physical abuse where a parent, mostly the mother, invents a story of illness in her child and often fabricates physical signs in the child to substantiate her story. This may lead to the child being admitted to hospital and having invasive, uncomfortable, and completely unnecessary investigations to try to find the cause of the symptoms, which have been fabricated. At times the fabricated illnesses can be life threatening,

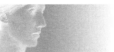

such as smothering, deliberate poisoning, or the injection of harmful substances into the child to produce the symptoms.

In all physical abuse cases the injury, serious as it might be, is an outward sign pointing to the need to assess the family so that the child can be protected. Treating the injury without investigating the factors that led to the injury will do little to protect the child. Follow-up studies of physically abused children show that, while the abuse ceases as they become older, they are more likely than other children to have difficulties at school, low self-esteem, and reduced ability to make meaningful friendships.

### Sexual abuse

This is the exploitation of a child for the gratification of an adult. Many factors are involved. These include the child's lack of power to resist the overtures of the abuser, the child's lack of understanding of the nature of the sexual activity, and the use of threats and coercion by the abuser.

Is this an abused and neglected child? (Picture reproduced courtesy of the NSPCC and posed by model.)

Sexual abuse is not a new phenomenon. In the Roman Empire boy brothels were popular in several cities and in Athens sexual abuse was such a problem that laws were passed so that private tutors could not be alone with their pupils. Kinsey's 1953 study of sexual behavior in women found that 9% of the sample recalled sexual contact with an adult before their 14th birthday. Not until the 1970s did child sexual abuse come to be widely discussed. It is not surprising that this widespread recognition could come only after an awareness of physical abuse. Once society became aware that parents could seriously physically injure their own children, it became possible to recognize the even greater taboo of child sexual abuse, including the fact that much of this abuse occurs within the child's own family.

### Who are the abusers

Contrary to earlier stereotypes, child sexual abusers are not seedy men in raincoats who lurk in dark corners. Sex abusers can be parents, relatives, teachers, neighbors, and child care workers. In fact, they can come from any field of work and from all socio-economic groups. About one quarter of abusers are strangers to the child. In the other three quarters the child knows the offender and in about half of these cases the offender is a member of the child's own family. Most sexual abusers are men, although studies suggest that about 5% are female.

The majority of sexual abuse cases are never reported. The incidence of reported cases which are substantiated is roughly 2 cases per 1000 children. This is in contrast to the true situation, where population studies, asking samples of adult females whether they had been sexually abused as children, have shown figures ranging from 6% to 62%. These wide-ranging figures reflect the variations in studies — some used narrow and others broad definitions of sexual abuse — and upper age limits have varied between 14 and 18 years. However, even the lower figures from these studies suggest that sexual abuse of children is common. Girls are more commonly abused than boys, who comprise about 20–30% of cases.

Most sexual abuse of children is not violent. It is a gradually escalating involvement between the victim and the perpetrator. For the perpetrator to have access to the child is not difficult if he is a family member or a person in a position of trust who has temporary care of the child. The perpetrator often engages the child in a 'game' which has some level of sexual activity and often will tell the child that this game is a secret. The adult's authority combined with bribes may convince the child that this behavior is acceptable. The sexual activity escalates and the child's secrecy is often gained by threats of retribution to the child or the child's loved ones if this behavior is revealed. The child may often feel a responsibility to protect the threatened family member, such as her mother, by complying with the perpetrator's wishes. This aspect of power on the part of the adult, sometimes combined with bribery, fear, confusion, and the desire to avoid a threatened catastrophe on the part of the child, explains why the sexual abuse often continues over several years without being detected.

A variety of factors lead to the discovery of the abusive behavior. There may be accidental discovery when the abuse is observed by another person. Sometimes the provocative sexual behavior that is seen in some sexually abused children may arouse suspicion. Sometimes the child will tell another child her 'secret' and that child tells an adult who takes the story seriously and informs the relevant authorities. In some cases there is a physical injury, such as bleeding, which arouses suspicions. School protective behavior programs, where children are told what sexually abusive behavior is, how to avoid it, and tell if it has occurred may lead to detection.

Families react in different ways after the disclosure of sexual abuse. Many are supportive of the child, arrange for appropriate professional assessment, and take steps to protect the child from further abuse. Others behave quite differently. The child may be punished for 'lying'. In some cases of intra-familial abuse the family may close ranks, refusing to believe that such a thing could happen in its family. There may be so much pressure on the child for disrupting what was outwardly a respectable family that the child may reluctantly agree that the abuse did not happen at all.

### Do children tell the truth?

In the past there has been a view that children are more suggestible than adults. Most recent studies show that for children over 5 years of age, their ability to recall events in which they were involved and their resistance to being misled by suggestive questioning are as good as those of adults. False reports of sexual abuse by children do occur but are rare, in the order of 1–2% of cases according to the best research, and are more likely to be from older children, often with disturbed backgrounds, where a story of abuse may be created to 'get even' with an adult. False stories of abuse by young children are more rare, partly because they usually do not have the knowledge of adult sexual behavior to be able to make a specific allegation. A far greater problem is the number of children who are sexually abused who do not tell about their abuse because of threats and fear.

### 'Repressed' memories

Recently the topic of sexual abuse has become further complicated by adults who claim to be recalling sexually abusive experiences from their own childhood which had been repressed in their memories. There is a concern that a proportion of these so-called 'repressed memories' may not be accurate, but instead may be a result of suggestions that the person's current emotional difficulties may be because of sexually abusive experiences in the past which have been repressed. It is possible for memories of childhood sexual abuse to be repressed and to surface in adult life, as shown by the small number of cases where a reliable third party has been able to corroborate the events that have been recalled. However, in most cases there is no corroboration and after so many years the truth or otherwise of these allegations is elusive, given the present state of knowledge.

There is a variety of theories to explain why some adults sexually abuse children. No single theory explains the whole problem. One simple, but incorrect theory is that child sexual abusers were themselves the victims of sexual abuse as children. However, if being abused was the only factor that led to a person becoming an abuser then, as most abused children are female, it would follow that most abusers would also be female, something which is clearly not the case.

Some theories suggest that abusers are arrested in their psychosexual development and so relate more readily to children in social relationships. Their low self-esteem, perhaps resulting from unhappy childhood experiences, may make it easier for them to feel powerful and in control while exploiting children.

There may be some difficulties in deciding whether a child has been sexually abused. By far the most useful is the story given by the child. A skilled interviewer who has an open mind whether or not abuse occurred can generally make an accurate assessment. Proving that abuse has occurred is more difficult as it is carried out in secret with no opportunity for corroboration by a third party. Physical evidence such as damage to the child's genitals may provide proof but is not present in some types of sexual abuse. Other behavioral indicators such as psychological symptoms may suggest that sexual abuse is a possible cause for these symptoms but this is not sufficient proof. The reliability of the child's story, supported by physical evidence when present, is the most useful way to make the diagnosis. It should go without saying that interviews of the child should be kept to a minimum to avoid distressing the child as well as to avoid suggestions that the child's memory may have been contaminated by the interviews. Such interviews should be performed by a skilled professional.

## FOUR CONDITIONS FOR SEXUAL ABUSE

It has been suggested that four conditions have to be met for the sexual abuse of a child to occur.

- The adult must have sexual feelings for the child. We do not know how many adults are sexually attracted to children, although, unless the other three conditions are met, abuse will not occur.

- The adult has to overcome his or her internal inhibitions against acting out the sexual feelings. Drugs, alcohol, or pornography may be used to help overcome these inhibitions.

- The adult must then overcome any external obstacles to acting out the sexual feelings. These restraints can be fairly easily overcome when the adult has close, unsupervised access to a child, such as by being a family member or being a person who is in a position of trust in caring for children.

- The adult has to be able to overcome the resistance of the child. Some children are needier and more vulnerable to the overtures of an abuser than others. Other children are bribed, tricked, or threatened into a sexually abusive relationship. Protective behavior programs which teach children how to be aware of and how to avoid sexual abuse are aimed at preventing this fourth factor.

Sexually abused children suffer in a variety of ways. In addition to the abuse itself, there is fear resulting from the abuser's threats as well as sexual confusion in many cases. A significant proportion of sexually abused children have low self-esteem, poor school performance, depression, and difficulties in interpersonal relationships. Often many of these difficulties persist into adult life.

### Emotional abuse and neglect

Emotional abuse may be regarded as an underlying characteristic of all forms of child abuse. Children who are physically injured by their parents or care takers and children who are sexually misused for the emotional gratification of an adult are also emotionally abused as a result of these acts which give the child the message that their value to the adult is not as a person but as something adults can use for their own satisfaction.

Although neglect and emotional abuse in children are common, they cause no physical signs and are subtler in their manifestations than physical or sexual abuse. As a result, this type of abuse may come to the attention of professionals less often.

It is not only parents who can emotionally abuse children. Emotional abuse can be caused by relatives, neighbors, and those who work in schools, hospitals, child care, detention centers, residential units, and organizations which care for physically or intellectually disabled children. Emotional abuse by the child's own parents is likely to be more serious.

The most common type of emotional abuse occurs when an adult refuses to show any affection, often combining this with constant denigration and belittling of the child. This behavior refuses to acknowledge the child's values and needs. Other forms of emotional abuse include preventing the child from forming friendships and mixing socially, corrupting the child by leading the developing child into antisocial or deviant behavior patterns, and terrorizing the child by constantly threatening with extreme punishment and making the child fearful. Parents who emotionally abuse children often have little idea of the child's normal developmental needs. They may be reinforcing child rearing behaviors that they learnt as children form their own parents.

Neglect is not the same as emotional abuse. Neglected children do not receive their basic need to be fed, clothed, loved, sheltered, and protected when their parents or society are unwilling to provide for these needs. Neglect should not be confused with poverty or ignorance. To label a family as neglectful when they fall into circumstances over which they have no control and no awareness of how to obtain help is unreasonable. Neglect can also include neglecting a child's needs for medical care such as immunization, for education, and for emotional and spiritual development. The emotional abuse and neglect which accompany many cases of physical and sexual abuse are more likely to be responsible for the adverse long-term outcomes seen in many abused children than the episodes of abuse themselves.

### Prevention

Child abuse is a complex and serious problem requiring multiple prevention strategies. These include providing new parents with practical support and education to develop the skills required to be a good parent. They involve teaching children how to protect themselves from sexual abuse and what to do should it happen. They also include the detection of abuse by training professionals who work with children and providing adequate treatment resources for children who have been abused, something which is an important step in breaking the cycle of abuse in the next generation.

Prevention also involves appropriate ways to deal with perpetrators ranging from treatment in some cases to imprisonment in others. Public education is necessary to create an environment where child abuse is seen as a serious problem which requires prevention strategies at a variety of levels. This may include a change in community attitudes so that it is possible to talk more openly about the causes of child abuse and neglect and the need to take a firm stand that child abuse in all its forms is totally unacceptable.

Although child abuse is unlikely ever to be eliminated, there is now sufficient understanding about its causes and prevention to be able to reduce its incidence significantly as long as there is a public, professional, and political will to do so.

### Global dimensions

In world-wide perspective, the public health problem of child abuse and neglect is enormous. In 1997, the United Nations Children's Fund estimated that there were roughly 250 million child workers in the world. This does not include an estimated 20 million abandoned children, living on the streets in cities and towns in Latin America, Africa, and Asia, eking out a living by begging, drug trafficking, and prostitution. In several war-ravaged parts of the world, children as young as 8 years are pressed into military service, often after their parents have been killed and they have been kidnapped. Parents with no other resources in some Asian and African nations sell their daughters into prostitution. The censuses in India and China show a deficit of several million females that can only have come about as a result of female infanticide, doubtless compounded by neglect of female offspring.

Children are the main victims of sanctions imposed on Iraq and the US embargo on trade with Cuba. In many countries in the developing world, disproportionate numbers of girls receive little or no education, so female literacy rates in these countries are substantially lower than those for males. Several million girls every year in some countries are subjected to the barbaric ritual of 'CIRCUMCISION' — female genital mutilation. All these categories of children may accurately be described as abused and/or neglected. Child workers engaged in tasks such as weaving carpets, stitching footballs, and making sports shoes; collecting fuel and tending cooking fires; foraging on garbage dumps, are deprived of education and robbed of parental care and affection. The United Nations Convention on the Rights of the Child proclaimed in 1990 that such deplorable practices must end, but in a world where poverty and warfare are so commonplace, this is easier said than done.                                    RKO

**CHILD HEALTH — HISTORY** In the Egyptian EBERS PAPYRUS, dating from the first half of the 16th century BC, there are sections on the diseases of infancy. In Indian and Chinese manuscripts, and to a lesser extent in the Talmud, diseases of children are described and discussed. HIPPO-CRATES (p 382) in his *Aphorisms*, notably in the fragment 'On teething', gives advice which persisted with relatively little change, from classical times down to the middle of the 16th century AD.

Rosen von Rosenstein, professor of medicine at Uppsala, Sweden, founded modern pediatrics as a medical specialty, writing, in 1765, the textbook entitled *The diseases of children and their remedies*. A private hospital for the treatment of children was opened in Vienna in 1787. After the Revolution in 1802, the French government founded a hospital for sick children (*Hôpital des Enfants Malades*) in Paris, followed by the founding of children's hospitals in Berlin (1830), St Petersburg (1834), and Vienna (1837).

In 1852 Charles WEST (p 175) opened the Hospital for Sick Children in Great Ormond Street, London, with the objective of cutting down the high infant and child death rates by improving the skills of the doctors, and also instructing mothers about hygiene and the general care of children, and training nurses. However, although pediatric hospitals provided centers in which medical and nursing skills could be fostered, it was soon evident that their contribution to falling death rates would be small. Indeed, hospital admission could itself engender epidemics of infectious diseases, often fatal. The solution was to be sought and found elsewhere in better public health.

**Books and journals**

In 1825 in the USA, William Potts Dewees, a professor at the University of Pennsylvania, published one of the first American texbooks of pediatrics. The American Pediatric Society held its first meeting in 1889, the *Archives of Pediatrics* having been founded five years earlier. The members of the society, like the contributors to the journal, were physicians with a 'special interest in the study of diseases in children'. Nevertheless, much time and space were devoted to infant feeding. Hygiene, public health, and child labor were recognized as appropriate subjects for discussion, but the doctors' chief concern was disease. The first American children's hospital was opened in Philadelphia in 1855, followed soon after by those in Boston and New York City. John Howland established the notable Harriet Lane department of pediatrics at JOHNS HOPKINS HOSPITAL (p 840) in Baltimore in 1912. In Japan the children's hospital of Tokyo National University celebrated its centenary in 1989.

Currently, some 60 pediatric journals are published, spreading good practice and reporting research findings although most important research is reported in only a few of these. One of the first of these was the *Jahrbuch für Kinderheilkunde*, first published in Germany in 1868, which subsequently became *Annales Paediatrici* and then evolved into the present-day *Pediatric Research*. Today, among the leading pediatric journals are *Archives of the Diseases of Childhood*, *Pediatrics*, and *Journal of Pediatrics*.

The real function of the children's specialists initially remained general medicine applied to the special age group that began at birth, although many years were to pass before the obstetricians relinquished their nominal responsibility for the newborn. When the special age group ends is still undecided, the onset of puberty being one obvious determinant. In the USA, however, pediatricians often care for patients until they are in the third decade of life, and pediatric cardiologists, for example, may continue to provide care jointly with general physicians for their patients with congenital heart disease through young adulthood. The development of adolescent medicine as a further specialization (so-called 'ephebiatrics') has only a limited following, except in the USA and Canada, where there are now adolescent medicine specialists in most large urban areas.

The introduction of effective immunization began with diphtheria toxin-antitoxin mixtures. During the 1920s, clinical trials were made on selected populations. One preoccupation was the risk of serum-sickness, a complication of immunization noted by von PIRQUET (p 32) in Vienna in 1905 and leading him to his conception of

## PIONEERS IN PEDIATRICS

George **ARMSTRONG** (1720–89). British physician. Employed as a pharmacist in Hampstead before training in medicine, he founded a charitable dispensary for children in 1769 which failed after 12 years through lack of funds. He may be regarded as the first British pediatrician. He wrote *An essay on diseases most fatal to infants* (1767).

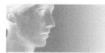

Denis John Wolko **BROWNE** (1892–1967). Australian surgeon. Invalided home after serving in Gallipoli, he graduated in Sydney, then traveled to Britain for postgraduate study. He was appointed in 1928 to the honorary staff of the Hospital for Sick Children, London, where he remained until 1957. Browne was the first surgeon to operate exclusively on children, and was a founder of modern pediatric surgery. He is remembered for his operations for hypospadias (a congenital deformity of the penis), harelip, and cleft palate and for his use of 'controlled movement' for clubfoot.

*(continued opposite)*

ALLERGY. The general adoption of active immunization took many years. Its introduction found the general public, and even the doctors, somewhat suspicious despite the century-long experience of SMALLPOX vaccination. Protection against tetanus and, to a lesser degree, against whooping cough (pertussis) became available, but not until the 1940s was the vaccine being offered in Britain accepted by the majority as safe and beneficial.

POLIOMYELITIS epidemics (first noted in 1910) swept Western countries as late as 1955 in Australia, inducing the sort of community panic which was associated with the BLACK DEATH and PLAGUES of the Middle Ages and leaving a trail of death and serious motor handicap. The problems posed by TUBERCULOSIS were different. Consumption had been recognized in classical times and tuberculous disease of the bone was diagnosed, with as much certainty as possible, in the third millennium BC. KOCH (p 455) identified the tubercle bacillus, publishing his research in 1882. Infection was spread by coughing and, less commonly, by drinking infected milk, and by the dawn of pediatrics tuberculosis had established itself as a disease of the community as well as of the family. Certainly, among urban populations almost every child (either as a baby or at some time before maturity) would encounter and be challenged by the tubercle bacillus. Some babies succumbed; others overcame the challenge, becoming sensitized, so that their response to further almost inevitable encounters led to an altered reaction. This, through the results of his tuberculin test, confirmed von Pirquet's belief in his concept of allergy.

At first a whole system of special clinics and dispensaries was aimed at treatment of the individual patient. Later, mass radiography led to early case finding, better segregation of open cases (patients with bacilli in their sputum), and a reduction in the sources of infection. Grandfather coughing by the fireside was removed and his opportunities for infecting his grandchildren were lessened. The discovery of an effective antibiotic (streptomycin) by Waksman in 1944 provided a final touch, but the rise in drug-resistant tuberculosis associated with the disease in people with HIV infection indicates that story of childhood tuberculosis is sadly not closed.

Although these developments neither originated in children's hospitals, nor directly involved pediatrics, they greatly influenced the health of children. At the same time, further research had put into the doctors' hands other antibiotics, so that most non-viral infections could be safely treated at home by family doctors or, if in hospital, within a much shorter time and with less resulting debility. These advances, with the reduction in tuberculosis, effective treatment of meningitis, and virtual disappearance of life-threatening acute gastroenteritis, osteomyelitis (inflammation of bone marrow), and rheumatic fever (with its tendency to cause valvular disease of the heart), reduced the demand for hospital beds and therefore for the hospital pediatrician of later childhood.                    FHM, RDHB, AWF

*See also* ANTIBIOTICS AND ANTI-INFECTIVE DRUGS; CARDIOLOGY; CARDIOTHORACIC SURGERY; CHILDREN – EXPERIMENTATION ON; GENERAL PRACTICE; POLIOMYELITIS; VIOLENCE

**CHILD HEALTH** Pediatrics or child health is the branch of medical practice which applies to infants and children. Nomenclature varies among different countries and institutions, and among different aspects of medical practice. The term 'child health' is sometimes used interchangeably with 'pediatrics'.

Pediatricans are doctors who spend the bulk of their time working with children. In several countries pediatricians provide the primary medical care of children, whether prevention or treatment. In Britain primary care for children is predominantly provided by general practitioners, and increasingly also their primary preventive care. Pediatricians in Britain work mainly in hospital inpatient and outpatient practice, although recently the number specializing in community pediatrics — community pediatricians — has increased appreciably. In the USA general pediatricians provide health maintenance, treat common illnesses, and coordinate for patients with complex disorders the consultations and treatments of pediatric subspecialists. Family practitioners also provide primary care for children in the USA, especially in rural areas.

Pediatricians, especially at university hospitals and to a greater extent in North America, have become specialized by disease or organ system, as in pediatric oncologist (cancer and leukaemia), pediatric neurologist (brain, nerve, and muscle disorders), and pediatric gastroenterologist (intestinal disorders). Neonatology is a numerically important branch of pediatrics, specializing in the disorders of the newborn. Pediatricians in the USA may be certified by the American Board of Pediatrics as competent in general pediatrics and also in one or more of 13 subspecialties.

For rare or complicated disorders, the chances of successful treatment are greater when pediatric expertise in the various specialties is available in 'tertiary referral' centers. These are usually university-associated children's units or hospitals, ideally in close proximity to obstetric departments (for complex neonatology) and specialized adult facilities — neurosurgery and cardiac surgery — with which their pediatric counterparts can co-operate. The success of such specialized children's centers is enhanced by the availability of pediatrically trained nursing staff and similarly expert personnel in physiotherapy, radiography, nutrition, and other support services, such as pharmacy. The availability of clinical laboratory personnel experienced in the range of disorders and the micro-methods appropriate to pediatric specimens is also important.

For more common conditions, facilities close to the patient's home allow integration of primary care and hospital services for effective treatment of patients with ASTHMA, pneumonia, or gastroenteritis, who need admission to hospital only sometimes, usually being safely treated at home. Such secondary facilities provide care for most hospitalized children and newborn babies; only those with severe disease or very low birth weight are referred to the tertiary center. These units also provide a useful focus for the provision of community pediatric services.

## Death and disease in childhood

In the industrialized world (where most pediatricians work) the complex and devastating interaction of malnutrition, infection, and poverty on children's health and survival has largely been abolished, but it is continuing over much of the poorer world . In 1997 some 40% of the 5.8 billion inhabitants of the world, or 2.3 billion, were younger than 20 years. In developing nations, the proportion of the population in this age group is greater. From 1955 to 1995, the global death rate of children younger than 20 years fell by two-thirds. By 1995, the annual global death rate for children younger than 5 years was 1720 deaths per 100 000 and for the ages 5–19 years, the rate was 210 deaths per 100 000.

World-wide, the leading causes of death before the age of 5 years are malnutrition, diarrhea, acute lower respiratory infection, prematurity, birth asphyxia, and MALARIA. In developed countries the leading causes of death in the neonatal period (first 28 days) are prematurity and congenital anomalies. Between 28 days and 1 year of age the leading cause of death is SUDDEN INFANT DEATH SYNDROME (cot death), followed by the later effects of congenital anomalies and by pneumonia and influenza. In children of 1 to 4 years old, accidents are the leading cause of death, followed by congenital anomalies, malignant tumors (neoplasms), diseases of the heart, and HIV/AIDS. Homicide — usually from violence within the family, CHILD ABUSE, or non-accidental injury — is also of importance. Except for congenital anomalies, these same causes are the leading ones for death of children aged 5–14 years.

An important component of child care, whether mainly provided by pediatricians, as in the USA, or by general practitioners and their nursing colleagues, as in Britain, is child health maintenance, including oversight of appropriate nutrition, growth, and development, and immunization against many childhood infectious diseases. Schedules for immunization during the first two years of life are available to protect against diphtheria, tetanus, pertussis, poliomyelitis, hepatitis B, *Hemophilus influenza* type b, measles, meningitis, mumps, rubella, and varicella (chickenpox). In less developed nations, children may also be immunized against TUBERCULOSIS, and they may be protected against neonatal tetanus by immunization of their mothers. Between 1974 and 1995 an effective campaign by the World Health Organization increased the world-wide immunization rate against common pediatric infectious diseases from 5% to 80% of children.

Other health maintenance functions include anticipatory guidance of parents; injury prevention, and hearing and vision screening for young children; screening for some heritable disorders such as phenylketonuria (INBORN ERRORS OF METABOLISM) and hypothyroidism (subnormal activity of the thyroid gland) in the newborn; management of behavior disorders, school adjustment problems, and school failure in older children; pre-participation examinations and counseling for sports participation; prevention of pregnancy and infection in sexually active adolescents; and counseling to prevent smoking and substances abuse.

Common diseases treated by physicians caring for children are upper respiratory infections (colds), otitis media (earache), gastroenteritis (vomiting and/or diarrhea), and epilepsy (seizures). Several chronic diseases are increasing in frequency in the developed parts of the world, including asthma, certain malignancies, obesity, and diabetes mellitus. These are multifactorial diseases in which environmental factors interact with genetic susceptibility. Other chronic diseases are single gene disorders, such as cystic fibrosis and muscular dystrophy, and are the current targets of research to replace the mutant gene responsible for the disease. The rapid pace of molecular genetics investigation is adding much new knowledge about pediatric diseases.

Pediatricians also care for and integrate the activities of consultants for children with developmental and post-traumatic disabilities, such as learning disability (mental retardation), Down's syndrome, cerebral palsy, and post-traumatic head injury. A group of problems sometimes known as the 'new morbidities' is becoming increasingly prominent. Very broadly defined, these problems include: smoking and substance abuse; anxiety, depression, and suicide; self-mutilation; injuries arising from violent acts; teenage pregnancy; and child and child sexual abuse.

(continued)

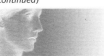

Charles **WEST** (1816–98). British physician. Born in London. West studied in Bonn, Paris, and Berlin, where he qualified in medicine. He failed in general practice in the City of London, so went to Dublin to study midwifery. He returned to London as physician to the Infirmary for Women and Children, Waterloo Road, and lectured on midwifery at the Middlesex Hospital and St Bartholomew's. In 1852 he founded the Hospital for Sick Children in Richard Mead's house in Great Ormond Street and was physician there for 23 years. Those who helped the foundation included Lord Shaftesbury and Charles Dickens.

Most medical care of children is given outside hospital. The average child in Britain sees a doctor (usually a general practitioner) four times a year, visits a hospital once every 5 years, and is admitted to hospital only once per childhood. Such hospital stay is likely to last roughly four days; it was three times as long in 1955.

### Community pediatrics

This has evolved in Britain to address medical issues which have historically been dealt with inadequately by general practitioners and by hospital-focused pediatricians. These include the surveillance for presymptomatic or early signs of disorder, by screening for conditions such as deafness, metabolic disorder, poor growth, and developmental delay. The balance of cost-benefit and inconvenience and timing of this have been given considerable thought. Health education and disease prevention, including advice on feeding babies, immunization, and advice on accident prevention have been other important roles of community pediatrics.

Child protection has become another important focus of work, in conjunction with the law courts and other social agencies attempting to improve conditions for children in families where violence or neglectful parenting puts the child's health or development seriously at risk, and has extended into the controversial area of abusive adult–child sexual interactions. The amelioration of the impact on the child and family of severe handicap is another important role, as is the overlapping task of health education, giving medical advice on the diagnosis and management of children who are performing unexpectedly poorly at school. Again, community pediatrics has a joint role with educational psychologists, social workers, and, of course, parents. Historically community pediatric services in Britain were provided as an aspect of local government. Over the past 20 years there has been a gradual but somewhat erratic evolution of services towards surveillance, prevention, and education, predominantly provided by the primary healthcare team of general practitioner and specialized nurses and health visitors. Handicap, specialized educational medicine, and child protection are predominantly provided by specialist community pediatricians, often working as part of a team with general pediatricians based on a district pediatric unit. In the USA the activities of British community pediatricians are generally recognized as a core responsibility of all general pediatricians. Specialized pediatric nurses provide a link between home-based and hospital-based treatments with other specialized nurses such as asthma nurses, diabetes nurses, or cancer nurses.                                    FHM, RDHB, AWF

## CHILDREN — EXPERIMENTATION ON

Children have a long history of participating in new treatments and taking part in trials of new vaccines and medical procedures. This history has been marked by exploitation of children, especially poor children, as well as important advances in medical knowledge that have benefited large numbers of children and adults. In the 18th century, because of their lack of exposure to SMALLPOX, children were among the first to undergo both variolation and VACCINATION in efforts to achieve immunity to the disfiguring and often deadly disease. In perhaps the best known experimental trial in the 19th century, a badly-bitten child, 10-year-old Joseph Meister, received the first human application of Louis PASTEUR's (p 620) rabies vaccine. In the early 20th century, pediatricians increasingly used children in orphanages and schools for the mentally disabled as research subjects. In 1914, New York pediatrician Alfred Hess argued that research at the Hebrew Infant Asylum was more reliable because the children belonged to the same stratum of society and had the same daily routine, enabling him to approximate 'conditions which are insisted on in considering the course of experimental infection among laboratory animals, but which can rarely be controlled in a study of infection in man'.

### Lübeck disaster

In 1930, a tragedy focused international attention on the participation of children in research. In Lübeck, Germany, administration of the Calmette (BCG) vaccine against TUBERCULOSIS to 250 children resulted in the death of over 76 infants. The public outcry prompted the German Ministry of the Interior to issue regulations concerning new medical treatments and scientific experiments on man (1931), including special protections for children under the age of 18. After 1933, when the National Socialists came to power, children were not exempted from concentration camp experiments. Physician Josef MENGELE (p 387) conducted extensive experiments on twin children at Auschwitz, and large numbers of mentally and physically disabled children were killed in the Nazi euthanasia programs.

During the Second World War, researchers in the United States and Britain used children in the development of new vaccines and treatments. In the USA access to institutionalized populations such as the children at the New Jersey State Colony for the Feeble-Minded enhanced investigators' applications for government funding. After the war, as the pace of clinical research intensified, pediatric investigators recruited children in hospital, orphanages, and schools. In some cases, physicians obtained parental consent for a child's participation in tests of a new treatment or procedure. In the 1950s, researchers at the Massachusetts Institute of Technology conducted nutritional studies on 'retarded' boys at the Fernald State School in Massachusetts. For the tests, which involved eating cereals containing low doses of radioisotopic iron and calcium, investigators obtained parental permission, but failed to disclose the use of radioactive isotopes and the absence of benefit for the children. (In 1998 the now grown child-participants and Massachusetts Institute of Technology reached an out-of-court financial settlement.) In what would become perhaps the most infamous pediatric research project of the 20th century, the hepatitis studies involving children at the Willowbrook State School in New York, infectious disease researcher Saul Krugman met with groups of parents to obtain their consent to study their children intentionally infected with the virus of hepatitis A.

More than consent was at issue. In the 1960s physicians Maurice PAPPWORTH (p 616) in Britain and Henry K. BEECHER (p 94) in the United States criticized the unnecessary risks incurred by children and others in the development of such techniques as cardiac catheterization and in studies of such diseases as hepatitis. In 1966, Beecher included the Willowbrook hepatitis studies in his article on 22 ethically suspect clinical researches. Pappworth's *Human guinea pigs* (1967) cited 21 published reports in which 'the special consideration due to children and babies because of their particular vulnerability and helplessness' was clearly lacking.

Since the 1970s there have been ongoing efforts in Britain, Canada, and the United States to forge workable guidelines for the ethical conduct of experimentation on children. No one disputes that research on children is important for the health of all children, but achieving this goal while simultaneously promoting the autonomy and welfare of child participants has been controversial. The participation of infants and children in research not intended to benefit them has proved especially problematic. Whereas some would prohibit non-therapeutic experiments on children which posed hazards to the participants, others have argued for an assessment of risks and benefits that would permit exposing children to minimal (and even greater) risk when the expected benefits to knowledge are considerable. Many of these discussions focus on the vagueness of such terms as risk—negligible, minimal, and more than minimal — and the assessments of benefit. In Great Britain and Canada, for example, physicians and policy makers have debated the permissibility of venipuncture in non-therapeutic research. Although children experience no long-term physical harm from the procedure, some worry about the potential for psychological harm to children who dislike venipuncture and undergo it for reasons unrelated to their own healthcare.

In addition to protecting child welfare, policy makers have sought to promote children's rights. Since the NUREMBERG CODE (1947), the voluntary consent of the individual has been a cornerstone of ethical experimentation. As a matter of law and tradition, children have been considered unable to exercise decision-making capacity, and parents have been asked to consent to treatment and research on their behalf. Adolescents and infants differ enormously in their abilities to understand, cooperate, and permit both research and treatment. In the United States, in an effort to maximize the child's 'voice' in research, current federal guidelines require institutional review boards to determine when children are able to assent (offer an affirmative agreement to participate) even though they are not legally able to give consent. There continues to be wide variation in practice; in the published literature, estimates for the child's capacity to assent to research range widely, from 5 years to 15 years of age. Guidelines issued by both the British Paediatric Association and the Council for International Organizations of Medical Sciences recommend that researchers, where possible, select older children rather than younger ones, because older children are presumably better able to protect their own interests.

The conduct of research with children continues to raise difficult ethical questions. Given the significant biological differences between children and adults and the fact that many drugs have not been tested on pediatric populations, the need for ongoing research involving children seems indisputable. The issue remains how to conduct ethically sensitive research using infants and children.    SEL

*See also* BIOETHICS; CHILD HEALTH; INFORMED CONSENT

**CHINA** Medicine in China currently combines western medicine, traditional Chinese medicine, and medicine of Minority with its own history in China. All of them have made great contributions to Chinese healthcare.

Traditional Chinese medicine has a very long history. The earliest medical work extant in China, the *Canon of internal medicine*, appeared about 300 BC. It dealt mainly with basic theories of traditional Chinese medicine and of acupuncture, including a variety of subjects, such as physiology, diagnosis, and treatment. Around 100 BC, Shen Nong's *Pharmacopoeia* emerged as the first specific work extant on materia medica. In 200 AD, the surgeon, Hua Tuo, successfully performed abdominal tumor excision under general ANESTHESIA with Mafeisan (powder for anesthesia). In 1076 AD, the government of Song Dynasty unified diagnosis and drug treatment in the creation of the National Bureau for the Administration of Medicine. Later, the government set up the Bureau of Imperial Physicians to take charge of medical education for as many as 300 students. According to the historical records, vaccines were developed as early as 1567. In 1578, Li Shizhen completed the *Compendium of materia medica*, which became a comprehensive summary of all pharmacological knowledge accumulated in China up to that time.

After 1840, some doctors raised the slogan of the 'combination of western and traditional Chinese medicine'. In 1955, the People's Republic of China established the Academy of Traditional Chinese Medicine and traditional Chinese medicine courses were included in medical colleges. Western medicine — first introduced into China during the 19th century — now has the predominant role in China. Meanwhile, Chinese have contributed to western medicine, such as the identification of chlamydia and the synthesis of bovine insulin.

The medicine of Minority with a history of over 3000 years is important for including China and Tibet, and has made many contributions to Chinese healthcare over the past two millennia. All forms are regarded as complementary to one other. Patients can choose which kind of medical system they use.

## Contemporary medicine

The medical and health service in China is a combination of non-profit service and paid service provided by the government and private components. Its priority strategies emphasize putting prevention first and relying on scientific and technological progress. The Chinese government has prioritized preventive medicine and the rejuvenation of traditional Chinese medicine and pharmacology, giving equal attention to both traditional Chinese medicine and western medicine, and to serve the needs of people in both urban and rural areas. Since the adoption of policy reform and increased foreign contact in the late 20th century, China's health services have been improving. Infant mortality and morbidity of certain infectious diseases have decreased dramatically. PLAGUE, KALA-AZAR, TYPHUS, relapsing fever, and sexually transmitted diseases, prevalent in the early 1950s, have been controlled. The prevalence of INFECTIOUS DISEASE has dropped and deaths from them, once ranked first among causes of death, have dropped to ninth. Cerebrovascular diseases, cardiac diseases, and cancers have been the leading causes of death in the past two decades. Some progress has been made in the control of epidemic diseases such as filariasis,

MALARIA, Ke-shan disease, and SCHISTOSOMIASIS, suggestive of significant advances in healthcare. Life expectancy has increased on average by over 30 years for both men and women over the past 40 years.

A task of prime importance in China's health services is to protect the health of women and children, who constitute two-thirds of the total population. With the promulgation by the State Council of the 'Provisional regulations governing the healthcare service of female employees' and the 'Regulations governing the labor protection of female workers', some special measures have been taken to protect women's health, especially during pregnancy and birth. General screening for common diseases of women has been carried out periodically in both rural and urban areas. As a result, a three-tier mother and children healthcare network has taken shape. Thanks to the systematic management of pregnant women in rural areas and regular healthcare services in urban areas, women's health status has improved and the maternal mortality rate fallen. In March 1991, the government signed 'the World declaration on the survival, protection, and development of children' and its plan of action in the 1990s. Moreover, the Ministry of Public Health formulated the 'National program for the control of four diseases among children' and the 'Healthcare system of nurses and kindergartens'. The Ministry has also helped in the control of rickets, anemia, pneumonia, and diarrhea and improved the nutrition and healthcare of infants and children. Additionally, the infant mortality has decreased and children's physical development has noticeably improved in rural and urban areas.

## Infrastructure of the healthcare system

To satisfy the people's medical and healthcare needs and control diseases, the infrastructure of the healthcare system combines a medical and 'epidemic prevention' system. The two systems are independent. The former comprises hospitals and clinics and the latter largely epidemic prevention stations. By now, State health organizations comprise a large part of healthcare organizations, of which private health organizations are only 3.6%. The health organizations founded by community, collective, and private groups are complementary to State organizations. According to a 1997 report, there were 15 219 hospitals at the county level and above, including 2 109 116 beds; 51 535 village hospitals including 742 400 beds; 506 sanitariums; 3984 clinics; 125 246 private hospitals; and 1893 specific prevention and cure institutions. In order to use health resources better, the Ministry has developed a stratified healthcare management since 1989.

(*continued on p 180*)

**Plate 1** Mammogram of breast cancer. At center right, a cancerous tumor appears as a yellow core with radiating contours of color.

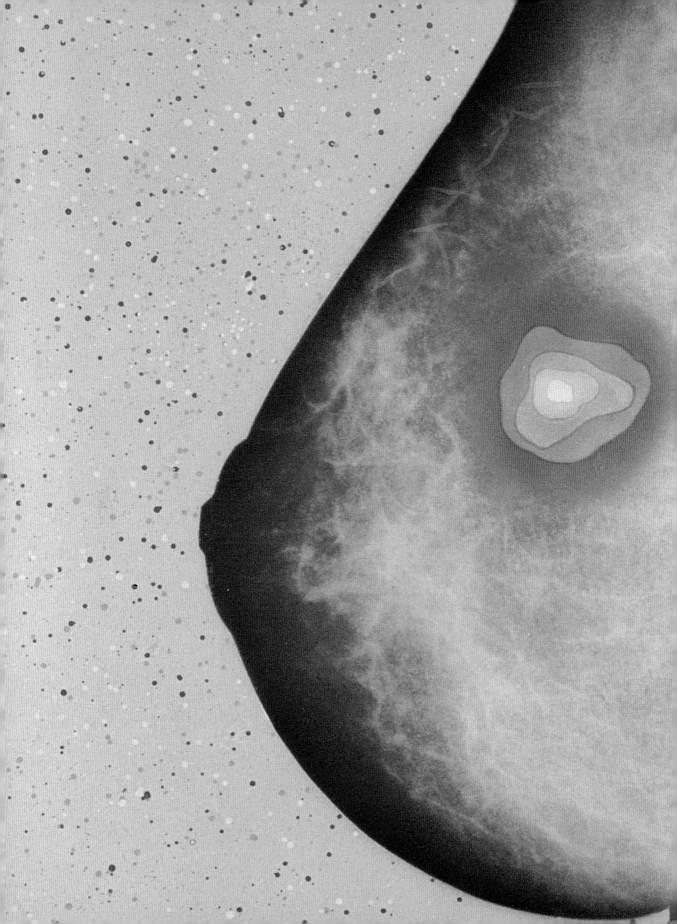

# LET THE TODDLER'S FIRST STEPS

*-lead to the*

# WELFARE CENTRE

GET EXPERT ATTENTION AND ADVICE BEFORE AND AFTER BABY COMES
ADVICE ON FEEDING-MILK OR SPECIAL FOOD
TRAINED NURSES WHO LIKE CHILDREN
DO WHAT THE DOCTOR TELLS YOU

USE YOUR HEALTH SERVICES

NORFOLK

Medical and healthcare systems concentrate on the rural areas because 80% of Chinese people live there. The most important aspects are setting up three-tier medicine prevention and healthcare institutes, cooperative medical care, and village doctors. There are now over 2000 county hospitals, 1900 county epidemic prevention stations, and 1700 county women and children healthcare stations. They are also centers of disease prevention and training for the development of primary healthcare in rural areas. Over 90% of villages have medical clinics.

### Healthcare personnel

According to 1997 statistics, the total number of medical technical personnel was 4 397 805.

In 1997, there were an average 2.14 beds for every 1000 persons in China: in cities, 3.49 beds for every 1000 persons, and in rural areas 1.57 beds. The average number of healthcare workers for 1000 people was 3.65 country wide — 5.29 in cities, and 2.37 in rural areas. There were 1.65 doctors and 0.99 nurses per 1000 inhabitants.

Like most developing countries, China is facing the problems of the shortage and low quality of health workers, limitation of health resources, and uneven distribution of healthcare personnel. The government has applied some strategies and measures to develop medical education to meet the needs of healthcare services.

- Developing all branches of medical education. The medical education system includes primary, secondary school, and higher education, with secondary school education first.

- Gradually distributing medical manpower evenly all over the country. The measures include directional enrollment, directional training, and directional assignment to rural areas, while increasing the number of courses related to rural healthcare and increasing the opportunities to practice in rural areas.

- Reform of education. Some medical universities have learned from educational models used in developed countries, such as problem-solving and student-centered techniques and the combination of different subjects and computer-assisted education. Some universities have also reformed course content.

There is now an integrated medical education system in China. There are 121 medical colleges and universities (including 30 colleges of traditional Chinese medicine). Eighty-four of these and 28 separate institutions can undertake the training of graduate students. In addition, there are 330 medical secondary schools; 1047 county health schools; 41 continuing medical colleges; and 174 secondary schools for training medical staff.

**Plate 2** Poster for a welfare center (1937) (Reproduced courtesy of the Mary Evans Picture Library/Bruce Castle Museum.)

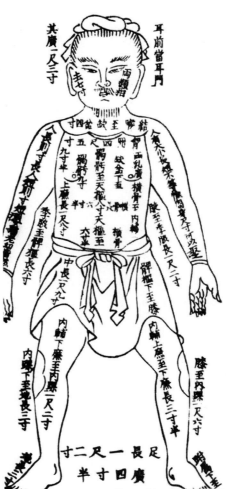

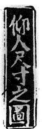

An illustration of a human figure from an early Chinese medical textbook. (Reproduced courtesy of the WHO/National Library of Medicine, Bethesda, MD.)

Medical education is directed by the National Education Commission and the Ministry of Public Health. The management of colleges and universities is under the leadership of a Communist Party committee in a presidential system. The academic committee, degree committee, and committee for administrative affairs of a school or college are consultative organizations for the college president. The length of schooling in colleges and universities is three years for diplomates, five years for bachelors, seven years for masters, and eight years for doctors. There are 10 medical tracks and 57 subjects in colleges and universities. The enrollment is organized by the National Education Commission and students take a common entrance examination. In 1997, for example, there were 70 425 recruits, 61 239 graduates, and 271 137 students in medical college and universities. There were 149 750 recruits, 119 313

(continued)

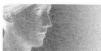

Norman **BETHUNE**
(1890–1939). Chest surgeon
and blood transfusion
pioneer. Sevice as a
stretcher-bearer from August
1914 to April 1915, when his
leg was damaged by shrapnel
at Ypres, was followed by a
return to medical school and
graduation in December
1916. Postgraduate study
was followed by a long spell
of tuberculosis at Saranac,
where he was an early
volunteer for pneumothorax.
At the age of 38 he joined
Professor Edward Archibald at
McGill in thoracic surgery.
With the outbreak of the
Spanish civil war Bethune
took a motorized service of
refrigerated blood to the
front. The Japanese invasion
of China in 1937 so angered
Bethune that he joined the
8th Route Army and by
the time of his death in
November 1939, had become
a legend to the people of
China.

graduates, and 425 225 students in medical secondary schools.

There are clear differences in healthcare financing between cities and rural areas. In cities, the patterns mainly include free medical service (provided by the government), labor insurance, medical insurance for employees, and juvenile and child medical insurance. In 1987 among urban citizens, 16.23% received free medical care; 45.64% had joined labor insurance; 24.18% received other forms of medical services supported by collectively raised money, and 11.95% paid for medical services out of their own pockets. These patterns of healthcare have had important roles in past decades. However, because of the shortage of money and problems in management, healthcare financing is now far from sufficient to meet the ever-increasing healthcare demands. Consequently, in 1994 the government established a new model of healthcare financing in some cities. In this, the medical expenditure of an urban citizen comes from a small portion of the salary and a large portion of public funds. In 1996, the Ministry of Public Health decided to promote this new model in other cities.

## Patterns of financing

Patterns of healthcare financing in rural areas include the predominant cooperative medical care, privately funded care, and other patterns. In the late 1940s, the government established the cooperative financing pattern based on personal need, mutual help, and community support. In the following decades, this was developed along with the agricultural cooperation movement. In this, the individual pays a large portion of the medical costs, the community a small portion, and the government provides necessary instructions and policies. By 1979, cooperative financing had covered more than 90% of villages. However, during the 1980s, this pattern failed to adapt to the rapid social and economic changes and was abolished in most rural areas of China. In 1989, only 4.8% of villages still maintained this pattern. In 1990, the coverage slowly rose to 10%. Only in the last few years has the cooperative financing pattern regained the government's attention. This occurred because of the reappearance of some problems (for example, bankruptcy of farmers because of illness) and the resurgence of some diseases once extinct or well controlled. Thus, the re-establishment and promotion of a rural cooperative medical care financing system have taken place. By the end of 1995, 64.2% of villages and 56.6% of the rural population in Jiangsu Province had joined cooperative financing. In Henan Province about 17% of population in 58 countries participated in the pattern. The government expects that by 2010,

the coverage of cooperative financing will reach 80% in rural areas of China.

## Leading public health problems

*Infectious diseases* Although the morbidity and mortality of infectious diseases in China have been remarkably reduced, the incidence of some infections remains high. The overall incidence of infectious diseases is above 500 per 100 000 people and the estimated number of patients is over 10 million. All of the diseases covered by the Expanded Program on Immunization have been effectively controlled. However, the control of other diseases has not been satisfactory. In fact, since many risk factors have not been eliminated, many new epidemics may occur in the future. A good example is the hepatitis A epidemic in Shanghai in early 1988, in which over 300 000 persons were infected within several months.

China is a high risk area for viral hepatitis. Hepatitis A, B, and C are widespread throughout the country, with a total incidence of over 1000 per 100 000 people. AIDS has also become a threat to China since its first identification in Beijing in 1985. In March 1998, the cumulative number of known HIV infections was 9960; however, experts estimated that the actual number of HIV infections in China exceeded 300 000, and was rapidly spreading.

*Parasitic diseases* The common types of parasitic diseases are schistosomiasis, malaria, filariasis, leishmaniasis, and hydatid disease, all of which are widespread throughout the country. At least 1 million people are suffering from schistosomiasis, and the disease is out of control in over 100 counties.

*Non-infectious diseases* There has been a gradual yet obvious change in the causes of mortality in China since the mid-1970s, now strikingly similar to those in developed countries. This is especially true in cities. Over 70% of deaths can now be attributed to non-infectious diseases such as HYPERTENSION, stroke, coronary heart disease, cancer, and DIABETES, all on the rise. In 1995, as many as 25.1% of urban citizens had one or more types of chronic disease. In rural areas, the percentage was 9%. Each year there are 1.34 million new cases of cancer and over 1.5 million people suffer a stroke.

*Endemic diseases* Endemic diseases are widely distributed all over the country, with perhaps the greatest diversity in the world. In rural areas, over 65% of counties have one or more types of endemic diseases, with the total number of patients around 36 million. In the whole country, more than 400 million people are now facing the threat of endemic diseases. At present, about 510 million people are living in iodine-deficient areas, almost one half of the global total.

*Occupational diseases* The main occupational diseases include pneumoconiosis, poisoning, and physical injury. Because of poor working conditions and the lack of effective protection, the prevalence of occupational diseases has been rising rapidly in recent years. Nearly 20 million workers still work in harmful environments, which are present in at least 700 000 enterprises throughout the country.

*Unhealthy life-style* Smoking has been steadily increasing in recent years, especially in the young. Among middle school students, 34% of boys and 4% of girls smoke. ALCOHOL consumption has also increased since the 1980s, as has alcohol dependence, with the age of the onset becoming younger.

*Population aging* A large population over 60 years old has emerged in many big cities and economically developed rural areas. In 2000, the total number of people over 60 was 130 million and made up 10% of the country's population. Nearly 30% of the aged are in poor health. Hypertension, coronary heart disease, chronic bronchitis, stroke, cancer, diabetes mellitus, and benign prostatic hypertrophy pose serious threats to the elderly, which at present make up 8% of the total population. KZ, YX, MLiu

*See also* HEALTHCARE SYSTEMS

**CHIROPRACTIC** Chiropractic originated in the United States, developed in 1895 by Daniel David Palmer, a lay healer. According to Palmer's philosophy of health, all living beings are endowed with what he called 'innate intelligence' (vital force), and this intelligence regulates all the vital functions of the body as it flows through the central nervous system. Palmer believed that correcting misalignments or subluxations of the spine enabled the nervous system to work optimally, and that the innate intelligence could then carry out its role of maintaining the body's health and equilibrium.

Chiropractors are also trained in separate colleges of higher education and are required to complete a full-time 4–5 year course. They are statutorily registered in Britain and in various States across the USA. They co-exist peacefully and constructively with the body of British medicine, but have had several dramatic and confrontational battles with the conventional medical profession in the USA. While most chiropractors are exclusively focused on the techniques of manual medicine, some see themselves as offering a broadly based complementary practice that

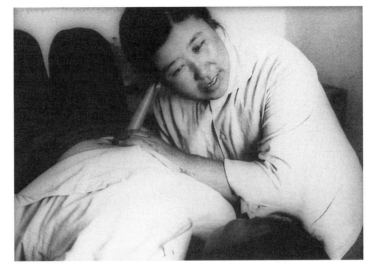

involves prescribing homeopathic and nutritional products, and indeed some who seem to adhere to Daniel Palmer's views that many ills can be diagnosed and cured by examination and manipulation of the spine.

There are various manipulative methods and techniques. These include manipulation of the soft tissues of the body; passive, gentle, and repetitive movement of a joint through its range of movement to free it from restrictions; a high-velocity, low-amplitude thrusting movement, or a low-velocity, high-amplitude, repetitive type of manipulation of joints; moving the affected part in the opposite direction to the

An old-style 'barefoot' doctor listens to the heartbeat of the unborn child. (Reproduced courtesy of the WHO/National Library of Medicine, Bethesda, MD.)

A chiropractor treats a patient. (Reproduced courtesy of the British Chiropractic Association.)

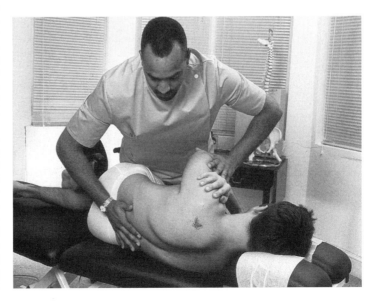

limitation of movement to relieve restricted tissues; contracting and stretching of muscles, and gentle manipulation of the bony structures of the cranium. In many conditions, particularly low back pain, there is overwhelming evidence that these approaches appear to be effective in both the short and long term. A characteristic shared by many chiropractors is manifest interest in their patients as individuals. They take pains to get to know their patients to a far greater extent than many orthodox medical practitioners.

GL

*See also* COMPLEMENTARY AND ALTERNATIVE MEDICINE

**CHRISTIAN SCIENCE** See RELIGIOUS SECTS

**CHURCH OF JESUS CHRIST OF THE LATTER DAY SAINTS (MORMONS)** See RELIGIOUS SECTS

**CIRCUMCISION** In males, circumcision is surgical removal of the prepuce or foreskin of the penis. As part of a coming of age ceremony or a religious rite, it dates back to preliterate neolithic society if not further into antiquity. It is still practiced in some tribal societies, for example, in New Guinea, with that connotation. Circumcision is performed as a religious ritual on the 8th day of life by the Jews, and usually in later infancy or childhood at varying ages before adolescence by Muslims. It is performed among Christians in some countries such as the USA and Australia, on a high proportion of male infants because of a belief that it enhances sexual hygiene, and because it has become customary (so sons must look like their fathers); but the medical and epidemiological evidence of the benefits versus the harms of the procedure is increasingly debated.

Female circumcision, or female genital mutilation, is different. This is a ritual procedure, grounded in tribal customs that appear to have originated in East Africa. It is practiced mainly in Egypt and African countries from Somalia and the Sudan to Sierra Leone and Kenya and among immigrants from these countries in Europe and North America.

### Genital mutilation

Genital mutilation is not related to or associated with any particular religion: it is performed on girls who are nominally Christian, Moslem, or believers in traditional African religions, mainly but not exclusively in rural villages. The custom is perpetuated as much by the women who have had this done to them as by their menfolk, fostered by their belief that no man will marry a girl without this proof of her virginity and purity.

Female genital mutilation may be classified according to the severity of the operation. It ranges from a minor procedure, an incision in the clitoral hood without loss of tissue, to a radical operation that includes amputation of the clitoris and labia minora, wide excision of much of the labia majora, and suturing of the raw surfaces to leave only a small hole for passage of urine and menstrual fluid.

Incision of the clitoral hood is a comparatively innocuous coming of age ritual for sophisticated urban girls, for example, in Nairobi. The incision is just enough to draw blood to provide proof that it has been done. In many other places where the custom survives it is a barbarous procedure. In cultures where the most extreme form of female genital mutilation is practiced, the operation is commonly performed on small girls aged from 2 to 10 years without anesthetic or antiseptics, so pain, shock, hemorrhage, and infection are severe, and death is not uncommon.

Survivors experience no pleasure and much pain on sexual intercourse, and childbirth may be very hazardous for both mother and infant. Obstructed labor may severely damage the bladder and rectum, not uncommonly with fistula formation and urinary and/or fecal incontinence. The foul smells resulting from this may lead to ostracizing of the woman or to her expulsion from the community. Safe delivery usually requires wide incision of the introitus. Other complications of radical female genital mutilation include keloid scars that deform the perineal region and chronic infection of the bladder and kidneys.

Despite western abhorrence for the practice, legal sanctions against it, resolutions against it by the World Health Assembly of WHO, and efforts to educate women about the harm it does, traditions in some cultures ensure that female genital mutilation continues to be perpetrated on several million girls every year in societies where it persists into the 21st century. These include not only the African countries where the custom originated but also immigrant groups from these countries in western Europe and North America.

JML

**CLINICAL CHEMISTRY** also called clinical biochemistry, chemical pathology, or biochemical medicine, is a branch of laboratory based investigative medicine. It arose from the physician's desire to enhance the clinical history and examination by more objective criteria, one of the earliest examples being the recognition of the sweetness evident in the urine of patients with DIABETES MELLITUS. Glucose is a reducing substance, and the chemists had a reagent (Benedict's reagent) which is precipitated by these substances,

# THE GREAT KILLERS: CHOLERA

Cholera is an acute bacterial infection (caused by *Vibrio cholerae* — a non-invasive bacterium called a vibrio or the 'comma bacillus') involving the small intestine. A disease clinically resembling (but not proved to be) cholera was described by early Indian, Greek, and Chinese writers. Alternative names are Asiatic, epidemic, or malignant cholera; the name (in English) is derived from *choler* (1561). The toxin, or poison, of this bacterium, when present at high concentration, produces a flow (secretion) of fluid and salts into the lumen of the intestine; this results in watery diarrhea which may be torrential (up to 20 litres in 24 hours) and rapidly causes severe dehydration.

Foci of infection have existed (and been endemic) for many centuries in south-east Asia. The 'natural home' of the infection seems to lie in the Ganges plain and delta; traditionally, the spread occurred along caravan and other trade routes. In the early 19th century, the infection broke loose from Asia and traveled in epidemic form along trade routes to many European and north American countries; six pandemics occurred between 1817 and 1923. Major epidemics ('Asiatic cholera') occurred in Britain in 1831–2, 1848–9, and 1853–4; less important ones were recorded in 1868 and 1893. Many thousands of people in several major cities were smitten by the disease. Contemporary accounts differentiated it from a milder diarrheal illness, to which the name cholera was also applied. Although the overall mortality was far less than that from earlier plague epidemics or other illnesses such as tuberculosis at the time, the rapidity with which the disease might take effect (within a few hours of the onset of symptoms) and the mystery surrounding its origin(s) (the miasmatic theory — bad air — of causation of disease reigned supreme) caused great national (and international) alarm. Between 1898 and 1907, 370 000 deaths were caused by this infection in India. The seventh pandemic (caused by the *El Tor* variant) began in 1961. In the 1980s the infection spread widely (predominantly in crowded refugee camps and city slums of famine-stricken countries) in African countries; Ethiopia and Sudan were particularly severely affected. By mid-1991 cholera was common in south and central America. Despite recognition of the cause of this infection and an understanding of appropriate management (see below), cholera continues to be a major source of death and disease in the world's developing countries.

A causative relationship with fecally-contaminated drinking water was strongly suggested on epidemiologic grounds by John SNOW (p 48) (and the Reverend Henry Whitehead) working in London's Soho. According to legend, removal of the handle from the Broad Street pump (from which the local populace derived its drinking-water supply) halted the 1854 epidemic in that locality but in fact the epidemic had already begun to decline. The causative organism, *V. cholerae* was discovered by Robert KOCH (p 455) while he was working in Egypt, in 1883.

## Types of organism

*V. cholerae* (which is killed by heating for 15 min) exists as several types: *V. cholerae* 01 (the cause of classic cholera); the *El Tor* variant (first isolated in 1906 at the El Tor quarantine station at Sinai); and *V. cholerae* 0139 (which first appeared in southern India in 1992 and has already found an ecological niche in the ponds, lakes, and rivers of Bangladesh). The *El Tor* variant may survive for longer periods in the environment compared with the classic organism; on the other hand, the former organism causes fewer clinical cases. Only in Bangladesh do the classical and *El Tor* variants co-exist today. The first outbreak to be caused by *V. cholerae* 0139 was recorded in Madras in October 1992; in December of that year, this organism was responsible for an outbreak of the disease in southern Bangladesh, and by April 1993 it had spread to Thailand. Other vibrio species also cause acute diarrheal disease in tropical countries; only on rare occasions have they been associated with extensive outbreaks.

Infection is caused by ingestion of the organism(s) through contaminated water or food (there is no animal reservoir of infection); the incubation period ranges from a few hours to five days. The dehydration, imbalance of salts in the body (with low blood concentrations of sodium and potassium), acidosis, and reduced blood volume consequent upon the acute watery diarrhea, may result in kidney failure — with a mortality rate ranging from 3 to 40%. Low blood pressure and a low blood glucose concentration are further

*(continued overleaf)*

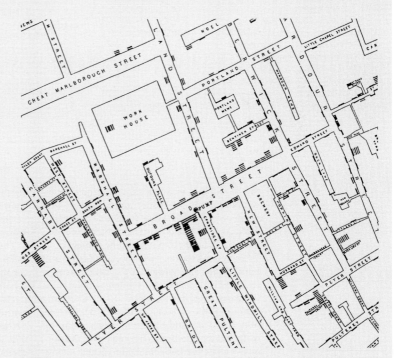

A spot map showing the location of cases of cholera in the epidemic in London in 1854. (From Snow, J. (1855). *On the mode of communication of cholera*, Churchill, London.)

*(continued)*

features. Vomiting, muscular cramps, and intense thirst follow; in a severe case, the affected person has by then become stuporous and comatose. As with all infective illnesses, a wide spectrum of levels of severity exists; 5–40% of people infected remain either without symptoms or only with mild ones. Unlike the causative agents of the 'enteric fevers' (typhoid and paratyphoid), persistent carriers of *V. cholerae* are extremely unusual.

Epidemiologically, in endemic areas of Bangladesh the infection shows seasonal peaks following monsoons; this phenomenon is considered to be related to an increase in growth of algae in saline, estuarine areas — after a monsoon. *V. cholerae* and zooplankton form a symbiotic relationship that enables the pathogen to survive indefinitely in contaminated water. National disasters, political upheaval, and refugee movements may spread the infection to new areas. The disease is not infrequently associated with cyclones and floods.

Diagnosis in endemic areas is usually presumptive. Under the microscope fecal specimens may show characteristic vibrios; bacteriological culture is required for confirmatory diagnosis.

Management consists first and foremost of rapid rehydration — usually by mouth (using an oral rehydration fluid); only in exceptional cases is an intravenous drip (first advocated in the 1831–2 outbreak) necessary. Most oral rehydration fluid preparations contain glucose to enhance the absorption of salt. Sucrose and rice-water-based solutions have also been used

successfully. Intravenous glucose may be required to counteract low blood glucose levels in children. The antibiotics tetracycline and doxycycline reduce the duration of diarrhea and excretion of *V. cholerae*; however, the organism may rapidly become resistant in an epidemic. Co-trimoxazole and furazolidone have also been used in individual cases.

Public health measures are required for long-term control; chlorination of water supplies, boiling of water (in households), and construction and maintenance of temporary latrines are imperative. Safe fecal disposal is also essential. Vaccines have no useful role in an outbreak; individual protection is not above 50–60%. Effective surveillance (with

identification of affected cases) is an essential component of cholera control. New vaccines (using genetic engineering techniques) are undergoing clinical trials; they may contribute to effective control of an infection which is likely (given experience in South America) to remain of considerable importance in tropical countries for many years to come. Infection with the classic organism gives no protection against *V. cholerae* 0139; a high attack rate of the latter in adults has recently been recorded in an epidemic in the Indian subcontinent.

GCCoo

*See also* CHANGING PATTERNS OF DISEASE IN THE 20TH CENTURY; INFECTIOUS DISEASES; WATER

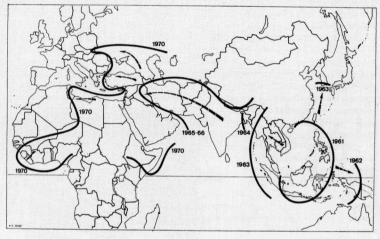

The spread of cholera, 1960–70.

the color of the precipitate depending on the concentration present. Other urinary tests were developed, of which testing for significant quantities of protein was of particular importance as a potential indicator of disease of the kidney.

For various reasons, urinary examination is of limited value and, given that the main carrier of (bio)chemically important substances is the blood (anticoagulated whole blood or its fluid after removal of the cells by centrifugation), devising tests based on known chemical reactions for many substances was the inevitable next development, with other body fluids (in particular, cerebrospinal fluid) following on. As the tests became increasingly used, the additional burden on ward-based staff became onerous, and small laboratories were set up to take over some of the chemical testing, the first in Britain being at St Thomas's Hospital in London. As parallel developments

were occurring in HEMATOLOGY and bacteriology (now MICROBIOLOGY), these laboratories tended to embrace the group of disciplines under the name of clinical pathology.

Thus, clinical chemistry may be defined as the estimation (assay) of (bio) chemical substances (or their components), including pharmacologic agents (drugs) and/or their breakdown products, in body fluids. Changes in the concentrations may be due to an increase or a decrease of those normally found, or appearance of a substance not normally found. The clinical chemist has to know the levels in **health** before he can understand the levels in **disease**. This is easy when a substance is virtually absent in health, for example, the overflow of derivatives of the amino acid, phenylalanine, into the urine of infants with one of the INBORN ERRORS OF METABOLISM known as phenylketonuria. Most substances measured to aid the diagnosis and/or treatment of disease are present in health, and these levels are defined by their so-called normal or reference range. These ranges are not absolute and, like biological variables such as height, they tend to conform to a Gaussian distribution. To complicate matters, some distributions are skewed. Reference ranges are wider than some might expect owing partly to biological variation, which includes such things as race, age, diet, sex, and posture. This has two components, individual (variation in glucose concentration during the day due to the ingestion of food is an obvious example) and inter-individual variation within the population being studied.

## Analytical variation

In addition, there is a laboratory component, analytical variation. This is affected by the way in which a specimen is taken and its subsequent handling, and thereafter by laboratory factors, which consist of:

- within-batch variation — repeated measurements of the same sample will show a Gaussian distribution, the curve being sharp with a narrow base for easily measureable substances present in large amounts and low and wide for substances difficult to measure and/or present in small quantities

- between-batch variation, in which factors such as small differences in reagents, equipment behavior, and the analyst's technique come into play. To assess the validity of a result, the clinical chemist must take account of both types of variation and has had to develop techniques which will not only indicate the degree of confidence to be placed upon the laboratory results, but will also assist in improving analytical performance.

One method of achieving this quality control is to send a sample from a designated center containing one or more analytes to all laboratories and feeding back a consensus value and other statistical data, which provide a long-term measure of performance. Another is including a sample of known analyte content with each batch of assays to obtain a measure of day-to-day performance. Measurement of an analyte (often referred to as a test) also has to take account of how specific it is as an indicator of disease and how sensitive it is. A high specificity means that only a small percentage of patients free of the disease in question would have an abnormal result, and a high sensitivity is when virtually all patients with the disease have an abnormal result. It follows that interpretation of results is no simple matter. Single measurements of one or more analytes is often inadequate, and it may be necessary to assay the analyte(s) over a period to follow changes in parallel with changes in the course of the illness.

## Enzyme activities

This can be exemplified by the measurement of the activity of an enzyme released into the blood after damage to an appreciable number of cells of an organ; the muscle cells of the heart contain important enzymes (biological catalysts of the vital reactions occurring within living organisms), for example, creatine kinase is released from heart muscle after the cutting off of the blood supply to part of the heart (a so-called heart attack). The enzymic activity in the blood rises rapidly, giving a peak usually in the first 24 hours and is usually back to normal after 72 hours. Another device is to cause change in an analyte level by stimulating a physiologic response and determining whether the response is appropriate. Examples are administration of glucose and then following the changes in blood and urine levels with time as a test for diabetes mellitus (the glucose tolerance test), and testing of an endocrine gland's ability to produce a hormone (another important mediator of cellular activity), for example, stimulation of the cortical hormones of the adrenal gland by administration of the anterior pituitary hormone, adrenocorticotrophic hormone, to assess the functioning of the cortical part of that gland. It will now be apparent that clinical chemistry covers a wide range of aspects and may make an important contribution to patient care. The hazards in interpreting the results show that it is, at best, an inexact science, and, if the results are inconsistent with the clinical findings, it has to be remembered the patient is always right and the clinician and/or the laboratory must think again.

## Growth of clinical chemistry

The growth of clinical chemistry was slow at first, and shortly after the Second World War an analyte such as blood glucose in major centers might be assayed in twice weekly batches. As the value of laboratory investigation, the development of new tests, and improvements in assays grew, problems of space and training new staff to be *au fait* with all the components of clinical pathology arose, and the individual subjects increasingly became relatively independent of each other. More and more analytes were requested daily, and inevitably for some of them they were sought out of hours leading to the need for an emergency service, albeit with a limited repertoire. By the mid-1950s the load for commonly requested assays such as glucose, urea, and the so-called electrolytes (sodium, potassium, chloride, and bicarbonate — important in monitoring cardiac failure, renal disease, and control of

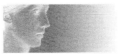
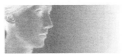

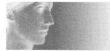
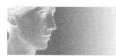
postoperative fluid replacement among others) was becoming too great to handle, particularly as they involved the use of cumbersome and temperamental equipment. This led to the development of new equipment to mechanize and speed up assays. In 1957, Skeggs in the United States introduced his continuous flow system, which was developed by the Technicon Corporation as the AutoAnalyzer. Initially modules were introduced to assay a single analyte, but it was not long before multichannel machines appeared which would assay twelve or more analytes on a single sample. Numerous other machines appeared on the market, some of which allowed batch analysis of specific analytes, using alternative sets of reagents for different assays; others were developed with an emphasis on smaller and smaller samples; and others to cover new assays being added to the standard repertoire. A notable example of the so-called discrete approach was the centrifugal analyzer, which speeded up reactions by carrying them out during centrifugation and required only small quantities of both sample and reagents.

### Growth in demand

Growth in demand has two components: more frequent use of existing assays and the arrival of suitable methods for measurement of clinically important substances. From the early days of half a dozen different tests, the list has grown to nearer 100 incorporating markers of all aspects of metabolism, from inherited disorders to diseases of major organs such as the liver and systems such as the endocrine system. Thus, the laboratory is faced with measurement of a huge variety of substances from the inorganic to the organic; the activity of biological catalysts (enzymes), hormones and their products; and many drugs and their metabolites. A teaching hospital laboratory, which measured its workload in hundreds per annum in the early 1950s, might have been undertaking over a million by the 1980s.

As so often happens, the solution to one set of problems leads to the appearance of new ones. For example, the multichannel analyzers were seen as having a potential for detecting symptomless disease as health screening became popular. Problems of interpretation were mentioned earlier, but if twelve analytes are measured on a single sample and 90% confidence intervals set for trying to differentiate between a normal and abnormal result it is apparent that by chance alone at least one analyte in the specimen is likely to fall outside those limits. Screening of this type, or even more targeted screening of specific populations such as the screening of infants for phenylketonuria, can be misleading unless the

tests used enjoy high specificity and sensitivity. Another problem was the need on rare occasions for an analyte which required uncommon and expensive equipment and/or particular expertise. Very small batches carried out infrequently are particularly prone to error, and for this and economic reasons designated centers had to be set up to carry out the assays — leading to an improvement in analytical reliability, but sometimes a delay in availability of the results. A different sort of problem results from the huge growth in testing.

There are three phases in any clinical laboratory's activity: the receiving of the sample (sometimes its collection as well), and being sure the sample is correctly identified so that the right sample is analyzed for a given patient and that the right results are attached to it; the actual analysis; and finally the reporting of the result to the clinician. Reports get mislaid or lost on occasions, so the laboratory also needs to keep a record for clinical, if no other, purposes. The value of serial results referred to earlier led to a desire for cumulative reports. In larger centers especially, data handling by traditional manual methods collapsed. Fortunately, by this time the mini-computer, as opposed to big mainframe systems, had appeared on the scene, so that in the late 1960s development and implementation of computer systems became yet another task for the clinical chemist. Reading the results from the Auto-Analyzer had become a tedious, and error-prone task, and the obvious next step was to use computers to do this as well. Refinements such as carrying out any necessary additional calculations and monitoring machines' analytical performance against internal quality control samples run at intervals during a batch of assays were soon to follow. The efficiency and productivity of the laboratories, although very commendable, are now in danger of overloading the clinician with data, with inherent risks of a vital result being overlooked. Furthermore, they have become very expensive to equip and operate, even despite some reduction in manpower after extensive automation.

The normal functioning of the cells, and hence the total organism, is disrupted in many diseases and the indicators, although many do not always produce a specific pattern of change. Monitoring and correcting the changes are vital after acute and severe threat to the integrity of the organism, for example, after major trauma, whether accidental or deliberate as in extensive surgery. Circulating concentrations of many substances reflect what is happening at cellular level. Cells cannot function properly without water or with either excess or inadequate concentrations of sodium and potassium; cells can operate properly only at or near physiologic hydrogen ion concentration (expressed as pH); adequate oxygen transport is essential. These critical factors are usually assessed as part of a group of tests: electrolytes and blood gases. Markers of organ function include urea and creatinine for the kidney; bilirubin, various proteins, and alkaline phosphatase for the liver; and measurement of their specific hormones with or without preliminary stimulation for the hypothalamus, pituitary, thyroid, and adrenal glands, in particular. Calcium, magnesium, phosphate, and alkaline phosphatase levels are measured in bone disease. Fatty substances (lipids, cholesterol, triglycerides, and their carrier proteins, and lipoproteins) give information about fat metabolism, important in assessing cardiovascular disease. High uric acid concentrations are found in gout.

### Inherited diseases

Most inherited diseases arise from a genetically determined absence or modification of a specific protein — excluding hemoglobin (see HEMATOLOGY), the protein is usually an enzyme controlling a synthetic reaction, so that the substance(s) from which the product is formed (substrate) accumulates and the product itself is reduced or even absent. Product, substrate, or enzyme activity may be assayed in body fluids and/or tissues. The consequent disorder in metabolism (amino acid, carbohydrate, lipid etc.) may have profound physical and mental effects, and, although the biochemical markers may be useful diagnostic tools, the emphasis has shifted to chromosomal studies (cytogenetics) and study of the individual genes to elucidate the nature and diagnosis of these conditions. Cancers (malignant tumors) affect many organs and the biochemical disturbances may be demonstrable by some of the markers already mentioned (for example, by spread of the disease into bone), by overproduction by the malignant cells of a secreting organ (such as insulin by pancreatic cells), or appearance in abnormal quantities of a particular protein (for example, alpha fetoprotein in tumors of the liver). Drug concentrations are measured to detect drug abuse or self-poisoning, or to monitor drug treatment to check compliance or achieve optimum therapeutic levels (for example, anti-epileptic drugs).

Clinical chemistry is a dynamic and demanding specialty, and advances elsewhere continue to impact upon it. Chemistry is no longer its base science. Physical, biochemical, immunological, and genetic techniques are now part of its armament. The enormous advances in molecular biology are shedding new light especially in inherited disease, and the ability to determine DNA profiles on minute samples not only of body fluids, but also tissues, adds another dimension. Parallel advances in our understanding of the immune system, and development of techniques to study it, have increasing application to the extent that specific immunological laboratories are not uncommon. Long ago, the chemical tests for phenylketonuria were replaced by a microbiological technique, the Guthrie test. Many hormones now are assayed by immunological methods. Automation and computing have been added. As clinical chemistry splintered from clinical pathology, so genetic and immunology laboratories have emerged. But the sister subjects have been affected by the various advances in a similar fashion, and the demarcation lines between these sub-specialties is becoming increasingly blurred.

Administrators are alarmed at the spiraling costs of the laboratory services, and clinicians are being made aware that unless they modify their demand there will be less money for direct clinical purposes. Already there are moves to bring the pathology disciplines back together, and as the underlying science becomes more complex it is perhaps inevitable that scientists, rather than medically-trained people, will control the laboratories. The other side of the coin is the increasing difficulty for clinicians, faced with continuing advances in their own discipline and an increasing number of patients, to keep abreast of the underlying science in the laboratories to be able to interpret for themselves the reported results. They will have to rely more on laboratory physicians, who, as the hematologists already have, will consequently be less in the laboratory and closer to the patient, whether in the community or hospital. The wheel seems to be turning full circle, and one wonders whether the next edition of this book will even show a separate entry for clinical chemistry. PDG

*See also* LABORATORY MEDICINE; ONCOLOGY; SCREENING

**CLINICAL INVESTIGATION** Most physicians will agree that 'clinical investigation' is the cornerstone of medical progress. However, opinion soon divides when people are asked to define what is meant by the term. Is it just investigation carried out by physicians? Or is it all investigation whose results are immediately applicable at the bedside? Or is it only investigation at the bedside? Or should we say that in modern times it is the same as numerical evidence by epidemiologic and statistical methods?

The father of experimental medicine, Claude BERNARD (p 102), was convinced that most of the time true experiments that showed causality and function could not be applied to patients — laboratory studies in animals were needed to see what an

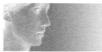
organ's function was. In his 1865 treatise on the principles of experimental medicine, however, he wrote that physicians could usefully apply pathophysiologic reasoning at the bedside, by mere observation. Observation was to him not just the haphazard collection of facts. It had the same rigor as experiments: one should think beforehand what observations were needed to prove what point, and then search where to find such observations. For example, a patient's illness could disclose something about the workings of an organ or organ system. The big division between observation and experiment was that the latter entailed a purposeful intervention to improve learning, while observation did not. Nevertheless, physicians could usefully mimic laboratory experiments by exploiting pathophysiologic 'accidents', and from time to time also by intervention. This logic of Claude Bernard was the basis of almost all clinical investigation in the first half of the twentieth century.

In his 1930s treatises on clinical research, the British cardiologist, Sir Thomas LEWIS (this page), incorporated the teaching of Claude Bernard into a wider vision. He accepted gracefully all the results of the studies in experimental medicine, but professed that by itself it was not sufficient, especially if it meant that the only worthwhile investigation was physiology on laboratory animals. Lewis delineated how all problems worthy of investigation in medicine are first found by observations at the bedside. Such observations are not only physiological, but may also have to do with signs and symptoms, with potential etiology (observing transmission), and heredity (observing familial patterns). Thereafter the problems might be taken to the laboratory — physiological, microbiological, or otherwise — even though the driving force of the investigation should remain clinical. Ultimately the results of either process, bedside or laboratory, should be applied and tested on a few patients at the bedside again. The first and the last part of this cycle, in which most modern physicians still believe, is certainly clinical investigation — but, again, what is its nature today?

Two things changed in the second half of this century. Firstly, pathophysiologic thinking about whole organs or organ systems, guided by bedside observation, ceased to be regarded as the seat of innovation in medicine. It was replaced by research, first at the cellular and later at the molecular level, usually called 'basic science'. This became more remote from the bedside, and at the same time it became unclear what 'clinical investigation' was. Did the mere fact that some leukemic cells came from a patient and that the chief of hematology was still the chief of the lab, make all consequent molecular investigation 'clinical'? Or was that only worthy of the name when the

molecular investigation tried to elucidate the mechanism of something that was observed in a patient? Or when the results might be applied to patients? Were clinical observations, apart from the crude overall fact that the patient had leukemia, still the driving force of these investigations?

The story of the discovery of the first 'molecular disease', sickle cell anemia, is sometimes told as if it had resulted from a sudden insight of biochemical genius. However, the story has some deeper roots. Before the molecular biologists could start their research, the disease first needed to be defined. Even if sickle cell anemia had probably existed for many thousands of years, its original description, first clinical genetic hints, and first crude laboratory observation (the transformation of red blood cells into sickle shapes when the oxygen concentration is reduced) came at the beginning of the 20th century. Only later could molecular biology step in: the problem was presented on a plate, and then the latter science added its genius. Almost all the success stories in molecular biology, whether in cystic fibrosis or the successive mutations that give rise to cancer of the colon from colonic polyps, are more or less similar. Academic physicians have adapted to the first new paradigm of the times: they have incorporated molecular biology in their research strategies, as an extension of the age-old pathophysiologic reasoning at the bedside.

### 'Numerical reasoning'

There was also a second change, however: the 'ascendancy of numerical reasoning'. The irony is that its original roots in medicine were older than Bernard's pathophysiologic thinking. '*La méthode numérique*' was introduced into the clinic in Paris in the 1830s by Pierre Charles Alexandre LOUIS (p 780). Even more ironic, this approach met with staunch opposition, firstly from clinicians, who thought that it would deal only with averages and disclose nothing about individual patients. Later, Claude Bernard became a strong opponent, given his ideas of experimental medicine, which looked for mechanisms and causes in carefully controlled animal experiments: numerical averages, he argued, would teach us nothing. Bernard even opposed the calculation of 'average values' on 24-hour urine specimens, stating that only the variation during the day (resulting from metabolic variation in other organ systems) would teach us something. Bernard cited with much approval the viewpoint of a chemist in Holland: that numerical reasoning amounted to watching how many people walk into a house and how much smoke comes out of the chimney. Such mere correlations would not teach us anything about causation.

Times have changed. While the opposition by Bernard and others was certainly successful in keeping numerical reasoning in clinical investigation out of sight for about a century, numerical reasoning came back in full force in the middle of 20th century. Firstly, there was the ascendancy of the randomized trial. Later, there was the rebirth of epidemiologic and statistical reasoning in clinical medicine, in studies of diagnosis, prognosis, and etiology (such as the link between cigarette smoking and lung cancer). Numerical reasoning has become the corner-stone of the type of clinical investigation that has led to EVIDENCE-BASED MEDICINE. It corresponds to the last part of Thomas Lewis's cycle: the application at the bedside that should finally show whether the new insights from the laboratory are worth anything. Today such investigations are fully guided by the numerical methods for which Louis originally planted the seeds.

Clinical investigation is nowadays richer than ever. It still starts with bedside observation, coupled to first laboratory insights on specimens taken directly from the patient and the first clues on the likely etiology. For example, the first papers on the acquired immunodeficiency syndrome (AIDS), published in a single issue of the *New England Journal of Medicine*, in 1981, already held almost all the seeds of what was to come later: the baffling immunodeficiency — somewhat like immunodeficiency caused by cytotoxic drugs but without any apparent cause; the epidemic nature of the disease; and the hints at the nature of transmission. After these initial observations work in the laboratory, by basic scientists, identified the virus causing the condition, determined its genetic make up, showed how it produced its efforts, and began work on specific drug treatment. Though no cure is in sight, such work has already improved the quality and length of lives of patients, and pointed the way to preventing the disease altogether.                          JPV

**CLINICAL TRIAL** See RANDOMIZED CONTROLLED TRIAL

## CLINICOPATHOLOGICAL CONFERENCE

This is a case conference at which the presentation and discussion of the clinical features and diagnosis precede description of the pathologic findings, the latter often based on the AUTOPSY. Although the conference may refer to a seminar in a hospital, the term is now often applied to the transcript of medical grand rounds and has achieved its world-wide popularity because of its publication in journals, such as the *New England Journal of Medicine*.

The earliest form of clinicopathological conference, that is, the first attempt at correlating clinical symptoms and signs with anatomic lesions, was the *De Sedibus et causis morborum per anatomen indagatis* written by Giovanni MORGAGNI (p 621) in 1761. Much later, around 1900, Walter CANNON (this page) at Harvard Medical School realized that didactic lectures in medical schools had their limitations and were a 'dreary and benumbing process'. He adapted the case system form of teaching from Professor Christopher Langdell, who had used them at the Harvard Law School in the 1870s. Based on a lecture Cannon delivered and an article he wrote in the *Boston Medical and Surgical Journal*, this system of teaching was introduced in Harvard Medical School. The conference as we know it today, is essentially the result of efforts by a clinician, Richard CABOT (p 190), who himself learned the approach from Cannon.

Cabot wrote books with case histories followed by a questionnaire on diagnosis, treatment, and prognosis, with the idea of presenting medicine in terms that would make readers think and to solve puzzles such as those that confronted them at the bedside. On realizing that clinicians were either unaware of or were uninterested in the differences between their clinical diagnoses and the post-mortem diagnoses, Cabot (along with the pathologist James Homer Wright) initiated weekly conferences in the Massachusetts General Hospital in 1910. Here, a clinician evaluated a patient whom he had seen before and tried to arrive at a diagnosis based on a logically thought out process. This was followed by the pathologist who described the post-mortem findings, which confirmed or negated the diagnosis. Such conferences were well attended and were so popular that from 1915 physicians around the world were sent printed versions of the discussions. The *Boston Medical and Surgical Journal* (later renamed the *New England Journal of Medicine*) started publishing a weekly report from the 12 July 1924 issue, which has continued almost without interruption. Since then numerous journals and hospitals have published or conducted such conferences as an educational tool or as a means of maintaining audit.

The main participants are the expert physician and a pathologist together with other specialists, postgraduate students, and undergraduate medical students. There are three sections in the published version of the clinicopathological conference. Firstly, the details of the clinical history and physical examination, followed by the laboratory and imaging investigations are stated. Next, the expert elaborates the various differential diagnoses for that particular patient. One by one, possible diagnoses are eliminated, with a detailed explanation. At the end, the working clinical diagnosis as well as the expert's opinion is stated. The pathologist has the final word as he expands on the gross and microscopic findings and the final diagnosis.

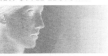

FOUNDER OF CPCs

Richard Clarke **CABOT** (1868–1939). American physician and sociologist. Cabot practiced in Boston on the staff of the Massachusetts General Hospital. His textbook of physical diagnosis was widely used and went through many editions. Cabot discovered 'ring bodies' in the erythrocytes of patients with anemia. He inaugurated the CLINICOPATHOLOGICAL CONFERENCE as a teaching exercise at his hospital. He became increasingly concerned with ethical and social aspects of medical practice and introduced the first social service department in an American hospital.

The conference has undergone minor changes with time. The findings of laboratory investigations and imaging are now given more importance compared with the emphasis on clinical findings in the past. Whereas the autopsy provided the final diagnosis in about 90% of cases in 1934, the corresponding figure was only 5% in 1994 — a result of better medicine and technology. Conventionally, however, the conference has ended with the diagnosis, a reflection of the times when diagnosis was all that mattered and treatment options were often limited and were empirical. Nowadays, the focus of discussion may also be on a special feature of the disease or some aspect, which may be of particular interest.

**Detective story**

The clinicopathological conference is the quintessential medical 'whodunit', with the physician playing detective. Faced with a maze of facts, some apparently insignificant, he has to link them together in sequence to arrive at a correct or reasonable diagnosis. Thus the conference depicts the logical chain of thought in the clinician's mind. There is no place for guesswork. Moreover, the clinicopathological conference illustrates only the scientific method of medicine and does not usually include softer aspects such as humor, ethics, or the history of medicine. In fact, a major criticism has been that these conferences are divorced from the humanistic and socio-economic aspects of disease and hence are artificial and theatrical. Its proponents, however, argue that the *raison d'être* of the conference is to illustrate the scientific aspects. Further, they point out that management of disease is based on the foundation stone of a proper diagnosis.

Selection of cases is of utmost importance. They must be neither run-of-the-mill, nor exotic cases which are unlikely to be seen again by the practicing doctor. Rather, they should pose a broad spectrum of differential diagnosis and stimulate thinking as well as impart information. Diagnosis is based on deduction and appropriate analysis of the facts at hand. The physician in the drama, by explaining the rationale behind his thinking, educates students and qualified physicians alike about the approach to a diagnosis as well as the salient features of the pertinent diseases.

Part of the appeal of the clinicopathological conference is that the reader has exactly the same facts as has the participating physician and hence can match his wits with the physician. Thus the conference reveals the interplay of clinical symptoms and anatomic/pathologic findings and teaches the art of thinking. Since the physician has to draw on his common sense and experience, in addition to a sound knowledge of disease, the conference has

served as an excellent teaching tool, emphasizing the importance of a well-taken medical history and investigation. As a form of continuing medical education, it is unparalleled.                    SAP

*See also* EDUCATION; GRAND ROUNDS; JOURNALS; PATHOLOGY

**COINS AND MEDALS** Medical numismatics is the study of coinage and medallary portraying health themes. Preserved in memorials as lasting as bronze are the portraits of doctors and medical scientists; records of great medical discoveries; commemorative events, such as the opening of hospitals and research institutions; and medallic prizes awarded by learned medical bodies. The international medical numismatic collection now exceeds 5000 different issues.

Any individual or organization may issue a medal. Yet numismatics has never reached any consensus on a concise definition of a medal. The name derives from the Latin *metallium*, meaning metal. Most coins are metal, but obviously coins are not medals. While any person is free to create a medal, governments universally reject the private manufacturer of coins. Hence medical subjects on coins are uncommon, governments remaining conservative in selecting only the most worthy medical practitioners and medical discoveries to be honored. One such example is Jan van Riebeeck, surgeon and founder (in 1652) of Cape Town. Millions of coins bearing his effigy circulated in southern Africa in the 20th century. Another example is the A$1 coin, issued in 1998 to commemorate the centenary of the birth of Lord FLOREY (p 52), a discoverer of the clinical effects of penicillin. Other coins of medical interest are the braille-embossed coins issued by Italy to facilitate the transactions of the visually impaired; and those issued to commemorate medical institutions of particular national significance, for example, the A$5 coin issued in 1998 to commemorate 70 years of the Royal FLYING DOCTOR Service. The intermediate between coins and medals are coin 'look-alikes', called tokens, almost always of metal and given as receipts. They might be reused as quasi-currency and medical themes abound. Examples include the 'touch-pieces' awarded by the British Sovereign, following the Monarch's 'laying-on-of hands', to cure the KING'S EVIL (tuberculosis) in suppliants who were chosen each year. Another poignant example are the coin receipts issued by The Foundling Hospital, London, from 1754, as an anonymous receipt to destitute mothers driven to leave their infants in a basket at the corner of Guilford Street and Lamb's Conduit Street.

In contrast, many medals record medical themes. Anybody is free to create a medal; and, relieved of the rigid government constraints which apply to coins, medical medals thus portray an extraordinary diversity of design and construction. Moreover, they were also made from clay, enamels, ceramics, and plastics. Josiah Wedgewood crafted several commemorative medical medallions in ceramics, including the effigies of Sir

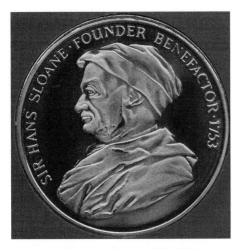

The Sir Hans Sloane Donor's Medal of the British Museum. This medal commemorates the life and work of Sir HANS SLOANE (1660–1753) (p 56), physician, towering patron of science, and the principal founder of the British Museum, London. This medal, struck in 1997, is an ongoing issue and is given as receipt for donations to support the work of the museum.

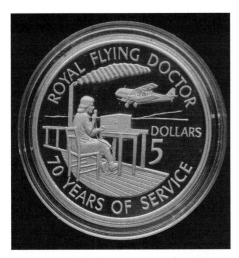

The Australian five dollar silver coin, issued in 1998, to commemorate the 70th anniversary of the Royal Flying Doctor Service of Australia. The reverse, shown here, portrays a Trager pedal wireless being operated by the wife of the owner of a cattle station in the far outback. In the sky is an aircraft flying on an emergency medical mission.

HANS SLOANE (p 56), Dr Richard Mead, and Dr Henry Pemberton. JHP

**COMMUNICATION** In parallel with the tremendous bio-technologic revolution that has been the centerpiece of medicine in the 20th century, communication in medicine, or more specifically, the doctor–patient relationship, has also undergone an unprecedented metamorphosis. The unilateral, hierarchical, paternalistic and authoritarian behavior that was the hallmark of physician communication is slowly being transformed into a relationship which is collaborative, autonomous, and patient-oriented. To appreciate the magnitude of this transformation more fully, this article reviews the historical context in which the patient–physician relationship has developed (the past), then discusses the current situation and understandings (the present), and finally entertains new alternatives and approaches (the future).

### The past

Despite the bleary-eyed mythic remembrances of older, wiser, benevolent, white-haired country doctors who could render everything from family therapy to appendectomies, a review of the history of modern medicine teaches us that physicians, for the most part, did not operate within a model of patient care that was collaborative or communicative. Modern medicine has its foundation in the study of patients with whom communication was not necessary and not even possible — that is, the study of cadavers. The academicians and scientific leaders of the earlier period (17th and 18th centuries) of the modern era of medicine were scholars of anatomy, dissection, and surgical pathology. Physicians studied and perfected their art on patients who were dead. Students of medicine were instructed in large halls, in which they viewed dissections of cadavers as they listened to anatomic recitations. In this context, the patient was an object and the physician was an objective, impersonal, observer–clinician striving to make sense of the inner workings of the human body and attempting to discover the cause and effect of disease on the human organs. Dr Sherwin Nuland, a medical historian, in his book, *Doctors — the biography of medicine*, describes the birth of modern medicine in the mid-1700s. He writes 'the anatomic concept of medicine… became the foundation of all subsequent medical thought… Henceforth, the human body was to be viewed as composed of a group of coordinated physical–mechanical structures… the key to the origin of every disease [was] to be found in some local disturbance of an individual organ. To seek out that local disturbance was to be the first commandment of the new medicine'.

Realizing this centuries-old tradition from which the doctor–patient relationship evolved, one begins to understand how we arrived at the present concept of doctors as doers and patients as passive and noncontributory participants. Over the years, various metaphors have been used to describe this model of patient care: the war metaphor, in which doctors are viewed as warriors waging battle against the enemy of disease and patients are seen as the hapless and helpless victims; the paternalistic metaphor, in which doctors are viewed as benevolent, prudent parents and patients as vulnerable and naïve children; the mechanical metaphor, in which doctors are viewed as skilled technicians and patients as damaged parts or malfunctioning machinery; and the traditional teacher–pupil metaphor, in which doctors are seen as erudite pedagogues holding all knowledge and patients as *tabula rasa* (empty-minded) recipients of this information.

### Voltaire's comment

'Doctors are men who prescribe medicine of which they know little, to cure diseases of which they know less, in human beings of they know nothing'.
                                        VOLTAIRE

The advent of anesthesia in the 19th century contributed greatly to the surgical treatment of patients, but it also reproduced the corpse-like patient with whom communication was not necessary and not possible. In the early 20th century, as our understanding of cellular and molecular mechanisms of disease evolved rapidly, physicians continued to ignore patients and focused instead on the science and technology of medicine. William OSLER (p 602), the 20th century father of modern diagnosis, noticed this trend and reminded his students that 'sometimes it is more important to know what patient a disease has than what disease a patient has'. In the 1920s, Dr Peabody, a young professor of medicine at the Harvard School of Medicine, became acutely aware of this problem of patient–physician communication. He had developed cancer of the stomach and at an early point in his career simultaneously became teaching doctor and dying patient. In one of the most quoted lectures in medicine Peabody cautioned his students that, 'the significance of the intimate personal relationship between physician and patient cannot be too strongly emphasized, for in an extraordinarily large number of cases both diagnosis and treatment are directly dependent on it...' and concluded with the memorialized dictum: 'the secret of patient care is in caring for the patient'.

### The present

Since Peabody's lecture there have been several pioneers who guided and advanced our understanding of the doctor–patient relationship, amongst them: two internists, Henry Richardson and George Engel, a psychiatrist, Michael Balint, and a physician–anthropologist, Arthur Kleinman. Richardson, a professor of internal medicine at the Cornell University Medical College, led a research study in the 1940s known as 'The Macy Project'. The purpose of this project was to investigate the interrelationship between a patient's illness and their family situation, and explore its implications for treatment. In conjunction with the anthropologist Margaret Mead, the research coordinator, Richardson hypothesized that a patient's illness, symptoms, and treatment outcomes were not isolated individualistic phenomena, but instead were somehow connected to and associated with what was happening in the patient's immediate environment — the patient's family. Dr Richardson and his group viewed the family, not the individual, as the 'unit of living' and thus as the 'unit of illness' and health.

In his book describing the Macy Project, *Patients have families*, Richardson concluded, 'The time is ripe for a coordinated attack on the problems of family adjustment in relation to the maintenance of health and the treatment of illness'.

The practical implication was that in order to effectively and efficiently treat the individual patient, clinicians must consider the effect that families have on patients' illness and the effect of illness on patients' families. Richardson's ideas were visionary. It is both surprising and unfortunate that his concepts have not yet been fully understood nor utilized by clinicians, healthcare planners, medical managers, and public health administrators. However, his work laid the foundation for family practice medicine and medical family therapy. His conclusions continue to inspire other researchers and clinicians to investigate further the obvious connection between illness, recovery, and family interactions.

In 1957, Michael Balint, the respected Tavistock Clinic psychiatrist, published a book entitled, *The doctor, his patient, and the illness*, which summarized his conclusions from years of research on the topic of doctor–patient relationships. He had initially recognized that, 'it happens not so infrequently that the relationship between the patient and his doctor is strained, unhappy, or even unpleasant'. In his book, he reveals an elegant concept — 'the doctor as pill' — the idea being that the physician and the relationship the physician creates with the patient is, to a large extent, the healing influence for the patient. He regarded the patient–physician relationship as the central and most essential component of medical work, regardless of what technical advances were being made in medicine.

In the introductory chapter of his book, Balint remarked that he was disturbed that this key component (the doctor–patient interpersonal interaction) of clinical work had not been more thoroughly researched and that 'no guidance whatever is contained in any textbook as to the dosage in which the doctor should prescribe himself, in what form, how frequently, what his curative and his maintenance doses should be…'.

He believed that, 'psychologically, much more happens in general [medical] practice between patient and doctor than is discussed in the traditional textbooks'. Based on years of studying the interactions between patients and physicians, he was also vexed by the 'shallowness of this self-reassuring advice… that experience and common sense will help the doctor to acquire the necessary skill in prescribing himself…'. His primary goal was to study the patient–physician relationship and to devise a 'new pharmacology' to instruct physicians in how to 'avoid certain processes in the doctor–patient relationship (the undesirable and unwanted side-effects of the drug 'doctor') which cause both the patient and his doctor unnecessary suffering, irritation and fruitless efforts'. His second goal was 'to describe diagnostic signs to enable the doctor to recognize these pathological processes…', and his third and final goal was 'to indicate what sort of therapy might be applied' by the physician to create a more mutually satisfactory and productive doctor–patient relationship.

## 'Two-person' medicine

One simple but little understood insight that he formulated was the expansion of a 'one-person' clinical encounter into a 'two-person' medicine. Because the 'doctor and patient are influencing each other all the time' he felt that it was insufficient to study the patient's responses without also taking into account the physician's thoughts, beliefs, and emotions. This particular idea may be misunderstood as countertransference. It is important to recognize, however, that Balint did not advocate an intrapsychic examination of physicians but rather a bona fide research of the dialog between patient and physician. Just as Richardson's work had brought the patient's family into the clinical picture, Balint's work brought the physician, and more specifically, the interaction between the patient and physician, into the clinical picture. Balint's work yielded many innovative and insightful concepts but his

greatest contribution to the topic was that he demonstrated and modeled the notion that the patient–physician relationship was accessible to study. The realization of this unprecedented accomplishment opened the door for the legions of researchers who were to follow in his footsteps.

In a landmark article published in the journal *Science* in 1977, entitled *The need for a new medical model: a challenge for biomedicine*, George Engel offered the world of medicine a new concept of patient care — the 'biopsychosocial model'. Engel was familiar with Thomas Kuhn's book, *The structure of scientific revolutions,* in which Kuhn points out that 'the time to rethink the appropriateness of a framework [paradigm] is when it progressively becomes less able to answer the questions asked of it'. For Engel, the inadequate paradigm was the biomedical model, which did not allow for the inclusion of the psychological and behavioral aspects of illness. Because the biomedical model did not recognize psychosocial and behavioral data, it was incapable of processing these phenomena. Therefore, it did not afford the physician or clinical scientist the opportunity to create necessary and useful information out of these data. Engel understood the entrenched bias long held by our dualistic and reductionistic scientific tradition. His goal was to eradicate this restrictive bias by applying the scientific method to the collection of the social and interpersonal data that are an integral component in the medical care of patients. To achieve this end, he proposed that we apply the rigorous scientific requirements of objective observation, inductive reasoning, hypothesis development and testing, and the unbiased, reproducible recording of data for the purpose of forming experimentally-based conclusions.

Engel held the strong conviction that the expansion of the biomedical model into a biopsychosocial model was essential for medicine to become more scientific. He also understood that physicians and biomedical scientists had been loath to accept the psychosocial sciences. Engel urged physicians to realize that the 'crippling flaw' of the biomedical model was that it did not allow them to realize and observe the obvious psychosocial phenomena that they were encountering daily. He argued that empathy and interpersonal understanding were not only important components of being a humane physician but were also a 'requirement for scientific work in the clinical realm'. He pointed out that clinicians, by the nature of their work, must function within the psychosocial realm — the manner by which we collect clinical data from patients during the medical interview is in fact a psychological technique; the technology by which we enact treatment, the physician–patient relationship, is a psychosocial process; and the aim of our efforts may be measured by the psychological and behavioral outcomes of our patients.

## Understanding the principles

In a similar vein to Balint, Engel understood the dialog between doctor and patient to be a powerful instrument of diagnosis and treatment. He believed that only through serious research efforts could we begin to understand the underlying principles of the patient–physician relationship. Once understood, these principles could then be used to instruct physicians in the most effective modes of dialog and interaction with their patients. Engel taught, mentored, and inspired an entire generation of clinician-scientists who would spend the next thirty years carrying out his vision of the scientific method applied to patient–physician communication.

There is one more person whose ideas irrevocably altered our understanding of patients, disease, and illness. In a 1978 *Annals of Internal Medicine* article entitled, *Culture, illness, and care*, Arthur Kleinman, a medical anthropologist, introduced the idea that disease and illness were two different entities. He acquainted us with the notion that disease is an abnormality in the structure and function of a patient's physical organs, whereas illness is the experience of human suffering during sickness. He then illustrated the point by observing that illness can and does occur commonly without the presence of an identifiable disease and disease can and does occur commonly without the presence of an identifiable illness.

Kleinman explained the concept of 'illness' as the manner in which an individual perceives, experiences, and copes with disease. This individual perception, he argued, was a reflection of larger social and cultural rules. Based on his and other anthropologists' cross-cultural studies, he began to see any single individual's illness behavior as a representation of the complex interaction of personal, family, ethnic, class, and larger cultural beliefs and reactions to disease. He proposed that it was these deeply held beliefs that guided our personal explanations, experience of, and reaction to disease.

Supporting Engel's notion of the inadequacy of the biomedical model, Kleinman, through his clear understanding of the undeniable difference between illness and disease, explained the limitation of the biomedical model. Because of its concern with diagnosing and treating disease, the biochemical model had not and could not allow for the recognition of patients' illness experience as a legitimate concern and as a legitimate area of scientific exploration. Simply stated, doctors were interested in curing disease and patients were concerned about the healing of their illness. A tremendous mismatch of explanations and expectations existed between the crossed purposes of patients and the formal healthcare system. It was this profound limitation of the biomedical model to which he attributed many of the current problems in healthcare. He believed that 'discrepancies between these views strongly affect clinical management and lead to inadequate and poor care'. In order to solve this problem, he reasoned that 'clinical science must investigate illness as well as disease; and clinical care should be directed at both'. On a practical level, he believed that for doctors and patients to communicate more effectively, the 'explanatory models' or 'health belief models' of patients, families, and physicians should be elicited, discussed, and negotiated in order to arrive at the most mutually satisfactory explanation and understanding of illness and disease. He also believed that patients and physicians should discuss their expectations about the mode or manner in which medical care was going to be delivered.

Both Kleinman's and Balint's work underscored the idea that patients' illness explanations take the form of a narrative or story. This concept revealed the existence of yet another mismatch of expectations between patient and physician. Physicians had been trained to forage for discrete pieces of data (such as symptoms) and to construct a medicalized 'disease story'. Patients, on the other hand, were interested in delivering their 'illness story' and not just spouting a meaningless list of physical symptoms. Patients wanted to discuss 'meanings' and physician wanted to hear 'facts'. This concept of the 'meaning of the illness' or role of the illness in patients and their families is derived, to a large degree, from Kleinman's work. He and many other socio-medical scientists who would develop the concept of the 'illness narrative' further proposed that a workable compromise be struck between patients' need to tell their illness story and physicians' need for specific disease oriented information.

Richardson had taught us that illness behavior is a function of the interpersonal complexities of family life. Balint had taught us that, in a sense, the physician becomes part of the family dynamic, at least in regard to health and illness, and therefore illness behavior is a function of not only the family dynamic but more comprehensively the patient–family–physician dynamic. Kleinman had taught us that illness behavior was not solely dependent on the specific patient–family–physician unit, but was also a function of the larger ethnic, historical, socio-cultural milieu from which the patient and the family derived its deep and often implicit beliefs, explanations, and rules concerning illness and health behavior. Engel had shed the light of scientific method on the topic of patient–physician communication. Thanks to the groundbreaking efforts of these individuals and many other early and mid-20th century psychosocial scientists and thinkers, the past three decades have brought a surge of research effort and attention to the patient–physician relationship. It would be impossible, in the context of this article, to review in detail the many achievements in this area over the past thirty years. A few comments can be made, though, regarding the most important aspects.

### Role of behaviors

Much of the work to date has focused on discovering and correlating which specific physician communication behaviors lead to improved patient–physician outcomes, and which lead to poor outcomes. The literature has clearly and repeatedly demonstrated that effective physician communication leads to enhanced patient satisfaction, increased patient participation in medical treatment and follow-up, improved patient adherence to treatment plans, enhanced physician ability to understand and diagnose illness — especially psycho-emotional illness — and improvements in patients' physical health outcomes. Additionally, ineffective and unsatisfactory physician communication has been directly correlated with an increased likelihood of patients and their families initiating malpractice litigation.

One of the central themes has been the issue of patient autonomy. Through their research, psychosocial scientists have come to understand and define autonomy and self-competence as basic human needs. It has been observed that the healthcare system, and the behavior of its agents, often erodes patients' sense of control over their bodies, their minds, and their behaviors. These researchers have proven that through the restoration of autonomy and self-competence, patients are more willing and able to participate as allies in their medical care. This increase in patient participation and the leveling of the traditional hierarchical doctor–patient relationship have been shown to lead to significant, measurable improvements in patients' health.

There has been detailed study of specific physician communication techniques and behaviors measuring physicians' verbal as well as non-verbal communication, much of it through the use of audio and videotaping of actual patient–physician encounters. These studies have yielded tremendous insights into how physicians and patients normally communicate with one another. Based on the results of these studies, others have attempted to demonstrate that effective communication behaviors can be taught to physicians. A number of these studies have met with mixed results but a few have demonstrated

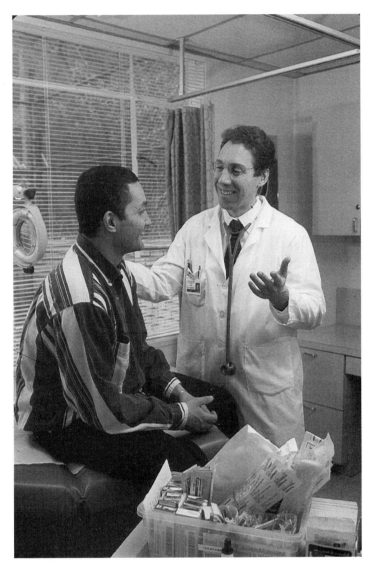

A physician discussing treatment options with a patient.

that even small investments and changes in physician behavior can lead to positive patient outcomes.

In 1994, C. Everett Koop, the former United States Surgeon General, commented that, 'if you talk to the people who receive healthcare, the number one concern is, "My doctor is not the kind of man or woman I want a doctor to be. He doesn't listen to me. Or when I talk to her, she doesn't understand me"'.

A recent flurry of international news articles and large public surveys have indicated the widespread demand for improved relationships with physicians and more humane healthcare systems. Physicians have also begun to describe their inability to establish meaningful relationships with patients and to discuss their own experiences of being dissatisfied patients. Despite the large strides made in our understanding of the doctor–patient relationship, we still have a long way to go.

## The future

One of the deficiencies in the research on patient–physician communication has been a lack of understanding as to how physicians benefit through enhanced communication with patients. We may speculate that physicians have much to gain. For example, the research on malpractice litigation indicates a clear advantage in terms of reduced risk of litigation as a function of improved physician communication skill. However, from an interpersonal perspective, there has been little research investigating physicians' benefits from the use of effective communication and relational strategies. In fact, since Balint's early descriptive work, it seems that physicians have been left out of the relational picture. The research over the past thirty years has focused on 'patient-centered' models of care. One might argue that this model swings too far in one direction, creating an unequal conceptualization of the patient–physician relationship. What seems to be missing is the understanding that we must work in a collaborative framework in which the focus is not on a patient-centered model, nor a physician-centered model, and not even on a communication-centered model, but rather on a patient–physician relationship-centered model. If physicians are to adopt new behaviors and participate willingly in new types of patient–physician relationships, there must be some definitive conclusion of what benefits and gains they stand to accrue. This is, as yet, a wholly unexplored and fertile topic for future research and investigation.

Another model of patient–physician communication that has recently re-emerged is the concept of patients as customers or consumers. Many physicians and patients seem to initially resist this concept. Upon further inspection, however, there are many shared similarities between the customer model and the patient-centered principles extensively discussed in this article. Regina Herzlinger, a healthcare economist, in her recent book entitled *Market driven healthcare*, argues that patients, as autonomous entities, require convenience of healthcare service, control or self-mastery of their healthcare, and information to make the serious decisions concerning from whom and which type of healthcare they will accept. The driving force and the expected outcomes of a customer-driven model, she explains, are the delivery of the highest quality, lowest cost healthcare service. Aaron

Lazare, in an article in the *Archives of Psychiatry* entitled *The customer approach to patienthood*, puts forth a 'customer-oriented' concept that sounds surprisingly similar to Kleinman's 'Explanatory model of illness'. Lazare states that physicians have been trained to respond to patients' physical complaints, and from these complaints physicians develop their own understanding of the diagnosis and treatment plan. He points out that physicians have never been instructed to inquire about patients' 'goals' (expected outcomes) of treatment or to elicit patients' 'requests' for how to go about attaining the desired treatment outcomes. Parallel to Kleinman's transactional methodology, Lazare recommends that physicians elicit these 'customer-oriented' understandings and then negotiate a mutually acceptable understanding with the patient (customer). In a similar discussion to Engel's thesis regarding the expansion of the biomedical model into a biopsychosocial concept, Lazare reasons that obtaining this information from the patient (customer) provides another source of diagnostic data from which to develop clinical hypotheses. As we compare and contrast the customer model of patient care with other patient-centered or collaborative models of communication the distinctions grow blurry and the models seem to merge. At the very least, this new model provides another fresh metaphor which, upon further investigation, might provide us with improvements in patient–physician communication and more humane healthcare relationships.

Much has been learned about patient–physician communication over the past century, but very little has been systematically applied. This is one of the most difficult and important hurdles to be overcome if healthcare is to become more humane and if we are to realize substantial improvements in patient–physician relationships. Individual physicians and patients no longer determine healthcare. Large healthcare organizations, hospitals, governmental agencies, insurance companies, and collective employer coalitions determine, to a large extent, the policies that govern the behavior between patients and physicians. The principles of the biopsychosocial model, patient autonomy model, explanatory models of illness, family-oriented care model, and patient/customer service model will come to naught unless they are applied on these larger healthcare systems levels. These relational models, as well as the effective communication techniques painstakingly described over the past thirty years of research, must be put into daily medical practice on an equal footing with advancements in biomedical science and large corporate economic incentives. This will be the greatest challenge for the future of communication in medicine — not to change individuals' behaviors but to develop and implement more humane policies that will govern the communication behaviors of all members of the healthcare system.                                    ZEN

*See also* DIAGNOSIS; EDUCATION; HEALTH-CARE SYSTEMS

**COMMUNITY MEDICINE** See PUBLIC HEALTH

**COMPLEMENTARY AND ALTERNATIVE MEDICINE** is a term that describes many differing and often unrelated treatments. These approaches have, collectively, been called unconventional, alternative, or fringe medical practice. According to the WORLD HEALTH ORGANIZATION, many such treatments are the traditional medicine on which two thirds of the world rely as their main source of primary care. Recent surveys from the USA and Australia indicate that enormous sums are being spent on complementary medicine. Its provision in the industrialized world is largely within the private sector, although in Britain availability and interest within the National Health Service are increasing. The situation in the USA is also changing as more medical insurance companies and health maintenance organizations offer complementary medicine as part of their managed care portfolio.

People seeking advice from complementary medical practitioners are often not gullible and ill-informed, but are seeking another approach to the management of their often intractable and chronic complaint. Furthermore, they have not necessarily abandoned conventional medicine. Two thirds of people seeking complementary medicine have consulted their primary care physician or hospital specialist first but found no solution to their problem. About one quarter of patients with chronic illness are concurrently receiving orthodox and complementary care. Many who attend such practitioners appear to know more about their own health than the general population. For instance, patients attending a homeopath are more likely than the general population to believe that a good diet, cutting down smoking, having time to relax and meditate, and sleeping properly are positive health maintenance measures. They also have more 'internal' beliefs about their ability to control their health and use complementary medical practitioners to facilitate egalitarian consultations about the management of their medical problems. Patients attending complementary medical practitioners generally approve their consultation style. Conventional physicians may have much to learn from the alternative medical professions, particularly in allowing patients to play an active part in the management of their own health.

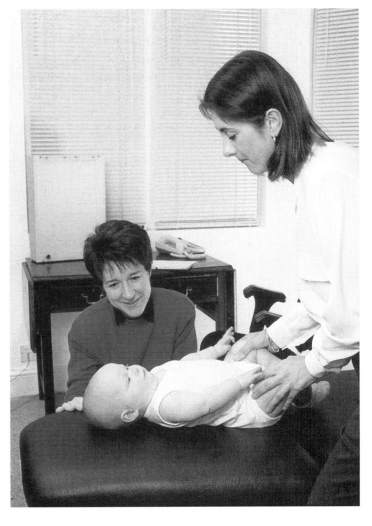

A chiropractor treating a baby. (Reproduced courtesy of the British Chiropractic Association.)

The increasing popularity of complementary medicine is therefore a complex issue, involving a variety of factors. Patient demand has triggered a desire for information about these therapeutic interventions, leading to the development of a plethora of journals, and undergraduate or postgraduate courses.

Until recently there has been little interest, motivation, or financial support for complementary medical research. Consequently, there has been insufficient evidence for the effectiveness of these treatments and the underlying physiologic mechanisms involved remain poorly understood. We undoubtedly need a more solid evidence base; such investment is either under way or being considered by most of the industrial nations and a clearer scientific picture should emerge over the next decade.                    GL

*See also* ACUPUNCTURE; CHIROPRACTIC; ENVIRONMENTAL MEDICINE; HERBAL MEDICINE; HOMEOPATHY; NUTRITION; OSTEOPATHY

**COMPUTERS** Nowadays a photograph of a doctor at her desk in the consulting room shows a computer keyboard and screen in the background more often than a stethoscope and blood pressure measuring machine. Computers truly are pervasive in medical practice. They have several uses:

- Computers store and retrieve clinical information in medical records. Financial and administrative records, appointment systems, also employ computers more often than pen, paper, and appointment-book in most modern hospitals and clinics.

- Computers can routinely process large amounts of data. Statistical summary details of hospital separations (that is, discharges and deaths) with diagnoses, length of stay, procedures, and outcomes can be processed and produced efficiently only with computers. Doing this manually would be prohibitively expensive.

- Computers aid clinical decision-making by applying simple logical rules. This is an application of artificial intelligence, whereby a large-capacity computer is programed to use the logic of the diagnostic process. Just as a computer can defeat a human at chess, fed the necessary facts, a computer can arrive at a correct diagnosis using systematic logic, and often reaching conclusions as reliable and valid as those of an expert diagnostician.

- Calculation of medication doses, radiation exposures, etc.; the assembly and interpretation of results of a batch of biochemical tests using an auto-analyzer; and a wide range of other routine procedures in medical practice, in hospitals, clinics, and even in solo general practice may be done more efficiently with computers than by humans.

- Interactive computer-based educational packages are widely used for self-instruction, continuing education, or distance-learning in medicine. An example of the many uses of computers in medical education is the Visible Human project, accessible on the World Wide Web. This is a three-dimensional visual image of a human body that can be used to teach anatomy.

- Almost all medical research requires computers to process and analyze the data, carry out the statistical significance tests, write up the results using a word-processing program, and even transmit the finished paper to the editorial office of a medical journal over the INTERNET, rather than entrusting it to the post.

In short, computers have become an indispensable feature of medical practice, medical education, and medical research, in the affluent industrial nations, as well as in some of the remotest outposts of civilization.

A computer consists of hardware and software. The hardware is a central processing unit, where microchips, fixed or hard magnetic disks, floppy or transportable and removable disks, and complex circuits, receive, store, and transmit electronic signals; a screen to display the information being dealt with; and a keyboard that the computer operator uses to send signals into the system. A pointing device, called a mouse, displays an arrow on the screen and is used to switch signals, change programs, block and move text, etc. The software is the set of computer programs for data input and analysis, to communicate with other computers over a network within a hospital or clinic or to the outside world through the internet, for wordprocessing, for image-drawing, and for many other applications.

### Sizes and shapes

Computers come in many sizes and shapes. Mainframe computers the size of a kitchen refrigerator, or a whole bank of such machines, are rarely seen outside the data-processing centers of large institutions. Modern hospitals and clinics function effectively with a bank of desktop computers, linked together in a local area network, so that their capacity can be shared. Many professional people have a laptop computer, which can pack a great deal of power and high-speed processing of information into a very small space. Handheld computers are operated by flashlight batteries; palmtop computers use a stylus rather than a keyboard. Both of these miniaturized devices can connect to the internet as well as store information needed away from the office. It is easy to recognize busy professional people in places such as airport departure lounges by their intent gazes fixed on the fluorescent screens in front of them. These, and their cellular telephones, enable them to communicate information back and forth via the internet, no matter where they may be in the world.

Isolated physicians are among those who make great use of these new technologies to transmit and receive complex clinical information over long distances. An important aspect, TELEMEDICINE, is used by doctors in remote areas to transmit and receive complex clinical information over long distances for computer assisted diagnoses and distance learning.

The advantages of computers in clinical practice are immense. All the pertinent facts about a patient may be neatly stored in a central location, where, after a password has activated the system and a few keystrokes made to enter identifying information, the pertinent details about a patient are accessible instantaneously to any member of the clinical team authorized to use the system. All can easily read it, and it is assembled in logical order, usually with the essential details, positive diagnostic findings, cautions about allergies to penicillin, etc, suitably highlighted for instant recognition. The fear that individual privacy can be invaded and confidentiality violated is less serious than with paper records stored in filing cabinets that can be rifled by unauthorized users more easily than a computer hacker can gain access to computerized medical records protected by well-designed passwords and an encryption system.

The disadvantages perceived by early generations of users (high installation costs, teething troubles during transition and staff training, lack of flexibility and adaptability as innovative computer programs are developed) have largely disappeared. Problems remain, however. A computer may 'crash', losing large amounts of stored information. It may be invaded by a virus that destroys or corrupts the software programs used to operate it. A computer virus is a self-replicating mathematical program or logic tree that is introduced to a computer on a floppy disk or over the internet. Once it has invaded, it can replace the existing software such as the operating system, with meaningless files that make the computer malfunction and become useless. For these reasons the essential information in the computer's memory must always be copied routinely and frequently to disks that are filed separately. The Y2K problem, like other millennial fears, did not materialize in any important public service computer system or network as all were suitably modified to circumvent the problem. However, many personal computers made before the late 1990s, that were equiped only to program the late two digits of the four-digit year do not accurately record dates, instead reverting to those of the 1980s or not registering dates at all.

The problem of rapid onset of obsolescence, especially of personal desktop computers, has not been solved. As soon as a medical practice, or a medical research team, invests in a new computer with seemingly limitless capacity, the manufacturers release a new, bigger, faster — and often cheaper — one. Moreover, software operating systems, wordprocessing programs, and protocols for transmitting files over the internet are frequently changed, allegedly improved, always using more computer memory than before, and therefore needing a more powerful system. This never-ending spiral of upgrading is constantly introducing barriers to easy communication when the intent ought to be to facilitate it. This leads to much lamentation and occasional allegations of a conspiracy on the part of hardware and software salesmen to extract the maximum from a gullible public; but it reflects the rapid rate of development and innovation in the subject. Perhaps it is a price worth paying for the benefits computers bring.                    JML

*See also* DIAGNOSIS; RECORDS

**CONTRACEPTION** About half of women aged 18–44 years in a western country such as Britain use some form of reversible contraception; 50% rely on the contraceptive pill, 25% use condoms, and 12% the intrauterine contraceptive device. About 8% rely on withdrawal (coitus interruptus); the remainder use the diaphragm, with or without spermicides, or the 'safe period' (rhythm method). The effectiveness of all these methods is measured using the Pearl Index — the number of unwanted pregnancies that occur during 100 woman years of exposure (normally fertile women having regular intercourse). The natural pregnancy rate (that is, the Pearl Index without any birth control) is about 80%.

### Natural family planning
Coitus interruptus relies on withdrawal of the penis before ejaculation; so the effectiveness depends very much on the male partner. The failure rate is 8–17%.

The rhythm method involves predicting the time of ovulation and avoiding intercourse seven days before and three days after. The time of ovulation can be pinpointed by monitoring the menstrual cycle for 12 months and using the longest and shortest cycles to predict the likely fertile period. Other factors that may be used to help identify the time of ovulation include the rise in basal temperature that occurs after ovulation, mittelschmerz (ovulation pain), and changes in cervical mucus. A recent introduction is the Persona system, which measures urinary hormone levels to calculate the safe days. The failure rate of methods which depend on identifying the fertile period is 2–20%.

### Barrier methods
Condoms are made of thin latex rubber and are usually lubricated, sometimes with spermicide. Problems include reduction in male sensation and breakage. The quoted failure rate is 2–15%.

The diaphragm consists of a rubber hemisphere in various sizes, surrounded by a spring to keep it in shape. The woman inserts the device before intercourse and removes it six hours later. Some practice is needed, and the failure rate (4–18%) declines with duration of use. Cervical and vault caps have similar features, but they are kept in position by suction rather than spring tension. All need to be combined with a spermicide.

Spermicides are substances that destroy sperm (for example, nonoxynol 9), and should always be used in combination with barrier methods. Quoted failure rates for spermicide alone are 4–25%.

The female condom (femidom) is a soft, loose fitting polyurethane sheath with a loose inner ring to hold it across the top of the vagina, and an outer ring outside the vagina entrance. The failure rate is 5–15%.

Although barrier methods are generally slightly less effective than the intrauterine device and hormonal contraception, they have the advantage of providing some protection against SEXUALLY TRANSMITTED DISEASES.

### The intrauterine contraceptive device

The intrauterine contraceptive device may be inert plastic or contain an active ingredient — such as copper (Multiload) — or a progestogen hormone (for example, Mirena). It is best suited to women who have completed their family. The device acts by stimulating a reaction in the lining of the womb. The copper component is spermicidal. The failure rate for intrauterine devices is 5% in the first year and 1–2% in subsequent years.

Absolute contraindications to the intrauterine device include malignant disease of the genital tract, vaginal bleeding of unknown cause, suspected pregnancy, active pelvic infection, and previous ectopic pregnancy. Higher expulsion rates occur at menstruation or in the first eight weeks after giving birth. The device should continue to be used until one year after the menopause.

The use of the device is associated with several possible, though unusual, complications. Heavy periods, intermenstrual bleeding, and painful menstruation may occur; these improve with use. The device may be expelled or, more seriously, may perforate the uterus. Extrauterine devices are removed by laparoscopy (using an operating telescope) or open operation. The risk of pelvic infection is highest in the first few months after insertion; its frequency in users aged under 20 is over 10 times that of 30–50 year olds. Treatment includes removing the device and giving antibiotics.

Of all pregnancies that occur with an intrauterine contraceptive device in place, 3–9% are ectopic, perhaps because these provide more protection against intrauterine than tubal pregnancies. The rates are lowest with copper devices and highest with progesterone containing devices. Perforation of the uterine wall occurs in 1 per 5000 cases. Patients should be instructed to feel for the device monthly and attend for 6-monthly check-ups. Mirena needs to be replaced every three years and copper devices every 3–8 years.

### Hormonal contraception

The combined contraceptive pill is used by 20–30% of all sexually active women. The classic combined pill contains estrogen (ethinylestradiol or mestranol) and progesterone (19-norsteroids such as norethisterone, norgestrel, ethynodiol, lynestrenol; and the newer generation compounds such as desogestrel, gestodene, and norgestimate). The earlier pills contained 50 $\mu$g estrogen, but current generations contain 20, 30, or 35 $\mu$g. Two types of preparations are commonly used: (1) fixed-dose pills (monophasic), in which estrogen and progesterone are taken in constant doses for 21 days followed by a seven-day pill-free period and (2) multiphasic preparations, which contain variable doses of progesterone and estrogen and allow the use of the lowest dose of both hormones capable of providing good cycle control; as a result, side-effects are minimized. The main action of the pill is to suppress ovulation (by suppressing secretion of hormones from the pituitary).

Correctly used, the failure rate of the pill is only 0.1%. However, true failure rates among married women average 3%, the discrepancy being explained by lack of compliance, including inconsistent use and missed pills.

In addition to preventing pregnancy, the pill has several well-established beneficial non-contraceptive effects. These include protection against ovarian cancer, endometrial cancer, salpingitis, ectopic pregnancy, benign breast disease, dysmenorrhea, and iron deficiency anemia. Less well-established are protection against osteoporosis, colorectal cancer, uterine fibroids, toxic shock syndrome, and rheumatoid arthritis. These beneficial effects are usually not well publicized. By contrast, side-effects are the subject of almost constant media attention. Despite this, the method has achieved widespread acceptance.

Prominent amongst the 'risks' is that of cardiovascular disease, including an increased incidence of myocardial infarction, stroke, and venous thromboembolism. It is now accepted that the pill is perfectly safe for healthy, non-smoking women of any age. That said, specific contraindications include smokers aged over 35 and, on grounds of prudence, women with a history of pulmonary embolism, deep venous thrombosis, sickle cell disease, porphyria, and jaundice, and those about to undergo major surgery. There is also some evidence that the risk of spontaneous blood clotting in the veins in young women may be slightly increased with the newer progestational agents (for example, desonorgestrel).

Metabolic effects include increased levels of triglycerides and low density cholesterol but decreased ones of high density cholesterol (that is, an unfavorable lipid profile). The new generation progestogens (such as desonorgestrel) cause fewer metabolic effects and lead to a rise in high density cholesterol and a reduction in low density cholesterol. The pill increases the risk of blood clotting, by increasing plasma fibrinogen and other clotting factors, but, none of these appears to be clinically relevant in low risk women.

Among the greatest concerns of users is that pill use increases the likelihood of cancer. Much of this concern is due to over-reaction by the media. The reality is that the incidence of several important cancers is reduced. That is not to say that there is no controversy — for example, the effect on breast cancer in early and late reproductive life is still being debated. But the overall picture is highly reassuring.

Some drugs can interfere with the action of the pill. Most notable of these are certain antibiotics (rifampicin, griseofulvin) and anticonvulsants (phenytoin). These may raise the level of liver enzymes, which increase the rate of breakdown of the pill components. Women taking such agents may need to increase to a higher estrogen pill if breakthrough bleeding occurs.

Progesterone-only pills contain either ethynodiol or norethisterone. These produce alterations in the endometrium and the cervical mucus. They have to be taken at the same time every day for three weeks of a four week cycle. The failure rate is 1–4%. The incidence of amenorrhea, irregular breakthrough bleeding, and functional ovarian cysts is increased compared with the combination pill.

***Post-coital contraception*** In the classic 'Yuzpe' regimen two pills each containing 50 $\mu$g ethinylestradiol and 250 $\mu$g levonorgestrel are taken within 72 hours of unprotected intercourse during the mid cycle and repeated after 12 hours. If the woman vomits treatment is repeated. The failure rate is 1%–2%. There are no published reports of death or serious illness after its use; the only contraindication is thromboembolism. An alternative is to insert an intrauterine contraceptive device up to five days after unprotected intercourse. The use of progesterone antagonists such as mifepristone will increase in the future.

***Injectable steroids*** include intramuscular depot preparations such as Dopo-Provera (a 17-hydroxyprogesterone derivative; 150 mg every three months) or Noristerat (norethisterone 200 mg every two months). The drug works primarily by blocking the surge in pituitary hormone secretion and thus suppressing ovulation. It also acts on cervical mucus and the endometrium. Side-effects include amenorrhea (up to 45% in the first year), irregular vaginal bleeding, and weight gain. Menstrual cycles and fertility return to normal within six months of the last injection.

The Norplant system for delivery of the levonorgestrel is effective for up to five years. The drug is sealed into six Silastic cylindrical capsules (each containing 38 mg) and implanted under the skin. The failure rate is 1%, but rates are higher in heavier women. Abnormal vaginal bleeding occurs in up to 40% of users within the first year, but improves with time. After removal of the implant, half of those wanting to conceive become pregnant within three months and 85% within one year.

Because compliance is not an issue, the failure rate is 1%. Overall, injectable progestins appear to be a highly effective alternative to the traditional pill, especially in women who may have a contraindication to an estrogen-containing preparation. There is no increase in cancer risk. The only reservation is whether there is a potential risk of osteoporosis.

***Immunological methods*** An immunological approach to contraception with a vaccine against the hormone human chorionic gonadotraphin is in clinical trial. Studies in animals suggest that the vaccine can block fertility at an early stage of pregnancy without significantly affecting the menstrual cycle.

***The male pill*** Despite extensive research into Growth hormone releasing hormone (GnRH) analogs, steroids, anti-androgens, and gossypol as potential male contraceptives, there is no method of suppressing sperm production without affecting libido.                    TGC

*See also* OBSTETRICS AND GYNECOLOGY

Nicolaus **COPERNICUS** (1473–1543). Polish astronomer, whose fundamental contribution to scientific thought changed for ever man's view of the universe. The Copernican or heliocentric theory of astronomy proposed a daily motion of the Earth around its own axis and a yearly motion around a stationary Sun, replacing the Ptolemaic or geocentric idea of the heavens which had hitherto held sway. Copernicus was born in Torun, in what is now eastern Poland. In 1491 he entered the University of Cracow, where he studied Greek and mathematics and first became interested in astronomy. Further education followed at Bologna and Padua (1497–1503), and it was during his four years at the latter university that he received his medical training; it has been said that in addition to his command of theology, mathematics, law, and astronomy, he mastered all the medical knowledge of his day.

**PIONEERS IN CONTRACEPTION**

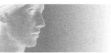

Marie Charlotte Carmichael **STOPES** (1880– 1958). British pioneer of contraception. Marie Stopes was trained as a botanist and in 1911 she was married for the first time. The marriage was annulled in 1916 for non-consummation and in 1918 she married Arthur Verdon-Roe, who was also interested in birth control. She founded the first contraceptive clinic in Britain in 1921. She wrote numerous books on sex and contraception; the first, *Married love* (1918), was translated into 13 languages.

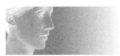

Margaret **SANGER** (1883–1966). American feminist leader, and world figure in the birth control movement. As a nurse in a poor district of New York City, Margaret Sanger became concerned about the problems of uncontrolled fertility in conditions of poverty. She became a leader in feminist causes, especially in education about methods of birth control. She established birth control clinics in the New York area, and was prosecuted for violations of the law and spent one 30-day term in gaol. Nevertheless she persisted, and founded the American Birth Control League in 1921. She wrote and published several books on birth control.

The subsequent development of the life and work of Copernicus is beyond the scope of the present note, except to record that following his return to Poland to settle permanently in Frauenberg (where his financial security was assured by a cathedral canonry) he undertook medical practice among the poor and needy of that city.

**CORONARY THROMBOSIS** See ATHEROMA; CARDIOLOGY; CARDIOTHORACIC SURGERY – HISTORY; DIET AND DISEASE

**CORONER** See FORENSIC MEDICINE

**COT DEATH** See SUDDEN INFANT DEATH SYNDROME

**CREATIVITY** is that attribute of the human mind characterized by originality and meaningfulness. It requires the ability to combine existing ideas, perceptions, experiences, and objects in different ways for new purposes. It is a person's capacity to produce new and original ideas, insights, inventions, or artistic products of scientific, technical, esthetic, or social value, the proceeds of a lively faculty of imagination. Unfortunately, these definitions are not precise enough to acclaim any individual output as creative. Judgement is subjective and communal, like beauty, lying in the eye of the beholder.

Only the juxtaposition of elements which produce a useful (beautiful, evocative, functional, revealing) product may be regarded as creative in any significant way, because random associations are serendipitous, not evidence of a human power. If a computer is programmed to solve a problem and a creative solution is thereby produced, who is its creator — the computer or the programmer? Or is the result no more than a child of chance?

Although there is some pattern in the production of creative ideas, inventors, artists, and scientists seldom know how their new ideas or novel combinations of old ideas arise. It is rare for anyone to be creative in more than one main aspect of endeavor. LEONARDO da Vinci (p 40)is an exception, but most others operated and created within one particular discipline.

Distinctions may be made between personal and historical creativity, and between creative insights and creative expressions. Examples of personal creativity are the deduction by Blaise Pascal that the angles of a triangle sum to two right angles, at a time that he was quite unaware of Euclid; and the insight that the mathematics subsuming Student's $t$-test and the chi-square are identical. Although these realizations may have been original, they do not constitute new knowledge and thus do not rank as historical creativity (the enunciation of the principle for the very first time), even though they indicate the existence of creative minds. Although Dean Inge considered that originality was no more than undetected plagiarism, there has to be a first time for any new idea.

Creative insights are, of course, more common than their expressions. Many of us have them on occasion, probably betokening a modicum of creative talent, but unless the insight is useful and recognized as such, is acted upon, and ultimately is realized, it remains latent. Only those with the added skills to follow through these steps will achieve the expression of their idea.

Lists of outstanding creative works will be as long and various as their authors choose. Darwin's theories of evolution; Clough Williams Ellis's model villages; Doric pillars; atonal music; Hemingway's prose style; William Pitt's introduction of the income tax; Shakespeare's neologisms; the sonnet and the limerick; the spinning Jenny and the ball-point pen; the Braille alphabet; proportional representation; the double helix of Watson and Crick; the moves in chess; cubism; Microsoft Windows; Kekule's conception of the benzene ring; the scansion of the prose of the King James Bible; the periodic table; James Watt's steam engine; the binary system; Mary Pratt's painted representation of plastic wrap; Buckminster Fuller's geodesic dome; the second fireplace in Frank Lloyd Wright's prairie houses; Mickey Mouse; Mahatma Gandhi and the concept of passive resistance; the machines of Heath Robinson and the harmonic rhythmicities in Disney's *Fantasia*; Bell's telephone; and the dance innovations of Martha Graham are some of the items on the list.

These creative activities may be categorized. They include the solution of a defined problem (Einstein, Fleming, Babbage, Watson, and Crick); the devising of an encompassing theory (Darwin, Freud, Einstein); the creation of a permanent work (Moore, Fuller, Pratt, Stravinsky, Magritte); the performance of ritualized work (Martha Graham, Lawrence Olivier, Glenn Gould, Disney); the creation of communication links (the translators of the King James Bible, Alexander Graham Bell, Braille); and societal intervention (Lloyd Wright, Gandhi, Pitt).

To define the element(s) common to these items construes creativity. The first element might be creative space; that is, there must exist the problem to be solved, or at least the opportunity to produce a novel association, within the compass of the individual possessing the skills to recognize the elements of the problem and in an environment permitting its solution. Thus

Gutenberg, familiar with each machine, combined the wine press and the die punch to make the printing press.

Second, the creative person must possess sufficient background knowledge in one (and probably in a second) discipline to allow the combination of disparate elements, and third, be motivated not just to recognize the significance of the new association but also to execute it. Fourth, there must be some pre- or post-hoc insight, often the aha! phenomenon, transcending deduction along logical, scientifically valid lines of argument; because deduction, the fruit of directed labor, results only in discovery, but not that knight's leap that switches paths to create novelty.

Creativity may be no more than the random generation and selective retention of ideas, but only a few have the ideas to start with. Such generation demands some knowledge of the subject and also that perspicacity that will lead to the enunciation or realization of an insight. Along the spectrum (from sheer chance through cultivated chance to systematized chance, fair bets, good bets, and certainties), creativity is usually a manifestation of cultivated chance. The individual, creative in one particular domain of accomplishment, requires the achievement of expertise in that and often another domain before being able to execute any truly creative work.

The searcher deliberately opens up to a variety of semi-random inputs, harvesting and refining the occasional useful connections. The creative person thinks, it is suggested, not just of actualities but of possibilities of varying payoff and promise. It is less the seed landing on the right soil, and more the soil finding, gathering, and nurturing the seed; as PASTEUR (p 620) remarked, 'Chance favors the prepared mind'.

The mental attributes of such a person have been discussed frequently, with few unchallenged conclusions. Personality factors are better at predicting creativity than are tests of divergent thinking; although low-focus thinking is a characteristic that has face value and schizoid, over-inclusive thought patterns may facilitate creative output. While superior intelligence is surely a desirable attribute, a cohort of 300 gifted children followed through two or three decades produced one Nobel prizewinner, but no subject considered outstandingly creative by the definition suggested above. Superior intelligence is probably necessary, but is by itself insufficient to predict creativity.

## Domains of intelligence

Various domains of intelligence are recognized, such as body-kinesthetic, intra- and inter-personal, visual-perceptual, linguistic, musical, and logical-mathematical. From the examples above, it may be seen that most creative people operate in two of these modes at a high level, but other characteristics have also been identified. They are often described as being energetic, demanding, difficult, and liable to manifest cognitive, affective, emotional, and social traits more appropriate to childhood — ascetic, masochistic, rebellious, self-seeking, tactless, intemperate, and exploitative. As an extreme, it has been suggested that a legacy of destruction and tragedy surrounds those that enter into the orbit of the creative individual, although, for most, cognitive and affective support systems are in place for them during their periods of distant creative exploration.

Great creators often appear to sacrifice some element of their personal life on behalf of their art. This is sometimes a Faustian bargain. Fortunately, more positive traits have also been defined in creative as opposed to non-creative students; they have been described as liberal, adventurous, tolerant, candid, spontaneous, flexible, and artistic. The characteristic mental process underlying creativity may be described as that fluency of thought allowing the generation of multiple theoretical associations between ideas not usually linked (a form of over-inclusive thinking). The larger the knowledge base is, the more creative such associations are likely to be. Their expression, however, depends upon the subject's ability to see the utility of the idea and his or her drive to carry it through to realization.

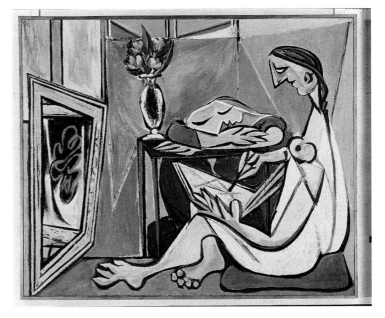

*The Muse* (1935), Pablo Picasso (1881–1973). (Musée National d'Art Moderne, Paris, France. Reproduced courtesy of the Bridgeman Art Library © Succession Picasso/DACS 2001.)

The left brain/right brain dichotomy has been considered to account for some aspects of individual creativity. The left half of the brain is certainly dominantly responsible for language and calculation, the right for visuo-spatial and musical functions, but to ascribe variously Yang and Yin, left/right, emotion/reason, intellect/intuition, analytic/relational is no more than the simplistic and unverifiable product of fertile imaginations. The conceptions of relativity and of the double helix must each have involved both logical mathematical and spatial intelligences; while Henry Moore's right hemispheric spatial gifts must have been complemented by left-sided praxis. Schnabel's pianistic brilliance required not only a remarkably developed sense of rhythm — he himself regarded his skills not in playing the notes, but in designing the pauses that he inserted between them — but also body-kinesthetic intelligence, which depends on bilateral motor skills. Yet the body's motor systems are but the messenger between the mind creating and the environment receiving.

Creativity may best be considered as multifactorial, relying upon intelligence, upon the ability to form associations between different domains of knowledge, and upon the ability to express these as an invention or product with societal value. No single cognitive attribute has been identified among the creative, but as far as forward planning and abstraction ability are regarded as a function of the frontal lobes of the brain, any ascribable localization must include these. The cerebral localization of the necessary knowledge base, imagination, drive, associative skills, and analysis of usefulness of the creative work is unknown and indeed may not be focally situated at all but rather a general factor relating to the functioning and interactions of all areas of the brain surface.

Thus creation, as defined here, is likely to be the result of knowledge, experiment, intuition, deduction, serendipidity, and play (as Frank Capra said, 'a hunch is creativity trying to tell you something'), fueled by innate drive, and realized within a facilitating environment.　　　WP-P

**CRITICAL CARE** The birth of critical or intensive care may be best described in the words of a young nurse who was present.

In the winter of 1953–4, I was a new registered nurse working at the University Hospital in Edmonton. The director of nursing asked me into her office one morning after my night shift. She asked me if I would go to the Royal Alexandra Hospital to care for the polio patients in their hastily created isolation and support unit. At that time our community lived in fear of the epidemic of polio, which was even worse

than the one of the previous year. The lack of effective treatment was frightening. No immunization existed. All we had to rely on was good nursing and isolation technique to prevent spread of the disease and to protect ourselves. Older married nurses, many of whom had children, volunteered to work in our jobs so that we could go. I agreed without hesitation. She looked across the desk at me for a long time and then said, 'Nurse you have just set a precedent. You are the first person on our staff to volunteer'.

Her sister, a student nurse, at the same hospital describes the first shift. 'We rode the bus to the isolation hospital in the dark and cold, watched as she took off her trench coat, tucked her scissors in her apron waist band, put on her cap, accepted the flashlight given to her and walked into the huge makeshift unit filled with iron-lungs. This was the extent of her orientation.'

Although circumstances and timing varied from city to city and country to country, similar situations occurred in the early 1950s in many parts of western Europe and North America. The huge load of critically ill, often paralyzed polio patients requiring breathing support and intensive nursing for all bodily functions, overwhelmed hospitals.

The contrast between these early days and the modern intensive care unit is striking. Then as now, intensive care was defined by the excellence of complete nursing support. Modern nurses receive extensive extra education and preparation, commonly over six months. This is a great advance from the preparation given to the early staff. Unlike the physicians, who dealt with those epidemics using only cuirass or 'iron lung' ventilators, or relied upon staff to ventilate patients manually with handbagging, the physicians of today can rely upon complex technology to monitor cardiovascular, respiratory, and other organ systems. Effective technology makes ventilation of failing lungs and dialysis for renal replacement therapy commonplace. This progress is due to the vision and innovation of a few remarkable people and the courage of many who worked in the units.

The polio epidemic in Copenhagen in 1952 provided the stimulus for what is generally accepted as the first development of the principles of intensive care. From 24 July to 5 December 1952, the Hospital for Communicable Diseases in Copenhagen admitted 2722 patients with polio. Of these, 315 had respiratory problems which required respiratory support. Weakness of respiratory muscles was worsened by pharyngeal paralysis and inability to clear secretions or swallow. This early care was given in tank or cuirass ventilators, often called 'iron lungs'. Patients were placed in a metal cylinder with only their heads protruding. Cyclical variation of the pressure in the cylinder assisted their breathing. Of the first 31 patients admitted with respiratory paralysis, 27 died within three days. The 32nd patient, a 12-year-old girl, was nearing a terminal state of respiratory failure. An anesthetist, Dr Bjorn Ibsen, was consulted by Dr H. C. A. Lassen. He called for a prompt tracheostomy, the insertion of a cuffed endotracheal tube in the orifice, and the initiation of manual artificial ventilation with a conventional to and fro system using a handbag. This improved oxygenation corrected the faulty concentration of blood gases and in the words of Dr Ibsen 'the patient had improved by the measures carried out by the anesthetist in the operating theater'. Subsequently the rapid organization of teams of manual 'ventilators' consisting of nurses, anesthetists, interns, and medical students provided manual artificial ventilation and care in shifts. The teams ventilated up to 70 patients simultaneously. The overall mortality rate using this technique was reduced from over 85% to less than 30%.

### Airway control

The essential aspects of care had been identified. Airway control to avoid aspiration was particularly important in those patients who also had pharyngeal paralysis. Physiotherapy, which included postural drainage, assistance to coughing, suctioning of secretions, and the use of humidified gases, allowed prolonged use of intubation with cuffed tubes. Perhaps most importantly, the idea of multidisciplinary collaboration was established.

Very quickly similar units developed in other centers of Europe and North America. In Canada the first respiratory failure unit specifically for polio was developed by Dr B. J. Sproule in Edmonton in 1952. Intensive care units soon followed and dealt with critically ill patients with a variety of diseases. In 1958 the respiratory unit at the Churchill Hospital in Oxford was opened; a multidisciplinary intensive care unit was opened at the University Hospital of Baltimore; a respiratory unit was started at the Toronto General Hospital. In 1961 the respiratory unit at Massachusetts General Hospital opened.

The insight and persistence of certain people enabled the available technology to be applied for the first time in a comprehensive organized fashion. Sir Robert Macintosh, professor of anesthesia at Oxford, interested Lord Nuffield, (William Morris) in the use of tank ventilators. Lord Nuffield was so impressed with these ventilators that he offered to build and donate such a ventilator to any hospital in the British Commonwealth which requested such a machine and would staff it. Experience gained in the use of these ventilators world-wide was reported. The comprehensive approach to care was developed when this technique was later applied to polio patients during epidemics. Rapidly, positive pressure ventilators were developed for use in intensive care units in response to the observed improved outcome with prolonged ventilation.

The demonstration of the first successful external defibrillator to restart the heart in 1956 by Dr Paul Zoll, and the development by Lown and co-workers of synchronized direct current cardioversion to treat recurrent refractory disturbances of the heartbeat, revolutionized the care of patients with myocardial infarction (a 'coronary'). It also created the need for continuous electrocardiogram monitoring in their care. In 1960 W. B. Kouivenhoven introduced the technique of external cardiopulmonary resuscitation. These developments taken together laid the foundation for effective coronary care units.

Although the first successful dialysis machine using heparin as an anticoagulant and cellophane as a filter was introduced by Willem Kolff in the early 1940s, widespread physiological support for acute renal failure using hemodialysis did not become widely available until the early 1960s. It then provided a tremendous advance in the effectiveness of intensive care therapy.

An early observation in the care of patients in these units was the essential role of maintaining an adequate circulation. Clinical assessment of ventilated and critically ill patients was frequently inadequate to adjust the fluids and drugs needed to support the circulation. In 1970 Swan, Ganz, and Forrester published a study in which 100 consecutive patients were assessed at the bedside using a catheter advanced through the use of an inflatable balloon at its tip to 'float' it through a major vein, into the right heart and into the pul-

Early pediatric intensive care unit. (Reproduced courtesy of the National Cancer Institute, Bethesda, MD.)

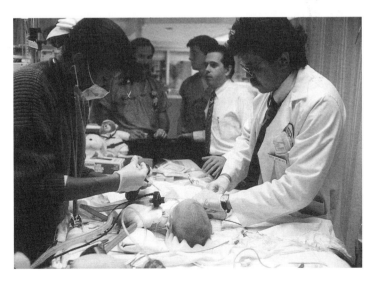

# CREUTZFELDT–JAKOB DISEASE AND BSE

Creutzfeldt–Jakob disease (CJD) occurs world-wide with an incidence approaching (and in some countries exceeding) one case per million population per annum. There are four forms of the disease: sporadic, with no known cause; familial, associated with mutations of the prion protein gene; iatrogenic, due to transmission of the agent via medical treatment — including the earlier treatment of small stature with human pituitary growth hormone and the use of human dura mater grafts; and new variant, which may be causally linked to bovine spongiform encephalopathy (BSE).

Sporadic CJD is characterized clinically by rapidly progressive dementia, involuntary movements of the muscles, and death, with a mean survival of about four months from the first symptom. It is mainly a disease of late middle age with a mean age at death of about 66. Patients with sporadic CJD aged under 30 at death are exceptional. Men and women are affected equally and epidemiological studies have not discovered significant evidence of clustering of cases to suggest an environmental point source of infection. Case-control studies have not shown any consistent risk factor for the development of the disease (except for a family history of neurodegenerative disease) and its cause is unknown. One hypothesis is that there is no environmental source of infection, and that the disease develops after the chance mutation of prion protein in the brain into the abnormal, autocatalytic, disease-associated form.

In contrast some years ago, one form of human prion disease, KURU, in New Guinea was transmitted from person to person through ritual cannibalism, by eating infected brain.

In 1996, a novel form of CJD, designated new variant CJD, was identified in Britain. This form of CJD was recognized as atypical because of the young mean age at death of 29, an unusual presentation with early psychiatric symptoms, and neuropathological features, including widespread florid plaque deposition, which had not been seen in CJD. There have now been over 100 cases of new variant CJD in Britain and three cases in France, and one in the Irish Republic. A causal link between new variant CJD and BSE was suggested by the occurrence of a novel form of human prion disease in a country with a potentially novel risk factor (in the form of BSE). Biochemical studies have shown that the pattern of the prion protein deposited in new variant CJD is distinct from sporadic CJD and similar to transmitted BSE. Transmission studies in laboratory mice have shown that the incubation period and distribution of

neuropathology following inoculation of new variant CJD are similar in mice to BSE transmissions from a range of animal species and distinct from sporadic CJD. This evidence provides strong support for the hypothesis of a causal link between CJD and BSE.

Bovine spongiform encephalopathy (BSE) is a fatal neurological disease of cattle first identified in 1986 in Britain, and called 'mad cow' disease by the media. Epidemiological research indicated that the likely source of this disease was transmission of an infectious agent through contaminated meat and bone meal in cattle feed. BSE was initially linked to

*(continued opposite)*

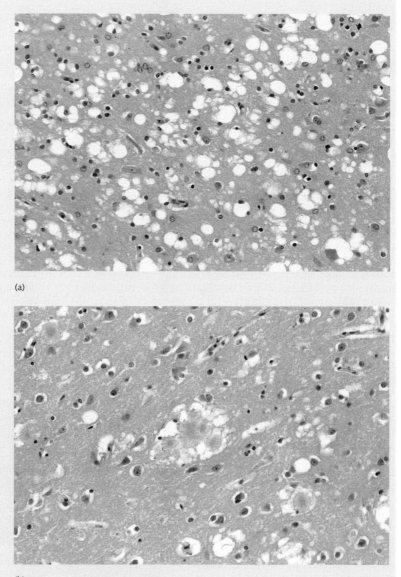

(a)

(b)

Microscopic view of brain tissue. (a) sporadic CJD, showing widespread spongiform change on staining with hematoxylin and eosin (H&E). (b) Using H&E in new variant CJD shows spongiform change and in addition (in the center of the picture) a florid plaque.

*(continued)*

other so-called prion diseases by the neuropathological appearances. Subsequently transmission studies in laboratory mice confirmed the presence of an unconventional transmissible agent, commonly now referred to as a prion (for proteinacious infectious particle). Prion diseases of animals including scrapie in sheep had been recognized for many years in several countries, but the occurrence of novel BSE-related diseases in exotic ungulates in British zoos and (in 1990) the domestic cat heightened public awareness and concern about the possibility of a risk to public health.

In 1988 legislative measures were introduced which banned the feeding of ruminant proteins, including meat and bone meal, to ruminants. Prion diseases are characterized by prolonged incubation periods and in BSE (with an average incubation period of about five years) this measure resulted in the epidemic peaking in 1992, with over 1000 cases a week being reported. The subsequent rapid decline in the number of cases meant that by 2000 only 45 cases a week were being reported. There have now been over 180 000 cases of BSE in Britain up to 2001, of which over 40 000 were in animals born after the ban. There is some evidence of maternal transmission of BSE from cow to calf, but currently no indication of horizontal transmission, for example, through contamination of pastures. Mathematical modeling of the BSE epidemic suggests that the disease will decline to low levels in the early years of the 21st century and may, perhaps, disappear.

Small numbers of cases of BSE have occurred in other countries, including Switzerland, Portugal, the Republic of Ireland, and France, presumably because of the export of contaminated cattle feed from Britain or through the export of cattle incubating the disease.

In Britain, the risk of BSE causing human disease was originally thought to be remote, in part because scrapie in sheep had not been shown to be causally linked to the human prion disease CJD. In 1989 legislative measures were introduced to minimize human exposure to cattle tissues that might contain significant levels of infectivity. The 'specified bovine offals ban' applied to all cattle, because some tissues may have contained infectivity even in apparently healthy animals. In prion diseases there is no test for infectivity before the onset of clinical disease, and there may be prion replication, particularly in lymphoreticular tissue, early in the incubation period. This measure, although not fully implemented, will have significantly reduced human dietary exposure to the BSE agent, but before 1989 there may have been fairly extensive exposure of the population. Surveillance of CJD was instituted in 1990 in Britain to identify any change in the epidemiological or other characteristics of this condition that might be related to the BSE epidemic.

The mechanism of transmission of BSE to the human population is presumed to be through the consumption of contaminated bovine food products in the 1980s. There is currently no evidence of an epidemic of new variant CJD, but a large future number of cases cannot be excluded. The occurrence of new variant CJD has had major political and economic implications and is estimated to have cost Britain £4 billion. One outcome has been a review of animal feeding practices in many countries, some of which have restricted feeding ruminant proteins to ruminants.

RGWil

*See also* CHANGING PATTERNS OF DISEASE IN THE 20TH CENTURY; INFECTIOUS DISEASES; KURU; NEUROLOGY

monary artery. For the first time, accurate measurements of right and left heart function, previously possible only in the cardiac catheter laboratory, could be made at the bedside. The impact of these initial observations and refinement of the technique has been enormous. The application, understanding, and use of data from hemodynamic monitoring have become an icon in the practice of critical care.

Although the development of intensive care units in modern western clinical medicine was in response to an epidemic illness that is now controlled, the principles applied in the care of the critically ill were so effective that intensive care became well established. Most hospitals moved quickly to create intensive care units. There was competing demand between vertical medical departments and visions for individual discipline or organ-system based intensive care units. The pressure for cost-effectiveness has led many centers to 'federation' and creation of multidisciplinary units where critically ill patients with medical, surgical, trauma, or other conditions are cared for by a dedicated team of intensivists, or critical care physicians. The staffing of modern intensive care units reflects its multidisciplinary endeavor. Physicians, nurses, respiratory therapists, dietitians, pharmacists, and nutritionists work together, each providing unique necessary input to the management of complex and desperately ill patients.

### Training

The unique nature of this activity is recognized in the creation of critical care training programs for physicians. These programs vary from country to country but usually require an additional two years of education subsequent to the completion of base specialty training in internal medicine, surgery, pediatrics, or anesthesia.

The emergence of intensive care as a separate discipline was heralded by the first world congress of critical care medicine, held in Britain in 1971, attended by 300 physicians, and since then a well-attended international event occurring every four years. By 1997, it was attended by over 2000 physicians. The effectiveness of critical care support has changed; much of the work is carried out by critical care attending physicians. Initially, they functioned almost entirely as healthcare providers. Now, responsible for admission and discharge policy to their scarce intensive care beds, they face the very difficult ethical issues of withdrawing or withholding of life support in circumstances where further support is futile. In addition, the extreme limitation on the availability of intensive care beds in some countries introduces excruciating decisions about who should be admitted. This is particularly true of countries with developing healthcare systems and many competing needs.

Nevertheless, critical care occupies a substantial portion of healthcare and hospital expenditures. This varies from 3% of all hospital beds (some European countries) to 8% (USA). Demand continues to increase as medical progress pushes the limits of the magnitude of disease treated and the need for physiologic support during treatment. Future success depends on the same commitment to patient care as that shown by the innovators who have been named, as well as the host of anonymous pioneers such as the young nurses in Edmonton in 1953–4.                    JDS

*See also* ANESTHESIA; POLIOMYELITIS

**CULTS AND QUACKERY** Just as heretics are unthinkable without the enforcement of religious orthodoxy by the churches, so quacks are essentially products of the development of medical orthodoxy seeking to define and enforce a single proper mode of medical practice: without regulars, no irregulars. In former centuries, at least, it makes more sense to distinguish orthodox medicine from quackery on the grounds of legal and professional exclusion, than in terms of the scientific standing or the success rate of treatments given. It would be historically misleading to imply that official medicine has always been competent whereas fringe medicine has been ineffectual or fraudulent. Unlike, perhaps, the regular profession, fringe medicine has always had notorious black sheep, from the huckstering mountebanks satirized by Ben Jonson and Molière to the 'toadstool millionaires' and 'medical messiahs' who swindled the public in modern America. Yet the regular profession has often appeared mercenary and domineering, and, until the 19th century, it could not reliably counter life-threatening diseases. It is little surprise that irregular healers retained their attractions.

In pre-modern times, the similarities between regular and fringe medicine were no less apparent than the differences. Both evolved a certain showmanship. Orthodox healers of former centuries cultivated a gentlemanly bedside manner, the use of Latin as mumbo-jumbo, the ancestor-worship of HIPPOCRATES (p 382) and GALEN (p 324), and grave rituals like urine-gazing — all these created the aura of the medicine man *within* the profession, by way of parallel to the quack's alligator, black cats, snakes, or canting neologisms. In centuries in which there was little efficacious *materia medica*,

psychological soothing and the placebo effect formed a major component of successful therapy amongst regulars and irregulars alike.

The boundaries between fringe and core medicine have been fluid and shifting. Certain fringe practitioners have sought to ingratiate themselves with the establishment, or at least to bask in its prestige, and many have called themselves Professor or Doctor, without proper justification. Orthodox medicine, for its part, has sometimes seen fit to assimilate fringe practices rather than lose patients *en masse* to marginal medicine. To some degree this happened in the Victorian age with MESMERISM; it may be occurring today with acupuncture. In short, the historical distinction between medical quackery and orthodoxy has been more social than scientific.

From medieval times, all major European nations developed systems of medical licensing, policed by the upper echelons of the medical profession and ultimately sanctioned by kings and governments. Guilds and corporations regulated entry into the profession, and medical oligarchies emerged, exercising a near monopoly of access to promotion, power, and favor, and aiming for a closed shop, to maintain professional standards and protect the public. Numbers were kept small, and fees correspondingly high. This strategy was certainly effective in stigmatizing and marginalizing other healers. But it rarely proved effective as a way of *suppressing* the unorthodox. For, until recently, there were never enough privileged practitioners to meet the overall demand for medical services, especially in rural areas and small towns. With regulars too distant or too expensive, common people had to resort to self-medication and to quacks.

Moreover, in centuries when disease was king and death omnipresent, not only the poor patronized irregular healers. In the case of severe disease, it made sense for all manner of sufferers to shop around. When Prime Minister Sir Robert Walpole found no relief in orthodox medicine for his stomach ailments and kidney stones, he had resort to the quack Joshua WARD'S (this page) much-touted pills. The physician Sir Hans SLOANE (p 56), who rose to become President of the Royal Society and chief endower of the British Museum, had a niece with a spinal deformity. When orthodox treatment failed, he called in the Epsom bone-setter and manipulator, Sally Mapp, who is said to have worked a cure.

Irregular healers have appealed in many ways. Sometimes their cures have appeared extremely modern. Others have been less disgusting and severe than orthodox medicine's heavy artillery of purges, bleedings, and vomits. Certain fringe practitioners, like some evangelical preachers, achieved fashionability. Wealthy invalids with time on their hands would want to sample novel treatments. In the 19th century, Viktor Preissnitz's health-farm hydrotherapy became chic amongst the European élite. In one year his patients supposedly included one royal highness, one duke, one duchess, 22 princes and princesses, 149 counts and countesses, 88 barons and baronesses, 14 generals, 53 staff officers, 196 captains and subalterns, 104 high and low civil servants, 65 divines, 46 artists, and 87 physicians. Hypochondriacs might be flattered by the assiduity and attention they received from a polished fringe doctor. Such unorthodox practitioners as Franz Anton MESMER (p 487) (the late-18th century inventor of hypnotism) and his contemporary James Graham (pioneer of sex therapy) were skilful showmen and actors. Advocate of vegetarianism, mud-bathing, and sexual rejuvenation, Graham combined a marvelous theatrical touch with a sure grasp of audience psychology. Graham presented himself as a high priest at what he called his Temple of Health at the Adelphi, just off the Strand, with a young female priestess who assisted, half-naked, 'at the display of the Celestial Meteors, and of that sacred Vital Fire over which she watches, and whose application in the cure of diseases, she daily has the honour of directing'.

Fringe benefits like Mesmer and Graham astutely addressed themselves to those problems that were the fancy packaging, appealing brand names, and particular ills of high society: ennui, anxiety, HYSTERIA, sexual incompatibility, depression, and nervous disorders. By being forced on to the margins, fringe practitioners were almost forced to exploit the opportunities and techniques of the marketplace in the era of expanding capitalism. The medical profession ensured the prosperity of those they proscribed.

## Public standing

Unlike licensed medical men, the irregular's fame came entirely from his standing with the public, not his peers. He had to sell his wares in the market. The arts of publicity were crucial. Some, such as the Prussian influenza-curer, Gustavus Katterfelto in the 1780s, exploited penumbra of magic, wonder, and wizardry: black cloaks, snakes, black cats, fuming potions, and electrical sparks. Mountebanks traditionally toured accompanied by monkeys and zanies. Some sought status in the public eye by making the most of being — of pleading to be — foreign and exotic. Thus 'Chevalier' Taylor, the 18th-century eye specialist, lectured in pidgin Latin which he confidently, but inaccurately, described as 'the true Ciceronian'. Others sought credit by drop-

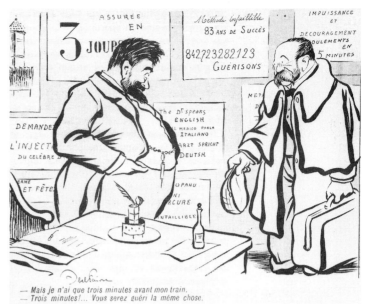

— Mais je n'ai que trois minutes avant mon train.
— Trois minutes!... Vous serez guéri la même chose.

ping the names of the powerful and famous. Bottles of 'Daffy's Elixir' had a label stating that 'The Elixir was much recommend to the public by Dr King, Physician to King Charles II, and the late learned and ingenious Dr Radcliffe'. Joshua Ward, the marketer of the famous 'Drop and Pill', won fame and public confidence after putting George II's dislocated thumb back in place. He also received the testimonies of celebrated men, including the novelist, Henry Fielding.

Quacks traditionally did their business through personal sales. Most were itinerant. The traveling salesman had the aura of mystery. He was elusive to the authorities. Having exhausted one market, he could move on. Increasingly, however, fringe healers settled down, relying upon the publicity apparatus of commercial capitalism, notably the newspapers. 'The Widow READ, removed from the Upper End of Highstreet to the *New Printing-Office* near the Market, continues to make and sell her well-known ointment for the ITCH', announced a Philadelphia newspaper in 1731. Newspaper advertising multiplied the potential market for quack preparations several thousand fold at a stroke. Their nostrums were often sold retail by newspaper publishers and offices.

Soon, some were trying Blitzkrieg advertising. James Eno was the first to use whole-page advertisements in the press for his fruit-salts. 'Professor' Thomas Holloway, who marketed cure-all pills in Victorian England, was spending £20 000 a year on advertising by the mid-19th

A quack claims he can cure a man in the three minutes before his train leaves. From a lithograph by J-A. Faivre, 1902. (Reproduced courtesy of the Wellcome Institute Library, London.)

century. He was the first world-wide advertiser. His name appeared on hoardings in London; it was to be found in newspapers of China, India, and Peru; it even appeared on the Great Pyramid in Egypt. Advertisements were usually festooned with testimonials and other forms of puffery. Quacks pioneered sales gimmicks, including fancy packaging, appealing brand names, and special offers.

Traditional quackery possessed many apparent advantages. It might appear cheaper than regular medicine. It could be more anonymous, important in the case of embarrassing complaints. Sometimes it appealed to nature. It claimed to conquer otherwise incurable diseases such as CANCER and TUBERCULOSIS. Not least, in an age in which women were excluded from regular practice, the presence of many women quacks in big cities doubtless appealed to female sufferers too embarrassed to take their gynecological problems to gentlemen surgeons.

Moreover, quacks exploited a psychological appeal, playing upon human unhappiness and unfulfilled expectations, the susceptibilities of the short, the fat, the inarticulate, the impotent, the aging, the unsuccessful, the shy, the spotty. Sometimes they have played upon fear and shame. Illness, pain, and debility are the wages of evil or ignorance, they claim. Such guilt-inducing ploys have obviously been particularly effective in the case of patients suffering from venereal diseases, from alcoholism, obesity, and psychological disorders.

In its individualist and itinerant form, quackery had peaked by 1800. Increasingly, the thirst for non-regular medicine has been satisfied since then by the rise of medical cults, espousing a philosophy of alternative healing, typically linked to specific religious and personal faiths, above all anti-professional, radical modes of self-help. With its appeal to natural and simple cures, HOMEO-PATHY, developed by Samuel HAHNEMANN (p 391) in late 18th-century Germany, was one of the first to enjoy a vogue. Hahnemann put forward the principle of treating like with like (for instance, fever-inducing drugs should be used in fever cases), and also believed in the efficacy of very small doses of exceptionally pure drugs, partly because, in his view, orthodox medicine habitually overdosed.

## Water cures

Water cures grew popular. WATER has had an enormous cachet as a cure on the medical fringes, regarded as an agent of cleanliness and purification, the matrix of life, and the symbol of baptism and rebirth. It has been deployed in fringe therapies in innumerable ways: pure fresh water has been drunk to cleanse the system; cold water baths have been used in hydrotherapy; sea water has been taken internally and externally; and, most commonly, healing mineral springs have been promoted. Within temperance and teetotal movements, water became medicinal.

The appeal of the fringe cults has been not just to relieve physical pain, but to make born a new person — even to put the world to rights. Their leaders have been moral, social, and political reformers, wanting to cure ills on the widest possible scale. Pain and suffering have been seen as the consequences of the radical misorganization of society and false values. Society needed to be cured along with the individual. Lydia Pinkham in 19th-century America offers a typical instance. Brought up in a QUAKER household, at an early age Lydia Pinkham embraced most liberal and humanitarian causes, including abolitionism and temperance. She dabbled with spiritualism and PHRENOLOGY, currency reform, and vegetarianism. She launched her own fringe medicine, the Vegetable Compound, quite expressly as part of her own feminist platform. She believed that male doctors were insensitive to female complaints. 'Only a woman understands a woman's ills', she contended. Testimonials from women using the compound confirmed the popularity of a medicine attached to a cause.

## Return to naturalism

Reacting against the early 19th century vogue amongst regulars for 'heroic physic', various health-reform causes sprang up, especially in North America, championed not by physicians but by lay people, disaffected equally with official creeds and regular medicine, and seeking to replace both with a unified, holistic philosophy of spiritual and bodily health, carved out of their own personal experience.

Amongst such sects as the Grahamites and the Thomsonians — both advocates of herbalism — certain convictions have been widely shared. These sects have argued that civilized man has brought disease upon himself by the 'fall' manifest in modern life-styles: urbanism, greed, speed, excessive meat-eating, and abuse of fermented liquor. By way of remedy, they advocated — on medical, moral, and religious grounds — a return to 'natural' ways of living — vegetarianism, sexual restraint, temperance (both general and specific), the abandonment of stimulants such as tea, coffee, and tobacco. They generally urged an end of artificial and synthetic drugs, trusting to God-given, natural herbal remedies. Homeopaths insisted upon ultra-pure medicaments, taken in minute quantities; Thomsonians and Coffinites restricted themselves to a few

*Plate 3* An assemblage of acupuncture models in a wooden frame. (Reproduced courtesy of Chave/Jennings/Tony Stone Images)

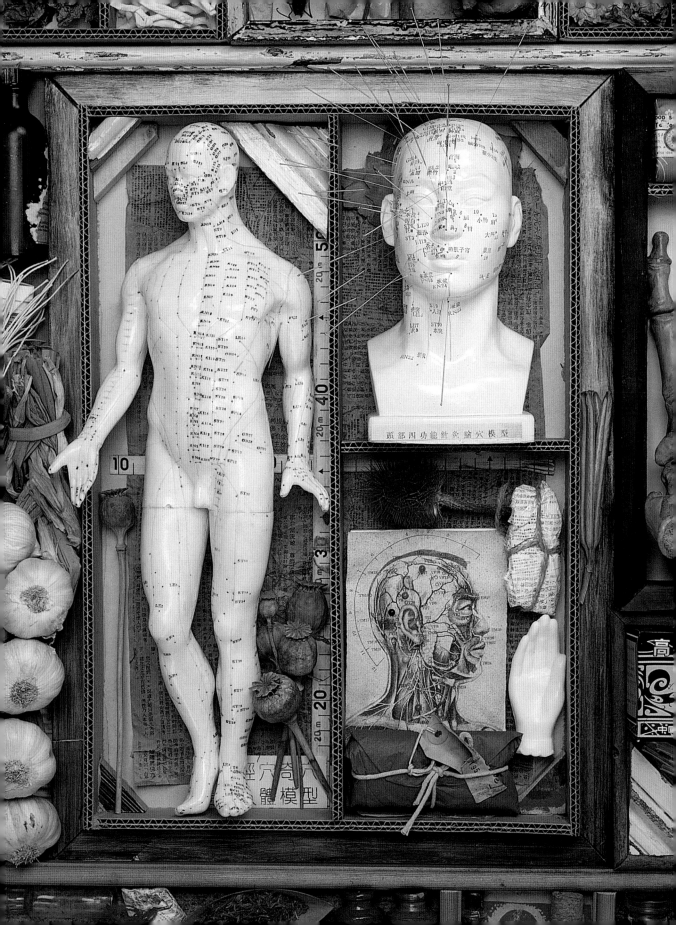

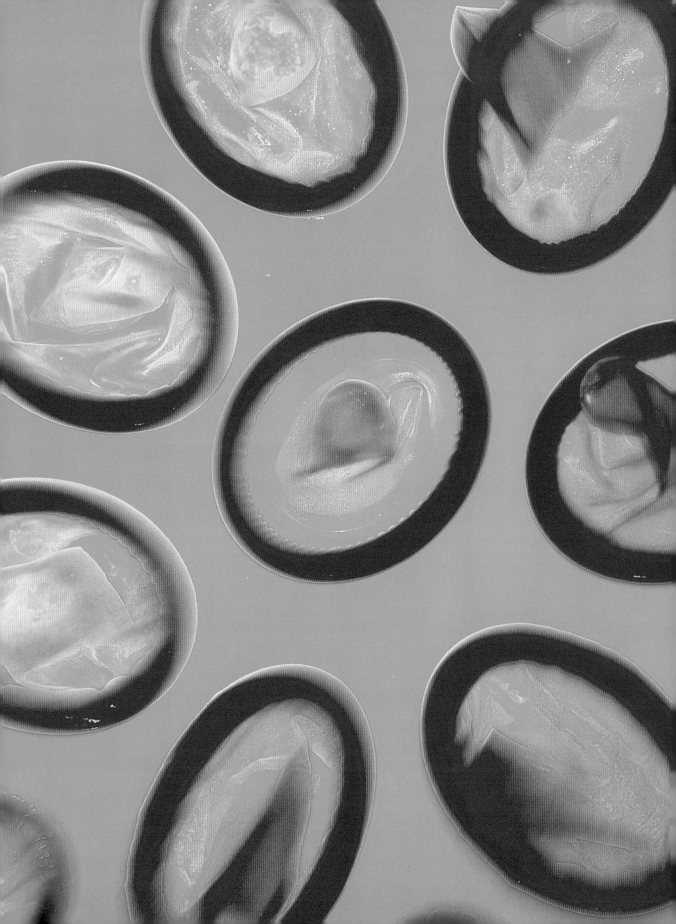

herbal preparations. Influenced by Swedenborgianism, some groups went a stage further, discarding medicines altogether, and trusting to the healing powers of nature, aided by the healing powers of water, prayer, self-control, and spiritual illumination.

The CHRISTIAN SCIENCE movement exemplifies many of these. Rejecting the strict Congregationalism of her parents, Mary Baker EDDY (p 713) spent much of her youth sick with non-specific nervous disorders. Regular physicians did her no good. Relieved by homeopathy she then undertook a self-healing process, the success of which, in 1866, led her to outline her own system, the creed of which declared that 'there is but one creation, and it is wholly spiritual'. Matter therefore was an illusion; hence there could be no such reality as somatic disease. As explained in her best-selling textbook, *Science and health* (1875), true 'mind healing' would dispel the illusions of sickness and pain. Proclaiming itself the new scientific medicine of the new age, Christian Science owed its high rate of conversions to the 'patient: heal thyself' confidence it inspired.

Especially in 19th-century North America, medical cults and fringe religion were typically interlinked. From their early days, both the Mormons and the Seventh Day Adventists voiced their antipathy to regular medicine, Joseph Smith recognizing only roots and herbs, and the Mormons, once in Utah, passing laws restricting the dispensing of most orthodox remedies ('deadly poisons'). Mormons, in particular, championed the constitutional right to resist compulsory smallpox VACCINATION. The Adventists, led by Ellen White, claimed a 'gospel of health', which particularly valued hydropathic cures. Their Health Reform Institute at Battle Creek, Michigan, was headed by John Harvey Kellogg (1852–1943), brother of the cereal manufacturer.

Why has the medical fringe enjoyed such a huge and lasting appeal? By being forced out of the élite world of medicine, fringe medicine was actually dumped in the most fertile seedbed of all: the capitalist market-place in the age of rampant capitalism (an arena which orthodox medicine, with its ethical and professional goals, chose to deny to itself). Moreover, fringe medicine often moved into an aspect of human experience and need largely abandoned by orthodox medicine and orthodox religion alike. Orthodox medicine increasingly treated just the body, in ways unintelligible to the patient. Orthodox religion made promises for an immaterial soul in the hereafter. By contrast, marginal medicine actually appealed to a sense of the whole person — the unity of mental and physical experience — and sometimes also to two other unities: the oneness of the person with the world, and the cooperation of patient and doctor. Quacks often spoke in languages that people understood.

RPor

*See also* RELIGIOUS SECTS

**CYSTITIS** See NEPHROLOGY

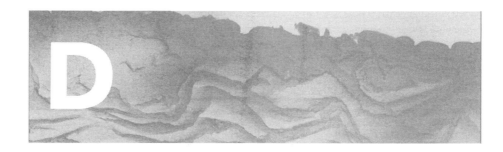

Sir Henry Hallett **DALE** (1875–1968). British physiologist and pharmacologist. After some years working with Paul EHRLICH (p 260), Dale joined the Wellcome Research Laboratories in 1904, where over a period of 10 years he established his reputation as an experimental pharmacologist. In 1914 he was made director of the department of biochemistry and pharmacology of the projected National Institute for Medical Research which was finally established in 1920; in 1928 Dale became its director. From 1938–60 he was chairman of the Wellcome Trust and from 1940 to 1945 president of the Royal Society. In 1936 he shared the Nobel prize in medicine with Otto Loewi for work on the chemical transmission of nerve impulses.

Dale's researches were mainly in experimental pharmacology. In his early years he showed that ergotoxin would reverse the hypertensive effect of adrenaline (1906) and he established the oxytocic effect of posterior pituitary extract (1909). From 1914–29 he worked on the active constituents in ergot and then on histamine and acetylcholine. In much of his research he was associated with Barger and they were the first to use the term 'sympathomimetic'. In his later years Dale was the dominating figure in medical research and a worthy spokesman for British science.

**ANOTHER FORM OF DANCE**

**TARANTISM** was an epidemic form of dancing mania prevalent in parts of Italy from the 15th to the 17th century. It was popularly supposed either to be caused by or to cure the effects of a bite of a spider.

**DANCE** Few people would have considered Rembrandt's great painting, *The anatomy lesson of Dr Tulp*, a good starting point for a ballet, but in 1964 it was brought to the stage by the American choreographer, Glen Tetley. He was working with an avant-garde company, Nederlands Dans Theater, and the combination of a famous Dutch picture and an unusual and controversial theme was appropriate for an arresting première in The Hague in the permissive 'sixties. The opening scene was faithfully reproduced, with the dead body on the dissecting table surrounded by the anatomist and various doctors and students, but that was the extent of the medical references. The rest was a flashback re-creation of the dead man's life with his mother, wife, and friends.

The grimmest balletic portrayal of the medical world came in Kenneth MacMillan's *Different drummer*. Based on *Woyzeck*, Georg Büchner's 1836 play, it showed a German private soldier of that time at the mercy of a half-crazed doctor who used him for callous experiments. MacMillan, always in his narrative works drawn to themes of misfits, outsiders, and perverse emotions, created a distressing picture of the mental and physical bullying of Woyzeck and its tragic consequences.

It was MacMillan who, in *The invitation*, first included a disturbing simulation of the rape of a young girl by a trusted man, and later extended his study of this into a gang rape on a dockland site in *The Judas tree*. In the last act of his *Anastasia*, doctors and nurses were featured when Anna Anderson's claims to be the Grand Duchess Anastasia led to her treatment as a psychiatric patient. Again, the medical staff as seen through her eyes were inhuman and heartless. Earlier in this ballet about the ill-fated Romanovs, hemophilia was poignantly indicated in the character of the little Tsarevich, his sudden serious attacks of bleeding, and the part played by Rasputin in their treatment. Fever and delirium brought about the final tragedy in MacMillan's *Manon*, in a tempestuous duet for Des Grieux and Manon as she died in the Louisiana swamps. In *Valley of shadows*, based on Georgio Bassani's *The garden of the Finzi-Continis*, a young man, Alberto, is mortally ill with leukemia. In *Mayerling*, MacMillan dealt with drug addiction, showing Crown Prince Rudolf injecting himself with a hypodermic syringe before he shot Mary Vetsera and himself.

Drug taking of a different kind, and treated romantically instead of realistically, occurred in 19th century St Petersburg in Marius Petipa's *La bayadère*, where Solor, mourning for the priestess Nikiya, smoked opium and dreamt that he was reunited with her in the Kingdom of the Shades. Nikiya had died from a snakebite — a chief priest had offered her an antidote, valiantly refused, in return for sexual favors. Another romantic drug-dreamer was the Poet in Frederick Ashton's *Apparitions*. To the exquisite accompaniment of music by Liszt, he crumpled up page after page of unsuccessful poems before taking a fatal dose of laudanum and entering a fantasy world. There, a beautiful woman in balldress, a hussar, a menacing monk, and a witches' sabbath, were part of his confusing hallucinations. The same theme served Léonide Massine in Berlioz's *Symphonie fantastique*, and in a production of *Swan lake* Peter Darrell revised the traditional story so that the Swan Queen was a drug-induced vision of Prince Siegfried's.

Drugs combined with drink were poor Bramwell Brontë's downfall, as seen in Gillian Lynne's ballet *The Brontës*. TUBERCULOSIS, of course, featured in that production, and also, less emphasized, in a short work, *Charlotte Brontë*, by Ronald Hynd. The same scourge of the time, naturally, played its part in *Marguerite and Armand*, Ashton's intensely lyrical ballet for Fonteyn and Nureyev based on *La dame aux camèlias*. Naturally, nothing too devastatingly clinical was attempted. The modern scourge, AIDS, has preoccupied both American and British choreographers — two recent British works have been Matthew Hart's *Dances with death*, in which the ensemble were dressed in white, for healthy, and red, for infected, blood. David Bintley's *The dance house* (for San Francisco Ballet), which in intention linked AIDS with medieval PLAGUES, again made its point mainly through design — some of the women's costumes were bisected by a broad red band from crotch to chin. In essence, these have been symbolic pieces, no more closely identified with medical problems than any of the lyrical tussles of older ballets in which a lover struggles with the figure of Death for the life of a doomed partner.

For most of the ailments and illnesses referred to in dance works, doctors play no part and, sadly, there is no trace of anyone depicting a doctor or a nurse as a helper and healer. Friar Lawrence was no doctor but, as a herbalist, in all versions of *Romeo and Juliet*, he provides Juliet with the clever potion that will counterfeit death. The scenario Nureyev adopted, taken more closely from Shakespeare, also introduced the Apothecary who — under the counter — sold Romeo a phial of poison in Mantua.

Somnambulism has provided a theme for one or two ballets, notably Balanchine's *Night shadow* — no one who has seen it forgets the wonderful dance of the unconscious lady with the candle, who wanders in on points and is gently manipulated by the Poet. An inability to speak occurred in *Mute wife*, based on Anatole France's story by Antonia Cobos, while Matthew Bourne's *Cinderella* for Adventures in Motion Pictures showed a speechless Cinderella suffering traumas after witnessing a murder. Both she, and her injured air pilot lover, were reunited and instantly cured in a psychiatric nursing home, where a doctor actually seemed to be asking her a few questions. Bintley's *Sylvia*, with a revised scenario,

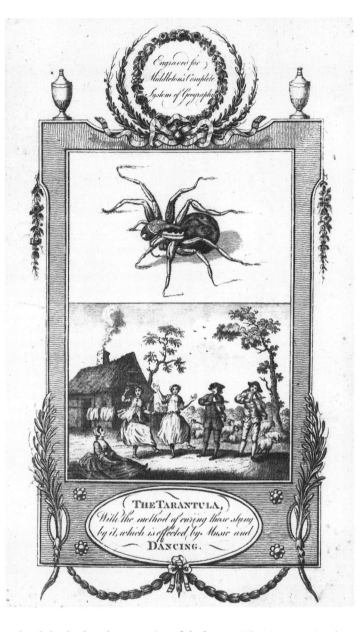

18th century engraving of tarantism. (Reproduced courtesy of the Wellcome Institute Library, London.)

replaced the death and resurrection of the hero Amynta with a spell of blindness, dealt with light-heartedly. During this, Amynta (supposedly) partnered Sylvia by touch only. He was visited by Eros posing as an optometrist (with white coat and head lamp), and later that playful god danced a solo as a wooden-legged pirate chief. More seriously, but in romantic terms, blindness (and death) finally afflicted the sylph in *La Sylphide*, when her mortal lover was deceived by the witch into giving her a scarf that robbed her of her wings, her sight, and her life. A very different attempt to treat the problems of blindness was

## THE OTHER DARWIN

Erasmus **DARWIN**
(1731–1802). British
physician and writer. Darwin
practiced in Nottingham,
Lichfield, and latterly Derby.
He was a man of great
energy with a powerful
intellect, but aroused
antagonism by being
imperious and irascible. He
was a friend of Samuel
Johnson and a member of the
Lunar Society of Birmingham,
which also counted Josiah
Wedgwood, Joseph Priestley,
and James Watt as members.
He was the grandfather of
Charles DARWIN (this page)
and Francis GALTON (p 285).
His publications were *the
loves of the plants* (1789)
and *Zoönomia* (1794).

## ORIGIN OF SPECIES, THE

is the classic work of
Charles Darwin, published
in 1859, in which he
proposed natural selection
as the main mechanism of
evolution. The full title
was *On the origin of
species by means of
natural selection, or the
preservation of favoured
races in the struggle for
life.*

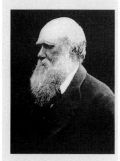

Charles Darwin
(1809–1882), author of
*The origin of species.*
(From the National Library of
Medicine, Bethesda, MD.)

made by Geoffrey Cauley in a short-lived ballet,
*La symphonie pastorale,* based on an André Gide
story of a blind young girl rescued by a clergyman. MacMillan, in a work for American Ballet
Theatre, *Winter's eve,* also dealt sensitively with
the harrowing theme of a blind girl in love with a
sighted man.

Insanity is always the stuff of drama. In the
romantic era, Giselle lost her reason in a celebrated 'mad scene', when she was betrayed by
Albrecht, and countless ballerinas have produced
personal interpretations of her tragedy. MacMillan
created a stark work called *Playground,* in which
all the characters were modern mental patients
and the leading role was a remarkable study of a
young woman with fixations about her cosmetics
and her handbag. A long and (it must be admitted) tedious ballet choreographed by Flemming
Flindt for the Royal Danish Ballet, *Caroline
Mathilde,* was enlivened by a powerful study of the
mad and epileptic King Christian VII of Denmark
— and here a doctor seemed to be in attendance.
Back in 1935 Ninette de Valois composed a masterpiece in *The rake's progress,* based on Hogarth's
series of pictures. The rake's dissolute life gradually brought him to lunacy, and the Bedlam scene
with which the ballet ends was as moving and
truthful a study of a group of men withdrawn
from sanity (and the helplessness of those who
love them) as has ever been put on stage.    KSW

*See also* ART; DR TULP (p 66); OPERA; TUBER-
CULOSIS

**DARWIN**, Charles Robert (1809–82). English
naturalist. The grandson of Erasmus Darwin,
Charles Darwin made abortive approaches to
medicine and to the church before finding his true
vocation through the influence of Henslow, the
professor of botany in Cambridge, and the writings of Alexander V. Humboldt. It was Henslow
who procured for him the post of naturalist to the
*Beagle,* and probably Humboldt's enthusiastic
accounts of South America which gave him the
firmness to overcome parental resistance to his
expedition. The observations which he made on
that voyage, and his subsequent reflections, led
him to the belief in evolution of species through
the mechanism of natural selection acting on
spontaneous variations. This theory was matured
during long years of semi-invalidism at Downe,
perhaps the most striking instance of 'creative
malady' described by Sir George Pickering; and it
was given to the world, partly because of similar
ideas communicated to him by A. R. Wallace, and
certainly without precipitancy, in November 1859.
In response to requests for an account of his
'success as a man of science, whatever this may
have amounted to', he drew attention to 'the love
of science, unbounded patience in long reflecting

over any subject, industry in observing and collecting facts, and a fair share of invention as well as
of common sense'.

**DEGENERATION** became a significant medico-
psychiatric diagnosis during the second half of
the 19th century that was applied not only to individuals, but also more generally to culture and
society, even to national populations as a whole.
Juxtaposed with concepts of regeneration and
collective fitness, the language of degeneration
entered significantly into European racial thought
(most notoriously in anti-Semitism), and was also
assimilated to varying degrees across the range of
the human sciences. None the less, even in the
hey-day of western imperialism and Orientalism,
such perspectives were always reversible. Thus, for
instance, historians have compellingly described
Chinese eugenic myths about the biological inferiority of the non-Chinese and shown that these
were never simply the product of western discourse. Moreover, degeneration was not only used
to describe extra-European 'races' (degeneration
*from* a European norm), but also to express the
disordered state of populations *within* its authors'
own societies. In Britain, specialist medical journals, including the *Lancet,* charted pathological
decline in rural hinterlands and within the great
cities, above all among the 'casual poor'. Emerging
Victorian medical concerns with nutrition and
social welfare were often inflected by — and
deflected into — the phantasmagoria of degeneracy. 'Nature' and 'nurture' were both seen to contribute to degeneration, although emphasis was
characteristically placed on the former.

### Cluster of ideas

Whilst in broad terms, the theme of degeneration
is ancient and culturally widespread, the specific
cluster of medico-psychiatric ideas described here
was decisively formulated by Dr B. A. Morel in
France just before the publication of DARWIN's
(this page) *The origin of species* (1859), and then
greatly extended by others after the collapse of
Louis Napoleon's Second Empire, the débâcle of
the Franco-Prussian War, and the renewed revolutionary events in Paris, 1871. Morel's *Traité des
dégénérescences physiques, intellectuelles et morales
de l'espéce humaine* (1857) was broadly Lamarckian
in flavor (it assumed the inheritance of acquired
characteristics); it drew upon a range of existing
ideas about racial variation and the environment,
but offered a new and appealingly broad synthesis. It assumed that myriad 'pathologies' could be
passed through the family tree, but that there
would be different forms in each generation.
Beginning from the enigma of cretinism (which
he divided into curable and incurable categories),
Morel posited a wider network of ailments,

amidst which the cretin was but an instance. Individual phenomena, which might have previously looked quite unrelated, were now considered to be symptoms of the underlying transgenerational condition. While he suggested that morbid families became sterile in a few generations, later commentators took issue with his reassuring expectation of extinction within degenerate lines. During the period of the Third Republic, the celebrated French psychiatrist Magnan developed this pioneering work, elaborated the technical vocabulary, and removed the most conspicuous traces of Morel's Catholicism: degeneration as sin, product of 'the Fall'.

### Shock waves

Although no single degenerationist text, Morel's included, produced shock waves — or a clash with orthodox religion — quite on the scale of Darwin's *Origin*, the argument and themes of the *Traité* had enduring importance within social and scientific thought for the remainder of the century, often in loose combination with Darwinism. Ideas from Morel, Darwin, Spencer, and others informed a major new tradition of thought on social delinquency, which frequently challenged assumptions about human free will (and thus brought it into conflict with the orthodox views of lawyers and churchmen). What came to be known as 'positivist criminology' involved a rejection of classical penology (as earlier developed by Beccaria and Bentham), which had been committed to viewing each subject as a potentially reasonable being, who could calculate right and wrong, and the personal price to be paid in the event of social transgression. In the influential if sometimes decided thought of Lombroso (the pioneer of this 'criminal anthropology') it seemed obvious that atavistic offenders could not 'calculate'; they had either regressed from, or not fully evolved to, the standards and mental capacities of the civilized and should thus be segregated or even eliminated altogether in the interests of the newly unified Italian nation. If Lombroso's brigands and other assorted villains were cast as spectacularly monstrous (handle-shaped ears, hairy faces, thick skins, etc.), others feared less visible forms of social morbidity, suspecting the presence of mutations and lesions inside the offender's body. Lombroso's works, such as *L'uomo delinquente* (1876), although always controversial, lay at the center of international debate about the nature of the criminal for several decades. Important international congresses were held in European capitals in and beyond the 1880s, where the so-called 'Italian School' and its swelling band of critics were pitted against one another in fierce and animated discussion of atavism, recidivism, and the pathological milieu.

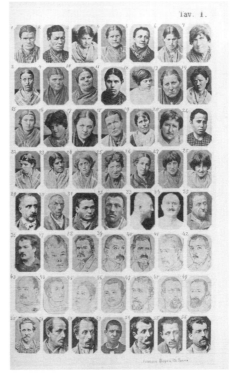

Some portraits from the Lombroso Museum of criminal anthropology now housed at the department of legal medicine in Turin. The drive to visualize degeneration and atavism was undoubtedly the most dominant of its tendencies. Lombroso and his followers produced a vast gallery of portraits, waxworks, photos, handwriting samples, painting, sketches and so forth. In Britain, Darwin's cousin Francis Galton even invented a composite photography machine to capture the essential image of the deviant, the Jew, and others. (Reproduced from Pick, D. (2000). *Faces of degeneration*, CUP.).

In psychiatry, criminology, and later, sexology, degeneration usually implied the helpless condition of the group: degenerates were enslaved by their organic state, the 'tyranny of their organization', as one specialist, the Victorian doctor, Henry MAUDSLEY (p 484), memorably declared. Not all commentators favored interpretations as pessimistic as those expressed in the later work of Maudsley (from *Body and will*, 1883, to *Organic to human*, 1916), nor solutions to crime problems as draconian as Lombroso's, but these basic ideas and models were extensively developed on both sides of the Atlantic. Detailed genealogical case studies of families in the United States — '*The Jukes': a study in crime, pauperism, disease and heredity* (1877) was the best known — appeared to confirm the inherited nature of antisocial behavior. Readers of Émile Zola's contemporaneous cycle of novels on the degeneration of the Rougon-Macquart family would not have been surprised by such gloomy American conclusions.

Degeneration was used to comprehend a bewildering range of physical, mental, and sexual conditions. Not infrequently, medical certificates of this period would begin 'dégénérescence mentale avec…' But solemn claims for the scientific validity of the word sat uneasily with its actual variability of use. It was, however, this very plasticity which had made it so durable a concept, albeit one

The skull of the brigand Vilella, which led Lombroso to dream in 1870: 'At the sight of that skull, I seemed to see all of a sudden, lighted up as a vast plain under a flaming sky, the problem of the nature of the criminal — an atavistic being who reproduces in his person the ferocious instincts of primitive humanity and the inferior animals. Thus were explained anatomically the enormous jaws, high cheek bones, prominent superciliary arches, solitary lines in the palms,... the desire not only to extinguish life in the victim, but to mutilate the corpse, tear its flesh and drink its blood. (Reproduced from Lombroso, C. (1889). *L 'uomo delinquente*, Turin.)

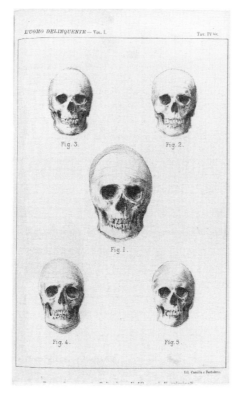

criminality, pathological emotions, and neuro-pathic families, and in Krafft-Ebing's frequently re-issued *Psychopathia sexualis* (1886).

## Anxieties

Anxieties about population decline (especially in France after 1871) or differential birth rates between classes (notably in late-Victorian and Edwardian Britain) were frequently conceived in terms of national degeneration; so too were contemporary tastes in fiction and philosophy. In criticism of the so-called 'Decadent' literary mood of the *fin de siècle*, the Hungarian emigré to Paris, Dr Max Nordau (better known perhaps as a key figure in the early history of Zionism) caused a stir in 1892 by publishing his outrageous compendium, *Entartung (Degeneration)*, in which many illustrious writers were severely diagnosed and condemned. In identification with, and sometimes derision of, these medico-psychiatric pronouncements, creative writers constantly engaged with the terms. Nordau's critics flippantly accused him of being degenerate himself, but the arcane nomenclature showed no sign of abating. The stories of, *inter alia*, Maupassant, Huysmans, Zola, or Conrad, the paintings of Ensor, the dramas of Ibsen, the philosophy of William JAMES (p 449) and Nietzsche are frequently unintelligible without some awareness of these powerful and intensely contested concerns. FREUD (p 321) was also deeply intrigued by — and increasingly skeptical of — such hereditarian models, particularly as associated with the 'Napoleon of the neuroses' who had initially so inspired him, Jean-Martin CHARCOT (p 401). But perhaps no personal appropriation of degenerationist classifications has quite the urgency or the personal poignancy of Oscar Wilde's reference to the theme in a letter to the Home Secretary. Jailed in 1895 for HOMOSEXUALITY, under the Criminal Law Amendment Act of the previous decade, Wilde sought clemency on the declared grounds that he was indeed a degenerate and therefore worthy of treatment rather than punishment. He cited Nordau and Lombroso's views of 'the petitioner' himself and remarked of his own sexual behavior: 'Such offences are forms of sexual madness'.

More important than the sheer quantity of degenerationist jeremiads was their shared acceptance of natural scientific authority. The fate of the individual and the ups and downs of western society at large were no longer discussed primarily as religious, philosophical, or ethical problems, but as the precise outcome of physical conditions and organic processes. The dry technical aura surrounding such emotive affairs was further perpetuated when Galton coined the term 'EUGENICS' (in 1883) to describe a putative science of racial policy, based on the model of animal husbandry, a

subject to an increasingly powerful critique by the 1890s. If it first implied a 'falling away from an ideal type' (however defined), it quickly came to cover a multitude of inherited ailments and sins, and had the potential to implicate the loftiest prince as well as the most down-trodden pauper. Precisely because of its discursive ambiguity, it could be deployed as a term by scientists, artists, and novelists of varying political sympathies (including considerable numbers who would have defined themselves as liberals and socialists). DARWIN (p 214) himself was troubled by the social risks of allowing the 'unfit' to breed (unlike on a good farm, let alone in the wild), but left it to more brazen followers, including his cousin, Francis GALTON (p 285), to consider more fully such implications. Versions of social Darwinism and degenerationism converged, as, for instance, in a book by an English scientist, Edwin Ray Lankester, *Degeneration: a chapter in Darwinism* (1880), where the problem of thriving parasites was taken to be a scientific as much as a sociopolitical issue of immediate concern. Titles such as *Degeneration amongst Londoners* (1885) or *Evolution by atrophy in biology and sociology* (1894) typified significant intellectual tendencies across *fin-de-siècle* Europe. Degenerationist labels and diagnoses multiplied still further in Charles Féré's series of works on

project of whose urgency he was in no doubt. He eventually sponsored a movement which gathered a varied membership in and beyond Edwardian Britain, most notably through Galton's energetic protégé, Karl PEARSON (p 782) as well as in the USA, continental Europe, Latin America, and so forth. Ideas of degeneration were increasingly institutionalized through academic posts, journals, congresses, legislative struggles, and conflicts in different countries, albeit to vastly varying degrees of success. It is not to be forgotten that the Nazi sterilization laws of the 1930s were in part modeled on much earlier debates on German eugenics, but also, crucially, on broader European currents of thought on race and degeneration, not to mention specific legislation introduced in various American states during the early decades of the century.

The theme of degeneration can be traced beyond 1914, not only with regard to psychiatric and cultural diagnosis, but also in terms of national self-definitions. The idea of the other side's biological degeneracy was deployed alongside 'civilization' and 'barbarism' in the propaganda battles of the Great War. But nowhere was the inseparability of such cant medico-moral terminology more ominously portrayed in our own 'age of extremes' than in Nazi cultural political rhetoric itself. The 'Degenerate Art' exhibition in Munich in the 1930s was a gruesome legacy of the form of cultural criticism pioneered in different circumstances by Nordau and company. The display was paralleled by an exhibition of approved German work. Although the history of the Third Reich and the Final Solution inevitably must shadow our reading of the entire earlier literature, it is important to recognize the quite different contexts in which degenerationist thought had originally been formulated, as also the political and scientific ambiguity of this investigation, at least until the First World War and perhaps well into the 1930s. Only in the light of the Holocaust has the language of degeneration and eugenics come to be so widely excoriated in western culture, exorcised from mainstream political discourse, although not so completely, even then, as has sometimes been supposed. To assume that it is extinct, or that it has always been a function of an exclusively German tradition, would involve a powerful and dangerous cultural amnesia.                                          DPi

*See also* HOLOCAUST

**DEMENTIA** See ALZHEIMER'S DISEASE

**DEMOGRAPHY** 'It is an obvious truth that population must always be kept down to the level of the means of subsistence': Reverend Thomas Malthus, 1798.

Future demographic trends are inherently uncertain, increasingly so the longer the time horizon. None the less, forecasts of population growth are more 'robust' than predictions of social or economic trends (such as marriage patterns, unemployment, or the stock market), because population change is generally less volatile and many determinants are already in operation. Demographic events have long-term 'knock-on' effects, current population numbers and trends being in large part predetermined by the fertility and mortality patterns of previous generations. These will, in turn, set the demographic scene for several decades to come.

### Historical trends

For almost all of human history since its start about a million years ago, population growth has been negligible. The population increased slowly, to 300 million in 1 AD and 800 million by 1750, taking 1600 years to double (Fig. 1). In the next 50 years population increased to 1 billion by 1800, and 1.7 billion people by 1900, almost double the number 100 years before.

The world population grew slowly until about 250 years ago because high birth rates were matched by high death rates. Any excess of births over deaths in normal years just about compensated for the exceptional loss in years of FAMINE, WAR, and epidemic bouts of catastrophically high mortality. European history best describes the demographic events of those times. When the BLACK DEATH struck in 1348, England's population of 3.7 million fell 20% in just three years, and by 1400 was 50% lower than it would have been if PLAGUE had not occurred. Life expectancy of 32–35 years in medieval England was reduced to under 18 years by the late 14th century. The main change in 16th and 17th century Europe was the disappearance of bubonic plague, with tuberculosis assuming ascendancy as the single most important cause of death till the mid-19th century. Checks to population growth in pre-industrial Europe also came from social constraints on procreation, notably through deferred marriage and low rates of marriage. These represented social responses to the availability of economic resources. Fertility in medieval Europe was, therefore, much lower than the physiological maximum, or the 20th-century birth rates seen in many developing countries.

It was Europe that first broke from the dire controls on population growth. The disappearance of the great killer diseases by the mid-18th century ended the near equilibrium between birth and death rates, leading to increased life expectancy and population. Increasing population at this time was as much a function also of changes in fertility, greater prosperity leading to

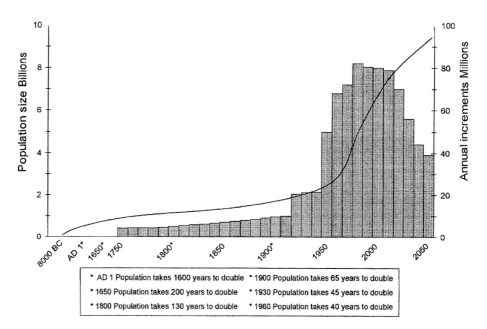

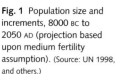

**Fig. 1** Population size and increments, 8000 BC to 2050 AD (projection based upon medium fertility assumption). (Source: UN 1998, and others.)

| | |
|---|---|
| * AD 1 Population takes 1600 years to double | * 1900 Population takes 65 years to double |
| * 1650 Population takes 200 years to double | * 1930 Population takes 45 years to double |
| * 1800 Population takes 130 years to double | * 1960 Population takes 40 years to double |

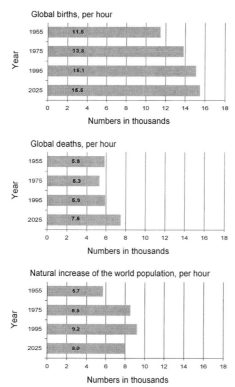

**Fig. 2** Global births, deaths, and natural increases of the world population. (Source: WHO 1998.)

rising birth rates through earlier and more frequent marriage and higher marital fertility.

This changing pattern in birth, death, and population growth rates since the 18th century is called the demographic transition. Large reductions in both fertility and mortality occurred in the now developed western world over the next two centuries, doubling life expectancy and halving fertility. Where the decline in fertility and mortality was simultaneous, as in France, population growth was modest. However, in most of the western world the decline in mortality preceded fertility decline, leading to faster population growth (Fig. 2). The dramatic declines in mortality in 19th-century Europe resulted from PUBLIC HEALTH measures, medical advances, and improvements in sanitation, personal hygiene, and housing and living standards. Improved survival was followed by the desire for smaller families, prompting the growing use of abortion and contraception (primarily coitus interruptus, since modern contraceptive methods were largely unknown then) and leading to declining birth rates. By the 20th century the situation had been reached where three pregnancies in a woman's life could produce the same level of population growth as six or more pregnancies in pre-industrial days.

Whereas in the developed western world the demographic transition occurred over two centuries, in the developing world the process has largely been condensed into the second half of the 20th century (Fig. 2). The nature of the transition has also been different, leading to unprecedented growth of world population. The rapid, widespread application of well-established and advancing public health and preventive technologies (such as immunization) even in poor, illiterate societies have led to precipitous falls in mortality in the populous, developing world. Although fertility declines have also followed, aided in many developing countries by governmental family planning programs, the fall has been slower and later than the fall in mortality. World population grew to 2.8 billion by 1955, a growth rate of 0.8% per annum, then by 1.8% per annum to 5 billion by the mid-1980s, and reached 6 billion by 1999, having taken less than 40 years to double.

However, the most rapid phase of world population growth is past. Growth rates and annual increments have been declining since the 1980s. The AIDS pandemic, and the return of killer infectious diseases such as malaria and tuberculosis, also moderated the significant mortality declines experienced by developing countries last century.

## Present situation

In 1996 the world's population stood at 5.8 billion, and was increasing by 1.4% — or 81 million — a year. This is equivalent to an hourly addition of over 9000 people (Fig. 2). High as this may seem, it is down from the peak period in the history of world population growth — the late 1980s — when 87 million were added each year. Some 80% of the world's population now lives in less developed countries and 85% of the global population increase is in Asia and Africa, with China and India alone contributing 35%.

The most important determinant of future population size now is the continuing decline in fertility in most world regions (Fig. 3). World fertility remained nearly constant at five births per woman until the 1970s, when it started to decline rapidly to the present three. This average,

however, conceals wide regional disparities that reflect differences in social and economic development and contraceptive use. Fertility varies from 1.2 births per woman in Italy and Spain, well below replacement level, to 6.4 in parts of Africa. However, virtually all high fertility countries are now experiencing declining trends. The most spectacular example is that of China, where the average number of births per woman fell from six to two in 15 years (Fig. 3), a demographic change that took 150 years in Europe. Given the time lag in demographic events, the decline in world fertility will not, however, mean a fall in the global number of births each year until after 2025. Hence the number of babies born each year will remain unchanged from the present 132 million (Fig. 4).

Compared with this, roughly 51 million people die each year, over 20% of them children under 5 years of age. About one-third of these deaths are due to infectious and parasitic diseases, primarily diarrhea, tuberculosis, malaria, respiratory infections, and AIDS), another one-third to circulatory diseases, and 12% to cancer. Again, there are wide mortality differentials, with infant mortality ranging from 7 per 1000 live births in western Europe to 108 in eastern Africa, and life expectancy ranging from 47 years in eastern Africa to 77 years in western Europe. Moreover, the rich–poor divide in health is widening. Child survival programs (immunization and oral rehydration therapy, in particular) implemented by governmental and international organizations in recent decades are starting to show significant effects on child mortality, reducing deaths from 21 million in 1955 to 10 million in 1997, and a projected 5 million by 2025. On the other hand, the AIDS pandemic and resurgence of (drug-resistant) malaria and tuberculosis will act as checks on the pace of future declines in

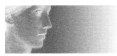
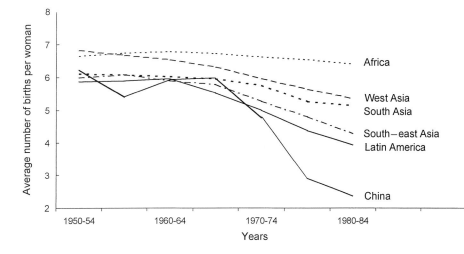

**Fig. 3** Fertility decline in the developing world. (Source: IIASA 1994.)

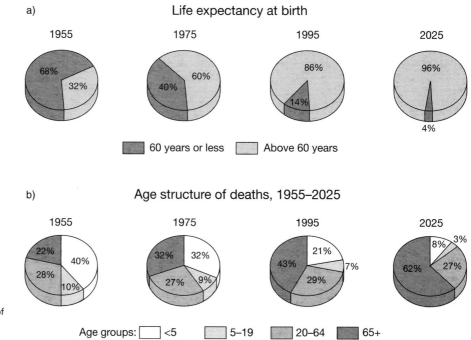

Fig. 4 Life expectancy at birth (a) and age structure of death, 1955–2050 (b). (Source: WHO 1998.)

mortality, particularly in sub-Saharan Africa, and chronic non-communicable diseases will assume a growing role in the developing world.

The most notable feature of population trends in the 21st century, resulting from the fertility declines currently underway, will be population aging — a familiar feature of the current demography of industrialized countries, but increasingly affecting the developing world also. Moreover, people will be living longer (Fig. 5). The result will be that the world's population aged over 60 will increase from 9% of the total in 1990 to 16% by 2030 and to 22% by 2050 (similar to the current situation in the 'oldest' region today — western

Europe), and to 30% by 2150. The mean age of the world's population will rise from 28 years currently to 40 years by 2050. China, in particular, will experience very rapid aging, because of the abrupt and large declines in fertility it experienced under its government's one-child policy. In only 35 years China will have a higher old-age dependency ratio that the United States, and there will be 274 million Chinese (20% of the total population) aged over 60, more than the total present US population. One of the biggest challenges of the 21st century — particularly in the poorer countries — will be how to finance healthcare of an aging population.

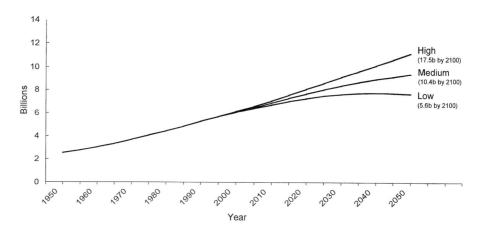

Fig. 5 World population size: past, and projections based on medium, high, and low fertility variants 1950–2150. (Source: UN 1998.)

Population aging is a function of population growth; hence assumptions about the latter will determine the pace of the former. Rapid population growth and rapid aging are considered undesirable, but they cannot both be avoided. The highest population growth scenario results in only moderate population aging, whereas the most conservative assumptions showing population leveling off imply very rapid population aging. Even intermediate scenarios combine substantial population growth (doubling of the population by 2050) with substantial aging (doubling of the proportion over 60).

## Demographic impact of HIV/AIDS

No commentary on future population trends would be complete without a discussion of the devastating impact of HIV/AIDS on the populations of some regions.

Of the 52 million deaths annually, about 2 million are attributable to AIDS. The World Health Organization estimates that by the mid-1990s about 20 million people had been infected with HIV since the start of the pandemic in the late 1970s, 1.5 million of them children. Over 90% of these cases occurred in developing countries: 11 million in Africa, 3.5 million in Asia, and 2 million in Latin America. The 24 countries where by 1994 over 2% of adults were HIV-positive are African, most in sub-Saharan Africa. Prevalence is highest in Botswana, Malawi, Uganda, Zambia, South Africa, and Zimbabwe — where 11–15% of adults are HIV-positive. Other countries with large and rapidly increasing numbers of HIV cases are India, Thailand, and Brazil. Under-reporting of HIV/AIDS is a serious problem, and hence these figures are subject to a large margin of error.

The United Nations, among others, has estimated the demographic impact of the HIV/AIDS pandemic. In India and Thailand there will be 22 million fewer people by 2050 as a result of AIDS. For Africa the figure is 52 million, 6% less than in the absence of AIDS. In the five worst affected African countries, mortality at the turn of the century would be almost 50% higher because of AIDS, and by 2050 there will be 13% fewer people as a result; however, high fertility in these countries means that their populations will none the less treble between 1995 and 2050 in spite of AIDS.

The impact of AIDS is greatest in young adults. In 1985–2005, deaths in adults aged 15–49 in the 24 worst affected African countries will be 43% higher as a result of AIDS. The speed of decline in infant mortality has also been adversely affected as a result of mother-to-child transmission of HIV infection, with infant mortality up to 50% higher in some African countries as a result of AIDS. Over the last decade and the next, there will be 2.5 million additional child deaths in

Africa, 9% higher than in the absence of AIDS. The World Health Organization anticipates that 'one of the biggest hazards to children in the twenty-first century will be the continuing spread of HIV/AIDS… the disease could reverse some of the major gains achieved in child health over the past 50 years.'

AIDS has had a dramatic impact on life expectancy in the worst affected countries in Africa; this will continue well into the 21st century. In several of these countries life expectancy has actually fallen since the 1980s, and in 2000 AD longevity was up to 20 years lower than it would have been in the absence of AIDS.

## Future trends

Although the most rapid phase of global population growth is now over (Fig. 1), and global fertility is falling, substantial growth in world population during the next half century is unavoidable. This is because past high fertility means that ever-increasing numbers of young women are entering the reproductive ages. Thus, even if the mothers of today have fewer babies than women had in the past, the overall numbers of births, and population, will increase for some time to come. Even if replacement level fertility were universal now, the built-in growth momentum means that world population will grow to 9.5 billion by 2150.

The United Nations has prepared three variants of population projections until the year 2050, assuming different levels of future fertility: high, medium, and low (Fig. 5). They yield population forecasts of between 7.7 and 11.2 billion by 2050. The medium variant (which assumes that fertility will come to stabilize at replacement level — just over 2 children per woman) is taken to be the most likely, indicating that world population will increase to 9.4 billion by 2050, a 62% increase over its 1996 level, with most of the increase occurring in the less developed regions. Under this assumption, the population will eventually stabilize at about 11 billion in 2200.

Population projections by the International Institute for Applied Systems Analysis incorporate a wider range of assumptions about future fertility, mortality, and migration patterns than the United Nations model; hence it produces a wider range of estimates. It forecasts a world population of between 8 and 15 billion by the middle of the 21st century. Its 'central' scenario reaches 11 billion, equivalent to the highest projection from the United Nations.

All the world's regions will grow with the exception of Europe, the only region projected to decline in population size over current levels. Europe's population in 2050 will be the same as it was 20 years ago, declining from its share of 22%

of the world population in 1950 to 13% in 1996 and to 7% in 2050.

Pierre **FAUCHARD**
(1678–1761). French dental surgeon, regarded as the founder of dentistry in France. He was one of the first to crown teeth, to make dentures, and to deal effectively with caries. He gave the first description of pyorrhea alveolaris. He published *Le chirurgien dentiste ou traité de dents* (2 vols, 1728), the first dental textbook.

(*continued opposite*)

## Sustainability

How many people can the earth support? Will finite resources determine the limits of population growth? Many distinguished minds have tried to estimate the 'carrying capacity' of our planet, the balance between natural resources and the number of people. The diversity of conclusions ranges from under 1 billion to 100 billion and higher. Some have argued that there are no limits to population growth, others that we have already passed the limits of sustainability and are on the way to ecological disaster.

The most influential commentator on the relation between population growth and resources remains the Reverend Thomas Malthus, whose work *First essay on population* was published in 1798 and developed further in subsequent writings. Malthus's thesis was that population growth would outstrip resources unless held in check by 'moral restraint' or 'positive checks' such as plague, famine, and war.

> Population, when unchecked, increases in a geometrical ratio. Subsistence increases only in an arithmetical ratio. A slight acquaintance with numbers will show the immensity of the first power in comparison of the second. By that law of our nature which makes food necessary to the life of man, the effects of these two unequal powers must be kept equal. This implies a strong and constantly operating check on population from the difficulty of subsistence. This difficulty must fall somewhere; and must necessarily be severely felt by a large portion of mankind.

Although Malthus's analysis remains a formidable exercise in political economy, it has not always been borne out by events. The undernutrition and famines seen in our times are largely man-made, not the result of agricultural limits on carrying capacity. However gloomy some of the prognostications of demographers, humanity has, in general, not merely survived, it has thrived. Global life expectancy is 68 years compared with 48 in 1955, and is projected to rise to 73 years by 2025. Food supply has more than doubled in the past 40 years, growing much faster than population growth, adult literacy rates have increased over 50% since 1970, and per capita gross domestic product has risen over 2.5 times in real terms in the past 50 years. Most of the world's children are now immunized against the main childhood diseases, although 2 million children still die each year from vaccine-preventable diseases. The gains have not been uniformly shared. Millions of the poorest and most needy have seen little if any improvement, and there remains a wide gap in life expectancy between rich and poor nations. But there are few countries today where longevity does not far exceed that of earlier centuries. The astonishing growth of world population last century was a triumph of man over his environment. The demographic history of world population has shown that the carrying capacity of the earth is not a constant, but a dynamic equilibrium determined not only by resources and the level of technology, but also by the ingenuity with which we shape our world-wide economic, social, and political arrangements.                    VSR

*See also* AFRICA; CHINA; FAMINE; WORLD HEALTH ORGANIZATION

**DENTISTRY — HISTORY** Although the origins of dentistry and dental care have been lost in antiquity, there is good evidence that dental disease has been widespread throughout human history. In Britain, dental ailments were being treated as far back as the Roman occupation (55BC–410AD). Scribonius Largus, the surgeon who accompanied Emperor Claudius in AD43, is believed to have treated dental ailments in addition to his surgical duties. A small instrument similar to the volsella (forceps) described by CELSUS (30BC) (p 806), found among the archaeological remains of the time, is regarded as being brought to Britain by Largus.

There is little evidence of any development of dentistry in Britain until the 14th century, although the Druids employed incantations and magic in an attempt to treat dental ailments, and members of religious orders dedicated to the healing of the sick included among their skills an ability to extract teeth. The early practitioners of dentistry were barbers and charlatans, who, dressed in picturesque clothing and with musical accompaniment to drown the anguished cries of their victims, succeeded in earning large incomes. In cities it was possible to find a physician or a surgeon to undertake extractions.

This was the situation in the developed countries throughout Europe. In less developed areas of the world, the tribal 'medicine men' carried out extractions but, as the major dental problem was inflammatory periodontal disease leading to loosening of the teeth, no particular skills were required.

In 1300 the Company of Masters of Barbery and Surgery was formed in the City of London. It comprised two groups: one was the 'tooth drawers', who, because of their poor training and crude methods, were held in scant respect. In 1540 a new company was founded under a Royal Charter granted by Henry VIII which united the Guild of Surgeons and the Company of Masters of Barbery and Surgery, to become the Company of BARBER-SURGEONS of London. This company did much to raise the standards of surgery but specifically failed to exclude 'the drawing of teeth' from its practice constraints. The company was dissolved in 1745 by Act of Parliament, enabling the emergence of the Company of Surgeons, which in 1800 became the Royal College of Surgeons of London and, in 1843, the Royal College of Surgeons of England. Dentistry in Britain and indeed many other parts of the world, owes the pattern of its evolution from a trade to a profession to this college.

During this period Pierre FAUCHARD (p 222) was pioneering dentistry in France and taking every opportunity to acquire and disseminate sound knowledge based on actual practice. In 1728 he published his two-volume classic, *Le chirurgien dentiste*, which heralded a new era, creating a profound impression on dental thinking throughout Europe and Britain.

By the middle of the 19th century there was a general realization throughout the western world of the need to raise the standards and status of dental practice. Mainly under pressure from members of the newly founded Odontological Society of London, the Royal College of Surgeons and the government finally acceded to the demands of the profession and successfully laid before Parliament the Medical Bill empowering the College to establish a diploma course, hold examinations, and award the Licence in Dental Surgery (LDS RCS Eng). The first examinations were held in 1860; soon afterwards similar diplomas began to be awarded by the Royal Colleges in Glasgow, Edinburgh, and Dublin. Not only were LDS diplomas the principal dental qualification in Britain, but many students from the British Empire, Commonwealth, and other overseas countries came to take the examinations.

Despite the availability of formal education leading to a prestigious qualification, there was still no control over unqualified practice provided that the practitioner did not call himself either a dentist or dental surgeon. In 1897, the British Dental Association was founded, its primary aims being to eradicate unqualified practice, encourage high standards of professional conduct, and promote research. It took 43 years to remedy the defects of the 1878 Act. The 1921 Dentists Act required everyone who practiced dentistry to be registered annually, though it did allow people who 'had been in reputable practice' but who were without a dental or medical qualification to register provided they satisfied the requirements of the Dental Board of the United Kingdom and were of 'good personal character'. Only recently did the last of the '1921 men' finally leave the Register. During its 36 years, the Dental Board, under the authority of the General Medical Council, was charged with maintenance of the Register, regulating professional dis-

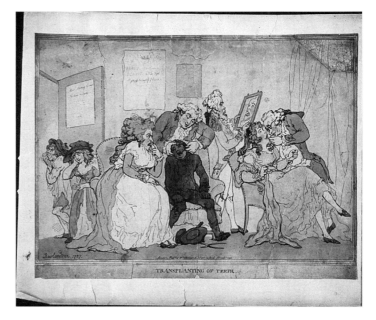

cipline and setting educational standards of the schools, dental health education, and the welfare of the schools and students.

The 1957 Act consolidated all previous Acts and authorized the founding of the General Dental Council, which established the independence of the dental profession, thus finally completing the transformation of dentistry 'from a trade to a profession'.

## Education

In 1699, L'École Dentaire in Paris became the first dental school to offer formal education in dentistry and very soon became an internationally recognized center of excellence. Such celebrated dentists as Fauchard and Bartholomew Ruspini, who practiced in London, were students there. The first school in the USA was the Baltimore College of Dentistry, founded in 1839.

Although the first dental school in Britain was not established until 1859, several London teaching hospitals provided courses of lectures on dental subjects. Among these courses were those of James Fox at Guy's Hospital and of John HUNTER (p 398) and William Rae at St George's. Several books appeared based on these lecture courses, the most notable being that by Hunter, *The natural history of the human teeth* published in 1771, which included not only his anatomical and pathologic descriptions but also details of his scientific investigations.

By the end of the 19th century nine dental schools had been established in Britain. The remaining seven were founded after 1900, the last being the Dental School of the Welsh National

18th century. A fashionable dentist's practice where teeth are being extracted from poor children in order to create dentures for wealthy people. Colored etching by T. Rowlandson, (1787). (Reproduced courtesy of the Wellcome Institute Library, London.)

*(continued)*

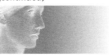

John **TOMES** (1815–95). English dental surgeon. As a house surgeon at the Middlesex Hospital, he invented a new type of dental forceps adapted to the different shape of the necks of the teeth. He was prominent in promoting the use of anesthesia in dentistry. Establishing a reputation as an authority, he published a course of lectures in 1845, a series of papers in the *Philosophical Transactions of the Royal Society*, and his *System of dental surgery* (1859). He was active in promoting the Dental Act of 1858, which introduced obligatory training and registration for all dentists. *(continued overleaf)*

(continued)

Greene Vardiman **BLACK** (1836–1915). American dentist. He advanced techniques of conservative dentistry by drilling out cavities caused by caries so that the shape held fillings in place, and by making a porcelain crown for front teeth which was screwed into a root cavity filled with gold.

School of Medicine in Cardiff, which was opened in 1965. Soon after the Second World War, the Postgraduate Dental Institute was founded at the Eastman Dental Hospital in London, to which dental graduates from around the world attend courses leading to postgraduate specialist qualifications.

However, during the last 20 years several factors have led to the closure and merging of some dental schools throughout the world. For example, in Britain the number of schools has been reduced from 16 to 12.

*Teachers* Until the early 1940s most clinical teachers were part-time practitioners who spent much of their working life in their practices. Their valuable contributions were mainly concerned with the practical skills of clinical dentistry, mostly treatment of the ravages of oral sepsis brought on by neglect. Students became highly skilled in tooth extraction under general and local anesthesia, and in giving short-lasting primitive anesthetics with mixtures of nitrous oxide and oxygen. Such has been the improvement in dental health in the western world that students now do not acquire these skills to a similar extent. The teaching of the preclinical subjects of anatomy, biochemistry, and physiology, was, as was the teaching of pathology and bacteriology, usually given with medical students.

During the late 1940s and early 1950s far-reaching changes took place in the dental schools, all of which in Britain became institutions within universities. Part-time staff were replaced by full-time career teachers, professorial chairs were established, and research, on a hitherto unprecedented scale, began to be conducted. As a result, dentistry rapidly became a clinical science, enabling teaching to abandon its long-standing empirical basis and assume an evidence-based character.

*Research* Dental research throughout the world has received tremendous encouragement from The International Association for Dental Research, which was founded in New York City in 1920. From its small, mainly US-based beginnings, the Association now comprises about 12 000 members from 90 countries around the world. A general session of the association is held annually in the US and, more recently, in other member countries. At the 1998 meeting in Nice, 3226 research presentations were made, ranging from immunology and microbiology to the everyday practice of dentistry.

The Association is divided into divisions and sections, each of which holds at least one scientific meeting a year. Abstracts of the papers presented at the general session and at divisional and section meetings are published in the *Journal of Dental Research*. By providing opportunities for research activity to appear in the public domain and thus be open to criticism and comment, the Association has, for almost 70 years, contributed enormously to the greater understanding of dental disease, raising the standards of dental teaching, and exerting a profound influence on the practice of dentistry throughout the world. MNN

*See also* BARBER-SURGEONS, COMPANY OF; PROFESSIONAL REGULATION

**DENTISTRY** Advances in dental practice have extended across the whole range of patient care and have included the development of equipment, instruments, techniques, and treatment procedures. New drugs are available which are invaluable in treating dental ills. Some drugs for the management of medical conditions can also profoundly influence patterns of dental treatment, of which the anticoagulants and corticosteroids are examples. Furthermore, the availability of new anesthetic drugs has made the traditional 'gas and air' anesthetic obsolete, and has largely taken anesthesia out of the hands of the dentist into those of the specialist anesthetist. Major advances have been made in treating inflammatory diseases of the gums: whereas 'pyorrhea alveolaris' (periodontal disease) was regarded as untreatable other than by wholesale extraction of teeth, much can now be done to control the progress of the disease and prevent its onset.

The prevalence of dental decay has dramatically declined in the western world over the past 20–25 years. Despite the tremendous increase in knowledge of the cause and natural history of this disease, the precise reason for its decline in prevalence is not clear. Decay is a disease of multi-factorial origin, and its prevalence is influenced by dietary factors, oral hygiene and fluorides, and others unidentified. However, this decline in prevalence has occurred in association with a general improvement in oral hygiene and the increased use of fluoride-containing toothpastes.

There have been many major advances in restorative dentistry. Among the more notable have been the development of vasoconstrictor local anesthetics, which have enabled virtually all dental procedures to be carried out entirely without pain. Furthermore, intravenously administered sedation enables the anxiety of treatment to be controlled in that remaining small minority of patients for whom dentistry is an anathema.

### Air-turbine revolution

As recently as 40 years ago students were taught to prepare cavities using a treadle powered drill and steel burrs, which rapidly became blunt especially when attempting to cut undiseased tooth substance. However, the electrically powered drill, later to be followed by the air-turbine, both of which drove tungsten-carbide and diamond burrs, overcame these problems. Indeed, the air-turbine, which became available during the 1960s, has revolutionized restorative dentistry, being described as capable of cutting tooth substance rather like 'a hot knife cutting butter'. The disadvantages of the air-turbine are that it generates considerable heat and requires a water coolant, which tends to obscure vision, and produces an irritating high frequency noise. More modern turbines have appreciably lower noise levels and frequently have an in-built fiberoptic light, which bathes the operating site with an intense local light.

There have been important advances in the materials used in the restoration of teeth. The gold materials have been alloyed to provide greater dimensional stability and easier handling, while the silver–tin alloys have been modified to provide faster setting times, greater strength, and easier handling. The safety of silver–tin alloys is under question despite the fact that 'amalgam' fillings have been used regularly for almost a century without concern. There are now non-metallic materials available which are esthetically excellent but whose durability falls considerably below that of the older metallic materials.

Perhaps the most important advance in restorative care has been the philosophical change in the approach to cavity preparation. Hitherto, with almost sacramental dogma, cavities were prepared following the principles laid down by G. V. Black at the beginning of the 20th century. Implicitly these principles involved the loss of considerable amounts of valuable sound tooth tissue to prevent recurrence of the disease. This 'extension for prevention' policy has now been discarded and, as a result, cavities are smaller, teeth are less likely to fracture, and fillings are kept well clear of the gum margins, thus contributing to the prevention of periodontal disease.

Another important advance has been the development of endodontics, which is concerned with treatment of diseased root canal and pulp chamber tissues. Improved materials and instruments, and the development of clinical and technical skills, together with a greater understanding of the biology of the root canal and associated structures, have encouraged the not unreasonable statement that 'no tooth ever need be lost'.

There have been equally important advances in prosthetic dentistry, not only in materials science (which includes new denture materials and more accurate impression materials), but, of perhaps greater importance, a more complete understanding of the physiologic principles of mastication and orofacial muscular activity. These advances have exerted a profound effect on the design of dentures, especially partial dentures, which are

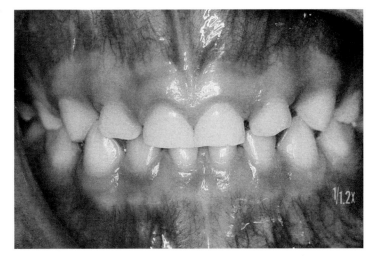

supported by the remaining teeth rather than soft tissues, with minimal, if any, hazard to the teeth themselves or the supporting tissues. A recent successful development, which is affecting the whole range of dental practice, concerns implants, which can replace individual teeth or contribute to the retention and stability of dentures.

Orthodontic practice has been greatly influenced by the increased understanding of the growth patterns of the facial skeleton. This work has been dependent upon computer analyses of considerable volumes of radiologically derived numerical data. The use of fixed appliances has become more widespread as a result of the availability of better adhesive materials. Improved patient attitudes towards orthodontics, together with greatly increased accuracy of prognosis, has considerably increased the popularity and demand for such treatment.

Healthy deciduous dentition of a three-year-old child.

Rampant decay of the deciduous dentition of a three-year-old child.

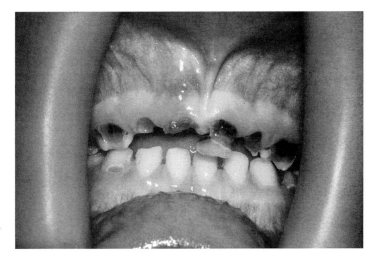

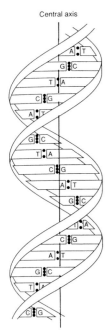

Central axis

The structure of DNA. The diagram is a model of the Watson–Crick DNA double helix. The two bands represent sugar-phosphate backbones of the two strands, which run in opposite directions. The vertical line represents the central axis round which the strands wind. The position of four nucleotide bases, C, A, T, and G, is shown, together with the hydrogen bonds (•) which link them together. (From Weatherall, D. J. (1985). *The new genetics and clinical practice,* 2nd edn. OUP.)

In many countries, Britain in particular, dentistry has evolved in very close relationship with medicine and enjoys an equal status as a sister profession. This relationship is particularly strong in the specialties of oral medicine and oral surgery, in which most, though by no means all, practitioners are qualified in both medicine and dentistry. Both subjects are regarded as mainly 'postgraduate' and owe their development to the tremendous advances made in virology, MICROBIOLOGY, IMMUNOLOGY, and PHARMACOLOGY. Many of the oral soft tissue diseases, hitherto treated by empirical procedures, can now be tackled rationally and with good prospect of success. Oral surgeons venture far beyond the removal of unerupted wisdom teeth, the enucleation of cysts, and the dental aspects of the management of fractures of the facial skeleton. They now undertake full care of patients with malignant disease, correction of congenital and hereditary defects, and the repair of disfigurement after trauma. Their work is carried out in close cooperation with the oncologist, the plastic surgeon, and the anesthetist.

### Postgraduate education

Gone is the old attitude that once qualified there is nothing else to learn. Indeed, today's view is that qualification is merely a stage in learning. Throughout the world there are dental associations, societies, and colleges dedicated to the task of providing dentists with the postgraduate education necessary for them to keep up to date with advances. University-based dental schools and colleges provide opportunities for postgraduate students to take courses leading to master's degrees and diplomas in clinical subjects. The need for continuing education is widely appreciated, especially among the younger practitioners.

The newly qualified dentist, on qualification, has a considerable career choice, which ranges from general practice, specialist practice, hospital practice, dental teaching, research, and practice in the community service or in the armed forces. The career patterns vary from country to country, but, with the possible exception of general practice, postgraduate qualifications are desirable if not essential.

### Conclusion

The past century and a half has seen dentistry change from a trade to a profession, and during the last fifty years it has undergone even further far-reaching changes. New materials and techniques have been introduced, pain during treatment is (or should be) a thing of the past, and gum disease is largely treatable. The most important advance, however, has been the change in attitude of the public towards dental health. There now exists an ever increasing desire to retain 'teeth

for life', a state that can now be accepted as a practical possibility. The future of dental practice is difficult to predict but better and more up-to-date dental care needs to be established in developing countries. There is evidence that countries in the western world are becoming increasingly aware of this need, but a properly coordinated approach is required. Whatever the future, undoubtedly dentistry will remain an exciting, challenging, interesting, and fulfilling profession which will continue to attract into its ranks young men and women of high intellect and practical skills.                                        MNN

*See also* WATER

**DEOXYRIBONUCLEIC ACID** is usually abbreviated to DNA. Its structure was elucidated, using X-ray diffraction, by M. H. F. Wilkins, F. H. C. Crick, and J. D. Watson in 1953, a discovery for which they later received the NOBEL PRIZE. It is composed of linear molecules found in chromosomes and some viruses, consisting of two interwound helical chains of polynucleotides (a nucleotide consists of a pentose sugar, a phosphate group, and a nitrogenous base derived from either purine or pyrimidine). In DNA the sugar of each nucleotide is 2-deoxy-D-ribose and the base is one of the following four: adenine (A), cytosine (C), guanine (G), or thymine (T) (cf. ribonucleic acid (RNA), in which uracil replaces thymine). The order of the bases determines the genetic code, each sequence (triplet) of three bases coding for one amino acid. Complementary base pairs (that is, the bases opposite each other on the two helical chains) are linked by hydrogen bonds.

DNA carries genetic information for all organisms except the RNA viruses. Each of the 46 chromosomes in human body cells consists of two strands of DNA, containing up to 100 000 nucleotides. Along each strand, about 1500 bases, on average, form a gene.

*See also* CELL AND CELL BIOLOGY; GENETICS, HUMAN; IMMUNOLOGY; MOLECULAR BIOLOGY

**DERMATOLOGY — HISTORY** Dermatology comprises all that is known about skin in health and disease. The skin around us is the one organ on which each of us makes daily observation, from the infant bemused by his rosy fingers, to the adolescent bewitched by acne, or the aged bemoaning wrinkles, everyone has an interest in the skin. For here is a canvas on which portraits appear, not only of aging but also of the specter of disease.

For centuries the skin was observed for signs of SMALLPOX, SYPHILIS, LEPROSY, and pellagra.

Physicians, surgeons, philosophers, and charlatans had little to offer in the way of understanding or treatment. But knowledge was to come from the ever branching paths of specialization. Robert Willan in Britain was the first to publish and classify portraits of skin disease. Further systemization came from Jean Louis Alibert in Paris as he taught his pupils to view each skin disease as a specific branch off a dermatologic tree. The third great center was in Vienna, where Ferdinand von Hebra represented the full flowering of the new discipline, dermatology, beautifully displayed in a 5-volume text. By the 1920s Josef Jadassohn brought out a magnificent 36-volume German encyclopedia detailing every aspect of the skin and its diseases. Today, the classic summary of dermatologic information is Rook's, *Textbook of dermatology*, now in its 6th edition. Library shelves groan with dozens of textbooks, scores of monographs, and over 200 dermatologic journals devoted to the understanding of the nearly 3000 identifiable skin diseases.

Description and classification represented the early achievement of this fledgling specialty. Little was known of causes and even less of specific treatment. Yet, during the 19th century a few select causes of skin diseases were discovered. In 1831 David Gruby showed that fungi can cause disease, and in 1834 François Renucci that scabies was due to a mite, confirming what the poor people of Paris knew in the 16th century when they picked these barely visible mites from their thread-like burrows in the outer skin. More insight was provided by the brave volunteers for experimental induction of disease, including smallpox, allergic contact dermatitis, and drug eruptions.

There was an important leap in knowledge when the microscope and the biopsy (a surgical sample) were used. The pathologist was able to see the skin in all its structural and cellular detail and study its derangements. At the same time, the new science of bacteriology provided understanding of infectious diseases, such as impetigo (a spreading infection of the skin) and boils. By 1906 a spirochete had been identified as the cause of syphilis, and in 1910 EHRLICH (p 260) found the 'magic bullet' for syphilis on the 606th trial of arsenical medications. It was a great advance in 1914 when Joseph Goldberger showed that pellagra was due to a simple nutritional deficiency. The specific missing vitamin, nicotinic acid, was not isolated until the 1930s.          WBShe, EDS

**DERMATOLOGY** Today, the disciplines of biochemistry, PHARMACOLOGY, cell physiology, IMMUNOLOGY, GENETICS, electron microscopy, internal medicine, and MOLECULAR BIOLOGY have each brought deepened understanding of both diagnosis and treatment in dermatology. We no longer look on the skin as a mere covering sheath. It is a dynamic organ, shimmering with countless biochemical syntheses and cellular messages.

The invisible part of the skin has become visible to the eye of the microscopist, using stains, immunofluorescence, and electron beams. It has also become visible to the biochemist and molecular biologist with their DNA probes, polymerase chain reactions, and chromosomal spreads. And in tissue cultures of skin cells the skin has become visible to the biologist, who listens to the conversations between these cells, via their cytokines.

The diagnostic grasp on skin disease has grown tremendously, so that the modern dermatologist can cite thousands of disease constellations, using the known landmarks of morphology, insights of an informed history, and a wealth of laboratory data. The blood may tell of hair loss due to anemia, skin dryness (xerosis) due to vitamin A deficiency, or ulcers due to lack of zinc. Antibodies in the serum confirm the diagnosis of pemphigus (watery blisters) and other blistering diseases, as well as lupus erythematosus (chronic inflammatory disease), scleroderma (chronic disease with thickening of the skin and scarring in the joints, digestive system, heart, and kidney), and Lyme disease (infectious arthritis). The urine may reveal that blisters on a dorsal hand eruption are due to porphyria cutanea tarda, or that facial

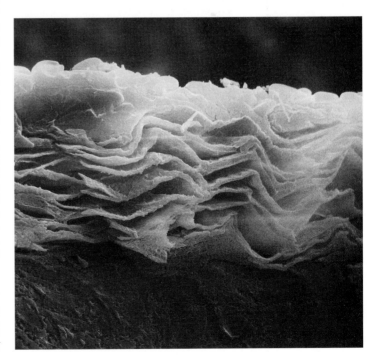

Dead outer layer of skin in cross-section using scanning electron microscopy, showing the protective flaky pie-crust structure of this stratum corneum (× 5000).

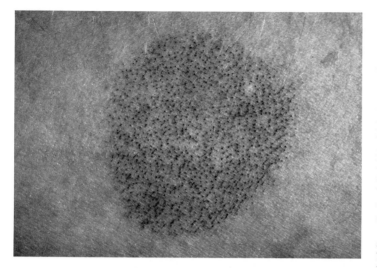

Sweat gland orifices on skin of forearms (stained surface view). There are 2 million of these eccrine glands (glands which pass their secretion down a duct), which cover the skin with water for evaporative cooling.

## EARLY DERMATOLOGIST

Jean F. **DARRIER** (1856–1938). French dermatologist. Born in Budapest, he went to Paris to finish his studies and, after graduating, specialized in dermatology. In 1889 he described keratosis follicularis (Darrier's disease), a congenital progressive wartiness of the skin, and in 1896 was the first to report pseudoxanthoma elasticum, a progressive degeneration of the elastic tissue of the skin and elsewhere. His textbook on dermatology, *Précis de dermatologie*, was published in 1909 and was subsequently translated into English, German, and Spanish and went through several editions.

flushing is coming from a carcinoid tumor. An X-ray film may disclose the lung cancer responsible for dermatomyositis (inflammation of skin and muscles), or a foreign body responsible for pain. The computerized tomography scan may identify a pancreatic tumor responsible for necrolytic migratory erythema (a shifting inflammation causing destruction of the skin).

The microbiologist may track the cause of a wasting nail to a superficial fungus, such as *Trichophyton rubrum*, or a linear chain of sores after a rose prick to the deep fungus, sporotrichosis. Tissue cultures may also identify an atypical mycobacterial infection from a swimming pool abrasion. Viral cultures help make the diagnosis of a type 1 or type 2 herpes simplex infection, or confirm the presence of chickenpox or shingles, caused by the varicella virus.

The most important diagnostic tool remains the biopsy, an excision of a tiny sample of diseased skin which gives the pathologist a cellular basis for diagnosis. This shows the outer cells (epidermis) separating in pemphigus, the accumulations of cells of metabolic disease, and the uncontrolled cell growth of malignancy, as in T-cell lymphomas. The dermatologists' tools include immunofluorescence using specific antibodies, specific stains for chemicals, such as iron or mucin, and electron microscopy for viruses. Emission scanning electron microscopy can detect and identify traces of foreign metal in skin biopsy specimens. The prenatal biopsy of skin allows identification of serious genetic diseases.

## Allergies
Dermatologists are able to identify specific challenges to the patient, ranging from controlled exposures to environmental inhalants and foods

to usage tests with drugs and cosmetic products such as toothpaste. The challenge test may be localized on the skin, in the form of a patch test, which exposes an area of skin to chemicals from work and hobbies, suspected of causing allergic contact dermatitis. Intradermal tests — with the actual injection of materials into the skin such as tuberculin, hormones, or other chemicals — may produce immediate or delayed reactions; scratch tests or prick tests, usually read after 15 minutes, give information about ALLERGIES such as hayfever, ASTHMA, and hives. Exposing patches of skin to sunlight or ultraviolet light is of great value in detecting photosensitivity problems, sometimes using the prior application of photosensitizing chemicals.

The treatment of skin disease has continued to advance ever since the early conquest of smallpox by vaccination. We have seen syphilis eradicated by penicillin, LEPROSY subdued by dapsone, and cancer of the skin totally excised by micrographic surgery. We have witnessed lymphomas of the skin, such as Alibert's dreaded mycosis fungoides, treated with topical nitrogen mustard and systemic chemotherapy. Precancerous skin lesions such as sunlight-induced actinic keratoses (skin thickening) are destroyed by freezing with liquid nitrogen or the simple application of 5-fluorouracil cream for a few weeks.

Relief is brought to photosensitive patients with antimalarial drugs (chloroquine), and to poison ivy victims with topical and systemic cortisone derivatives. The discovery in 1950 of the universal anti-inflammatory action of cortisone has been of benefit to millions of people suffering with dermatitis of all kinds.

Pharmaceutical research has accomplished much more for dermatologic treatment. By studying 1500 derivatives of vitamin A, one was found (isotretinoin) to be dramatically effective in suppressing sebum formation (an oily substance secreted by sebaceous glands) and treating severe scarring cystic acne. An analog, retinoic acid, is similarly helpful in the topical treatment of comedonal (blackheads and whiteheads) acne. Much excitement was created when it was discovered serendipitously that long-term topical use of retinoic acid can erase wrinkles. Recently, an ointment containing a vitamin D analog, the sunlight vitamin ($D_3$, calcipotriol), has proved effective in treating psoriasis, long known to respond to ultraviolet light. It is truly 'sunlight in a salve'.

The powerful therapeutic effect of sunlight can be enhanced by administering photosensitizers internally or externally. This is the basis for the popular PUVA treatment, which uses oral or topical psoralens and the UVA band of ultraviolet light. More recently, other photosensitizers such as porphyrins have been used with UVA light to destroy skin cancers; this is known as photodynamic therapy. Certain skin conditions, including lymphomas, are treated by irradiating the patient's blood as it flows through a bypass outside the body.

Perhaps the greatest boon to dermatology has been the parade of antimicrobial agents for bacterial disease, beginning with sulfanilamide in 1937. The early antibiotics, penicillin and tetracycline, were followed by the wide-spectrum compounds, erythromycin, quinolones, and cefalosporins, now in their third generation of derivatives. Even greater fire power has been provided by antibiotics which can be given intravenously. Skin infections, formerly chronic or even fatal, now yield to intravenous ceftriaxone. This is likewise true for foci of infection, which influence skin reaction patterns such as psoriasis, erythema nodosum (painful red lumps in the skin), and lichen sclerosus et atrophicus (thin, shiny skin).

Skin diseases due to fungi felt the first blow when the oral antibiotic griseofulvin, effective against dermatophytes, was introduced in 1959. This was followed by ketoconazole in the early 1980s, effective against a wide variety of fungi, including yeasts. With ketoconazole, oral thrush, cutaneous candidiasis, and chronic paronychia (infection around nails) became easier to treat, as did the yeast-driven seborrheic dermatitis (a type of eczema). Even in a shampoo, ketoconazole has given relief to those suffering from dandruff. More recently, three additional oral antifungals have been marketed: fluconazole, itraconazole, and terbinafine. Fungal infections of the toenail, present mainly in adulthood, can now be cured with these medications.

The antiviral agents, acyclovir and its derivatives, valacyclovir and famciclovir, are 'wonder drugs', specifically engineered and synthesized to inhibit the herpes simplex virus responsible for cold sores (herpes simplex). In higher doses these are effective for treating shingles (herpes zoster) and chickenpox caused by the same varicella virus as shingles. Immediate oral treatment may help avert years of post-herpetic pain in older patients.

For parasitic infections, ivermectin is the crowning glory. A single dose of this drug can eradicate the 'seven-year-itch' of scabies (infestation by the itch mite). Gone is the need for head to toe applications of lindane lotion or sulfur ointment. Ivermectin is also effective in eliminating helminthic (parasite or worm) infections in the skin, such as strongyloidiasis and onchocerciasis. Another anti-parasite drug, thiabendazole, provides equally exciting results in treating other parasitic infestations and their cutaneous sequels,

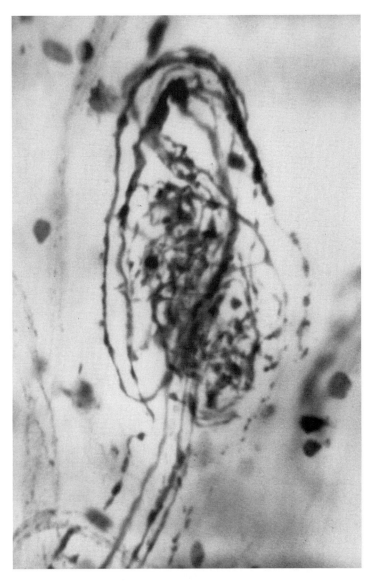

such as the itch of pinworms, or 'swimmers itch' from the blood fluke schistosome cercaria. The louse, responsible for the transmission of so many diseases (such as typhus) down through the centuries, can be eradicated by a new synthetic agent, permethrin.

Brilliant flashes of success in modern treatment have come from pimocide, an 'orphan drug' which effectively eliminates the delusions of some patients that they are infested with parasites. The other major success for treating psychocutaneous problems is seen in the treatment of compulsive hand washing. Here the drug of choice is fluoxetine, which acts by interfering with the neurotransmitter, serotonin.

Specialized nerve ending in skin for the sensation of touch: Meissner corpuscle.

## Surgery

Dermatologic surgery for skin lesions has advanced to the precision removal of just the lesion, and now includes advanced plastic patterned excisions and the Mohs technique for histologic tracking of skin cancer during the actual operation. Excessive sweating (hyperhidrosis) in the armpits may be eliminated by excision of the affected skin or through laparoscopic surgery on the sympathetic nerve ganglia (keyhole surgery on the nervous relay stations overlying the backbone). For those who prefer to avoid surgery, superficial injections of botulinum toxin into the skin give long-term help by blocking the nerve endings to the sweat glands. The same injections are uniquely helpful in treating palmar sweating. Botulinum toxin can also eliminate ominous brow wrinkles by paralyzing the underlying skin muscles. Other surgical techniques include hair transplants for baldness and liposuction for skin contour control.

Laser surgery has permitted exquisite skin resurfacing, replacing the mottled and wrinkled aged skin with the bloom of fresh, youthful skin. Most remarkable with lasers has been the essentially scarless elimination of disfiguring superficial hemangiomas (blood vessel growths), called port wine stains. Lasers are now used for removing a variety of skin growths, undesired hair, and tattoos.

Indeed, nowhere has there been a greater impact of technology on clinical dermatology than with the laser. Scarcely 30 years ago, the carbon dioxide laser was introduced as an optical beam scalpel permitting bloodless surgery. Today, the pulsed dye laser, with its precision yellow beam of 585 nm wavelength, allows truly selective destruction of the fine blood vessels of vascular birth marks. With pulses of 450 microsecond ($\mu$ sec) the thermal destruction is limited to the oxyhemoglobin within the vessel and scarring is avoided. Similarly, selective photothermolysis of another mode is used in destroying pigmented lesions such as moles, age spots, or tattoos. Here, lasers such as the Q-switched ruby laser are used; this emits a red light (695 nm) in ultra short bursts of 40 $\mu$ sec targeting only the undesirable pigment. Before the remarkable specificity of the modern lasers, one could only excise or destroy the entire affected area of skin, with subsequent scarring.

Cosmetic procedures in dermatology have not been limited to surgery. Both the vitamin A derivative, tretinoin, and alpha hydroxy acids, derived from fruits, have proved helpful as creams to erase many of the signs of photoaging. Several hundred commercial versions of the latter fill our pharmacy shelves. More rapid results are achieved by acid peels carried out by the dermatologist. People may still feel old, but they need not look that way.

Now there are two choices for combating hereditary hair loss: locally applied minoxidil solution and the oral drug, finasteride. Minoxidil was discovered serendipitously when it was observed that some bald men grew hair while taking this drug by mouth for treatment of high blood pressure. Finasteride is a synthetic inhibitor of the male hormone, androgen, long known to induce male pattern hair loss. Unfortunately, these drugs are not effective in everyone. Once hair growth has been induced, maintenance of growth requires continuation of the drug.

## Malignant tumors

Malignant skin tumors have become the most deadly problem of the skin. Their prevalence has increased in the United States almost threefold in the last four decades (and other countries, particularly Australia, could report the same). One major risk factor is ultraviolet radiation, but others include easily sunburned 'fair' skin, a family history of skin tumors, and the presence of melanoma precursors, dysplastic and congenital nevi (moles). People must become aware of these moles and monitor their own skin for any changes in them. Early detection and removal of superficial tumors lead to high cure rates, whereas melanoma that has spread distantly is virtually incurable. Australia, a land of sunshine and melanomas has taken the educational lead in popularizing sun-avoiding behavior, as well as protective creams and clothing, surveillance of moles, and removal of suspect lesions. Only in this way can fatal malignant melanomas and other skin cancers be averted. Such 'sun-smart' behavior affords the additional cosmetic benefit

Hair removed from unwashed armpit and placed on agar shows immense growth of bacteria in 48 hours: It is these bacteria which produce the distinctive body odor and thus account for the entire deodorant industry.

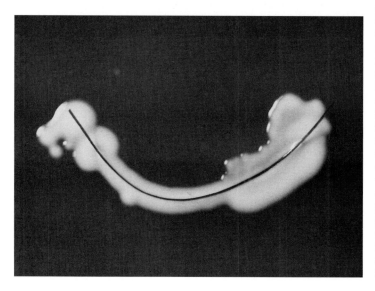

of a reduction in wrinkles and the age spots of photoaging.

Just as SYPHILIS was once in the domain of dermatologists, who recognized ulcers and the various secondary syphilitic rashes, today the AIDS virus may first be recognized by the skin specialist. HIV infection may appear as an innocent red spot (Kaposi's sarcoma), a whitening of the sides of the tongue, or a dismaying display of warts, molluscum contagiosum (bumps due to viral infection), or bacterial infections.

A similar display of recalcitrant viral, bacterial, and yeast infections of the skin is seen in patients with organ transplants, whose general immunity has been intentionally suppressed by drugs to prevent rejection of the organ. Thus, 77% of kidney transplant patients develop warts. Seeing these patients, as well as the rare individual born with an immune deficiency, is evidence that skin health requires the continuous presence of an effective cellular and humoral immunity. The newest supportive treatment is an injectable immunoglobulin (antibody), helpful in a variety of skin diseases associated with immunodeficiency.

With the growing awareness of AIDS has come greater interest in other SEXUALLY TRANSMITTED DISEASES, including syphilis, herpes simplex, warts, and molluscum contagiosum. Genital warts are very common and of major concern because of their association with genital and cervical carcinoma. Although warts do not greatly differ in clinical appearance, nearly 100 different types of human papillomavirus (wart-causing virus) have been isolated from them. This 'wart typing' is based on DNA hybridization techniques and has revealed that type 16 is most commonly associated with squamous cell carcinoma.

The skin may act as a window to internal disease. We may see the cutaneous metastasis (secondary tumor) of internal tumors, the butterfly rash of systemic lupus erythematosus, or the pyoderma gangrenosum ulcers of ulcerative colitis. We can look for the seborrheic eruption of histiocytosis, the yellow nails of pulmonary disease, and the thickened skin of systemic scleroderma. The skin also tells us of genetic disorders, from abnormal fingerprints to the dry rough scaly skin of congenital ichthyoses, to the daunting blisters of epidermolysis bullosa and photosensitivity of xeroderma pigmentosum. Here, the hope of the future rests with GENE THERAPY, in which flawed genes are either repaired or replaced. It is the ultimate in cellular transplants.

With greater knowledge about skin diseases has come awareness that an identifiable disease does not necessarily have a single cause. For instance, hives (urticaria) may have almost as many causes as there are patients suffering from it. Indeed, many skin diseases which are morpho-

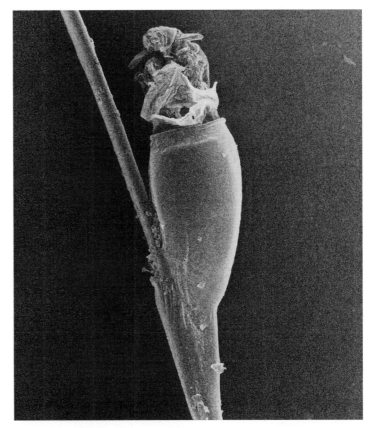

The birth of a louse: note the head emerging from a nit glued to a scalp hair (scanning electron microscope).

logically unique clinically, such as erythema multiforme, lichen planus, and contact dermatitis, represent reaction patterns. They require detective work to discern the cause in a given patient. To this end, a complete history of all that comes into or around the patient is essential. The focus is on drugs, 'bugs', foods, and environment, any of which may be responsible for cutaneous disease. In addition, a patient deserves a careful medical review, since some skin changes herald internal diseases such as diabetes mellitus, kidney disease, cancer, or raised blood lipid concentrations leading to heart attacks. The search is a serious one, since elimination of the cause may be the only cure.

Formerly resistant skin ulcers can now be cured with a variety of advances in wound healing. These include increasing the blood flow using pentoxifylline, controlling infection with antibiotics, accelerating the renewal of the skin surface with platelet-derived growth factor, and grafting laboratory grown artificial skin.

Great as the advances of dermatology have been therapeutically, the future holds a continuing challenge. There is still no specific drug to combat itch. There is no systemic antiviral drug to treat the common wart. Nor do we have a 'magic bullet' for psoriasis. Somewhere, in some laboratory, in some clinic, in some researcher's mind, the answers are to be found. Until then, patients will continue to search the internet, where an ever-expanding web of anecdotal and alternative therapies will enchant them. Never have we had such a wealth of information at our fingertips, and never has skin and its portraits of disease been so well displayed.          WBSHE, EDS

*See also* AIDS; ANTIBIOTICS AND ANTI-INFEC-TIVE DRUGS; SEXUALLY TRANSMITTED DISEASES

**DETECTIVE STORIES** There are several reasons for considering the detective story in a serious medical work.

Some doctors have written excellent detective stories. The first among equals was Sir Arthur Conan DOYLE (p 233), with his main character Sherlock Holmes and the assisting Doctor WATSON (p 233). The latter, however, seems to be placed in the story only to show Sherlock Holmes in a good light, given that Watson's contributions are not much to brag about.

R. Austin Freeman (1862–1943) created a detective who was a qualified doctor, a lawyer, and a criminologist — and based it on real life. His doctor, E. Thorndyke, was modeled after a professor, Alfred S. Taylor. But Thorndyke lived his fictional life in the shadow of his much greater colleague, Sherlock Holmes, and never really gained esteem in the same way. The humorous (medical) writer Richard Gordon has explained it in this way: 'Sherlock Holmes was a doctor in all but qualifications, Dr Thorndyke is a Sherlock Holmes in all but literary genius'.

Josephine Bell (1897–1987) had two careers: medicine and writing. After studying at Cambridge, where she stroked the first Newnham boat, she worked at University College, London, but left medicine in 1954 to devote her time to writing. Many of her detective novels have been reprinted subsequently, such as *The port of London murders*, *Easy prey*, and *Curtain call for a corpse*.

The Swedish psychiatrist, Ulf Durling, is regarded as one of the foremost authors of detective stories in Sweden. His first book, *Old cheese* (1971), is a locked room mystery as well as a medical murder. In this, the murderer mixes an antidepressant drug with his victim's antihypertensive medicine, gives him Chianti to drink and old cheese to eat. After retiring for the night and locking his hotel door, the victim eats the food, drinks the wine, and then takes what he thought was his regular medicine. But the effect of such a combination is to raise the blood pressure high enough to cause a fatal brain hemorrhage.

Secondly, there are a few doctors in fiction who are also detectives. Dr. John E. Thorndyke has already been mentioned, while forensic pathologists must be regarded as a variant of general medical detectives. Dr. Kerrison in P. D. James's *The death of an expert witness* is not only a forensic specialist but turns murderer when he is threatened by losing his children in a divorce case. One of today's best-known forensic pathologists is the beautiful but hard-boiled doctor Kay Scarpetta, created by American author Patricia Cornwell. In a recent appearance, in *Unnatural exposure* (1997), the murderer uses a mutated pox virus to create a fatal smallpox-like disease.

A third reason for discussing the detective story here is to learn how mistaken some authors can be in using medical situations wrongly. Thus Dorothy L. Sayers used a medical adviser who gave her

Dr Watson watches while Sherlock Holmes examines the evidence in *The valley of fear* by Arthur Conan Doyle (1914). (Reproduced courtesy of the Mary Evans Picture Library.)

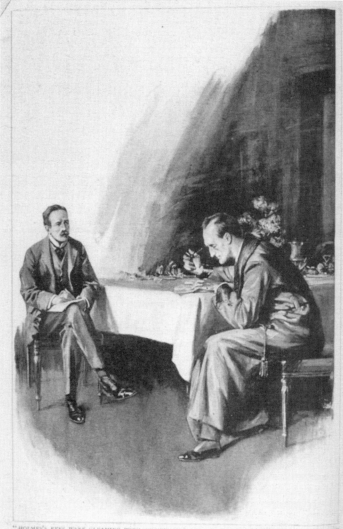

" HOLMES'S EYES WERE GLEAMING WITH EXCITEMENT, AND HIS THIN, NERVOUS FINGERS TWITCHED AS HE COUNTED THE WORDS—" DANGER,' ' HA ! HA ! CAPITAL ! PUT THAT DOWN, WATSON.' "

'Lesefrüchte' — the fruits of his reading. Nevertheless, he had no medical experience whatsoever. (He appears under his pen name as a co-author of *The documents in the case*; otherwise he is totally anonymous.) The first error in her books I heard of during my student years was when my professor of pathology said: 'Air might kill a person — but not in the small amount used by Dorothy L. Sayers.'

In Sayers's first book, *Whose body?*, the murder is committed by a famous surgeon and neurologist — an interesting combination — who eventually confesses: 'I struck him heavily with the poker just over the fourth cervical vertebra — it was delicate work, calculating the necessary force to kill him without breaking the skin — but my professional experience was useful to me. Do British medical schools and hospitals teach such skills? I can assure you that the Swedish ones do not.

It is in the next Sayers's novel, *Unnatural death*, that the 'air-lock in the feed' is found, a term borrowed from vintage motor cycles, which Sayers loved to ride. The murderess is a nurse who uses a hypodermic syringe of 1–2 ml to inject one dose of air into the blood stream, far too small an amount to kill a person.

In *The unpleasantness at the Bellona Club* the error centers on the dose of digitalis. The old general could not have been killed by the dose mentioned — and Mr Swain, the old taxi driver, probably would not have been observant enough to give this textbook description of cardiac insufficiency: 'Very faint, 'e seemed, and a vary bad colour, sir, breathing, 'eavy and blue-like abatah the lips'.

*The nine tailors*, generally regarded as the best of Sayers's books, tells about change ringing. The victim is bound and confined in the bell chamber of a church while no fewer than 15 840 Kent treble bob majors are rung. Even if noise today is one of the worst forms of pollution, nobody would die even from such prolonged and strong sound — though they might go crazy.

Fourthly, medical detective stories might illustrate how to use — or not to use — medicines and drugs. Agatha Christie spent several years in both world wars as a nurse in hospital pharmacies and learnt much about drugs and doctors' behavior. Her Hercule Poirot is heard to say: 'There was a time when you would have considered all poisoning un-English, a device of foreigners'. But POISONING — English or un-English, U or Non-U — is being used by nearly half the murderers of Dame Agatha. She uses a wide variety of poisons, physiological substances, therapeutic medicines, and alkaloids from plants and animals — I have counted at least 20 different poisons identified by name in her books. All of them might not have worked as well as indicated in the text — I doubt whether digitalis resists

boiling — but morphine and barbiturates seem safe enough, as does cyanide mixed in champagne or poured into antiallergy inhalors. Strychnine is used several times, as is arsenic — 'they soak fly paper, you know' — as well as taxine from yew berries; coniine from spotted hemlock, and aconite from monkshood. Interestingly, many years later a modern and very promising drug for treating advanced ovarian carcinoma is derived from the yew tree. Agatha Christie does not like today's doctors, or their medicines: 'The young doctors are all the same. They take your blood pressure and whatever's the matter with you, you get some kind of mass produced variety of new pills. Pink ones, yellow ones, brown ones. Medicine nowadays is just like a supermarket, all packaged up'. She nostalgically dreams herself back to her own youth: 'I remember so well in my young days, the black mixture and the brown mixture (the cough mixture that was) and the white mixture and Doctor So-and-So's mixture. People did not mix those up nearly so much'.

## Doctors and their foibles

Detective stories also convey one view of what doctors are like. Agatha Christie learnt not only about drugs but also about doctors, and their foibles and prescribing habits. In fact, one might hear Miss Marple say of her creator in *A Carribbean mystery* that: 'She's got a thing against doctors'.

Christie is not impressed by their prescribing: 'Doctors seem to follow one another in prescribing like a flock of sheep'. She does not believe them when they are giving legal testimony: 'Medical evidence — doctors indeed — innocents, that's what they are', not to talk of their ethics: 'Moran blabbing about his patients — you never know what things will come to next'.

Baroness (P. D.) James was married to a doctor, who died many years ago, and she served for many years as a hospital administrator in the British National Health Service, learning about medicine and doctors. She caricatures doctors — with a considerable dose of good humor — and there are ironic comments on doctors in almost all her books, more in the earlier ones.

The doctor making his round on the very first page of *The black tower* was: 'gift wrapped in invisible foil and immune to the chance winds, frosts and ungentle fingers which would mar more vulnerable professions'. In *The skull beneath the skin* she states: ' "Doctors could be wrong"— Sir James, MD, did not privately believe that he personally could be wrong. His assertion thus was a conventional gesture to modesty'. But not all doctors are modest: in *Shroud for a nightingale* we read: 'Vanity, Mr Dalgleish, is a surgeon's besetting sin as subservience is a nurse's'. Back to *The black tower*, in which Commander Dalgleish had

## AUTHOR AND HIS CREATION

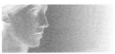

Sir Arthur Conan **DOYLE** (1859–1930). British physician and author. After unsuccessful practice in Southsea, Hampshire, Doyle turned to writing. His most successful novels were those recounting the adventures of Sherlock Holmes, an amateur detective, whose character was said to be founded on that of Joseph Bell, Doyle's distinguished teacher of surgery in Edinburgh. The first of these stories was *A study in scarlet* (1887). His later years were devoted to spiritualism. (*See also* AUTHORS, DOCTORS AS).

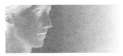

Dr **WATSON** is the companion, friend, foil, and chronicler to Sherlock Holmes in the much-loved stories of Sir Arthur Conan Doyle. Dr Watson's medical practice was variously 'quiet', 'never very absorbing', or 'could get along very well for a day or two'.

## A PALE HORSE

Reading a detective story might save life: *The British Journal of Hospital Medicine* (1977) told the story of a critically ill child who had been flown in from Qatar to England. Nobody understood the clinical picture until a nurse suggested that it might be thallium intoxication. The reason for her suggestion was that while keeping watch over the sick child she was reading Agatha Christie's *A pale horse*, in which a series of thallium intoxications occur. The title *A pale horse* stems from the Revelation of Saint John the Divine in the Bible — The pale horse with its rider, the name of whom was Death *(Revelations 6:8)*.

## COMPLEX PROCESS

The complexity of the diagnostic process is due to several factors. First, the extraordinarily varied presentation of disorders — many symptoms and signs are non-specific, appearing in numerous disorders. Further complexity is introduced by the way the patient reacts, which greatly modifies disease expression: a variety of types of host resistance and psychological factors affect the latter, sometimes substantially, including even the patient's own culture.

just escaped from a diagnosis of acute leukemia to that of an entirely benign glandular fever. He had been presented with a sentence of death: 'communicated by grave looks and a false heartiness as well as by a superfluity of clinical tests' — and later: 'with a sentence of life, pronounced with less sophistry!' *The black tower* has more of doctors than any of the other books. P. D. James goes on to state: 'Now that death had replaced sex as the great unmentionable it had acquired its own prudency; to die when you had not yet become a nuisance and before your friends could reasonably raise the ritual chant of "happy release" was in the worst of taste'. Sir James always hoped that 'the patients should realize in their good time that they were dying', evidently not to embarrass him with difficult questions.

In *Devices and desires* she gives an irresistible description of a forensic pathologist, Dr Anthony Maitland-Brown: 'He was an elegant and extraordinary handsome man, over six feet tall, who had once in youth — so it was rumoured — been told that he looked like Leslie Howard and spent subsequent years sedulously promoting that image. He was amicably divorced, comfortably well-off, and well able to indulge in his twin passions of clothes and opera. In his free time he escorted a succession of young and extremely pretty actresses to Covent Garden and Glyndebourne, where they apparently got an extra frisson of knowing that the elegant hands which poured their wine or helped them out of the Mercedes were commonly engaged with more bizarre activities'.

Finally, a good detective story might have a therapeutic effect, diverting its reader's attention from more worrying matters.          LEB

*See also* AUTHORS, DOCTORS AS; FORENSIC MEDICINE; LITERATURE

**DIAGNOSIS**, identifying the disease or other circumstances responsible for the patient's complaints (that is, his or her illness), has been the basis of clinical practice for millennia. It not only points the way to management strategies and allows the formulation of prognostic estimates, but permits categorization of clinical experience, recognition of patterns of presentation of various disorders, and recognition of new clinical entities. The time-honored sequence of progressive collection of the relevant clinical facts through the history and physical examination and the orderly application of various laboratory and other ancillary procedures has come under pressure in recent years from two sources. Firstly, is the appearance of many complex technologies which are widely perceived to offer shortcuts to identifying the process producing the patient's illness. Secondly, is the variety of time constraints derived from market forces that have resulted in shortened hospital stays

and the introduction of cost constraints in choosing and applying diagnostic tests and procedures. Both of these factors have increased the extent to which the diagnostic process, even in patients requiring hospitalization, is conducted in ambulatory care facilities, often by clinical teams different from those responsible for hospital care.

### Differential diagnosis

The process whereby the clinician sifts through the various possible causes of the patient's complaints is, ultimately, an exercise in the reduction of uncertainty. The clinician begins with maximal diagnostic uncertainty and, through a process of hypothesis generation and inductive reasoning, attempts to reduce this to a minimum. Absolute diagnostic certainty is unattainable, and undoubtedly the quest for diagnostic certainty can be carried too far. In addition, certainty is rarely necessary for effective treatment; clinicians generally proceed with this when diagnostic confidence is reasonable or when the urgency of the situation demands action on the basis of something less. Moreover, the patient's response to treatment is often a test of the diagnostic hypothesis on which the clinician is acting. Efforts in pursuing diagnostic certainty through excessive and often redundant testing incur excessive costs and expose patients to needless risk. In general, the closer one approaches certainty in diagnosis, the smaller is the likelihood that the information provided by a given additional test will add substantively to the diagnostic process. Nevertheless, repetition of tests already obtained is common: one study in a large teaching hospital found that of early repeats after a normal initial result for ten commonly used tests, a weighted mean of 40% were redundant. If such tests had not been performed the annual reduction in patient charges at this hospital would have been over US$900 000.

Diagnosis rests upon clinical observations of several types. The most time-honored, and still the most powerful and productive, are the medical history and the physical examination, in which clinical data are gathered from the patient at the time of the initial or subsequent encounters. Despite the extraordinary panoply of diagnostic technologies, some 88% of diagnoses in primary care are established by the end of a brief history and some portion of the physical examination. In one study 56% of patients in a general medical clinic were assigned correct diagnoses by the end of history-taking, and 73% by the end of the physical examination. The accuracy and yield of these basic procedures depend on how carefully they are carried out. The experienced clinician has learned to make history-taking an efficient, directed, interactive process with the patient. One of the chief benefits of experience is its ability to assign weights,

# DIABETES MELLITUS

Diabetes Mellitus is a chronic non-communicable disease, which, if inadequately treated, leads to a plethora of complications of two main types: microvascular disease in the eyes, kidneys, and nerves, which may cause blindness, renal failure, and foot ulceration; and macrovascular disease (atherosclerosis), which makes diabetics at least three times more likely to have heart attacks and strokes and twenty times more likely to have a leg amputated.

The disease was known in antiquity, when Aretaeus of Cappadocia described it as:

A wonderful affection not very frequent among men, being a melting down of the flesh and limbs into urine...The kidneys and bladder, the usual passageways of fluid, do not cease emitting urine and the outpouring is profuse and without limit...The development of this disease is gradual, but short will be the life of the man in whom the disease is fully developed. Emaciation proceeds quickly and death occurs rapidly.

In the 17th century the sweet taste of diabetic urine was noted by Thomas Willis and in 1776 Mathew Dobson of Liverpool evaporated a sample and was left with a residue which looked and tasted 'like brown sugar'. In 1815 the French chemist Chevreul identified the sugar in the blood and urine as grape sugar or glucose. The organ primarily affected was elusive. Aretaeus thought that it was the gastrointestinal tract, GALEN (300 AD) (p 324) the kidney, Richard Mead (1740) the liver, and CULLEN (18th century) (p 129) a disease of the brain and nerves. By 1850 the focus had moved to the liver as the result of the work of French physiologist Claude BERNARD (p 102), who suggested that sugar absorbed from the gut was converted in the liver into glycogen which constantly replenished the sugar in the blood during fasting. Another experiment of Bernard seemed to implicate the nervous system. He found that in animals damage in the region of the 4th ventricle of the brain caused glycosuria and, although this was transient, the condition became known as piqûre diabetes. The main investigative tool in the 19th century was the AUTOPSY and frustratingly, this usually yielded normal findings although occasionally gross disease of the pancreas was found.

The role of the pancreas was confirmed in 1889, when Minkowski and von Mehring found that removing it surgically in dogs was followed by severe diabetes. In 1893, Laguesse suggested that the pancreas produced a hormone which controlled carbohydrate metabolism and that the source

of this was the curious groups of cells, described in 1869 by Paul Langerhans, which he called the islets of Langerhans. For 30 years a series of reputable investigators failed to isolate the anti-diabetic hormone, but this was finally achieved in 1921 in Toronto by Frederick BANTING (p 236) and Charles BEST (p 236). The aftermath of this epoch making discovery was marked by bitter wrangling between the main proponents and disputes about the priority of the Rumanian physiologist Nicholas Paulesco. The 1923 NOBEL PRIZE was awarded to Banting and his boss J. J. R. Macleod, who, although an acknowledged authority on carbohydrate metabolism, had only been peripherally involved. Banting announced publicly that he would share his prize with Best, whereupon Macleod decided to do the same with the chemist J. B. COLLIP (p 267), who had been involved in purifying the extract. Paulesco had published two papers less than a year before Banting and Best which clearly showed that he had isolated an active pancreatic extract. However, he did not 'cure' any human patients with it.

By the autumn of 1922 insulin was being produced in commercial quantities and it was soon clear that it was, as one patient described it, 'a force of magical activity'. Its most dramatic effect was seen in young people who had been reduced to skin and bone by a starvation diet and were resurrected. At first it was thought that insulin might cure diabetes but it soon became obvious that patients would have to inject themselves several times

a day for the rest of their lives. What was not foreseen was that in time these young patients would develop complications and that insulin had converted an acute fatal disease into a chronic one with long-term complications. Diabetic eye (retinopathy) and nerve (neuropathy) changes had been described in the 19th century but because they were seen only in the middle-aged or elderly patients were thought to be due to atherosclerosis. Once insulin had enabled young diabetics to live for 20 years there were reports of a steadily increasing frequency of retinopathy and kidney disease. A paper in 1950 described 50 young people who had developed diabetes before 1924, of whom a third had died at an average age of 35. Equally worrying was that among the survivors there were 'ominous signs of hypertension, azotemia, and proteinuria' (high blood pressure and kidney failure). The cause of these complications was not clear, with some holding that they had a genetic basis unrelated to diabetes whereas others thought they were the result of a toxic effect of high glucose levels in the blood; insulin treatment could not then and still cannot restore a state of complete metabolic normality. There was considerable circumstantial evidence that the metabolic hypothesis was correct but the issue was not finally settled until 1993 by the Diabetes Control and Complications Trial, which showed that over a 10-year period those with the best blood sugar control had a 50–70% lower rate of complications.

Apart from the introduction of long-acting insulins, the first in 1935, no major changes

(*continued overleaf*)

Many diabetics are required to inject daily with insulin. (Reproduced courtesy of Leland Bobbe/Tony Stone Images.)

(*continued*)

took place in the management of diabetes between 1925 and 1970. By contrast, on the scientific front it was the stimulus for Nobel prize-winning work. In 1956, Berson and Yalow introduced the immunoassay for insulin, and extension of this technique revolutionized endocrinology. In 1956, Sanger reported the complete amino acid sequence of insulin, an achievement which had a catalytic effect on research in many other subjects. In 1972 Dorothy Hodgkin reported the 3-D structure, which paved the way for producing and modifying the insulin by genetic engineering.

Since 1880, when the French physician Lancereaux divided diabetes into *maigre* (thin) and *gras* (fat), it was evident that there were at least two types. The thin type, now called insulin-dependent or type 1, predominantly affected young people, and in the 1970s it was shown to be an autoimmune disease in which there is highly selective destruction of the insulin-producing beta cells. An important genetic risk factor lies in the human leukocyte antigen (HLA) genes on the short arm of chromosome 6 but environmental triggers are almost certainly involved. The incidence of type 1 diabetes varies as much as 30 fold between countries and in Europe appears to be doubling every 20 years. Attempts to produce an artificial pancreas to cure the disease have failed. Pancreas transplantation is a desperate solution, usually carried out only in patients who also need a kidney transplant. In the long-term, prevention seems likely to come from some form of immunomodulation.

In all populations the *gras* form of diabetes, also called type 2 or non-insulin dependent diabetes mellitus, is much more common. This is particularly true in developing countries, where it was catapulted from an extreme rarity at the beginning of the 20th century to a significant cause of death and disability. The prevalence varies very widely from virtually zero in Inuits and traditional living Melanesians in Papua New Guinea to highs of over 30% in Pima Indians and Nauruans. The Republic of Nauru is a coral island in the Pacific where exploitation of phosphate deposits has led to great wealth. Before 1954 diabetes was virtually unknown but it now affects a third of those over 20 and two thirds of all adults over 55; it causes a quarter of all deaths. The onset is approximately 20 years earlier than in Europeans. Migration studies suggest that non-insulin dependent diabetes increases when adverse life-style factors, such as lack of exercise, obesity, and a diet high in refined foods, interact with genetic susceptibility. Explosions of diabetes, like those in Nauru,

have been seen in most Amerindian tribes, as well as in Mauritius, India, and China. In 1997 the World Health Organization forecast that between 1995 and 2025 the number of diabetics in South-East Asia would increase from 8.5 to 19.5 million and that the number in Africa would treble.

The cause of type 2 diabetes is unknown; it is likely to be a syndrome with many different causes. Heredity is important and in one unusual subtype called 'Maturity onset type diabetes of the young' at least five different genetic defects had been identified by 1998. Most patients with type 2 diabetes have a combination of insulin resistance and insulin deficiency and the question is which is the chicken and which the egg. There are two polar views: the first is that insulin resistance is the primary defect and that diabetes does not develop provided that the pancreas can produce enough insulin to overcome it. Eventually, pancreatic exhaustion leads to insulin deficiency and a self-perpetuating vicious cycle in which glucotoxicity further impairs insulin secretion. The second view is that there is an inherited defect of the beta cell, which has no clinical consequences until insulin sensitivity is reduced by obesity, age, drugs, illness, or other factors. Whichever of these views is correct, type 2 diabetes mellitus is a multimetabolic disorder in which high blood sugar concentrations are usually accompanied by high blood pressure and abnormal lipid levels; the latter may be as or more important than blood sugar in causing the macrovascular disease which underlies most of the premature mortality in this type of diabetes mellitus. GA, RBT

*See also* DIET AND DISEASE; FATNESS AND THINNESS; NUTRITION

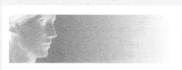

Sir Frederick Grant **BANTING** (1891–1941). Canadian orthopedic surgeon and physiologist. After qualification he served with the Canadian Army Medical Corps in France from 1916–18 and was awarded the Military Cross. He subsequently trained as an orthopedic surgeon, but occupied his spare time in research in J. J. R. Macleod's department of physiology. It was here in November 1921 that, working with Charles H. BEST, he isolated insulin. For this work Banting and Macleod were awarded the NOBEL PRIZE for 1923. In 1939 he became head of the medical research committee of the National Research Council of Canada. He was killed in an aircraft crash when flying to Europe in 1941.

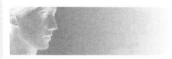

Charles Herbert **BEST** (1899–1978). Canadian physiologist. While still in medical school he collaborated with Frederick BANTING in experiments leading to the isolation of insulin. The NOBEL PRIZE was awarded for this work, to Banting and to Macleod (head of the department in which the research was done). Banting shared his award with Best. Later in his career Best conducted other successful pieces of research: discovery of histaminase (an enzyme which degrades histamine), recognition of choline as a dietary factor, and purification of heparin.

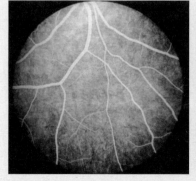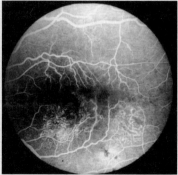

This fluorescein retinal angiogram in (a) a non-diabetic and (b) a diabetic of 15 years' duration. In the lower sectors, note new vessel formation. (Reproduced with permission from Laycock, J. F. and Wise, P. H. (1996). *Essential endocrinology*, OUP.)

or valences, to clinical data. Similar weights are assigned by the experienced clinician to findings of physical examination. These basic procedures are extraordinarily powerful, if carried out well, not only offering important diagnostic information, but often providing reliable insights into the probable generic nature of the patient's disorder, the organ or organ system involved, the physiologic derangements that have resulted, the pace of the process as well as its extent or degree, the urgency of the situation and its probable outcome. In recent years rigorous training in bedside examination has been eroded, in large measure because of increasing dependence on technologic procedures.

## Collecting and analyzing facts

Fundamentally, diagnosis involves two basic procedures: collecting the facts and analyzing them. In assembling the facts the choice of technologic diagnostic procedures should be based upon preliminary diagnostic formulations, derived from the history and the physical examination. Each test procedure should be performed to answer a specific diagnostic question. Ordering many laboratory examinations unselectively is inefficient and costly, possibly exposing the patient to unnecessary risks, not only from the test procedures themselves, but also from the misguided therapeutic interventions that may follow from the diagnostic hypothesis they generate. Further, such test ordering patterns undermine the diagnostic process and expose it to unnecessary inaccuracy.

Beyond these considerations, tests must be selected with understanding and appreciation of their functional characteristics; namely, sensitivity, specificity, positive and negative predictive values, and likelihood ratios. In general, diagnostic accuracy is heightened if the physician has reliable information on the prevalence of the disorders in the population from which the patient comes.

A systematic approach to diagnosis is essential, and involves assigning orders of importance, or clinical weights, to the facts most likely to be relevant to the patient's disorder. Thereafter central features or findings are selected, around which the differential diagnostic process can be oriented. Each candidate disorder is examined for the specific features of this case, comparing them with the variety of clinical hypotheses generated by the clinical problem. In this way, the most likely diagnosis — that is, the one that best explains the clinical features in the patient — is selected. Diagnostic formulations must be modified frequently, and sometimes changed altogether, as the patient's illness evolves.

In many instances despite intensive early investigation substantial diagnostic uncertainty remains. Thoughtful consideration of the unfolding course of the clinical process may then be considered an additional diagnostic test. The nature of a puzzling disorder may become clearer as new symptoms or physical findings appear, or as new data from the laboratories or other ancillary studies become available. Even when the diagnosis seems clear, the experienced clinician will continue to review the diagnosis and watch for the emergence of possible complications or for evidence that the disorder is responding or not responding to treatment. As new facts appear, the clinician must evaluate them in a diagnostically unbiased manner, assigning them appropriate weight. It is as unwise to attempt to force new information into an uncomfortable fit with the working diagnosis as it is to allow the isolated, discordant result of a laboratory test to shake a diagnostic formulation that seems sound on every other basis. Finally, despite all the modern diagnostic techniques, AUTOPSY examination frequently shows findings unsuspected during life: in roughly 10% of such instances this knowledge would have altered treatment and potentially changed the clinical outcome.

In office practice, standardized questionnaires are often used to shorten physician–patient encounters (in the interest of maximizing the number of patients a physician can see in a session of finite duration). This is an 'efficient' process in many ways, ensuring that all the relevant questions are asked. But it does not allow for subliminal signals patients may transmit in a face-to-face encounter, and erodes the base of the personal relationship and the trust that patients often must have in their doctor as healer of their ills.

## Recent developments

Research in the diagnostic process has sought to strengthen the evaluation of diagnostic test procedures, to link computer-based information management with clinical decision-making, and to formalize the process of clinical decision-making. Central issues include reintroduction of rigorous training in bedside skills and in diagnostic analysis, the introduction into medical education, training programs, and clinical practice of more selective use of modern technologic capacities, and validation of new technologic procedures in diagnosis before they are adopted in widespread fashion.                                JABaro

*See also* CLINICAL INVESTIGATION; EVIDENCE-BASED MEDICINE; STATISTICS

**DIALYSIS** See NEPHROLOGY

**DIET AND DISEASE** The pattern of people's food intake is one of the major determinants of disease. For some diseases the influence is subtle. Poorly nourished people are most likely to develop pathology when tuberculosis bacilli enter their body but

'The Reun cretin' from the Reun model book *Reuner Musterbruch* produced by the Cistercian Abbey at Reun (near Graz) Austria, and dating from 1215. This model book covers everything that an educated 'clericus' of the 13th century had to know. The cretin has a large trilobed goiter with the third lobe strung over his left shoulder. His right hand clutches at a frog (possibly for healing) and his left hand holds the 'fool's scepter' in order to make the mental deficiency clear. (From Merke, F. *The history and iconography of endemic goitre and cretinism*, MTP Press, Lancaster.)

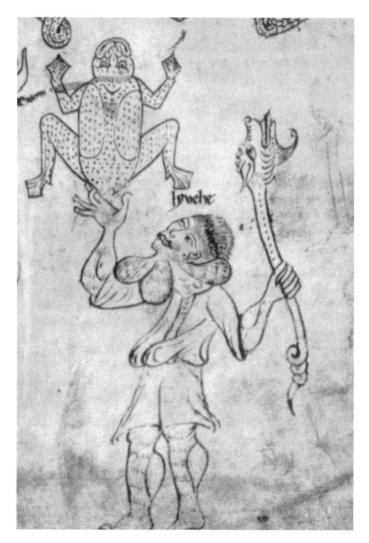

exactly why has not been clearly defined. For some other diseases inadequate diet is a major cause. Powerless people, especially children in developing countries, generally suffer. The big nutritional deficiency diseases are FAMINE, protein-energy malnutrition, iodine deficiency disorders, vitamin A deficiency, and nutritional anemias.

In famine, adults as well as children are starving. Malnutrition is extensive. People sell their few assets to try to buy food. Practically all social and economic structures break down and there may, as a last resort, be mass migration of the sufferers. If there is a crop failure today, relief food can be flown in by generous donor countries and nongovernmental organizations but this can only happen if the food crisis is officially acknowledged and the aid can be brought in safely. Severe famines nowadays are usually the result of war.

## Protein-energy malnutrition

This might be better called energy-protein malnutrition. Children under 5 years old are the main victims. They have higher nutritional requirements and depend on adults to provide adequate food for them. Mild to moderate protein-energy malnutrition affects many more children than severe protein-energy malnutrition. There is wasting or, less commonly, stunting. Marasmus (extreme wasting) is the more common severe form than kwashiorkor, in which there is edema with skin and hair changes, in a miserable child with loss of appetite. Usually the need is for traditional local foods. Cereals are not pure carbohydrate. They contain enough protein if they are not refined or diluted.

## Iodine-deficiency disorders

These affect around 200 million people in inland, often mountainous areas, the Himalayas, the Andes, parts of China, Africa, and Papua New Guinea. Here the original iodine has been leached out of the soil by heavy rainfall or glaciation so if people rely on locally grown foods the human diet is lacking in iodine. People have enlarged thyroids or *goiters*; where the deficiency is severe some babies develop abnormally, with mental deficiency and dwarfism (*cretins*). Elimination of iodine-deficiency disorders is a WORLD HEALTH ORGANIZATION priority: this is mostly achieved by iodization of the salt that people use with their food.

## Deficiencies

The most obvious effects of vitamin A deficiencies are on the eyes of young children. The conjunctiva becomes dry and thickened. The cornea can be involved with loss of vision. This eye disease, *xerophthalmia*, occurs mostly in South-East Asia. Where it occurs, trials have shown that vitamin A supplements can reduce the severity of respiratory infection and gastroenteritis in the community, presumably by correcting subclinical deficiency of vitamin A, the 'anti-infective vitamin'.

Unlike other deficiency diseases, anemias occur in affluent as well as poor countries. Iron is needed to make hemoglobin in the red blood cells. When iron is lacking the red cell count goes down — there is *anemia*. Iron is lost from the body by bleeding. Iron deficiency affects women between 15 and 50 years because they lose iron during menstruation – some lose more than others — and also during pregnancy. Iron in meat is better absorbed than iron in vegetable foods. Folic acid deficiency and vitamin B12 deficiency may also cause anemia but these are not so common.

Other diseases are related in part to eating too much. 'They are as sick that surfeit with too much as they that starve with nothing' (Shakespeare: *Merchant of Venice* I, II, 6). The most important diseases of affluence related to nutrition are OBESITY, DIABETES, coronary heart disease, and two cancers: of the large intestine and of the female breast.

## Obesity

Throughout the western world and in the rich minority in developing countries, obesity is an increasing problem. Authorities agree that obesity starts when body weight (in kilograms) divided by height squared (in meters) exceeds 30. Two conditions are leading to the increase in obesity: a great variety of delicious foods, relatively inexpensive and freely available, coinciding with decreasing opportunities to engage in muscular exercise. Obesity is uncomfortable and in the west may have social disadvantages. It increases the risk of degenerative disease, especially diabetes mellitus.

In diabetes mellitus the blood glucose (sugar) level is too high. There are two varieties. In the less common, type 1, insulin production from the pancreas is insufficient. It starts in young adults. Change of diet is used in treatment but diet is not agreed to be causative. In type 2 diabetes insulin is produced but there is resistance to it in the tissues. Obesity is the best known predisposing cause of this *maturity onset diabetes*. Weight reduction and increased exercise improve type 2 diabetes if the patient can be persuaded to stick with them.

## Coronary heart disease

One or more of the small coronary arteries that provide blood to the heart muscle become narrowed by atherosclerosis. Atherosclerosis can affect arteries elsewhere in the body but the coronaries are critical because the heart has to keep beating (about 37 million times a year). Cholesterol is the most characteristic substance that accumulates in atherosclerosis. This is derived from cholesterol in low-density lipoprotein in the blood. The classic risk factors for coronary heart disease are a high blood cholesterol, cigarette smoking, and high blood pressure. Blood cholesterol can be lowered by cutting down dietary saturated fat and body weight; increasing polyunsaturated fat and fiber. 'Statin' drugs are more potent but expensive. The classic risk factors account for about only half the incidence of clinical coronary heart disease. Other factors are still being discovered, including raised plasma homocysteine and oxidation of low-density lipoprotein-cholesterol. It may be possible to improve these by dietary change using more folate and more vitamin E respectively.

## Cancers of the large intestine and of the breast

These cancers are associated with a western lifestyle, including diet. Our concepts of the role of diet in their development rest mainly on epidemiological associations and are still very insecure. It looks as if animal fats (and inactivity) increase the risk of large intestine cancer while insoluble fiber (such as wheat bran) and brassica vegetables may be protective. There is even less certainty about the role of diet in development of breast cancer. An association of national fat consumption and breast cancer has long been described, but in the large prospective study of 89 000 US nurses, fat intake did not emerge as a risk factor. An interesting suggestion being investigated at present is that weak plant estrogens (*phytoestrogens*), found particularly in soya bean products, might be protective. Breast cancer incidence in Japanese, who eat soya products regularly, is less than one-third that in transatlantic countries. AST

*See also* ATHEROMA; CARDIOLOGY; ENDOCRINOLOGY; FATNESS AND THINNESS; HEMATOLOGY; NUTRITION; VITAMINS

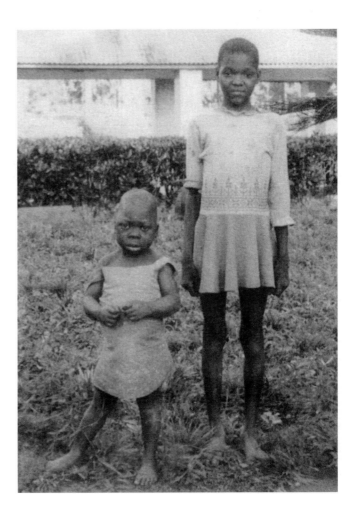

A myxedematous cretin girl from Zaire aged 9 showing gross dwarfism compared with a normal girl of the same age. (From Delange, F. et al. (1972). *Journal of Clinical Endocrinology and Metabolism*, **34**, 1059–66.)

# THE GREAT KILLERS: DIPHTHERIA

Diphtheria is an acute and dangerous INFECTIOUS DISEASE, primarily of young children, affecting the nose, throat, and larynx, and occasionally superficial wounds. The name derives from a characteristic grey necrotic false membrane which forms in these areas (*diphthera* was the skin of the goat on which Jove wrote the destiny of man), and which may produce symptoms and signs of obstruction.

The condition is due to the bacillus *Corynebacterium diphtheriae*, which produces a powerful toxin. Although the infection remains local, the toxin, carried in the circulation, may affect the heart, causing myocarditis and heart failure, and the peripheral nervous system, causing degeneration of the nerves with variable paralysis, which may involve respiratory muscles and cause respiratory failure.

The incidence of the disease has been greatly reduced since the mid-1950s by prophylactic active immunization; this is now normally carried out in the first year of life with diphtheria toxoid (modified toxin) combined in a triple vaccine with tetanus and pertussis vaccines. Treatment of the disease, now rare in the West but returning in RUSSIA, is urgent. It includes antitoxin administration, penicillin, and sometimes tracheostomy.

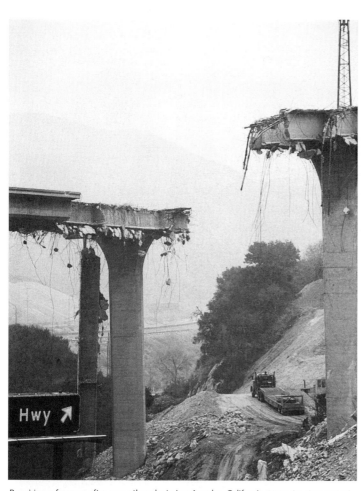

Repairing a freeway after an earthquake in Los Angeles, California. (Reproduced courtesy of Deborah Davis/Tony Stone Images.)

**DISASTERS** are events that totally disrupt the lives of a number of people, ranging from a small group caught in a fire to a whole community obliterated in an earthquake.

Volcanoes and earthquakes are the main causes of natural disasters. Flooding, high winds, famine, epidemics (including animal), and insect (locust) invasion now appear more as consequences of human action through environmental depredation, war terrorism, or global warming. Transport accidents, pollution, industrial and structural accidents are direct consequences of human action. Some disasters affect communities (floods, air raids), some affect groups of workers (on an oil rig, or in a factory fire), travelers (rail or air crash), passers-by (terrorist bomb), or people gathered together for a purpose (stadium disaster). The victims comprise the survivors of the event, those who were witnesses but not in personal danger, and others who learned of the event through the media, or who came on the scene later to find loved ones killed or injured.

The phases of human reaction are similar to those following bereavement:

- *Shock and apathy* People wander aimlessly, expressing little emotion, and do little to protect themselves from further danger.

- *Reaction* After hours or days, according to the severity of the event, grief and intense distress are expressed at the losses, both human and material. There is an intense desire to tell one's story, often over and over again. There is also a pressing need for explanation, somehow to make sense of the event. In the western world the explanation is generally sought in terms of the shortcomings of some human authority; in traditional cultures metaphysical explanations may be sought. At this time the survivors are very vulnerable and suggestible, and need to be kept away from those (some politicians and reporters) who would exploit them. Many of the survivors and witnesses sleep badly, show signs of depression and anxiety, and some will display acute distress for several weeks. They need gentle emotional support, preferably from people known to them. Sedative medication may help.

- *Recovery* If the experience has not been too horrific, if the losses have not been too great, or if the community has not been devastated, people can be expected to begin recovering after a month or two, and slowly return to normal life within about a year. Continuing emotional support is important, as the need goes on after the excitement of the disaster has passed. Survivors of transport accidents, for example, may return anonymously to their communities, often with great and unrecognized needs.

● *Post-disaster reactions* Ideally all these should be dealt with by people expert in treating post-trauma states. Depression, anxiety symptoms, panics at anything reminding the survivor of the disaster, are common in the early months; so also is heavy drinking. POST-TRAUMATIC STRESS DISORDER, a serious condition, may appear after about a month.                 GB

*See also* FAMINE; GLOBAL ENVIRONMENTAL CHANGE; TRAUMA

**DISASTER MANAGEMENT** Whether a disaster is natural (earthquake, flood, hurricane), or man-made (factory explosion, chemical spill, airplane crash in a populated area), or associated with violent conflict, certain essential services must be deployed to deal with it. In most developed nations there is a formally constituted authority with plans in place ready to manage any kind of disaster. These services usually include police, fire departments, hospitals, public health services, local government officials, the media (especially radio and television stations), and the military. Local government officials (mayor, town councillors, elected members of legislatures) may also be members of a local or regional disaster planning group. The money to pay for these services comes mainly from national treasuries, often after a national leader formally declares that a disaster has occurred; additional funds come from voluntary donations and several forms of insurance.

Floods, hurricanes, and earthquakes often make dwellings uninhabitable, and temporary shelter must be found for many people. Some, perhaps including children, may have become separated from their families and may be frightened and anxious. Information, reassurance, and action to reunite scattered family members, as well as to provide them with shelter, are therefore a priority. Food must be provided and communal kitchens set up to cater for displaced people, who may be temporarily housed in public meeting halls or tents on sports grounds. Washing and toilet facilities for displaced people are also needed. All these services must be coordinated, preferably by experts in disaster management. Most nations train and regularly retrain key staff members of the relevant sectors (police, fire, medical, ambulance personnel), and have an established plan to cope with unexpected disasters. Sometimes, as with floods on densely settled alluvial plains and earthquakes in geologically unstable regions, disasters are predictable, although their exact location and timing may not be.

The established fabric and infrastructure of organized society may be disrupted. In widespread floods, road and rail communication is impossible and local airports may be under water. Evacuation of large numbers of people to temporary shelter must be coordinated. If many thousands of people must be moved out of danger rapidly, military forces and transport are often pressed into service. Earthquakes may sever transport and communication routes and destroy many dwellings, often trapping people indoors. Survivors must be extricated quickly, which requires heavy lifting equipment and the use of transport vehicles to move the equipment where it is needed.

In floods and earthquakes, sewage treatment plants are incapacitated and water supplies become contaminated. Decomposing dead bodies of humans and animals pose an additional threat. Local, regional, and national public health services have a responsibility to protect vulnerable populations against fecal–oral and other epidemic diseases.

Natural disasters are usually self-limiting in duration: the floodwaters subside, the hurricane passes, the drought breaks and rains fall again, the earth stops shaking. Man-made disasters associated with violent conflict may continue for many years or even decades. The most prominent aspect of this kind of disaster, ever present on our television screens, is the endless flow of refugees and displaced people. Some, such as the Palestinians displaced when the state of Israel was established, are permanently uprooted and require resettlement elsewhere — though often not before they have had to spend years or even decades in refugee communities.

This aspect of man-made disasters introduces other elements, such as the need to provide ongoing rather than interim emergency medical care, schooling for children, work for able-bodied adults, more permanent housing than tents, and secure water supplies and sanitation services. Since the end of the Second World War, there has never been a time when the world-wide number of victims of this kind of prolonged man-made disaster has fallen below 15–16 million, and usually it is over 20 million; a further 30–50 million people are permanently or long-term displaced populations within the borders of their own country. The medical problems and social and healthcare needs of these unfortunate people are met as best as may be achieved by staff of the United Nations High Commission for Refugees and by volunteers who work for non-governmental organizations and missionary societies. It is a sad comment on our times that the need for these services never ends.                 JML

**DISEASES** See CHANGING PATTERNS OF DISEASE IN THE 20TH CENTURY

**DISPENSARIES** The word 'dispensary' is used today to describe a place where drugs are stored and medicines are made up according to prescriptions. However, in the past, it described a medical institution in Britain which provided free medical

**FOUNDER OF
DISPENSARIES**

John Coakley **LETTSOM**
(1744–1815). British
physician. A protégé of John
FOTHERGILL (p 695), he
founded the General
Dispensary in Aldersgate in
1770 and the Medical Society
of London in 1773.

care for the poor. The difference between hospitals and dispensaries was simply that the dispensaries had no inpatient beds. They were outpatient institutions, sometimes designed to look like small hospitals. Physicians attended at stated times to see the sick poor, and visited the homes of patients too ill to travel to the dispensary. Most dispensaries employed a housekeeper and a paid resident APOTHECARY.

The management of the dispensary fell to the treasurer because the dispensaries, like the voluntary hospitals on which they were modeled, depended on voluntary subscriptions. An appointment as an honorary physician to a dispensary (which occasionally included a small honorarium) was not as prestigious as an appointment to a hospital, but was nevertheless much sought after by aspiring young physicians. Through the dispensaries, these physicians became intensely aware of, and wrote about, the extent of disease and misery within the homes of the urban poor — a fact of the times from which most hospital physicians and physicians in private practice were shielded (as some hospital specialists still remain today).

The dispensary movement began as part of the remarkable philanthropic impulse of the 18th century. The historian M. C. Buer wrote in 1926 that 'The crown and glory of 18th century medicine is that it first attempted to bring such knowledge as it had to the service of the mass of the people. The rich physician, pampering to the imagined ills of the wealthy, has been taken as typical of his age, but he is common to all ages; the new figure was the dispensary doctor risking his life daily in the disease-ridden hovels of the poor'. The QUAKER physician, John Coakley LETTSOM (this page), a compassionate man, started the dispensary movement when he founded the General Dispensary in Aldersgate Street in London in 1770. It was seen to be so successful that by 1800 another 15 dispensaries had been opened in London, and 22 in the provinces. The great advantage of the dispensaries was their cheapness compared with hospitals, and the fact that they were able to treat thousands of patients a year compared with a few hundred in the hospitals. For instance, the Liverpool Dispensary treated 13 000 patients in 1796. In London the Finsbury Dispensary provided care for 4000 in 1808 including 1500 home visits.

For the most part, dispensaries treated medical cases leaving all but the most trivial surgical cases to the hospitals. But the scope of care provided by the dispensaries was far from uniform. Some, such as the Westminster General Dispensary and the Sussex Dispensary in London, not only treated medical and surgical cases but also had very active lying-in (maternity) departments. There were also lying-in dispensaries or charities responsible solely for providing services for the delivery of poor women in their own homes. Of all the outpatient charities, the lying-in charities were the most successful, achieving very low rates of maternal mortality compared with the dreadful mortality of the LYING-IN HOSPITALS.

There were also poor law dispensaries and provident dispensaries, where poor families were required (for the good of their souls) to pay a small fee in return for medical care, and there were dispensaries for special diseases. There was a small dispensary for children (the Dispensary for the Infant Poor) in the 18th century but it was feeble and lasted only a few years. The first proper children's dispensary (the Universal Dispensary for Children) was established in London in 1816. It changed its name and location several times, moving to a site in Waterloo Bridge Road. Charles WEST (p 175) was one of the physicians at this dispensary, but when he failed to persuade the management committee (in 1849) to open wards and turn the dispensary into a hospital for sick children, he resigned and founded Britain's first children's hospital in Great Ormond Street, which continues to this day.

The dispensary movement began to fade gradually in the late 19th century, and rapidly when the National Insurance Act of 1911 enabled working men — the mainstay of the dispensaries — to visit a general practitioner free of charge. As numbers attending dispensaries diminished, many closed and only a few remnants were in existence when the National Health Service was introduced in 1948. In their heyday, the dispensaries provided an extensive network of medical care for the urban poor. Many kept detailed records, providing the single most important source for historians with an interest in the statistics of illness amongst the poor in that period. IL

*See also* BRITAIN; HOSPITALS

**DISPOSAL OF THE DEAD** At the edges of this life, the questions are childlike, existential: where do we come from, where are we going, how long till we get there, have we lost our way? The Neanderthal widow hovering over her man — a great lump of protein gone still in a way she had never seen in him before — knew that she would have to do something. She could leave the cave to become his tomb. Or she could dig a hole or build a fire or shove him over the hill or into a ditch or a swamp or the sea. But there would be an effort to budge or bury or burn him up, something involving the larger muscles. She put flowers in his grave, so 20th century archeologists deduce that she missed his presence. Looking up or down or out or into the flame or the hole — whatever void she would consign him to — she would ask herself a version of the overwhelming questions.

What comes next? Why is he cold? Is that all there is? Can it happen to me?

These questions shaped many enterprises: poets, priests, philosophers, of course, but also undertakers, sextons, shamans, and sin-eaters. Likewise stonemasons and cabinet makers, singers of praise, and anyone who traffics in sadness and wonder, or sells their fashions and accessories.

First among the signs of civilizing impulses found in the ancient landscape were the graves. Before we found the killing tools and kitchenwares and bones, we found the cairns, dolmens, and crematoria — those deliberate heaps of stone that said our kind was here before. We buried our dead or burned them before we discovered alphabets or farming. At first the impulse was, no doubt, olfactory. The urge to dispose of the dead was practical — they smelled bad, harbored sickness, didn't work, and were troublesome in other ways. It soon became clear something would have to be done.

Ceremony and ritual and liturgical speech bespoke an evolving sense that something more was needed — something for the living and the dead.

The funeral followed as the subtle notions of memory and a Maker and an afterlife made noises in the collective mind of man. The relationship between bodies in motion and at rest, the quick and the dead, the former and present and future tense, informed this ancient and honorable agreement that we witness and keep track of our own, not because it matters to the dead, but because the dead matter to the living. Thus, before we quit the dead, we have our say at our wakes and funerals. We shake our fists in their faces — the dead, the gods, the fates. We sing their praises. We take our leave at our own pace, dirge-like, slowed by the sorrow, we process between the cities of the dead and the cities of the living. We range between the good laugh and the good cry. Life goes on.

A thousand years before the pyramids were built, a society otherwise unknown to us spent three or four generations building the white quartz mortuary mound at Newgrange north of Dublin. The stone they used was not local. Boats were built to bring huge boulders north, up from Wicklow by the Irish Sea and up the River Boyne, then uphill to the point that overlooked the valley. A cave was hollowed out of the hillside, a tunnel dug into the round interior. There the dead were burned, their bones stored in stone bowls and jars in surrounding chambers. This singular enterprise required visionary leadership, personnel management, a division of labor. Hunters, gatherers, planters and harvesters, cooks and caretakers, boatsmen, haulers and high priests — all the makings of a civilization were engaged to build a kind of city of the dead. And 5000 years later, what is left are the stones. The white face of the

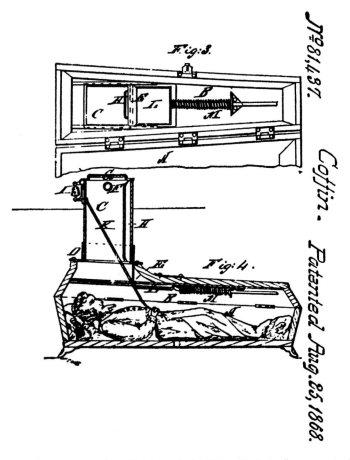

Device to allow a prematurely buried person to pull a rope and signal a bell above ground. (Reproduced courtesy of Dover Publications, Inc.)

mound can be seen for miles through the Irish mist, a monument to the makers' vision and muscular will. And as testimony of their intelligence, a portal in the stoneface was built that lets the light in one day a year to illuminate the inner chamber on the winter solstice. Such deliberate stones are found all around the planet — the efforts of mortals to put on immortality.

The Egyptians embalmed for the long haul, figuring that the soul would need the body back some day. Nothing was spared in the preparation of the dead body for its long wait for reanimation. Eviscerated, soaked in salt, perfumed, wrapped in linens, placed in coffins and sarcophagi and pyramids — the care of the dead was handled by a professional class of priests, artisans, and embalmers. The Greeks believed in a disembodied afterlife adrift in the Elysian fields of glory. They buried and burned their dead with ceremony, as did the Romans, who washed and anointed and waked their dead before elaborate processions bore them out of town to the grave or pyre, where paid wailers shrieked and beat their breasts and tore out their hair in payment of the emotional tax the living were calculated to owe the dead. The early Hebrews rent their garments, shaved their beards, and went barefoot as signs of bereavement and lamented their dead in elaborate dirges. They buried their dead in caves and trenches and reasoned that an unburied body meant the disconsolate soul would wander on earth and in the netherworld. Cremation was forbidden except as punishment. But for the early Scandinavians the burning of the dead both freed their spirits from their bodies and kept them from returning to haunt the living. The great Viking ships set adrift to burn with their eminent dead suggested that these northern Europeans like their Mediterranean neighbors understood death as a journey and adventure.

It is the same in tombs and columbaria everywhere — this effort to name our losses and quiet the adverbials: who, what, where, when, how, and why?

**Why do we dispose of the dead?**
We dispose of the dead for a variety of reasons. Bury them to bury the smell of putrifying flesh, and we provide food for worms, beetles, bacteria. Then the great chain of being brings the protein back in the fullness of time for future humans. The soil of France after the Great War of 1914–1918, nourished by all those fallen soldiers, yielded bountiful harvests as well as human skulls or thigh bones. Burial is sound ecology. Burning isn't, although it does kill germs. Leaving the bodies for carrion birds to feast till nothing remains but dry bones also makes sense in a hot dry climate — it is sanitary and ecologically sound.

In most societies, the priest, pastor, rabbi, or shaman stands between the living and the dead and tries to make some sense of these mysteries. Thus the witch-doctor or archbishop has managed access to the necropolis. But throughout this century both the church and the cemetery have been secularized. The marketplace and mega-mall are contagious. Theology has given ground to therapy and sin has been replaced by self-esteem. The job is not to do good as much as it is to feel good about one's self.

The newly dead today, like the newly dead before them, are laid out for the living to see. In North America they are washed, embalmed by arterial and cavity injections with formalin-based solutions to provide a temporary preservation, enough time to get the dead back home from distant travels (this method of embalming became common during the American Civil War) or the living relatives back from their far-flung lives. Hairdressers and cosmetologists, the Sunday best the dead are dressed in, the flowers we surround them with, the music we pipe into well-appointed funeral parlors, none of these can hide the stillness that separates the dead from the living.

At the same time cemeteries and churches have both begun to sound increasingly like golf courses. Forest Lawn and Heritage and Oakland Hills and Willow Creek all sound vaguely like portals of heaven, God's little acres, and good golf links. And since folks began to spend their Sundays on the back nine, the comforts of faith have been a little lost. Gone are the certainties and blessed assurances. In the face of death we must, too often, reinvent the wheel, rolling our own orthodoxies, *à la carte*, off the religious and spiritual buffet.

What is done when a death occurs is relative. By whom it is done and for what reasons are issues to be considered. For most of the 20th century, just like most of history, the funeral has served to dispose of the dead and articulate the meaning of death to the living survivors. Thus, the wakes and ceremonials observed by early cultures came to this century pretty much intact. The fashions change but the fundamentals remained. There is the body, the box, some ritual articulation of a common faith, the burial or burning, and the commisery and commemoration. Custom often gives way to convenience, meaning to cost-efficiency, public grief to private treatment. In a century of changes we have seen the shift from public funerals and private sex to public sex and private funerals. A culture that buried its dead and burned its trash now does landfill and crematoria.

The burning of the dead in the western world is, for the most part, a fashion of the 20th century. Because the pagan Romans did it, the early Christians first disapproved then later disallowed it. Fire was thought to be punitive, wasteful, associated with shame. In trouble with God, the vexed soul was cast into the fires of hell or purgatory. Hindus and Buddhists proclaim that fire purifies, frees the spirit from its corporeality, reunites the soul with its Maker. In such cultures, cremation is public, ritually observed, celebratory, metaphorically correct. In the west, encumbered as we are by our traditions, too often cremation is a way to dispose of the dead and to distance them from the living — an effort to deal with death by not dealing with the dead body; more of a disappearance than a disposition. In 21st century America and Europe, cremation is seen not as an alternative to earth burial but as an alternative to a funeral. More and more a death in the family is regarded not as a spiritual, social, or existential event but as a retail one and cremation is viewed less as a way of disposing of the dead properly than as a way of avoiding costs associated with a funeral — fiscal, spiritual, and emotional. Since the last half of the 20th century, the dead have been alienated from the living; the disposition of the dead body has increasingly become a practical nuisance, a chore assigned to death care professionals disassociated from the community and familial impulse to mourn and remember or to articulate some doctrine of an afterlife. A memorial service — a ceremony without the dead body present — has become the memorial equivalent of a baptism without the baby or a wedding without the bride and groom.

The burning of bodies in the west has become fashionable not for sacred but for secular reasons. Cremation renders the dead more like the living in a post-modern, post-industrial, wishfully post-mortal world. Ashes, unlike corpses, are portable, scattered, mobile and minimalist, divisible and dismissible, cost-efficient, commemoratively neutral — the grain of sand in a psychosocial desert where less is said to be somehow more. No longer grounded to the family plot, the cremated remains of the dead enjoy, as they did in life, a variety of choices. And for surviving family they occupy that ever-shifting ground between some-thingness and nothingness. They can be more icon than debris, more remnant than essence. Cremation gives the living options, too. A portion may be scattered in a favorite fishing hole or sand trap. A portion placed in a columbarium in the center-field fence of one's local baseball team. Another bit cast into a memorial paperweight or bookend or egg-timer — some homey applica-tion — and still another pinch placed in a memo-rial pendant to be worn, say, as an ankle bracelet by a devoted daughter or former paramour; the downsized, upmarket, high-fashion, low-cost, user-friendly version of the Taj Mahal.

Still more amazing is the New Age variation on tree or sky burial (long the standard practice among Native Americans and certain Tibetans), whereby instead of scavenger birds to pick the bones clean, the dead are launched with digitally reconstructed and enhanced images into the vast abandon of cyberspace, where they occupy their memorial webpages with links to other family members and friends in cyber-cemeteries of their own where surfers and browsers might pay their random respects. Links to on-line chat groups form a community of grief support unencum-bered by geography so that bereaved parents, new widows, and adult children of the newly dead can network with others of their kind in real time in the great void of grief.

The dead and the living require witnesses — some testimony to the fact of their being. Disposing of the dead, when we take part in such sad duties, provides such witness. Whether they are buried or burned or blasted into space, the dead don't care. The living do. The efforts of the living to keep track and to distinguish seem at once both noble and futile. The letters fade, the trees that bore our dead aloft fall down, the ashes are scattered, the pyramids are plundered, the graves are overgrown. Eventually, however, the efforts link us to those of our kind for whom the dull math of mortality — we all die — is not enough. They seek some meaning beyond the grim equations, beyond the black and white calculus of being and ceasing to be.                                             TL

**DOMESTIC VIOLENCE** See ABUSE OF OLD PEOPLE; AUTOPSY; CHILD ABUSE AND NEGLECT; FORENSIC MEDICINE; VIOLENCE

**DREAMS** A dream is an experience of living in a fantasy world during sleep. In a dream we meet others in familiar or unfamiliar places, we have conversations, see things, touch things, experience emotions, and we have human interactions. The man blind from birth dreams like the rest of us except that he sees nothing in his dream, for he does not know what it is to see. In the dream we are removed from present reality, separate themes are condensed together, the identity of people is displaced one for another, one person or object symbolizes another or several, and associations may be based little upon logic but instead upon, for example, assonance: the dreamer in whose room the name 'Robert' was repeatedly spoken later described dreaming of a distorted rabbit.

The seemingly unfettered and primitive quality of thinking during dreams has given them appeal for painters and poets, for philosophers and cranks. The possibility of some kind of function for dreaming has repeatedly provided oppor-tunities for unverifiable theories in terms of hydraulics, magnetism, radar, or computers, depending upon the fashion of the age. Around the world and throughout history dreams have often been thought of as times when the soul is freed from the body, so to mingle with supernat-ural agents and thereby receive guidance for the future, either explicitly or through symbols.

In the 19th century books abounded to enable the layman to interpret dreams and forecast the future. Medical thinking during the same period by such men as Maury in France, Stekel in Germany, FREUD (p 321) in Austria, and JUNG (p 676) in Switzerland, moved on into the next century and saw dreaming as a time in which the individual's true personality was laid bare, his conscience quelled, and his individual passions and fears revealed to the discerning interpreter.

The 1960s saw an increase in research into dreaming, as a mental process arising from a bio-logical substratum. In Chicago, Dr Nathaniel Kleitman led younger research workers to investi-gate, first in infants and then in adults, what came to be known as rapid eye movement (REM) or paradoxical sleep. During sleep, and about every 50 minutes in the infant and every 100 minutes in the adult, the eyeballs would begin to jerk hither and thither, and this would continue for 10, 20, or

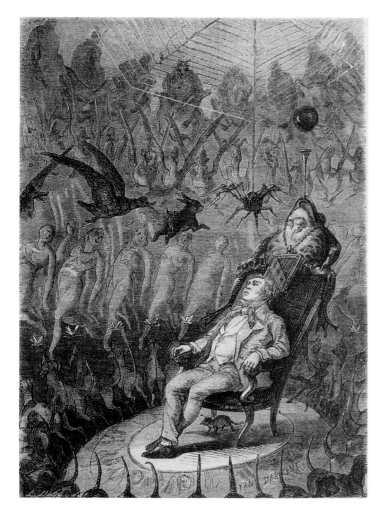

Ether-induced dreams. Early 19th century sketch showing French journalist Granier de Cassagnac after inhaling ether. (Reproduced courtesy of the Mary Evans Picture Library.)

ately after the eyes had just jerked were compared with awakenings during REM sleep after 30 seconds of eyeball stillness and the question was, 'What was the last experience in your mind before you were awakened?' When the eyeballs had been quiescent, mental life had merely been as in non-REM sleep, whereas accompanying the moments of jerking of the eyeballs mental life appeared to show peculiarly dream-like qualities, as if these were suddenly injected into mental experience simultaneously with the jerking movements.

## Deprivation of REM sleep

At first there had been a tendency to write as if dreaming and REM sleep were one and the same. Deliberate selective awakenings at the start of each REM period led to selective deprivation of REM sleep and the procedure was called 'dream deprivation', while the compensatory catch-up of REM sleep when undisturbed sleep was subsequently allowed was said to indicate a 'need to dream'. Dreams are the time when we all are insane, and it was even rashly claimed that without our dreams we would go insane. Time brought a reappraisal. Selective deprivation of REM sleep certainly led to later compensation by extra duration of REM sleep, but no one went insane. We need to sleep, we need REM sleep, and, who knows, we may also have psychological needs during sleep as we may while awake. But so far no one has succeeded in designing an experiment to show specifically whether we need the mental experience of the dream, as opposed to needing the physiological functions of sleep. What is realized is that we can dream at any time of the night, and not just during REM sleep; especially we dream when first falling asleep or at the end of the night. REM sleep is the richest time for dreams, but it is not the only time for them.

It also became clear that everyone dreams, and for a large part of the night, and that if dreams are not promptly recalled by awakenings at appropriate times, almost nothing of them remains stored in the memory. The dream a patient may report represents only a tiny fraction of total dreaming. Another fact that had to be acknowledged was that, as had been known from alarm clock awakenings 70 years earlier, most dreams are dull, tedious, and jumbled replays of ordinary life: only a few are spiced with symbols of our earthy urges. In the popular mind at least, Freudian dreams meant sex in disguise. Most dreams are not like that, but Freud would have been pleased that today we still do not understand why REM sleep is always accompanied by penile erection in men and enhanced vaginal blood flow in women, and why it is only in REM sleep that spontaneous orgasms (wet dreams) occur. It should be added that the rapid eye movements, like the simultaneous face

30 minutes, with bursts of several eye movements at intervals of seconds or a half minute. Could it be that here was the dreamer looking around at his dream world?

When sleeping volunteers were wakened from REM sleep and asked, 'Were you dreaming?', on 80% of occasions they answered, 'Yes'. When wakened from non-REM sleep, they usually answered, 'No'. Even people who claimed never to dream were then found to do so, though sometimes they would choose to call their rich sleep fantasies 'thinking'. Time brought refinement: if sleepers were instead awakened and asked, 'What was passing through your mind?', 80% of awakenings from REM sleep still elicited a description, but so did 60% from non-REM sleep. The descriptions of the former category were the more copious and the descriptions were of richer, dafter, more 'dream-like' mental events, while non-REM sleep provided duller, more everyday content. Awakenings during REM sleep immedi-

and finger twitches, may correlate loosely with vigorous events of the dream life, but it has not been possible to sustain the idea of the eye movements as movements for looking at dream pictures.

The new techniques for eliciting dreams through the night brought a research fervor that has now died away and attention has been again directed to other dream experiences. There are the sensory shocks of drowsiness, such as a sudden feeling of impact after falling, a flash of light, a musical chime, an electric feeling through the body, or sometimes all simultaneously. There are the brief dreamlets of drowsiness, known as hypnagogic hallucinations, most of which are immediately forgotten. There are night terrors and there are nightmares, historically associated with an overpowering demon in the form of a horse. The night terror is a phenomenon of non-REM sleep, running in families, usually arising in the early night, most common in youth, and usually with a brief unelaborated fear of being trapped, strangled, or devoured, often accompanied by a shriek and a stumbling out of bed. The nightmare comes later in the night, as a long, continuous, and anxious dream during REM sleep, experienced at any age, and accompanied, as reality is neared, by awareness of a complete inability to move. Both night terrors and nightmares are more usual at times of life when daytime anxiety is running high, but both occur sporadically as normal features of normal people.

There is no sharp dividing line between being awake and being asleep, and likewise there is no sharp division between the characteristics of day dreams and those of night dreams. REM sleep and its dreaming come about every 100-minutes in the night, as a manifestation of a biological rhythm that is also detectable during wakefulness. If adults are given a dull environment for hours at a time, their restlessness, their spontaneous eating, and their day dreaming wax and wane according to the same 100 minute rhythm. Dream experiences are the product of a mind working inefficiently and so they intrude also, with visions, voices, or delirium, when there is sleep loss, fever, alcohol withdrawal, dehydration, loss of the normal balance among electrolytes in the body fluids, or loss of the reassurance given by customary surroundings. So it is that the febrile child, the elderly lady in hospital at night, or the shipwrecked mariner may all wander in the mind in a half-waking dream.   IO

*See also* SLEEP

René Jules **DUBOS** (1901–81). American microbiologist. Born in France, Dubos came to the New Jersey Agricultural Experiment Station for graduate study in soil microbiology. In 1928 he began a lifelong association with the Rockefeller Institute (later Rockefeller University). Initially in the department headed by O. T. Avery, he used his experience with soil organisms to find species capable of degrading pneumococcal polysaccharides. This goal was achieved, but the products were too toxic for therapeutic use; nevertheless, the results gave encouragement to others who developed such important products as penicillin and streptomycin. In the latter half of his career Dubos became a respected and effective philosopher and interpreter of biomedical subjects, writing a series of widely read books.

*See also* SKEPTICS

**DWARFISM**, or smallness, is shortness of stature that is less than the third percentile for children of the same age and racial origin. There are many causes. It may be secondary to many general disorders when they occur in childhood before growth is complete, for example, those associated with malnutrition, malabsorption, low cardiac output, hypoxia (low blood oxygen levels), and kidney failure. Hormonal disturbances may be responsible, such as hypothyroidism, hypoparathyroidism, or gonadal dysgenesis; or precocious puberty can cause premature fusion of the epiphyses. Smallness may be due to primary abnormalities of the bones.

The most important group for diagnosis and treatment are those resulting from failure of normal action of human pituitary growth hormone. This may be due to panhypopituitarism, an iatrogenic cause for which is prolonged corticosteroid treatment for rheumatoid arthritis or asthma. The deficiency may be selective for human pituitary growth hormone, resulting in the pure or 'perfect' dwarf. Except in those where end-organ unresponsiveness is responsible (as in African pygmies), the logical and effective treatment is administration of human pituitary growth hormone itself, provided it is begun early enough, that is, before the epiphyses have fused.

*See also* CARDIOLOGY; CHILD HEALTH; ENDOCRINOLOGY

**DYSLEXIA** See LANGUAGE

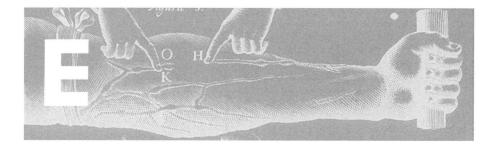

## ENT (EAR, NOSE, AND THROAT SURGERY) — HISTORY

ENT is a specialty of the early 20th century, when the separate disciplines of otology and laryngology were joined together. Otologists were surgeons, whereas laryngologists were physicians who also treated diseases of the nose and chest.

Early otological treatment was empirical and did not reflect the advances in anatomy, physiology, and pathology.

### Early treatments

Eustachian tube catheterization (1724), myringotomy or piercing of the ear drum (1801), and early attempts at mastoidectomy (removal of air cells from the bone behind the ear) (1774) were to remain the main surgical treatments until the middle of the 19th century when anesthetics and antisepsis were introduced.

The origin of laryngology, by contrast, may be traced to that day in September 1854 when Manuel Garcia, a singing teacher, at last achieved his lifelong ambition to view his own larynx with a mirror. Nevertheless, Benjamin Babington, a physician at Guy's Hospital, London, probably performed the first laryngoscopy with his 'glottiscope' in 1829. These observations were applied clinically by Ludwig Türck and Johann Czermak, who effectively founded the discipline of laryngology. The first university clinics of both otology and laryngology were established in Vienna in the 1870s.

Until Friedrich Voltolini introduced the oxyhydrogen incandescent light (1859) and later Thomas Eddison invented electric light (1879), it

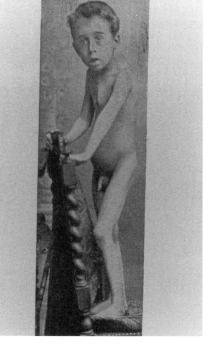

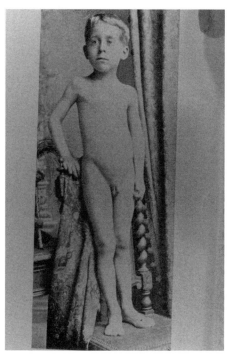

(a) A boy aged four and three-quarters suffering from adenoidal hypertrophy showing the characteristic expression, attitude, and deformities of the chest.
(b) The same boy aged five years and four months, from whom the adenoid had been removed seven months previously. (From St Clare Tomson and Negus, V. E. (1948). *Diseases of the nose and throat,* Cassell and Company Ltd.)

(a)

(b)

was possible to view the hidden structures of the ear, nose, and throat only by daylight or with a candle. The traditional otologist's concave mirror with a central perforation to look through appeared in 1841, firstly as a hand-held device but later worn on a head band (1855). Carl Nylen of Sweden introduced the monocular operating microscope in 1921 but modern microsurgery of the ear became possible only with the first binocular operating microscope for otology by the Zeiss Optical Company (1953). Fiberoptic light sources, developed by Hopkins in 1954, heralded a new era of endoscopy and flexible fiberscopes used to examine the nose, nasopharynx, larynx, and pharynx in outpatients have in many instances prevented the need for hospital admission.

The 20th century witnessed unparalleled change. At its opening, brave attempts were made to perform skillful surgery under primitive anesthesia, without antibiotics. The stimulus of two world wars led to immense advances in technology and with them greater opportunities to explore new and resurrect old surgical procedures. The discovery of antibiotics saw an end to acute mastoiditis and the major complications of inflammation of the middle ear, as well as a decline in TONSILLECTOMY and adenoidectomy operations.

In rhinology a greater understanding of IMMUNOLOGY and the function of the nose has expanded the knowledge of ALLERGY and led to more conservative nasal surgery. The complications of sinus infection have become rare. The discovery of radium by the CURIES (p 556) in 1898 and its first application to malignant disease by Danysz in 1903 led to the development of RADIOTHERAPY. Coupled with cytotoxic drugs this has reduced much of the potentially mutilating surgery of the head and neck. The emphasis on reconstruction after extensive removal of malignancy has been aided by the introduction of skin and muscle flaps (1960s), which have enhanced functional and cosmetic rehabilitation.

Audiology has become a specialty in its own right and the complex tests of hearing and balance, together with the investigation and treatment of deaf children and elderly people, are managed by audiological physicians. The early audiometers were derived from two inventions: the induction coil in 1849 by Emil de Bois Reymond and the telephone in 1876 by Alexander Graham Bell. The thermionic valve was pioneered by J. A. Fleming and Lee de Forest at the beginning of the 20th century and was rapidly developed during World War I. It was incorporated into the Western Electric I A audiometer (1922) designed by the American E. P. Fowler. Valves were replaced by transistors in the 1950s and at the same time printed circuits were introduced. The transistor has since been superceded by the micro-

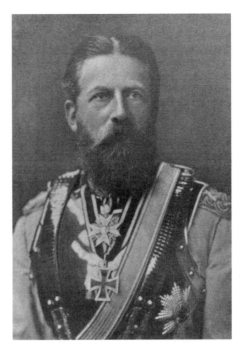

Crown Prince Frederick of Germany at Queen Victoria's Jubilee on 21 June 1887. Earlier in the same year he had complained of hoarseness and was found to have a growth on his left vocal cord which was subsequently diagnosed as cancer. The famous English laryngologist Sir MORELL MACKENZIE (p 253) was requested to manage his care. The Crown Prince became the Emperor Frederick III but soon died of the tumor, for which Morell Mackenzie was blamed. (From Scott Stevenson, R. (1946). *Morell MacKenzie: The story of a Victorian tragedy*, Heinemann, London.)

chip. Hearing aids, too, have benefited from similar advances and have now entered the digital era.

During the last thirty-five years, although still calling themselves otorhinolaryngologists — head and neck surgeons — individual practitioners have tended to subspecialize into otology, head and neck surgery, rhinology, phonosurgery, facioplastic surgery, otoneurosurgery, and pediatric otorhinolaryngology. Each of these subspecialties has its own societies and specialist journals.

The inevitable problems of the cost of a service have to be addressed and this varies from country to country, but the need to be conscious of the standards and quality of care offered should be paramount. The otorhinolaryngologist should also realize that most advances are still not yet available to roughly 70% of the world's population.      NW

## ENT

### Otology

The virtual disappearance of the emergency cortical mastoidectomy, frequently performed in the past with hammer and gouge, with the arrival of antibiotics led to an awareness and dominance of the lesser degrees of middle-ear disease such as otitis media with effusion. Although not a new condition, the term 'glue ear' was introduced only in 1960 and the first grommet or ventilation tube of the modern era was reported in the USA by B. W. Armstrong (1954). The grommet aims at equalizing pressure on either side of the eardrum and allowing resolution and absorption of

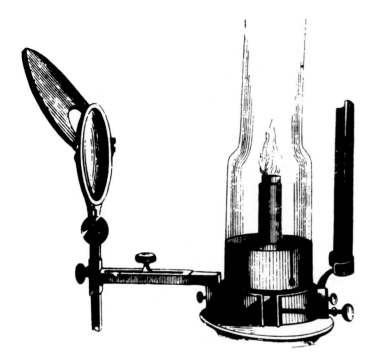

Fauvel's oxyhydrogen lamp with reflector. Charles Henri Fauvel (1830–96) favored this lamp, as did Morell Mackenzie.

FAMOUS NAMES IN ENT

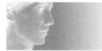

Sir Willian Robert Wills **WILDE** (1815–76). Irish surgeon and antiquary . He practiced in Dublin as an ophthalmologist and otolaryngologist. He was the father of Oscar Wilde and husband of 'Speranza', the poet.

(continued on p 252)

the middle-ear effusion. Drainage of the fluid and insertion of the grommet are now said to be the most common operation performed under general anesthetic in the western world. Acute infection of the middle ear is treated by the family doctor.

Training in the use of the operating microscope and increased knowledge of the underlying pathology of middle-ear disease have led to a reduction in the need for radical surgery. With advances in anesthetic techniques producing ideal otological operative conditions the emphasis today is on reconstruction of the middle ear rather than removing parts. Tympanoplasty techniques include repairing the ear-drum and restoring continuity of the three ossicles of the middle ear.

Otosclerosis results in fixation of the third ossicle (the stapes or stirrup) bone and reduced sound transmission to the inner ear. Attempts at the beginning of the 20th century to remove the stapes (stapedectomy) resulted in failure and loss of inner ear function. An alternative approach, fenestration of the lateral semicircular canal, to short circuit the otosclerotic focus by conveying sound through the canal to the inner ear, gained popularity in the 1920s and '30s. Perfected by Julius Lempert in New York, it remained the technique of choice until Samuel Rosen, also of New York, by chance rediscovered stapes mobilization (1952) by touching the bone to assess its fixation before proceeding to a fenestration operation under local anesthesia. There is a sudden restoration in the patient's hearing, though lasting improvement is

achieved in only a quarter of patients. This finding and the arrival of the binocular microscope served to reawaken interest in stapes surgery. John Shea of Tennessee re-established stapedectomy (1958) and replaced the bone with a nylon replica. Nowadays a tiny (0.8 mm) hole is drilled in the stapes foot-plate (stapedotomy) and the continuity of the ossicles is restored by interposing a plastic or metal piston between the second ossicle (the incus or anvil) and the stapedotomy, thus offering patients an excellent prospect of long-term improvement in hearing.

Endolymphatic hydrops, or Menière's disease, produces the three debilitating symptoms of deafness, tinnitus, and vertigo. Its cause is unknown, and a wide range of drug and surgical treatment techniques has been developed. In cases not responding to drugs the choice of surgical treatment rests between operations which are designed to relieve the patient of vertigo and to retain hearing (saccus decompression first described by Georges Portmann of Bordeaux in 1926), cutting the vestibular nerve (described by R. H. Parry in 1904), or abolishing the balance mechanism if there is no remaining useful hearing (translabyrinthine or total labyrinthectomy, first described by F. H. Quix of Utrecht in 1912). Each of these techniques has been refined by modern microsurgery and the recent introduction of endoscopy of the posterior cranial fossa has reduced the morbidity of vestibular nerve section. The balance mechanism may also be abolished with drugs such as gentamicin — a simple method that carries only a small risk of damage to the hearing.

Collaboration between the otologist and the neurosurgeon enables the removal of tumors arising in the space between the temporal (ear) bone and the base of the brain, the most common of which is a vestibular schwannoma, which invariably presents with one-sided hearing loss.

Our hearing ability probably starts to decrease early in life, and severe hearing impairment, often with tinnitus, is now an important cause of social deprivation in the elderly. In addition, many drugs damage the inner ear producing permanent profound deafness. This situation combined with the desire to help prelingually deaf children led to research into cochlear (hearing organ) implants. The concept of electrical stimulation producing the sensation of hearing in the deaf was not new. Alessandro Volta placed metal rods in both his ears in 1800 and connected them to a source of electricity. He apparently heard the sound of boiling water before losing consciousness. The modern advances in cochlear implantation were led in the 1960s by groups in many countries and the technique — a team effort of otologists, audiological technicians, scientists, and teachers of the deaf — is now well established.

In the last few years many deafness genes have been identified, and both the HUMAN GENOME PROJECT and DNA 'chip' technology will eventually help us to understand inner ear development and the mechanisms necessary for hair cell repair and regeneration. Perhaps we should be able to supplant hearing aid technology in the management of deafness.

## Audiological medicine

Not all otologists wish to be surgeons, and the need for complex tests of hearing and balance, together with investigation and treatment of deaf children and elderly people, led to the emergence in the 1970s of a new specialty of audiological medicine.

Before the late 19th century, hearing was tested using either the human voice or various mechanical devices, such as the watch, tuning fork, whistles, or acoumeters. The main weakness of all these methods was the lack of quantitative measurements. The first audiometers, in which sounds of various intensity were produced electrically, appeared only after the key inventions of the induction coil and telephone. The term audiometer was first used in 1879 by David Edward Hughes and his clinical collaborator Benjamin Ward Richardson. Present complex computer-driven audiometers can not only test hearing subjectively but can also objectively assess hearing at all levels from the cochlea to the temporal lobes (where hearing is appreciated in the brain), thus differentiating between sensory (cochlea) and neural hearing loss. Objective tests are particularly useful in determining the ability to hear in newborn babies, as this is impaired in about 1 in 10 000. Kemp (1978) discovered oto-acoustic emissions (sounds made within the ear) and the ability to capture these sounds has led to a complex test of hearing for 'at risk' babies.

Dramatic progress has been made in developing hearing aids. The bulky battery pack body-worn aid, available in Britain free of charge with the inception of the National Health Service (1948), soon gave way to smaller transistor postaural aids (1955). Miniature circuits and microchips made available even smaller 'in the ear' or 'in the canal' devices. Attention is now drawn to developments in signal processing, and the introduction of the 'digital' age of sound will help overcome the complaint that hearing aid users have difficulty in understanding speech against background noise. A major improvement in the rehabilitation of patients with sensorineural deafness has occurred with the creation of hearing therapists.

## Rhinology

The arrival of antibiotics reduced the necessity for radical surgical procedures for major sinus disease. Thereafter rhinology amounted largely to straightening the nasal septum but not reshaping the nose, washing out the sinuses, removing nasal polyps with a snare, and operating to eradicate chronic maxillary sinusitis.

Three important factors have led to a resurgence of interest in rhinology. First, developments in immunology have enabled differentiation between allergic rhinitis and the more common vasomotor rhinitis. Steroids applied to the lining of the nose have provided a suitable non-surgical treatment. The modern rhinological clinic is now staffed by both an immunologist and a rhinologist. Secondly, a much greater understanding of the anatomy, physiology, and pathology of the nose and sinuses led Professor Walter Messerklinger of Graz, Austria, to place an emphasis on the anterior ethmoid air cells as the key to effective sinus drainage and aeration (1967). The development of computerized tomography by Sir Geoffrey Hounsfield (1969) and the reintroduction of sinus and nasal endoscopy (originally conceived

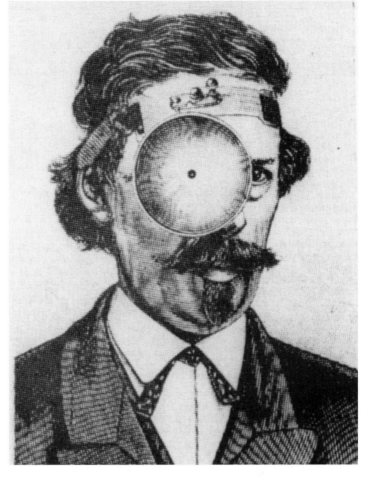

Kramer's mirror. Wilhelm Kramer (1801–75) preferred to use sunlight to examine the tympanic membrane but used artificial illumination with an argon burner fitted with a screened opening through which light was reflected into the external auditory meatus via a concave mirror.

(continued)

**Anton Maria VALSALVA**
(1666–1723). Italian
physician and anatomist.
Valsalva was a pupil of
Malpighi and became lecturer
in anatomy in Bologna,
where he taught Morgagni.
His *De aura humana tractatus*
(1704) contains an excellent
account of the anatomy of
the ear in which he names
the Eustachian tubes. He first
described the aortic sinuses
(sinuses of Valsalva).
Valsalva's maneuvre provides
a simple test of circulatory
function.

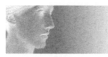

**Adam POLITZER**
(1835–1920). Hungarian
physician and otologist. He
described the cone of light
seen in the normal eardrum,
and the hearing, on
swallowing, of a tuning fork
placed centrally on the
forehead in only the normal
ear. Still in use is his bag used
for inflating the middle ear
through the Eustachian tube.

(continued opposite)

by M. Reichert (1902) and Alfred Hirschmann (1903) together with Etienne Escat (1911)) using fiberoptic endoscopes heralded the era of functional conservative endoscopic sinus surgery. Thirdly, the shrouds of mystique surrounding facioplastic surgery, in particular, rhinoplasty, have been removed largely by the work of the American Academy of Facial Plastic and Reconstructive Surgery, founded in 1964, and the European Academy of Facial Surgery (the Joseph Society), founded in 1977. This has led to the logical involvement of ear, nose, and throat surgeons in the former domain of the plastic surgeon.

## Laryngology, head and neck surgery, and phonosurgery

Laryngology was originally practiced by physicians, who learnt to remove small lesions of the larynx and adjacent pharynx using the mirror and curved forceps. Any larger lesions required a general surgeon. Sir Felix Semon was appointed in 1882 as the first laryngologist to St Thomas's Hospital, London, and was fortunate to have as a colleague Sir Henry Butlin (1843–1912), a general surgeon, who shared an interest in throat diseases. Together they promoted the operation of laryngofissure for early cancer of the larynx, which was the most common tumor of the head and neck. By 1928 Sir St Clair Thomson could report only two operative deaths and a 76% three-year survival in 74 patients.

The first total laryngectomy for cancer was performed in 1873 by the general surgeon Professor Theodor BILLROTH (p 518) at the ALLGEMEINES KRANKENHAUS, VIENNA (p 352). The patient survived the operation and lived for a further seven months. The chief complication of the early laryngectomies was aspiration of food and drink into the lungs. By severing the larynx from the trachea and suturing it to the skin Themistokles Gluck, in 1881, resolved this major problem such that by the early 1920s good results were being reported throughout the world. Both Gluck and his colleague Soerensen knew of the importance of removing tumor spread in the lymph nodes at the neck at the same time as removing the primary tumor, but in 1906 the American George Washington Crile promoted the operation of *en bloc* removal of the cervical glands with the primary tumor.

In Britain, the move in the 1930s was towards developing radiotherapeutic techniques to treat primary laryngeal cancer. After World War II greater complexity in dosage, field size, and avoidance of skin damage and inflammation of the mucous membranes all resulted in radiotherapy becoming the first line of treatment for early disease. Surgery was held in reserve for failures and more advanced tumors.

Carl Gussenbauer developed a voice prosthesis (1874) for use by Billroth's first laryngectomy patient. By 1900, Nicholas Taptas of Constantinople rehabilitated a patient using a direct connection between the tracheostomy tube and a deliberately created pharyngeal fistula, enabling the patient to speak by occluding the tracheostomy cannula with his finger. This was the forerunner to the tracheo-esophageal puncture and valved prosthesis introduced by Eric D. Blom and Mark I. Singer (1980), now the most frequently used form of voice prosthesis.

Over the last thirty years the surgeon laryngologist has gradually evolved into the head and neck surgeon capable of managing, often in collaboration with the radiotherapist, medical oncologist, neurosurgeon, and other experts, malignancies of the head and neck with the exception of the eye and the brain. Plastic reconstructions of the pharynx, larynx, and oral cavity using stomach transposition, myocutaneous flaps, and microvascular anastomoses have succeeded in providing patients with acceptable levels of appearance and function after the most radical of operations. The feasible limits of excision have now been reached, and further progress lies in the realm of molecular biology as a new approach to cancer treatment.

Paradoxically the laryngologist has on the whole been interested only in gross lesions of the vocal folds rather than voice abnormalities. Further advances in endoscopy, with either rigid or flexible fiberscopes, combined with reliable stroboscopy and the means to analyze the quality of voice, have led to a greater understanding of vocal function. By working closely with speech therapists and teachers of voice and singing the laryngologist can participate in diagnosis and treatment and is able to offer a delicate form of microlaryngeal surgery (phonosurgery). This not only permits excision of minute lesions of the vocal folds but also encompasses vocal fold medialization techniques, thus enabling restoration of the voice.

## Pediatric otolaryngology

Pediatric otolaryngology as a specialty was first promoted in 1938 by Danielowitz of Warsaw, Poland. Removal of the tonsils and adenoids, once the mainstay of ear, nose, and throat surgery, has shown a welcome decline in popularity, coincidental with an appreciation that recurrent upper respiratory infections may be how a child acquires immunity. The practice of intubation of preterm infants with chest problems led to the development of subglottic stenosis and with it a range of surgical corrective procedures. Perhaps the pediatric otolaryngologist's best contribution is in the management of congenital abnormalities of the ear, nose, and throat, where specialized facilities and skills have reduced the risks of treatment.

Few specialties have undergone such dramatic development within the past three decades as otorhinolaryngology — head and neck surgery. The specialty has taken advantage of the new advances of each decade, whether in endoscopy, microsurgery, the use of lasers, cytotoxic drugs, flap reconstruction, or the microchip. Today's otorhinolaryngologist can offer his patient a wide range of skills in diagnosis and treatment.    NW

*See also* SPECIALIZATION

**EATING DISORDERS** probably first arose when eating became more than just an activity designed to satisfy energy needs; maintain body temperature; move, grow, and survive through puberty to the time of reproduction, and care of replacement offspring. The origin of such eating disorders is as shrouded in mystery as the biology of human evolution is itself; for nobody knows if our remote ancestors were carnivores or herbivores or, like the chimpanzee, opportunistically both. But nature, recognizing the vagaries of food supply, endowed humans with the ability to store food as fat while supplies are plentiful, to be used for energy stores, hibernation, and, in the case of the female, reproduction during times of famine.

Our more recent ancestors also exhibited such forethoughtful behavior and probably recognized its value. Gorging was commonplace. Breughel's peasants were often rotund (and jolly). In the 14th century intelligent man doubtless consumed as much as possible of his strenuously garnered grain and meat in the autumn before marauding brigands and armies would take it away from him. THINNESS was an indicator of feebleness, disease, or even untrustworthiness. A degree of FATNESS was prized as evidence of strength, wealth, health, and contentment. Only excessive fatness would have been an encumbrance, hampering mobility and generating inertia. Yet even in those times continued excessive eating may have relieved boredom, protected against depression, and resolved ambivalences within relationships that might otherwise have progressed to defection and separation. Thus the neurotic basis of obesity was born.

As food became more plentiful, eating acquired a social value and the need for gorging no longer existed. Still, fat tends to accumulate in girls at puberty for the purposes of reproduction, ultimately representing around 25% of female body weight and serving to attract the male. But puberty also represents many other stresses and needs for adaptation, of reviewing aims and renegotiating relationships, of coming to terms with one's sexuality, and of maintaining robust self-esteem. If not well enough handled, these stresses may cause early maladaptation, some expressed as an 'eating disorder'.

Thus, teenagers experience puberty as a confusing process and some increasingly feel out of control. Girls may attribute this to their emerging 'fatness' and strive, usually unsuccessfully, to diet. The wish to be thinner lies at the root of eating disorders, and may manifest itself as anorexia nervosa (a retreat from pubertal growth itself). It may otherwise spill over into bulimia nervosa, or the smothering protective inertia of obesity.

At the heart of anorexia nervosa is the search for security; the sense of relief from panic and its origins. It is not a new disorder. It may have arisen as long ago as neolithic times as the pubescent girl, subject to endless pregnancies and early death, may have associated such growth with food and sought relief through abstention from it. The ancient ascetics may also have suffered it beneath their defiant facades, as may some hunger protesters. Some of those attracted to dance, gymnastics, or athletics may likewise have this hidden tendency. Byron may have had it, being able to concentrate creatively only when secure within it. For the majority, starvation demands that thoughts of food alone occupy the mind.

Anorexia nervosa is the most severe of the mental illnesses, having a potential mortality of around 20% by the age of 40. Chronic sufferers may develop severe physical, social, and psychological handicaps. Suicide is common. Natural remission occurs in perhaps two-fifths of those with the fully fledged condition. The assessment and treatment processes described below can increase recovery to 70% at 5-year follow-up and reduce mortality to 4% at 20 years. The first task for the clinician trying to help the sufferer from anorexia nervosa is diagnostic; the syndrome and the underlying concerns about body shape may be self-evident or hedged round with denial. The maturational problem is the most important issue, often denied and requiring special skill to identify. Current family battles over food and eating are secondary and not greatly informative. Trust and skill are crucial for a favorable outcome. As many as 50 hour-long psychotherapy contact sessions with the sufferer and family may be needed, coupled with support and occasional hospital admission at times of crisis.

Bulimia nervosa is a severe eating disorder occurring at normal or above normal body weight, driven by the need to binge eat in the face of a powerful aversion to perceived fatness. Vomiting, and laxative and diuretic abuse are the core features, together with the binge eating and the associated distress (low self-esteem). Behavioral programs to mute the ingestive abnormalities, coupled with psychotherapy, are the preferred therapeutic approach, rendered easier by the greater degree of motivation to achieve change. Again predominantly a female disorder in the

(*continued*)

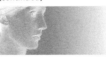

Sir Morell **MACKENZIE** (1837–92). British laryngologist, Mackenzie was appointed physician to the London Hospital in 1873. He developed an interest in diseases of the throat and retired in 1876 to found the Throat Hospital in Golden Square. He became expert in the use of the newly devised laryngoscope and acquired a large practice in laryngology. In 1887 he was called to Berlin to see Crown Prince (later Emperor) Frederick III. On the basis of a negative biopsy he declared that he did not have laryngeal cancer. This view was opposed by the German surgeons; events proved Mackenzie wrong and he defended himself in undignified pamphlets which earned the censure of the Royal College of Surgeons.

### EBERS PAPYRUS

The best preserved of the four principal medical papyri in existence (the others being known as the Berlin, the Hearst, and the EDWIN SMITH papyri). It was found between the legs of a mummy in a tomb near Luxor, advertised for sale, and acquired by Professor Ebers in 1872. The papyrus (dated about 1550 BC) describes the elaborate pharmacopoeia possessed by the ancient Egyptians, listing such preparations as pills, pastilles, snuffs, gargles, inhalations, ointments, poultices, bandages, suppositories, and enemata.

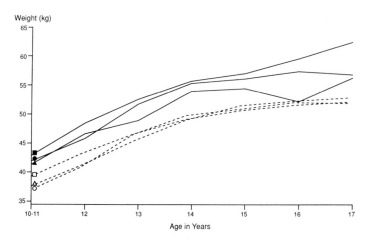

Weight (kg)

Age in Years

A study of 2000 schoolgirls in London 1972 (△), in London 1988/90 (○), and 800 schoolgirls in Ottawa, Canada, 1990 (□). The girls' actual mean body weights (—) vary in the three populations, especially in the mid to late teens (note especially the dip at age 16 in the 1972 London population, suggesting that low body weight eating disorders were more prevalent at the time). In contrast, the preferred mean body weights (----) of these three populations were remarkably similar. This unchanging view of desirable body weight/shape suggests that powerful biological forces underlie it, which may relate to the pubertal process and the ambivalence which many teenage females have long felt towards it. (Reproduced courtesy of the *Postgraduate Medical Journal*.)

clinic, it remains speculative how akin was debauched Roman feasting or is the Friday night male syndrome of binge drinking and vomiting. People with bulimia nervosa, who also have a propensity to develop avoidant reactions to strain, may slip into alternating episodes of anorexia nervosa and bulimia nervosa. Thus Byron, when unable to sustain the anorectic avoidant posture, would find himself propelled into bulimia nervosa. At such times his despair and self-loathing were paramount.

True bulimia nervosa, especially in its more multi-impulse ridden form, may be more common these days. It erupted in the clinical arena in the 1970s. At that time, social structures and boundaries were dissolving (the 1968 student revolts were symptomatic) and apparent new 'freedoms' such as the availability of the contraceptive pill and the acceptability of the drug culture arrived. 'Fashion', often implicated causally in the eating disorders, is surely more a mirror of such cultural changes than the driving force. Meanwhile, whereas anorexia nervosa reflects the penultimate biological solution to existential turmoil, bulimia nervosa reflects a default of self-regulation while remaining engaged in the chaos of such turmoil. The self-reinforcing avoidant position of anorexia nervosa is the most dangerous. Ten years later those with bulimia nervosa have more often naturally recovered. Emerging coping skills and constructive life events within the ongoing fiery furnace of biological maturity have facilitated maturation and sufficient self-regulation to get by. The number of chronic cases and related deaths are significantly less than in anorexia nervosa.

It is as easy to underestimate the suffering generated by these psychopathologically driven body weight and shape disorders as it is to overlook their true underlying psychopathology, so often denied — at least by the anorectic. One opts instead to call the syndrome an 'eating disorder',

as one might mistakenly diagnose and label pneumonia or lung cancer a 'cough'. AHCri

**ECOLOGY** See GLOBAL ENVIRONMENTAL CHANGE

**EDUCATION — HISTORY** The history of medical education is that of healing and of some exceptional personalities, who taught by example, and whose cumulative legacy continues in the modern medical profession. In ancient Mesopotamian cultures illness was a punishment inflicted by malevolent deities, and exorcist remedies were found in places of worship and the functions of their priest-doctors. Learning medicine was part of a religious process, with faith and belief as the foundations of power and influence over health. Among the Sumerian gods Nabu was the deity of science, including medicine, and the temple erected to honor him contained a medical school. The development of systems of cuneiform writing on clay tablets in Sumeria around 3000 BC was crucial to record and transmit knowledge of human biology, illness, and forms of treatment. Access to the accrued knowledge and skills was protected by the practitioners, who determined who could become a doctor, and their preferred transmission of skills was to their own children. The priest-doctors of the temples attended to the rulers and nobility, with a secondary class of healers, the barbers, performing surgery, including the branding of slaves. Their rules of conduct derived from religious ritual, and these became established as codes of practice.

The medical traditions of Mesopotamian cultures were reiterated and developed further in Egyptian, Greek, Hebrew, early Christian, and Islamic societies. By 1500 BC there were complex documents, such as the EBERS PAPYRUS that resemble modern medical texts. Egyptian doctors were instructed by the papyri how to examine a patient, seek physical signs of specific maladies, treat, and prognosticate.

Magic, prayers, incantations, and supernaturalism were essential to medical practice for many centuries, until the addition of scientific reasoning that followed emergence of Greek philosophy in the 7th century BC. Observation, measurement, and thought based on experience characterize the writings in the 70 books that are attributed to HIPPOCRATES (p 382). Some of his works appear as pithy teaching directed at students of medicine, as in the Aphorisms — for example, 'Spinal deformity often co-exists with cough and tubercle of the lungs'. Many centuries later, GALEN (p 324) contributed numerous works in anatomy and physiology that complemented the clinical writings of Hippocrates among the foundations of medical learning in Europe for over 1000 years.

Greek works were translated into Hebrew and Arab languages by Christian sectarians driven from the Byzantine Empire. By the 8th century, hospitals, libraries, and medical schools had been developed by Islamic cultures. A hospital built in Baghdad in the reign of Al-Rashid (786–809) contained a major medical school.

Arab culture spread as far as Sicily and Spain and influenced the early medieval centers of medical learning in SALERNO (p 448) and MONT-PELLIER (p 319). Salerno was of particular importance as one the first secular schools of medicine, including women as students and teachers, something not seen again in Europe for another seven centuries. Other great universities were established in the Middle Ages — Paris (1110), BOLOGNA (1113) (p 447), Oxford (1167), and PADUA (1222) (p 447); these centers combined libraries of medical texts, scholars, and international repute. The language of teaching was Latin, the universal language of the educated people of Europe, and this allowed students from many countries to converse.

The association of medicine and religion had continued throughout the Middle Ages, with medical libraries being lodged in monasteries. Cathedral schools of medicine existed, for example, at Chartres, around AD 1000. The Christian hospitals arose as philanthropic institutions, caring for the old, the homeless, and the disabled. They acquired medical roles from the early part of the second AD millennium. Notable among these was the Holy Christ Hospital in the university city of Montpellier, a model that spread across Europe. In later years, the management of the religious hospitals changed hands from religious orders to municipal administrations.

In the Renaissance there was rapid growth of population and of conurbations, setting the stage for the physical proximity and later affiliation of universities and hospitals. It also saw the collectivism of practitioners, as in the establishment in Britain of the first of what became medical and surgical royal colleges, when the barbers and surgeons of Edinburgh were granted a charter in 1505.

### Diffusion of university-based education

Some of the new European universities of the 16th century were particularly important in the rise of university-based medical education — notably, LEIDEN (p 257), Edinburgh, Koenigsburg, and Dublin. Teaching methods began to improve. Montanus of Padua introduced bedside teaching in 1545, an idea that was carried to Leiden by a Dutch doctor, Heurne. Hermann BOERHAAVE (p 121) of Leiden was a seminal figure in the history of medical education, a physician who combined theory, clinical practice, and bedside teaching in a sequential curriculum. His fame as a

teacher spread across Europe, and among his many international pupils were founders of the important medical schools of Edinburgh and Vienna.

British medical education in the 17th and 18th centuries was centered on Oxford, Cambridge, and Edinburgh. The last was founded in 1583, and its chair of medicine established in 1685, with the involvement of the Royal College of Physicians of Edinburgh, by Robert Sibbald, who had studied in Leiden. It was staffed by others who had also studied at Leiden, including MANRO (p 41), Rutherford, and Whytt.

The Edinburgh medical school was the most productive in Europe for several decades, and attracted many Americans who later established their own medical schools — Shippen and Morgan (who established the College of Philadelphia curriculum in 1765) and Benjamin RUSH (p 726) (whose work established medical education at the University of Pennsylvania). At Edinburgh the language of instruction was English, rather than Latin, and the degree of Doctor of Medicine was granted after attendance for three terms of lectures and submission of an acceptable thesis. Oxford and Cambridge required a BA degree for admission, attendance for three years of lectures in Latin, after which a Bachelor's degree in medicine was granted. Their degree of Doctor of

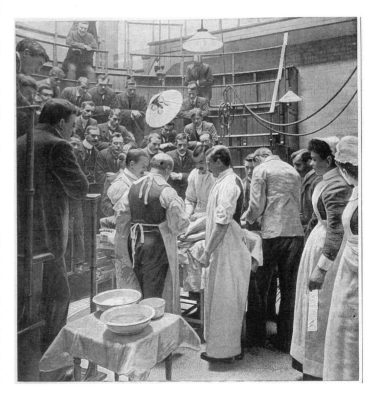

An operation at Charing Cross Hospital, London, in 1900, watched by students and colleagues. (Reproduced courtesy of the Mary Evans Picture Library.)

Medicine required seven further years' practice, presentation of a thesis, and examinations.

### Teaching hospitals and private medical schools

The Royal Infirmary of Edinburgh was established in 1738 and was a resource for the medical school. Although the Radcliffe Infirmary (1770) and Addenbrooke's Hospital (1776) were established in Oxford and Cambridge, respectively, the two universities did not take advantage of the clinical environment to give practical education in medicine, as was then happening in so many other European university centers.

Hospitals in London became increasingly important as medical schools during the 18th century, and their number trebled with establishment of the Westminster, Guy's, the London, and Middlesex hospitals. The wards were walked by medical and surgical apprentices as well as independent fee-paying pupils. A dissecting room for the study of anatomy was built at St Thomas' Hospital in 1730, where also many Cambridge students were taught clinical medicine by Richard Mead. In 1783, at the London Hospital, William Blizzard proposed a full range of medical lectures to accompany walking the wards. He persuaded the hospital to build a lecture theatre and this venture was later described as England's first medical school of university type. Students attended for courses in medicine, surgery, and other subjects. On being given a certificate of attendance or proficiency, they presented themselves at Cambridge or another university for an MD degree.

Private medical schools flourished in England and several other European countries. In 1767 William HUNTER (p 88) organized a private school in Great Windmill Street, London, with an auditorium, library, several dissecting rooms, and a museum. Similar endeavors arose in provincial cities, sometimes in hospitals and sometimes in private houses close to the hospitals. Teaching of medicine as a private enterprise also existed in France before the Revolution, with lectures in Paris and Strasbourg being delivered by university professors wishing to augment their income.

Private medical education was the norm in the USA by the early 19th century. The commercial medical schools took as many applicants as possible, offered little or no clinical instruction, and graduated their students without examination. In 1830 most American doctors had served an apprenticeship of variable duration but had not attended any organized lectures. By 1830 there were also rural medical schools, perhaps half of all the schools, giving craft training to rustic youths. All of these schools were legally empowered to grant medical degrees that exempted the holders from the majority of state licensing examinations.

The historical legacy of some older universities continued into the 19th century. For example, entry to Oxford and Cambridge required affirmation of the Articles of Faith of the Church of England. Seeking to have a medical school to which they could send their children, non-conformists established a school at the North London Dispensary. Later this school migrated to University College Hospital, which was associated with the University of London, established in 1827.

### State regulation of practice and education

State involvement or control of medical education had been present in the Middle-Eastern city-states of ancient times. By the time of the Chinese T'ang dynasty (598–907) medical institutions and medical schools were supervised by the state. In Japan, there was state interest in medical education under the Taiko code of AD 702 that required the construction of a university with a medical school in the capital city and a medical college in each province. In Europe it was not until the 19th century that the proliferation of medical schools created pressure towards greater regulation and social control of the production and safety of doctors. The regulatory environment in Britain was haphazard, with medical and surgical qualifications being granted by universities, the Royal Colleges, or other colleges and teaching hospitals. A reform movement sought better regulation of entry to the practice of medicine and the London Society of Apothecaries led the way, empowered by The Apothecaries Act of 1815. The Apothecaries required apprenticeship to a general practitioner for five years, attendance at lectures, and success in a written examination (oral examinations had prevailed in universities since the Middle Ages). The Apothecaries Act had also rendered Scottish degrees invalid in England. After much further debate the Medical Act of 1858 created the General Medical Council, under the Privy Council, and required registration of all medical practitioners, whether apothecaries, surgeons, physicians, or combinations or these. It abolished regional licenses, and required minimum criteria for medical licensure that would be valid throughout Britain.

### Clinical methods and laboratory science

The content of the medical education changed most rapidly in the 19th century. The early part added diagnostic clinical methods, the middle saw the introduction of routine laboratory tests, and the end had ROENTGEN's (p 873) discovery of X-rays. Percussion and auscultation were refined and promulgated as clinical methods in medical schools. Teaching of physical diagnosis became a more important and respected part of medical education and, at the turn of the century, William

OSLER (p 602) wrote of the need for a systematic approach. 'Physical diagnosis is to be learned only be experience; 'tis not an inheritance; it cannot be revealed. Learn to see, learn to hear, learn to feel, learn to smell, and know that by practice alone you can become expert'.

During the second half of the 19th century, there were spectacular advances in medical sciences achieved through research methods, consolidating the importance of the universities as both repositories of medical learning and the cradle of new knowledge. In Britain, medical research was generally a minor academic activity of practicing doctors. In Germany the approach was more committed to full-time research scientists in universities and teaching hospitals. Several new scientific journals were established by these German workers, who understood the academic value of publication.

American doctors began to look towards Germany rather than Britain for their model of medical education. The JOHNS HOPKINS UNIVERSITY (p 840) medical school in Baltimore was inaugurated in 1893, with its four major founding figures in medicine and surgery — Osler (p 602), HALSTED (p 746), Kelly, and Welch, creating a thoughtful new pattern of education. Their four-year curriculum minimized the importance of didactic lectures, promoted active independent learning, and in the later years combined scientific and clinical teaching, with students serving as supervised clerks and dressers. Welch had studied in Germany with Ludwig and Cohnheim, and cherished research and scholarship. Later he was an advisor to the ROCKEFELLER FOUNDATION, established in 1901, that soon turned its attention and its financial resources towards the faltering health of American medical education. In 1910 it sponsored Abraham FLEXNER'S (p 258) highly influential study of medical schools in the USA, and his epic report that embraced the German-inspired Johns Hopkins model. In England, Haldane chaired a parliamentary Royal Commission on university education, commencing in 1909, at which both Flexner and Osler testified on medical education. Osler had by then moved from Baltimore to the Regius Chair of Medicine at Oxford — he said to the commission 'we need an invasion of the hospitals by the universities'. RL

*See also* APOTHECARIES; FOUNDATIONS; PROFESSIONAL REGULATION

**EDUCATION** During the 20th century the dominant drivers of change in medical education were the rapid advances in biological sciences and the socio-economic pressures from the structural needs of publicly funded or corporate health services. These influences led to great changes in medical education and in the educational environment.

Medical schools admitted more students, and many more women. Medicine remained a highly favored career; most medical schools had more applicants than they could accept. In the competitive selection process, all medical schools sought students with high academic ability, able to grasp the scientific complexities of medicine. Other traits of character and achievement were also sought, derived from contemporary judgement of the qualities thought to be desirable in future doctors. In most European schools admission was in the late teen years, after completion of secondary education; North American medical schools developed as graduate schools, requiring a first university degree in a science or a discipline related to healthcare.

How many students should be admitted to medical schools was the subject of much debate. The advent of publicly funded or communal healthcare systems and advances in medical knowledge were followed by increased demands for more medical services, and hence for more doctors. Planning for the required number of doctors was confounded by many variables, including the long period of time necessary to train them, varying estimates of the needs for generalists *vis à vis* specialists, and migration of trained doctors. Some British doctors, for example, emigrated to other English-speaking countries, to be replaced by graduates from the Indian subcontinent and later from other countries of the European Union. The increased number of women doctors also affected the popularity of some pathways of postgraduate training, as fewer women wish to enter the major acute specialties such as orthopedic surgery.

In response to growing public expectations, additional medical schools were established in several countries in the 1960s and 1970s. Medical immigration was another reason for establishing new schools in some countries that wanted to become self-sufficient in producing their own doctors. Such new medical schools were often located in centers of rapid population growth or in young universities where new ideas in medical

STUDENTS OF EDUCATION

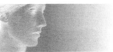

Simon **FLEXNER** (1863–1964). American microbiologist and research institute administrator. Flexner studied microbiology and pathology under W.H. Welch at JOHNS HOPKINS (p 840). While serving on a special commission in the Philippines he discovered a strain of dysentery bacillus which was long known by his name. He served briefly as professor of pathology at the University of Pennsylvania, and then accepted appointment as the first director of the newly formed Rockefeller Institute in New York City, a post which he retained until 1935. There he attracted a group of able biomedical investigators, and provided conditions for them to work effectively. His fame rests chiefly on his superb talent as dirctor of a research institute.

*(continued overleaf)*

## LEIDEN

Leiden owes its pre-eminence in the history of medical education to three factors: an early emphasis on clinical teaching, the acceptance of students of any religious denomination, and two inspired teachers — Franciscus Sylvius and Hermann BOERHAAVE (p 121). Clinical teaching was started in about 1636, with two wards in the Caecelia Gasthuis, a charitable institution, being chosen to house six male and six female

patients who were demonstrated at lectures. Starting to lecture in 1701, Boerhaave was appointed professor in 1714, being the most influential teacher in Europe until his death in 1738. In particular, Leiden's liberal and modern practices were copied elsewhere, as at Edinburgh, where from 1741 students themselves took the initiative in ensuring that the study of patients was integral to their training.

(continued)

Abraham **FLEXNER**
(1866–1959). Flexner had no
formal training in medicine,
but prepared himself for a
career in education at JOHNS
HOPKINS UNIVERSITY,
Baltimore (p 840), then
founded a private boys'
school in Louisville, Kentucky.
This became highly sucessful,
but he gave it up and went
abroad in 1905 to study
psychology. While in
Germany he wrote a small
book that was highly critical
of American colleges and
contrasted them unfavorably
with the German universities.
This book attracted the
attention of Henry S. Pritchett
of the Carnegie Foundation
for the Advancement of
Teaching, and he persuaded
Flexner, in 1908, to undertake
a study of medical education
in North America. The
resulting *Flexner report* was
published in 1910. In 1930 he
published another book,
*Universities,* and partly
because of this he was invited
to become the first director of
the Princeton University
Institute for Advanced Study.
See *also* ACADEMIC
MEDICINE

education were a means to create an institutional identity. New schools could innovate and experiment in education in a manner that was often difficult in the conservative environment of long-established institutions. Such was the case in schools such as Southampton and Dundee in the United Kingdom; Maastricht in the Netherlands; Southern Illinois and New Mexico in the United States; Newcastle and Flinders in Australia; and McMaster and Calgary in Canada. Other new medical schools were established, not to increase the overall number of doctors, but to produce doctors to serve in remote or sparsely populated rural areas — for example, in Tromsö in Northern Norway and in West Virginia in the United States. The social aspects of medicine were emphasized in a new medical school in Michigan called the College of Human Medicine.

## Changed environment

The environment in which medical education took place changed. Initially it was more centralized in universities and teaching hospitals, later becoming less centralized. The marriage of medicine and universities flourished throughout the century, usually in large urban teaching hospitals. There was enthusiasm to seek new medical knowledge through research in the university setting, then to be applied as rapidly as possible in the nearby teaching hospital. In the United States, medical schools had varied greatly in their capacity to provide scientific education, until the report and recommendations of Abraham FLEXNER (this page) in 1910 for the Carnegie Foundation for Advancement of Teaching. With this background medical curricula in Europe and North America increasingly emphasized a solid scientific foundation as a prerequisite for clinical education. Later, in the final decades of the century, there was concern that large tertiary care teaching hospitals with their complex technology and highly specialized services were not the most appropriate environment for teaching medical students, most of whom would eventually practice primary care. Concern about educational context, as well as the increased numbers of students, brought about greater use of district general hospitals and smaller community clinics as teaching venues. General practice and primary care flourished into a major academic discipline, giving balance to the predominance of teaching by hospital specialists that was the norm until the 1960s.

## Evolution

Medical curricula evolved throughout the century. The traditional sequence was a departmentalized curriculum in which basic sciences preceded clinical education. Development was usually piecemeal, in the sense of each department being responsible for its own segment of the curriculum. The number of science departments that were contributory to medicine expanded; anatomy, physiology, and pathology were joined by bacteriology, biochemistry, pharmacology, and others. As science advanced, the volume of knowledge to be memorized by a student became vast and unmanageable, and was sometimes resented for apparent lack of relevance to clinical practice. This problem was often dealt with by altering the sequence and organization of the curriculum, requiring a shift in administrative philosophy from departmental planning to a non-departmentalized or interdisciplinary approach. Not having the burden of tradition, it was opportune for the new medical schools to accomplish this and to become leaders in innovative curricular design. Reorganization of the existing pre-clinical curriculum into functional body system units, such as the cardiovascular system, allowed earlier introduction of clinical content so that, for example, the clinical features of peptic ulcer disease could be taught with the anatomy, physiology, and pharmacology of the gastrointestinal system. A related strategy was that of building a small multi-discipline course around a common symptom or clinical presentation such as headache.

Expansion of medical education in the second half of the century helped to generate diversity in educational methods. Teaching of facts by lectures was regarded as passive, inefficient, and less enduring than actively stimulating students to seek knowledge. The stimulus to learn could be created as a problem to be solved in the informal setting of a small group of students where the teacher gives guidance instead of direction. This pattern of cooperative small group learning was adopted in medical education some years after it had been used in primary schools. The logistics of medical education in the setting of problem-based learning are more elaborate and more expensive in use of staff time than the traditional didactic lecture. Most teachers in medical schools had been educated in the conventional manner, and it was often necessary to have them instructed in the value and conduct of small group teaching.

Clinical competence, the academic goal of medical education, comprises a trinity of scientific knowledge, professional attitudes, and clinical skills. In the medical curriculum, acquisition of knowledge was the most straightforward to plan. Professional attitudes were demonstrated by example or by role modeling of clinical teachers in their practice, as had happened from the time of HIPPOCRATES (p 382). This remained the preferred method to instill professional values and humane behavior, although medical BIOETHICS became a small formal part of some medical curricula. It was realized that teaching of the third element, clinical skills, was often haphazard and unpredictable in the less structured clinical part of the curriculum. During clinical attachments, the role of the doctor in communicating with patients, performing physical or mental examination, and guiding patients was to be observed and emulated by students. However, the extent of what could be learned would depend on which patients were available in clinics or hospital wards at the time. Students would see the work of experienced clinicians, but conversely it was uncommon for a student to be directly observed and coached by the clinical teacher.

## New methods

Several new methods were developed for learning and examinations, such as use of videotape recording for teaching and assessing communication skills. This would allow students to review their performance with an expert, and sometimes see themselves as they might appear to the patient. The recording could be with an actual patient or with an actor trained to give a standardized portrayal of an illness. Medical skills' laboratories were developed, comprising consultation rooms equipped for videotaping, models, or manikins to learn procedures such as pelvic examination, actors to work as standardized patients, and sometimes real patients with stable chronic illnesses. Thus clinical skills could be taught and examined in conditions not subject to the service needs of teaching hospitals or to the happenstance of which patients had been admitted on a particular day. The concept was similar to the flight simulator used in training and periodic re-assessment of aircraft pilots — techniques could be taught, practiced, and tested without endangering the safety or dignity of sick patients.

Two forward-looking authoritative reports strongly advocated reform of medical education — *Physicians for the twenty-first century: general professional education of the physician*, published in 1984 by the Association of American Medical Colleges, and *Tomorrow's doctors*, published by the British General Medical Council in 1993. Both reports were critical of traditional medical curricula and proposed adopting many of the curricular innovations pioneered in the new medical schools. Their recommendations included fewer lecturers, less didacticism, encouraging independent self-directed learning, small group learning, and teaching of communication skills. The two reports stimulated curricular reform in long-established medical schools. Often the key to institutional change is recognition that there must be reasonable limits to the content of the medical curriculum, that there must be the will sometimes to discard material honored only by time, and

that the quality of learning may be more important than the quantity.

General aspects of medical education were influenced by external criticism from patients, health economists, and government health departments (and also commercial health maintenance organizations in the United States). Deficiencies in the performance of doctors were often attributed to what 'should have been taught in the medical school', with consequent pressure for change. The most frequent cause of complaints against doctors was that of poor communication with patients, giving impetus to improved instruction in those skills. More difficult were the cost-constraints of health services in many countries, and the recognition that discretionary treatment decisions by doctors had profound economic implications. Departments of public health in medical schools became more actively involved in the epidemiology, biostatistics, and economics of healthcare analysis. Students were expected to have some knowledge of the comparative efficacy and costs of different interventions, and EVIDENCE-BASED MEDICINE was advocated as a new approach. It had long been taught that each clinical problem could be solved from basic principles through intellectual analysis and personal experience, and management grounded in a rational scientific method would follow. Now teaching was to emphasize evidence derived from published experience of many similar patients, proved by scientific trial methods and supported by critical appraisal of medical literature.

Education itself became an academic discipline in some medical schools, and the scientific thinking that university staff were accustomed to use in their research was applied to their role as teachers. Medical education was sometimes seen as a process in which changes in curricula were designed as experiments in which the outcomes should be assessed. Experts in educational psychology were appointed to medical schools, especially in North America, with the intent of better understanding the mental processes of medical experts, then to purify the best methods and to use the principles to enhance the production of good doctors. This alchemy-like approach turned out to be too simple. Much effort was expended to analyze diagnostic methods and medical problem-solving ability, with the perhaps predictable conclusion that the processes vary according to medical experience and specialty, and from illness to illness. Hypothetico-deductive clinical reasoning, with collection of facts, induction and testing of hypotheses, and recursive analysis, was used as the basis of teaching problem-solving skills in medical schools. It was found that expert doctors often used short cuts in

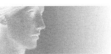
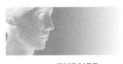

this complex process, using clinical pattern recognition and learned illness scripts, which require more experience of medical practice than is to be expected of a junior medical student.

The involvement of educational psychologists in medical education enhanced the analysis and refinement of examinations. Essays and oral clinical tests were found to be inconsistent, with the examiner sometimes being a major variable in the results rather than the candidate's ability. Examinations with good statistical reliability were seen to be fair to candidates and useful in giving feedback about the effectiveness of teaching. Multiple choice examinations became popular. Their clinical analog was the multiple station examination, in which each candidate would be watched performing a series of clinical skills tasks and be assessed by a pre-determined check-list of required functions. The medical skills laboratories were of particular value in these clinical examinations, with their resources of standardized patients.

Interest in the outcomes of different patterns of medical school education also increased. Outcome could be assessed in simple quantitative measures of number of doctors produced, the practice careers that they chose, and their location or type of medical practice. Qualitative outcomes were more difficult to evaluate, particularly in attempting to demonstrate differences in the skills or career success of graduates of traditional and new curricula. The changes in curricula had been stimulated by criticism from outside the medical profession and opinions from within rather than being based on firm evidence of comparative effectiveness.

### Measuring outcomes

Conclusive evidence of general superiority of the new forms of medical education was elusive. This was to be expected, given the complexity of medical education. Measuring comparative outcomes of medical care provided by the graduates of different types of program is extremely difficult, given the heterogeneity of illness in patients and the many variables in postgraduate education. Variation in performance of graduates of different types of curricula might be related to different policies in medical school admission, and some students might select their school because of its curriculum. After a quarter of a century of innovation and experimentation in medical education there was no evidence that the graduates of medical schools with new curricula were less able doctors than their colleagues from other schools. Follow-up studies suggested that the graduates of innovative medical curricula eventually were more satisfied and less critical of their education than the graduates of traditional curricula.

The growth and proliferation of specialization also changed the structure of the medical profession. Accordingly, medical schools and universities diversified from producing undifferentiated graduates to specialized postgraduate medical education and continuing medical education. A medical degree, once the starting point of an independent professional career, evolved into a milestone on a journey into further medical education and training. Career paths were often chosen as the result of formative experience in medical school. Many medical schools introduced unstructured periods into the curriculum, during which students could elect to gain experience in disciplines or countries of their own choice, and broaden their concepts of different types of medical practice.

During the final decade of the century there were rapid and extraordinary advances in electronic information technology. The storage and retrieval of clinical information could be automated and accelerated, and medical knowledge could be accessed via the internet from almost any point of the globe. Electronic editions of medical journals became instantly available and allowed rapid searching that previously would have taken hours or days. The efficiency of learning and the application of the evidence-based approach would be enhanced by the new technology. Of particular interest were the potential implications of the electronic repositories of medical knowledge, hitherto acquired through arduous study, and of great value to the practice of medicine, being in the public domain.

At the end of a century of evolution and change the scope of medical education had grown enormously. Society's expectations of the skills and humanity required of the medical graduate remained much the same as they have been down the ages. Most doctors still considered it a privilege and pleasure to teach their younger colleagues and support the education of future members of the profession.     RL

*See also* COMMUNICATION; PROFESSIONAL REGULATION; SPECIALIZATION

Paul **EHRLICH** (1854–1915). German hematologist, immunologist, and pharmacologist. Born in Upper Silesia, Ehrlich studied at the Universities of Strasbourg, Breslau, and Leipzig, from where he was awarded his medical degree in 1878. He then worked as clinical assistant at the University of Berlin, becoming head physicain at the CHARITÉ (p 354) and then professor. In 1886, suspecting he had pulmonary tuberculosis, he resigned from the hospital and spent two years resting in Egypt. He returned to Berlin three years later and in 1891 joined the new Institute for Infectious Diseases, to develop an antitoxin for diphtheria. By 1892, Ehrlich, with Emil von Behring, had produced the antitoxin, which in clinical trials achieved great success. In 1899, moving to direct the Institute for

## EDWIN SMITH PAPYRUS

One of the four principal medical papyri in existence (see EBERS PAPYRUS). It was discovered in 1862 at Thebes by Edwin Smith, an American Egyptologist, and bequeathed by him to the New York Academy of Medicine. It records 48 case histories classified according to the organ affected, and describes various injuries affecting men.

Experimental Therapy in Frankfurt, he continued to work on antibody formation. Using animals for experimentation he also investigated cancer, trypanosomiasis, and syphilis. Ehrlich used organic chemicals on a trial and error basis, determining their efficacy in destroying the pathogens. In this way he discovered the arsenical compound, salvarsan or 606, which he found to be effective against syphilis and trypanosomiasis, and it is for the development of this that he is best remembered. In 1908 he was awarded, jointly with Elie Metchinkoff, the NOBEL PRIZE for physiology or medicine for his work on serum therapy and immunity.

**ELEPHANT MAN** Joseph Merrick (1862–90) came to medical notice in Whitechapel, in the East End of London, when he was advertised to the public by a Victorian showman for display, as 'the great freak of nature' and 'half a man and half an elephant.' His story, told by Sir Frederick TREVES (this page) in *The Elephant Man and other reminiscences* (1923), made him a subject of perennial clinical, historical, and social fascination. As a young surgeon and some 40 years before he wrote his moving account, Treves befriended Merrick at a time when he had become destitute; he persuaded the authorities of The (now Royal) London

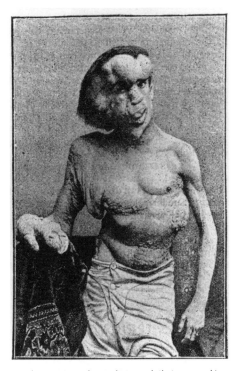

Joseph Carey Merrick in a photograph that appeared in the *British Medical Journal* on 19 April 1890. (Reproduced courtesy of the Wellcome Institute Library, London.)

Hospital to offer him a permanent home, where he was sheltered from public gaze and where kindly friendship and support were available. The explanation for Merrick's extensive deformities of bone and skin resulting in his grotesque appearance is still a subject of debate; most authorities think it was an atypical neurofibromatosis (multiple benign tumors of nerves), while others think that he showed features of a rare tissue disorder named Proteus syndrome in 1983.

The diagnostic enigma is, however, of little relevance in the context of Merrick's humanity, fortitude, and dignity, which underlie the pathos of his story. For centuries many unfortunate individuals with physical aberrations were displayed in shows and fairs to satisfy ghoulish curiosity. Ironically it was the belated discouragement of such displays that ended Merrick's precarious and demeaning career as an exhibit. The Elephant Man's story and its interpreters are considered in detail in two recent books: *The true history of the Elephant Man* by M. Howell and P. Ford, revised and illustrated edition, 1983; *Articulating the Elephant Man, Joseph Merrick and his interpreters* by P. W. Graham and F. H. Oehlschlaeger, 1992. In 1980 a film was made of the story.          DDG

**EMBLEMS** The most widely accepted emblem of medicine is a staff (or rod) with a snake entwined around it. In ancient Greece and Rome the staff and serpent were associated with the god of healing, ASCLEPIUS (Aesculapius, Asklepios) (p 721), the divine physician. In early statues of Asclepius the rod and serpent were represented separately. Epidauros, COS, and Cnidos were notable centers of the cult of Asclepius, where the priestly order of Asclepiadae practiced the healing arts, in which herbs and sacred serpents found application. The serpent, which sloughs its skin, was venerated as a creature of renewal and rebirth; the staff conveyed notions of resurrection and healing and was sometimes shown sprouting leaves. From being a classical attribute of Asclepius, the staff and serpent became the symbol of medicine.

The caduceus in Greek mythology was a herald's wand used by messengers of the gods, especially Hermes (Mercury). The caduceus bestowed health and prosperity and, by some accounts, its touch turned objects into gold. It was originally represented as a rod ending in two prongs twined into a knot; later the prongs were replaced by two serpents with heads that met at the top. Sometimes a pair of wings was attached to the top of the staff, signifying the fleetness of Hermes as a messenger. The caduceus came to be a token of peace, as well as a symbol of trade and prosperity. The association of the caduceus with medicine began in the Renaissance and probably stemmed from symbolism used in alchemy. From

**PATRON OF ELEPHANT MAN**

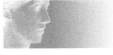

Sir Frederick **TREVES** (1853–1923). British surgeon. Treves trained at the London Hospital, to which he became surgeon. A renowned teacher of anatomy until 1893, served as consulting surgeon to the Army in the South African War (1899) and to the Royal Family, Treves operated on King Edward VII for acute appendicitis on 24 June 1902, which led to the coronation being postponed. He was the author of several textbooks as well as books of travel and *belles-lettres*. He was also the holder of a 'master mariner's ticket'.

# PHARMACOPOEA
## AMSTELREDAMENSIS,
### OF
## AMSTERDAMMER
## APOTHEEK,

In welke allerlei Medicamenten, tot
Amſterdam in 't gebruik zynde,
konſtiglyk bereid worden.

*Als ook*

Derzelver kragten en manier van Ingeven.

*Negende Druk, Vermeerdert en Verbetert.*

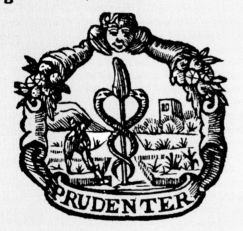

PRUDENTER

*t'AMSTERDAM,*

By GERRIT DE GROOT,
Boekverkoper op de Heilige Weg. 1736.

The title page of *Amsterdam pharmacopoeia* (9th edn, 1736) also shows the caduceus as a printer's vignette, with the staff taking the form of a spatula, whereby this sign became a pharmaceutical emblem.

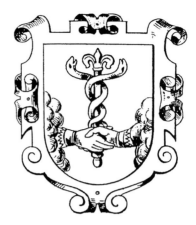

The caduceus, held by two clasped hands, appears on the title page of the first English book on tropical diseases, *The cures of the diseased in remote regions* by George Watson, published in London in 1598.

1516 a modified caduceus was printed in medical books published by Froben of Basel. Though the caduceus has long been accepted as a device to represent medicine, it is the staff and serpent of *Asklepios* which have the more ancient and authentic claim to be the emblem of medicine.

Purists lament substitution of the staff of Asclepius by the caduceus. Witty and learned essays occasionally appear in journals that care about the history and traditions of medicine, expounding on the provenance of the staff and serpent as the legitimate emblems of medicine, rich in the symbolism of healing and fertility. They disdainfully point out that Hermes was a cheat and a liar, so the caduceus signifies these unlovely qualities. It is an entertaining argument, but the caduceus (which was for a time the symbol of the British Medical Association as well as that of the US Army Medical Corps and many other medical organizations) is too firmly established in medical and lay minds to be displaced.

Many other emblems are associated with medicine and its institutions. The RED CROSS and the Maltese Cross of the Order of St John of Jerusalem have long been associated with first aid and emergency medical transport (the RED CRESCENT being a counterpart in Muslim countries); crosses of other colors are used by medical insurance agencies. Stylized logos, the wheelchair symbol for handicap, and initial letters such as H for hospital, have become ubiquitous symbols. Large hospitals often have a range of readily recognizable and memorable symbols intended to make it easy for patients to navigate their way

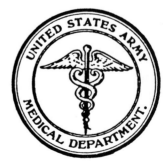

The caduceus of Mercury became the official insignia of the US Army Medical Department in 1902.

from the outpatient department to diagnostic services such as X-ray and hematology laboratories. Specialists' colleges and academies have armorial bearings, often taking part or all of these as an emblem on stationery, etc. — for example, the Royal Society of Medicine has a sprig of the herb all-heal that is reproduced on ties, scarves, and other articles that it sells to its Fellows.     DDG

**EMPIRICISM** was one of the post-Hippocratic schools of medical thought and practice. Unlike the Dogmatists, with whom they were coeval, the Empiricists rejected theory and based their system on observation and experiment. Symptomatology and therapeutics were the two major components of their approach, the latter being further subdivided into pharmacology, surgery, and dietetics. Despite the modern ring to this, empiricism later became synonymous with ignorance, unscientific thought, and quackery.

*See also* EPISTEMOLOGY

**ENCYCLOPEDIAS OF MEDICINE** Historical pride of place under this heading must go to the famous *Naturalis historica* of Pliny the Elder (AD 23–79) dealing with man and healing as well as other parts of natural science. Pliny claimed that it contained 20 000 facts culled from 200 authors. It was, moreover, an encyclopedia in the true and original sense, that is, a work arranged for systematic study rather than occasional reference, as are the alphabetical encyclopedias of today.

Although the feat has sometimes been attempted in the past (for example, *Cyclopaedia of practical medicine* (1834–5)), no modern work exists with full claim to the title, although several large and definitive TEXTBOOKS are available for such subdivisions of the whole as internal medicine, surgery, pediatrics, and so on, and some of the general English language encyclopedias (for instance, *Britannica, Chambers', Everyman*) give adequate coverage to most medical topics and major biographies. Perhaps closest come the important medical dictionaries (*Dorland, Black, Stedman, Taber, Butterworth, Blakiston, Wiley*) and the *British pharmaceutical codex*.

*See also* BOOKS AND LIBRARIES; TEXTBOOKS

**ENDOCRINOLOGY — HISTORY** In 1855, Claude BERNARD (p 102) discovered that glucose was synthesized in the liver and secreted into the portal vein. He described this secretion as 'internal', to distinguish it from bile, the 'external' secretion of the liver. The same year Thomas Addison described a syndrome caused by destruction of the adrenal glands, usually by TUBERCULOSIS, which was soon named 'Addison's disease'. Shortly after, Charles Édouard BROWN-SÉQUARD (p 708) found that the adrenals were essential to life.

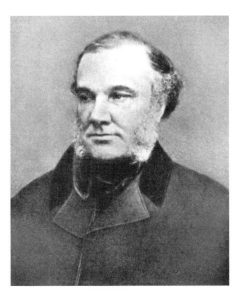
Thomas Addison (1795–1860)

Goiter and cretinism had long been attributed to iodine deficiency. In 1871 Hilton Fagge proposed that cretinism was due to congenital absence of the thyroid. In 1873, his colleague, William Gull, described an adult form, later named myxedema by William Ord. In 1883 Theodore Kocher found that total thyroidectomy caused 'cachexia strumipriva', which resembled cretinism in children and myxedema in adults. The same year Felix Semon proposed that all these states were associated with thyroid deficiency.

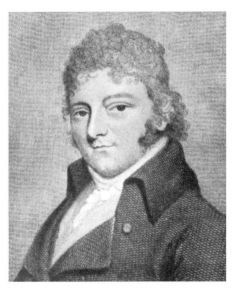
Caleb Hiller Parry (1755–1822).

**EARLY ENCYCLOPEDIST**

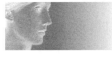

Peter Mark **ROGET** (1779–1869). Anglo-Swiss physician and savant. After serving as physician to Manchester Infirmary from 1805–8, Roget moved to London and became a lecturer at the Great Windmill Street School in 1809. He was physician to the Northern Dispensary and the Millbank penitentiary. Roget was one of the founders of London University and secretary of the Royal Society from 1827–48. He made many contributions to the *Encyclopaedia Britannica*, but his main claim to fame is his *Thesaurus of English words and phrases* (1852), of which there had been 76 impressions by 1983.

Soon total thyroidectomy in animals was found to cause tetany, which was often fatal, and myxedema in the survivors. The parathyroid glands, discovered by Ivar Sandström in 1880, were studied experimentally in the 1890s by Eugène Gley and others, and the acute effects of thyroidectomy were recognized as due to their simultaneous inadvertent removal. Tetany sometimes followed thyroidectomy in patients for the same reason.

Exophthalmic (toxic) goiter was described by Caleb Parry, and reported posthumously in 1825, and later by others. In 1884 Ludwig Rehn reported relief by thyroidectomy and proposed that thyroid overactivity caused the toxicity. Thyroid hyperplasia in this condition was described by Edward Greenfield in 1893.

In 1886 Pierre Marie described acromegaly, which he attributed to pituitary insufficiency. It was soon found that acromegaly and gigantism were often associated with pituitary tumors, and it was suggested that both were caused by excess of a pituitary growth factor.

In 1889 Brown-Séquard, then aged 72, claimed to have rejuvenated himself with injections of canine testicular extracts. This stimulated great interest in internal secretions. In 1893 he claimed that extracts from the testes and other tissues were beneficial in many serious diseases and that bovine testicular extracts were particularly effec-

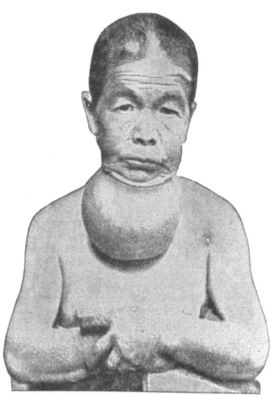

Goiter in a cretin. (From Rolleston, H. (1911). *The endocrine organs in health and disease*, OUP.)

tive. This 'alternative therapy' was accepted uncritically by many, and 'organotherapy' was exploited for 40 years. Clinical endocrinology, which began to emerge at this time, was unfortunately confused with it and achieved respectability only many years later.

In 1891 George Murray injected an extract of sheep's thyroid into a woman with myxedema. She recovered and in 1892, treatment by mouth proved equally effective. This was the first form of endocrine replacement therapy to be used.

At this time, it was suggested that Addison's disease, like hypothyroidism, resulted from deficiency of an internal secretion, and in 1893 George Oliver made an adrenal extract. He and Edward Schäfer found that it caused hypertension and stimulated the heart when injected into dogs. In 1897 the active constituent, named 'adrenaline' in Britain and 'epinephrine' in the United States, was prepared by John Abel and Albert Crawford. It arose from the adrenal medulla, which consists of nervous tissue, was identified as a catecholamine, and synthesized; but was ineffective in Addison's disease, which is caused by adrenocortical deficiency. It was the first product of a ductless gland to be characterized chemically.

## Hormones

In the 19th century the nervous system was thought to co-ordinate most bodily functions, and Bernard considered that it maintained 'la fixité du milieu intérieur'. Ivan PAVLOV (p 729) emphasized nervous reflexes, but at the end of the century internal secretions were also seen to contribute. In 1893, Gustave-Édouard Laguesse suggested that the islets of Langerhans in the pancreas produced an internal secretion, whose absence caused DIABETES MELLITUS. He described this secretion as 'endocrine' (Gk to secrete internally) to distinguish it from the 'exocrine' (Gk to secrete externally) digestive juices, secreted by the acinar cells into the pancreatic duct.

Schäfer, with Oliver, obtained a vasoactive extract from the pituitary. In 1895, he wrote that some glands (liver and pancreas) with ducts had internal and external secretions, while others (thyroid, adrenals, and pituitary) had internal secretions only.

In 1902 William Bayliss and Ernest Starling, found that acid in a denervated loop of jejunum caused secretion of pancreatic juice. An extract of jejunal mucosa injected intravenously acted similarly, but intravenous acid had no effect. These findings required the operation of a chemical, not a nervous, reflex, and Bayliss and Starling proposed the name 'secretin' for the hypothetical chemical messenger. They conceived it as a product of the intestinal mucosa, conveyed by the blood to the pancreas, where it stimulated exocrine secretion. In

1905 Starling proposed the name 'hormone' (Gk to excite) for such substances. Hormones, or chemical messengers, were produced in particular organs, passed into the blood, and influenced cell processes in distant organs.

## Normal form and function

Soon new hormones and their glands of origin were identified, and their properties and related clinical syndromes studied. The effects of castration in animals and men had been known since prehistoric times, being described by ARISTOTLE (p 64) in the 4th century, BC. The gonads were recognized as endocrine glands after 1910, when earlier work on the testes, which had been strangely overlooked, came to light. In the middle of the 18th century John HUNTER (p 398) had found that, after orchidectomy, the secondary sex characters of cockerels could be maintained by implanting their own testes. In 1849 Arnold Berthold had confirmed these findings and concluded that the testes acted through the blood. Comparable experiments on the ovaries after 1910 provided similar results.

Gastrin, which stimulates gastric acid secretion, was obtained from the stomach by John Edkins in 1905, while a renal extract, later named renin, was found to raise the blood pressure. The effects of adrenaline were similar to those of sympathetic nerve stimulation, and the post-ganglionic nerves were called 'adrenergic'. Then, in 1911, Walter Cannon described how the hormone adrenaline was secreted in response to anger and fear, and prepared the body for 'fight or flight'. Iodine proved essential to normal thyroid function, and a thyroid hormone, which controlled general metabolism, was purified in 1914. In the 1920s it was identified as tetraiodothyronine, synthesized, and named 'thyroxine' by Charles Harrington. In 1922, insulin extracted from the pancreas revolutionized the treatment of diabetes, and renewed interest in clinical endocrinology. The parathyroids were accepted as endocrine glands in the 1920s, when it was found that tetany, after parathyroidectomy, was accompanied by hypocalcemia, and that both were relieved by injection of parathyroid extract or calcium.

## Pituitary hormones

Apart from the pituitary and the adrenals, both of which had two parts, it was thought that each gland secreted only one hormone. However, events soon caused this view to change. Total removal of the pituitary gland in animals proved fatal, but subtotal removal caused atrophy of the thyroid, adrenal cortex, and gonads (its target glands). A general growth-promoting extract (growth hormone) was obtained from the anterior pituitary by Herbert Evans in 1921. In the next two decades this lobe was found to secrete several trophic peptide and protein hormones. Two regulated somatic growth and lactation, by growth hormone and prolactin, respectively. Others stimulated the target glands. In 1931 Langdon Brown described the anterior pituitary as 'the leader in the endocrine orchestra'. In 1928 the posterior lobe was found to contain vasopressin, an antidiuretic, and oxytocin, which stimulates the uterus and the breasts. The sex hormones, secreted by the gonads, control sexual development and reproduction, and in the 1930s were all identified as steroids, synthesized, and found to restore secondary sex characters in hypogonadism. The Leydig cells secrete an androgen, testosterone. Graafian follicles in the ovaries produce estradiol, an estrogen, and the corpus luteum secretes progesterone.

Adrenocortical extracts were obtained in the 1920s, and the active principle was named 'cortin'. In 1930 a more potent preparation maintained the lives of animals from which the adrenals had been removed and of patients with Addison's disease. The main function of these hormones, which are also steroids, was thought to be the control of electrolyte metabolism, and a weak mineralocorticoid, deoxycorticosterone, was extracted in the 1930s. The quest was led by Edward Kendall and by Tadeus Reichstein. In the 1940s, however, cortin was found to influence carbohydrate and protein metabolism; to have anti-inflammatory properties; and to protect the body from stress. In the late 1940s the potent glucocorticoids, cortisol and its analog cortisone, were extracted and synthesized. Cortisone was used clinically in 1948, and revolutionized the treatment of adrenal insufficiency and rheumatoid arthritis. A strong adrenal mineralocorticoid, aldosterone, was discovered by James Tait and Sylvia Simpson and by Reichstein in 1952–5.

In 1926 Cannon had coined the term 'homeostasis' to describe the process by which the body maintains its internal stability. The crucial role of hormones became apparent when, from the 1930s onwards, increasingly complex systems of negative feedback control were discovered. The role of the hypothalamus, the *conductor* of the endocrine orchestra, proved crucial. The study of metabolism in general was made easier by the use of radioisotopes, the first of which, radioiodine, was introduced in 1938 to investigate thyroid function.

Four important hormones had now been discovered, whose balanced actions controlled general metabolism. Insulin and cortisol are vital, while thyroxine and growth hormone are essential to health, but not to life. In 1952 a second thyroid hormone, triiodothyronine (the active form of thyroxine), was discovered. Many other hormones, working in concert, regulated particular physiological systems.

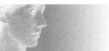
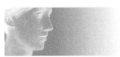

In 1953, two achievements boosted the study of endocrinology. First, Frederick Sanger analyzed insulin; and this was rapidly followed by the analysis and synthesis of other peptides and proteins. Second, James Watson and Francis Crick described the structure of DNA, and gave a great impetus to MOLECULAR BIOLOGY and GENETICS.

Hormones had long been measured by insensitive bioassays, but chemical methods were gradually introduced for thyroid hormones and for steroids. In 1959, Solomon Berson and Rosalyn Yalow invented a radio-immunoassay for insulin, which simplified and improved its measurement. From the 1960s similar assays were developed for other peptides, and proteins, and most hormones.

At the same time, the pancreas and gut were found to contain another diffuse neuroendocrine system, of which the islets of Langerhans and the chromaffin and other epithelial cells formed the principal part. About a dozen amines, peptides, and proteins were designated as hormones, although only insulin is vital. Some, including somatostatin, are also present in the central nervous system.

By the 1970s, newly discovered features of hormonal synthesis, storage, release, transport, and modes of action could be described in general terms. Some hormones were endocrine, in the original sense, some paracrine (acting locally), and some autocrine (self-regulatory) in their effects, and two main modes of action had been discovered. Some interact with receptors on the cell membanes, while others form complexes with receptors in the cytoplasm.

### Mechanisms of endocrine disease

Three main types of endocrine disorder were found — namely, hypofunction, hyperfunction, and dysfunction. All glands may be affected in at least one of these ways, and some in all three. Diseases of glands that secrete several hormones exhibit many complex combinations of features.

Hypofunction results from the failure of glands to secrete their normal products, as in Addison's disease. Hypopituitarism, due to compression of the pituitary by tumor, or an inadequate blood supply causing wasting away and reducing the function of its target glands, was described by Morris Simmonds in 1914. Iodine deficiency was confirmed as the principal cause of simple goiter in 1918 by David Marine. In 1939 Harold Sheehan found that maternal hemorrhage after birth was the commonest cause of pituitary infarct (death of part of organ due to failure of its blood supply). In 1956 Deborah Doniach and Ivan Roitt discovered autoimmune disease as a cause of thyroiditis, and later it was found to cause other endocrine diseases. In the 1950s and 1960s enzyme defects, due to INBORN ERRORS OF METABOLISM, were recog-

nized as causes of goitrous cretinism and adrenal virilism; and around 1960 abnormalities of the X and Y chromosomes were found to cause the syndromes of hypogonadism described by Henry Turner in 1938 and Harry Klinefelter in 1942.

Hyperfunction is excessive secretion of the normal products of glands by tumors or hyperplasia, as in hyperthyroidism, Cushing's syndrome, and hyperparathyroidism. Dysfunction results from hyperplastic or neoplastic lesions secreting hormones that are uncharacteristic of their cells of origin. For example, tumors or hyperplastic lesions of the adrenal cortex may secrete androgens, and bronchial tumors may produce vasopressin.

### Investigation of endocrine disease

Until the 1930s endocrine diseases were diagnosed mainly on clinical grounds and by non-specific qualitative analyses. X-rays had been used for the anatomical diagnosis of pituitary, thyroid, and adrenal disease since the 1900s. Measurement of the basal metabolic rate, developed in the 1910s, provided an index of thyroid function. In 1928 Selmar Ascheim and Bernhard Zondek developed a biological assay of urinary gonadotrophins for the diagnosis of pregnancy. Quantitative measurements and dynamic assessments of the effects of stimulation and inhibition of glands were introduced in the 1930s. Chemical measurement of hormones and their metabolites followed. These included thyroid hormones in the 1940s, and adrenal steroids and catecholamines in the 1950s. Radio-immunoassays were adopted for clinical purposes in the 1960s. Surgical exploration and biopsy of glands were used in the early days, but were largely abandoned, except for needle biopsy of the thyroid.

### Treatment of endocrine diseases

By 1900 natural products, surgical operations, drugs, and hormone replacement therapy had all been used effectively to treat thyroid disease. In 1907 radiotherapy for pituitary tumors followed. The discovery and synthesis of hormones and their analogs then led to reliable treatment of many deficiency states. The highlights were insulin (1922), sex hormones (1930s), cortisone (1948), and recombinant peptides (1980s). Transplantation of animal glands proved useless. Human grafts were tried also without benefit, except for pancreatic and islet cell transplants.

Treatment of hyperfunction requires surgical operations, radiotherapy, and drugs, alone or in various combinations. Surgery has always played an important part in the treatment of thyroid, pituitary, islet cell, gonadal, parathyroid, and adrenal lesions. Radioiodine was first used for thyroid diseases in 1942. Drugs which blocked the secretion of hormones, especially in the thyroid and the adrenal cortex, were developed later, as were other drugs, such as the adrenergic blocking agents, which antagonize the actions of hormones on the tissues.

Three endocrine diseases merit individual attention.

*Toxic goiter* Toxic goiter was named hyperthyroidism by Charles MAYO (p 841) in 1907. The goiter was usually diffuse, affected young adults, and was accompanied by nervous symptoms and abnormally rapid heart rate. In another form, described by Mayo's colleague, Henry Plummer, the patients were older, often had nodular goiters, did not have protruding eyes (exophthalmia), and suffered cardiac complications. Partial removal of the thyroid was the first effective form of treatment, but the mortality was high and recurrence was common. By 1910 Thomas Dunhill appreciated the need for subtotal removal, and obtained better results.

Iodine treatment had been used for toxic goiter, as for simple goiter, but with less benefit. However, in 1923 Plummer found that it greatly reduced the mortality if given preoperatively. Iodine, with subtotal thyroidectomy, became the standard treatment for twenty years.

In 1942 radioiodine treatment was introduced, and the next year antithyroid drugs were used effectively, either alone or as preparation for operation. Within a few years thyroidectomy, radioiodine, and antithyroid drugs were all used and reduced the mortality of the treated disease almost to zero. Later a beta-adrenergic blocking drug was found to relieve some acute features of hyperthyroidism very rapidly.

In 1956 a pathological long-acting thyroid stimulator was found in the blood of thyrotoxic patients by Duncan Adams and Herbert Purves.

*Hyperparathyroidism* In 1891 Friedrich von Recklinghausen reported a condition of osteitis fibrosa cystica, known by his name. Features included high urinary and blood levels of calcium, renal stones, and muscular weakness. Parathyroid adenomas were later recognized, but were thought to result from the bone disease, not to cause it. In 1925, however, Felix Mandl removed an adenoma from such a patient, with rapid relief, confirming that it was due to hyperparathyroidism. The disease had been diagnosed only in patients with bone disease until 1932, when Fuller ALBRIGHT (p 265) began to find hyperparathyroidism in patients with renal stones only. For over thirty years many cases were found in this way, but the disease was regarded as rare. Most patients responded well to operation, but some died later from kidney failure and HYPERTENSION. In the 1960s routine screening for serum calcium often revealed high levels, and many patients with early disease were recognized and treated, with good results. By 1965 it was estimated that one in every thousand members of the population in the USA had hyperparathyroidism. Usually only one of the four parathyroid glands is diseased. Preoperative localization of the lesion has been attempted, but experienced surgeons identify them best and cure most patients with one operation.

*Cushing's syndrome* In 1912 Harvey CUSHING (p 537) described a case of 'polyglandular syndrome' and, in 1932, reported other similar patients, many of whom had basophil pituitary tumors and bilateral adrenal hyperplasia. He proposed the name 'pituitary basophilism' for this condition, which soon, however, became known as 'Cushing's disease'. The role of the pituitary was uncertain, but it was suggested that the basophil adenoma secreted an excess of corticotrophin. Pituitary irradiation was sometimes effective, but half the patients died within five years. In the 1940s treatment by partial adrenalectomy was attempted, but the patients died from adrenocortical failure. In 1948, however, after the identification of cortisone, it was used effectively for the treatment of adrenal insufficiency, and James Priestley undertook radical adrenalectomy, under cortisone cover, with good results. Some patients with adrenocortical tumors had the clinical features of Cushing's disease, and those with benign lesions were cured by their removal. Overdosage with cortisone caused the features of Cushing's disease, and the term Cushing's syndrome was applied to all such patients, whatever the cause. The role of the pituitary remained unclear until about 1960, when it was found that all the patients with Cushing's disease had tumors, often microadenomas, secreting corticotrophin, which could then be measured. In the 1960s and 1970s pituitary micro-surgery was developed, and most patients were treated effectively by removal of the gland.

### Contraception

CONTRACEPTION using hormones was achieved with some success in animals in Austria in the 1920s, and then forgotten. In the 1950s Gregory Pincus pursued the matter and, by 1957, managed to suppress ovulation in women for as long as desired, with oral synthetic estrogens and progestogens. The process was reversible. Within a decade 'the pill' was used effectively, in various forms, by millions of healthy women, world-wide, to prevent pregnancy.                    RBW

**ENDOCRINOLOGY** is the study of the regulation and function of the endocrine glands and the action of hormones secreted by them. The word 'endocrine' derives from the Greek and was

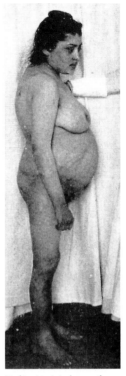

Cushing's original case of pituitary basophilism. (From Cushing, H.(1912) *The pituitary body and its disorders*, J. B. Lippincott Company, London.)

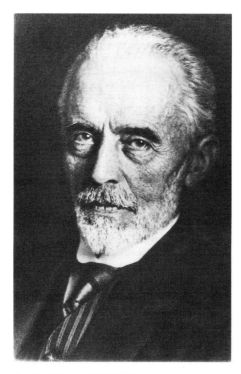

Theodor E. Kocher (1841–1917).

first used in 1913 to describe glands which secrete substances into the blood, unlike the 'exocrine' glands, which release their products through a duct. The concept of 'internal secretion' had been developed earlier and the term 'hormone' for 'chemical messengers or effectors' was introduced in 1905. The major endocrine glands — pituitary, thyroid, parathyroids, gonads, and adrenal — each produce one or more unique hormones, whose synthesis, structure, and mode of action have been largely defined. The boundaries of endocrinology, however, have been greatly extended with the discovery that many organs and tissues other than the specialized glands also secrete their own hormone. For example, the kidney secretes erythropoietin, which promotes the production of red cells, and the left atrium of the heart releases atrial natriuretic factor, which increases excretion of sodium by the kidney. Some widely dispersed tissues also produce hormones which may have a specific target: for example, fat secretes leptin, which acts on the hypothalamus to reduce appetite. Tissues may also release hormones and growth factors, which may be 'autocrine' (self-regulatory) or 'paracrine' (regulating processes in cells adjacent to the producer cells). Most common endocrine diseases are a result of either hormone deficiency or excess due to gland failure or overactivity, respectively.

Hormones may be divided into two categories — namely, 'peptides' (small proteins), or chemical messengers such as 'steroids' (derivatives of cholesterol) and thyroxine. All are synthesized in specialized cells, where they are stored until released in a controlled fashion. Hormones may have a single target organ or may affect many different tissues. Peptide hormones do not enter their target cells but bind to specific receptors on the cell surface; this binding leads to receptor activation and initiation of complex signaling pathways, often culminating in modulation of gene activity. In contrast, steroid hormones and thyroxine enter cells and bind to intracellular receptor proteins with the resulting complex interacting directly with DNA to regulate target gene function.

Hormone secretion is closely regulated. At its simplest there may be a direct connection between the end product and regulator (for example, parathyroid hormone acts to increase the concentration of calcium in the blood, but in turn its secretion is inhibited by calcium and normally an equilibrium is maintained). The most complex hormonal regulatory systems are integrated by the hypothalamus in the brain, acting via the pituitary gland, to control the function of the thyroid, adrenals, and gonads. Both the size and hormone output of the latter glands are determined by individual hormones (thyroid-stimulating hormone, adrenocorticotrophic hormone; the gonadotrophin luteinizing hormone and follicle-stimulating hormone), produced by distinct cells in the anterior pituitary. The hypothalamus regulates the secretion of the pituitary hormones by producing its own stimulatory or inhibitory hormones, which it releases into small blood vessels linking it directly to the anterior pituitary. The hormones of the thyroid, adrenals, and gonads act to inhibit the production of regulatory factors at both the hypothalamus and pituitary. The whole operates as a negative feedback control system, but the hypothalamus is also able to impose rhythmicity (for example, circadian or ovulatory cycles in women) and to integrate environmental influences with the control system.

### The hypothalamus and pituitary

The hypothalamus is not only an important regulatory center but produces a range of small peptide-releasing and release-inhibiting hormones, which control the anterior pituitary. Two hormones, arginine vasopressin and oxytocin, are made in the hypothalamus and are transported through nerve fibers to the posterior pituitary, where they are stored until released. Arginine vasopressin acts on the kidney to conserve water; its release is evoked by thirst and may be induced by falls in blood pressure. Oxytocin is released during childbirth, when it causes uterine contraction, and by suckling, when it causes milk ejection.

Tumors and other destructive lesions of the hypothalamus can cause a variety of endocrine disorders, mostly because of secondary failure of anterior and posterior pituitary function. Arginine vasopressin deficiency results in production of large volumes of urine, a condition known as diabetes insipidus, and is treated with a synthetic analog of this peptide.

The pituitary gland is divided into two anatomically distinct parts, anterior and posterior. The gland is anatomically and functionally connected to the hypothalamus of the brain. Another important anatomical relation is to the optic chiasm, which lies immediately above; tumors of the pituitary gland expanding upwards may cause visual-field defects. The posterior pituitary is an outgrowth of the hypothalamus. The anterior pituitary comprises different cell types which produce six peptide hormones: follicle-stimulating, gonadotrophin luteinizing, thyroid-stimulating, and adrenocorticotrophic hormones as well as growth hormone and prolactin.

Growth hormone induces production of another peptide, insulin-like growth factor I, from the liver, and both are essential for growth. Growth hormone secretion is enhanced by hypothalamic growth hormone-releasing hormone, but the hypothalamus also produces a hormone (somatostatin) which inhibits secretion of growth hormone. Growth hormone deficiency is a rare cause of growth failure; it is most often due to inability to produce growth hormone-releasing hormone, sometimes due to a hypothalamic tumor or a failure of pituitary growth hormone synthesis. Growth hormone deficiency is treated by injections of genetically engineered synthetic growth hormone. Excess production of growth hormone and insulin-like growth factor I before puberty results in gigantism, and, after puberty, in acromegaly. Patients with acromegaly characteristically have coarse features, large hands and feet, thick greasy skin, and enlargement of the internal organs. Gigantism and acromegaly are due to benign tumors of growth hormone-producing cells; the treatment is surgical, although drugs and radiotherapy may ameliorate the condition.

Prolactin promotes lactation. It has no known function in men or in women other than in the puerperium. The regulation of prolactin synthesis is unusual in that its secretion is usually suppressed by the hypothalamus; therefore, while hypothalamic disease results in general pituitary failure, it is associated with an increase in prolactin output. Increased prolactin secretion may cause inappropriate lactation (galactorrhea) and may interfere with the regulation of gonadotrophin luteinizing and follicle-stimulating hormone secretion, producing amenorrhea and infertility in women and decreased libido in men. Small prolactin-secreting tumors are common in women and may be treated with drugs or surgery.

Adrenocorticotrophic hormone, which regulates the adrenal cortex, is a peptide of 37 amino acids cleaved out of a larger precursor peptide, part of which also affects the pigment cells of the skin. Thus over-production may be associated with abnormal pigmentation, whereas suppression results in a failure to tan on exposure to sunlight. Over-production of adrenocorticotrophic hormone by small pituitary tumors stimulates the adrenal cortex, leading to excess secretion of steroid hormones and is one cause of Cushing's syndrome (see below). Treatment is by surgery, radiotherapy, or drugs. Adrenocorticotrophic hormone deficiency is usually part of general pituitary failure and is treated by giving adrenal steroids.

The gonadotrophins, luteinizing, follicle-stimulating, and thyroid-stimulating hormones are structurally similar. Pituitary tumors secreting thyroid-stimulating hormone and causing thyrotoxicosis are very rare. Tumors secreting fragments of gonadotrophins are not uncommon but are usually 'functionless', not being associated with distinct hormonal syndromes, although they may enlarge to cause visual abnormalities or pituitary failure (hypopituitarism) through compression of the optic chiasm or pituitary gland, respectively.

Hypopituitarism is a partial or complete failure of pituitary endocrine functions manifested by primary failure of arginine vasopressin production or secondary failure of the thyroid, adrenals, and gonads. It may be caused by tumors arising in the pituitary or in surrounding structures or follow surgery or radiotherapy to tumors. Other causes of hypopituitarism are thrombosis of blood vessels connecting the hypothalamus and pituitary following post-partum hemorrhage (Sheehan's syndrome) and autoimmunity. Treatment of hypopituitarism aims at replacing hormone deficiencies. However, the need to correct growth hormone deficiency in adults with hypopituitarism is controversial.

### The thyroid gland

The thyroid gland lies in the neck across the front of the trachea. It produces the prohormone thyroxine and its active derivative triiodothyronine, which regulate the level of metabolic activity in many tissues. Thyroxine contains four atoms of the trace element iodine and necessarily the thyroid gland can capture and store iodide from the blood. Dietary deficiency of iodine results in a failure of thyroid hormone synthesis, with the consequent increase in thyroid-stimulating hormone leading to enlargement of the thyroid gland (goiter). Maternal iodine deficiency in pregnancy impairs brain development in the fetus, causing mental retardation (cretinism). World-wide, iodine deficiency is a major public health issue, with an estimated 200 million people affected.

Disorders of the thyroid gland are a common cause of endocrine dysfunction; they are more common in women than in men, and in England about 4% of women will develop a disorder of thyroid hormone production with 10% exhibiting an enlargement of the gland. In England such thyroid disease, often with goiter, is most commonly the result of an autoimmune process, with antibody-mediated tissue damage or alteration in function causing gland failure or overactivity. Elsewhere in Europe the development of thyroid nodules secondary to iodine deficiency is still common. Benign and malignant tumors of the thyroid are not rare. Any thyroid swelling is regarded as suspicious until its nature is defined, usually by obtaining cells by needle aspiration, after which some require excision. Most thyroid cancers are curable by surgery with or without adjunctive treatment with radioactive iodine.

Thyrotoxicosis is the clinical state induced by overproduction of thyroid hormones, resulting in increased metabolism in most tissues, while hypothyroidism is the converse situation. Thyrotoxicosis, which is often episodic, may be treated either with drugs to block hormone production or, if persistent, by destruction (with radioactive iodine) or removal of part of the gland (surgery). Hypothyroidism is simply treated with thyroxine, which is converted in peripheral tissues to the active triiodothyronine.

### The adrenal glands

The adrenal glands lie above each kidney and consist of two parts: an outer cortex and inner medulla. The adrenal cortex produces steroid hormones: cortisol, which affects carbohydrate and protein metabolism and reduces inflammation, and aldosterone, which controls sodium and potassium balance by regulating their excretion via the kidney. The size of the adrenals and cortisol secretion are both determined by adrenocorticotrophic hormone from the pituitary, whereas aldosterone secretion is independently regulated by the extra-pituitary renin-angiotensin hormone system. An excess exposure to cortisol causes Cushing's syndrome, characterized by obesity, plethoric moon-face, thin skin, muscle weakness, and fatigue. This picture is most often due to administration of large doses of steroids for non-endocrine disorders, but may result from adrenocorticotrophic-hormone producing tumors or tumors of the adrenal cortex. Overproduction of

aldosterone (Conn's syndrome) causes high blood pressure or weakness, and may be due to a tumor or over-development of the secreting cells. Treatment of these conditions is determined by definition of the cause. Destruction of the adrenal cortex (by autoimmunity, infection, or tumor deposits) causes Addison's disease, which is usually insidious in onset with non-specific symptoms of fatigue, anorexia, and weight loss, with skin pigmentation due to excess adrenocorticotrophic hormone synthesis. The disorder is treated by replacement therapy with synthetic steroids. The adrenal medulla is a specialized part of the autonomic nervous system and releases catecholamines (adrenaline and noradrenaline) in response to stress. Catecholamine-secreting tumors (pheochromocytoma) are a rare cause of hypertension or paroxysmal headaches and palpitations; most arise from the adrenal medulla.

### The gonads

The gonads, ovaries and testes, are endocrine glands producing sex steroid hormones as well as, respectively, ova and spermatozoa. The hormones, estrogen in the female and testosterone in the male, largely determine the physical and emotional changes at puberty and maintain the secondary sexual characteristics (such as breast development and body shape in women, and beard growth and musculature in men) and libido throughout adult life. The production of both is determined by the hypothalamic-pituitary system. Pulsatile release of gonadotrophin-releasing hormone from the hypothalamus regulates the differential secretion of luteinizing and follicle-stimulating hormones.

The ovulatory cycle in women reflects a complex sequence of hormonal events: at the outset follicle-stimulating hormone stimulation progressively increases estrogen production, initially from several but later from one dominant ovarian follicle; the latter grows rapidly towards mid-cycle, producing a further rise in estrogen which triggers a sudden surge in luteinizing hormone secretion which is followed, 36 hours later, by ovulation from the dominant follicle; the follicle then forms the corpus luteum which produces another steroid, progesterone, as well as estrogen; the corpus luteum has a limited life of 10 days, at the end of which progesterone and estrogen production fall, which is the signal for initiation of the next cycle. If the ovum is fertilized, the conceptus produces human chorionic gonadotrophin, a hormone similar in structure to luteinizing and follicle-stimulating hormones, which stimulates the corpus luteum, maintaining progesterone production necessary for the continuation of pregnancy. During the cycle estrogen and progesterone both prepare the uterus for implantation of the fertilized ovum; if this does not occur the late-cycle fall in these hormones results in spasm of the uterine blood vessels, shedding of the tissue lining the uterus, and menstruation. Infertility may be due to failure of any component in this pathway. Treatment of infertility in the woman requires precise definition of the cause. The modern practice of reproductive endocrinology often involves the hormonal manipulation of the cycle. The female menopause occurs when the supply of potential follicles is exhausted, with consequential fall in estrogen production.

In the adult male, testosterone is produced in the Leydig cells of the testis, under the stimulus of luteinizing hormone. The production of spermatozoa is controlled by testosterone and follicle-stimulating hormone, and is a continuing process.

In both men and women sexual development and fertility may be abnormal because of chromosomal abnormalities (commonly in a woman loss of an X chromosome, resulting in Turner's syndrome; or in a man the presence of an additional X chromosome, causing Klinefelter's syndrome), failure of embryonic gonadal development, and genetically determined resistance of tissues to gonadotrophins or sex steroids, or abnormal synthesis of these hormones. These various conditions, most of which are rare, may not be obvious at birth and may become apparent only because growth or puberty, or both, are delayed.

### The parathyroid glands

There are four parathyroid glands, which lie behind the thyroid. They produce parathyroid hormone, a peptide hormone which in conjunction with vitamin D acts to control the level of calcium in the blood. Parathyroid hormone releases calcium from bone and increases the retention of calcium by the kidney. The secretion of parathyroid hormone is inhibited by a rise in calcium in the blood. Vitamin D, although present in food, is mostly produced in the skin following exposure to sunlight, and is another steroid hormone. Dietary or skin vitamin D is inactive, but it is processed first in the liver and then in the kidney (under the influence of parathyroid hormone) to the active steroid, which increases calcium absorption from the intestine and is essential for normal bone formation. Lack of vitamin D causes rickets in children or softening of the bones (osteomalacia) in adults. Excess parathyroid hormone or vitamin D results in a rise in calcium in the blood, which may cause non-specific symptoms. Small parathyroid hormone-secreting tumors arising in one of the four parathyroid glands are not uncommon; they may be excised surgically.

### The endocrine pancreas

The endocrine pancreas comprises clusters of cells (islets of Langerhans) distributed throughout the exocrine gland. The islets comprise specialized cells producing the hormones insulin, glucagon, and somatostatin. The former two hormones are concerned with carbohydrate metabolism; insulin is discussed under DIABETES MELLITUS. Somatostatin is also found in the hypothalamus and is a representative of an expanding class of small peptide hormones involved in the regulation of gastrointestinal function, which also act as messenger substances in the nervous system. A further example is leptin, produced by fat cells, which regulates appetite by modulating hypothalamic levels of neuropeptide Y.

### Endocrine manifestations of cancer

Although hormones are generally produced by specialized cells, their genes are present in all tissues. Malignant transformation of a cell may result in the aberrant expression of such a gene and the unregulated production of a hormone from an unusual site. Syndromes of 'ectopic hormone production' are well recognized — for example, cancers of the lung producing either adrenocorticotrophic hormone or arginine vasopressin. The high blood calcium associated with some cancers may be due to the synthesis of a gene product, parathyroid hormone-related peptide, which is not normally expressed.     VKKC, RHim

*See also* DWARFISM; GIANTS; REJUVENATION

**ENVIRONMENT** See ENVIRONMENTAL MEDICINE; GLOBAL ENVIRONMENTAL CHANGE

**ENVIRONMENTAL MEDICINE** Environmental medicine is concerned with individual maladaptive responses to environmental substances manifesting as disease. Such responses may or may not be immunologically mediated, are characteristically chronic and cyclic, and may affect one or more organ systems, although multiple involvement is usual. Adverse responses may develop after prolonged or excessive environmental exposure; infection, physical, chemical, and emotional stresses are common triggers. Techniques of avoidance and neutralization of the responsible environmental stressors in air, food, and water form the basis of treatment.

This approach to the diagnosis and management of illness has generated much controversy. Terms such as 'food allergy' and 'food intolerance' are used differently by conventional allergists and environmental physicians. Some of the claims and cures promoted by environmental physicians are not supported by adequate evidence, but some of the criticisms levelled at environmental physicians seem to ignore the available evidence, and interested readers may have to form their own opinions.

Albert Rowe of Oakland, California, has been called 'the father of food allergy'. He made many contributions to ALLERGY in general and to food allergy in particular; his first publication on allergy appeared in 1922 and his last book in 1972. In 1928 he first described the diagnostic use of elimination diets.

Herbert Rinkel of Kansas City in the 1930s, described masked food sensitivity and how to use unmasked food reactions diagnostically. Later he also described the therapeutic use of rotation diets and the use of intradermal testing techniques.

In 1924, under pressure from European allergists and immunologists, the definition of allergy became restricted to immunological reactions between antigens and antibodies. From then allergists were divided into those who went along with the new definition, and those who took a broader view and continued to study non-immunological reactions.

There are important differences between food allergy and food intolerance. Environmental physicians define *food allergy* as an adverse response to food in which there is evidence of an abnormal immunological reaction mediated principally by the protein in the blood known as IgE. *Food intolerance* is a reproducible, unpleasant, and adverse reaction to specific foods, for which there is no complete immunological or biochemical explanation, and is not IgE-mediated. Food intolerance is not psychologically based and may be validated clinically; it forms the basis of environmental medicine's approach to dietary management.

Food intolerance does not follow a specific dietary pattern. While it is possible to show that conditions such as migraine, irritable bowel syndrome, and rheumatoid arthritis may respond to food avoidance, the exact foods will vary from individual to individual. Food intolerances are almost invariably multiple; usually there are one or two 'major' foods such as wheat or milk, and several 'minor' foods such as chocolate, tomatoes, potatoes, or onions. An environmentally oriented medical history differs from the standard medical history in several ways. The main complaint is minimized, in view of the many symptoms the illness produces. Medical events are recorded chronologically, instead of being divided into the present and past histories, because of the importance of preserving sequential events. Personal–environmental relationships are emphasized. The two factors involved are the individual susceptibility and the environmental challenges to which the person is reacting, which combine to cause a reaction. The medical history is interpreted in terms of specific adaptation in the presence of individual susceptibility.

The diagnostic methods specific to environmental medicine include:

- The elimination diet and challenge testing with food.

- Challenge testing with chemicals: after a period of avoidance, this may be performed using serial dilutions given under the tongue, or injected into the skin, or by inhalation of known concentrations. Placebos should be included when testing.

- Coca pulse test: was originally described by A. F. Coca (1942). Speeding or slowing of the pulse by over 10 beats per minute after eating a food or exposure to a chemical (after a period of avoidance) is taken as a positive response, indicating sensitivity to that particular food or chemical.

- Provocation-neutralization testing: entails the intradermal injection of small volumes of specific dilutions of foods, inhalants, or chemicals to which the patient may be sensitive. Double-blind, RANDOMIZED CONTROLLED TRIALS indicate that this technique may have real value in both diagnosis and treatment.

- Leukocytotoxic testing: live white blood cells are exposed to a range of foods and chemicals. The presence or absence of damage caused to these cells is an indicator of the presence of food and chemical sensitivities. The evidence for the value of this technique is, as yet, incomplete.

The value of environmental medicine in chronic illness will continue to be challenged until an evidence base emerges to underpin its concepts and claims. It is important for those who wish to criticize environmental medicine to look at the scientific literature that supports at least some of the claims made by those who espouse this approach.                                   GL

**EPIDEMIOLOGY — HISTORY** Epidemiology, as other natural and biomedical sciences, has developed throughout history. Empirical observations led to inferences, generalizable statements, and rational explanations of the observations. This sequence took about 2000 years, from classical Greece to post-Renaissance western Europe. The science expanded and flourished like other medical sciences in the late 17th century, and when it adopted logical reasoning and statistical methods, it reached early maturity in the late 19th century. Since then it has extended its reach into all the clinical disciplines that were undergoing proliferation and expansion at the same time.

The science began with the observations and inferences of physicians–priests of the Hippocratic school (5–4th centuries BCE). The Hippocratic text, *Epidemics*, was based on observations that must have been collated, perhaps counted, to provide a basis for generalizable statements — the foundation on which all science is based.

Epidemics, such as the PLAGUE described by Thucydides that struck Athens at the end of the first year of the Peloponnesian War (429 BCE), were terrifying natural disasters defying rational explanation. That plague and those described in the Old Testament were attributed to the wrath of God, the work of evil spirits, or other supernatural forces, but the concept of contagion may have been at least partly understood, because those societies shunned people with LEPROSY.

The numbers of victims of epidemics were seldom counted, although the Romans, and the Egyptians before them, did count the numbers of their people in censuses for tax-gathering and military purposes. The development of numerical methods was the next logical step in the advancing science of epidemiology.

In medieval and early Renaissance Europe, parish registers kept BILLS OF MORTALITY, a record of deaths with some facts about the mode of dying. These Bills of Mortality enabled John Graunt, a London haberdasher, amateur scientist, and Fellow of the Royal Society, to compile the first quantitative work on epidemiology and vital statistics, the *Natural and political observations … on the bills of mortality* (1662). Graunt showed the relationship of death to rural or urban residence and how it varied between males and females. He made the first analytic study of health-related events — namely, deaths due to plague and other causes. William PETTY (p 219) followed with *Political arithmetic* (1687), a basic work on demography, another essential source of information on the health of populations.

In the next 200 years, physicians and others in several European nations expanded the frontiers of understanding about the impact of disease, injury, and disability on groups of people. In Italy, Bernadino RAMAZZINI (p 583) wrote *De morbis artificium diatriba* (*On the diseases of workers*, 1700). Although he gave no numbers, this was simple descriptive epidemiology.

Thomas Bayes, an English clergyman who was fond of gambling, wrote an *Essay towards solving a problem in the doctrine of chance*, published posthumously in 1763. This work enunciated mathematical concepts that have proved crucial in the logical analysis of epidemiological data, especially in clinical epidemiology, where Bayes's theorem is applied to evidence to establish the likelihood of diagnoses being correct, an essential component in clinical reasoning and decision-making.

In France, Pierre-Charles-Alexandre LOUIS (p 780), a physician who was proficient in mathematics, began to make comparisons between groups of patients treated by bloodletting, which was then the orthodox treatment for many conditions, with other groups of patients treated by different regimens, showing that far from improving the outlook, bloodletting often made matters worse. Louis's main contribution was a series of observations and statistical analyses of groups of patients with TUBERCULOSIS, *Recherches anatomico-physiologiques sur la phthisie* (1825). This laid the foundations of statistical analysis that were soon developed further.

Louis attracted disciples from other countries, including William FARR (p 780) from London and Oliver Wendell Holmes from Boston, so that his statistical methods soon took root in Britain and in the United States. The stage was set for the next great leap forward in the emerging science of epidemiology — the marriage with statistical methods on which almost all further advances henceforth were dependent.

In the second half of the 19th century epidemiology advanced rapidly in England, mainly because of the work of two towering figures, John SNOW (p 48) and William Farr. John Snow accomplished much in his short life. He was a general practitioner in London, a pioneer anesthetist (he administered chloroform to Queen Victoria at the birth of two of her children), and an amateur epidemiologist. Using at first only logical reasoning, he proved that the CHOLERA epidemics ravaging Britain and western Europe could not be caused by a miasma emanating from rotting vegetation (the popular theory at the time) but must be due to a transmissible agent. In 1854 he studied an epidemic in London, and showed that it was caused by something in the drinking water from a particular pump in Broad Street, Soho. In a larger epidemic in South London he collected information about the sources of drinking water and related this to death rates, which were strikingly higher in households that obtained their water from the Southwark and Vauxhall water company, downstream in London, compared with the Lambeth company upstream, where the water was cleaner (see Table). Snow's work, *On the mode of communication of cholera* (1855), is as useful today as when it was published — it is a model of logic and epidemiology.

William Farr was appointed the Compiler of Abstracts in the office of the newly established

Cholera mortality in London, 9 July–5 August 1854

| Source of water | Houses supplied | No of deaths | Death rate per 10 000 |
|---|---|---|---|
| Southwark and Vauxhall | 40 046 | 286 | 71 |
| Lambeth | 26 107 | 14 | 5 |
| All others | 287 345 | 277 | 9 |

William **BUDD** (1811–80).
British physician and
epidemiologist. After five
years in practice with his
father he moved to Bristol in
1847, where he was
appointed physician to the
Bristol Royal Infirmary. He
established the method of
spread of typhoid fever by
studies in his own practice
and in 1866 showed that the
cholera epidemic in Bristol
could be controlled by
hygienic measures.

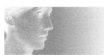

Major **GREENWOOD**
(1880–1949). British
epidemiologist. After
qualification Greenwood
studied under Karl PEARSON
(p 782). In 1917 he became
director of the division of
medical statistics in the newly
established Ministry of
Health and in 1928 the first
professor of epidemiology at
the London School of
Hygiene and Tropical
Medicine. He was one of
the pioneers in introducing
statistics to medicine and
published important works
on epidemics, infectious
diseases, and experimental
epidemiology.

Registrar General of England and Wales in 1839.
He occupied the position for over 40 years, and in
a series of beautifully written annual reports, he
described and commented upon many statistical
and epidemiological methods that have since
become standard. He was a member of the
London Epidemiological Society, a group of
doctors and others who read papers to one
another about the innovative work they were
doing to explain and control the great epidemic
diseases that afflicted the new industrial cities and
towns of 19th century Britain. Farr was a pioneer
in the detailed analysis of vital statistics as a rich
source of insights into the health of population
groups that could be distinguished from one
another, by the town in which they lived, their
occupation, and their living conditions. In collaboration with his Swiss friend Marc d'Espigne, Farr
developed the first comprehensive classification of
diseases and causes of death. The *International
statistical classification of diseases and related
health problems* (1991) is the 10th revision of the
system that began in the 1890s, based on the Farr–
d'Espigne classification. Farr's many other original contributions to the evolving science of epidemiology included development of the first
mathematical models to explain the natural
history of epidemics. His life's work was published in a posthumous collection, *Vital statistics*
(1885).

### Mathematical theories
In the late 19th and early 20th century, epidemiologists such as Stallybrass and Hamer were preoccupied with efforts to develop mathematical
theories to explain the spread of epidemic
diseases. Their concepts were consolidated by
Ronald ROSS (p 481), who identified the mosquito
responsible for transmitting MALARIA and created
a mathematical model of malaria epidemiology.
Such mathematical models have proved useful in
planning, conducting, and evaluating campaigns
to control malaria and other communicable diseases. This approach has gained new impetus
since the 1980s, with efforts to control the spread
of HIV infection.

Another approach was 'experimental epidemiology' which is associated with the name of
Major GREENWOOD (this page) and others. This
was based on observations of captive colonies of
rats, mice, or rabbits selectively exposed to infection, and clarified many uncertainties about the
relationship of infectivity to population size and
density, infectivity of the causal organism, development of resistance due to natural or artificially
acquired immunity — work that had obvious
applications in control of communicable diseases.
Greenwood was responsible for introducing
greater logical rigor into epidemiology at the

same time that the statistical methods of Ronald
Fisher were advancing biostatistics. Greenwood
also emphasized the importance of the host–
agent–environment nexus in communicable
disease epidemiology and control — a concept
that soon proved to be valid for non-communicable conditions too. Greenwood's work is
recorded in his many publications, particularly
*Epidemics and crowd diseases* (1933).

Until the mid–20th century, epidemiology was
preoccupied with infectious diseases, especially
those able to cause epidemics. By the end of
World War II, two new problems were challenging
epidemiologists. First, the pattern of disease was
shifting away from the era of infection. Methods
were needed to investigate possible causes of new
epidemics — coronary heart disease, cancer, and
traffic-related injury and death. Secondly, new
preventive and therapeutic regimens were being
discovered to deal with some ancient scourges;
it was necessary to find out as rapidly and reliably
as possible whether new and often expensive
antibiotics could cure tuberculosis, or if new vaccines could protect against poliomyelitis and
other dangerous infections.

Two innovations proceeded in parallel: the use
of large-scale RANDOMIZED CONTROLLED
TRIALS of new vaccines and drugs to treat tuberculosis and other serious diseases; and epidemiological studies to identify the causes of chronic
and non-infectious conditions such as cancer
and heart disease. In the third quarter of the
20th century, spectacular progress was made in
these uses of epidemiology. Randomized controlled trials, some with very large numbers of
subjects, proved the efficacy of streptomycin and
isoniazid to control tuberculosis, of polio and
other vaccines, of mood-altering drugs to treat
emotional disorders, and of many others. These
studies sensitized epidemiologists to the ethical
imperatives of human experimentation, especially to the need to respect human dignity and
autonomy.

Case-control and cohort studies, described in
the adjoining article, clarified the causes of some
important varieties of cancer. Everyone now
knows that cigarette smoking causes lung and
other cancers. This knowledge has come entirely
from epidemiological studies that have made the
word epidemiology familiar to all who read newspapers and watch television. Similar methods
have been used to identify risk factors for coronary heart disease, and to investigate a wide
range of other diseases whose causes had hitherto
remained mysterious. The development of record
linkage systems made possible the study of very
large numbers of people, millions rather than
hundreds or thousands, over prolonged periods,
decades rather than years.

## Role of computers

In the final quarter of the 20th century, these methods were refined and their analytic power considerably enhanced by COMPUTER-based methods of data-processing and analysis. A useful approach was to collect results from many studies carried out under closely similar circumstances, and to analyze the aggregate results, a procedure known as meta-analysis. Although this has some pitfalls if all studies are not closely comparable, it is a valuable way to add to the power of analysis, especially when it is desirable to identify the best way to treat conditions that are rare enough so that no single center can accumulate the many cases required to confer adequate statistical power.

During this period, epidemiology began to undergo the same process of specialization and fragmentation as other branches of science and medicine: pediatric, psychiatric, cardiovascular, and many other varieties of disease or body-system-oriented epidemiologists have appeared; other epidemiologists evaluate the working of health services, study traffic-related injury and death, study human behavior (such as smoking and risk taking), or make comparisons across cultural and national boundaries, seeking factors shared in common as well as differences that could explain the varying impact of disease and premature death: why, for instance, do Japanese women seldom get breast cancer compared with Swedish, Scottish, and American women, amongst whom it is common? Yet another variety of epidemiologist has come to the discipline with a background in statistics and mathematics, introducing advanced statistical reasoning and methods.

## Clinical epidemiology

Another important development is the rise of clinical epidemiology, which has flourished and indeed dominates population-based varieties of epidemiology in some places. Clinical epidemiology is the application of the methods of epidemiology in a clinical setting, to solve problems of patient care. This has introduced the methods and procedures of epidemiology to specialist clinicians, and, since these are the main teachers in medical schools, this has meant that young doctors emerge from medical school with understanding and insights that previous generations of doctors often lacked. The most important contribution of clinical epidemiology has been the concept of EVIDENCE-BASED MEDICINE, expounded in a book with this title by Sackett and others, published in 1996, and, sign of the times, available on-line on the World Wide Web. Closely related to this is the work of the Cochrane Collaboration — named in memory of the British epidemiologist A. L. ('Archie') COCHRANE (p 79)

— a world-wide network of collaborating centers that collect, review, and publish critical commentaries on clinical trials that are the essential evidence on which clinical decision-making is based. This has transformed clinical medicine from what was sometimes a rule of thumb approach based on opinions and received wisdom, into a more rational, logical process. If the essential compassion and human touch are retained, modern medical practice, enlightened by these epidemiological insights, can confer on sick people a better chance of smooth recovery from serious illness than would have been their lot in the days before this marriage of epidemiology to clinical medicine was consummated.

Computers and the internet have fostered other advances too. The INTERNET makes possible the instantaneous world-wide notification of a case of a disease of PUBLIC HEALTH importance such as plague, and — as in other aspects — facilitates discussions among epidemiologists all over the world, who can join open-ended internet-based discussion groups, thus becoming part of a true global community of scholars.                    JML

*See also* AUDIT; STATISTICS

**EPIDEMIOLOGY** Originally epidemiology meant the study of epidemics but nowadays it encompasses the study of all varieties of illness and injury as they affect defined groups of people. Epidemiologists seek to identify, count, measure, and control all diseases, injuries, and causes of premature death in relation to associated inherited and environmental factors. Epidemiology is the basic science of PUBLIC HEALTH. It is a particular way of thinking about diseases and their causes that is not merely quantitative or numerical but also rigorous, logical, and very well connected to other disciplines.

## Connections

Epidemiologists draw upon information and ideas from a wide range of sciences, technologies, crafts, and occupations. Some connections are obvious, for instance, with vital statistics, biostatistics, MICROBIOLOGY, and IMMUNOLOGY, and with all kinds of clinical medicine from pediatrics to geriatrics, from family practice to neurosurgery. Less obvious connections include the social and behavioral sciences, agricultural sciences and animal husbandry, natural sciences such as physics and chemistry, and topics as diverse as engineering and town planning, educational institutions, law enforcement agencies, communications technology and the media, and many more. Probably, no other branch of biomedical sciences has so many interconnections with such a diverse range of other human activities, and all of these connections are fruitful.

### Rates

The fundamental feature of epidemiology is comparison of groups of people. For the comparisons to be valid it is necessary to convert raw number to rates. A rate is a fraction: the numerator is the number of people affected by the condition of interest, and the denominator is the number of persons in the population 'at risk' of experiencing this condition. A multiplier is used to express the rate per thousand, hundred thousand, million, etc. Rates are also used to calculate the risk to individuals or groups of experiencing an event, such as the occurrence of cancer, a heart attack, or traffic injury. When rates are examined the epidemiologist can compare and contrast particular kinds of people whose environment or behavior differ from one another, or look for differences at specified times, or in defined places such as counties or cities. The observed differences are the basis for inferences about reasons, or are used to test hypotheses, for instance, about a putative cause of a particular type of cancer.

### Uses

The first use of epidemiology is to investigate epidemics. Studying trends over time enables us to determine whether the health of the population is improving or deteriorating, and in what ways. 'Community diagnosis' means assessing the nature and variety of health problems afflicting the population, such as addiction to tobacco, the prevalence of domestic violence, and the proportion of elderly people living alone in what were once family homes. Epidemiology can tell us if health services are working efficiently. Another application is assessing risks, for example, of smoking, being overweight, or working in certain industries or occupations. When attempting to assess the total impact on society of a common disease, it is important to identify all variations in the way it can present. For example, coronary heart disease may be threatened by the presence of precursors such as raised serum cholesterol concentration and enlarged left ventricle (of the heart) or it may be 'silent' and revealed only by an abnormal electrocardiogram, or by scars in the heart muscle detected at autopsy. Alternatively, it may present clinically as angina, a mild coronary thrombosis, or as an instantly fatal acute myocardial infarction (that is, an overwhelming heart attack).

Identifying syndromes, 'lumping and splitting', is discovering that seemingly different diseases are manifestations of the same disease, or that conditions which are seemingly all cases of the same disease are in reality due to different causes. For instance, TUBERCULOSIS and SYPHILIS may mimic many other diseases; and apparently identical cases of hepatitis may be caused by several kinds of viruses that invade the body in different ways and therefore require different kinds of control measures. The most valuable use for epidemiology is the search for causes of diseases and, related to this, ways to control them and evaluate control measures. Another use is evaluation of symptoms and signs: what is the probability that headache and impaired eyesight, backache and weakness in leg muscles, pain and tenderness in the lower right abdominal region, etc., are due to each of the most common known causes of these symptoms and signs? Clinical decision analysis, application of EVIDENCE-BASED MEDICINE, and development of clinical practice guidelines are the main uses of clinical epidemiology, discussed later.

### Methods

Epidemiological methods are observational, analytic, or experimental.

***Observational epidemiology*** begins with surveillance of populations, using many varieties of vital and health statistics — death rates, arranged by age, sex, locality or region, and cause of death; information on notification of infectious diseases of public health importance; information obtained from registries for diseases such as cancer; hospital discharge statistics; and imaginative use of many varieties of existing information about defined population groups. For example, schools and many employers keep records of absences due to illness, sometimes with information about the reasons for these absences; the police keep records of calls to settle domestic disturbances and damage caused by vandals, which are useful indicators of 'social pathology' such as local variations in the frequency of domestic violence, alcohol abuse, or broken families.

Inferences based on the observations of descriptive epidemiology may generate hypotheses that are then tested by analytic epidemiological study.

***Investigating epidemics*** An epidemic is the occurrence of numbers of cases of a disease clearly above normal expectations. Observational and analytic epidemiology blend in investigation of epidemics. The investigation requires scrupulous attention to detail in gathering information about all the cases of the condition, including mild and inconspicuous cases as well as those with florid manifestations, and must include information about associated factors such as diet, occupation, living conditions, and unusual recent experiences. Particular attention is paid to the 'index case', that is, the first identified case of the condition. In infectious disease epidemics this might be the one that introduced the infection into the affected community. Information is gathered about healthy people in the same community, aimed at discovering why they have not been affected. Laboratory tests are used to confirm the diagnosis, to identify the pathogenic organism, toxic chemical, or other noxious agent that caused it, and to measure immunological responses among both sick and healthy people. Analyzing all this information often clarifies the nature and cause of an epidemic, and points the way to control measures.

Investigation of epidemics may be tedious and painstaking, even a seemingly boring routine task; but more often it is as exciting as detective fiction. An epidemic of TYPHOID in 1965 in Aberdeen, Scotland, was traced ultimately to a contaminated tin of canned beef from Argentina that had been cooled in a river adjacent to the canning works; as the pressure inside the can fell when it cooled in the polluted river waters, the typhoid bacilli were sucked into the can through a minute hole. Techniques of molecular biology, notably DNA typing and identification of biomarkers, have enhanced the precision of epidemic investigation. It is possible to identify and trace exactly the passage of an infectious agent such as the gonococcus through a group of infected people, and to determine how certain cancer-causing agents actually induce cancers. Many books and articles in the popular press and in medical journals have been written about investigation of epidemics (such as Berton Roueché's stories in the *New Yorker*, collected in several anthologies).

***Epidemiological surveys*** Epidemiologists often study all the people, or a representative sample of them, in an entire community or country. The diverse aims of surveys include assessment of dietary intake and nutrition, dental health, vitamin deficiency states, physical fitness, prevalence of smoking, use of habit-forming drugs, respiratory function tests, evidence of anemia, high blood pressure, mental and emotional health, and many other ways in which the people of a community or country differ from one another. In the USA, national health surveys that cover these and other characteristics of the population have been conducted continuously since 1957. Information gathered in national surveys is used to plan and evaluate health services and has led to much further research in which possible reasons for observed differences are more thoroughly investigated.

***Analytic epidemiology — case-control studies*** Observant doctors who take careful medical histories from their patients have often been able to make connections between present disease and past exposure. Percivall Pott described cancer of the scrotum in 1775, observed that it occurred in chimney sweeps, and deduced its relationship to coal tar lodged many years earlier in the creases of the scrotal skin. Normal Gregg, an ophthalmologist in Sydney, Australia, saw many babies with congenital cataract in 1940 and recognized the connection to the epidemic of rubella that had affected their mothers in early pregnancy.

The case-control study is an extension of medical history taking, in which individuals, usually patients with the condition of interest (the cases) are compared with other people who resemble them in such respects as age and sex, but do not have the condition (the controls). The histories of exposure to suspected risk factors of persons in the two groups are compared and analyzed in search of statistically significant differences. Sometimes only small numbers of cases are needed to identify significant differences in the past history of exposure to specific risk factors, thus making the case-control study a particularly suitable way to search for causes of rare diseases. The discovery that a rare form of liver cancer was associated with occupational exposure to vinyl chloride required only four cases; the fact that expectant mothers' use of estrogens during pregnancy can cause cancer of the vagina many years later in their daughters was based initially on a case-control study of eight cases.

Case-control studies may be flawed, mainly because of biases that are often difficult or impossible to eliminate, but they are none the less a valuable method of investigation, because they can be carried out rapidly and at relatively little cost. The findings can be confirmed or refuted by more rigorous research methods.

***Analytic epidemiology — cohort studies*** A more powerful analytic method of epidemiological study is to identify individuals exposed to varying levels of risk in a large population, and observe over a period the rates at which they fall ill or die of the condition of interest, calculating the illness or death rates in relation to their levels of exposure to the risk factors of interest. This method requires study of large numbers, often many thousands of people, over a prolonged period, perhaps years or even decades. It is therefore expensive. Some cohort studies have become famous. Framingham, Massachusetts, is the setting for cohort studies of coronary heart disease that began in 1954 and have continued ever since. In 1951, Richard Doll and Austin Bradford HILL (p 381) began a cohort study of lung cancer in relation to smoking habits of British doctors; this too has continued, and is yielding valuable information on the risk of many other kinds of cancer and of coronary heart disease, as well as lung cancer, in relation to smoking.

It is possible to obtain results from a cohort study without waiting many years, if facts exist about varying levels of individual exposure to risk at some time in the past, and information about health or causes of death at the present time can be obtained for all members of the studied population. A record linkage system facilitates this approach.

*Record linkage* is the process of relating information in two or more sets of records, often collected years apart and sometimes by different agencies or organizations. A record linkage system immensely enhances the power of epidemiological studies to reveal details about the long-term relationships between causes and effects. The natural history of diseases varies from those where exposure to a disease agent has an immediate consequence, to others where the exposure may not lead to overt disease until decades later, or even not be expressed until the next generation. We have only recently begun to understand some of these subtle connections. For instance, infant development seems to be related to the occurrence of high blood pressure and heart disease many decades later; the nutritional status of girls and young women can influence the health risks in adult life of their progeny. The relationship of exposure of the developing fetus to diagnostic X-rays (very small doses of ionizing radiation) during early pregnancy, and the occurrence of childhood cancer, and abnormal development in childhood and adolescence, have been investigated in several cohort studies using record linkage, one of which used over three quarters of a million records of X-rays taken during pregnancy, in hospitals in the New England states. Such a study is expensive, but less so, and less time-consuming, than it would have been if it had begun with the original X-rays and followed the outcome among the liveborn offspring for the next 20–30 years. A necessary prerequisite for record linkage is a system for precise identification of individuals, such as a unique number for each individual, or the use of a phonetic method to identify names, accurate information about birth dates, birth place, etc. The preservation of old medical records is another necessity. Guardians of privacy who advocate the destruction of records once they have fulfilled the immediate purpose for which they were collected, have resisted development and use of record linkage systems. In the EUROPEAN UNION a draconian Directive was drafted that would have made record linkage studies impossible in any of the nations of Europe. Epidemiologists and others who use record linkage systems have the utmost respect for personal privacy and protection of confidentiality; they were able to demonstrate not only the immense benefits of record linkage but also that there has never been an instance of serious violation of confidentiality or of harm to individuals or communities as a consequence of personal information falling into unauthorized hands.

### Experimental epidemiology

In the early 20th century 'experimental epidemiology' meant observing the passage of infectious micro-organisms in colonies of experimental animals and the effects of interventions on the transmission of infection. Such experiments are rare now. Experiments in which the investigator studies the effects of intentionally altering one or more factors related to the course of a disease, are now commonly performed on humans rather than experimental animals, using a randomized controlled trial design.

### Clinical epidemiology

Epidemiological methods that were developed to study health problems in communities or large populations have been modified to suit clinical conditions, where they are applied to study small numbers or even individual patients. This approach is transforming patient care into a more logical and rigorous scientific process than it used to be. Clinical epidemiology is becoming the basic science of clinical medicine in the same way as classical epidemiology has long been the basic science of public health. Every aspect of the clinician's task — the diagnostic process, choice of treatment regimen, and predicting and evaluating outcomes — can be improved by the application of clinical epidemiology.

Two essential features of clinical epidemiology are clinical decision analysis and evidence-based medicine. Clinical decision analysis is a derivative of operations research and game theory that involves identifying all available choices and the potential outcomes of each, at every stage in the series of decisions that must be made about all aspects of patient care. For example, having diagnosed coronary heart disease the attending physician must decide whether this particular patient is more likely to benefit from surgical intervention or a medical regimen. The evidence needed to make this decision is contained in reports of randomized controlled trials; hence evidence-based medicine is an integral part of clinical epidemiology. The Cochrane Collaboration assembles and reviews the nature and quality of published evidence from randomized controlled trials on all aspects of patient care. This network has played an important part in making evidence-based medicine, and the epidemiological studies on which the evidence is based, the keystone of high quality medical care all over the world. This is the most important contribution that clinical epidemiology has made to clinical medicine.

JML

*See also* CLINICAL INVESTIGATION; RANDOMIZED CONTROLLED TRIALS; STATISTICS

**EPILEPSY** See NEUROLOGY

**EPISTEMOLOGY** Knowledge is a representation of facts and concepts organized for future use, problem solving, and understanding wider questions. Epistemology is the branch of philosophy concerned with the study of the theory of knowledge and how we come to recognize knowledge, its nature, scope, limits, and possibilities.

When we speak of 'medical knowledge' we imply that it is different conceptually from other knowledge. Most studies of knowledge are general, or are focused on a specific topic such as science, or a discipline, such as astronomy or physics. Medical knowledge is more complex, combining diverse aspects of knowledge which contribute to understanding the human condition and how it is altered by physical and emotional disorders. Thus medical knowledge takes knowledge from the sciences, the arts, the social sciences, and the humanities; studies of personal relationships; and studies of healers and healing. It also explores the way physicians use knowledge and concepts to solve problems within the very personal patient encounter.

Discussion of the epistemology of medicine tends to focus on one aspect, the scientific knowledge, as if medicine was a science, with less attention to the knowledge and skills applied to practice, decision-making, and the humanistic side of medicine. However, medicine is not a science: it is a caring profession that *uses* science as one aspect of the caring for patients. It also uses science to advance the understanding of illness and suffering. Medicine was caring for the sick thousands of years before science became a prominent aspect, so a discussion of knowledge in medicine must recognize a broader view.

Because medical knowledge comprises knowledge from many disciplines, a fundamental and coherent foundation of medical knowledge is difficult to enunciate, except for two key features: it is derived from many disciplines, and it incorporates the concept of critical thinking, testing of theories, and change. Knowledge in medicine is better understood by the *theory of coherence*, where belief and knowledge are based on other beliefs and knowledge, with coherent relationships that help explain each other. E. O. Wilson talks of *consilience*, or the 'jumping together' of knowledge and theories from different disciplines to create a common groundwork of explanation.

It has been easier for medicine to relate knowledge within the various sciences than it has been to link the sciences and the humanities, but that is the more important challenge. It is particularly important when all aspects are becoming increasingly specialized, posing greater difficulties for the easy sharing of ideas. The increased specialization, the narrower training of the specialists, and a reductionist focus in research has yielded much information and incredible discoveries, but it has

made it less likely that the larger philosophical aspects of the endeavor will be explored with the same intensity.

**Beginnings**

Medicine began as a *belief system*: beliefs ingrained in a society, with the expectation that they would have permanence. In even the most primitive communities there was an understanding why there were tragic events such as floods, famine, sickness, and death. Spirits or gods, sorcery, taboos, magic, or the influence of another person with powers might visit tragedy and suffering on a village or on an individual. The teachings of elders, passed from generation to generation, showed how to counteract, modify, or negotiate the influences of those powerful forces. Healers or shamans who used special magico-religious powers would be called on to modify the influence, negotiate with the spirit, or understand the nature and reason for the event. There was a concept of cause and a reasonable response, a therapy. As long as the tragic events were explained by a belief system, there was no need for change in those beliefs, and, indeed, any new ideas would be heresy, and the heretic punished or banished.

Healers might become *authorities*, and their words and their recommendations not only highly regarded by the society and by their students and followers but by later generations. HIPPOCRATES (p 382) and the Hippocratic writings of his school in Greece in the 4th century BC did not deny the role of gods in illness, but felt that observation of the afflicted could tell more about the nature, the progress, and the prognosis of a symptom or an illness and whether intervention would be successful. Various schools developed with different philosophies and approaches, but the role of authority, such as Hippocrates, gave credibility to a body of knowledge, and his views were accepted for the next 1500 years. Only centuries later would new authorities such as GALEN (p 324) and PARACELSUS (p 617) bring different viewpoints, but then their views would last for centuries if they were not challenged.

By the Middle Ages medical knowledge was a mixture of the recognized authorities, influences from the rising medical schools of SALERNO (p 448), BOLOGNA (p 447), MONTPELLIER (p 319), Paris, Oxford, and Cambridge, and writings from Jewish, Arab, and Chinese medicine, and from local folk medicine. The authorities for physicians of 1390 are well outlined in Chaucer's description of the Doctor of Physic, one of the pilgrims in *The Canterbury tales*. The Doctor was said to be well versed in the writings of Hippocrates, Rufus, Discorides, RHAZES (p 59), Hali, Galen, AVERROES (p 768), AVICENNA (p 60), Constantine, Bernard, and John of Gaddesden, showing a wide reading of authorities over a span of 1800 years.

Change as a feature of medical knowledge developed with the advent of the scientific method. The beginnings were slow. Francis Bacon (1561–1626), perhaps the most influential thinker of the Enlightenment, put aside the Greek approach to logic, philosophy, and classical learning and substituted inductive reasoning, which became the basis of the scientific method. He called for an observation of nature, gathering facts, and noting patterns. He accepted that creating new knowledge was a dynamic phenomenon continually refined and changed and growing. René Descartes attempted to find a unifying basis for knowledge by taking a skeptical view of any statement to find what could be free of question or doubt.

### Learning from experience
The philosopher John Locke (1632–1704), a physician by training and the first of the British Empiricists, believed that knowledge came from experience, and that such experience added more and more information towards a whole that could never be achieved, but is constantly sought. Locke felt that we are born with our minds a clean slate upon which experience writes. However, how we recognize that what we learn from experience is true might require intuition or experiment. What constitutes relevant experience constantly changes, and differs in various cultures and traditions. Relevant experience and how that experience is perceived vary if the physician is in Ayurvedic, Chinese, or western medical tradition, for instance. For many centuries the experience of physicians has been accorded high regard as a method of achieving and recognizing medical knowledge. Even today experience can hold a high place, sometimes even when there is some contrary evidence, or when others have a different experience and conclusion. Beginning the statement with 'In my experience...' still has great force. This high regard for experience as a basis for knowledge suffers little from the observation throughout the history of medicine that experience may be faulty, as with the centuries-old therapy of bloodletting, the heavy dosing with mercury, the routine removal of tonsils, and prolonged bed rest for myocardial infarction, childbirth, stroke, and acute back pain, to mention only a few. Even Hippocrates noted the problems of experience when he said of medicine, 'Life is short, the art long, opportunity fleeting, experience treacherous, judgement difficult'.

In medicine it is important to clarify what is based on belief, and what is based on substantial evidence. As far back as Plato there were debates on distinguishing belief from knowledge. Modern writers such as C. S. Peirce and Sir Karl Popper would argue that we cannot prove something to be true, but only to be false, and our confidence in the correctness of a theory is based on the ability of the theory to withstand criticism and rigorous testing. This also implies that every idea should be challenged, and our system of knowledge should be open to criticism, with the expectation that our concepts may be shown to be false, and replaced by better ideas and new theories.

Popper stated that science, and we would include medical science, grows, not by accumulating more and more evidence, but by posing more and more questions, analyzing problems and posing tentative solutions, conjectures, hypotheses, and through careful testing, analysis, and trials, eliminate errors. The vigorous testing of ideas and theories and the rejection of those found to be in error are how science and medicine advance.

### Paradigm shift
The historian of science, Thomas Kuhn, indicated that important shifts in our understanding might occur by the acceptance of some new concept, and this could be such a powerful change in our thinking, which he called a *paradigm shift*, that we would not see things the same afterwards. Later we would forget how powerful the old competing beliefs had been, and we might wonder how people could have believed those old views. Such shifts in thinking occurred in medical knowledge with the discovery of the circulation by William HARVEY (p 363) and the approach to diagnosis with the invention of the stethoscope by LAËNNEC (p 461). These may seem deceptively simple in retrospect, as we could all make the same observation in a few moments by manipulating the veins on our forearm with a finger, or rolling a sheet of

An important paradigm shift. Illustration from Harvey's *De motu cordis*. (Reproduced courtesy of the National Library of Medicine, Bethesda, MD.)

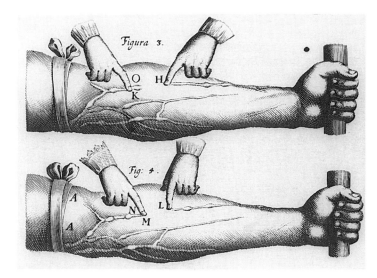

paper into a tube and using it to listen to someone's heart. However, these new ways of thinking changed how we saw the body and its function in health and disease. With a new understanding there was then a need to know more about the anatomy and physiology of the body to understand disease. Other important shifts occurred with the germ theory of the 19th century, and the concepts of the social determinants of health in the 20th century.

The expanding knowledge in medicine easily overwhelms the practitioner, so that methods of managing information are necessary. An early method of managing medical knowledge was to evolve systems of classification of disease, adopted from botany, and enthusiastically pursued in the 17th century. Crude as they may have been, often including symptoms as diseases, these classifications helped physicians place diseases in a structure, a framework, that helped organize approaches to treatment, at a time when ideas of diseases were complex and conflicting. Classification gave the impression of a systematic body of knowledge that gave medicine the status of a profession. Although the enthusiasm for classification has waned, it may be seen in any textbook, or in the DSM-4 classification of psychiatric disease. We also group seemingly disparate appearing diseases under umbrella concepts such as immunological disease, collagen vascular disease, myopathies, or vasculitis. Much effort is made in subdividing the various diseases and syndromes that come under these headings. The philosopher Kant was cynical about physicians becoming confident about naming and listing of diseases, however, and chided, 'Physicians think they do a lot for a patient when they give his disease a name'.

The experimental method, the hallmark of the sciences, formulated eloquently for medicine by Claude BERNARD (p 102) in the last century, was based on making a hypothesis and then designing an experiment to test it. The hypothesis may be fanciful but the experiment should be rigorous and able to answer the question, and the results must be assessed dispassionately. But knowledge does not progress just by adding more and more facts on top of the old ones. Popper rejected inductivism and logical positivism as the basis for the continual development of knowledge in favor of a trial and error. He felt that the method of conjecture and refutation was the characteristic of all rational discourse. A scientist puts forward statements, constructing hypotheses, and tests them step by step by observation and experiment. Although theories that stand against severe criticism are preferred, such survival does not attest to its justification, confirmation, or reliability. Thus a theory that has survived for a long time may still be rejected later when other knowledge and more

robust theories develop and explain things better. All knowledge in medicine is conjectural and thus fallible. No theory should be regarded as beyond criticism and even rejection. The object is not to pursue certainty, but to recognize that science is fallible and knowledge grows by constantly challenging, criticizing, and testing theories and beliefs. The view that knowledge in medicine and science is fallible has become the dominant paradigm of the 20th and 21st centuries. A second paradigm has been the abandonment of the traditional 'true belief' theory of knowledge, replaced by a concept that justification of truth is impossible.

The idea of shifting paradigms explains important changes in the overarching philosophical or scientific thinking in science and medicine. Paradigms are 'universally recognized achievements that for a long time provide model problems and solutions to a community or practitioners'. Kuhn felt that scientific activity could be divided into 'normal science' or 'revolutionary science' (Big Science). Normal Science occurs within an overarching scientific paradigm and works within it, explaining phenomena in terms of the paradigm. To Kuhn this was puzzle solving, putting pieces together within the paradigm which is characterized by a high level of consensus about theories and beliefs. In normal science the paradigm is not tested, and research is pursued to determine an adequate fit within the paradigm. But all puzzles are not solved, and when more and more phenomena do not fit, there is pressure to determine a new paradigm that accounts for the questions not answered by the old paradigm. Kuhn felt that competing scientific paradigms were incommensurable, and since the ideas and language are different in each paradigm, a decision about which one to accept is made, and this tends to be a bandwagon effect rather than a rational and reasoned argument.

## Pattern recognition

Margolis believed that cognition was based on *pattern recognition*, and that shifting from a paradigm, in science or in medicine, requires us to shift our patterns of mind to another pattern overcoming barriers in our thinking. In shifting our thinking to a new pattern, it is not so important how big the *barrier gap* is but what are the critical barriers within the gap that make it difficult to make the shift in thinking. How revolutionary a new idea or paradigm is may depend on how different it is from rival theories, or how difficult it is to put into practice. New theories often look ridiculous, and the critical sense of physicians and scientists may be very effective in blocking change. Although most ridiculous new ideas are indeed ridiculous, the one in a hundred that can be shown to be a good idea gives physicians the reputation of usually blocking new ideas, even though medicine is characterized by change. As Swift said, 'When a true genius appears in the world, you may know him by this sign, that the dunces are all in a confederacy against him'. But new ways of thinking do happen, and the critical barriers to seeing a disease process, or a scientific theory, or a new treatment in a completely different way continually occur.

Knowledge does not always come in a planned way. New knowledge may come by SERENDIPITY, as unexpected findings often appear when looking for something else. The skill is to recognize and capitalize on these unexpected discoveries, as Alexander FLEMING (p 50) did when a contaminant ruined the bacterial growth in a Petri dish, leading to the discovery of penicillin.

Medicine is a balance of the sciences and the humanities, but the state of the methods and approaches to the humanities is less well formulated. Many would argue that the holistic approach of the medical humanities should not be subjected to the objective, reductionist approach of the sciences, as the humanities and the humanistic aspects of medicine deal with the human condition and social phenomena that are formulated in qualitative rather than quantitative terms. Suffice it to say that, although the pursuit of knowledge in the medical sciences would benefit from more holistic approaches to large questions, the humanities would also benefit from a more rigorous approach to inquiry with more objective and quantitative measurement.

Some would say this whole discussion has a male perspective. Feminist philosophy criticizes the current approach to belief and knowledge, as the male viewpoint had laid most store in objectivity over opinion, of reason over emotion, of facts over belief, of masculine over feminine, with little recognition that they are all part of the whole. They would argue, and with good reason and evidence, that the attitudes to illness, to disease, to treatment — especially the care of women with illness — has been from a masculine point of view. It raises the question of whether there are different versions of knowledge and truth. How do we deal with an aspect of medicine as seen by a male or female clinician, a nurse, and patient, a medical anthropologist, a medical economist, a social scientist, or a molecular geneticist? Is it none of the above but a composite of them all, or is there a more central truth, with these being pieces of that whole?

### Knowledge and belief

How do we regard knowledge in relation to belief? Experience shows that knowledge may be in error and belief may be later shown to be true. Current methods in medicine of subjecting ideas to scrutiny include research to accumulate data, effective statistical methods, the randomized clinical trial, systematic reviews including meta-analysis, and organization of such reviews under the Cochrane Collaboration. This has given rise to the concept of EVIDENCE-BASED MEDICINE, which sets standards of evidence and then assesses how these can be applied to evaluate the strength of evidence in support of a theory, a treatment, or an approach. Although it may be traced back to the development of statistical approaches to medicine in Paris in the mid-19th century, this movement has gained great momentum in the last decade. Many healthcare systems are requiring evidence for everything they pay for, and this has led to the mythical but commonly quoted figure that physicians have evidence for only 30% of what they do, implying that the other 70% is based on belief. This fails to differentiate between biomedical knowledge as facts, in contrast to the knowledge used in complex decision-making. Although the randomized clinical trial is a laudable concept, there are important aspects of medicine that are difficult to subject to a clinical trial, although they may be important, and this philosophy tends to reject issues that have not been tested or are difficult to assess. Also, the focused and pristine design of a clinical trial does not necessarily represent the reality of patients in a physician's practice.

The physician uses complex knowledge in decision-making. There is knowledge from the patient, not just about the symptoms and signs but the context, the setting, the inter-relationship, the family, and the community and social setting. The physician also uses knowledge from study and literature, and from experience that is brought to bear on the questions. Thus the expanding knowledge in medicine is not the issue for the physician: it is the relevant knowledge that can be effectively and usefully brought to bear on the important issues that patients bring, and broader issues related to the community and society.

The adage that medical knowledge doubles every ten years has little meaning to the physician, who measures expansion of knowledge in terms of what will improve the care of patients in her or his practice. Any knowledge may lead to further knowledge and discoveries. There are many instances of an obscure piece of data in an obscure journal published years ago becoming the crucial step that led to the major advance.

Much has been said of the variable success of incorporating new knowledge into the practices of physicians. Sometimes this happens incredibly fast, such as the use of anesthetics, as the tangible result was obvious and immediate. Sometimes this happened slowly; despite the importance to the success of the British Navy, the published results of James LIND's (p 854) discovery of the treatment of scurvy were not accepted or put into place for fifty years because of the power of conflicting views about the cause of this disease. Although Lind's case is an exception, usually a surprising new concept, a paradigm shift, may occur faster if there is an obvious action and outcome resulting. LISTER's (p 473) antisepsis took decades because physicians had to deal with the acceptance of the germ theory first. The critical sense used by physicians, so important in advancing knowledge, may also inhibit acceptance, especially if the new knowledge does not fit accepted concepts and views. However, in a very short time physicians changed from believing that duodenal ulcers were due to stress to treating them with an antibiotic for an infection by *Helicobacter pylori*.

Because knowledge in medicine comes from many disciplines, the challenge will be to have a view and a medical training that allows recognition of potential contributions from sciences, social sciences, and the humanities, and to balance and integrate these so that knowledge in one aspect informs the other aspects. Each class of medical students is told that half of the knowledge they will be taught will be out of date in ten years, but unfortunately even the teachers don't know which half. Physicians also comment that, just as we shake our heads at the silly practices of the past physicians, later generations will be amused and appalled at some of the things we do, although we aren't yet sure which ones. These comments just underline the understanding that medical knowledge will always continually change and advance.                                   TJM

**ERRORS** Medical errors are acts of omission or commission that may cause harm to a patient. Such errors are receiving increasing publicity and demands for accountability. They include incidents such as fatal chemotherapy overdoses, mastectomies on the wrong breast, amputating the wrong leg, dismissing symptoms of meningitis as a benign headache, sending patients with chest pain from the emergency department to die of a myocardial infarction, or not diagnosing abdominal pain later found to be metastatic cancer. Such headline grabbing cases may lead to investigations, disciplinary measures, or malpractice suits.

Yet, given a moment of honest introspection, most experienced physicians can recall treatment errors or missed diagnoses, often brought to their attention only later, by a pharmacist's call or by the unfolding of the patient's illness. Though mostly of little ultimate consequence, especially if the prescription is corrected in a timely manner

or if the disease treatment is not critical, they bear an important connection to the sensational newspaper cases. For, while the public is relieved to learn that the surgeon who didn't know right from left was fired, how will we rid medicine of these troublesome and all too common errors?

The answer is increasingly to be found in applying the disciplines of human psychology, epidemiology, industrial engineering, and quality improvement theory to the problem of errors in medicine. Improvements in medical practice may depend on understanding that errors, while often invisible, are ubiquitous (see Table). When meticulously sought out by looking at detailed reviews, many of these errors have reported frequencies of 15–40%. Rather than representing isolated individual lapses, most errors can be traced to failures of process. Predictably occurring events call for error reduction strategies. Understanding where such strategies might best be targeted can be guided by insights from several decades of work in both medical and non-medical settings (such as aviation safety). Careful analysis of the various causes of errors offers important lessons for prevention and improvement:

● Examining individual incidents is a powerful way of understanding what happened when things go wrong. Drawing on the tradition of morbidity and mortality conferences, inquiries should be conducted so as to probe deeply, not to fix blame, but to understand the root causes of an adverse event. Although in the past such discussions seldom went beyond the case at hand, it is essential to identify patterns and integrate such inquiries into larger organizational strategies of learning and improvement.

● Many errors occur in the interactions between different components of the system — interfaces between laboratory and pharmacy, or doctors and pharmacists. In hospitals numerous prescriptions are written annually for potassium supplements while a raised serum potassium level sits in the laboratory computer. Demanding that each person do their job more carefully (that is, memos or threats imploring doctors to check laboratory results before refilling potassium prescriptions) represents a 'low-leverage' strategy. Re-engineering the way people, departments, and other system components (for example, interfaces between laboratory and pharmacy computers) communicate and coordinate to make these interfaces more error-proof, yields greater dividends.

● Mistakes seldom occur because of a single slip. Rather, multiple lapses contribute to these undesired outcomes. The term 'latent failures' has been applied to the multiple weaknesses in the

**EPONYM**
The name of a person used as part of the name of a disease, syndrome, anatomical feature, etc. (e.g. Bright's disease, Pott's fracture). The doctor, or doctors, associated with an original description or invention are the most frequent to be so honored, but a few diseases are named after patients (e.g. Christmas disease) or places (e.g. Marburg disease).
See *also* MISNOMERS – EPONYMOUS

Types and causes of medical error

| Types of medical errors | Causes |
| --- | --- |
| **Diagnosis** | Information transfer/availability |
|   Misdiagnosis | Lack of knowledge/training |
|   Missed diagnosis | Reliance on human memory |
|   Delayed diagnosis | Failure to recognize warning signals |
|   Erroneous diagnostic work-up strategy | Distraction |
|   Failure to obtain, act on, or follow-up laboratory result | Poor communication among providers |
| **Drug treatment** | Suboptimal communication between patient and providers; failure to listen |
|   Prescribing | Cognitive errors/biases |
|     Drug for patient known to be allergic | Failure to seek advice; ask questions |
|     Contraindicated due to underlying condition | Over-stressed system (staffing, pace, fatigue) |
|     Dosing error, miscalculation | Lack of continuity/familiarity |
|     Name mix-up | High-risk situations/drugs |
|   Dispensing | Failure to appreciate clinical urgency |
|     Wrong drug dose | Work station/engineering design (visual cues, lighting, labeling) |
|     Delay or failure to give | Information systems; poor design, over-reliance, misleading information |
|   Administration | Equipment failures |
|     Wrong dose, route | Failure to adroitly respond once complications arise |
|     Wrong patient | Organizational culture (denial of problems, disempowered workers) |
| **Procedural** | Fear inhibiting reporting, investigating, and learning |
|   Wrong procedure/organ/patient | Guilt, blame |
|   Erroneous indications, patient selection | Overconfidence; failure to appreciate uncertainties, risks |
|   Technical slip; poor technique in procedure performance | Failure to learn from past mistakes |
|   Delayed treatment | Lack of accountability: to patients for mistakes, for learning. |

practice environment that contribute to errors. These combine with 'active failures' committed by individuals such as physicians or nurses who come in direct contact with the weaknesses in the system. One recent investigation of a fatal medication error (1.5 million units of benzathine penicillin given intravenously to a neonate) uncovered over 50 latent failures leading to the erroneous infusion; had any one of them been prevented the fatal reaction could have been averted.

● Aiming for an organizational culture where errors are openly acknowledged, reported, and dealt with in a non-punitive fashion represents a critical departure from traditional approaches. This change is needed to get beyond the *status quo* of denial, blaming others, and perfunctory and meaningless under-reporting. As health workers' entire professional identity revolves around avoiding harm to their patients, many experience extreme feelings of guilt when such harm occurs. Encumbering the processes with self-inflicted or legally-assigned guilt is unlikely to be productive enough to induce the large-scale changes needed to prevent errors. Only an environment safe for actively seeking out, reporting, and addressing mishaps can effectively reduce error.

● Reporting of errors needs to take on a new character. Letting physicians and others commit and learn exclusively from their own mistakes is an inefficient and inhumane approach. Reporting must be purposeful — not just for counting events, discharging reporting mandates, or even comparing institutions or providers (so-called report cards). Instead, reporting should delineate a critical communication pipeline connecting front line workers with the institution's leadership. Communication should flow (in the language of the re-engineered aircraft cockpit) against the authority gradient, such that each employee's experiences are heard and valued. By turning up the volume of this communication lifeline, near-misses may be heeded and future errors averted. Separating signal (true problems warranting interventions) from noise (false alarms) becomes a central scientific and statistical challenge.

By focusing on three key aspects — process redesign, implementing basic prevention strategies, and overcoming obstacles — many healthcare organizations have demonstrably reduced errors, thereby saving lives and money. Despite their appealing simplicity, each of these approaches challenges entrenched reflexes to blame and deny. But adopting a proactive posture would, perhaps more than any other single activity, would enhance and justify public confidence in medicine, and ensure progressive improvements in patient care.                    GDS

*See also* ADVERSE DRUG REACTIONS; AUDIT; DIAGNOSIS; MISADVENTURE

**ESTHETIC SURGERY** See PLASTIC SURGERY

**EUGENICS** The naive view of eugenics is embodied in the (probably apocryphal) remark of Isadora Duncan to George Bernard Shaw about a child with her looks and his brains (and his riposte saying that it might have his looks and her brains). While emerging as, if not a science in its own right, a highly scientized discourse, in the late 19th century, its roots can be seen in age-old concepts of 'like breeding like' and centuries of animal husbandry.

Eugenics is often supposed to have been a conservative and oppressive doctrine from its inception, reaching its logical culmination in the excesses of the German Third Reich, leading to a backlash against the entire notion until modern genetic engineering reintroduced it as a more insidious agenda. This is only one story, depending a good deal on hindsight, about an idea (rather than an ideology) which had a strong appeal across the political spectrum, being embraced by Spanish anarchists and Russian Bolsheviks as well as by German and Italian fascists, British liberals, and Scandinavian social democrats. Its appeal owed much to its association with modernity and the promises of science. While eugenic ideas certainly had much influence during the 20th century, what 'eugenics' meant in any particular context and at any given moment varied enormously. About the only common meaning would be an emphasis on the importance of biological factors within a population and their conscious manipulation for the better well-being of state and society. Related concepts which emerged around the same time, their meaning strongly overlapping with eugenics but not coterminous with it, were 'racial hygiene' and 'puericulture'.

The term itself was coined by Sir Francis GALTON (this page), polymath scientist and cousin of Charles DARWIN (p 214), in his 1883 *Inquiries into human faculty*. He defined it as 'that science which deals with all influences which improve the inborn qualities of a race; also with those which develop them to the utmost advantage'. Galton had a pre-Mendelian view of the mechanisms of heredity, as operating in a straightforward like-begets-like fashion. Many early eugenic arguments were based on the assumption that desirable and undesirable characteristics — physical, mental, and even moral — were transmitted in this unproblematic way. Some convinced eugenicists, for example, Galton's disciple Karl PEARSON (p 782), believed that too little was known about heredity to determine what policies should be followed to improve 'the race' and that research, not propaganda, was the priority, a note of caution seldom heard among those accepting the theory. The complexities of Mendelian GENETICS took some time to have any impact on eugenic thinking.

In terms of policy, eugenics had two facets: 'positive' and 'negative'. On the one hand, the 'fit' should reproduce themselves at (at least) replacement rate. On the other hand, the 'unfit' should be discouraged from perpetuating themselves. Some hardliners argued that sanitary science, and the implementation of social welfare policies, were by their very nature dysgenic: but few argued for dismantling existing public health provisions. The problem was therefore to provide some counterweight to the noticeable decline in family size among the 'better' classes, and to find some means to curb the reckless fertility of the lower orders.

As taken up and embodied in the British Eugenics Education Society (founded in 1907), eugenics appeared to appeal to an established (male) meritocracy. It might, however, be used more critically and subversively to assert 'nature' versus 'culture' and attack economic and social arrangements militating against eugenically desirable matches. Some feminists added a eugenic slant to attacks on the iniquities of the marriage system, suggesting that genuinely free female mate choice would improve a race degenerating under existing patriarchal arrangements, a recension also found in the Spanish anarchist version, along with a rhetoric of sexual reform.

Although to Galton eugenics was explicitly and inherently about innate hereditary qualities, the term was used much more loosely in connection with a wider conglomeration of ideas and anxieties. In some countries (for example, France and parts of Latin America), and for some individual exponents, heredity as a concept was still strongly inflected with neo-Lamarckian ideas about the inheritance of acquired characteristics. In the early 20th century there was frequently confusion between strictly hereditary defects and those brought about by congenital factors (most powerfully epitomized in the ravages of congenital SYPHILIS), resulting in a rather blurred concept of 'good breeding', which drew many into the eugenics movement.

### Varied policies

Policies advocated or undertaken in the name of eugenics varied greatly according to highly specific local contexts and were subject to the

**FOUNDING FATHER**

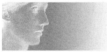

Sir Francis **GALTON** (1822–1911). British eugenist. A QUAKER who was for a short time a medical student, Galton later was interested in heredity and 'improving the race'. He was the founder of the study of 'eugenics' and responsible for developing 'anthropometry and biometrics'. He described the individuality of fingerprints in 1893.

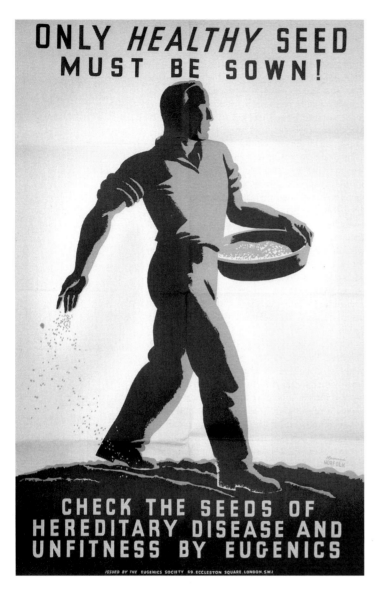

# ONLY *HEALTHY* SEED MUST BE SOWN!

## CHECK THE SEEDS OF HEREDITARY DISEASE AND UNFITNESS BY EUGENICS

ISSUED BY THE EUGENICS SOCIETY 69 ECCLESTON SQUARE.LONDON.S.W.1

*Healthy Seed* poster: this poster, which from the address given and the style would appear to have been produced during the 1930s, conveys a message of negative eugenics. (Reproduced courtesy of the Wellcome Institute Library, London.)

accepting that Mendelian genetics rendered the whole concept a good deal less simplistic, and taking into account scientific developments in other disciplines, such as nutrition, which indicated that important environmental factors still had to be addressed.

While eugenics was believed to have fallen into disrepute because of the abuses of the Nazis (which could be seen to have roots in policies of the preceding Weimar Government), it has recently been a cause of scandal that several nations (such as Sweden) have, until extremely recently, sterilized sections of their population under laws originally passed for eugenic purposes. Meanwhile recent developments in genetics have led to the resurgence of the belief that 'it's all in our genes' (including criminality and sexual orientation) and that science can, potentially, manipulate genetic material to make everyone into good and healthy citizens. It is also argued that developments in prenatal screening are reintroducing a crypto-eugenic agenda, presented in terms of individual 'choice'.

LAH

*See also* HOLOCAUST; SCREENING

**EUROPEAN UNION — HISTORY** In 1957, the leaders of six European countries signed a treaty in Rome to establish a European Economic Community. Over the next 40 years the community developed from a common market of six into a European Union (EU) of 15 countries and 372 million people. The single market is now a massive trading block, comparable in size to the USA. In January 1999, despite division and doubt, European monetary was realized when 11 of the 15 EU member states adopted the euro as a common currency.

1999 was to prove a testing year for the EU. The entire staff of one if its key institutions, the European Commission, resigned after the exposure of fraud, mismanagement, and nepotism. Turnout for the European Parliament elections reached an all time low. War in Kosovo showed, yet again, the EU's inability to speak with one voice on foreign policy and defence issues. The difficulty in realizing the EU's next ambitious goals of political union and Eastward enlargement to include up to 11 more member states was underlined.

To understand how EU legislation has affected the health sector and its potential to do so, for better or worse, it is helpful to understand how 'Europe' works. This article looks at how the community was established and describes its key institutions (which occupy a seventh of the total office space in Brussels) and their involvement with health. The second article focuses on the main effects of the EU on medicine.

pressures of contingent circumstances, such as the perceived expense of social welfare during economic crises. Eugenic actions, undertaken by the state, argued for by propagandists, promoted by voluntary bodies, or put into practice by various health professionals, might include restricting immigration, calls for premarital health examinations, sterilization of the 'unfit', research into birth control, legalization of abortion, maternal welfare measures, and even (in some Latin American nations) miscegenation to create a new racially mixed type. Even as the Third Reich was taking power in Germany, there was a shift in Anglo–American eugenic circles from the old 'mainline' eugenics to a new 'reform' eugenics,

In 1948, after the appalling devastation of the First and Second World wars, the Congress of Europe marked the first step towards the reconciliation of former enemies and the establishment of economic, political, and cultural union in Europe. Four years later France, Germany, Italy, Belgium, the Netherlands, and Luxembourg united to form the European Coal and Steel Community. This was an historic act, for it was the first time that key industries had united across national boundaries. By 1957, the same six countries signed the Treaty of Rome and established the European Economic Community or 'Common Market'. Years of political machinations followed, until finally, in 1973, a reluctant Britain, along with Denmark and Ireland, threw in its lot with 'Europe'. In the 1980s Greece, Portugal, and Spain joined followed a few years later by Finland, Sweden, and Austria.

In the late 1970s and '80s the impact of 'Europe' was felt throughout the member states as a steady stream of 'opinions', 'recommendations', 'decisions', 'directives', 'regulations', and other missives emerged from the Brussels institutions. Couched in long-winded 'Brussels speak' and laced with indecipherable acronyms, they were not designed to obfuscate but were undoubtably difficult to grasp. European journals and periodicals helpfully published glossaries of what the various terms and acronyms meant, but many organizations and individuals struggled to follow the draft legislative proposals. Disenchantment with 'Brussels and its bureaucrats' was widespread.

The first time 'health' formally appeared on the European agenda was in the Maastricht Treaty, which was signed in 1992 by the leaders of the then 12 member states. The treaty established a program for economic and monetary union and created the framework for a common foreign and security policy, and for cooperation in justice and home affairs. Within the small print, in the obscurely worded 'Article 129', provision was made for the community to protect and promote public health and to integrate health into other community policies.

Although the EU institutions have become more familiar over time, and all are now committed to 'transparency', it is still not easy to understand exactly how they function and interact. The internet has revolutionized access to information though. Through the main EU web site *www. europa.eu.int* it is now easily possible to find out about 'Europe' and its day to day business. Despite this, Chambers' 1966 description of the EU as a 'Kafkaesque labyrinth' still rings true.

Over time the interaction and balance of power among the three main institutions, the European Commission, the European Parliament, and the European Council of Ministers, have changed, but they remain the key players. A fourth institution, the European Court of Justice, is the 'guardian and ultimate interpreter' of the European treaties. There are also several important consultative bodies such as the Committee of the Regions and the Economic and Social Committee.

### The European Commission

Charged with implementing the EU treaties, the Brussels-based commission has the right to propose legislation. It also monitors and reinforces the laws adopted by the Council of Ministers. It has a staff of around 16 000 people, many of whom are translators and interpreters, for business is routinely conducted in 11 different languages. The staff work under a president and 19 commissioners, who are appointed, not elected. It reached its legistive peak in 1990, under Jacques Delors, when the single market program was accepted.

Jacques Santer, Delors's successor, promised 'to do less but better' but lacked either the strength or vision to instigate change in what was widely described as a faceless, cumbersome, unnaccountable organization. On 15 March 1999 a damning report on the commission from an independent committee, set up by the European Parliament, was published. The parliament was triumphant but, before it could use its newly acquired power to sack the commission, Mr Santer and his entire staff resigned.

The debacle shook the commission to the core and further damaged 'Europe's' credibility. It was obvious that root and branch reform was essential. Those in positions of responsiblility in the commission had to be made accountable for the action of their staff and openness and transparency to become the rule not the exception. After a short but uneasy hiatus a new commission president, Romano Prodi, a former prime minister of Italy, was appointed. Committed to reform and showing more force and determination than some expected, by mid-September 1999 Prodi had elected his new team of 19 commissioners and embarked on organizational change. Most significantly for those concerned with health, he appointed (and the parliament approved) the first ever commissioner for health, David Byrne, a former Irish attorney general. Although Byrne's portfolio is wide and encompasses consumer affairs, which are likely to dominate his agenda, his appointment holds promise that the EU may begin to work in a more coordinated and effective way on health.

Historically many different departments, or Directorate Generals as they are known, have been responsible for implementing policies which have an impact on medical practice and public health.

The powerful agriculture directorate, for example, has had infinitely more effect on health than the commission's small, poorly resourced public health unit. Messages about limiting fat intake and raising fruit and vegetable consumption have cut little ice with policy makers acting in the interests of farmers, whose livelihood depends on the production of dairy products. The EU ban on tobacco advertizing was hailed as triumph, but it sits oddly next to policy which ensures that tobacco growers get substantial EU subsidies.

Under a strengthened clause in the latest European treaty, the 1997 Treaty of Amsterdam that came into force in 1999, the EU now has a stronger mandate to take action to protect public health and to ensure that the health impact of community policies is taken into account. The extent to which Byrne and the new environment commissioner, who has also defined health protection as a priority, will be able to stand up to the economic and political power of the departments convened with trade, industry, agriculture, and transport remains to be seen. By the millennium, however, health lobbyists were expressing cautious optimism.

### The European Parliament
The European Parliament started life in 1952 as the common assembly of the European Coal and Steel Community. Members (MEPs) were appointed rather than elected up until 1979, when the first direct elections to what was then called the European Parliament were held. Over the next two decades the parliament grew steadily in size, power, and influence.

Its main role is to exercise democratic control over the commission. It cannot draw up laws, but it can amend or even reject bills put forward by the Commission. In addition, it shares almost equal control over the EU budget with the Council of Ministers. Under each successive European Treaty the parliament's hand has been strengthened, and as result it is surrounded by lobbyists, specialist interest groups, and representatives of non-governmental organizations. These (together with an inevitably large media following) have been dubbed the 'Eurosphere', where getting a word in the right MEP's ear has been honed to an art form.

Despite its transition from 'talking shop to body with bite', as an article in *European Voice* put it, the parliament has two major problems. Firstly, it operates from two homes. One is in Brussels and one in Strasbourg; both are new, massive, hugely expensive, glass edifices. Meanwhile its secretariat is in Luxembourg. MEPs and their retinues have to traverse Europe (on generous expense accounts) like restless lemmings. Secondly, it is not trusted or respected by many of the citizens it rep-

resents. In 1979, 63 per cent of the electorate voted at the European elections; in 1999 the turnout was only 49 per cent. *The Economist* warned that this 'Euro-apathy' was a rebuke not only to parliament but to the entire European enterprise.

Within the European Parliament, most of the health issues are dealt with by the Committee on the Environment, Public Health, and Consumer Policy. It is through debate in this committee, and in plenary sessions of the parliament, that most health-related legislation and non-legislative reports are dealt with. Health issues are also regularly discussed in an informal 'Health intergroup' of MEP's with a special interest in health.

### The European Council of Ministers
This name is given to the meetings of groups of ministers from national governments who regularly get together for a few days to agree on policy, adopt legislation, and make various declarations. The composition of the Council and the frequency with which it meets vary. The Foreign Affairs, Finance, and Agricultural Councils meet once a month; other, less high-profile Councils, including the Health Council (made up of - member states' health ministers), meet less often. In between the major meetings the detailed working of intergovernmental business is carried out in Brussels by the 'permanent representatives' of the member states. Most of these are diplomats, who act as 'proxies and problem solvers' for the different national governments.

Over the years, the European Council has gained in ascendency, and the importance of each country's tenure at the top (the presidency by tradition rotates from country to country every six months) has become an important component of national diplomacy. Heads of states usher in their presidencies by widely publicizing their priorities for action at EU level. At the end of this term, during which the country holds the initiative on EU affairs and hosts a series of high profile meetings, a summit is held to discuss what has been achieved and to set out the agenda for the next six months.

In the 1980s and 1990s the Council came under heavy fire for not being close enough to most issues, for conducting business behind closed doors, and for rubber stamping agreements brokered by 'faceless civil servants in Brussels'. But, as EU affairs have slowly and steadily become more integrated and central to national concerns, heads of state and their ministers have assumed a much more hands-on role and the power of their representatives in Brussels has been reined in. In addition, increased transparency has resulted in better understanding of the Council's affairs and the complex system of weighting which is used in decision-making. As the EU is set to enlarge, the mechanics of the latter are being widely debated and a trend to take more decisions by majority rather than consensus seems inevitable.

## The European Court of Justice

Often confused with the European Court of Human Rights in Strasbourg, the European Court of Justice in Luxembourg is concerned with enforcing European rules. This is no easy business, for EU law is often more honored in the breach than the observance. By the late 1990s Brussels watchers were lampooning the status quo. In a lighthearted article in *European Voice* 3–9, Geoff Meade noted (in September 1998) that 'Never before in the history of the European Union have so many member states been in the dock at the European Court of Justice at the same time, accused of breaching the laws of Euro-land'. The problem he quoted a court official as saying is that 'You have no idea how complicated it is. You've got to give governments time to amend their national legislation to comply with European law and sometimes they run into all sorts of bureaucratic and political problems. And then we have to prompt them a bit with some legal stuff'. But judicial wheels grind slowly and the Court is often criticized for being slow, secretive, and undemocratic.                                          TJLR

## EUROPEAN UNION — IMPACT ON MEDICINE

Initially the impact of the EU on medicine was confined to spin off from legislation aimed at establishing the free movement of goods, services, people, and capital. The EU has never sought to interfere with the funding and organization of healthcare at national level. Indeed, under its commitment to subsidiarity (roughly translated as, don't do anything at community level which is better done at national level), it is expressly prohibited from doing so.

The first sign that the EU was interested in health issues at all was in the appearance of the public health clause in the Maastricht treaty. Although this triggered some debate, if little passion, about what a European public health policy should look like, the five-year public health program that was set up to run from 1993–98 was unambitious. It consisted of eight 'vertical' programs promoting collaboration and research in communicable disease, AIDS, cancer, health promotion, drug abuse, accidents and injuries, rare diseases, and diseases related to pollution. Collection of EU health data for comparative studies was instigated along with measures aimed at ensuring the safety of blood for transfusion and self-sufficiency within Europe.

In 1998, the Commission publicly acknowledged that these programs had had only limited impact. It was also evident that producing annual reports on the integration of health requirements in EU policy would not persuade those departments whose policies had adverse effect on public health to alter direction. By the end of 1999, a new public health strategy was being hammered out and a commitment made to tackle health determinants through health promotion and disease prevention and to react (more) quickly to potential health threats. There was also agreement about the need, if not the methods, to do health impact assessments of community policies along the lines of the now mandatory environmental impact assessments.

While the public health programs may have had little impact on the health sector, single-market legislation relating to medicines, health insurance, medical devices, and health and safety has. EU data protection legislation is also strong and has been criticized by some for hampering epidemiological research. Legislation on public procurement ensures that major capital projects, such as building new hospitals, are open to competition throughout Europe. EU legislation has also affected doctors.

## Free movement and convergence on training

The medical profession has not been quick to see the relevance of 'Europe', especially at the beginning. The Treaty of Rome guaranteed the freedom of every EU citizen to work, set up business, or provide services in any member state. A commitment was also made to work towards mutual recognition of professional qualifications. In 1975 the 'Doctors' directive' was formally adopted, which allowed mutual recognition of basic medical and medical specialist qualifications. This was followed by a directive for mutual recognition of general practitioner training in 1986. Similar directives were adopted for nurses, dentists, midwives, and pharmacists. The directives each set out minimum criteria for education and training, based primarily on length of training rather than its content or quality. They also established mutual recognition of qualifications and freedom of movement of professionals throughout the European Economic Area.

In the wake of this legislation, there was concern that medical migration might take place on a large scale and upset the balance of medical manpower and the nature of national practice. These fears have been largely unfounded, however, partially because of professional conservatism and also because of ignorance about the options and the bureaucratic, cultural, and language barriers that had to be overcome. Over the years these various barriers have been reduced by the creeping process of Europeanization and it has become more

## RECIPROCAL MEDICAL CARE

Under Regulation 1408/71 any national of one member state visiting another may be reimbursed for the cost of medical treatment if they become acutely ill away from home. The caveat is that this must be for 'treatment of a new problem', or a 'genuine exacerbation of a pre-existing condition' arising during their visit. There are also reciprocal agreements with other countries in Europe such as Norway, Poland, Romania, and Iceland. Being reimbursed for non-acute care is also possible, provided that the appropriate authorities, for example, in Britain the District Health Authority and the Department of Health, sanction it.

In practice, cross-border treatment for non-acute care is not big business but it is growing. A landmark European Court judgement in April 1998, which went in favor of two people who claimed for the costs incurred in one member state — one for purchasing spectacles and the other for orthodontic treatment — without first getting authorization from the insurance providers in their own member states, set the precedent. Shopping around for the cheapest drug, for example, across national boundaries may become common practice for it could save money for both individuals and insurance companies. In addition, it may allow people to receive treatment in one member state that is not reimbursable in their own. Debates about drug pricing, priority setting, and rationing are beginning to take on a European dimension.

common for health professionals to work in another member state. The migration has been dependent on where the jobs are. Countries such as Germany, Belgium, Italy, and Spain which have tended to overproduce doctors because the number of students enrolled in medical schools has in the past not been limited, have been major exporters of junior doctors. Other countries, notably Britain, have failed to train enough, and as a result have large contingents of EU-trained medical graduates. Despite the fact that their training has been different and their language skills are variable, their right to work is not questioned.

The fact that the training for specialist qualifications in some EU countries was, until recently, shorter than in Britain and the practical experience gained was less resulted in the UK failing to allow some European specialists to work at the same level as they had in their own country. But in 1992 the European Commission threatened to take the British government to the European Court of Justice for not observing the law on mutual recognition of qualifications. As a result a lengthy report by the Chief Medical Officer of Health resulted in a major upheaval in postgraduate training to bring Britain in line with 'Europe'.

UK junior doctors now complete specialist training and are added to the list of recognized specialists in a much shorter period of time than before. The down side, some claim, is that they lack the experience of their 'old style trained' peers and face uncertainty in finding definitive posts. In time, the long-standing work of both the European Union of Specialists and the European Union of General Practitioners to harmonize not just the length but the quality of specialist training and of continued medical EDUCATION will iron out more of the differences between doctors trained in different member states — but they face an uphill struggle. The differences that exist reflect appreciable and well-entrenched differences in healthcare organization, health beliefs, medical practice, customs, and cultures. If EU expansion, to include Central and Eastern European states, is realized, as planned, the effect of free movement and mutual recognition of qualifications will present more challenges and spur further change.

### Professional working patterns

The 48-hour working time directive, which came into force in October 1998, did much to focus attention on the unacceptably long hours worked by many doctors. At present, junior doctors in training are exempt from its provisions, but steady lobbying by the Permanent Working Group of Junior Doctors of the EU is likely to overturn this exclusion. Maternity and more

recently paternity leave are also increasingly being protected by EU law. As a result, hospitals in Britain and elsewhere have had to introduce new patterns of working, with the introduction of shift systems to accommodate junior doctors working fewer hours and having more time off during their training. Consultants' work patterns have also changed; as back-up by juniors has been reduced, they have had to assume more of the burden of acute care.

### The pharmaceutical industry

Prescribing patterns and drug prices in the member states vary widely but the steady progression of single market legislation has brought convergence on labeling, packaging, the conduct of clinical trials, advertising, postmarketing surveillance, patenting, and drug licensing. The European Medicines Evaluation Agency, which operates from London's Canary Wharf, has been operational since 1995. Its authority to grant EU-wide approval has revolutionized drug licensing. Instead of having to seek individual approval from each member state, pharmaceutical companies may now submit a single dossier to the authority and, once approval is obtained, market their product throughout Europe. In time, convergence over drug pricing, availability, and classification is inevitable. Similar convergence may be expected with over-the-counter medicines and homeopathic products.

### Research and development

One of the original aims behind the creation of the European Community was to bring the countries of Europe together so that they could compete effectively against the USA and Japan. Collaboration on research was one means of effecting this. In the early 1980s the so-called 'framework' program was set up to coordinate research. After the Treaty of Rome was signed in 1957, research and development became a priority, and since then expenditure on research programs has steadily increased. As much of the money is directed towards promoting coordination and collaboration between different research groups working throughout Europe as it is towards funding individual projects.

Total expenditure on the third framework program, which ran from 1990–1994, was 5700 million ecu (£3972 m); of this, 133 m ecu went towards biomedical and health research. The fifth framework program, operating between 1998–2002, has an overall budget of 14 000 m ecu. Of this, 2239 m is budgeted for a program to 'improve the quality of life and management of living resource', under which food, nutrition and health, control of infectious disease, health and the environment, the 'cell factory', and research on the aging population are included (details may be found on the website http://www.cordis.lu/fifth/home.html).

## Environmental issues

Public concern about environmental threats and about their possible impact on health is now high. What in the 1980s were deemed extremist views about pollution and climate change have now become mainstream concerns. In response the EU set up an ambitious five year environmental and sustainable development program. Surprisingly perhaps, the European Union was a key player at the third United Nations Convention on Climate Change in Kyoto in 1997 in backing an agreement to reduce the collective global emission of greenhouse gases by 5.2% by 2008–12 and the pledge to reduce emissions across the Union by 8% over the same time.

Opinion on the scale and nature of the adverse effects on health of climate change brought about by emission of various pollutants is a huge subject in its own right, but along with national and international monitoring centers the European Environment Agency collects data and disseminates information. The familiar problem of the lack of comparability of much of the data has had to be tackled. In addition, the agency produces regular reports on how the agricultural, transport, and manufacturing sectors in the member states have responded to EU policies and action programs.

## Communicable disease surveillance

Exchanging information at European level about trends, clusters, and outbreaks of infectious disease has always made sense and was one of the spurs behind the establishment of the public health unit in the European Commission. After Maastricht, when cooperation to control communicable disease became enshrined as a priority, the major European institutes concerned with national surveillance started to work together to facilitate the exchange of information and skills. Proposals to do this by building yet another large and expensive European institution — an observatory for communicable disease surveillance — were sensibly dropped in 1998 in favor of promoting and enhancing networks of electronic networks among key centers.

Institutes with particular interests and skills have taken the lead on different diseases. The Communicable Disease Surveillance Centre at Colindale, in the UK, for example, is the coordinating center for enteric infections and is responsible for collating and disseminating relevant data to other national centers, identifying trends and outbreaks, and alerting countries which have not identified problems. In addition to the various disease-specific networks, data are

also being collected on antibiotic resistance, where the National Institute of Public Health in Bilthoven, in the Netherlands, took the lead.

National variations in terminology, classification, and laboratory practices are steadily being ironed out as exchange has progressed. Common training programs, such as the European Interventional Epidemiology Training Programme, are bringing the goal of common European standards closer. Cooperation and exchange have not, however, been confined to Europe. In 1996 the US President, Bill Clinton, and the President of the European Commission, Jacques Santer, signed an accord on global surveillance and response, and since then there has been a steady growth in global exchange and cooperation in the investigation of disease outbreaks.

## Combating drug abuse

In the 1980s concern about the rising level of drug abuse throughout the member states prompted a variety of joint European initiatives. These included a 'Community action program on the prevention of drug dependence', legislation geared at preventing money laundering, and the establishment of a 'Eurocentre' to collect data on the prevalence and pattern of drug misuse. The European Monitoring Centre for Drugs and Drug Addiction was established in Lisbon in 1995. Its role is limited, in that it is essentially a repository for data, not a policy-making body, but it does play a part in combating the problem by identifying good practice and priorities for action. It works closely with national centers in the member states and the European Commission, in addition to Europol and the various international bodies concerned with drug abuse. Each year it produces an annual report, which provides an epidemiological overview and information about the various demand reduction measures that have been taken and the cost-effectiveness of various anti-drug strategies.

## Conclusions

Quantifying the effect of the EU on the healthcare sector is impossible. For every concrete example, such as the standardization of pacemakers or urinary catheters, there is an intangible one where the benefits cannot be measured. How, for example, do you measure the benefit of the EU-supported exchange and cooperation among hospitals, medical schools, and universities? European Union-funded programs, such as the Socrates–Erasmus Program to promote exchange of teachers and students, and the Leonardo da Vinci Program supporting exchange between healthcare professionals, have unforeseen spin-offs. Health telematics is another huge domain where there has been extensive collaboration. Electronic healthcare records, common European health cards, international data exchange, and the plethora of high-tech TELE-

## CONDITIONS JUSTIFYING EUTHANASIA

- There must have been a voluntary and well-considered request from the patient.
- There must be unacceptable, unendurable, and hopeless suffering.
- An independent physician must have been consulted beforehand.
- The procedure to be followed must be laid down in a detailed written report.
- Other relevant disciplines (for example, social workers) must have been consulted.
- The physician must be present or easily reached during euthanasia.
- Euthanasia must be carried out meticulously from a medical–technical point of view.

In the 1985 report of the State Committee on Euthanasia, these recommendations were slightly amended but remained essentially unchanged. In March 1987, the Dutch Health Council formulated the requirements for meticulous euthanasia anew. These now read as follows:

- The medical practitioner must have informed the patient about his or her present situation, the expected further course, and any possible ways of affecting it.
- The medical practitioner must be convinced that the patient submitted and maintains his request for euthanasia voluntarily and after careful consideration.

(*continued opposite*)

MEDICINE projects — the scope and potential for co-operation and exchange if not total harmonization are endless.

The greatest challenge facing the EU, however, is undoubtably European enlargement. To join the 'club', applicant countries need to meet stringent requirements. In its turn, the EU, and its institutions, will have to metamorphose into a more transparent and workable entity. Considerations other than health will continue to dominate its business for the foreseeable future. But striving to create greater equality between western Europe and the poorly resourced member states of central and eastern Europe (with their notably worse morbidity and mortality) is a challenge to rise to. For what is the European dream about, if not that?　　　　　　　　　　　　TJLR

**EUTHANASIA** For centuries, the Netherlands (with which this article is largely concerned) has been famous world-wide as a country that was wrested from the sea, with dykes, windmills, people in wooden shoes, great paintings, and large fields of tulips. During the past quarter of a century, this picture has changed. The Netherlands is increasingly known abroad for sexual freedom, liberal views on drugs, and the so-called free and uncontrolled practice of euthanasia. Especially the last, however, is unjustified, as we show clearly below in a review of 25 years' experience.

The discussion on euthanasia in the Netherlands flared up in 1973. In February of that year, a woman physician was accused of having terminated her mother's life the year before, after her mother had emphatically requested her to do so because she had an incurable disease. The physician received a suspended sentence of one week's imprisonment, and in its judgement the court also formulated, for the first time, the requirements which would have to be met for meticulous euthanasia. The judge also expressed the opinion that Dutch physicians need no longer feel compelled to prolong the lives of their patients under all circumstances. Following this judgement, the discussion on euthanasia rapidly gained momentum.

### What is euthanasia?

Euthanasia concerns the very essence of a person's being, life and death, the right to self-determination, the competence of the physician and the patient to judge, and the perception of the severity of human suffering. It is no wonder that it is almost impossible to give a definition of euthanasia with which everyone can agree and which will not offend anyone.

In the past, a distinction was usually made between passive and active euthanasia. Passive euthanasia meant that the attending physician decided to stop or refrain from treating the patient, while instituting palliative measures to alleviate suffering, whereas in active euthanasia, the physician himself administered the fatal medication. This distinction is no longer made. 'Euthanasia' now means the intentional termination of life or the intentional interruption of procedures intended to prolong life by a physician. This means that the patient must be fully competent mentally; newborn infants, children, and mentally incompetent adults do not fall under this definition. A distinction is still made between several procedures that resemble euthanasia, such as stopping giving food and fluids and the termination of a medically futile procedure. If the patient performs the act with materials provided by the physician, one speaks of assisted suicide.

### Legislation concerning euthanasia

Euthanasia is a very emotive subject, and everyone has an opinion on it, which need not necessarily agree with the consensus in society. Strikingly the prevailing opinions and decisions taken in the various levels of the population have not been in step. Four groups may be roughly distinguished: the population (and hence also the patients), physicians, experts in (medical) law, and politicians. It has been shown that an individual, a special interest group (the Dutch Society for Voluntary Euthanasia has played an important part in the discussions), or a part of the population can change its opinion from year to year. In 1973 the Royal Dutch Medical Association, for example, was still vigorously opposed to euthanasia. In 1984, however, this association felt compelled to depart from the standpoint it had always held and formulated the conditions under which a physician would be justified in performing euthanasia. The initial recommendations, which were later confirmed in legal procedures and which are still valid are given in the box.

Even if these requirements for meticulousness had been fulfilled, until November 2000 euthanasia remained a criminal offence, although in practice the physician who performed it usually was not punished. In 1984, the Supreme Court of the Netherlands attempted to find a solution for the physician who faces the dilemma of wishing to fulfill the patient's request to put an end to severe and irreversible suffering while, on the other hand, feeling bound by the Hippocratic OATH in which he or she has sworn always to try to preserve the lives of patients. According to this recommendation, the physician can claim *force majeure* and a conflict of duties, as a result of which the physician has become involved in an emergency situation. In the practice of euthanasia, however, it remains essential that the physician should be able to prove that the requirements for meticulousness have been fulfilled.

Until November 2000, however, all attempts to remove euthanasia from the Criminal Code failed. In 1984, for example, a Bill was submitted in which euthanasia would be legalized if the physician had acted in accordance with the requirements for meticulousness described above. As a result of the sharp religious and political divisions in the Netherlands, this Bill was not passed. In 1986, in an attempt to break the political deadlock, the Dutch government produced a very carefully formulated 'Tentative legislative concept', whose intention was to take the discussion on euthanasia a step further. In June 1994 a political compromise was reached in which euthanasia remained a criminal offence, the requirements for meticulousness were not elaborated further, and the physician was furthermore compelled to report every case of euthanasia (at the patient's request) or termination of life (without a request).

### Implementation of the guidelines

In 1995, the Dutch ministers of Health, Welfare, Sports, and of Justice ordered an evaluation of the reporting procedure to determine two outcomes: whether the goals for which the procedure had been set up were being reached and whether there were significant differences between the current implementation of the reporting procedure and that in 1990, when a similar investigation had been carried out. This evaluation involved interviews of a random sample of 405 general practitioners and specialists, as well as a written questionnaire circulated among the attending physicians involved in a sample of 6060 deaths selected from the death certificates submitted to the Central Bureau of Statistics for August–November, 1995. For both investigations, procedures were developed which guaranteed total anonymity of both the physicians and the deceased. The percentage of the total number of deaths that resulted from euthanasia was 2.3% in the interview study and 2.4% in the death certificates study. Assistance with a suicide had been given in 0.4% and 0.2% of deaths, respectively. These results agreed with those in 1990. In 0.7% of the cases, the patient's life had been terminated without specific request. A more intensive treatment of pain and/or other symptoms, probably resulting in earlier death, had been given in 14.7% and 19.1% of the cases, respectively, and in 20.2% of the total number of deaths a procedure intended to prolong life had either been stopped or not been started.

In all of the medical decisions concerning the end of life, with the exception of the termination of or decision to forgo a procedure intended to prolong life, cancer was the most frequent cause of death. The percentage of the instances of euthanasia and assistance with suicide which had been reported had increased from an estimated 18% in 1990 to 41% in 1995. Although this is a clear increase, these figures also mean that an estimated 60% of all instances of euthanasia were still not being reported. Cases of euthanasia without a specific request from the patient were reported very rarely.

In 1997, since the government's compromise with a reporting procedure had been shown in practice to be poorly adhered to by the attending physicians, the government proposed that every case of euthanasia should be judged by one of five regional committees consisting of physicians, ethicists, and legal specialists. Thus it was hoped that, even though euthanasia would continue to be a criminal offence, there would be more distance between the physician and its possible legal consequences.

Finally, the situation was clarified when in 2001 the Netherlands Parliament legalized euthanasia, though still under stringent conditions.

WHt, AJO

*See also* BIOETHICS; INFORMED CONSENT; PALLIATIVE CARE

**EVIDENCE-BASED MEDICINE** Medicine has long been characterized as an art as well as a science, but there has been a surprising lack of insight into the nature of the link between the two: How is science translated into the art of medicine? How do physicians keep up with new advances? How do physicians assess the validity and applicability of new evidence? The evidence-based medicine movement arose from the observation that new scientific data are often applied to patient care in an uneven and haphazard manner. Physicians may read medical journals, but not immediately apply what they have learned to their practice, in part because numerous studies that address a clinical question may arrive at conflicting conclusions. Physicians may reach their own conclusions based on what they happen to read, or learn about at continuing medical education courses, or they may rely on 'expert opinion' by assuming that experts have a more thorough knowledge of the evidence and the judgement to determine how best it should be applied.

With the rise of evidence-based medicine in the 1980s, expert opinion began to be questioned. Several key studies showed that experts were not always abreast of the most recent advances in medical research and were often selective in the evidence they relied upon. Proponents of evidence-based medicine believed that clinicians could evaluate the evidence for themselves and developed a systematic way for clinicians to deal with the information explosion in medical research.

*(continued)*

● If the patient is no longer able to express his wishes, but has previously submitted a written request for euthanasia, then this request may be looked upon as the expression of the patient's will, provided the medical practitioner is convinced that the request was made voluntarily and after careful consideration, and that there is no other solution to the critical situation in which the patient now finds him/herself.

● The medical practitioner must have consulted another medical practitioner who can be considered competent to render an independent judgement.

● The medical practitioner must record the procedure actually followed in a written report including at least the following: (a) the facts and circumstances referred to under points 1 to 3, inclusive; (b) the name and point of view of the other medical practitioner whom he/she consulted. This report must be retained for at least 5 years.

● If the patient is under 16 years of age, then the medical practitioner may not take any decision regarding the request for euthanasia until he has discussed, with the patient, whether or not the latter has weighty and well-found objections to involving his or her legal guardians in the decision. The patient's legal guardians must be involved in the decision unless, in the opinion of the medical practitioner and after having consulted an expert on the subject, the patient has weighty and well-found objections to such involvement.

Evidence-based medicine focuses on how science should be integrated into the art of patient care. It exposed the unscientific way that information transfer often occurred and offered what was claimed to be an 'evidence-based' alternative. This alternative was a framework to assess and critique medical research. Designed to empower the practicing clinician, evidence-based medicine has offered sobering insights into the quality of much of the current published scientific literature, provoked higher standards in clinical research, and has begun to illuminate the nature of knowledge development in medicine.

Evidence-based medicine has been defined by David Sackett, an Oxford professor, and colleagues as 'the conscientious and judicious use of current best evidence from clinical care research, in the management of individual patients'. Thus, when a question arises in clinical practice (such as 'Should medical therapy be recommended to prevent myocardial infarction in a 45-year-old woman with a moderately raised cholesterol level, who is otherwise at low risk for heart disease?'), advocates of evidence-based medicine advise that clinicians pose the seminal question: 'What is the evidence?' and follow three basic steps:

- access the best and most recent evidence

- evaluate it, and, if the evidence is found to be valid

- apply it to future treatment recommendations.

This three-step approach was thoroughly described for various types of clinical questions in a landmark series of articles published in the early 1990s by the Evidence-Based Medicine Working Group.

To access the best and most recent scientific evidence, advocates of evidence-based medicine have promoted the use of electronic databases, such as MEDLINE and EMBASE. They have popularized the use of search strategies and given generic suggestions for how to find one or two key articles from a literature search to address a specific clinical question. Although the initial search may identify hundreds of articles, use of evidence-based medicine protocols (including a preference for the use of RANDOMIZED CONTROLLED TRIALS and well-specified clinical outcomes) often narrow down the search to a few choice studies.

While it is fairly straightforward to undertake this assessment with one article, what if the targeted search strategy comes up with numerous randomized controlled trials that address the same question, have similar patient populations and outcome measures? Such redundancy in medical research is not unusual. This led to a natural part-

nership with other trends in medical research and information management at the time: the rise of systematic reviews and meta-analysis.

Authors of systematic reviews employ a methodical approach to analyze and combine the results of numerous studies on a particular topic to answer a clinical question that is based on the best available evidence. Results may be combined qualitatively or, in cases where study designs are similar enough, quantitatively. When results of numerous studies are mathematically combined, the systematic review is referred to as a meta-analysis.

There has been an exponential rise in the number of systematic reviews published in the past decade. The method of systematic reviews is still under development and methods vary among researchers. One of the leaders has been the Cochrane Collaboration, an international initiative to 'prepare, maintain, and disseminate systematic reviews of the effects of healthcare'. It has been likened to the HUMAN GENOME PROJECT with respect to its implications for medicine and medical research. It espouses evidence-based medicine principles and has made important contributions to synthesizing current research information, notably in such disciplines as obstetrics and neurology.

## Repercussions

The effects of evidence-based medicine have been widespread, profound, and, in some cases, disturbing. It has been increasingly incorporated into undergraduate medical education to the extent that learning search strategies for accessing recent evidence from electronic databases is considered a basic skill development in the first year of medical school. Critical appraisal skills are being integrated into the undergraduate medical curriculum. Evidence-based health policy is increasingly embraced at all levels of government. In short, it has become a new standard.

One of the more sobering effects of evidence-based medicine is that it has disclosed how much published research is of dubious value. By developing a system to 'sift through' the abundant scientific literature, evidence-based medicine is implicitly identifying many research studies that have important methodologic flaws, casting doubt on the validity of their findings. Most well-targeted search strategies will eliminate over 95% of published articles on any particular clinical question. For example, proponents of evidence-based medicine have established 'levels' of evidence, where randomized controlled trials are 'at the top' and, when available, suggest that studies with other types of research design be ignored. This has evoked outrage from some sectors in the research community; evidence-based medicine has certainly not been embraced by all.

Although proponents of this approach may seem imperious, the method of critical appraisal has revealed that much of the published medical literature is flawed, and that even the best evidence is often limited. As earlier noted, physicians who use the three-step evidence-based medicine approach can address answers to clinical questions if the identified studies pass the critical appraisal tests. More often than not, however, none of the studies pass all the tests — what then? For example, can the results of randomized controlled trials that were carried out only on men be applied to women? What if studies on a new treatment for a chronic disease were conducted for only 6–8 weeks — can a physician be confident about its long-term effectiveness on this basis? Another common dilemma arises when a study shows a very small, but statistically significant difference; is this clinically significant? Physicians faced with these situations still have to use their 'best judgement' to decide whether to base their therapeutic recommendations on this type of limited evidence. This is disturbingly akin to 'expert opinion' — the very thing evidence-based medicine was developed to avoid.

The greatest irony, however, is that it is itself based on surprisingly little evidence. If one poses the seminal question of 'What is the evidence?' for the validity of critical appraisal questions, the response is far from definitive. In the original series of articles, no justification or rationale — let alone evidence — was offered for the choice of critical appraisal questions. Certainly the questions appear to have 'face validity' — research methodologists would probably agree that these questions would identify weaknesses in a study design and therefore reveal threats to the validity of the findings. But are these the most important questions? Are any other questions equally or even more relevant?

There are some threats to the validity of studies that evidence-based medicine does not emphasize. In classic EPIDEMIOLOGY, for example, there are six criteria for inferring that an association might be causal: biologic plausibility, specificity of the association, consistency of the association, a temporally correct association, strength of the association, and a dose–response relationship. In the article on assessing non-randomized studies (often conducted to identify causation), only the last three of these six criteria are identified — why? No explanation was offered. Evidence-based medicine generally does not emphasize the importance of sample size calculations — a critical methodologic step to ensure adequate statistical power. Evidence for the validity of evidence-based medicine is sadly lacking.

The Evidence-Based Medicine Working Group has acknowledged that 'there is no correct way to assess validity'. Although the questions they pose are undoubtedly useful, there is no assurance that they are the only useful questions, nor that they are the most revealing. More important, there is no evidence that identifies the *relative weight* of each critical appraisal question. Thus, if a study does not meet one critical appraisal criterion, can the results still be valid? Generally, if no better study is available, then such results are accepted. This is the application of logic, not science. If a study does not meet two critical appraisal criteria, is it less valid than a study that does not meet a third? We do not know and logic cannot help. Again we fall back on expert opinion and making the best of the currently available evidence. This is an especially difficult problem in meta-analysis methodology; there is no comprehensive and valid method of giving relative weights to numerous flaws among studies with different weaknesses.

## Implications

Evidence-based medicine has not only revealed the limitations of scientific research; it has done nothing less than bring into question the very nature of scientific evidence. It touches upon the EPISTEMOLOGY of medicine — how is knowledge established? In doing so it has renewed efforts towards improving the rigor of scientific research.

There are definitive signs that evidence-based medicine has already been effective in improving the quality of medical research. Systematic reviews have abundantly identified common methodologic flaws in research design, as well as gross redundancies and gaps in addressing specific clinical questions. These are increasingly hard to ignore when considering future research directions. Systematic reviews are rapidly becoming the current standard for gathering and assessing evidence on which to base clinical practice guidelines.

Improvements in the reporting of research have been stimulated by this methodologic research. In 1996, the Consolidating Standards of Reporting Trials (CONSORT) Statement provided a checklist for the reporting of randomized controlled trials. It used evidence for its reporting criteria whenever possible, as well as a bit of what they called 'common sense' when no empirical evidence was available. The CONSORT Statement has been adopted by dozens of medical journals worldwide. Research into how to assess the relative weights of different studies when the results are combined in systematic reviews should be forthcoming.

Although evidence-based medicine was designed to help physicians deal with the massive amount of research that has been published, its greater contribution may be in promoting a deeper appreciation of how limited medical knowledge actually

## CRITICAL APPRAISAL

Evaluation of clinical research studies, often referred to as 'critical appraisal', is at the core of evidence-based medicine. It consists of looking for any threats to the validity of a study (such as bias that might arise from non-randomization, incomplete follow-up of patients, or inappropriate outcome measures); evaluating the certainty of the results (for example, determining whether the effect size has both statistical and clinical significance); and considering the applicability of the results to the current clinical question (for example, by examining whether the study population had relevant clinical characteristics).

To apply the example on p 294 to the final step, if a physician finds the key article on cholesterol-lowering medication and determines that it is free of bias and the study was conducted on a patient population that included 45-year-old women with similarly raised blood cholesterol levels, and the results showed a substantial reduction in myocardial infarction in a reasonable follow-up period, then the physician can confidently use this evidence to recommend the medication.

is. This has stimulated renewed efforts to improve the quality of research and identified the need to develop more rigorous research methods. In the meantime, *how* physicians apply scientific evidence to caring for patients remains, to some degree, an art.                                        PH

*See also* AUDIT; HEALTH ECONOMICS; JOURNALS; STATISTICS

**EXECUTIONS** By the end of the 20th century 106 countries had abolished capital punishment but almost as many continued to impose it — notably in Asia, Africa, and the Americas. In the United States the death penalty was used again in 1976 after the Supreme Court reinstated it and issued rules under which its application was constitu-

The electric chair at Sing Sing prison, New York State. (Reproduced courtesy of the Mary Evans Picture Library.)

Electric Chair, Sing Sing Prison, N.Y.

tional. In 2000, 85 people where put to death in the United States — 40 in Texas — all but five by lethal injection, and currently capital punishment is permitted in 38 states and also for certain federal crimes. Objectors to capital punishment have long maintained that application of the death penalty is uncivilized, revengeful, and barbaric — especially in the occasional bungled execution, such as when an electrocuted prisoner burst into flames or intravenous lines could not be inserted or maintained. It has also been argued that capital punishment does not deter crime but may actually promote it. Although 62% of persons executed in 1999 were white, it has also been suggested that a disproportionate number of minority members are being executed. Longstanding concerns about mistakes being made and innocent persons being put to death recently came to the fore when DNA testing revealed several instances in which death row inmates were shown not to have committed the crime, and several states have suspended the use of the death penalty pending further study. Yet polls in the United States have repeatedly found that more than 60% of people support the death penalty. Supporters point out that the death penalty has generally been imposed only for particularly heinous crimes, against children or women, with rape, and for mass murderers. Thus there was overwhelming support of the execution of the Oklahoma City terrorist bomber Timothy McVeigh, responsible for 168 men, women, and children dead and another 700 injured; and there was even considerable support for a proposal to show the execution in June 2001 on public television.

On general principles one would not expect health professionals to have a role in executions, although it was Dr Joseph GUILLOTIN (p 297), a physician, who developed a machine that he believed would be more humane than other methods of execution used at the time. But the issue of doctor participation came to the fore with the introduction of the lethal injection, when several state and federal authorities in the United States promulgated rules requiring medical professionals to be in attendance. This ran into vigorous opposition from medical (and also nursing) groups, which as early as 1980 passed resolutions prohibiting participation of doctors in executions. This view has generally prevailed over an opposing opinion that doctors have a moral duty to ensure that executions are carried out humanely and painlessly, especially since the procedures used in executions do not require the skills of a doctor.

Since 1991 the American Medical Association, the Medical Society of New York, and several other medical societies have issued guidelines clarifying what constituted participation. Activities thus defined included selecting injection sites; starting intravenous lines; preparing or maintaining execution fluids or devices; consulting or supervising lethal injection personnel or rendering technical advice; prescribing pre-execution drugs; attending, observing, or witnessing executions as a physician; monitoring vital signs during executions (including monitoring electrocardiograms); performing medical examinations during executions to determine if the prisoner is dead; providing psychiatric information about fitness to be executed; and soliciting or harvesting organs for use in transplantation. Determining that death has occurred during an execution also has the potential to require doctors' involvement, as in the case of a prisoner not dying immediately and the doctor having to signal that the execution process must be continued.

### Non-participatory activities

Activities not regarded as participation were: serving as a witness in criminal trials, advising about competence to stand trial, and relieving suffering or offering treatment at a convict's request, such as performing an emergency operation on a death row inmate, since this would prolong life, even though only for a short time. Certifying death after another person has determined or pronounced death is permitted, since it would not involve the doctor in the actual process of execution, nor would the carrying out of an autopsy following execution. These guidelines, now generally accepted, are consonant with the medical profession's mission to relieve suffering, prolong life, and do no harm.

Executions and other extreme forms of judicial punishment in many other countries display mankind's barbarous nature, and not infrequently involve members of the medical and related professions. In Islamic states that observe Shari'ah law, amputation of the hand (sometimes also the contralateral foot) is, it is claimed, a 'humane' punishment for theft because it is carried out by someone with medical training, under local anesthesia. On the other hand, few modern forms of execution are as barbaric and inhumane as stoning to death, the punishment meted out to adulterous women in Afghanistan under the Taliban regime.   GD

*See also* BIOETHICS; INFORMED CONSENT

## EXTREME ENVIRONMENTS

Our surroundings may be hazardous. If we disregard such things as smog or other harmful substances, breathed in, eaten, or drunk; dangerous animals; plant POISONS and toxic chemicals there still remain several purely physical causes of harm. Volcanoes, earthquakes, and fires represent significant hazards to people by reason of the enormous amounts of energy they liberate but we are concerned mostly about less violent causes of harm.

### Force and energy

The damage that physical forces inflict on the body is related to two things: the total amount of energy supplied, and the speed with which this energy is released. The human body has very limited capacities for absorbing or dissipating energy. The important events that expose people to massive amounts of energy are earthquakes and fires, but explosions due to LANDMINES or to terrorist bombs are all too common and also liberate large amounts of energy quickly. Land mines in particular have caused hundreds of thousands of civilians to lose limbs and made it difficult for many to earn a living. It is hard to find a more unpleasant modern example of physical forces on the body, although transport accidents account for more deaths worldwide.

Death is increasingly likely as speed increases, as the amount of energy produced is related to the square of the velocity, that is, twice the speed gives rise to four times the energy. This is even more considerable if very high speeds are involved; the effect of a high-velocity bullet hitting a limb can be literally shattering, causing widespread damage to tissues and fragmentation of bone, for which amputation may be necessary.

In the following examples of other types of physical effect, similar but smaller energy changes are the ultimate cause of damage, although not all changes are as severe or as sudden as the explosion of a landmine and some disorders are due to the body's response to damage or its attempts at repair.

*Vibration* Vibration may be involved in producing motion sickness, particularly when the whole body is affected, as in fighter aircraft. When localized, for example, to the hands of those using vibrating tools, it may lead to 'white fingers'. This condition is due to spasm of the smaller arteries of the hands.

*Motion-sickness* Seasickness is the best known form of motion sickness but perhaps not the most common, for many people are affected by motion in cars or buses. The organs that detect motion, called the semicircular canals, are situated in the inner ear. Disturbance of the fluid within them leads to the characteristic vertigo, nausea, and vomiting. It is possible to become conditioned to motion. Most people will not be affected by seasickness after three days, but some are made quite helpless and never seem to adapt.

Drugs may control motion sickness but may have unpleasant side-effects, such as dryness of the mouth, making swallowing difficult. Because it is hard to produce a standard dose of motion, testing such drugs is often inconclusive. As a result, the effectiveness of such remedies is largely a matter of personal judgement. When drugs are necessary, they need to be taken before any exposure to

## HUMANE MACHINE

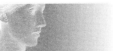

Joseph Ignace **GUILLOTIN** (1738–1814). French physician. Guillotin was a member of the commission investigating MESMER (p 487). After the Revolution he became the deputy for Paris in the Estates General. Guillotin suggested that it would be more humane to use some kind of machine rather than an axe for judicial decapitation. His idea was well received and Dr Louis, secretary of the Academy of Surgery , was ordered to design an instrument. It was first used to execute Pelletier, a highwayman, on 25 April 1792. Guillotin was a founder of the ACADÉMIE DE MÉDECINE.

motion. This is easily managed when boarding a plane or ferry, but not so easy in a shipwreck. Many ships now carry inflatable life-rafts, which are more easily launched than rigid lifeboats but have the disadvantage that their motion in the sea is violent. Most occupants suffer from severe motion sickness and will be unable to help themselves. A recent development, which may be useful, is the administration of drugs through the skin with a small patch, rather like a sticking plaster.

## Sound

NOISE is a cause of deafness and has led to regulations designed to protect hearing in noisy working conditions, either by limiting exposure or by using ear protection. The use of ear defenders when using a chain-saw is sensible and, incidentally, a good example of preventive medicine. However, not only chronic exposures cause damage. Temporary deafness may be caused by the sound levels reached in discos; while the very loud sounds of explosions or of gun fire may cause permanent damage.

## Light

The direct effects of sunlight (really of ultraviolet radiation) on relatively unpigmented human skin include sunburn and development of melanin pigment (tan). Sunlight is good for us in moderation but may be harmful in excess, especially for people with little natural melanin pigment. Without sufficient ultraviolet radiation exposure, we may not be able to synthesize vitamin D and may develop rickets in childhood or osteomalacia in adult life. However, adverse effects of excessive exposure to ultraviolet radiation include non-melanoma skin cancer, malignant melanoma, ocular cataract, and reduced efficacy of cell-mediated immunity (because the Langerhans cells in the dermis, which produce T-cells vital to immune defences, are damaged by high doses).

In the stratosphere, the action of solar radiation produces ozone from atmospheric oxygen. Ozone has a protective effect on the biosphere and its human inhabitants, protecting all living things from exposure to dangerously high doses of ultraviolet radiation flux, especially the extremely short wavelength radiation. Certain man-made chemicals, including chlorofluorocarbons and artificial fertilizers containing bromine, may destroy stratospheric ozone. In 1985, the effects of this destructive process were observed in a hole (actually extensive thinning) of the stratospheric ozone layer over Antarctica during the Southern Hemisphere spring. The hole has recurred every year and is getting larger. Since 1990 a similar region of seasonal thinning has been observed in the Northern Hemisphere, and is associated with increased surface-level ultraviolet radiation flux. Weather forecasts in Canada, New Zealand, Australia, and Britain, and some other countries, routinely include advisory messages about safe sun exposure times during the seasonal thinning.

*Lasers* are coherent beams of light. They are used in eye surgery, as the heat they give up on contact with tissue may be very finely controlled. Lasers have been used to reattach the retina, where this has become detached, and also to alter the curvature of the eyeball in those with excessive short-sight.

## X-rays and ionizing (nuclear) radiation

Radiation is beneficial as well as having potentially harmful effects. It is used in the diagnosis and treatment of disease, and similarly small doses of nuclear radiation are of value in clinical medicine to trace the working of the body systems. Small and usually harmless amounts of radiation exist in the environment, as natural radiation is given off by certain rocks and minerals. An example is the radioactive gas, radon, that may be detected in houses built from granite. There is an enhanced risk, albeit small, attributable to radon exposure inside dwellings.

Many regions of the world have climates that are intolerable from the physiologic point of view, yet people live there. The way in which they achieve this is by cultural and behavioral adaptation. Shelter and clothing produce a microclimate that changes less than the outside conditions. This allows physiologic mechanisms to operate within their tolerance limits.

## Heat and cold

*Hot climates* Body temperature is constant at about 37°C (98.4°F), and is actively controlled within a range of a few degrees. There is usually a balance between the heat produced in the body from food and the heat loss from the body in various ways. This balance may be upset, either by the addition of heat energy from outside or by greatly increased heat loss. There is then a net gain or loss of heat. A gain in heat causes a rise in body temperature (hyperthermia) and a loss causes a fall in temperature (hypothermia). Within narrow limits, these may be offset by sweating or shivering but body temperatures below 25°C or above 43°C may be fatal. The inability to sweat may lead to a rapid rise of body temperature known as heat stroke. A consequence of prolonged continuous sweating may lead to loss of salt from the body resulting in heat cramps. Extremes of temperatures, on the surface of the earth, range from about −88°C to +57°C and survival in such conditions depends almost entirely on adequate protection — for Inuit in the High Arctic, where temperatures may fall to −50°C, and for desert Bedouin, where they may exceed 50°C.

***Cold climates*** In countries where severe cold weather conditions are common, individuals learn how to avoid the more extreme forms of injury such as frostbite; this usually occurs accidentally. In temperate climates, such as Britain, the sea around our coast is cold enough, even in summer, to cause hypothermia and death within a few hours, if immersed unprotected. The fresh water of ponds, rivers, and canals in winter is usually colder than the sea.

An estimated two-thirds of fatal naval casualties during the Second World War died of drowning or exposure. At 15°C most unprotected survivors will die within six hours; the importance of finding them within this time is obvious. In polar waters survival times are much shorter, death normally occurring within the hour.

Much thought has gone into providing some sort of insulation that can be put on quickly before entering the water but more thought needs to be given to the entry itself. Jumping into water from a height of only 10 m may be a painful and dangerous experience.

A less common type of cold injury, first well recognized in the First World War, is trench or immersion foot, now commonly referred to as non-freezing cold injury. This is not like frostbite, in which tissues are damaged by being frozen. Cold, particularly wet cold, may affect the tissues directly by damaging nerves. It may also damage blood vessels, causing constriction of small arteries and even clots within the vessels. Fortunately, many cases recover completely but minor symptoms such as patches of numbness may persist.

## Electricity and magnetism

Lightning strikes, at potentials of thousands of volts, cause a few deaths each year but even household electricity at only 110 or 240 volts (domestic voltages in the USA and Britain, respectively) may produce a fatal shock. There were 27 deaths in England and Wales from accidental electrocution in 1990. Such accidents are particularly likely if the current passes across the body, when it may stop the heart beating. Dry hands or gloves and shoes with rubber soles protect. The outdoor use of electricity for grass- or hedge-cutting requires the fitting of a residual current device. These detect the leakage of electricity through the body to earth and switch off the current within milliseconds, preventing serious shock. Minor shocks may cause only surface burns, particularly if the hands are dry.

Minor shocks from static electricity are common in cars. The shocks may be prevented by touching a metal surface before leaving the car seat.

Indoors in low humidity conditions, walking on carpets made of artificial fiber generates large static electric charges that can create sparks several centimeters long on touching metal, such as doorknobs. The shock is quite painful on the fingers but can be discharged relatively painlessly by earthing the charge — that is, touching the door knob, with the back of the hand or the knuckles, which are less profusely supplied than the finger tips with sensory nerve endings.

Theoretically the magnetic fields caused by the flow of current through overhead power lines might affect the weak electrical activities within human cells. In spite of campaigns to expose the harmful effects (such as the allegation that these include childhood leukemia), careful studies have failed to find evidence that living under such power lines affects health.

## Air pressure

***Low pressure*** The air above the surface of the earth is acted on by the force of gravity. This makes it more dense at sea level and less dense at high altitude. The standard pressure exerted by this mass of gas, usually referred to as atmospheric pressure, is 101.325 kiloPascals (kPa), but other units such as atmospheres (atm), Torricelli (Torr), and millibars (mb) are occasionally still used instead. The higher one climbs, the less the barometric pressure and at a height of 5800 m it is roughly halved. At the summit of Mount Everest (8847 m) the pressure is about one third of an atmosphere. The gases which form the atmosphere are: nitrogen 77.9%; oxygen 20.4%; argon 0.9%; carbon dioxide 0.03%, and water vapor present in variable amounts. If air is breathed at such an altitude, the oxygen pressure is equivalent only to about 6.3% of 1 atm. This is why high altitude climbers often breathe oxygen instead.

This dependence of oxygen pressure on height is the reason for the pressurization of aircraft. Most civil aircraft are pressurized to give a cabin pressure equivalent to an altitude of 2000 m (80 kPa). Passengers sit at an altitude equivalent to that of Everest while breathing at the slightly reduced oxygen pressure of about 16% of 1 atm.

A potential fatal complication of low oxygen concentrations in the inspired air is pulmonary edema. This condition, which may attack climbers, particularly those not used to altitude (high altitude pulmonary edema, or mountain sickness), leads to increasing difficulty in breathing, because of the lungs filling with fluid. The cure is to descend to lower altitudes as soon as possible.

***High pressure*** Divers and pressure workers are both exposed to raised pressures, either in the sea or within tunnels or caissons. Each 10 m that one

descends in the sea increases the pressure by an atmosphere. These increased pressures have several side-effects.

One effect, noticeable at ten atmospheres, is a distortion of the voice. This 'Donald Duck' sound is due to the increase in density and hence the speed of transmission of sound within the vocal apparatus. In diving using mixtures of helium and oxygen, special devices have been developed to decode this distorted speech. At depths of 100 m (300 ft), the nitrogen gas contained in air exerts an effect resembling that of a narcotic drug. This was first noticed as several persistent but ill-defined problems. Divers at these depths were unreliable, sometimes seemed to have hallucinations, and often did not complete their tasks. The reason for this behavior was discovered in 1936 and the solution was simple: to breathe a mixture of oxygen with some other gas which was not narcotic. It is now known that nitrogen, argon, krypton, xenon, and neon all have narcotic properties, whereas helium and hydrogen are much less narcotic but may lead to other disturbances such as tremor.

**Oxygen use** Although essential to life, oxygen at raised pressures is poisonous to a wide range of organisms. For humans, the level at which this effect first occurs is at about 2 atm. It shows itself as generalized convulsions. Convulsions under water are particularly dangerous and have led to deaths. Prevention involves calculation and judgement. To avoid oxygen poisoning, one must avoid breathing oxygen at a pressure above 2 atm but to avoid asphyxia one must breathe over 10% of 1 atm.

The pressure of oxygen inspired when diving depends on the total pressure. This in turn depends on the depth. Using a 20%–80% mixture of oxygen and nitrogen (air) therefore allows one to go to a limit of 100 m or 10 atm, for at this depth the oxygen pressure is 2 atm. If one was to breathe pure oxygen this limit would be reached at only 10 m or 2 atm. Diving over a range of depths obviously requires using more than one breathing mixture, which must consist of oxygen in combination with another gas or gases, usually helium, or helium and nitrogen.

**Decompression** Decompression means passing from a higher to a lower pressure. Decompression illness has an indirect cause, for raised pressures cause gases to dissolve in the blood and tissues of the body. When the pressure is reduced too quickly, these gases come out of solution and form bubbles. These bubbles cause decompression sickness (also commonly called the 'bends'). Prevention is by decompressing gradually according to a regimen that depends upon the depth and duration of a dive.

The most soluble of inspired gases is carbon dioxide and the next oxygen. However, mechanisms exist in the body to transport and exchange these gases. There is no such mechanism for nitrogen. The body does not, however, consist entirely of water and, importantly, the solubility of nitrogen is some five times greater in fatty tissues. At a pressure of 1 atm the human body has dissolved in it some 800 ml of nitrogen, more in obese persons. Thus obesity is important in selecting personnel as this amount of gas is sufficient to cause decompression sickness in military air crew or in space walkers, who may be exposed to reduced pressures. Prevention in these cases is by breathing oxygen before being decompressed; this washes out the dissolved nitrogen.

The severe effects of decompression include deafness, paralysis, damage to knee or hip joints, and death. The prompt re-application of pressure, usually in a pressure-chamber, is essential to prevent or treat these severe effects. Worse outcomes may be expected with delay or inadequate recompression.                                    EEPB

*See also* MOUNTAINEERING; TRAUMA

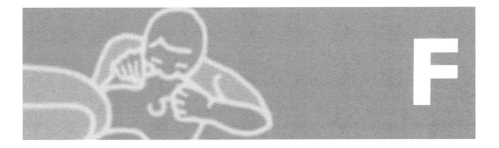

**FAMILY MEDICINE** See GENERAL PRACTICE

**FAMINE** is a serious shortage of food affecting a region or a large group of people over an extended period of time, resulting in hunger, suffering, and a marked increase in the death rate. There is something apocalyptic about famine. It suggests a calamitous visitation in the face of which mankind can only suffer helplessly. But there is a notable counter-example in the BIBLE. Joseph interprets the Pharaoh's dream as foretelling seven years of plenty followed by seven years of drought. Joseph is then commissioned by the Pharaoh to undertake what we would call food security measures. In this way, an impending famine is turned into a potential shortage, which is effectively met by building up strategic stocks of grain. Perhaps famines, or most of them, have always been preventable, provided timely action was taken to meet them. But, more commonly, famines have reflected a rather passive frame of mind, as seen in the tendency to blame the non-availability of food, rather than the absence of timely action to remedy the lack.

Famines are not simply caused by lack of food. During the Great Irish Famine of the 1840s, food was actually being exported from Ireland, and throughout the Great Bengal Famine of 1942, there were large food stocks in the state of Bengal. What caused famine in both cases was the people's inability to secure or acquire food. In simplest terms, they had neither the money to purchase food, nor the political power to command it. They quietly starved amidst plenty. The distinguished economist, Amartya Sen has shown convincingly that 'entitlement' and not availability is the crucial factor in whether or not people eat. In addition, he makes a striking observation. Democracies, he asserts, do not have famines. In other words, he goes beyond purely economic analysis to talk about 'the political economy of hunger', which suggests that hunger is not just an economic proposition concerning scarcity, but rather a political issue of who gets what, when, and how.

Historically, famines have been attributed to a sudden growth in population, generating an increase in demand that could not be met. Malthus summarized this proposition in typically 18th century rationalist terms. He speculated that if populations continued to grow geometrically, while food production grew arithmetically, there would soon be a gap between the population's requirements and the availability of food. Malthusian predictions of population growth have largely come true, but food production has more than kept pace with the population and today there is enough food in the world to feed every man, woman, and child. Yet, famine persists.

### In the midst of plenty

The paradox of famine in the modern world is that it occurs in the midst of plenty, despite tremendous willingness, at least at the humanitarian level, to assist people facing disastrous shortage of food. Although hundreds of millions still continue to lead lives of chronic hunger and malnutrition, the more acute and traumatic cases of starvation do not fail to elicit an international response: the news media penetrate the remotest parts of the globe, and it might be assumed that no population or group in peril would go unnoticed; the world community is willing to respond generously to the images of suffering that television can bring into our living rooms, and mobilize the necessary resources; organizations such as the World Food Program of the United Nations and a host of non-governmental organizations specializing in food aid are able to deliver food to the hungry quickly and effectively. It seems therefore that all the conditions necessary to banish famines exist. Then why do famines persist?

Our ability to respond to the threat of famine has increased dramatically, both at national and international levels. One of the best examples of national measures to overcome famine comes from India. Long subject to drought and famine, India now commands large strategic stocks of grain, thanks to improved agricultural production. This, combined with an admirably vigilant system of detecting early signs of famine, has rendered that scourge obsolete. In 1987, when the monsoons failed in India, a massive drought gripped large portions of the sub-continent. Yet India was able to cope with the effects of the crop failures that ensued without appealing for international assistance. The best recent example of international measures is the prevention of famine in Southern Africa. In 1992–3, the region suffered a massive crop failure as a result of the El Niño effect. Southern Africa, normally a food exporter, had to import over eleven and a half million tons of food, at an estimated cost of $4 billion, to avert a catastrophic famine. Only unprecedented regional co-operation combined with international assistance could cope with such a challenge. This was assured through collaboration between the Southern Africa Development Community, the donor community, the UN, and the affected states. Although each Southern African country chose its own approach to drought relief, government, UN agencies and non-governmental organizations pooled efforts, resources, and expertise to avert a disastrous famine.

Thus famines may be averted whenever national governments are sufficiently concerned about the welfare of their most vulnerable populations (as in a democracy), or where international action can be mobilized to avert a food disaster. The exception to this rule are cases where democratic concerns for the welfare of the people are absent, or where humanitarian access is denied to people in peril. It is still possible therefore to identify two particular sets of circumstances under which famines occur: under authoritarian regimes, and where political turmoil prevents humanitarian action.

Authoritarian regimes tend to hide the sufferings of their people from the outside world. This was the case in China during Mao's Great Leap Forward. The distortions imposed by that policy on the Chinese economy resulted in a catastrophic fall in farm production. Unwilling to believe that his revolution could fail, Mao hid this disaster not only from the outside world, but himself went into a form of denial. Provincial officials made wildly optimistic reports, anticipating their master's desire for good news. As a consequence, between 1958 and 1962, over thirty million people died in the famine that resulted. Perhaps a similar tragedy is unfolding in North Korea. The country has historically kept to itself, and does not welcome foreign intervention. In the face of agricultural and ecological disaster, its government continues to constrain access, and has found it difficult to admit that famine conditions prevail. It is a characteristic of such regimes that they can very easily stage-manage visits of outside dignitaries, who return from their tours to declare that they saw no evidence of famine. This is what happened in China in 1959; and this is what has tended to happen in North Korea. All signs suggest that a very considerable famine has been underway there since 1995. Similarly, modern complex emergencies also constrain humanitarian agencies from gaining access to large sections of affected populations.

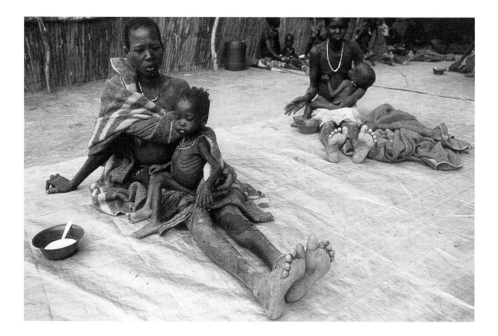

Malnourished women and children at a therapeutic feeding center in southern Sudan. (Photo: World Food Program/L. Gilbert.)

This is particularly true in areas considered to be in revolt against the central authority and where food aid is caught up in the politics of the region. It is not so much availability or entitlement but access that is the problem: how to ensure access to southern Sudan, for example, where, fueled by drought and war, famine returned to the Bahr el Ghazal province in the summer of 1998. While the international community was willing to airlift massive quantities of food aid to the region, access was either denied by the authorities or large parts of the south were rendered inaccessible owing to the conflict. Crucially, the Government of Sudan imposed a flight ban on much of Bahr el Ghazal during March 1998, crippling efforts to distribute seeds and tools at a critical time in the planting season.

### Balancing needs

The dilemma for authoritarian regimes or countries in civil conflict is how to balance the food needs of their people against what they perceive to be the tendency of the outside powers or opposition forces to capitalize on their vulnerability. For the donors, it must be a great temptation to push the political agenda in return for humanitarian assistance, especially if they consider that vital interests of economic or military security are at stake. Multilateral aid, provided through the United Nations, for example, is supposed to insulate such assistance from overt political influence. However, even multilateral assistance can become politicized if donors insist that 'their' resources not be used in aid for countries they do not approve of, or conversely, that their assistance go only to countries that they happen to favor. A pure humanitarian need does not always evoke a pure humanitarian response.

From an unavoidable calamity, famine has become a preventable disaster, taking place only when help is denied because of political considerations. An important question today is how to strengthen the reach of humanitarian assistance in areas affected by war or civil conflict; not that all would be well if access were secured. Even were this to be the case, international response would still be rather superficial — tending to respond late; to give too little; to pull out too early; or to pay scant attention to the fundamental causes of disaster. MHyd

**FATNESS AND THINNESS** In natural settings, moderate fatness in humans and other vertebrate animal species, particularly occurring on a seasonal basis, is an asset. Fat deposition is nature's way of banking surplus energy for mobilization in needy times. Over most of human history to be plump and sleek has been the cherished prerogative of society's privileged class. Some cultures deliberately fatten their rulers or their marriageable young women. European painters from Rubens to Renoir have portrayed naked corpulence as a symbol of fertility and sexual attractiveness. This widespread

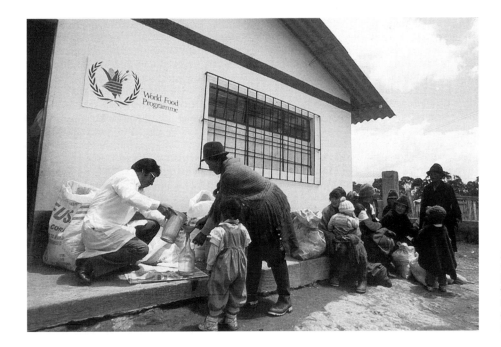

Mothers receiving food rations in return for bringing themselves and their children for care at health clinics in Equador.
(Photo: World Food Program/ R. Jones.)

cultural preference for fatness has origins in the prehistory of human ecology, in which hunter-gatherer food supplies were, in general, marginal. Indeed, food supplies have been precarious for most of human existence, with survival prospects finely balanced against the risks of famine and infectious disease.

Human biology, culture, and behavior have all therefore evolved over hundreds of thousands of years towards boosting the intake and storage of food energy. We have, in consequence, a biologically-based strong craving for 'survival foods' — energy-dense foods such as high-fat organ meats or depot fat from animals and sugar-laden foods such as honey. Biblical promises of good times referred to 'the land of milk and honey' or to 'the fat of the land'. In cultures everywhere, food and over-eating are central to celebration and festivity.

Given this evolutionary background, some genetically-based variation in tendency to obesity between individuals is to be expected. Indeed, studies of adoptees, twins, and intra-familial patterns of body weight indicate a genetic influence on obesity. This, however, should be viewed as a predisposing, not a determining characteristic; the critical determinant is the 'environmental' imbalance between energy intake and energy expenditure. Likewise, there may well be some differences between major population groups as a function of differential selection pressures in their ancestral populations in relation to the metabolic handling of energy. The role of genetic influences on body weight, both among and within populations, remains uncertain and controversial.

Among hunter-gatherers and in traditional human societies the three-way balance among the craving for survival foods, the limited food supplies, and the physical energy expended in obtaining food has meant that body weights fluctuate within a moderate range. Excessive weight gain in these situations is rare. Some additional homeostatic control of body weight comes from metabolic and hormonal pathways that stimulate eating and fat deposition in the underweight while constraining them in the overweight.

It is a remarkable feature of contemporary human ecology that, during the past half-century, we have ruptured this age-old balance. Urbanized human populations everywhere in the world are now rapidly becoming fatter. The explanation is simple: humans are taking in more energy than they are expending. Processed foods have become more energy-dense; consumer tastes (molded by modern advertising) have changed; and levels of physical activity have declined. The adverse public health consequences of this recent epidemic of obesity will become increasingly evident.

## Definition of obesity

'Obesity' is usually defined by the ratio of body weight to height-squared, the body mass index. In Britain the proportion of people who are obese (that is, body mass index exceeds 30) has doubled over the past decade and is now about 15%. In the USA the figure is higher, and approaches 40% in some segments of the population. In urbanizing populations in Third World countries the proportion is also rising rapidly. In Thailand, for example, the prevalence of childhood obesity increased by an estimated 35% over just two years in the rapidly westernizing city of Hat Yai.

Epidemiological studies have consistently shown that obesity entails markedly increased risks of high blood pressure, coronary heart disease, stroke, non-insulin dependent diabetes mellitus, various cancers (such as breast cancer, large bowel cancer, uterine cancer), and musculoskeletal disorders. Some recent evidence indicates that the rising prevalence of obesity may have contributed to the widespread rise in prevalence of asthma. There is, in general, no clearcut threshold for these increases in risk; in western populations the risks increase progressively as the body mass index rises above a figure of 25. Life expectancy decreases (that is, overall mortality rates increase) with increasing adult body mass index, particularly above 25.

## Central and peripheral obesity

Researchers have begun to clarify the difference between 'central' (or visceral or abdominal) obesity and that of 'peripheral', buttocks-hips-and-thighs, obesity — that is, the 'apple shape' versus the 'pear shape'. Central obesity is the major hazard to health. There is some evidence that certain populations may be constitutionally (presumably genetically) predisposed to central obesity — South Asians, for example. This pattern of body fat deposition appears to be associated with metabolic disturbances such as increased insulin resistance and altered metabolism of corticosteroids. Those metabolic changes then increase the risks of diabetes, raised blood pressure, and heart disease.

Nevertheless, healthy and moderately fat (but non-obese) persons may gain little in health or life expectancy by reducing weight. Indeed, there is some counter-evidence. For example, while overweight women are at increased risk of gallstone disease, that risk increases even further if such women undergo a marked reduction in weight. Some research indicates that adults undergoing weight loss may experience an increased risk of heart disease and overall mortality but other research does not. Perhaps the safest course, so long as extremes of body weight are avoided, is to maintain stability in adult body weight.

In general, dieting does not eliminate fatness. Individuals may lose weight under intensive (and expensive) regimens of weight loss, but they usually put it on again within two years. This does not mean that some individuals are unalterably 'fat'; rather, it means that obesity is a collective social problem. It reflects an imbalance in a society's culture and behaviors that makes it nigh-impossible for many individuals to break ranks: 'Obesity is a disease of society, and not of the individual'. Within developing countries, there is typically a positive correlation between individual or neighborhood affluence and body mass index. However, within developed countries, particularly among women, the reverse typically applies: the poor are more obese.

Meanwhile, fashions of body shape in western society, especially in females, change cyclically. In the 1990s, emaciated pubescent super-models helped spawn extreme dieting patterns in suggestible teenagers. There appears to have been an increase in the frequency of abnormal food-denial behaviors, often culminating in anorexia nervosa and bulimia. The risk to health from this extreme thinness is well known; young people occasionally die from self-imposed starvation. Minor levels of thinness, on the other hand, carry few risks to health — so long as future food supplies are guaranteed. Studies that have taken adequate account of smoking and of early (sub-clinical) disease, both typically associated with thinness, have found no increased risks of serious disease and mortality in lean persons of below-average body weight.

To complicate the story, evidence is accumulating that body weight at birth and in infancy may affect long-term risks of adult diseases. Somehow suboptimal fetal development, resulting in low birthweight, affects the lifelong 'setting' of various metabolic mechanisms that subsequently manifests as increased adult risk of DIABETES, high blood pressure, and coronary heart disease. However, much of that increase in risk is confined to those who begin life underweight and then become overweight in adulthood. Meanwhile, some other evidence shows that high birthweight and rapid weight gain in childhood foreshadows increased risks of certain cancers in adulthood, especially breast cancer in women.

The overall conclusion that emerges is that, to minimize the risks to health, not only is it desirable to avoid excessive gain or loss of weight in adulthood, but lifelong avoidance of such change is also desirable. Moderate variations in body weight around the healthy average have negligible health consequences. After all, part of the long prehistorical and historical experience of humans,

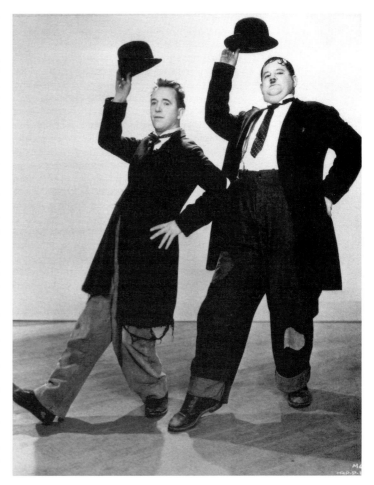

living in a variable environment, has been to fluctuate moderately in bodyweight. Within those moderate limits, human metabolic flexibility enables satisfactory adjustment — and maintenance of good health.                    AJM

*See also* DIET AND DISEASE; EATING DISORDERS; NUTRITION

**FIBROMYALGIA** See RHEUMATOLOGY

**FIRST AID** Everyone ought to have some knowledge of first aid. Lives can be saved in an emergency if bystanders know what to do about sudden cardiac arrest; spinal cord damage with permanent paralysis of the limbs may occur if someone with a fractured spine is moved carelessly; people may bleed to death, or choke on their own vomit if no one knows how to minimize harm until expert medical care is available. Boy scouts and girl guides, police, firemen, ships' captains, airline cabin staff, designated workers in

The thin and the fat. Stan Laurel and Oliver Hardy. (Reproduced courtesy of The Hulton Getty Picture Collection Limited.)

many industries, school teachers, and many in other walks of life are required or expected to have some knowledge of first aid and the relevant practical skills. Courses are offered to all and sundry, and advanced courses to selected groups, by organizations such as the St John Ambulance Brigade and the RED CROSS/RED CRESCENT.

First aid did not begin to become organized until the late 1700s — though a manual had been published as far back as 1633 (Stephen Beadwell's *Helps for suddain accidents*) and subsequently ready-made medicine chests appeared for sale. In 1767 some European cities — Amsterdam, Hamburg, Paris, St Petersburg, and Venice — formed humane societies to restore the apparently drowned. London followed in 1774, and, though not a founder member, John Coatley LETTSOM (p 242) was to be associated with it for the rest of his life. Over a century later, in 1887, the St John Ambulance Brigade announced its intention of training volunteers from the public in 'aid to the injured' at public events, a role they have continued in Britain and internationally ever since.

The most essential, practical, life-saving skills are cardiopulmonary resuscitation; the Heimlich maneuver; arrest of serious bleeding; ensuring that an unconscious person has a clear airway; immobilizing the spine, especially the neck, when a fracture or severe whiplash injury is suspected; and the management of burns and shock. It is easier to manage the less dangerous but distressing mishaps such as a foreign body in the eye, insect and animal bites, poison ivy rash, and a host of other everyday events when those dealing with them have some knowledge of what has to be done. Such people are also able to minimize the harm and prevent mismanagement of injured or ill persons. It is important to know what not to do, as well as what is necessary.

Cardiopulmonary resuscitation can and does save many lives. A person who has suddenly collapsed and is pulseless should immediately be positioned flat on the back on a firm surface. The airway should be inspected to ensure there is no blockage. The first aid worker administers mouth-to-mouth resuscitation by pinching the nose and blowing his own breath gently but firmly into the mouth of the victim. This is combined with intermittent firm rhythmical thrusts with the heel of the hand on the lower part of the breastbone. The timing of the mouth-to-mouth breathing and of the rhythmical pressure on the breastbone mimic approximately normal heart and breathing rates. The Heimlich maneuver can dislodge an obstruction, such as inhaled food or vomit, from the upper airway. The first aid worker stands behind the victim, clasping the victim firmly about the upper waist; he clenches both fists and thrusts

suddenly and forcefully into the upper part of the abdomen just below the margin of the ribs. The resulting sudden increase in pressure forces air out of the lungs and can dislodge the obstruction from the upper airway.

Both cardiopulmonary resuscitation and the Heimlich maneuver can fracture ribs if too much force or pressure is applied, especially to frail elderly persons, whose bones may be rather fragile.

A person with a suspected fracture of the spine, who is at risk of having the spinal cord damaged and thereby suffering an irretrievable permanent paralysis, must be kept absolutely still, immobilized until suitable splinting or purpose-designed padding is obtained. It requires several attendants to move the victim, whose head, neck, and body must be kept immobile while being moved.

Severe bleeding is best tackled by firm pressure over the bleeding point, or on the artery supplying that part of the body. Prolonged use of tourniquets should be avoided as these may cause paralysis or gangrenous limbs.

Suspected or known fractures and dislocations should be immobilized with splints and bandages.

The details of all these and many other useful first aid methods and procedures can be found in St John or Red Cross manuals that are widely available and also on the World Wide Web.

It is desirable, some would say it is essential, to have an elementary first aid kit in the home, and another in the car. This contains bandages, 'Bandaids', sticking plaster, disinfectant, and burn ointment, perhaps an anti-allergy remedy. It should be inspected and replenished with fresh supplies at regular intervals.                    JML

*See also* TRAUMA; VIOLENCE

**FLEXNER REPORT** In 1908 Abraham FLEXNER (p 258) was asked to report on the state of medical education in North America. Initially he spent some time observing the system at the JOHNS HOPKINS medical school (p 840), which he chose as a model; he then set out to visit about 160 'medical schools' in the USA and Canada. The *Flexner Report*, published in 1910, was harshly critical in pointing out specific deficiencies, both educational and financial, in many schools, emphasizing inadequate laboratories and libraries for the students; it urged the importance of close affiliation with a university. This provoked a sensational reaction, and within a few years many private schools he had described were obliged to close. The general scheme he advocated — beginning with strong foundation in basic science, then studying clinical medicine in an atmosphere of critical thinking, with incorporation of the medical school in a university if possible — was widely accepted not only in North America but

## Emergency Care Guide

**Call 911 for immediate help in life-threatening situations.**

### CPR*

Place victim flat on back on a hard surface.

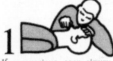

**1** If unconscious, open airway. Lift chin, tilt head.

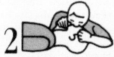

**2** If not breathing, pinch nose, cover mouth with your mouth. Give 2 full breaths.

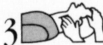

**3** Check carotid pulse. If pulse absent, begin chest compression.

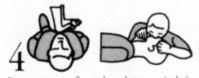

**4** Depress sternum (breast bone between nipples) 1½" to 2". Give 15 rapid compressions, followed by 2 full breaths. Continue until emergency help arrives

### First Aid for Choking

**Conscious Victim**

**1** If the victim can speak, cough or breathe, do not interfere.

**2** If the victim *cannot* speak, cough or breathe, give upward abdominal thrusts. Repeat until item is expelled or person can breathe.

**If Victim Becomes Unconscious**

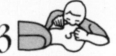

**3** Lift chin. Tilt head back. If not breathing, pinch nose, cover mouth with your mouth. Give 2 full breaths.

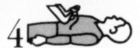

**4** If unsuccessful, give 10 quick upward abdominal thrusts.

**5** If unsuccessful, try finger sweep to remove object. Repeat steps 3 to 5 until emergency help arrives.

Two lifesaving first-aid procedures that everybody should know how to apply (CPR* = cardiopulmonary resuscitation).

also in British and European medical schools, a report on which he published in 1912 (see p 6).

*See also* ACADEMIC MEDICINE

**FLYING DOCTORS** After the success of powered flights in 1903, doctors soon exploited the aerial domain both for their own transport to their patients and for aeromedical evacuation. The first doctor to fly was Dr Constantinos [von] Economou, a Romanian-born doctor of Greek (Macedonian) heritage. He was one of the first aviators in Europe; while still a medical student in Vienna he undertook pioneering work in aeronautical research. He is best known for his 1917 description of lethargic encephalitis, or von Economou's disease as it came to be called. He was the first pilot to fly in the Austro–Hungarian Empire; and in 1914 enlisted as a volunteer in the flying corps. A 1976 Austrian stamp commemorates his pioneering contributions to neuropathology, clinical neurology, and aviation medicine.

Mail was carried in the air long before patients; and the first US air mail service was established on 15 May 1918 with a triangular run between Washington, Philadelphia, and New York. If passengers and mail, why not patients? In 1919, the Australian Inland Mission quarterly publication, *The Islander*, published an article on the potential of outback aviation; and in 1920, in the same publication, the Reverend John Flynn published a milestone paper — 'Sky doctor — why not?'.

By 1920, Dr Frederick Archibald Michod was flying regularly in the Queensland outback, visiting remote cattle stations and properties to give medical care. Based at the hospital which he had established in Longreach, he occasionally used his pioneering aircraft as an aerial ambulance. Together with Hudson Fysh, Fergus McMaster, and Paul McGinness he was one of the founders of QANTAS (Queensland and Northern Territory Aerial Services), and was appointed a foundation director in 1920. One of the first emergency mercy flights, specifically targeted as a flying doctor flight, was undertaken by Dr William Trethowan, who was flown by Charles (later Sir Charles) Kingsford-Smith from Perth to Carnarvon in 1922, a distance of 525 miles. That first flying doctor performed an emergency tracheostomy on the daughter of the District Medical Officer, Dr Hemsted.

The first outback flying doctor service was established by a legendary Presbyterian minister, the Reverend John Flynn, who in 1912 founded the Australian Inland Mission to spread the gospel and to provide hospitals and education in remote districts of Central Australia. Ministers of religion, so often acting as doctors in the outback, traveled by camel and horse and later used trucks. The dream of an aerial medical service remained unrealized, however, until the technology of the aircraft themselves developed, and an effective outback communication system could link doctors and their patients across vast regions of the hitherto communication-silent outback.

By 1925, 20 years after the development of sustained, powered flight, emergency medical flights were common in Europe; and many doctors had been airlifted and patients carried on the emergent transcontinental routes. The long-distance carriage of patients was recorded in Spanish planes, in this era, on the Madrid-Manila run. Nations with vast outback distances, particularly those of central Africa, Canada, and Australia, used aircraft on an *ad hoc* basis to carry the sick and wounded and the doctors who treated them.

The initial, informal flight of the Aerial Medical Service, a unit established within the Australian Inland Mission, was successfully completed on 2 August 1927, when Dr George Simpson, with Mr Norman Evans as pilot, flew from Mt Isa in north-west Queensland to retrieve an injured stockman.

## Pedal wireless

The essential ingredient in the establishment of a flying doctor service was the invention of the pedal wireless (radio), which enabled contact between a central medical base (and its pilots) and patients in the remote outback who were without power or telephone. The invention of the pedal wireless was the work of the South Australian electrical engineer, Alfred Traeger. It revolutionized communication in remote regions of many countries of the world, being a simple, inexpensive device using electricity generated by bicycle pedals. Pedal wireless was portable enough to be used at homesteads, mission stations, and mining camps. Initially aircraft were de Havillands (DH-50A), mostly chartered from emergent airline companies. In Australia, the first formal Flying Doctor flight (17 May 1928) was in a plane chartered from the newly established QANTAS Airways from the township of its origin, Cloncurry, in north-west Queensland (with Kenyon St Vincent Walsh as doctor and Arthur Afflick as pilot). In 1998, the Royal Flying Doctor Service of Australia operated 38 aircraft from 16 bases in Australia, employing 35 doctors, 83 pilots, and 14 radio staff. Like flying doctor services in many countries, 90% of its work is now to establish healthcare clinics in remote sites, particularly serving indigenous peoples. In Australia, this unique aerial medical service covers two million square miles or two-thirds of the Australian continent.

At the beginning of the 21st century, many countries are served by flying doctors. They include outback clinics in rural Mexico served by the Flying Doctors of Mercy, a volunteer service based in Santa Ana, California. There are several examples in Africa, for example, the flying doctor clinics of north-western Kenya, served by the Flying Doctor Service, which bring primary healthcare, vaccines, family planning, advice, and emergency trauma care to the Turkana people, a Nilotic tribal group of central Africa. In northern Canada, the government-run flying doctor service is critically important for doctors to reach isolated patients and for medical or obstetric emergencies to reach hospitals in the south. Dramatic advances in the

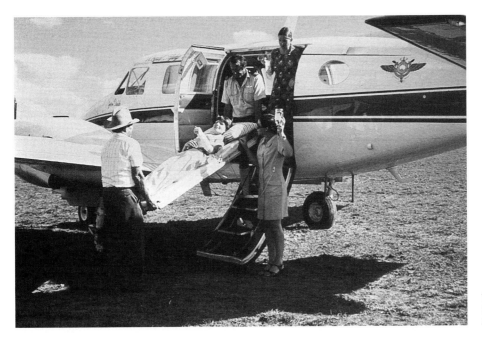

The Royal Flying Doctor Service on a mission in inland Australia.

technology of the last decade of the 20th century, particularly global satellite positioning devices and hand-held satellite telephones, mean that all patients of the future will be 'as close as the phone' to their doctor, irrespective of their location on the planet.                                                    JHP

*See also* AUSTRALIA; TELEMEDICINE

**FOOD AND DRUG ADMINISTRATION** of the USA (FDA) began just after the Second World War, when the first edition of the *Requirements of the United States Food, Drug and Cosmetic Act* was subtitled *A Guide for foreign manufacturers and Shippers.* This outlined legal requirements for importers. The FDA now enforces the laws enacted by US Congress concerning foods, drugs, and cosmetics. Before marketing it is necessary to obtain prior approval of new drugs from the FDA, and it exercises stringent control on imports. If a drug is marketed and turns out to be dangerous there are powers of recall of stocks, wherever they may be. Manufacturers of drugs in the USA have to be registered with the FDA. The objective is to ensure the wholesomeness of food and the safety and efficacy of drugs available to the public. The remit covers not only these but also labeling, directions as to use, appropriate warnings of adverse effects, advertising, and the prohibition of misleading statements. Drug manufacture and containers have to conform to standards laid down by the FDA. Biological products, cosmetics, animal products, medical devices, and electronic devices are subject to its control. It forms an excellent safeguard for the US consumer, though, as with any bureaucratic machine, it is sometimes pilloried for being over-cautious and making mistakes, and inevitably taking too long to reach decisions.

**FORENSIC MEDICINE** The description of 'forensic medicine' covers a wide spectrum of professional interests and, in fact, deals with any aspect of medicine which has an interface with the LAW.

The practice of clinical medicine itself gives rise to a legion of legal problems; foremost amongst these is medical malpractice and negligence. There is also a wide range of ethical and legislative matters, intertwined with a veritable jungle of administrative regulations which impinges on every aspect of the practice of medicine. The disposal of the dead, drug safety and regulations, consent, professional secrecy, disciplinary procedures, transplantation, compensation, reports, certificates, and a host of other matters confront doctors during their daily practice.

Many subspecialties contribute to forensic medicine, the major division being between those that are 'clinical', that is, they deal with the living patient, and those that are 'pathological', concerning the dead body — although a number, such as forensic serology and toxicology, span both groups.

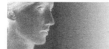
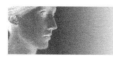
Historically, the oldest section of forensic medicine — forensic pathology — is certainly the one that gains most public attention, almost solely because of its central role in the investigation of homicide, although forensic pathology has a far wider range of interests than murder. Certain types of death attract legal investigation, whether they occur in a jurisdiction with a coroner, under a Procurator-Fiscal system as in Scotland, or a Medical Examiner system, which is increasingly used throughout the USA.

## The coroner system

Central to the work of the forensic pathologist in Britain is the coroner system (excluding Scotland, which has a somewhat similar Procurator-Fiscal system).

The coroner was established in AD 1194, as part of the fund-raising activities following the massive ransom required for King Richard I. The original wide fiscal duties have contracted down to a responsibility for the investigation of sudden deaths, although determinations on treasure trove remain a legacy from medieval times.

The modern coroner —who was introduced into many parts of the world, including the USA, during the British Imperial period — is usually a lawyer, but may be a doctor, some of whom also have a legal qualification. He is employed by local government, but functions under the Coroner's Acts and Rules laid down by Parliament. His basic function is to investigate all deaths that cannot be satisfactorily certified by physicians in the usual way.

These include deaths:

- where no doctor was in attendance during the last illness or within 14 days before death
- where the cause of death is unknown or the body unidentified
- due to industrial POISONING, VIOLENCE, neglect, ABORTION, drugs, or ALCOHOL
- during surgical operation or before recovery from anesthetic
- during police or prison custody

Over a quarter of the 600 000 deaths recorded annually in England and Wales are reported to coroners, and, in the majority of cases, the coroner will request an autopsy.

About 80% of such cases are due to natural disease, where deaths can be disposed of by the coroner by simple documentation, but the remainder, which prove to be unnatural, must be the subject of a coroner's inquest.

An inquest is a public court inquiry (in certain circumstances with a jury of at least eight persons), to determine by means of a 'verdict' or 'finding', precisely 'where, when, and by what means' a person came to his or her death.

Accidents and SUICIDES form the greater part of inquests, but medical mishaps, drug or drink deaths, industrial diseases, and a range of less common conditions are also dealt with.

Where death is due to criminal action, the coroner adjourns the inquest until any criminal proceedings are completed. If no suspect is charged, then an inquest is likely to return a verdict of 'unlawful killing'. In recent years, the coroner has lost his power either to commit a person for trial or to impute criminal or civil liability, so that his jurisdiction is now confined to a fact-finding inquiry, which, however, may be used as the basis for further action in other courts.

## The forensic pathologist

When a death thought to be caused by murder or manslaughter is discovered by the law enforcement agencies, the forensic pathologist is usually called in at an early stage. Where suspicious circumstances exist, the pathologist will be summoned to the scene of the death and will examine the body *in situ*, a most useful way of obtaining the best impression of what may have occurred. Many such deaths turn out to be innocent, in that the pathologist can declare them to be caused by accident, suicide, or even arising from natural causes; but where obvious or suspected crime has occurred, meticulous investigation takes place at the locus of the death. The pathologist will relate the position of the body to any blood splashes, marks upon adjacent structures, and the immediate environment of the body in a way that he could never do several hours later in the mortuary. He will study the clothing, especially if it is soiled, disarranged, or damaged, and interpret this in the light of his later autopsy findings. The presence of trace evidence upon the body may be vital and, with his non-medical forensic science colleagues, he will retrieve and evaluate any foreign material upon the body, which might have been lost if the body had been transported from the scene before expert examination.

The detective officers wish to know the identity of the body and often the best estimate of the time of death. The latter is extremely difficult, and much forensic medical research has been directed towards this problem. The body temperature falls after death from the normal 37°C and, theoretically, back-calculations from the temperature of the corpse at the scene should give the number of hours since death. Unfortunately, so many variables distort this calculation that any hope of accuracy is in vain. The initial temperature may be considerably higher or lower than 37°C, through fever, exposure, brain damage, etc. The physique, clothing, posture, age, and other intrinsic factors alter the rate of cooling, as do obvious environmental conditions such as air temperature, wind, rain, snow, and sun.

The identity of a body may also be an insoluble problem. Although most persons found dead are identified by relatives or friends, some victims of homicide may have been deliberately concealed to allow decomposition to render them unidentifiable. Sometimes mutilation or even dismemberment adds to the difficulties of identification, as does long immersion in water. Sometimes the body is partly or wholly skeletalized. The pathologist uses his anatomical and even anthropological skills to try to arrive at the correct identity. The following questions must be answered where possible. Is it human? Fragments or skeletal remnants may pose difficulties in this respect. If human, is it male or female? Depending on the state of preservation, anatomical differences in the organs and bones give the answer where obvious appearances cannot be relied upon. What is the age? In infants, children, and young adults the size and maturity of the bones can give accurate results, but in middle age and beyond only specialized techniques can get nearer than decades as units of estimation. What was the stature? Where intact, direct measurement is possible, although the corpse varies by several centimeters from the live height. Where only limbs or bones are available, anatomical formulae may allow approximate calculations to be made. The race may be vital, especially in these days of ethnic mobility.

The last, but vital, question is 'What is the personal identity?' All manner of features may assist, such as scars, old operations, deformities, tattoos, industrial stigmata (scars of industrial injury), head and beard hair, old fractures seen on X-ray, blood groups, teeth and dental work characteristics, signs of obvious pregnancy, old injuries, fingerprints, sinus patterns, etc.

Once the scene of death has been thoroughly examined by pathologist and forensic scientist, the body is removed to the mortuary and an AUTOPSY started. Many of the techniques mentioned above will be continued here, as the clothing is carefully removed and preserved for laboratory examination.

The pathologist makes a careful external examination of the body, which in cases of death by violence may be of more use in interpreting the nature of the trauma than the internal examination. However, it is the latter which more often reveals the exact mode of death. Any contributing factors, such as pre-existing natural disease, and the contribution of alcohol or drugs, are also evaluated. Blood and other body fluids and tissue samples are usually retained for analysis, and samples of tissues are commonly taken for later microscopic examination.

Modern advances in forensic techniques have added to the repertoire of the pathologist, who is no longer confined to mere inspection of morphological changes. Histochemical procedures may assist in determining whether wounds were caused before or after death and similar techniques may determine whether a heart attack, too recent to be detected by the naked eye or by classic microscopical methods, may have contributed to death.

In a criminal death, the pathologist has to interpret wounds, head injuries, gunshot wounds, stabbing, and more rarely poisoning, before preparing a report, which will be used by the prosecution in any subsequent criminal trial. Commonly, a second autopsy will be conducted by another pathologist retained by the lawyers defending an accused person. This second pathologist, although it is rare to discover much to dispute in the physical findings, may well have a different interpretation of those facts and may give testimony in court as to his opinions upon the findings, if they benefit the defence.

### Sudden and/or unexpected deaths

The pathologist seeks to discover the natural disease causing death and to exclude any unnatural process, including criminal action. About 80% of English coroners' cases fall into this category. The autopsy reveals the true cause of death in all but a few occult conditions, and this assists the governmental agencies responsible for constructing mortality statistics in increasing greatly the accuracy of their tables, for it has been shown repeatedly that causes of death given by doctors without the benefit of autopsy are incorrect in about half of all cases, the error being substantial in a quarter. In western countries, coronary heart disease and other degenerative conditions of the cardiovascular system account for the great majority of sudden deaths.

The most common cause of death in industrialized countries in men between the ages of 15 and 30 years is accident. Deaths due to road-traffic accidents now assume almost epidemic proportions in Europe and America, and are especially serious as they tend to involve healthy active people in the productive period of life. Forensic pathologists perform autopsies on the victims of traffic, domestic, and industrial accidents with several objects in mind. The cause of death and, more importantly, the mechanism of death are determined. Many accidents are unwitnessed or seen by persons with a confused recollection of the events. The pathologist's findings can help to reconstruct the accident, with consequent help to both the legal consequences and to preventive measures. For instance, the mandatory use of crash helmets for motorcyclists and seat-belts for motorists arose substantially from the findings published by pathologists.

(continued)

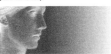

William **PALMER** (1824–56). British physician and poisoner. Palmer was trained at St Bartholomew's Hospital, London, and practiced in Rugeley, Staffordshire. He was found guilty on circumstantial evidence of poisoning his wife in 1854, and his brother and his friend James Parsons Cook in 1855. He was believed to have murdered thirteen persons in all.

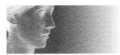

Buck **RUXTON** (fl. 1935) British medical practitioner and murderer. Ruxton killed his wife and nursemaid, then dismembered their bodies in a bath, extracted some of their teeth, cut off ears and parts of the face, as well as finger tips, all to make recognition difficult. The parts of the two bodies were distributed widely on moors near Edinburgh. The forensic investigation was brilliant in reconstructing the two bodies as the parts turned up. The mode of dismemberment showed that the person responsible must have had medical and anatomical knowledge since joints were neatly disarticulated and features were removed to make identification difficult. Search of Ruxton's house revealed hair and bloodstains in the bathroom and on various parts of the stairs, and human remains in the drainage system. Ruxton was found guilty of murder and was hanged.

Domestic accidents are almost as common as road accidents, and again the autopsy may reveal hidden or unexpected causes from disease or toxic states in the victims of falls, electrocution, fires, etc. The legal consequences include criminal charges, civil actions for negligence, and substantial insurance claims.

In industrial situations, the legal consequences are even more likely, with relatives and trade unions naturally keen to obtain the maximum compensation both from national schemes, as in the scheduled industrial diseases, and from the employers, via negligence actions for both injuries and disease. Coal-worker's pneumoconiosis from dust, asbestos and asbestos-related cancer, heart disease allegedly brought on by exertion, and a host of other claims make the autopsy upon a presumed industrial death most essential.

Although public and medical attitudes have changed radically in recent years, suicide still carriers a stigma. In Britain, changes in the law have made it no longer a crime to commit or attempt to commit suicide, and the coroner's procedure has been modified to make the investigation more discreet than hitherto, although undesirable publicity about what is basically a mental illness still occurs.

The task of the pathologist is to confirm the mode of death, to detect suicide where it is unsuspected or has been concealed, and to exclude criminal action. In addition, it must be separated from those masochistic exercises in men, which are accidental deaths, but which have been frequently mistaken for suicide in the past. The mechanism of death, especially if it be by an overdose of drugs or other poison, must be fully investigated. The prime function of the forensic pathologist here is to ensure that other modes of death are excluded so that an unwarranted verdict of self-destruction is not arrived at mistakenly. On some occasions this might wrongly invalidate a recent life insurance policy.

Death may be associated with medical treatment. When death takes place during, or soon after, a surgical operation or major medical procedure — or under an anesthetic — the case is almost always the subject of a medicolegal investigation. A forensic autopsy, coupled with a full appraisal of the clinical history, is important not only in interpreting the chain of events, but may also assist in preventing similar tragedies in the future. Where allegations of medical, surgical, or anesthetic malpractice are made, then the full autopsy findings are indispensable in getting at the truth. Similar importance attaches to deaths from untoward drug reactions and other mishaps in medical care, which all too readily lead to litigation.

Deaths in custody, whether in police hands or in prison, tend to be emotive events, often leading to accusations of mistreatment or neglect by the custodians. A full investigation, of which the autopsy is an indispensable part, is necessary to allay — or occasionally to confirm — these allegations

## Infant deaths

Deaths of infants are not medicolegal cases *per se*, but many proceed to forensic autopsies because of other factors. The most common cause of infant mortality after the first week of birth is the 'cot' or 'crib' death, more accurately known as the SUDDEN INFANT DEATH SYNDROME. Still little understood, it is probably due to immaturity of the respiratory control system, but a detailed autopsy is necessary to exclude other causes and to allay some of the self-recrimination that always attaches to the parents, who may think that death was due to smothering or some other untenable explanation.

Another less common cause of infant death is CHILD ABUSE, the so-called 'battered baby syndrome', and again the forensic medical investigation must exclude or confirm signs of repeated injury. Stillbirths are often examined forensically to differentiate them from deliberate infanticides. Deaths of mothers after abortion, now much rarer through extensive birth control and medical terminations of pregnancy, must be investigated if there is any doubt that the miscarriage was due to anything other than natural causes.

Other conditions requiring the attention of the forensic pathologist include deaths from self-neglect: chronic alcoholism and drug abuse have increasingly come into this category in western countries and have reached epidemic proportions in many large urban communities. In Britain a marked increase in both acute and chronic alcoholism has occurred in the past decade. Some 700 000 alcoholics are known to doctors, of whom a significant number die from the metabolic effects of long-term drinking, as well as from accidents, fires, and intercurrent infections brought on by their condition. The pathologist is often faced with these deaths, as well as those of abusers of many drugs and, latterly, youthful 'glue sniffers', who may suffer sudden death from the effects of inhaling the fumes of organic solvents.

In all these problems, and many others, the forensic pathologist has a wide range of ancillary disciplines to call upon for specialist assistance.

## Forensic odontology and toxicology

A young offspring of forensic pathology is odontology, the application of dental expertise to legal matters. The major contribution of the forensic dentist is in the field of identification, either in individual cases or in the mass disaster, especially aircraft crashes. The dental expert carefully records all the dental data from an unknown corpse and compares this with the dental records made during life, which can give a positive identity as good as that given by fingerprints, as long as ante-mortem data are available. Much of the evidence for the identification of Adolf Hitler, Martin Bormann, and Eva Braun, for example, was based upon dental characteristics.

Another task for the forensic odontologist is the matching of teeth and bite marks in assaults and murders. Marks upon the skin — and sometimes even on foodstuffs such as cheese or apples — can be matched with the dentition of a suspect, using tooth spacing, notching, and other characteristics.

Again a long-standing partner of pathology, the science of the detection of poisons is a vital adjunct to the pathologist. Although homicidal poisoning has declined greatly in advanced countries — perhaps in large measure owing to the efficiency of the toxicologists — the role of these specialists has increased greatly in relation to environmental, accidental, and self-poisoning. The experts in this topic are now almost exclusively chemists rather than doctors, and the complexity of their analytical methods has developed in line with the advances in scientific technology in general. However, the pathologist still has an interpretive part to play in fatal poisoning, as the actual laboratory findings on toxic levels in body tissues are often difficult to relate to the mechanism of death. A large proportion of the toxicologist's work now relates to therapeutic substances, and the distinction between medicinal administration and overdose may be difficult to evaluate.

Other disciplines that the forensic medical expert may need to call upon at times include anatomists and anthropologists, where skeletal remains need intensive study. Radiologists co-operate in these investigations on bones, and also have an important role in X-raying the victims of suspected child abuse and in searching for foreign objects at autopsy, especially firearm missiles and bomb fragments. Photography and video are also used extensively, for both teaching purposes and the recording of evidence; many pathologists are themselves proficient photographers, and many forensic scientists are expert document examiners, skilled, for example, in detecting forgery.    BJK

*See also* MURDER; TRAUMA; VIOLENCE

Michel **FOUCAULT** (1926–84). French philosopher and historian. Arguably the most influential intellectual of the last generation, Michel Foucault paid particular attention to medicine (understood in its widest sense). Thus his influence did much to shape today's critical

thinking about medical knowledge, power, and the body. A surgeon's son, he received his philosophical training at the École Normale Supérieure in Paris. Later he did voluntary service in organizations assisting mental patients, and this bred in him highly a critical outlook on the scientific agendas and methods adopted by the medical and psychiatric professions. His positions, in many ways, coincided with those embraced by anti-psychiatry. While distancing himself from Marxism, Foucault was to be lastingly concerned with the mechanisms of domination.

His first major work was *La folie et la deraison: Histoire de la folie á l'age classique* (1961), a much abridged translation of which appeared under the title *Madness and civilization: a history of insanity in the age of reason* (1965). Brilliant but demanding, this work turned the standard 'whiggish' history of PSYCHIATRY on its head. Instead of tracing, as was conventional, a progression from neglect to care, from ignorance to science, from brutality to therapy, Foucault maintained that psychiatry had never actually 'freed' the insane. Rather it had secured them in institutions and within the straitjacket of its own diagnostic categories. In medieval times, lunatics had been accepted in society and had had a voice of their own, their own truths to tell. First the rise of madhouses and then the discipline of psychiatry had excluded the insane and silenced them. So-called 'humanitarian' currents within psychiatry — notably the 'moral therapy' which had emerged around 1800 through PINEL (p 77) and the York Retreat, and the later development of PSYCHOANALYSIS and psychotherapy — were in reality more menacing bastilles of the mind.

If *La folie et la deraison* surveyed therapeutic structures from an essentially Romantic standpoint, drawing upon the insights of Rousseau, Nietzsche, and Artaud, *The birth of the clinic: an archaeology of medical perception* (1973) tendered a less visionary but more compelling analysis of the transformation of medical theory and practice from the late 18th to the mid-19th century. Through the development of the 'medical gaze', associated with the prestigious practice of pathological anatomy as conducted in the huge Paris hospitals, clinical medicine abandoned its old dependence upon patient-centered, subjective diagnosis. Instead, it had become disease-based in its search for truth, and exploiting new diagnostic technology (notably the stethoscope) and the routine conduct of the post-mortem.

The notion of a 'gaze' through which experts would exercise objective professional control (*savoir/pouvoir*; knowledge/power) became central to Foucault's thinking in the 1970s. It found further expression in *Discipline and punish: the birth of the prison* (1977), which explored the transformation of the prison and similar panoptic institutions around the turn of the 19th century. Foucault drew attention to the intensification of power which arose from the foresaking of brutal punishments directed against the criminal's body (whipping, torture, executions) and their replacement by such subtler controling mechanisms as solitary confinement, work discipline, and constant surveillance, all aimed at monitoring the mind or psyche.

The changing fate of the body under regimes of power was a theme central also to Foucault's final, biggest, and unfinished project. This was a history of sexuality, initially announced as a six-volume enterprise. In the first volume, *La volonté de savoir* (1965), translated as *The history of sexuality* and subtitled *An Introduction* (1979), he once again turned the standard historiography on its head. The approved telling of the history of sex — a stirring tale of Freudian liberation from traditional Christian and Victorian prudish repression — was, he argued, self-serving and self-deceptive. In truth, the powers which had traditionally policed sex, far from repressing and silencing it, had actually 'produced' it. This it achieved largely through the creation, via sexological theories, of such identities as the hysterical woman, the homosexual man, and the pervert. As ever, he repudiated 'essentialist' or biologistic readings, insisting on the 'discursive' nature of sexual reality.

Subsequent volumes examined sexuality in antiquity, when it was primarily understood and regulated in terms of what were called the 'techniques of the self'. This reflected Foucault's growing preoccupation with the history and understanding of the body in general, and with the possibility of an 'esthetics of the self' as an alternative to the modern ascription of identities, disease categories, and diagnostics by the professions, with their claims to scientific authority.

Foucault's outlooks were characterized not just by a repudiation of naked power but by a distrust of the Enlightenment and modern faith in the emancipatory powers of reason, science, and liberal individualism. He regarded humanism as an illusion and error — the remnants of an ideology shattered by the decentering of man accomplished by the theories of DARWIN (p 214), Nietzsche, and FREUD (p 321). Proclaiming in addition 'the death of the author', he sometimes wrote as if he believed that 'mankind' should be treated primarily as a category posited by overarching structures of discourse and language — explaining why he has commonly been associated with Structuralism and Postmodernism. Critics have accused Foucault of being wilfully bleak, and his critiques of the liberal professions, including medicine, have been judged unbalanced

and even paranoid. As for himself, he considered his stance to be dictated by ruthless honesty. RPor

**FOUNDATIONS** The Greeks and Romans established foundations and they have existed since the Middle Ages in Europe and the Arab world. There are now hundreds of these entities scattered around the globe differing widely in auspices, purpose, size, and complexity. Many support biomedical and health related research but some confine their grants to a single disease, locality, or type of care. However, only in the 20th century did wealthy industrial magnates create the largest of these, with their independent boards and professional staffs. Medical and health matters, the subject of this review, have benefited enormously from their largesse but overall education and agriculture have been the major recipients.

Financial support for individuals and institutions is the usual means for achieving each donor's objectives, as interpreted by successive generations of trustees and staff. When the two are combined, their influence is greatest but diverse forms of mentoring by foundation officers have also been influential. In the academic world the apostolic power derived from the original philanthropist is usually of greater currency than mere money. To fritter away either on ephemeral schemes advanced by dedicated enthusiasts or tackle too many problems simultaneously (what the foundation world calls 'scatteration') is to deplete intellectual and pecuniary capital. Foundations can succumb readily to such demands when they lack a sense of history and clear visions of needs and opportunities based on careful analyses of root causes; few have escaped such temptations from time to time.

Over the decades foundations have had an important influence on biomedical research, patient care, and health services organization. Interests and accomplishments vary; the seven foundations with the longest records in medical philanthropy are: Milbank, Carnegie, ROCKEFELLER (p 316), Commonwealth, Kellogg, Josiah Macy Jr, and WELLCOME (p 316). Their more recent and often larger counterparts have yet to generate similar accomplishments.

From its inception the Milbank Memorial Fund, established in New York in 1905, has supported epidemiology, demography, and economics as essential population-based disciplines for illuminating health, medical, and social problems and policies. To disseminate concepts, methods, and research bearing on these matters the fund has published since 1923 the widely respected *Milbank Quarterly*. This small foundation has contributed greatly to, for example, delineating the extent of

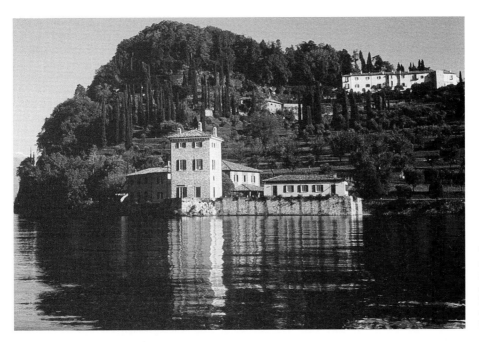

The Villa Serbelloni at Bellagio on Lake Como, used by The Rockefeller Foundation for conferences and for scholars in residence. (Reproduced courtesy of The Rockefeller Foundation.)

community mental health distress and the adequacy of needed services; analyses of fertility and nutritional influences on health and disease; and health manpower studies in Latin America. More recently the fund has had an important program supporting clinical epidemiology in American medical schools based on postgraduate education of young clinicians at the London School of Hygiene and Tropical Medicine.

Health policy reviews constitute Milbank's latest investment. Panels composed of representatives of the public and private sectors 'evaluate and synthesize information about an important issue in health affairs … and determine the implication for policy'. Findings are used to stimulate further 'research that could lead to practical responses to important questions about policy'.

Andrew Carnegie's many endowments included two that influenced the course of medicine throughout the 20th century. The Carnegie Foundation for the Advancement of Teaching, established in New York in 1905, supported Abraham FLEXNER'S (p 258) landmark study, *Medical education in the United States and Canada*, in which he argued that medical schools should be university-based with full-time faculties dedicated to science-based research, education, and patient care. The second entity, the Carnegie Corporation of New York, established in 1911, has had interests in health that have focused primarily on children.

Most of their grants have been to American institutions, but a small percentage has been to others in present or former British Commonwealth countries.

An important contribution was the early funding in collaboration with the Commonwealth Fund of the innovative Clinical Scholars Program. Over 600 young clinical faculty have received postgraduate education in epidemiology, economics, the social sciences, and health services research. The goal is to develop a cadre of physicians equipped to organize and assess health services to meet individual and collective medical needs appropriately, effectively, and efficiently.

The Rockefeller Foundation, established in New York in 1913, is recognized widely for its enduring international interests in medicine. The budget devoted to these has varied over the decades but the commitment persists and John D. ROCKEFELLER'S (p 316) credo continues to guide its policies: 'The best philanthropy involves a search for causes and an attempt to cure evils at their source'. His own early donations included initial support for the JOHNS HOPKINS UNIVERSITY (p 840) and the Rockefeller Institute for Medical Research (now Rockefeller University). Among the global scourges whose control or amelioration was funded in the earliest years by his foundation were hook-worm disease, MALARIA, SCHISTOSOMIASIS, and especially YELLOW FEVER, for which a vaccine

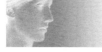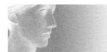

## BEHIND FOUNDATIONS

John Davison
**ROCKEFELLER**
(1839–1937). American industrialist and philanthropist. Soon after the first US oil well was drilled in Pennysylvania he began to invest in oil production enterprises, building refineries, and distributing the products. He founded the Standard Oil Company of Ohio in 1870. This expanded over the nation, and included other manufacturing and transportation interests, which yielded immense wealth to him. About the end of the century he turned his attention to philanthropy, and on the advice of his friend and clergyman, Frederick T. Gates, founded the Rockefeller Institute for Medical Research in New York City in 1904. Later he established the General Education Board and the Rockefeller Foundation, agencies which contributed to biomedical research, medical education, and control of world health problems, such as malaria, yellow fever, and malnutrition.

Sir Henry Soloman
**WELLCOME** (1853–1936). Anglo-American patron of science and medicine. With his compatriot, E. M. Burroughs, he founded the pharmaceutical firm of Burroughs Wellcome in 1880. In 1924 he endowed the Wellcome Trust. He was naturalized a British citizen in 1910 and elected fellow of the Royal Society in 1932.

was developed in 1935 by Max Theiler, later a NOBEL PRIZE recipient.

Warren Weaver, a long-time staff officer (1932–59), and for his last five years vice-president of natural and medical sciences, encouraged 'the application of the whole range of scientific tools and techniques, and especially those which had been superbly developed in the physical sciences, to the problems of living matter'. He coined the term 'molecular biology'. It has dominated medical and biological research and education to this day. Academic medicine's single-minded emphasis on disease mechanisms has brought enormous benefits to mankind, but it has been associated with diminished concern for optimal patient care and large imbalances in medical manpower and health services systems.

### Population-based research

The foundation has long recognized that, in addition to laboratory research at the molecular level of disease and clinical research with patients, population-based research, in which patterns of disease, behavior, and environmental influences are studied in communities, is also necessary. So great were the needs to improve the public's health and so great was neglect of these needs by medical schools that in 1918 the Rockefeller Foundation embarked on an important new initiative to establish schools of public health apart from schools of medicine. The Johns Hopkins University was first, followed by a second in 1921 at Harvard, and then 22 more in 17 North American, European, Latin American, and Asian countries. Much good resulted and the population-based disciplines flourished as never before.

International fellowships, 'backing brains' of potential leaders, as one Rockefeller trustee put it, have been a continuing foundation tradition since 1914. The subsequent careers of thousands of academic physicians and medical scientists worldwide have justified fully their selection for these prestigious awards. Examples of other foundation grants were to H. W. FLOREY (p 52) for developing clinical uses of penicillin; to Wilder PENFIELD (p 138) for the establishment of his world-renowned Montreal Neurological Institute; for creation of the first ultra-centrifuge; for early work on the mass spectrometer; and for the establishment of full-time departments of psychiatry in prominent North American medical schools.

A 20-year Rockefeller program launched in 1963 sought to strengthen leading universities in Africa, Latin America, and South-East Asia, including support for their medical schools. Establishment of community health clinics in rural areas provided educational venues to which students were assigned with the intention of broadening their perspectives and fostering community medicine. More recently

the foundation supported a network of university laboratories in the developed world for fundamental research on the great neglected diseases (diarrhea, acute respiratory infection, iodine deficiency, etc.) that kill millions in the developing world. A second initiative, joined by the WORLD HEALTH ORGANIZATION and the United Nations Children's Fund, was a global campaign to immunize and protect the world's children against preventable diseases that also take a heavy death toll.

The longest running and largest investment yet made by the Rockefeller Foundation is in the ongoing International Clinical Epidemiology Network. Conceived in 1978, it seeks to restore the population perspective to medicine alongside the molecular and clinical. About ten young clinicians, statisticians, economists, and social scientists from medical schools in the developing world are trained to the master's level in the concepts and methods of epidemiology in six universities in Australia, Canada, and the United States. Under the sponsorship of a recognized leader in their own medical school, usually the dean or a clinical department chair, the fellows establish a clinical epidemiology unit. In 1998, this rapidly enlarging network consisted of 52 units in 25 countries that conducted research directed at deploying science-based interventions and medical resources in ways that optimize their impact on the entire populations served. At regional and global meetings, often with the International Epidemiological Association (also supported since 1954 by the foundation), members and colleagues present research findings and discuss educational and policy innovations.

Not all the foundation's officials have agreed with its decisions. Alan Gregg, long-time legendary officer, and for his final five years vice-president for medical sciences, observed that the two worst mistakes the Rockefeller Foundation ever made were establishing schools of public health apart from the mainstream of scientific medicine in medical schools and backing Freudian PSYCHOANALYSIS as the 'scientific' underpinning for psychiatry.

In 1959 the Villa Serbelloni in Bellagio on Lake Como was bequeathed to the Foundation as an international resource for conferences and residencies awarded competitively to scholars, artists, composers, scientists, and others, including many physicians. Bellagio conferences bearing on medical matters include those credited with launching the Green Revolution, population control, the World Bank's interest in health and nutrition, and the global International Clinical Epidemiology Network. Others have addressed specific diseases or aspects of healthcare, especially problems in developing countries.

The Commonwealth Fund, established in New York in 1918, with a mandate 'to do something for the welfare of mankind', has strongly supported medical and related activities since its inception. Child welfare and health were its earliest concerns. These were broadened to include rural health problems in America and support for state health departments and community hospitals. The latter paved the way for the 1946 Hill-Burton Act, which supported aggressive hospital building throughout the United States. At the end of the 20th century the unintended consequences were an over-supply of hospital beds and an unduly expensive hospital-based healthcare system.

Other fund investments have included support of George N. PAPANICOLAOU (p 740) for development of his life-saving test for cervical cancer and, more recently, of the first hospice in the United States. Rational integration of medical care was pioneered in the United States by the Commonwealth Fund's support of the Rochester Regional Hospital Plan that linked six leading urban hospitals with 20 smaller ones in surrounding communities. In the 1960s Case Western University, supported by the Commonwealth Fund, carried out the first complete medical curriculum revision since Flexner's report. Changes adopted sought to integrate the basic and clinical disciplines and to bring students into contact with patients in their first year of medical education. Similar programs and objectives in several other medical schools sought to develop so-called comprehensive medicine.

### Supporting sabbaticals

Probably the Commonwealth Fund's greatest impact was its support over 30 years of some 340 American Commonwealth Fund Fellows in Medicine, who were exposed to other ideas, disciplines, and cultures during sabbaticals spent largely in Europe. The roster reads like a 'who's who' of academic medicine's leaders in the United States. Another program supporting innovations in hospitals to make the staff and services more 'patient-centered' has changed attitudes and emphases in many health service entities. In recent years the fund's focus has broadened to include more explicit attention to the problems of the elderly, women, children, and minorities in obtaining medical services. Healthcare policy studies are of increasing interest to the fund and its international Harkness Fellowship program now brings young scholars from Britain and the Antipodes to the United States for study and discussions with their counterparts.

The W. K. Kellogg Foundation, established in Battle Creek, Michigan, in 1930, was to 'use the money as you see fit so long as it promotes the health, happiness, and well-being of children'. Its earliest Michigan Community Health Project opened health departments, began screening programs for children, and trained public health nurses for home visits in many of that state's poorer counties. Later the foundation's interest spread to improving the education of physicians and other health workers in Latin America. The main focus in the 1950s and 1960s was support of university-based education for health services and hospital administrators. In recent years the theme of community development has been prominent, including efforts to encourage health services directed at meeting the needs of entire communities through support of what is referred to as comprehensive community-oriented primary care. More specifically, Kellogg's grants support the building of formal partnerships between schools of public health, health departments and community health services agencies.

### Relief of suffering

The Josiah Macy Jr Foundation, established in New York in 1930, was directed by the founder to 'devote its interest to the fundamental aspects of health, of sickness, and methods for the relief of suffering'. It has supported activities such as biomedical research, psychiatry, faculty development, and minority student recruitment. About 70% of the Macy Foundation's awards have been made for innovations in the education of physicians.

Macy is best known for its long tradition of publishing the findings of influential conferences on a wide variety of medical topics. Several of the most recent have dealt with the problems of improving understanding of the synergistic roles of medicine and public health, especially in the education of medical, public health, and nursing professionals.

The Wellcome Trust, established in London in 1936, has a long history of funding biomedical research in Britain and is now the largest non-governmental source of such support in Europe. Investigators and their institutes studying tropical diseases in developing countries are a special focus. Another important beneficiary continues to be the former Wellcome Institute for the History of Medicine in London, though this now comes under The Wellcome Trust and has changed its affiliation. In 1993 the Wellcome Trust established a completely independent American counterpart, the Burroughs Wellcome Foundation, in the Triangle Park, North Carolina. It too supports biomedical research in the United States and Canada, especially that by young investigators.

In 1948 the Pew Charitable Trusts were established in Philadelphia to 'contribute to the public's health and welfare and strengthen the communities in which we live'. For almost three decades their grants were given anonymously but gradually policies and procedures were formalized as national interests emerged and its first annual report was issued in 1979. Among Pew's most important recent initiatives has been the continuing support of a health professions commission that examines the opportunities and challenges related to the education, distribution, and practice arrangements of physicians, nurses, dentists, and others. The Health of Populations Program, jointly funded with the Rockefeller Foundation, supports projects to re-direct medical education, so that physicians understand the need to provide appropriate care for all citizens through more balanced deployments of ambulatory primary care, hospital-based tertiary care, and other caring modalities.

The Henry J. Kaiser Family Foundation, established in Menlo Park, California, in 1948, is among the large foundations devoted exclusively to health. It has supported conferences and analyses of a wide range of health policy issues; and applied research to define and measure public health problems, demonstration projects, and communication activities. One of its more influential publications, *Dear doctor* by Charles E. Odegaard, president emeritus of the University of Washington, argued forcefully that all physicians should listen attentively and 'carefully' to what patients experience and require; attributes that seem in short supply today.

## Scientific study of man

The Ford Foundation, established initially in 1936 for local philanthropic purposes in Michigan, was transformed in 1950 on receiving the proceeds from huge Ford family estates into a very large entity based in New York with vast global programs. Population growth and food supply, especially in developing countries, as with Rockefeller and Kellogg, have been major concerns that impinge on health and disease. Its program 'the scientific study of man' has included matters relating to health. Over the decades the foundation has supported projects to help the disadvantaged, minorities, children, adolescents, and the elderly, especially in the developing world. Under the umbrella title of Human Development and Reproductive Health, the Ford Foundation currently funds activities that address social, economic, and cultural factors influencing sexuality and reproductive health.

The Wolfson Foundation, established in London in 1955, is one of the largest in the United Kingdom. Since the Wolfson Foundation's inception it has supported many scientific and medical activities including centers and institutes dedicated to biomedical research and to education.

The Nuffield Trust (formerly the Nuffield Provincial Hospitals Trust), established in London in 1940, has played a significant part in the evolution of health services in both the United Kingdom and the United States. For over four decades the Nuffield Trust has published volumes on the organization, financing, and evaluation of healthcare. These reports, based on conferences, seminars, lectures, and research sponsored by the trust, have defined problems, raised questions, set standards, and advanced ideas about health services that transcend national boundaries.

The Robert Wood Johnson Foundation, established in Princeton, New Jersey in 1972, is the largest American philanthropy devoted solely to supporting domestic research and educational activities designed to improve access, costs, quality, and management of health services. It does not support biomedical research. During its first quarter century many facets of the country's abundant healthcare problems have been tackled. The continuing clinical scholars program, mentioned earlier, has been a major undertaking. Competitive awards for clearly defined programs are an innovative approach to grant-making pioneered by Johnson. Emphasis on primary care and the training of generalist physicians, physician assistants, and nurse practitioners has been a long-standing theme. Others include support for projects focused on minority medical education, children, the elderly, substance abuse, HIV/AIDS, so called 'managed care', health policy, and hands-on experience with the United States Congress for young physicians.

The Edna McConnell Clark Foundation, established in New York in 1974, devotes about a quarter of its budget to supporting research and clinical strategies for controlling tropical diseases in developing countries. Other programs focus on children's problems, including their health.

The John D. and Catherine T. MacArthur Foundation, established in Chicago in 1978, is the most recent and one of the largest. Health matters are no longer a major focus but in the past MacArthur has funded work in mental health and tropical diseases. It is perhaps best known for its 'genius awards'. Of the few given to physicians, one to Curtis G. Hames deserves special note. As the principal in the only family practice in a rural Georgia county, Hames recorded meticulously the genealogical and medical histories of his patients and over many decades froze specimens of their blood and urine. His trove of integrated individual personal data and specimens from the great majority of those living in a stable defined population has been mined by investigators from several countries. Their studies provide insights into the web of causality and the natural history of disease that have not been emulated in primary care practices since the contributions of Sir James MACKEN-

ZIE (p 332) and Will PICKLES (p 332) in the United Kingdom.

Other foundations, often with a long history, have made important niche contributions: the King's Fund (London, 1897) in health policy, healthcare quality, and public health; the John A. Hartford Foundation (New York, 1929) in aging, geriatrics, and health information; the Ittelson Foundation (New York, 1932) in mental health research; the William T. Grant Foundation (New York, 1936) in health of children, adolescents, and youth; the Novartis Foundation (formerly the Ciba Foundation, London, 1947) in support of medical and scientific conferences and short-term residencies for overseas scientists; the Charles A. Dana Foundation (New York, 1950) in neurosciences; and the Aga Khan Foundation (Geneva, 1967) in community-based healthcare in developing countries.

The roughly US$1.5 billion dispersed by American foundations is a trivial contribution compared with that country's US$1 trillion annual expenditures on health matters. For Britain the comparable figures are about US$500 million and US$180 billion. Foundation awards may make a substantial difference, as the record shows, and they often precede much greater support from government agencies. Small grants from a prestigious foundation may bestow recognition and kudos on the recipients far in excess of those derived from government grants or individual donations. Skill in conferring such recognition is a determinant of a foundation's impact on paradigms, policies, and practices that pertain to matters medical.          KLW

*See also* RESEARCH INSTITUTES

**FOUNDLING HOSPITALS** were established in many countries, especially in the 18th century for children abandoned by their parents. This was commonplace in an age of poverty and deprivation when many families were too large. Babies were left in maternity hospitals and the mothers could not be traced or were vagrants. Thousands of children were simply left in the streets to fend for themselves or became 'objects of charity', and the mortality among them was appallingly high. One of the more famous was The Foundling Hospital of London founded in 1739 by the sea captain Thomas Coram, whose heart was wrung by the plight of these unfortunates. Coram's Fields in London are where the hospital was once situated.

**FRANCE — HISTORY** The formal teaching and practice of medicine in France effectively began in the city of MONTPELLIER (this page). St Bernard reported that, from 1153, people went to Montpellier for healthcare. In 1220, 30 years before the

university began, the first great school of medicine was founded there, with a chancellor at its head. The school of medicine was the first in Europe and students came from many countries. The most famous physicians and surgeons were de Villeneuve and Mendeville (who was Philippe le Bel's physician and wrote a treatise on surgery and Guy de CHAULIAC (p 320), who wrote a treatise entitled 'Grande chirurgie'. Mendeville and Guy de Chauliac had different approaches: the former recommended suture of wounds; the latter thought that wound suppuration was preferable. A second school of medicine was created in Paris in 1270.

In the succeeding centuries many famous Frenchmen illuminated the history of medicine, notably Ambroise PARÉ (p 320), the great surgeon who achieved much outstanding work, author of the famous sentence 'I dressed his wounds, God healed him'; Jean Fernel, who studied and taught physiology; la Mettrie and his work, 'L'homme machine'.

During the French Revolution, schools of medicine were closed and medical journals forbidden. As with all other professions, the art of healing could be practiced by anyone. Medicine was in a parlous state. But, after Robespierre's fall, a physician named Foucroy protested and obtained permission from the Convention to re-open three faculties (Paris, Montpellier, and Strasbourg), with the creation of chairs and professors paid by the state. The 'medicine of observation' developed, with the increasing practice of dissection. The state ordered the appointment of professors of clinics in hospitals. Childbirth became a medical discipline, and Baudelocque was given a departmental chairmanship in Paris. He created the Port-Royal maternity hospital, which is still well known. Teaching was in French in place of Latin, and the Church no longer had authority over faculties and hospitals.

Notable figures in this intermediary period were PINEL (p 77), head of the first French psychiatric school, who delivered mental patients from chains, and Bichat, who identified the various tissues of the human body. Corvisart, Napoleon's physician, used percussion in thoracic disease. LAËNNEC (p 461) perfected auscultation, studied tuberculosis, and died after contracting the disease. He was a monarchist and a religious man; hence he was severely criticized by Broussais, a republican and an atheist of violent character. Bouillaud demonstrated the relationship between rheumatism and cardiac inflammation.

At the beginning of the 19th century several French physicians enhanced the reputation of French medicine, and surgeons such as LARREY (p 796), Desault, and Dupuytren created a brilliant surgical school.

## MONTPELLIER

Montpellier, in the south of France, is famed in medicine for carrying the torch of learning, especially during the difficult years of the 13th and 14th centuries leading up to the Renaissance. Its medical school probably began in the 12th century and may have been inspired by SALERNO (p 448). Geographically the university was placed between Italy and Spain, where much of the Arabic tradition in medicine remained. Many famous doctors studied there. John of Gaddesden, who became professor at Oxford in the 14th century, was one of them. So was Guy de CHAULIAC (p 320), who became physician and chaplain to Pope Clement VI at Avignon, and made contributions to surgery, including the invention of a rope suspended over the patient's bed by which they could lift themselves up. Other students and visitors were Andrew Boorde, who became physician to Henry VIII, and wrote *The Breviarie of Health*; PARACELSUS (p 617); Sir Thomas Browne; Sir Theobald Turquet de Mayerne, who became physician to James I; Thomas SYDENHAM (p 721); and Desgenettes, who became physician to Napoleon. The medical school still flourishes.

## FRENCH FIGURES

Guy De **CHAULIAC**
(c. 1300–68). French surgeon.
De Chauliac was the most
eminent surgeon of the 14th
century, and a writer of great
learning. His book *Chirurgia
magna*, written in 1363, was
first printed in 1498 and was
regarded as authoritative for at
least a century afterwards. In it
he advocated early excision of
cancer, the treatment of
fractures with slings and
traction, and operations for
hernia and cataract. He had
many distinguished patients,
including Jean of Luxemburg,
the blind king of Bohemia
(1336), Pope Clement VI
(1342) at Avignon, and his
successors Innocent VI and
Urban V.

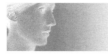

Ambroise **PARÉ** (?1510–90).
French surgeon. After working
as a barber-surgeon's
assistant, at the age of 19
Paré moved to Paris as a
resident surgical student at the
Hôtel-Dieu. In 1536 he
became a master barber-
surgeon and joined the army.
He served intermittently for
the next 30 years. He
acquired a reputation for skill,
judgement, and probity in
both the court and the army,
Probably the greatest surgeon
of the 16th century, Paré
revolutionized the treatment
of wounds, abandoning the
use of the cautery for simple
dressings. He recommended
ligature of the vessels, devised
many types of prosthesis, and
advocated massage. The son
of an artisan, he knew no
Latin and wrote in the
vernacular, but, in spite of this
and the opposition of the
professors of the Sorbonne, he
was elected to the Collège de
S. Côme in 1554.

*(continued opposite)*

Through Magendie and, above all, Claude BERNARD (p 102) an experimental revolution followed, with the study of many aspects of human physiology, including the recognition of the endocrine glands and the concept of function of the different organs. Bernard's *Introduction á la médecine expérimentale* (1865) became the standard reference work on physiology.

At the same time, the great epidemic diseases, mainly smallpox, cholera, tuberculosis, and typhoid fever gave rise to increasing concern for public health. Hygiene chairs were founded in every faculty. The French Academy of Medicine was founded in 1820 by Louis XVIII, with representatives of all human health disciplines: physicians, surgeons, pharmacologists, veterinarians, physicists, and chemists. Thus, in the 19th century, with so many scientists, clinicians, or researchers, France had achieved a prominent role in European medicine.

Soon afterwards, research in laboratory medicine began to develop. PASTEUR (p 620) disproved the concept of spontaneous generation, very popular at this time, identified the cholera germ, and, most important of all, carried out the first vaccination against rabies. He received many distinctions and honors and became famous throughout the world as a benefactor of mankind. In 1888, the Institut Pasteur was built with public grants and research activity has continued there ever since.

Research in chemistry promoted important therapeutic developments. Pelletier and Caventou identified emetine and quinine, digitalin was discovered by Nativelle, and Pravaz perfected the use of syringes. Advances were also made in human physiology. Marey studied human gait; Chauveau, cardiac contraction; Poiseuille and Potain, blood pressure. Because of the work of Pean, visceral surgery became a routine procedure.

Clinics continued to develop rapidly through the teaching of highly qualified clinicians such as Dieulafoy. Duchenne was interested in paralysis, and described a disease later called Duchenne's disease (muscular dystrophy). CHARCOT (p 400) had enormous prestige and founded a great neurological school to study several diseases later named after him. Together with Dejerine, Pierre Marie, and Babinski, Charcot ranks among the great pioneers of neurology in France. Broca was also prominent in studying aphasia. Esquirol was one of the first psychiatrists. In yet another field, Orfila created a reliable school of legal medicine, the only one in Europe. Venereal diseases were observed by Ricord and Fournier among others.

At about this time, some physicians also became interested in preventive medicine, and

DUNANT (p 706) created the private organization called 'la Croix Rouge' (the RED CROSS). In 1896, Imbert in Montpellier and Beclére in Paris were the first to use X-rays in clinical practice, and Beclére organized training in radiology in Paris. Later, Pierre and Marie CURIE (p 556) discovered radium.

Meanwhile, the Institut Pasteur had become a great center for biological research. In 1921, the introduction of a vaccine against tuberculosis (BCG) by CALMETTE (p 621) and Guérin was an important development. A student of Pasteur, METCHNIKOFF (p 412) inaugurated the first steps in immunology, and was soon followed by Fernand Widal and Charles Richet. D'Arsonval contributed new knowledge in medical physics. Nicolle and Deve made important contributions to parasitology.

In 1902, in France, several new laws introduced an important new system of public health, hygiene, compulsory protective inoculations, social security, and the foundation of an international office of public health.

During the second part of the 20th century, many advances were made in medical knowledge and techniques. They include a vaccine against poliomyelitis (Lépine 1954), the discovery of the human leukocyte antigen system (Dausset 1958), the relationship between Down's syndrome and chromosome 21 (Turpin and Lejeune 1959), advances in the clinical treatment of mental diseases (Delay and Deniker 1952), new developments in nephrology (Hamburger), and the introduction of organ transplantation.

In 1958, at Robert Debré's instigation, the practice of public medicine in university hospitals was, for the first time, controlled by law. According to law, physicians must comply with three tasks, namely, patient care, medical education, and research. Great hospitals became centers of training and research. Two systems of medicine, public and private, became more or less smoothly complementary.

In 1968, following serious student unrest, the official university organization was modified; chairs were changed into flexible professorships and hospital physicians into hospital practitioners. For the first time, faculties became teaching and research units (Unités d'enseignement et de recherche, UER) and later units of training and research (Unités de formation et de Recherche, UFR). The medical curriculum was extensively modified. The former system (*externat* and *internat des hôpitaux* — externship and internship) was replaced by a system which is supposed to be more democratic, with no '*externat*' examination, but an '*internat*' examination with a limited number of places in specialized medicine and an 'internship' in general medicine for all students.

GSer, OB

**FRANCE** The present medical system is very complex. There are private hospitals or clinics and public hospitals, called university hospitals in towns where a university is situated and regional hospitals in other towns. There is also an intermediate system in private, non-profit hospitals. The practice of private medicine requires the degree of doctor in medicine. In public medicine postgraduate students are appointed assistant residents, university lecturers, '*chefs de cliniques*' (assistant professors for 2 years, renewable), hospital practitioners (either full-time or part-time), and professors of the university at three levels (first class, second class, exceptional, and with other levels in each class).

Hospital healthcare is run by an administration called '*l'assistance publique*' (public healthcare) with a general manager appointed who cannot be a medical practitioner. The UER manager elected as dean of the school of medicine is responsible for university medical teaching and postgraduate education. The medical council of the hospital has an advisory role alongside the manager of '*l'assistance publique*'.

Graduate and postgraduate examinations are organized in the UFR under the control of professors. The '*concours d'internat*' varies according to modalities which are increasingly modified towards a regional organization. University hospital practitioners or professors are nominated by the National Council of the Universities, which includes elected and appointed members organized in sections and subsections.

The National Institute for Medical Research (INSERM) runs several laboratories partly related to, and situated in, the university hospital system; the managers of units are sometimes independent. In the same way, a number of research laboratories of the National Center for Scientific Research, are staffed by university hospital practitioners.

The 'order of physicians' (*ordre des médecins* — the regulatory authority) is divided into a national order and regional orders, and deals mainly with the legal and ethical aspects of the medical profession.

### Training and research

Training sessions are organized by regional associations, providing postgraduate medical training to give practitioners up-to-date information on medical knowledge and new techniques. The practice of private medicine is not age limited, whereas in hospitals the age limit is 65 years.

Research activity is well developed in several centers concerned with major current medical problems. The health and social security system ensures social protection. The state is responsible for legislation and bears overall responsibility for healthcare. This responsibility is divided between two ministries: the Ministry of Health and the Ministry of Education, which is responsible for the university-level education of health professionals. Recently, a ministry of high-level education and research has been created, which carries the responsibility of defining the priorities in various subjects of research, of following major advances, and of adapting and modernizing medical education.

The system of health funding, the '*sécurité sociale*', in France is based mainly on a private institution placed under Health Ministry control, and is divided into three branches: health, family, and aging. The resources consist of employees, and employers, taxes (90%), and French government contribution (10%). The first branch of *sécurité sociale* is in charge of health funding and comprises different *caisses* according to the occupations of the contributors (farmers, independent, minors, government employees, and so on).

Although rather complicated and non-homogeneous among the various *caisses*, this organization allows free access for all to either public or private hospitals or clinics, whatever the frequency, and the free choice of referring oneself either to any general practitioner or specialist. The patient is re-imbursed by the *sécurité sociale* for about 75% of health expenses, and pays for about 20%, directly or via private insurance. For chronic or expensive disease (such as cancer, severe heart disease, severe neurological disease, or AIDS) the system allows a 100% re-imbursement, whereas for symptomatic drugs, only 40% is re-imbursed. In some cases, the patient pays only for the part not covered by the *sécurité sociale*. The poor do not have to pay for their health expenses.

This idealistic system (accessibility, efficacy) has been dampened by harsh reality: the French health expenses are the second highest world-wide and efficiency is not optimal. The health funding system faces a chronic deficit. Taxes increase progressively, and the *sécurité sociale* re-imbursements decrease continuously. Reforms trying to promote the reduction of health costs have been implemented successively, being the last step before a total ceiling on health costs and the switch from a public system to profit-based private systems.                                        GSer, OB

*See also* HEALTHCARE SYSTEMS; PROFESSIONAL REGULATION; RESEARCH INSTITUTES

Sigmund **FREUD** (1856–1939). Austrian psychoanalyst. Freud was born on 6 May 1856 in the Moravian town of Freiberg, 150 miles north-east of Vienna. His mother, née Amalia Nathansohn,

*(continued)*

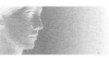

Jacques René **TENON** (1724–1816). French surgeon and ophthalmologist. Tenon joined the army as a surgeon in 1744 and later acquired renown as an anatomist and an ophthalmologist, describing several structures in the eye, including the fascial sheath of the eyeball (Tenon's capsule). In 1788 Tenon published a series of memoirs on Paris hospitals revealing their overcrowding, their squalor, and the total disregard for sanitation. These led the authorities to undertake great improvements.

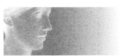

Antoine Laurent **LAVOISIER** (1743–94). French chemist. Lavoisier studied law until his interest in chemistry was aroused by attending a course of lectures by Rouelle in 1762. In 1775 after a meeting with Priestley he realized the significance of Priestley's 'dephlogisticated air', which he renamed 'oxygine' in 1787. He showed that the amount of oxygen absorbed by the body was increased by eating, by physical work, and at low temperatures. He was guillotined in May 1794.

*(continued overleaf)*

(continued)

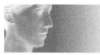

**Julien Jean César LEGALLOIS** (1770–1814). French physiologist. During the revolution Legallois worked in hospital while still a student and was a leader of a movement supporting the Federalists. An early experimental physiologist, he showed that respiration was controlled from the medulla oblongata (1812). He was much impressed by the importance of maintaining an adequate arterial blood supply to the tissues and this led him vigorously to oppose bleeding as a form of treatment.

was his father's third wife; and Sigmund was the first and favorite of her eight children, one of whom died in infancy. His father, Jacob Freud, was a penurious wool merchant. In 1859 the family moved briefly to Leipzig, and in 1860 settled in Vienna. Freud continued to live and work in Vienna until 1938, when the Nazi occupation forced him to emigrate to England. He died in Hampstead on 23 September 1939, just after the beginning of the second world war.

Although the family was Jewish, Jacob Freud neglected religious observance, and Sigmund never practiced the Jewish religion. In spite of this, his Jewish identity was a central feature of his personality: he attended meetings of his local Jewish society, and he made few friends who were not Jews. Throughout his life, he remained sensitive to anti-Semitism, which, in the Vienna of the 1860s and 1870s, was being fueled by an ever increasing stream of Jewish refugees from Eastern Europe.

The young Freud was so evidently gifted that his family were convinced that he would achieve something remarkable. They took trouble to ensure that the *Wunderkind's* studies were undisturbed, and when he complained of his sister's practicing, banished the piano from the apartment. At the age of 9, he became a pupil at the so-called 'Sperlgymnasium', where he was first in his class for seven years, and graduated *summa cum laude*. In addition to a thorough grounding in Latin and Greek, he learned French and English, and taught himself the rudiments of Spanish and Italian. A glance at his library in the Freud Museum in London shows that a high proportion of his books are in English. He began to read Shakespeare at the age of 8, and Shakespeare and Goethe remained his favorite authors.

### Student years

Freud enrolled in the medical department of the University of Vienna in the autumn of 1873. His initial interest was in zoological research, and from 1876 to 1882 he worked as a research assistant in the Physiological Institute of Ernst Brücke. Freud was strongly attracted by science, and might well have spent the rest of his life in research if he had been able to afford to do so. But poverty and his wish to marry forced him to complete his medical training, and, in April 1886, he opened his medical practice in Vienna.

The young Freud was, and remained, serious, dedicated, and ambitious. He exhibited many obsessional traits of personality, being meticulous, scrupulous, self-controlled, and reliable. As might be expected, he was notably neat in his dress and general appearance. Even when short of money, a barber attended him daily. Freud was an extremely hard worker, and had both an eye and a ear for detail. Anyone reading his paper *The Moses*

*of Michelangelo* cannot fail to be impressed with his powers of observation. It was the same when he listened to his patients. He based his interpretations on discrepancies and details from the patient's flow of talk which his sharp ear detected, but which the patient had not noticed.

Obsessional personalities are prone to superstition. Freud retained an irrational belief in the significance of certain numbers which he considered to be related to the date of his death. He also half-heartedly believed in telepathy. He was a compulsive collector of antique statuettes, which crowded his desk and shelves in such numbers that not one could be individually appreciated.

The story of Freud's life from the end of the 19th century until his death is the story of psychoanalysis. *An autobiographical study* (Standard Edition, XX) is devoted to his discoveries, and tells little about himself. At the age of 67, he developed a cancerous condition of the palate, which required over 30 operations, and which led to his death at the age of 83. Freud's Achilles' heel was smoking. Although he knew that his cigars exacerbated his cancer, he was unable to abandon the habit.

### Abandonment of science

The most puzzling feature of Freud's personality was his abandonment of science. He claimed to be a scientist, but psychoanalysis was largely built upon Freud's subjective perceptions, and its hypotheses are retrospective, cannot be used for predictions, and are insusceptible of scientific proof. Moreover, psychoanalytic theory is based upon a small sample of the Viennese upper and middle classes. Psychoanalysis is best regarded as a hermeneutic system which is designed to explain mental phenomena historically; that is, in terms of their origins. But Freud was dogmatically convinced that his interpretations were right; that he had discovered the origin of neurotic symptoms; and that art, religion, anthropology, and almost every other human endeavor could be explained in psychoanalytic terms. Like gurus who promote a religious belief system, Freud believed that he had discovered 'the truth'.

His erstwhile friend and collaborator, Josef Breuer, wrote of him: 'Freud is a man given to absolute and exclusive formulations: this is a psychical need which, in my opinion, leads to excessive generalization.' Breuer was right. Although Freud was personally tolerant and kind, both to his patients and within the family, he was intolerant of any kind of disagreement with his ideas, which only he was allowed to modify or revise. This rigidity led to the distressing defections from the psychoanalytic movement which so disfigured it in the early days. Among the rebels were Adler, Stekel, Jung, and Rank. But those who were content to sit at the feet of the master found him both impressive and lovable.

Freud remains an important, charismatic figure in the history of ideas; a great writer, and an innovator of such significance that he is often linked with DARWIN (p 214) and Marx as one of the three original thinkers who most altered man's view of himself in the 19th and 20th century.

A Sto

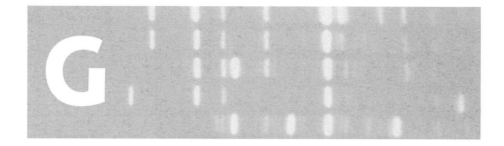

# G

**GALEN** (AD 129–199). Greek physician. Born in Pergamum, Galen studied first in the local temple of Aesculapius, then in Smyrna, Corinth, and Alexandria. He returned to Pergamum, where he practiced medicine and was appointed surgeon to the gladiators. In 161 AD he went to Rome, where, despite hostility from the citizens, his skills in diagnosis and treatment led to his introduction to many influential people, and he was soon made physician to the new emperor, Marcus Aurelius. Around 166 AD Galen returned to Pergamum but, after two years, was recalled to Rome, where he remained until his death. He was a prolific writer on philosophy and literature as well as science. His medical writings were based on experimental and direct observation and incorporated the traditions of HIPPOCRATES (p 382), Plato, and ARISTOTLE (p 64), and included the humoral theory. He was skilled in anatomy and physiology, deriving much of his understanding from meticulous observations of animal dissections, and focused much of his research on the nerves, heart, lungs, and pulse. He directed attention to the prevention of disease and maintaining a healthy equilibrium of the body through diet, exercise, rest, and hygiene; he also developed an elaborate system of therapeutics using plants and herbs. Galen's doctrine remained an authority on medicine for some 1400 years.

**GASTROENTEROLOGY — HISTORY** The study of the gastrointestinal tract in health and disease did not exist as a discrete specialty until the late 1920s or early 1930s. This is not to say that such diseases were neglected in the past: gastroenterologists have been at work since antiquity. The pharaohs of ancient Egypt employed a physician whose job was to keep the royal anus healthy, the 'Physician of the Clyster'. Hieroglyphs from Egyptian tombs clearly depict proctoscopy, the earliest known form of gastrointestinal endoscopy. The desire to 'look inside' prompted many innovative designs for endoscopes over the centuries — usually rigid tubes dependent for their optics on candlelight and mirrors — that led in the last hundred years to semiflexible and then truly flexible instruments using optics and, recently, computer 'chip' technology.

Until the mid-19th century, physicians saw gastrointestinal diseases that were largely infectious, which they were virtually impotent to treat: infectious diarrheas (or dysenteries), the most lethal being CHOLERA, parasitic infestations of the gut (such as hookworm), tropical diseases involving the liver (e.g. YELLOW FEVER, MALARIA), TUBERCULOSIS, and SYPHILIS. Nutritional disorders and alcoholic liver disease were also common. Significant abdominal trauma (sharp, blunt, or surgical) was almost uniformly fatal, as was severe pancreatitis before modern intensive care. Esophageal and rectal strictures were treated with dilators long before contrast radiology and endoscopy could accurately define them. The term 'bougie' used to describe dilators for esophageal, urethral, and other strictures, is a corruption of the Arabic name for a town in coastal North Africa (now Algeria) which was the world center for candle making in the 14th century AD. Candles have been used to dilate strictures for 600 years or more.

Hepatology — the study of liver diseases — had an early start, too. The liver has long been known to have amazing powers of regeneration, as reflected in the legend of the ill-fated Titan, Prometheus: his punishment for stealing fire from the Gods was to be chained to a rock and have his liver eaten away every night by an eagle, only to have it grow back again by day. In some African cultures, the liver (and not the heart) is regarded as the seat of the soul, giving rise to seemingly bizarre sentiments such as 'I would lay down my liver for you'.

Gastrointestinal anatomy has been studied systematically since the Renaissance, Ruggerio Oddi describing his eponymous sphincter as long ago as the mid-1600s. The gastrointestinal tract was a favorite of the great physiologist, Claude BERNARD (p 102), who studied the 'pancreatic ferments' and their role in digestion over 100 years ago. Abdominal surgeons of the late 1800s, such as Theodor BILLROTH (p 518), made enormous strides when general anesthesia (1846) and antisepsis (1870) for the first time gave patients a

fighting chance of surviving open abdominal surgical procedures, such as excision of the gallbladder and relief of mechanical bowel obstruction. In Vienna, the Billrothstrasse is a grateful city's way of thanking its local hero. Although Pasteur's germ theory was not quickly accepted, despite clear evidence (for example, SEMMELWEISS (p 479) and puerperal fever) that cleanliness keeps surgical patients alive, the pioneers of abdominal surgery showed the benefits of antisepsis so dramatically that it paved the way for phenol and its less irritant successors in all operating rooms. Sadly, these advances were too late to save US President James A. Garfield, who was shot by an assassin on 2 July 1881. He took 80 days to die, during which he underwent several operations in a vain effort to recover the bullet. Even Alexander Graham Bell was called in to try to locate the elusive bullet with a device similar to a modern mine detector. Garfield's death from overwhelming sepsis was widely blamed on his physicians' dirty hands and unsterilized surgical instruments. Even his assassin, caught at the scene and later hanged, denied that he had actually killed Garfield: 'The doctors did that,' Charles Julius Guiteau said, 'I simply shot at him'.

By the close of the 19th century, the foundations of gastrointestinal surgery had been laid. However, much physiology and pathophysiology remained obscure. Despite the continued empiricism of medicine, fewer people were dying from infectious diseases, thanks largely to major public health initiatives.

Another public health initiative early in this century addressed a major cause of chronic diarrheal illness associated with dermatitis and, eventually, dementia affecting the poor — namely, pellagra. This disease was common in slum communities and in asylums and prisons, where the diet was poor. Dr Joseph Goldberger of the US Public Health Service did not believe the prevailing theories that pellagra was infective or hereditary and managed to eliminate it from an orphanage in Missouri by bringing in meat, eggs, and vegetables. He also managed to induce pellagra in a group of prisoners by restricting their diet. In 1929 — after Goldberger's death — Dr Conrad Elvehjem of the University of Wisconsin discovered that a vitamin called nicotinic acid — or niacin — could cure pellagra.                                    JBai

*See also* DIET AND DISEASE; NUTRITION; VITAMINS

**GASTROENTEROLOGY** In the early part of the 20th century, gastroenterology is described as having been 'an amorphous collection of facts and fancies, usually unsubstantiated by clinical or scientific proof'. The physician's resources for investigating gastrointestinal disorders were

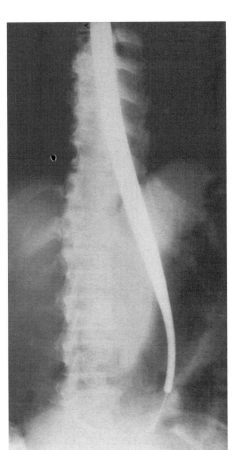

This chest X-ray shows a barium-impregnated, tapered, esophageal dilator which has been advanced over a guide wire to dilate a stricture. This application of endoscopy has made the business of managing esophageal strictures safer and more predictable than in the past, when the procedure was often done 'blind'. The earliest esophageal dilators were wax candles, and their alternative name, 'bougie', is a corruption of the name of a North African town (Bougia), which in the 14th and 15th centuries was the medieval world center of candle making.

severely limited: the stools could be examined for blood; there were a few simple blood and urine tests; stomach contents obtained by passing a tube through the nose could be tested for hydrochloric acid; rigid proctoscopy afforded a limited view of the anus and rectum; and the stomach and colon could be evaluated with contrast (barium) radiology. Cross-sectional body imaging (such as ultrasound, computed tomography) was half a century away. The word *abdomen* comes from the Latin, 'to hide': before cross-sectional imaging, the abdominal contents truly remained hidden until exposed by the surgeon at laparotomy (incision into the abdominal cavity).

Many of the advances in diagnosing and treating gastrointestinal diseases have resulted from radiological and endoscopic imaging. Although contrast studies still have a major role in radiology, cross-sectional techniques have revolutionized the doctors' view of the abdominal contents. Computerized (or computed) tomography has achieved remarkable resolution and sensitivity, such that subtle abnormalities can now be detected. It has largely replaced injecting the

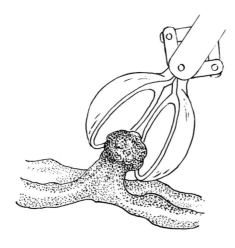

The so-called 'hot biopsy technique' for removing sessile polyps seen during endoscopy. Once the cups of the forceps are closed over the polyp, current is applied to cut off the polyp and cauterize the base. The arrows show current dissipating into the adjacent tissue. This technique prevents bleeding after polyp removal.

arteries supplying the intestine before taking X-ray films to visualize solid tumors of the gastrointetstinal tract and seeing whether they could be removed. For example, if the superior mesenteric artery or portal vein is encircled by tumor then cancer of the head of the pancreas cannot be removed.

Taking advantage of the abundance of hydrogen in the human body, magnetic resonance imaging relies on spinning protons to create computerized tomography-quality images without the use of ionizing radiation. Magnetic resonance imaging often provides complementary data to computerized tomography and is especially useful for visualizing lesions within the liver. The ability to opacify the body's arteries — arteriography — has greatly helped in localizing gastrointestinal bleeding sites, which can often be closed off using a variety of materials to promote blood clotting.

So-called 'interventional radiology' allows access from the outside to the bile duct system when endoscopic methods fail or are unavailable, and percutaneous needles and catheters guided by ultrasound or computerized tomography are used to drain fluid collections in the abdomen.

Direct and indirect tests of gastrointestinal structure and function have had a major impact on diagnosis. Percutaneous liver biopsy (obtaining a sample of liver tissue by passing a needle into the liver) has elucidated many disorders of that previously mysterious organ. Measuring hydrogen or radio-labeled carbon dioxide in expired air is the basis for various breath tests. Because changes in the breath reflect altered digestion and absorption, these tests offer non-invasive ways to study the function of the small bowel and pancreas. Breath tests can also diagnose and monitor the treatment of *Helicobacter pylori*, an organism recently identified as the principal cause of duodenal ulcers and a risk factor for adenocarcinoma (cancer arising from the glands) of the stomach.

The *Helicobacter* story is a vivid example of how a new theory — or paradigm — is required to overthrow long-established dogma. Despite overwhelming evidence that duodenal ulcers frequently relapse despite long-term suppression of gastric acid, and the observation that some ulcers healed with antibiotic treatment, the medical community was slow to accept that this disease could be due to an infection with a germ. Although the 'no acid, no ulcer' theory has been superseded, the brilliant work of pharmacologists who developed drugs to inhibit acid secretion should not be forgotten. Sir James Black, who synthesized over 800 agents before identifying the first clinically useful histamine-2 (H2) receptor antagonist, made the lives of ulcer and acid reflux sufferers immeasurably better long before the *Helicobacter* story unfolded.

Innovative pharmacology has given us many drugs that are useful in managing gastrointestinal disorders, ranging from resins that bind bile acids to treat choleretic diarrhea, to prokinetics (motility-stimulating drugs) (such as cisapride), synthetic gut peptides, antiviral therapy (interferon) for hepatitis B and C infection, and chemotherapeutic agents effective against gastrointestinal tumors. None of these would have been possible without well-funded basic research and carefully conducted clinical trials, activities we accept as routine today but which were uncommon before World War II.

### Transformation into specialty

What transformed gastroenterology into a specialty? The answer depends on one's historical and geographical perspective. In the 1930s, several institutions in the USA, including the MAYO CLINIC (p 840), the JOHNS HOPKINS UNIVERSITY (p 840), the University of Chicago, and Mt Sinai Hospital and Medical School (New York), set up gastroenterology programs. These recognized the importance of an increasing body of scientific knowledge in this specialty, the identification of discrete diseases caused by infectious agents, and the potential of semiflexible endoscopy. Nutritional factors and the diseases caused by their deficiency were identified and became treatable, these studies being accelerated by the privations of World War II and the terrible conditions endured by many prisoners of war. After the Second World War, the National Institutes of Health were established, with gastroenterology coming under the umbrella of the Institute for Arthritis and Metabolic Diseases in 1956. The expansion of gastroenterology has continued with increasing support for biomedical research. Kirschner has identified no fewer than 10 factors bringing gastroenterology into the mainstream of advancing scientific thought: (1) a growing body of scientific knowledge; (2) technological improvements; (3) public support for research and training; (4) physician acceptance of controlled trials; (5) support by philanthropic organizations; (6) the growth and influence of academic medical centers; (7) National Institutes of Health-supported research and training; (8) the growth and influence of scientific societies; (9) the growing global scientific information network; and (10) increasing public awareness of gastrointestinal disorders.

The 1980s and early 1990s saw an explosion in specialty training in gastroenterology in the USA. This was doubtless fueled by the promise of financial rewards from endoscopic procedures in specialist practice. A similar phenomenon was seen in cardiology, the other 'interventional' medical specialty.

In the USA, where 'specialism' has flourished more than in any country, gastroenterology has experienced a trend towards subspecialty 'differentiation': current subspecialties include esophagology, the management of acid-related disorders and *H. pylori* infection; nutrition, hepatobiliary, and pancreatic disorders; inflammatory bowel disease; motility (including irritable bowel syndrome); and hepatology (including transplantation of the liver). Gastrointestinal oncology has evolved as a hybrid subspecialty requiring a multidisciplinary team, including oncologists, gastroenterologists, surgeons, radiotherapy specialists (radiation oncologists), interventional radiologists, etc. Undoubtedly in certain disorders, subspecialty care improves the outcome, including survival, but, as it often involves advanced technology or treatment, it is usually expensive. Reliably successful liver transplantation

and immune therapy (with interferon) for hepatitis B and C have greatly enhanced the status of hepatology as a subspecialty of gastroenterology, as treatment for previously incurable disorders is now available.

Outside the USA, subspecialism in gastroenterology is uncommon; only a handful of physicians in Europe (and probably as few in Asia and Australia) successfully limit their practice to managing esophageal or hepatobiliary and pancreatic disorders, although many more advertise themselves as 'therapeutic endoscopists'. As tremendous technological advances in endoscopy began in the mid-1970s gastroenterologists in Europe tended to split into 'traditional' and 'lumenal': the gastroenterology establishment was suspicious of endoscopy and those who made their career 'pushing scopes'. Sadly, there are still pockets of anti-endoscopy prejudice, especially in major academic centers. However, the reality is that endoscopy has become the cornerstone of modern clinical and research gastroenterology. The technology (endoscopes and their accessories) is continually improving, with ever better access for diagnostic and therapeutic procedures. The boundary between minimally invasive endoscopy and surgery has become increasingly blurred. Miniaturization has resulted in 'miniscopes' for exploring the small bowel and the ducts of the pancreas and biliary tree. It will not be long before self-propelled robot endoscopes will be exploring the inside of the gut and peritoneal cavity under remote control, perhaps identifying and destroying early cancers and making running repairs as they go. Optical coherence tomography and reflectance spectrography will allow 'optical biopsies' with vastly greater sensitivity and specificity than are currently available from conventional forceps biopsy.

### Application of molecular biology

The application of molecular biology to the diagnosis of gastrointestinal disorders has great potential. Card tests of stool — similar to those currently used to detect occult blood — may soon be used to detect pathogens within minutes, saving tedious microbiological culture that may take days to provide an answer in infectious diarrhea. Rapid bedside tests — perhaps using polymerase chain reaction technology — may also detect subtle cell surface and DNA abnormalities that signal evolving colon and other gastrointestinal cancers. The great advances that have been made in understanding the gut mucosal immune system will result in immune modulation treatment for many diseases, especially inflammatory bowel disease and gluten-sensitive enteropathy (celiac disease). Work on the genetic basis for common gastrointestinal diseases, including malignancy, should help us to identify groups of individuals at high risk, for whom intensive screening or specific prophylactic treatment may be available. Drugs that control fibrosis (fibrogenesis — scarring) in the liver and pancreas and blood vessel formation (angiogenesis) in tumors are being developed. Preventing the deposition of fibrous tissue in chronic diseases of the liver and pancreas would greatly alter the natural history of cirrhosis and chronic pancreatitis. As tumors require new blood vessels to grow, inhibition of the process by which this occurs (angiogenesis) has major therapeutic potential in oncology.

Some successes with small bowel transplantation offer hope to patients with acquired short bowel syndrome and a variety of rare congenital disorders. Perhaps the largest population of patients with a gastrointestinal disorder remains the most poorly served: chronic functional abdominal pain — formerly 'irritable bowel syndrome' — is poorly understood and lacks specific treatment. However, gut peptide research has produced potent agents controlling motility and pain perception that appear to offer at least a subset of these patients hope of symptomatic relief. The future of gastroenterology as a specialty seems assured, despite the current turmoil over who will pay for ever more advanced technology. Well-designed outcomes research studies will determine what is cost-effective and quality improvement data, which audit physician effectiveness, should tell us whose services are worth paying for. JBai

*See also* EPISTEMOLOGY; IMAGING; RESEARCH INSTITUTES; SPECIALIZATION

**GENEALOGY** is the study of descent from a progenitor, and the enumeration and compilation of ancestors, their chronologies, and their biographic details, in the natural order of succession. Genealogy answers the first of the three great questions of all humankind — Where have I come from? (The other two being: What am I doing here? and Where am I going?)

The standard tool of the genealogist and the medical geneticist alike is the compilation of the family tree, sometimes called the kindred or pedigree. The study of kindreds applies not only to people, but also to institutions. Thus the Royal College of Surgeons, for example, can trace its ancestry from several early craft guilds of BARBER-SURGEONS. Family trees have within them information not only of important sentimental and medical value, but of legal and religious significance as well.

Genealogists compile family trees by the documentation of oral history, and by research of primary documents including birth, marriage, and death certificates. Wills, military service records, shipping lists, and court records are other examples of primary source documents indispensable in the compilation of extended kindreds. Medical terminology has changed dramatically over recent centuries. Older medical terms found during genealogical research of death certificates, for example, often include such diagnoses as 'falling sickness' (epilepsy), 'scrofula' or 'phthisis' (tuberculosis), or 'struma' (enlargement of a gland or organ, especially that of the thyroid gland). Diagnoses from old military records sometimes including the designation 'LMF' (lack of moral fiber), which has been more recently labeled neurasthenia and is now realized to include many cases of BATTLE NEUROSIS or POST-TRAUMATIC STRESS DISORDER.

Diseases cluster within families and are transferred by single genes carried by one or both parents (monogenic inheritance), by major chromosomal abnormalities (such as balanced translocations), and by the cumulative effects of several genes each individually of smaller effect (polygenic inheritance). Single gene diseases are relatively rare — the birth incidence of achondroplastic dwarfism, cystic fibrosis, or muscular dystrophy, for example, is each measured in only one case in every several thousand live births. By contrast, the major medical diseases of the 20th and 21st centuries — heart disease, hypertension, strokes, cancers, asthma, and dementia — all cluster within families. Each such polygenically-determined disease depends not only on familial genes raising or lowering an individual's threshold of risk, but on the presence of environmentally-determined agents which raise or lower the clinical threshold for the disease to manifest itself.

Each of us is a product of our genes, good and bad; and the effect, on these fundamental units of heredity, of the environment in which we grow and develop and live. For some things which are features in family trees — such as intelligence and personality and hair color — the genes are very important indeed. For others — like our waistlines, how well we do in exams, and the number of children we choose to have in our family — the environment is of much greater significance. The environment changes over time and varies from place to place; and includes the societal environment, which varies with fashion and custom. In family trees, genealogists see many genetic traits, such as the risk of disease, preserved because of the dominant importance of genes, especially those which cause monogenic disease. By contrast, changes in the physical environment follow such things as the emigration of a progenitor or variations in local custom or fashion or new medical discoveries. Such influences modify themes such as the number of conceptions in the average sibship, infant mortality rates, changes in life expectation, or the average height of individuals within a family. Medical and social details within an individual family tree often tell the story of the cultural evolution of humankind. Over the past 150 years the average height of members of the population has been increasing, not because of any change in genetic structure but because of changes in the environment. The secular trend in increasing height is some 3 millimeters per decade, which means in practice that the average height of children is almost one centimeter taller than that of their parents.

## Establishment of lineage

The establishment of lineage is a fundamental human desire both in the personal and in the societal sense. At the pragmatic level, to give a knowledge of one's family tree is sometimes of the greatest importance, especially in those instances where inherited diseases are occurring. Everyone should know the health details of their own family tree, a compilation spreading centrifugally to include at least a knowledge of one's third-degree relatives. First-degree relatives share one-half of their genes in common such as parents, children, and full siblings. Second-degree relatives share one-quarter of their genes, on average (for example, uncle–aunt and nephew– niece relationships and those of grandparent– grandchild). Third-degree relatives share one-eighth of their genes in common, an example being the relationship of first cousins.

In the last decades of the 20th century the hobby of establishing the chronology of personal family trees became hugely popular, especially in nations (such as the USA, Canada, Australia, and New Zealand) whose dominant populations emanated from colonial stock far removed from their geographic roots. The fulfillment that comes from knowing one's lineage is very old. In the Judaic–Christian religion, the importance of knowing one's family lineage was recorded in neolithic times. In Psalm 68 (verse 6) for example it is noted that for those without lineage 'God sets the solitary in families'.

The world's great cultures have all enshrined in holy lore genealogical progressions which establish not only the lineage of great prophets but also the first beings of the world. The family tree of the ancient Greek deities is complex, full of polygamy and incestuous unions which include the cultural origins of the history of the healing arts. In the Judaic–Christian tradition, lineages comprise a significant part of the basic doctrine in the book of *Genesis*. From Adam to Noah (in *Genesis* 5) twelve generations are listed by name; and in the pedigree of Shem (*Genesis* 11) the 'begats' run to 20 generations. The world's oldest surviving culture, that of the Australian Aboriginal Peoples, records a number of lineages emanating from the Rainbow Serpent.

Each individual has two parents, four grandparents, eight great-grandparents, and so on. At the time the Domesday Book was compiled (AD 1085), each individual living today has some $2^{30}$ potential ancestors, a vast theoretical number (more than a billion) greatly exceeding the population of the whole of Europe at that time. In fact, a greatly reduced number of ancestors spawned the population and most of us share common ancestors who lived at that time, their genes being inextricably mixed within relatively few generations. Almost everybody of Anglo-Celtic ancestry today can claim common genes with any others who had their origins, and inevitably their ancestors, in that

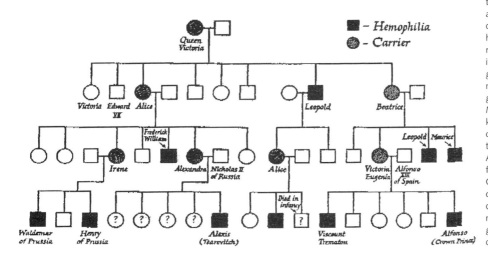

An abridged family tree of the Royal families of Europe illustrating the medical significance of genealogical study. Hemophilia (a bleeding disease) is caused by an X-linked recessive gene. Only males are affected, but females in such kindreds may be carriers. This family tree shows that Queen Victoria must have been a carrier of the hemophilia gene, although she herself was completely normal. None of her ancestors or lateral relatives had hemophilia; and it is highly likely that the gene either started as a new mutation in her or in the gonads of one of her parents. Males (within affected kindreds) who are normal cannot carry the gene and therefore cannot pass it on. As the present British Royal family is descended from Queen Victoria's second child (Edward VII), himself completely normal, this means that the hemophilia gene cannot be present, by descent, in the family.

Longfellow in *Hiawatha* described the importance of genealogy in Red Indian culture. He described the origins of writing as a result of the need to record genealogies:

> On the grave posts of our fathers Are no signs, no figures painted: Who are in those graves we know not,
> Only know they are our fathers. Of what kith they are and kindred, From what old, ancestral Totem, Be it Eagle, Bear or Beaver, They descended this we know not, Only know they are our fathers.

geographic part of the world. The concept that all people are ultimately of the one family saw its most extreme expression in the doctrine of the Familists, an extremist Christian sect derived from the Anabaptists of Delft in 1540.

The discovery in 1975 of restriction enzymes, which would cut DNA into tiny identifiable fragments opened the way to the absolute determination of parentage. Many hundreds of DNA fragments can be prepared from the blood or other cells of any individual; and each of these fragments in turn has sub-variations of pattern. At the beginning of the 21st century, this DNA technology is enabling family trees to be compiled independently of oral or written records, ushering in a new era of medical and legal genealogy. This DNA technique has led to 'familial' relationships being established not only for individual men and women, but for whole racial groups. By comparing such patterns from different 'racial families', the times of whole population migration and the degrees of inter-mixing of the world's peoples have been established.

There are two particular themes in genealogy which can be of great practical interest to family members. The first of these is the phenomenon of consanguinity, or the result of offspring from marriage between blood relatives. All cultures today forbid, both in secular and religious law, the union between first-degree relatives. In many countries consanguinity between second-degree relatives (for example, uncle–niece relationships) is not only permitted but regarded as socially desirable. In India, consanguineous relationships account for some 28% of unions, with 32% in Iran and more than 50% in the Yemen. Consanguinity simply concentrates genes, both good and bad (from the medical point of view). Consanguinity has family and societal advantages in that it prevents the dispersal of an ancestor's estate; it keeps precious familial culture and custom relatively intact and is a phenomenon regarded by many proud families as literally keeping desirable physical and intellectual traits 'within the family'. In western cultures, the closest degree of consanguinity permitted by secular law is that of first-cousin union. Union between first cousins doubles the risk of producing a child with a significant medical condition; but, provided there are no identifiable diseases within a family, the absolute risk of producing a child with a disability or abnormality is raised only from 2% (the baseline risk) to 4%. Most couples regard this latter still as a small risk.

### Types of descent

A second important practical theme emanating from genealogical study is the phenomenon of descent. This applies to the way in which a

society, or individual families within it, determines the inheritance of property and power. Religious descent (as in Judaism) comes from the maternal parent ('one always knows who one's mother is but not always one's father'). The inheritance of property is culture-specific in the context of laws of descent. Although patrilineal inheritance was enshrined in law in many western countries until the early decades of the 20th century, matrilineal property descent has been the norm for millennia in parts of India, and remains so today in those cultures and that of the Sepik region of Papua New Guinea.

In societies of patrilineal descent where wives and children within families adopt the family surname of the father, family names tend to die out. This is because males and their genes (and therefore their successors) are less fit, in the genetic and familial sense, than females. The male: female birth ratio is 106:100; but males show a differential mortality at all ages. Genealogists encounter this phenomenon constantly, where 'the male line dies out', and with it the male family surname. The oriental tradition of not using family names in a trans-generational sense, and the recent (late 20th century) phenomenon of western women preserving their own name after marriage, means that the gradual loss of surnames will become less common in the future. It will, of course, make the work of genealogists more difficult.

Genealogists answer the question 'Where have I come from?' with great enthusiasm. The answer gives to many a feeling of perspective and a feeling of continuity in the great scheme of things. For many, the perspective of one's kindred often helps in the answering of the second question, 'Why am I here?' and for some helps to define the future part of life.                    JHP

*See also* DEOXYRIBONUCLEIC ACID; GENETICS; 'ROYAL MADNESS' AND PORPHYRIA

**GENERAL PRACTICE** When historians reviewed the first 50 years of the National Health Service in BRITAIN, the story of 'general practice' was widely regarded as a success. General practice may be best described as what general practitioners do, even if that is extremely varied. Extracts from a fuller definition are helpful. 'The general practitioner is a licensed medical graduate who gives personal primary and continuing care to individuals, families, and a practice population, irrespective of age, sex, and illness; it is the synthesis of these functions which is unique … He will include and integrate physical, psychological, and social factors in his consideration about health and illness. He will undertake … chronic, recurrent or terminal (care) … . He will practice in co-operation with other colleagues, medical and non-medical …'.

This review is written from the background of general practice in Britain. The systems designed to provide primary care services to populations vary hugely in detail from country to country. However, irrespective of where 'primary care' is practiced and how it is organized, this definition of 'general practice' describes the common purpose everyone hopes to meet.

Medical graduates doing similar work in the USA and Canada are usually called 'family physicians' in recognition of their aspiration to care for whole families rather than just individuals.

Yet it is a paradox that, while this model of an essentially personal and continuous system of providing care is being adopted in health services world-wide, politicians, health service planners, and social commentators in Britain are increasingly describing this service as 'primary care', which indeed reflected the title entry of 'primary medical care' in the last edition of this companion. The choice of terms is more than an issue of semantics. Those who use the term 'primary care' see this as a logical descriptive term for care tiered from self-care, through primary care, on to secondary and tertiary care. Traditionally British general practice has controlled access to all specialist care except accident and emergency care, and care of patients with sexually transmitted diseases or dental disorders. But increasingly breaks in this pattern have been seen — such as opticians referring to ophthalmologists, and patients having direct access to healthcare from, for example, community based nurses, pharmacists, and complementary medicine practitioners — many medically qualified. Those providing complex secondary or tertiary care services (care of diabetic children, and for some malignancies) also increasingly encourage patients to make direct contact when 'primary care' type problems arise.

Perhaps equally significant is the economic debate whether doctors represent an over-qualified or over-expensive facility for providing services which are offered by nurses or care assistants in remote or less affluent societies elsewhere in the world. Prominent British general practitioners have advanced the case for general practitioners becoming consultants for groups of primary care professionals in the general practice setting, caring for patient lists of 5000 or more as against current averages of between 1500 and 2000 according to area. Thus far, patients both in Britain and in developing countries have shown a preference for direct access to doctors, and the economic case for substituting doctors with nurses falls when nurses take longer to consult than do doctors, and seek higher rewards as they adopt medical roles.

Whichever term is preferred, in Britain and for the foreseeable future, 'general practice' seems likely at least to describe the locus where personal and population centered primary care services will be based and co-ordinated.

## Workload

There are some 30 000 principals (partners or single-handed practitioners) in general practice in Britain now compared with less than 20 000 at the start of the National Health Service 50 years ago. Average lists have thus fallen from over 2500 per doctor to around 1800. Most doctors now work in partnerships, with only 10% (compared with nearly 50% in 1948) in a single-handed practice. 30% of principals are women. The role of assistants in general practice has greatly diminished, and this is no longer the route to principalship and partnership. Most practices are now based in purpose-built or modernized premises.

The 'average' British general practitioner consults with around 130 patients per week, 90% of these consultations being in the office ('surgery'). The average patient consults four times per year. The peaks of consultations are in infancy and old age, and for women in the child-bearing years. Two-thirds of patients consult in any one year and 95% over five years. There is one birth and one death for each doctor each fortnight. Nearly all births and most deaths take place in hospital.

*Morbidity* General practice has generated many publications on the content of its workload. Some come from individual doctors studying their own workload, some from single projects designed to survey specific local issues, and some from a periodic national study of morbidity. All studies are subject to variations in the way data are collected and the way doctors label the problems which patients present. This is particularly apparent for psychological problems, where estimates of proportions of consultations range from 5 to 50% depending on the source consulted, and reflecting varying perceptions of what constitutes a psychological problem.

In general, around 40% of adult consulting patients present with a new or acute problem and 25% with a continuing health problem. Some 10% present with an emotional problem, 5% with a social problem, and 10% with an administrative problem; 10% of patients consult for advice on matters to do with health rather than illness, or for a repeat prescription; 25% of patients consult because the doctor has asked them to return; 25% have more than one problem they wish to discuss.

Preventive medicine and health promotion activities are divided between opportunist care at

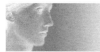

Sir James **MACKENZIE**
(1853–1925). British
physician. Mackenzie entered
general practice in Barnsley,
Yorkshire, in 1879, and
started clinical research at
once. He analyzed cardiac
irregularities with the
'polygraph' which he devised.
In 1902 he published *The
study of the pulse* and in
1908 *Diseases of the heart*.
Mackenzie came to London
in 1907 and in 1910 was
appointed lecturer at the
London Hospital. In 1918 he
returned to Scotland, where
he founded the Clinical
Institute at St Andrews.

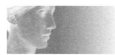

William Norman **PICKLES**
(1885–1969). British general
practitioner. The first
president of the Royal College
of General Practitioners,
Pickles practiced for 53 years
in the village of Aysgarth,
Wensleydale, Yorkshire. His
book *Epidemiology in a
country practice* threw
original light on the spread of
infection in a rural district. He
knew everyone in Aysgarth
and, with his wife, kept
meticulous records. There is
an admirable quality of
simplicity in his research
methods and writing. His
book survives as a classic.
'There is something in country
practice which breeds
content'.

consultations (particularly for advice on smoking
and weight) and organized care at clinics (particularly for children and well-women), which is
increasingly managed by health visitors and
nurses.

*Change* The general practitioner's job has
changed with changing patterns of disease and
evolving systems of care. For example, recent
years have seen an increase in work (in some areas
very substantial) due to problems of drug abuse
and AIDS/HIV disease, and more patients now
than formerly with complex psychological problems talk more openly about difficulties in relationships, including experiences of CHILDHOOD
ABUSE. Expectations about the monitoring of
continuing health problems have increased substantially. Hospitals are devolving or sharing care
for patients having routine treatment (anticoagulants) or illnesses previously treated as
inpatients (chemotherapy).

*Interfaces* About 5% of consultations are followed
by a referral to hospital — mainly to outpatient
departments. A similar number of consultations
leads to a laboratory investigation. The pattern of
referral has been affected by fund-holding; for
example, some orthopedic referrals are now
substituted by direct referral to physiotherapy,
often within the practice. Emergency referral is
unpredictable and influenced by patterns of out-
of-hours cover. In one year for a single doctor,
about a dozen patients have a myocardial infarction; three or four have appendicitis; and six
patients develop a new malignancy, half being
cancer of the lung. One person has bacterial
meningitis every seven years.

Doctors prescribe medicine at around 60% of
their consultations. The average patient receives
eight prescriptions per year, half through repeat
prescription systems. The consumption of
medicine averages out at one day's treatment with
a drug every day throughout a lifetime of 70
years. The cost of prescribed medicines is greater
than the cost of providing the rest of general
practitioner services.

## Working patterns

A strong feature of general practice has been the
clinical independence of its practitioners. This
has both accommodated and led to very different
styles of organization and provision of service,
some of which reflect attitudes to work and
beliefs about the place of medicine in health
and society.

The length of time spent at consultations is a
proxy for these issues. The average length of a
British general practice consultation is around
8 minutes, shorter than in many European and

American settings but longer than in countries
with developing health services. Doctors at the
faster end of the distribution (averaging five
minutes per consultation), when compared with
those at the slower end of the distribution (averaging 10 minutes per consultation), are less likely
to deal with more than the principal presenting
symptom. Thus slower doctors attend to a larger
element of existing co-morbidity, are more likely
to explore psychological and social issues (35% of
consulting patients may have a possible psychiatric condition) and to offer advice on health promotion matters. In short, slower doctors practice
more holistically than faster doctors. Reference
back to the job description of the general practitioner suggests this may be one definable
'quality-of-care' issue.

The etiology of fast and slow consulting is both
complex and interesting. Doctors who are more
rather than less patient centered are more likely
to consult more slowly, and more likely to book
fewer patients per hour at their surgeries. For
them, the problem arises when their booking
systems do not match their preferred working
styles and they run late (often very late). The
consequent need to consult faster to catch up
confuses their patients, changes the content of the
consultations, and promotes dissatisfaction
amongst patients and stress among doctors.

## Context

Discussion of clinical medicine tends to assume a
simple linear connection among diagnosis, treatment, and outcome. However, the medicine of
general practice is in many ways 'context
dependent'.

*Structure, contracts, and incentives* The shape of
British general practice has been significantly
altered by two contractual changes (apart from
the introduction of the NHS itself in 1948). In
1966 important changes (the 'Charter') encouraged and enabled the formation of group
practices and the employment and attachment
of nursing, administrative, and clerical staff.
In 1990 new requirements shifted general
practitioners in the direction of more screening
for health problems, increasing preventive
services (including immunizations), and improving management of continuing care of selected
health problems. The capitation elements of
remuneration were reduced and rewards for
achieving targets and delivering specified services
were increased.

Contemporaneously to, but separate from the
1990 contract changes, the 'NHS Reforms' created
an internal market in healthcare, in which
primary care 'purchased' secondary care from
hospital 'providers'. General practices became
entitled to hold funds to purchase services with.

Fund-holders used this opportunity to introduce quality standards into secondary care contracts (including limits on waiting times, requiring consultation opinions, and specifying agreed discharge patterns). Fund-holders also purchased specialist services to be provided within the community or in their own practices, reducing the revenue available to secondary care provider institutions. The initial restricted range of services open to fund-holders was enlarged in a series of 'total purchasing pilots', which were still being evaluated when a further range of reforms was announced to take effect in 1999.

In these, the internal market was formally discontinued. Aggregates of general practices serving communities of 100 000 will control their own budgets to provide community-based services including prescribing and staffing budgets. (In Scotland, however, such groups will have influence over a 'joint investment fund', through which to negotiate the shape of agreed secondary care services. It is not yet clear whether this element of the budget will be token (small) or considerable — a decision which will considerably influence whether the market concept has been discarded or simply re-designated.)

***Teams, groups, records and information technology, guidelines and evidence-based medicine*** As described above, practices increasingly work in groups to provide services to populations, consultations with individual patients being thus a part of a system rather than the whole of it as was the case when the NHS was launched. Practices are supported by community nurses (district nurses and practice-based nurses) and by health visitors (responsible for health maintenance rather than disease management). Patients have direct access to those services in many practices. In some practices nurses work as nurse-practitioners, replacing some doctor-based consultations, and in many practices nurses and doctors share care for conditions such as asthma, diabetes, and hypertension. Larger practices, often sharing premises, may employ or have access to other services including psychiatric nursing, physiotherapy, and social work. Midwifery services are generally shared with a local specialist unit. The concept of specialist consultant services (for example, dermatology or psychiatry) in the community has been piloted but appears not to be cost-effective and seems unlikely to be developed widely.

The increasing focus on providing care for populations has placed new emphasis on the organization of information both in practices and at area management scale. Paper records in many general practices are poorly organized and uninformative; however, teaching practices must have summarized and chronologically ordered records in order to be approved. Collecting meaningful data is, however, handicapped both by the frequent difficulty in identifying the real and complete reasons for patients' attendance, and by problems summarizing the sometimes obscure logic applied by doctors to the management of consultations.

Computers are obviously a substantial asset in indexing summary demographic and clinical data. The information they contain can reflect only the material they are provided with and even advanced information technology has not yet proved able to help with the complexities of truly holistic routine clinical practice. There is, however, growing evidence that the use of information technology improves the processes of care for patients with problems amenable to algorithm-based management.

The use of clinical algorithms and guidelines has generated enthusiasm among some doctors, but resistance from others. Their strength lies in the management of straightforward organic illness presentations where clearly defined and relatively immediate outcomes can be expected. These conditions are more commonly the province of hospital medicine than of general practice, in which the complex interaction of physical, social, and psychological problems, and the importance of behavioral outcomes (increasing understanding and improving coping and self-care strategies), complicate their application and reduce their relevance.

***Education and training*** The general practitioner of 1948 would have had neither undergraduate nor postgraduate education or training in or about general practice; would have no qualification or certification indicating competence to practice in the discipline; and would not have been able to, or have had to, undertake relevant continuing education after becoming a principal. Today, all medical students in Britain have been taught in and about general practice. Three years of approved vocational training have been a prerequisite to become a principal since 1982. All new principals have to satisfy a test of minimum competence and most new principals now sit and pass the Membership examination of the Royal College of General Practitioners. Taking part in continuing education attracts some remuneration, and the quality of that education is monitored by postgraduate supervisors.

***Institutions and governance*** General practitioners have always jealously defended their autonomy. As a profession, they have been unwilling to accept a necessity to pass an examination before entering practice, have resisted various contract proposals designed to increase services required as part of 'general medical services', and have been reluctant to undertake systematic audit as a part of routine practice. Part of the history of these positions reflects institutional tensions between the British Medical Association's General Practitioner Committee (which included a trade union function in its activities) and the Royal College of General Practitioners, founded in 1952 with the explicit purpose of improving quality in general practice and seen by many doctors at that time as élitist and as a threat to their autonomy. The Royal College has explicitly promoted both quality and audit, but has been reluctant to promote its examination as a compulsory route to principalship.

At the end of the 20th century, the general climate of public opinion, openness and accountability of professional groups became a major national issue, affecting medicine as much as any other activity. Safeguarding public safety and ensuring professional standards have been the province of the General Medical Council, a body which — although substantially democratized in recent years by elections and the inclusion of lay members — is still seen as overly protective of doctors. 'Clinical governance' is seen as the mechanism through which management (on behalf of the public) will assure the maintenance of appropriate standards of competence in and of service from the professionals who provide care, and the current challenge to professionals and the institutions representing their various disciplines is to deliver a package of proposals which will achieve this. Both (re-)accrediting practices and (re-)certifying doctors seem likely to figure prominently in discussions.

*Research and development* Given the inherent autonomy of general practitioners, and the necessity to 'tolerate uncertainty' in their day-to-day clinical practice, not surprisingly research took a low profile in the discipline's activities for many years. Exceptional individual leaders came together in the early years of the Royal College to create a national facility for research in the discipline, centering on several specialist research units, with networks of supporting doctors peripherally. The slow early growth of departments of general practice with a principal commitment to developing research gathered pace after 1970, and there is now a substantial research base and many publications throughout Britain. However, general practice — both as a service and as an academic discipline — has been disadvantaged compared with hospital clinical disciplines in terms of infrastructure support, critical mass, breadth of disciplinary base, and access to resources to maintain and develop successful program-based research teams.

The agreement of the NHS to provide some academic support money to underpin both teaching and research infrastructure in 1992 represented an important landmark and further improvements since have provided welcome additions. The creation of the 'National primary care research and development centre' in Manchester has ensured an important opportunity for the discipline, and an official report has embodied a wider set of proposals, implementation of which would place primary care in a much healthier research and development position than previously.

### Overview
The achievement of holistic care requires the ability to separate and prioritize content, and this depends to some extent on the way practitioners approach their work. This in turn is influenced by the context — both immediate and longer term — of their consultations. When the context is hostile, preferred working styles are compromised and the process of care is constricted. There is also accumulating evidence that the achievement of best outcomes is helped when continuity is good and that access — both to care and to continuity — is better in smaller than in larger groupings of doctors. Thus, although big may be better at delivering many services to populations, small may be better when it comes to care for the individual at a consultation.                    JHow

*See also* EDUCATION; EVIDENCE-BASED MEDICINE; HEALTHCARE SYSTEMS

**GENE THERAPY** is the ability to introduce genes into the body to cure or alleviate inherited or acquired diseases. Theoretically, it should be most effective in cases where the locus of a disease has been pinpointed to a single gene (such as sickle cell disease, Huntington's disease, or combined immune deficiency disease). However, it may well

Woman having her blood pressure taken by her general practitioner. (Reproduced courtesy of the Science Photo Library.)

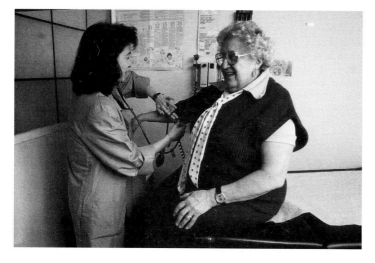

be useful in other disorders. The possibility of gene therapy arose from the biomedical revolution. This began with the elucidation of the double helical structure of DNA in 1953, to be followed by several important steps deciphering the mechanisms through which genetic information in DNA is transcribed into RNA and translated into protein; the cracking of the genetic code; the rise of recombinant DNA technology; and the development of the capability to rapidly sequence purine and pyrimidine bases (nitrogen-containing compounds) of genetic material, thereby allowing for the manipulation and manufacture of specifically 'designed genes.'

As evidenced by the large investment by the PHARMACEUTICAL INDUSTRY as well as by governments, gene therapy is viewed as having almost unlimited potential. However, over 200 clinical trials conducted by 1997 led a US panel of experts to conclude that there was no unequivocal evidence of any example of success. Nevertheless, gene therapy could become an exciting method of treatment, analogous to the antibiotic revolution for infectious diseases.

The success of gene therapy depends on the ability to introduce genes into living organisms to replace or augment faulty genes. The ideal situation will be the introduction of a gene through an appropriate vector which can be targeted to a designated site, be it an organ or a group of cells. The vector, containing this 'transgene', should be taken up in sufficient numbers and the gene incorporated into the genetic machinery of the cell such that it will be expressed for long periods of time.

The most immediate challenge for gene therapy lies in effective gene delivery. The gene may be delivered into the body or to cells in culture, which are then returned to the body. Three different methods of gene delivery have been explored: the use of viral vectors containing the transgene, the direct injection of DNA itself or combined with other substances (such as cationic lipids or polylysine), and the use of electroporation, which seems to alter the cell's membrane to allow DNA to pass through it. Current opinion is that the best method will involve using viral vectors designed to integrate into the cell of choice.

The ideal vector should be in high concentration allowing many cells to be infected. It should be easy to produce, and able either to integrate in a site-specific location in the host chromosome or to be maintained in the cell outside this. It should target specific cells, and its transcription unit should respond to manipulation of its regulatory units. Finally, there should be no immune response triggered by the vector. No vector having all these properties has yet been developed.

Viruses with some or many of these properties are the DNA-adenoviruses and the adeno-associated viruses, both of which show promise. Retroviruses (RNA viruses) also are being investigated. They share the problem of being non-infective for non-dividing cells, but might be used to infect cells in culture, which could subsequently be re-introduced to the body. Recently, Lenti-viruses (a type of RNA virus, the best known being the human immunodeficiency virus, HIV), which have the desirable capacity of infecting both dividing and non-dividing cells, have emerged as candidates for vector design. However, all current gene delivery strategies have been plagued by three problems: inefficient take-up of the transgene; transient expression of the transgene; and host response to the vector.

In combined immune deficiency disease, patients have a problem that affects only one gene, which is inactive for the enzyme adenosine deaminase (ADA), resulting in an inability of both T and B lymphocytes to function normally. Accordingly, such patients have had to spend their lives in sterile bubble-like chambers. The introduction of functioning ADA genes should relieve the problem and cure the disease. In the first trial of gene therapy allowed by the US National Institutes of Health and Food and Drug Administration, two children were given the ADA gene by a retrovirus vector inserted into isolated living cells, which were then returned to the body. However, ethical reasons required administration of ADA mixed with polyethylene glycol as an adjunct, thereby making ultimate interpretation of this experiment ambiguous. Five years later, one of the two children had 25% of the normal levels of ADA and had improved, whereas the other patient was unable to synthesize any active ADA.

Another problem in which gene therapy is being explored is in treating coronary artery occlusion by angioplasty. Before the use of stents to keep blood vessels open, the initial success of the mechanical procedure was about 90%, but within 3–6 months about one-third of these patients developed sufficient recurrence of the arterial narrowing or blockage (restenosis) to require additional angioplasty or bypass surgery. The major cause of the restenosis was found to be proliferation of smooth muscle cells at the site of vascular injury. A hypothesis was made that insertion of genes to repress cell proliferation would inhibit restenosis. Such a gene is the retinoblastoma gene, which is deficient in retinoblastomas (a malignant tumor arising in the eye), allowing the tumor cells to proliferate. Thus, viral-packaged retinoblastoma genes were inserted into animals and shown to inhibit restenosis. A similar strategy might prove to be successful in treating cancer.

Another form of gene therapy lies in 'genetic medicine'. In one approach, anti-sense oligo-nucleotides (synthetic RNAs) are designed to penetrate cell membranes, react with and bind to the specific mRNA (messenger RNA) of a pathogenic virus (or other pathogen), and thereby disable the ability of the cell to help produce the gene-product protein. Properly designed, such therapies could be very powerful, not only in treating infectious diseases, but cancer and other diseases (such as psoriasis) as well. Recently, an anti-sense oligonucleotide against a cytomegalic virus was found to be useful in treating cytomegalic retinitis, an eye disease induced by the virus. This anti-sense oligonucleotide is the first anti-sense to be approved for use by the US Food and Drug Administration, which licensed it in September 1998.

Another strategy representing the use of a 'genetic medicine' is using DNA as a vaccine. DNA from a foreign organism such as a virus (for example, HIV) is introduced into the cell, resulting in transcription and translation of the DNA to yield a foreign protein. The foreign protein is then treated by the cells as would be any foreign protein, ultimately eliciting an immune response directed against the protein coded for by the introduced DNA.

However, although gene therapy has had greater success as a concept than as a reality, the problems encountered in its development appear resolvable. Almost certainly any new edition of this book will attest to the potential of gene therapy becoming a reality. DAC

*See also* GENETICS, HUMAN

**GENETICS, HUMAN — HISTORY** The study of heredity touches on every aspect of clinical practice. It is likely to become a subject of prime importance for research and practice in the new millennium.

Until the middle of the 19th century thoughts about heredity were extremely confused. It was believed that a preformed embryo was encapsulated in the mother's ovum and that an ill-defined influence from the father galvanized things into activity. The 'preformation' theory is summarized by Bowler as follows: 'The theory of pre-existing germs held that all organisms grow from miniatures or "germs" created by God at the beginning of the universe, stored one within the other like a series of Russian dolls. The first woman, Eve, literally contained within her ovaries the whole of the rest of the human race, generations after generations of miniatures packed one inside the other, each waiting for an act of fertilization to give it a chance to grow … The male semen merely provided the stimulus that triggered off the expansion of the outmost miniature.'

It followed that if the germ defined an individual, their characteristics depended on what God had created, not on anything transmitted from the parents. Even after the discovery of sperm the preformation hypothesis was not abandoned and some held that an individual was preformed in the sperm, and only nurtured by the mother. The long struggle between ovists and spermists continued throughout the 18th century, and, although medical scientists started to recognize that disease might occur in successive generations of a family, a reasonable understanding of these observations had to wait for over 100 years.

**Two major advances**

In 1889 Walther Flemming, a German anatomist, discovered thread-like objects in dividing cells which absorb color from particular dyes. Flemming called these structures 'chromatin' and later they became known as chromosomes. When a cell divides (by a process known as mitosis), chromosomes appear to divide and identical copies are passed on to the next generation of cells. The notion that they might contain hereditary information was developed by the German zoologist August Weismann. Although his ideas were vague, he developed one critical concept. If the hereditary material from both parents resides in chromosomes, and is mixed in a fertilized egg, the egg ought to contain twice as much as the parental cells; in every succeeding generation it would double. Clearly this cannot happen. In 1887 Weismann reasoned that during cell division in eggs and sperm the amount of hereditary material is reduced by half. This reduction division became known as meiosis.

These ideas were extended by the American biologists Walter Sutton and Edmond Wilson, work which led to a clearer picture of how

A packaging cell containing a packaging-defective retrovirus allows one round of infection of the target cells by the vector carrying the new DNA. Thereafter the vector cannot infect further cells because it does not carry genes for the viral protection coat.

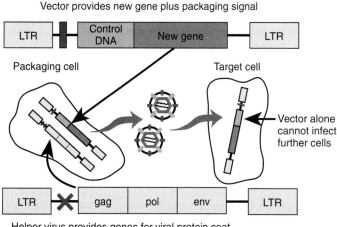

Vector provides new gene plus packaging signal

| LTR | Control DNA | New gene | LTR |

Packaging cell

Target cell

Vector alone cannot infect further cells

| LTR | gag | pol | env | LTR |

Helper virus provides genes for viral protein coat but is packaging defective

chromosomes are inherited. Except during the formation of gametes — that is, ova or sperms — cells divide by mitosis, which is preceded by doubling of each pair of chromosomes. This ensures that the two daughter cells each acquire a set of chromosomes identical to the parental cell, a state which is called diploid. On the other hand, during gamete formation cell division occurs by meiosis, to give progeny with half the number of chromosomes, that is, the haploid state; fertilization restores cells from the haploid to the diploid state.

The other main advance during the 19th century was the discovery by Gregor MENDEL (p 486) that inheritance of certain factors follows two simple mathematical rules.

The true significance of sexual reproduction and meiosis became apparent only during the early part of the 20th century, after a brilliant series of breeding experiments using the fruitfly *Drosophila* by Thomas Hunt Morgan and his colleagues. When maternal and paternal chromosomes become closely wound round each other during meiosis it is possible for genes to pass from one to the other by a process called crossing over, or recombination. Mendel's laws had described only the patterns of inheritance of individual genes, but Morgan's group in the USA and William Bateson in Britain realized that if two genes are on the same chromosome, and particularly if they are close together, they will tend to be inherited together. The genes are then said to be linked. The closer together a pair of genes are on the same chromosome, the less chance they will have to cross over. Hence, Morgan reasoned, the number of crossovers is a measure of the distance between genes. These seminal ideas led to the production of maps of genes on chromosomes, work that involved many linkage studies and the application of complicated mathematical models for their analysis. From the work of Herman MÜLLER (p 338) it also became clear that genes can change their structure — that is, undergo mutation — and that this process may be speeded up under certain conditions, such as the exposure of cells to radiation.

These studies in the USA were mirrored by equally important developments in Britain, where for the first time, statistical methods were used to study the behavior of genes in populations. The work of biometricians such as Ronald Fisher, J. B. S. Haldane, and Karl PEARSON (p 782), as well as clearly distinguishing between simple Mendelian inheritance and more complex hereditary systems under the control of many different genes, paved the way for the amalgamation of Mendelism and Darwinism, which formed the basis for modern evolution theory.

DJW

**GENETICS, HUMAN** Human genetics was developed in Britain in the second half of the 19th century. It was driven by the ideas of Francis GALTON (p 285), who was interested in improving the human species by selective breeding, work summarized in the first edition of his book *Hereditary genius*, in 1869. Although much of Galton's later thinking about genetics was confused — because unlike Mendel the traits in which he was most interested did not follow simple patterns of inheritance — he was the instigator of quantitative human genetics. And those who followed him, particularly Karl PEARSON (p 782) and Ronald Fisher, and J.B.S. Haldane, laid the foundations of quantitative genetics and, later, of population genetics.

Biochemical genetics was also born at about this time through the work of Archibald Garrod. In his book *Inborn errors of metabolism*, published in 1909, Garrod described several rare diseases which he thought were due to inherited defects in the body's chemical pathways. Garrod did not immediately appreciate the true genetic significance of his observations. He noted, however, a high incidence of parental consanguinity in some of his families and William Bateson pointed out to him that this is precisely what would be expected if the conditions he was describing were inherited in a Mendelian recessive fashion. Garrod had, in effect, laid the basis for the understanding of the genetic basis of biochemical individuality, a concept he later expanded to explain individual susceptibility to common disease.

Human genetics flourished in England during the first half of the 20th century. When Francis Galton died in 1911, University College, London, was left sufficient money to establish the Galton eugenics professorship and department of applied statistics, which included the Galton and biometric laboratories. Although some of its early work was related to eugenics — that is, the improvement of the population by selective breeding — it also established the scientific basis for human genetics. Work carried out at the Galton Laboratory (which became the Mecca for workers from all over the world just before and just after the Second World War) placed human pedigree analysis on a firm statistical basis, established the first genetic linkages in man, and laid the basis for the study of genetic disease.

Knowledge about the cellular and biochemical aspects of human heredity also advanced rapidly during the first half of the 20th century. Laborious studies of cultured cells gradually led to the conclusion that human beings have 46 chromosomes; 22 pairs are autosomes; the other pair are the sex chromosomes. The latter were designated X and Y, terminology derived from earlier work on the chromosomes of

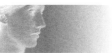

(continued)

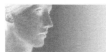

Herman Joseph **MÜLLER** (1890–1967). American geneticist, Müller was born in New York City and educated at Columbia University. The early part of his scientific career was spent at the University of Texas, where he carried out fundamental studies on genes, gene mutations, genetic linkage, and genetic recombination. His work on the production of gene mutations in *Drosophila* by X-rays was later to bring him the NOBEL PRIZE for medicine (1946). In 1933, at the age of 43, he left the USA for Moscow, becoming the senior geneticist at the Institute of Genetics of the Academy of Sciences of the USSR. Four years later he went to the Institute of Animal Genetics in Edinburgh, before returning to the USA. His later years were marked by involvement in controversial issues; he proposed the establishment of a sperm bank to perpetuate the genetic characteristics of outstanding men, and he was an early opponent of the use of nuclear weapons.

*Hemiptera* by Edmond Wilson. Females have two X chromosomes, males one X and one Y sex chromosome.

Another advance in cytogenetics — that is, the study of chromosomes — was the discovery that when chromosome preparations are stained with dyes (in particular, quinacrine mustard or Giemsa), they show alternate light and dark banding regions. Chromosome banding was an invaluable advance for identifying individual human chromosomes, in both health and disease. The first congenital defect found to be associated with an autosomal chromosome anomaly in humans was Down's syndrome; in 1959 Lejeune examined the chromosomes of nine 'mongoloid' children and found that in each case there were 47 chromosomes. The discovery of many other human cytogenetic abnormalities followed.

### Color blindness

The first gene to be assigned to a human chromosome was for color blindness, found to be on the X chromosome by workers at Columbia University in 1911. Another 57 years were to pass before a gene was localized to anything but the X chromosome; a particular blood group was assigned to chromosome 1 by a team in JOHNS HOPKINS UNIVERSITY (p 840) in 1968. For the next 20 years progress was very slow in assigning human genes to chromosomes, largely because there were so few markers for linkage studies. By 1976 at least one gene had been assigned to each of the 23 autosomes, yet by 1987 at least 1215 genes had been assigned, 365 of which are known to be the site of mutations causing disease. This remarkable period of progress stemmed from the use of new mapping techniques, first involving the fusion of human and animal cells, and later from advances in the recombinant DNA field.

### Human biochemical and molecular genetics

Human biochemical genetics evolved in the post-war period and took a considerable step forward with the discovery by Linus Pauling and his colleagues that the hemoglobin of patients with sickle cell disease (a severe inherited anemia in which the red blood cells assume a sickle shape) migrates at a different rate in an electric field (that is, on electrophoresis) to normal hemoglobin. A protein moves under these conditions depending on its charge, which in turn reflects its amino acid composition. This suggested, therefore, that sickle cell disease results from an inherited structural variant of hemoglobin.

In subsequent years many human proteins were examined by electrophoresis and every one turned out to be polymorphic; that is, there were genetically determined structural variants. In many cases these changes were harmless, but in others these were associated with abnormal function or stability of the protein and hence with disease. Many single gene disorders were found to be due to the synthesis of an abnormal enzyme or protein and it was possible to relate the particular structural changes to abnormal function or stability.

It was discovered in the late 1940s that genetic information is encoded in deoxyribonucleic acid (DNA). In 1953 James Watson and Francis Crick proposed a structure for DNA. Their model, which subsequently turned out to be correct, consisted of a double helix made up of two chains of nucleotide bases wrapped around each other and supported by backbones of simple sugars and phosphates.

There are four bases, adenine (A), guanine (G), cytosine (C), and thymine (T). Because of their particular shapes, A always pairs with T, and C with G; the bases, and the chains or strands, are linked by relatively weak chemical bonds. This structure makes it clear how genetic information is passed from cell to cell and from generation to generation. When a cell divides the two halves of the double helix come apart and each acts as a template for the synthesis of a new chain of nucleic acids; because of the rules of base pairing this has to be identical to its predecessor.

The information encoded in DNA by virtue of the order of nucleotide bases along its strands is used to direct the structure of proteins, the building blocks of all living tissues. Proteins consist of long strings of amino acids (peptide chains), which fold into complex three-dimensional shapes that are vital for their wide-ranging functions. Since there are only 20 naturally occurring amino acids it follows that the extraordinary diversity of proteins, ranging from the tough keratin of our skin and hair, through the soluble hemoglobin in our blood to the miriad of different enzymes that drive our body chemistry, depends on the particular order of amino acids in their constituent peptide chains. A gene is a length of DNA that encodes the structure of a particular chain of amino acids, together with the additional bases required to regulate its activity. The genetic code is a triplet code; that is, three nucleotide bases for each particular amino acid.

DNA is not directly concerned in making proteins but stays in the nucleus of cells directing these operations. When a gene is to be activated, or transcribed, one of its DNA strands is copied into a mirror image molecule called messenger RNA. This undergoes several chemical modifications while in the nucleus and then moves into the cytoplasm, where it acts as a template, or workbench, for the construction of proteins. Since it is a mirror image of the gene on which it is copied, it faithfully transmits the triplet genetic code for this purpose. Different amino acids are brought to the template attached to molecules called transfer RNAs, each of which has three bases, or anticodons, that are compatible with particular triplet codewords for the amino acids that they transport. When they reach the template they find the appropriate place by codon/anticodon base pairing. The messenger RNA is read from left to right. Once the first transfer RNA is in place the amino acid attached to it forms a chemical bond with the second amino acid after the second transfer RNA has ensured it too is in the appropriate place. The peptide chain is then two amino acids long. This process continues from left to right across the template until the peptide chain is complete. To make sure that things

happen in the right place, there are specific 'start' (initiation) and 'stop' triplet codons.

The analytical tools developed during these fundamental studies have had direct relevance to the characterization of human genes, in both health and disease. It turned out that the two strands of DNA can be dissociated and reassociated, by heating and cooling, for example. This reannealing reaction is highly specific and under the right conditions will occur only between DNA strands, or DNA and messenger RNA strands, that have identical or almost identical base sequences. Thus, to find a particular gene buried away in a large amount of DNA, a length of DNA or RNA with an identical sequence is constructed so that it will anneal to the gene but not to the rest of the DNA. This is the principle

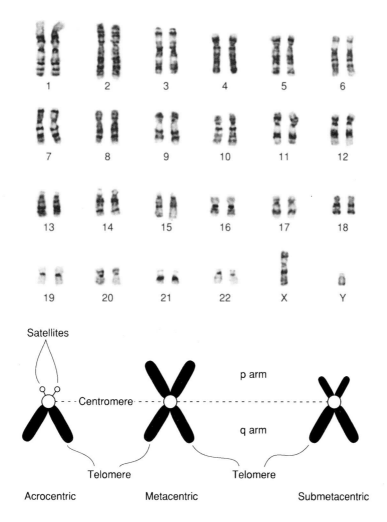

Human chromosomes. (a) The normal human male karyotype. The chromosomes are identified by their size, banding patterns, and position of the centromere. Trypsin-Giemsa banding. (Kindly prepared by Dr J. Jonasson.) (b) The anatomy of human chromosomes. (Both diagrams are reproduced from Weatherall, D. (1991). *The new genetics and clinical practice*, 3rd edn, OUP.)

behind constructing gene probes to find genes of particular interest.

## Restriction enzymes

Another advance was the discovery of a family of bacterial enzymes called restriction endonucleases, or restriction enzymes, which cleave DNA at particular sequences of bases. Thus it was possible to fractionate human DNA into pieces of predictable structure and size. This led to the development of human gene cloning which is based on the principle of inserting pieces of human DNA into an appropriate vector, that is, another DNA molecule capable of replicating in a bacterial cell. The first cloning vectors were plasmids, simple organisms that live and replicate

in the cytoplasm of bacteria. If DNA is fractionated and the plasmid DNA is cut with the same enzyme, and the mixture treated in a way that favors reassociation of the DNA fragments, some of the pieces of human DNA will be incorporated into plasmids. These now recombinant vectors are then inserted into bacteria, where they replicate independently from the bacterial DNA. Thus it is possible to generate what are called 'gene libraries' — fragments of DNA representing almost the complete human genome growing on bacterial plates. Genes that are being sought can be identified from particular colonies by hybridization with radioactively labelled gene probes. Once human genes could be grown in bacteria in this way they could then be isolated

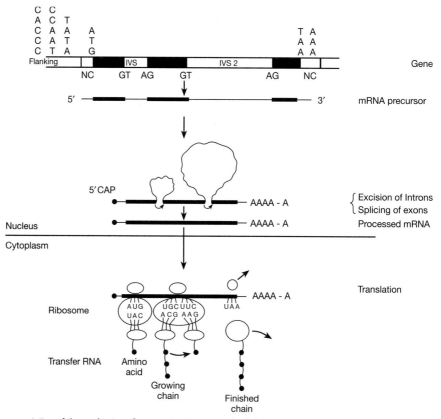

A representation of the mechanism of gene action. Genes are divided up into coding regions, or exons, and lengths of DNA of unknown function called introns (intervening sequences or IVS). In the gene that is shown here there are three exons shaded in dark and two introns shown as open boxes. The sequences at either end of the gene are involved in gene regulation. When the gene is transcribed, a large messenger DNA precursor is produced. While in the nucleus this undergoes processing, during which the intron sequences are removed, the exons spliced together, and a tail of adenoic acid residues (A) are added. The now definitive messenger RNA moves into the cytoplasm, where it acts as a template for protein synthesis. Amino acids are moved to the template on transfer RNAs, each of which has three bases which identify the appropriate triplet codons on messenger RNA. The growing peptide chains are transferred along the messenger RNA on the ribosomal subunits. There is a start codon (AUG) and a stop codon (UAA), indicating the beginning and end of chain analysis.

and their structure determined. Subsequently various ingenious cloning vectors were developed, some based on bacteriophage (bacterial viruses), others on yeast.

By using these techniques it was possible to isolate human genes and to introduce them into different cell lines, and later into animals, and to learn how they are regulated. Thus it was feasible to persuade human genes to make their products in bacteria, opening up a completely new approach to the production of therapeutic agents.

But the technology of the molecular era had even more important implications for the development of human genetics. In particular, it provided an opportunity for developing maps of the entire human genome. It is estimated that there are about 50–100 000 genes distributed among the 23 pairs of human chromosomes. In 1927 J. B. S. Haldane reasoned that if it were possible to map 50 or more inherited characters, that is, to place them in the appropriate position on their chromosomes, they could be used as markers for predicting whether children would inherit genes for important diseases. The idea was beautifully simple.

Supposing we wish to find the gene for a particular trait but know nothing about its location or function. First we must select a gene whose location is known and which can be identified in a simple way — a blood group, for example. If families are studied, and if the two genes are linked, they will always pass together through successive generations; depending on how close they are we may encounter some recombinants, but we should still be able to obtain some indication of their distance from each other. Of course, if they are not linked, they will segregate independently in different generations. Until the DNA era the problem with this approach was that very few markers could be used for linkage studies. However, the new DNA technology provided a wealth of linkage markers.

Normal people vary considerably from one another in the structure of their DNA. Much of this variation reflects single base changes that can be identified by particular restriction enzymes and that give different length DNA fragments after digestion. These restriction fragment length polymorphisms offer invaluable linkage markers. Even better, it turns out that there are regions of DNA, usually consisting of repetitive sequences, which vary widely in their length between different individuals. These highly variable regions provide very informative linkage markers; and there are even more common and variable repetitive regions of DNA called microsatellites. All this genetic variability in the structure of DNA has provided a rich source of markers, whose existence has transformed modern human genetics.

## Linkage analysis

Linkage analysis has led to the discovery of many human genes, some involved in important diseases. By searching for segregation of these disorders with particular linkage markers, it has been possible to identify the particular chromosome involved and then to pinpoint the position occupied by the abnormal gene. Linkage studies of this type may land geneticists many millions of bases away from the particular gene they are searching for. However, by some ingenious developments in molecular biology it is possible to 'walk' or 'jump' along chromosomes and, with some luck, to identify the particular gene responsible for a disease.

Having found a gene, the next step is for the geneticist to sequence it and then to make an educated guess about the likely protein structure of its product, based on its DNA sequence. This new approach, originally called reverse genetics and later renamed positional cloning, has led to the identification of the product of the genes involved in many human diseases for which the cause was not known and has already provided some understanding of their function and how this is affected by the mutations causing these diseases.

These remarkable successes, together with other improvements in mapping technology, have spawned the HUMAN GENOME PROJECT. Essentially this involves generating both genetic and physical maps of the entire human genome. A genetic map will consist of linkage markers spread at convenient lengths along all the human chromosomes. In essence, it will be like a road atlas that shows the position of towns along roads. The physical map, on the other hand, will describe the details of the roads, that is, the complete base sequence of the entire human genome. This will be no mean task. It is estimated that it is made up of three thousand million bases, and when fully sequenced, the information will fill approximately 13 volumes of the size of the *Encyclopedia Britannica*. Nevertheless, the preliminary phase of the project was completed in 2000.

## Medical genetics

Although originally medical genetics was confined to the study of single gene disorders and developmental abnormalities due to chromosomal defects, more recently it has touched on every aspect of clinical practice. It is now realized that many of the common diseases of western society, which seem to result from our life-styles or the new environments that we have created, also have an important genetic component. Furthermore, it has become apparent that the genetic machinery of cells may be damaged during our lifetime; this has bred a new discipline called somatic cell genetics, which has implications for a better understanding of cancer and, possibly, aging.

*Single gene disorders* In the clinical geneticist's bible, *Mendelian inheritance in man*, Victor McKusick lists over 4000 diseases which are either definitely, or very likely, the result of the action of a single mutant gene. These diseases are transmitted through families in a way which follows Mendel's laws of inheritance. As discussed earlier, of our 23 pairs of chromosomes, 22 are called autosomes and the other pair are the sex chromosomes; women have two X chromosomes while men have an X and a Y chromosome. Diseases may be transmitted on the autosomes or on the sex chromosomes. In dominantly inherited disorders affected persons are heterozygous for the abnormal gene, that is, a defective gene inherited from one parent is sufficient to cause a disease — thus one half of their offspring will be affected, regardless of their sex. On the other hand, the disorder is not transmitted by unaffected members of the family. Autosomal recessive disorders are manifest only in individuals who have inherited a defective gene from both parents. These conditions require a double dose to produce a disease. The parents, or carriers, do not show the disease and their offspring have a 25% chance of being affected.

Some defective genes are carried on the X chromosomes. In X-linked recessive disorders, only males are affected and the condition is transmitted through healthy female carriers, who pass on the disorder to half their sons, while half their daughters are, like them, carriers. Some extremely rare genetic disorders are transmitted on the Y chromosome; in this case the disease is passed directly from father to son. These Mendelian forms of inheritance of single gene disorders are illustrated opposite.

By using the new techniques of molecular genetics it has been possible to characterize the different varieties of mutations that underlie single gene disorders. Most of these conditions are heterogeneous, that is, more than one mutation can cause the same disease. For example, the common genetic blood disease, $\beta$ thalassemia, has been found to result from nearly 200 different mutations. Cystic fibrosis, Duchenne muscular dystrophy, and many other genetic diseases are equally heterogeneous at the molecular level.

There are also many different types of mutations. In general, they either lead to the production of an abnormal protein product, or to a reduction of the amount produced. Mutations that alter the structure of a protein, called missense mutations, lead to the insertion of the wrong amino acid in a peptide chain. Many varieties of mutations exist that cause a reduced output of a gene product. In some cases entire genes are lost, or deleted. In others, single base changes scramble the genetic code in various ways so that messenger RNA cannot be used as a template for synthesizing normal proteins. Many genetic diseases result from mutations which interfere with the processing of the messenger RNA while it is still in the cell nucleus. And yet others are caused by mutations that interfere with the initiation or termination of protein synthesis on the messenger RNA template.

Fortunately, most single gene disorders are extremely rare and their frequency reflects the mutation rate in human beings. There are exceptions, however. For example, the recessively inherited blood diseases, sickle cell anemia and thalassemia, are extremely common in many tropical countries; in some parts of the world over half of the population may be carriers. It turns out that such people are more resistant to the ravages of MALARIA than those who do not carry genes for these blood diseases. Because they are protected, they tend to survive and have more children. The frequency of these genes therefore increases in these populations until it is balanced by the loss, through death, of homozygotes — those who have received a gene from both parents and therefore have a severe form of anemia. This form of natural selection is called balanced polymorphism. It is currently believed that the very high frequency of the gene for cystic fibrosis in north European populations may have followed the same mechanism, though the selective factor is not known in this case.

Many recessive disorders can now be identified in carriers, either by simple biochemical tests or by DNA analysis. Couples who are both carriers for recessive diseases have the option either not to have children, to adopt, or to take the risk of having an abnormal child. DNA technology offers another possibility. By removing a small piece of tissue from round the fetus, a technique called chorion villus sampling, it is possible to analyze fetal DNA for many monogenic diseases and to offer termination of those pregnancies in which the fetus has received an abnormal gene from both parents. Although this approach was also feasible using amniotic fluid as a source of cells for biochemical or cytogenetic analysis, the DNA era has greatly increased the number of conditions that can be identified antenatally.

*Chromosome disorders: cytogenetics* Each of the human chromosomes can now be identified with certainty using banding techniques. When describing chromosomal pathology, cytogeneticists refer to the appearance of the chromosome during a phase of mitosis, called metaphase, during which it is in a particularly compact state and can be

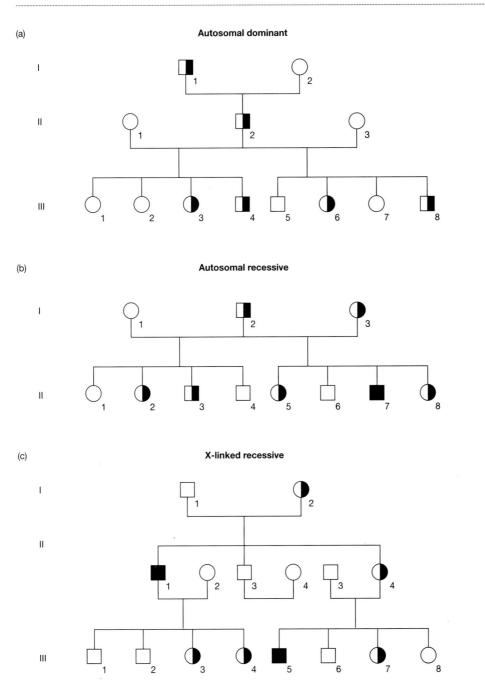

(a) **Autosomal dominant**

(b) **Autosomal recessive**

(c) **X-linked recessive**

Pedigrees illustrating different forms of monogenic inheritance. ○ represents male and □ female. In the family showing autosomal dominant inheritance the open symbols represent normal individuals and half-shaded are carriers (non-affected) and fully-shaded are affected. Note that in the family showing X-linked inheritance, in the third generation the daughters but not the sons of the affected male II-1, are carriers; among the children of the female carrier, II-6, half the sons are affected and half the daughters are carriers. (From Weatherall, D. (1991). *The new genetics and clinical practice*, 3rd edn, OUP.)

examined easily under the light microscope. Each chromosome is composed of two halves called sister chromatids. The chromatid halves are separated from each other along their lengths except at one point, the centromere, where they are joined. The centromere divides chromosomes into two unequal regions, which are called short and long arms, *p* for short and *q* for long. The total number of chromosomes per cell is described by an Arabic number and, if relevant, the sex chromosome constitution is indicated by one X and/or Y for each sex chromosome. Thus the normal male chromosome constitution, or karyotype, is written 46, XY, and a normal female 46, XX. If there is an extra chromosome, its number is preceded by plus, if one is missing by minus. For example, trisomy 21

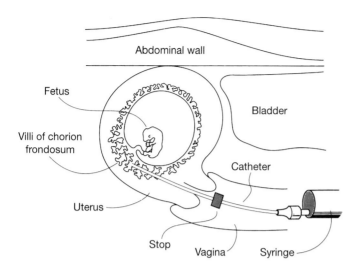

Abdominal wall

Fetus

Villi of chorion
frondosum

Bladder

Catheter

Uterus

Stop

Vagina

Syringe

The principle of chorion villus sampling to obtain trophoblast tissue for fetal DNA analysis. (Reproduced from Weatherall, D. (1991). *The new genetics and clinical practice*, 3rd edn, OUP.)

associated with chromosome changes. For example, a form of chronic leukemia that affects adults is almost invariably associated with a particular chromosomal abnormality called the Philadelphia chromosome after the city in which it was discovered. In this case there is usually a translocation between chromosomes 9 and 22.

Modern cytogenetics has made particularly good use of the new tools of molecular biology. For example, it is possible to persuade fluorescently labeled gene probes to hybridize on chromosome spreads and hence to localize the position of genes directly. By using a battery of different probes with different fluorescent labels, literally to paint the chromosome, it is possible to learn more about chromosome structure. These remarkable techniques, backed up by more advanced forms of microscopy, have transformed the subject.

*Genetic factors in common diseases; multifactorial inheritance* It has long been known that many common diseases, including heart disease, high blood pressure, DIABETES, the major psychoses, rheumatic disease, and others, have an important genetic component. However, epidemiological studies have shown that these conditions may all be precipitated by various environmental agents. Thus they reflect a complex interaction between nurture and nature. Since they rarely follow a Mendelian pattern of inheritance, susceptibility or resistance is thought to reflect the action of several genes. They are therefore called multi-genic, or polygenic, diseases.

One approach to estimating the importance of the genetic component of a disease is to study its occurrence (or concordance) in monozygotic (identical) compared with dizygotic (non-identical) twins. Clearly late onset, insulin resistant diabetes (type 2 diabetes) is, for all intents and purposes, a genetic disease, whereas the role of genes in ischemic heart disease, causing heart attacks, is small.

By using DNA analysis for linkage studies much progress has been made in determining some of the genes involved in these polygenic systems. For example, early onset diabetes (type 1 diabetes) is clearly associated with particular polymorphisms, that is, DNA base variations, of the genes of the human leukocyte antigen (HLA-DR) system and of another locus which appears to be close to the insulin gene. The human leukocyte antigen (HLA-DR) gene family, best known for its role in tissue typing for organ transplantation, is an important player in the body's immune system which identifies foreign invaders, or antigens. Possibly particular genetic variants of this system make it more likely that when we

(three chromosomes 21) is written 47, +21. Extra material on a chromosome arm is indicated by plus; for example, $14q+$ means that there is extra material on the long arm of chromosome 14. Similarly, a deletion is indicated by a − sign.

The frequency of chromosomal abnormalities at birth is about 5–6/1000. Of these, about 2/1000 are due to variation in the number of sex chromosomes, 1.7/1000 to variation in numbers of autosomal chromosomes, and 1.9/1000 to major chromosomal rearrangements. These anomalies account for 60 or more different clinical disorders. Among the more common and best defined are mongolism or Down's syndrome (trisomy 21), Edwards's syndrome (trisomy 18), Klinefelter's syndrome (sex chromosomes XXY), and Turner's syndrome (Xo — a sex monosomic disorder). Trisomies usually result from fertilization of gametes carrying two copies of a particular chromosome; in Down's syndrome the gamete carries two copies of chromosome 21. Such abnormal gametes result when homologous pairs of chromosomes fail to separate at the first or second division of meiosis, a phenomenon called non-dysjunction.

Diagnostic cytogenetics was originally confined to the analysis of children with congenital anomalies or mental retardation, and their families. However, it is now used widely in prenatal diagnosis programs for the identification of Down's syndrome, particularly in mothers at high risk. Cytogenetic analysis can be carried out after chorion villus sampling or on cells from amniotic fluid obtained later in pregnancy. Cytogenetics is also finding important applications in other disciplines, particularly in the diagnosis of cancer

encounter a particular antigen (a virus, for example) we mount a mistaken attack on our own tissues, in this case the pancreas; the result is diabetes. Several different enzyme variants concerned in glucose metabolism have been found in families with type 2 diabetes of unusually early onset. And polymorphisms or more extensive structural changes of several different families of genes concerned with cholesterol or lipoprotein chemistry have been found to be associated with an increased likelihood of developing coronary artery disease. The long-term objective is to define the important genes involved in susceptibility or resistance to these diseases to learn more about their underlying cause and, hopefully, to be able to define high risk individuals and establish preventive measures early in life.

*Somatic cell genetics and cancer* Although a few forms of cancer can be traced through families in a way that suggests the action of a single gene, in most cases this is not possible. However, it is now apparent that many cancers result from mutations of oncogenes — that is, a family of genes which, in health, regulate cell proliferation, maturation, and differentiation. Oncogenes can be abnormally activated in various ways, including single nucleotide base changes, amplification of their number, or translocation on to different chromosomes. When this happens cells may divide and spread in a disorderly way and become cancerous. It is also clear that some cancers result from the recessive inheritance of single genes, the action of which may become unmasked by various mechanisms, all of which have in common the inactivation of the normal partner, which, until this happens, can suppress the action of its abnormal allele. Although such loss of tumor suppression activity was originally thought to be restricted to some rare childhood tumors, it is now clear that it occurs in many common cancers, including of the lung, breast, bowel, and bone.

It is currently thought that the generation of cancer involves at least two genetic changes, and often many. For example, colon cancer seems to require the acquisition of mutations in at least six different oncogenes. This new branch of genetics promises to yield valuable advances in both the diagnosis and management of cancer.

Molecular genetics and cell biology have, therefore, brought together the disciplines of oncogenes, cytogenetics, and environmental studies of cancer to yield the beginnings of a coherent story of how most common cancers occur. As already mentioned, we may be born with a defective oncogene and a second mutation may occur which generates a cancer. But this is unusual. Much more commonly mutations of oncogenes probably result from the action of environmental agents, or mutagens, that can damage our DNA during our lifetime. These may come from the external environment or from the numerous chemicals generated during normal metabolism, which, if not inactivated, may also damage DNA. Some cancers result from critical chromosome disruptions such as deletions or translocations. Here, the site of the chromosome break or translocation may involve an oncogene which may become abnormally activated through being damaged or transported to another chromosome.

*Diagnostics and therapeutics* Recombinant DNA technology offers many possibilities for diagnosis and treatment. Probes that identify parts of the genome of micro-organisms promise to transform diagnostic microbiology. Similar techniques are finding wide application in diagnostic PATHOLOGY and FORENSIC MEDICINE. For example, studies using the hypervariable region gene probes have shown that each human being has a unique pattern, or DNA fingerprint. Despite early technical setbacks, DNA fingerprinting is now being used widely in forensic medicine. DNA is relatively stable and can be extracted from many different sources, even bones buried for thousands of years.

Recombinant DNA technology is also important in the pharmaceutical industry. It is possible to isolate human genes for a variety of functions and to insert them into micro-organisms to direct the synthesis of human products. Recombinant human proteins made in this way — such as erythropoietin, growth hormone, and insulin — are already in clinical use. A wide variety of different growth factors has also been produced — for example, to stimulate different cells of the bone marrow to treat patients with bone marrow failure. Recombinant DNA technology is also being used to produce vaccines and blood clotting factors.

*Gene therapy* Ever since the first experiments in which DNA was transferred between species, it has been realized that it should, eventually, be possible to correct certain genetic diseases in this way. Broadly, there are two ways in which this could be accomplished. First, a gene could be injected into a fertilized egg known to contain a defective counterpart. In this case the injected genes would be disseminated among all the organs of the growing fetus, including the gonads (ovaries or testes). In later life, the 'foreign' gene would therefore be passed to future generations. This form of germline GENE THERAPY has been banned in many countries. An alternative, somatic gene therapy, is different in principle. Here, a gene is inserted into a particular cell population and hence it does not become incorporated into the gonads

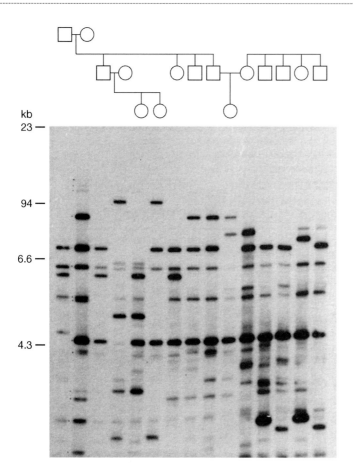

kb
23 —

94 —

6.6 —

4.3 —

Genetic fingerprinting. The patterns are from the individuals shown in the pedigree; each member is above his or her respective track.

and then internalized. Although this avenue has many attractions, it is difficult to be sure that the gene will not be damaged in its passage across the cell wall and into the nucleus of the cell.

A more attractive notion is to try to correct genetic diseases using another of nature's ways — by site-directed recombination. Here the idea is to line up a disease gene with a normal counterpart and encourage them to change places. This *tour de force* has been achieved in several systems, but so far it has not been possible to scale up the procedure to make it sufficiently efficient for use in the clinic.

Despite these problems there are genuine advances, and it seems certain that these will become part of clinical practice in the foreseeable future. Its first applications may well be in cancer, where short-term objectives are desired, controlling the growth of cancer cells, or even destroying them. But to correct genetic diseases, a great deal more will have to be learned about how genes are regulated, the best type of vectors with which to transfer them into appropriate cell populations, and whether, in their new home, they could have deleterious effects on the genome of the recipient.

### Broader issues in human biology

Molecular genetics is providing invaluable information throughout the whole of human biological research. Molecular approaches to population genetics are telling us how genes have become disseminated throughout populations and why particular genetic diseases are so common in some racial groups. Because our evolutionary history is written in our DNA, the comparison of DNA sequences, among different human populations and between humans and their nearest evolutionary ancestors, is providing important information about our place in the evolutionary tree and about how human populations have evolved and diverged. As this work develops it may have important implications for clinical medicine, in particular with respect to genetic susceptibility or resistance to important environmental factors responsible for some of the major killers of rich societies.

Human molecular genetics is also making important contributions to understanding development. It is helping to characterize some of the important genes concerned in different stages of human development and the complex mechanisms whereby genes are regulated at various stages. Again, this work promises to have important medical applications for understanding developmental abnormalities. Finally, molecular and cell biology combined with new approaches to human genetics is starting to make some inroad into the problems of aging and behavior.

and is not passed on to future generations. Hence, in principle, this approach is little different to organ transplantation.

Several problems still have to be overcome before somatic gene therapy can be successful. First, a particular target cell must be isolated. Ideally this should be a cell which renews itself. Most blood cells, for example, have only a finite survival. They are the product of a small population of bone marrow cells called stem cells which have the capacity for self-renewal. Therefore the aim of gene therapy for blood disease would be to insert genes into a reasonable number of stem cells. The next problem is how to insert the gene. This can be done directly by several physical methods but none of them is very effective. A second approach has been to use nature's way and to attach genes to retroviruses, viruses that have the ability to insert their genetic material into that of the host. Though it is possible to transfer genes in this way, it is difficult to achieve a high level of efficiency and there is no control over where the gene ends up in the genome. Another method is to attach genes to molecules identified by surface receptors on cells

There are likely to be important developments in genetics and it promises to lead the way towards understanding many of our intractable diseases.

**Ethical issues**

When human genetics was pioneered in Britain in the 19th century by Francis Galton and his followers, it was closely linked with EUGENICS — the improvement of the human stock by encouraging breeding by those who were considered to be the more acceptable members of society. Indeed, the development of human genetics, in both Britain and the USA, and elsewhere, was closely tied up with the eugenics movement right up to the beginning of World War II. After the war, and the realization of what had been perpetrated by the Nazi movement in the name of eugenics, this concept fell into disrepute.

In the second half of the 20th century, particularly after the molecular era and our increasing ability to dissect and manipulate DNA, fears of a recrudescence of the eugenics movement have been voiced. But, although modern clinical genetics is totally different in its attitudes to those of the eugenicists of the early part of this century, undoubtedly our increasing ability to manipulate our genes has brought with it some new ethical problems.

The increasing ability to identify different genetic traits in fetal life, and to terminate pregnancies which might be associated with severe disease after birth, has raised the important issue of what is 'abnormal'. Few question the right of parents to choose whether or not to have children with severe malformations or other life-threatening diseases, but there is an increasing tendency towards a desire for perfection, and it is not clear where this will all end. Indeed, some question whether society has a right to terminate pregnancies for any genetic disability. Similarly, there has been considerable debate about whether it is appropriate to alter the genetic make-up of an individual by gene therapy. While it is generally agreed that somatic gene therapy does not raise any serious new ethical issues, it is widely held that germline therapy, because it alters the genetic make-up of future generations, opens up new concerns.

Our increasing ability to identify the traits for genetic disease in unaffected individuals also raises problems. Sometimes it may be necessary to carry out a family study to see if a person is at risk for having a condition such as Huntington's disease which occurs only in middle life. One person in the family may want to know but to find out it may be necessary to study others who do not. Should our genetic make-up should be made available to insurers and employers? As we start to gain knowledge about genetic susceptibility to common diseases such as heart attacks and cancer, it may make it very difficult for some people to obtain insurance. Particularly in societies in which medicine is fully privatized, this might preclude many individuals from obtaining adequate medical care.

As more is learnt about our genetic make-up, and rapid screening methods are developed, there will be the temptation to carry out large-scale population screening for certain genetic diseases. This has the risk of causing considerable worry and stigmatization, and, if not backed up by adequate counseling, can have a demoralizing effect on society.

The commercialism of the human genome is also a problem. Should human genes be the subject of patents? Who owns our genetic material? Is it appropriate for companies to sell genetic screening services by mail order unaccompanied by genetic counseling?

These are all practical issues which are with us now. But even broader fears have been expressed, which again relate to the eugenics movement. If we learn which genes are involved in certain traits, aggression or artistic skills, for example, will there be a tendency in the future to try to hand-choose our children for particular characteristics? To what extent could this new power be used politically?

Most new branches of medical practice have, at least for a while, been the subject of considerable concern. Modern molecular genetics is going through the same phase. Many countries have set up licensing or other monitoring authorities to cover certain aspects. If these problems are adequately debated, those aspects of modern molecular genetics which are of genuine benefit for society should be allowed to develop; they have the potential to revolutionize clinical practice in the future.                    DWea

*See also* BIOETHICS; INBORN ERRORS OF METABOLISM; MOLECULAR BIOLOGY

**GERIATRIC MEDICINE — HISTORY** The commonly expressed idea that old age and its associated diseases and disabilities are recent phenomena is a misapprehension. Several of the world's ancient texts refer to the infirmities of old age. One of the most poignant allegorical descriptions of the disabilities of later life can be found in Chapter 12 of *Ecclesiastes.* HIPPOCRATES (p 382) noted urinary difficulties, constipation, apoplexy, pruritus, cataracts, hardness of hearing, and joint pains as being common in later life.

Because it is assumed that life expectancy at birth must have been low in ancient times, the 'old men' of the ancient writers are sometimes presented as being only in their 40s. This is to misunderstand the implications of life expectancy in undeveloped communities, where the deaths that reduce life expectancy take place in infancy and childhood. Once individuals have passed those early years, their fitness will be high because of the intense process of natural selection they have successfully survived. Old age, as we would now define it, is well documented in Classical Greece. Sophocles died at 91, Euripides at 78, Plato at 87, all still active, and Isocrates committed suicide at 98 when his political hopes came to naught. Agesilaus, King of Sparta, died in his 80s on the way back from commanding an active military campaign in Egypt.

Ancient writers speculated that senescence might to be due to desiccation or to loss of heat, but Francis Bacon was the first to propose anything that we would now recognize as a scientific approach to geratology. He outlined a program for observational research linking longevity with environmental and life-style factors that gives him an excellent claim to the intellectual fatherhood of both modern EPIDEMIOLOGY and geratology. An empirical approach to the clinical medicine of old age did not emerge until the 19th century. CHARCOT's (p 400) lectures on the *Diseases of old age*, translated into English by William Tuke in 1881, provided a detailed description of some of the common diseases of later life. G. M. Humphry published in 1889 a survey of 900 people aged over 80, the first essay in the epidemiology of the health and social circumstances of older people in a general population.

The term geriatrics was coined by I. L. Nascher, an Austrian immigrant to the United States. His textbook *Geriatrics: the diseases of old age and their treatment* was published in 1914. Although the American Geriatrics Society was founded in 1942, geriatrics as a medical specialty did not prosper in the USA. It was, however, one of the first fruits of the British National Health Service in 1948, and was based on the pioneering work of Marjory Warren at the West Middlesex Hospital in the 1930s. She had taken over responsibility for what had been an old WORKHOUSE hospital full of heavily disabled and socially disadvantaged patients, most of whom were elderly. Dr Warren worked to improve the hospital's facilities and the morale of its staff as well as to provide better care for its patients. She noted that many elderly patients consigned to the long-stay wards were capable of a better life if offered proper medical diagnosis and rehabilitation. During the Second World War, Warren published seminal papers advocating the recognition of geriatrics as a medical specialty, the provision of geriatrics units on all general hospital sites, and teaching in geriatrics for all medical students. Many visitors from elsewhere in Britain and from overseas visited Warren to learn from her methods, and she was invited to lecture in Canada, Australia, and the USA.

The National Health Service allocated responsibility for the old workhouse (municipal) hospitals, in which most long-stay elderly patients were confined, to the same health authorities as the traditionally more privileged charity hospitals. These latter had previously concerned themselves only with acute and curable illnesses and with the 'deserving' poor. With support from medical officers in the Department of Health the specialty of geriatrics was created to discharge a range of responsibilities that were essentially new to established medicine. Unfortunately, partly as a consequence of the old divisions between municipal and charity hospitals, for some years the new specialty was regarded as one to which only those doctors who had failed to make careers for themselves in more desirable specialties could be recruited. Fifty years on, geriatrics now flourishes as the largest specialty of adult hospital medicine in Britain. The corresponding psychiatric specialty of psychogeriatrics is a more recent creation but is also now providing specialist care in most districts of Britain.

In Britain, geriatrics is a hospital-based specialty with close links with community agencies. Three main models of geriatric service have evolved. In the traditional model, geriatric departments are restricted to patients referred to them for assessment, rehabilitation, and long-stay care. In the age-defined model, geriatric departments are run in parallel with general medical departments for younger adults, and provide all hospital medical services for patients above a specified age. In the integrated model, geriatricians work as members of multi-specialty teams of consultants providing acute hospital care for patients of all ages. In all three models, geriatric services offer specialist rehabilitation, day hospital, outpatient services, home visiting, and some long-stay care in addition to acute care. Respite care is also provided, in which elderly patients can be admitted on scheduled or occasional short-term stays to help in supporting informal carers.

Geriatrics is a recognized specialty in many countries, although not all have followed British models of practice. In North America the emphasis has been on geriatric assessment units or teams taking responsibility for selected older patients from other specialties for rehabilitation and resettlement in the community. RANDOMIZED CONTROLLED TRIALS of these North American models have shown their superiority to conventional hospital care for older patients in terms of cost-effective improvements in well-being and survival.

## Academic and research developments

The first journal concerned with the medicine of old age appeared in Germany in the 1930s and today there are many specialist journals in the discipline. Academic departments of geriatrics began to appear in medical schools in the 1960s, and are now widespread. Several national societies of geratology or geriatrics have an interest in fostering research. The International Association of Gerontology provides an umbrella organization, within which workers from the clinical, social, and biological disciplines can meet simultaneously every four years.

In the early 1940s the United States National Institutes of Health established a gerontology unit in Baltimore that became the Gerontology Research Center in 1966. In 1974 the National Institute on Aging was established under the directorship of Dr R. N. Butler, whose influential book *Why survive? Growing old in America* had stimulated great public and political concern about the inadequacies of medical and social provision for the growing numbers of aged people in the electorate of the USA. The institute provides dedicated funding to intramural and extramural research in all aspects of aging. As a specific scientific endeavor, aging has received little dedicated funding in other countries.                    JGE

## GERIATRIC MEDICINE (GERIATRICS) is a

specialty of medicine concerned with the care of old people. A related term, gerontology, was coined to designate the scientific study of aging but is etymologically incorrect as it implies study restricted to old men (γέροντες). The correct term for the study of old age (γῆρας) and aging is geratology. Social geratology is concerned with the social processes that affect aging and older people, biological geratology deals with the biochemical processes that cause senescence.

## The nature of aging

Senescence is defined by a progressive loss of adaptability of an organism as time passes. As we grow older, the homeostatic mechanisms on which our survival depends generally become less sensitive, less accurate, slower, and less well sustained. Sooner or later we encounter some challenge to which we can no longer mount an effective response and we die. A rise in mortality rate with age is therefore the biological hallmark of aging. In the human this rise begins around the age of 11 to 13 and apart from perturbations due to violent deaths in early adult life is continuous and nearly exponential thereafter. Measures of the prevalence of chronic disease and disability and use of health services also show a continuous and broadly exponential relationship to age throughout adult life. There are no discontinuities in later life to provide any biological justification for separating the elderly from the rest of the adult human race.

We age at different rates, so that differences between individuals increase with age. Although, on average, functional abilities decline with age, some individuals aged 80 will still be performing within the normal range for 30-year old people. It is important that medical treatment of older people should be based on an assessment of their individual capacity to benefit, not on their age.

There are some general characteristics of disease in later life. The longer we live the more time we have to accumulate diseases and disabilities and multiple pathology is common among old people who fall ill. Interactions between diseases and their treatments are a frequent source of difficulty in geriatric medicine.

Because of loss of adaptability, diseases may have a non-specific presentation. Inflammatory responses may be slower, and the perception of some forms of pain may be reduced in some older people. Pneumonia may therefore present as a delirium before signs are apparent in the chest; a heart attack or a perforated duodenal ulcer may present as sudden collapse or disorientation without pain. Loss of adaptability also results in rapid deterioration of an older patient if correct treatment is not instituted. Furthermore, there will be a high incidence of secondary complications of the disease and of its treatment. For all these reasons older people who fall ill need urgent access to the best of modern diagnostic and therapeutic facilities, and they will often need more investigations than do younger adults to establish an accurate diagnosis.

Most younger adults have sufficient functional reserve to recover spontaneously from illness; more old people will require a specific program of rehabilitation to return them to their former levels of function. Loss of adaptability also makes a person more vulnerable to the environment. Depressing or frightening surroundings in hospital can demoralize or confuse an older person. At home there may be an 'ecological gap' between what old people can do and what their housing demands of them. They may not be able to get upstairs to the only toilet in the house, or may not be able to reach a telephone to call for any help they may need. Good quality care has to bridge such gaps, by improving the patient's function (therapeutic intervention) or reducing the demands of the environment (prosthetic intervention).

The bridging of ecological gaps requires a multi-professional team with knowledge of the range of services available in hospital and community. Specialist geriatrics teams have a core membership of doctor, nurse, occupational

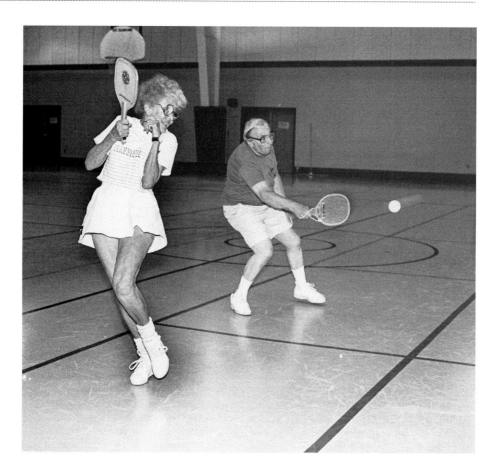

Aging may be healthier and more enjoyable if it is active rather than inactive.

therapist, physiotherapist, and social worker, and this team should be concerned in preparing vulnerable old people for discharge from hospital. This ensures the cost-efficient use of resources that is one of the responsibilities of a geriatric medical service.

### Components of human aging

The study of human aging usually starts with the differences between young and old people, but there are three sources of differences between young and old apart from aging. Because of selective survival people who reach old age will be different from those who died in middle age. This has been shown for some genes affecting susceptibility to disease but selective survival is also related to life-style and personality.

If aging is characterized by loss of adaptability it will be shown in the response of individuals of different ages to the same challenge. The organization of society can be such, however, that older people are presented with more severe challenges than face the young. Twenty years ago, one example of this differential challenge lay with

British housing policies which led to old people, at risk of hypothermia because of age-associated changes in metabolism, living in colder houses than those of younger adults. Differential challenges can now be found in the health services, where old people on average receive worse treatment than do the young. This has been documented in the USA in comparisons of the time spent by doctors in taking a history from patients of different ages and in the quality of treatment offered to cancer patients. In parts of Britain older patients have poorer access than the young to treatment for kidney failure and heart disease.

Cohort effects are most prominent in mental functioning in societies, such as the USA and Britain, which have been changing rapidly over the century. 'Intelligence' takes different forms in different cultures and the society for which older people were educated was very different from that in which the young are now raised.

### True aging

True aging is caused by interactions between intrinsic (genetic) and extrinsic (environmental and life-style) factors. In some lower animals single genes with a powerful effect on lifespan have been identified but in humans lifespan and aging rate seem to be determined by the actions of many genes. The intrinsic aging rate is largely determined by the effectiveness of the body's systems for detection and repair of damage to cells and their components.

The importance of extrinsic influences on aging lies in the scope for prevention and reversibility. Evidence is accumulating of the benefits of life-style change in middle life and old age both in recovering lost function and in retarding further deterioration. Courses of physical exercise by old people can improve muscle strength, and giving up smoking can reduce coronary heart disease risk even in late life. Among several age-associated changes or diseases thought at one time to be due to intrinsic aging but now known to have significant extrinsic determinants are vascular disease, high blood pressure, loss of muscle bulk and strength, osteoporosis and fractures, high tone deafness, and most cancers.

However, extrinsic factors may also have an irreversible impact, particularly in early life. The effect of childhood calcium intake on bone mass may prove to be one example. Susceptibility to some diseases with a significant effect on longevity may be determined partly before birth, through dietary and life-style influences acting on pregnant women,

The numbers and proportions of older people are increasing in both the developed and developing world. Over half of the world's population of people aged over 65 now lives in developing countries, where they may face particularly difficult circumstances. During economic development, agrarian cultures break down and traditional forms of family support for old people may be disrupted by industrialization, migration of young families to urban centers, and changes in cultural values. Economic development rarely provides the services necessary to replace the traditional social structures it destroys.

Two processes lead to the aging of populations. The first is demographic transition. When a nation reaches a certain stage of economic development its infant and child mortality rates start to fall steeply but it takes another generation for mean family size to fall commensurately. An unusually large cohort of survivors from childhood is therefore released into the population, eventually to become old. At a later stage of economic development mortality rates in middle and old age will also fall, so increasing the numbers of survivors into old age. This can arise because of a general improvement in health so that the new survivors into old age will be fitter than their predecessors. Alternatively, better health and social care may lengthen the survival of people with chronic illness and disability so that older people become less fit. Both effects are operating but the balance differs

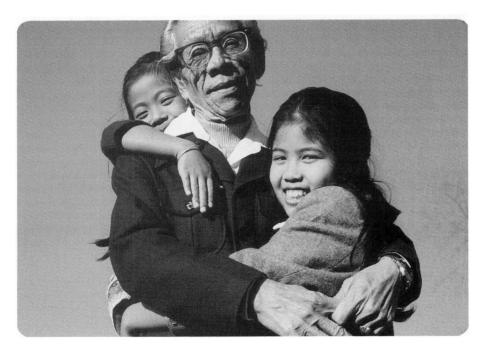

Both young and old benefit from the embrace.

between countries and between diseases. There are no reliable data for Britain but studies from the USA show that over the last decade older people have become fitter and have had less need of long-term health and social care. This is probably partly owing to improved life-style and partly to the prevention of disability by rational use of healthcare.

Declines in mortality in middle age are producing increasing numbers of people who fall into the category of the Third Age. The Third Age citizen is one who has completed his or her main career and perhaps raised a family but from the age of 55 or so has 20 or more years of potentially enjoyable life ahead. There is increasing concern about a lack of social planning, including means for preventing poverty and ill-health, for this large population group.

### The future

The immediate future of the medicine of old age will be dominated by the provision of appropriate care for the increasing numbers of elderly people in the world. 'Appropriate' in this context must include ability of the recipient to benefit (clinically appropriate) and availability of resources (economically appropriate). As technology advances, health interventions become less challenging physiologically and therefore clinically appropriate for older and frailer people. Economic constraints will mean that ethical questions relating to rationing of healthcare will have to be debated. In the longer term further ethical problems may arise if prolongation of maximum life-span becomes possible through genetic manipulation. It is likely that the central issue will be seen not as prolongation of life but rather as preventing age-associated disabilities. JGE

### GERMANY, AUSTRIA, AND SWITZERLAND

The present Federal Republic of Germany (FRG) was forged in 1990 through the union of West Germany (which comprised 62.7 million inhabitants and 11 states, or *Länder*, including West Berlin), and the German Democratic Republic (GDR), or East Germany (which had been a centralized state of 16.4 million inhabitants and which now consists of five additional federal *Länder*). The diametrically opposed forms of political organization in East and West Germany after 1945 gave rise to two completely different healthcare systems. Since 1990 all legal and administrative precepts of the old West Germany have also applied to the five new *Länder* created on the territory of the former East Germany, but a number of important dissimilarities still exist and must be kept in mind in the following account. The total population in 1996 was 81.9 million.

The Republic of Austria with its current borders has existed as a federal state essentially since 1918, when the Hapsburg monarchy collapsed after the First World War. The country consists of nine *Länder* (provinces, or states) and a population of 8.1 million (1996). Switzerland, largely unchanged since the 16th century, has been a federal state since 1848, is composed of 26 cantons, and has a population of 7.2 million (1996).

In the 9th and 10th centuries, what eventually came to be known as the Holy Roman Empire emerged from the partitioning and gradual dissolution of the Carolingian empire after Charlemagne's reign. As Christianization in Europe proceeded, the empire extended further and further eastward, chiefly along the Baltic coast, throughout the 12th century. In the 14th century, its dominions stretched nearly to present-day St Petersburg, encompassing what is now Germany, Austria, Switzerland, the Czech Republic, eastern France, the Low Countries, and parts of northern and central Italy.

In 1291, three of Switzerland's original cantons formed a league that became the nucleus of the Swiss Confederation. It grew in the wake of the Reformation and was virtually independent of the empire from 1499 on. Exacerbated by the wars of the Reformation in the 17th century, devolution of the Holy Roman Empire continued until approximately 300 principalities, dioceses, and free imperial cities existed within its borders. Austria remained the single major power and ruled vast territories of southern Europe for hundreds of years. Besides Austria, Saxony and Bavaria were the only German-speaking regions of relative note in terms of wealth and population. Not until the rise of Prussia in the course of the 18th century did the Hapsburg monarchy of Austria have to contend with a military and political rival as well. After liberation from Napoleonic supremacy in 1814, Prussia gradually grew to become the predominant and, in the 1860s, the prevailing political force in the unification of Germany.

Wars fought under this Prussian leadership shifted Germany's political boundaries repeatedly. They expanded northwards towards Denmark in 1864 and westwards towards France in 1870–71, culminating in the German Empire, often called the Second Reich (empire) to indicate its descent from the Holy Roman Empire of medieval times. In the First World War this Reich, too, spread eastwards — into Polish, Czech, Slovak, and Russian regions.

The end of the First World War saw the disintegration of the multi-ethnic Hapsburg empire. It was carved into several independent states, Austria itself becoming a republic with borders much as they are today. The defeated

### ALLGEMEINES KRANKENHAUS, VIENNA

This was founded in 1794 as a result of the 18th century development of the 'Old Vienna School' of medicine. The energy of the pathologist Carl Rokitansky, appointed prosector in 1832, complemented on the clinical side by Josef Skoda, made this the world center for studies in pathological anatomy and clinicopathological correlations during the 19th century.

German Empire also vanished and was superseded by a republic in 1918 and, in 1933, the Third Reich.

In the reorganization of Europe after the allied victory over Germany in the Second World War, considerable areas of the Third Reich in the east were ceded to, and subsequently integrated into, the Soviet Union and Poland. These regions, which no longer have German-speaking population groups, became indisputable parts of those two countries upon the signing of the peace treaties formally ending the Second World War. The two German states established in 1949 each existed as a part of its respective postwar power bloc, the capitalist West and the socialist East. The border between the blocs separated West and East Germany and, for a time, divided the world in half.

## A brief history of medicine

Medical activity goes back as far as our first human ancestors, a fact deduced from the 100 000-year-old bones of *Homo sapiens neanderthalensis*, some of whose remains have been discovered in Germany. Humans wounded or crippled when young were able to survive for up to 60 years of age, although they undoubtedly required intensive care and help both during their affliction and long thereafter.

The earliest documents from German-speaking areas show that the Benedictine canons of the 6th century required all monasteries to have rooms especially set aside as an infirmary. Ground plans of the monastery at St Gallen, dated to the 9th century, designated such sick rooms, along with a separate kitchen, separate bath, a herb garden, physician's quarters, and a building for bloodletting.

In the 12th century, after the monasteries had been the main centers of medical activity for centuries, intense discussion of clerical medical activity was prompted at several councils, because of the moral danger posed by operations performed by physicians. From 1215 on, clerics were prohibited from performing surgery and were denied even the right to receive medical training. For centuries thereafter, theoretical medical studies at the university were strictly disassociated from the various surgical techniques, which were not practiced by physicians. Simultaneously, the functions relating to the further development of medicine passed from the clergy to the temporal schools of classical medicine in the universities being founded at that time.

One cannot overestimate the impact of serious epidemics, above all, the PLAGUES. The first great wave of plague reached Germania in the 6th century AD. The second plague epidemic in central Europe, which raged between 1347 and 1532, coincided with a 30% mortality rate in the population as a whole. As in Nuremberg and Strasbourg in 1349, it led, among other things, to fanatical pogroms directed primarily against the adherents of the Israelite faith, who were held responsible for the calamity. Other INFECTIOUS DISEASES, particularly LEPROSY, led to the banishment of many people. In the 14th century, there were centers in Constance and Cologne to which people diagnosed (in effect, condemned) as having leprosy were obliged to travel in order to be committed to special hospitals for life. Hospitals were established and run throughout the German-speaking realm as far as Elbling on the Baltic Seas (in today's Poland), mostly by the knightly orders that originated during the Crusades.

The first German universities — Prague (1348), Vienna (1365), and Heidelberg (1386) — offered formal medical studies lasting 4–5 years, though the courses consisted solely of theoretical lectures. In the hospitals, however, physicians had no significance whatsoever for centuries to come. Not until the 16th century do records indicate the presence of permanently employed hospital physicians. Before that time, few towns had their doctors look after hospital patients as well, and even then just occasionally.

In medicine, the renaissance of the sciences in the 16th century is inseparably linked with the name of Andreas VESALIUS (p 846), who came from a family originally from Wesel on the Lower Rhine. He traveled throughout Europe during his years of study and, at 30 years of age, continued to do so as personal physician to Charles V and, later, to Philip II. He can be regarded as the father of modern anatomy, and hence of knowledge about the morphology and structure of the human body.

One of Vesalius's key contemporaries in medical thought was a man from the Swiss town of Einsiedeln, Theophrast von Hohenheim, known as PARACELSUS (p 617). Paracelsus became an outspoken critic of the traditional concept that the maintenance of health depended upon the harmony of the four bodily HUMORS — blood, phlegm, choler (yellow bile), and melancholy (black bile). At one point he served as town physician in Basel, and was active for some time in various cities in southern Germany, Switzerland, and Austria between Nuremberg and Vienna. Challenging long-unquestioned notions about the origins of diseases, he advocated the *experimenta ac ratio* — personal experience and one's own thinking.

The medical breakthroughs crucial to the further development of the subject in the German-speaking world came from Vienna in the latter half of the 18th century. They included the

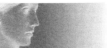
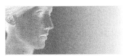

## CHARITÉ HOSPITAL, BERLIN

The Charité Hospital, now the teaching hospital of the Humboldt University of Berlin, dates from the early 18th century. PLAGUE then threatened the capital and a building was erected in front of the Spandau gate to serve as a reception center for the anticipated victims. When the threat did not materialize, the building became successively a workhouse, a military hospital, and a hospital for the poor. The original structure was replaced in 1797, and reconstructions, renovations, and additions to the buildings took place at intervals throughout the 19th century and into the 20th century. Meanwhile the Charité was establishing itself as the leading center of medical science in the German-speaking world and one of the most important in Europe, positions it continued to occupy until the Nazi regime in the 1930s. Great names of medicine associated with the Charité during this period include Johannes Mueller; Emil Dubois-Reymond; Rudolf VIRCHOW (p 853); Albrecht von Graefe; Wilhelm Griesinger; Robert KOCH (p 455); Ludwig Traube; Augustus Bier; Ferdinand Sauerbruch; Friedrich Krause; and many more.

regular observation of patients, the continual examination and pathological–morphological tracking of the clinical course of diseases, and discriminating diagnostic methods using technical aids. Yet another contribution by Viennese medicine came from the obstetrician Ignaz SEMMELWEISS (p 479). As the first person to realize that dreaded childbed fever (sepsis) coincided with infections conveyed by a physician's hands, he developed the basic principles of asepsis.

One of the pre-eminent bases for homeopathy, a widely practiced tenet of medicine in Germany, is vitalism's concept of health and disease, which constituted the climax of 18th century experiments in theoretical medicine. It was substantiated by the Thuringian Christoph Hufeland, a personal physician at the royal court in Berlin in the early 19th century and chief physician of the Collegium Medico-chirurgicum which predated Berlin's university.

### Birth of the modern hospital

The century of the Englightenment, the era of enlightened absolutism, also marked the birth of the modern hospital. The advent of this new philosophy, in which medicine was deemed a servant of the state, can be seen as the occasion for the building of the first state hospitals, such as the CHARITÉ (this page) in Berlin in 1727. The new state health institutions also assisted the universities in teaching. In addition, medicine promoted the health of people working in the burgeoning manufacturing sector. The fundamental elements of healthcare and social welfare were laid down as 'medical policy' by the Viennese physician Johann Peter Frank.

The principles of physiology as an empirical science are associated with Johannes Müller and in the school of thought in Berlin. Berlin was also home to Rudolf VIRCHOW (p 853), who pioneered the modern concept of pathological processes — by emphasizing that diseases arose not in organs or tissues in general but in their individual cells — and tirelessly campaigned for socially responsible health policy derived from medical knowledge. Another figure from the international heyday of medicine in Berlin was Robert KOCH (p 455), who discovered many pathogens of prevalent diseases and did more than anyone to establish the science of bacteriology.

In the early 1880s, protracted disputes with a strong labor movement led the chancellor of the German Reich, Otto von Bismarck, to initiate uniform social legislation aimed at providing workers with extensive accident protection, healthcare, old-age insurance, and disability benefits. In the health policy of many countries today, it still serves as a model of comprehensive social welfare.

### The organization of healthcare

*General* The healthcare systems of Germany, Austria, and Switzerland have many features in common. Unlike many countries of western Europe, they are not state-run. Instead, they are based on statutory social insurance — the government itself has little political authority and responsibility for shaping it directly. By virtue of the federal system, a number of those competencies lie with the states and cantons and with local authorities. The independence of the lower administrative echelons is greatest in Switzerland and least in Austria.

The most sweeping statutory and state-monitored social insurance is in Austria, where it embraces 99.8% of the population. The system is both compulsory and comprehensive, guaranteeing broad coverage in case of illness. The system has 19 sickness funds, which are regionally and directly responsible above all for a few large hospitals and a small number of professional units, and which are run by the beneficiaries themselves. In Germany 90% of the population has statutory health insurance, which is carried by 775 health sickness funds (1996). The majority of the remaining population is also covered against costs and risks to income in case of illness. In Switzerland only 30% of the population, including the sizeable group composed of all foreign workers who have temporary residence permits, are compulsory members of one of the some 375 recognized sickness funds created for this purpose, but 95–98% of the Swiss are protected by some sort of health insurance. Unlike their counterparts in Austria and Germany, however, Swiss patients must carry a substantial share of the costs directly: 10% of all outpatient medical charges and costs of medication as well as other fees, and all benefits in kind for accidents and dental treatment. The expenses of hospital services in particular must be met by optional supplementary insurance.

This article focuses mainly on the healthcare system in Germany. However, apart from the characteristics already mentioned, the situation in the other two countries does differ in important respects. In Austria, for example, inpatient and outpatient healthcare are not strictly differentiated, as is the case in Germany. On the whole, the medical associations in Austria have less influence on the structure of healthcare than they do in Germany, so most hospitals are able to give professional medical treatment to outpatients. Similarly, most Swiss hospitals can help treat outpatients. One peculiarity is that medication can be dispensed by the practicing physicians themselves, whose number is growing. In 1981 one-third of Switzerland's private physicians accounted for approximately 20% of the sales of medicaments in the country. The strong position of the chemical and pharmaceutical industry is considered responsible for this.

In Germany, government facilities represent only a tiny share of the healthcare institutions, which are customarily set up and run by private or independent non-profit (charitable) organizations. All outpatient care is handled exclusively by private physicians. Among them the number of specialists compared to the number of general practitioners has become proportionally bigger: all physicians 74 486 (1960)–287 032 (1998); private physicians total 42 618 (1960)–124 621 (1998); among them general practitioners 27 592 (1960)–44 953 (1998) and specialists 15 026 (1960)–80 118 (1998). Now the ratio is officially 40:60, but is thought to be at least 50:50. From 1998, new initiatives started to change this ratio.

The public health service is left with supervisory and preventive functions. One of its supervisory responsibilities is to monitor all health institutions for compliance with hygiene regulations, building codes, and other provisions. The public health service is also concerned with monitoring infectious diseases and, increasingly, with gathering data for the health-assessment reporting being developed in the *Länder*. A great defect of the manner in which data are presently gathered is that no relationship can be established between, for instance, mortality and living conditions. One of the central prevention-oriented responsibilities of the public health service is to give check-ups to pre-school and school-aged children, as well as to support and promote health awareness.

*Funding* Healthcare funds are raised by legally established provident institutions, namely, those dealing with statutory health insurances, statutory accident insurance, statutory retirement insurance, and statutory unemployment insurance. In essence, these institutions arose from the disputes between the state and the labor movement during the industrialization of Germany in the later half of the 19th century. Since its advent in the 1880s, the social safety net has been extended to nearly all occupational groups. By the 1960s practically 98% of the population had total coverage. Either for reasons of occupational status or because of income that falls below an income-adjusted threshold set annually by the government, 90% of the population is covered by statutory health insurance. All unemployed family members are insured as well. An additional 9% of the population is either entitled to total state health coverage as civil servants or is voluntarily insured by statutory or private health insurance. Health-insurance benefits cover:

- all treatment by physicians and dentists
- drugs, with a mandatory additional payment of up to about 10%
- dentures, up to about 50%
- medication and adjuvants, between 90 and 100% of the cost (for example, physiotherapy, spectacles, and artificial limbs)
- hospitalization, up to 100%
- sickness benefits, up to about 70% of the patient's income (in cases of protracted illness, disbursement begins on the day that the patient's salary is no longer paid by the employer — for most employees, after 6 weeks.)

Total expenditure on health benefits has soared in recent decades, but its percentage of Germany's gross national product has remained about the same. This developed from 69 674 (1970) to 192 836 (1980) to 303 700 (1990) million DM (DM 2.90 = £1) for the former western part. For Germany as a whole it rose from 378 913 in 1991 to 469 573 million DM in 1994, whereas the percentage of GNP has remained about 9.2 since 1980. Within the named sums the parts of the compulsory sickness funds in 1970 were 24 712 (in 1980 88 427, in 1989 127 579, in 1995 217 352, (for former West Germany) and for the whole of Germany in 1995 262 823 million DM.

The current discussion of health policy revolves mainly around four problems:

- The volume of outpatient services is steadily increasing because the number of physicians has continued to grow, whereas the population at large has not.
- The inordinately high percentage of specialists among physicians is leading to an excessive number of unnecessary and expensive diagnostic and therapeutic measures.
- Physicians are prescribing too many drugs whose effectiveness has not been proven, whose effects are even classified as detrimental, or whose use by the patient is altogether negligible.
- The health-insurances system is burdened by the growing share of old people who can no longer look after themselves adequately. They do not actually need long-term medical treatment but are hospitalized anyway for lack of other facilities (such as affordable accommodation designed to permit care for elderly occupants). This issue is to be solved by the introduction of insurance, designed specifically to provide for such care.    US

*See also* HEALTHCARE SYSTEMS

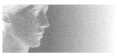
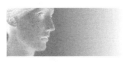

## SPECIALIST CARE IN GERMANY

It is clear from the statistics that the specialists outnumber the general practitioners, and that this disproportion has swelled with the vast increase in the total number of doctors, and the static population growth. Because all patients have free direct access to all private physicians, much family-doctor care is undertaken also by specialists. A large percentage of internists were allowed to work as family doctors, though their postgraduate education was not relevant. Pediatricians, gynecologists, and, to some extent, orthopedic surgeons, dermatologists, and psychiatrists, take care of patients who in other healthcare systems are cared for by family doctors. Private physicians own their own practices, including all the equipment, and are the employers of the personnel working for them. All private physicians caring for patients covered by statutory sickness funds are part of the Association of Sickness Fund Physicians, an organization administered by the physicians themselves. The Association of Sickness Fund Physicians monitors the bills written by the physicians and pays the individual physicians for their services, using a schedule of fees to distribute the total lump sum allocated to it by the sickness funds. This system of payment, which is based essentially on compensation for individual services rendered, has been heavily criticized in recent years because it has been shown to inflate the volume of medical services in relation to the number of licensed physicians. At the end of 1992, physicians were practically unrestricted in setting themselves up in private practice. Since then they may only obtain a license to care and to be paid for patients of the statutory insurance system when they take the place of a doctor giving up practicing and when they have had at least 3 years of postgraduate training.

### Hospital care

The hospitals solely responsible for inpatient care are organized by three main groups of institutions: public (cities and local communities), independent non-profit (such as Church-affiliated organizations and the German Red Cross), and private. For historical reasons, the share of hospital beds represented by each of these three groups varies in the German *Länder*. Whereas public institutions account for the biggest share in the *Länder* of northern Germany and those of eastern Germany (that is, the GDR until 3 October 1990), independent, non-profit institutions constitute the largest share in western and southern Germany. In 1995 the total number of general hospitals (including maternity, excluding mental health and rehabilitation) and beds were: 2081 and 564 624, out of which 56% of the beds belonged to public, 38% to charitable, and 6% to private institutions.

Except for the 35 university hospitals, hospitals give outpatient treatment in emergencies only. Under certain circumstances, psychiatric care and outpatient operations are possible (for cost reasons). In recent decades the number of hospital beds has steadily declined, for medical innovations have provided ways to treat many diseases satisfactorily on an outpatient footing. The numbers of inpatients treated per 1000 inhabitants were in 1970 154.0 and in 1995 201.0, hospital beds per 10 000 inhabitants in 1970 112.0 and in 1994 97.0, average length of stay (in days) in 1970 24.9 and in 1997 11.0, average utilization of beds in in 1970 88.5% and 1997 80.7%.

The hospitals are financed through the 'dual system': construction and capital costs for major equipment are covered by the government, provided that the hospitals are included in the hospital supply plan administered by the health minister of the *Land* in question. In each *Land* this schedule is reviewed and readopted every few years. It contains the state's input on the need for beds in the individual specialties as projected on the basis of demographic development, primarily age cohorts, and the other healthcare institutions involved. A hospital's running costs (salaries and non-durable medical supplies) are met by the hospital allowance to be paid by the sickness funds. This allowance is a lump sum paid per bed per day of hospital confinement, and is normally the same for all departments of the hospital. It is negotiated between the representatives of the hospital associations and the statutory sickness funds. The hospital must document its ordinary business expenses so that the sickness funds can approve the allowance for the following calendar year.

**GIANTS** are those adults whose height exceeds 2.0 m (80 in), or children who exceed the mean height for their age by three standard deviations or more. They either represent the extreme end of the normal distribution curve, or are suffering from an endocrine abnormality, usually pituitary gigantism. To judge from the list of those exhibited in London during the 19th century and therefore presumably authentic, giants rarely exceed 2.44 m (8 ft) in height (Chang Woo-Goo, the Chinese giant from Fychon, who was exhibited in 1865 and again in 1889, was 2.49 m (8 ft 2 in)). Reports of greater stature are of course legion, for example, Goliath at 6 cubits and a span was 3.40 m (11 ft 3 in) (but only if the cubit is accepted as 0.53 m (21 in) and a span 0.23 m (9 in)); and Eleazer, sent to Rome by Vitellius, was over 3.66 m (12 ft, 7 cubits).

In Greek mythology giants were the sons of Ge, who heaped Ossia on Pelion to scale the walls of Heaven and dethrone Zeus; with the aid of Hercules they were defeated and entombed under Mount Etna. In Scandinavian mythology giants were evil beings dwelling in Jötunheim and able to control their stature at will. The giants of nursery mythology (for example, Galligantus, Blunderbore, Bellygan) were little better.

### GLOBAL ENVIRONMENTAL CHANGE

Humanity is confronted by several interlinked changes in the global environment with potential far-reaching implications for health. These changes include global warming due to the accumulation of greenhouse gases; the depletion of stratospheric ozone by compounds such as chlorofluorocarbons; and widespread changes in land use such as increasing urbanization and deforestation.

The Intergovernmental Panel on Climate Change, a major international scientific collaboration of over 2000 scientists, has produced several publications describing the magnitude, causes, potential impacts, and mitigation strategies for climate change. Climatologists on the panel estimated that mean global temperatures rose between 1 and 3.5 °C in the course of the 20th century, which is proportionally much greater than that experienced by humanity over the last 10 000 years. The magnitude of the changes was greater nearer the poles than near the equator.

There is evidence that global temperature is already increasing: data on surface temperatures around the world between 1979 and 1994 suggested an average warming of 0.17 °C per decade. Ten of the twelve hottest years in the 20th century occurred after 1985. In 1998, the global surface air temperature was the highest ever since records began in 1860. The driving force for climate change is the increased concentrations of greenhouse gases in the atmosphere, largely owing to the increased use of fossil fuels but also to changes in land use, particularly deforestation. The global total emissions of carbon rose from around 3 million metric tons in 1751 to around 6400 million metric tons in 1995, with the bulk of the contribution from industrialized nations. Emissions might increase sharply as industrial development rises in China and India, which rely on soft coal for fuel. The atmospheric carbon cycle is tipped further out of balance by slash-and-burn clearing of tropical rain forests in Brazil, Indonesia, and South East Asia, further aggravating greenhouse-induced global warming.

Climate change is likely to have several implications for health. These are both direct (the effects of increased heatwaves and weather extremes) and indirect (for example, the impact of changes in temperature and rainfall on vector-borne diseases and water-related diseases). Indirect effects also include potential reductions in food supply in some critical regions, particularly Africa, and sea level rise of around 50 cm by the end of the 21st century, threatening some small island states and populations living in deltaic regions (for example, in Bangladesh). Changes in the availability of water and food together with a rise in the sea level could all contribute to increased numbers of environmental refugees in the next century.

Though the indirect effects of climate change on health are likely to far outweigh the direct effects, more is known about the latter, such as those caused by heatwaves in urban centers. Cities are particularly vulnerable because the urban heat island effect produces higher temperatures than in the surrounding rural areas. Studies of heatwaves have shown a transient increase in deaths, particularly in the elderly, in a range of cities around the world. The data from the USA are particularly extensive, but studies have also been undertaken in several European cities, in Shanghai, China, and in Cairo, Egypt. Some of the excess deaths during heatwaves occur in people who are already in poor

health and whose deaths are brought forward a short time. Probably, however, fewer than half of the deaths can be explained in this way. Populations acclimatize to hot conditions, so that death rates from heatwaves tend to be lower in cities in the southern USA compared with cities in the north. Although air conditioning may reduce the adverse effects of heatwaves, this necessitates increasing use of energy, which further contributes to the greenhouse effect. In temperate countries it has been suggested that climate change might reduce the excess mortality that occurs in the winter months, but this is still controversial.

### Effects of climate change

Climate change may affect the distribution of several vector-borne diseases such as MALARIA, dengue fever, YELLOW FEVER, LEISHMANIASIS, and tick-borne encephalitis. Changes in rainfall and temperature may affect the life cycle of plasmodium species and the mosquito vectors and lead to an extended range of anopheline mosquitoes and a wider distribution of malaria. Early effects might be seen particularly at the boundaries of areas where malaria is endemic — for example, at high altitudes in Africa. Flooding due to heavy rains in some parts of the world might disrupt sewage systems and increase the incidence of crypto-sporidiosis and leptospirosis. Decreased precipitation in other areas might reduce the availability of potable water, leading to an increased frequency of diarrheal diseases or diseases such as trachoma (eye infection) which can be controlled by regular hand washing. Globally the demand for freshwater increased six fold between 1900 and 1990, out-stripping population growth by a factor of two. In 1995–6 over one billion people did not have access to an adequate supply of safe water for household consumption, and about 20 countries were suffering from water scarcity, defined as an annual per capita availability of 1000 cubic meters or less. The number of counties experiencing water scarcity is predicted to rise in the 21st century, and the availability of water in countries already in this position is likely to decline further.

There has been much interest in the effects of oscillations of the equatorial Pacific Ocean current on health. El Niño (the baby) is the Spanish term to describe an anomaly in the flow of ocean waters in the Eastern Pacific, replacing nutrient-rich cold water off the west coast of South America by warm upwelling ocean water poor in nutrients. El Niño refers to the Christ Child and received its name because Peruvian fishermen noticed that the warming of the coastal waters tended to occur around Christmas. It has been known for many years that El Niño Southern Oscillations led to sharp declines in fisheries along the Pacific coast of South America. Since 1960, such

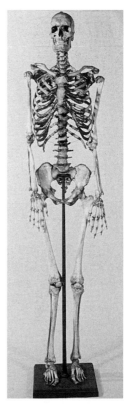

The skeleton of the giant Byrne. (Reproduced courtesy of The Royal College of Surgeons of England.)

oscillations have occurred every 3–5 years on average and are associated with changes in weather in many other parts of the world (teleconnections), such as East Africa, parts of Asia and Australasia, and Central and South America. The longest single El Niño period on record occurred between 1990 and 1995. This was followed by an even greater oscillation in 1997–8. There is developing scientific evidence that the apparent increase in frequency is related to global warming.

Many studies demonstrate significant associations between the El Niño cycle and human health. It may cause dramatically increased or decreased rainfall in different parts of the world and is associated with substantial increases in the global number of persons affected by natural disasters, particularly drought. The 1997 El Niño was associated with forest fires in Indonesia and Brazil. In association with the fires in Indonesia, dramatic increases in visits to hospitals for respiratory diseases in Malaysia have been documented. The fires have been caused mainly by human activity, burning the forest to clear the land for planting, and the lack of seasonal rains causing them to spread widely. Over the same period there was destructive flooding in South America, particularly in Ecuador and Peru. A large outbreak of Rift Valley fever, a vector-borne disease principally affecting livestock, occurred in Kenya and Somalia during severe flooding in 1997 and affected some 89 000 people. Increases in malaria with El Niño events have been recorded in Colombia, Venezuela, Pakistan, and Sri Lanka, for example. Dengue fever in some Pacific islands has been linked to the El Niño cycle, and some researchers have also suggested links between CHOLERA outbreaks and El Niño cycle. For example, the major outbreak in Peru starting in 1991 was associated with an event and in 1997 there was an increase in cholera in the Horn of Africa associated with heavy rainfall and flooding. There was also an increase in cholera in South America, particularly towards the end of 1997 and in early 1998. In 1998 the worst floods for over 100 years struck Bangladesh and China, while in the USA and Canada severe heatwaves led to widespread forest fires.

Measures to predict and prevent disease outbreaks related to El Niño are increasing. In several countries links are being forged between the national meteorological office and the health and other sectors which may be affected by El Niño to promote a rapid reaction to impending or evolving El Niño events.

### Ozone depletion
Stratospheric ozone depletion first became evident in the 1970s, and in the early 1980s the 'Antarctic ozone hole' was discovered. In the Antarctic, depletion is most pronounced in September and October. In 1996 an ozone hole of at least 10 million square kilometers persisted for over 80 days and since the early 1990s the northern polar region has also shown considerable ozone depletion. This extends as far south as Northern Europe and North America. As a result, an increasing proportion of solar ultraviolet is reaching the earth's surface. Impacts on human health include an increase in the incidence of skin cancer in light-skinned populations. The evidence is strongest for non-melanoma skin cancers but melanoma incidence might also be affected. It might also increase the frequency of eye lesions, such as cataracts, although there is still scientific debate on this topic, and is thought to cause suppression of the immune system with currently uncertain effects on health. Although the Montreal protocol to phase out substances which deplete the ozone layer is generally perceived as an international success story, it may be many years before the level of stratospheric ozone returns to its 'natural' level, and recent concern is that global warming might lead to further increases in stratospheric ozone depletion. In addition, there is continuing illegal manufacture and export of chlorofluorocarbons in some countries.

Land use is dramatically changing around the world. For example, urbanization, which began in Europe and North America in the last century, is spreading rapidly to the rest of the world. In the late 1990s roughly 45% of the world's population lived in urban areas and by 2025 the proportion may have risen to over 60%. More developed regions are 70–80% urbanized compared with 35% of the population of the less developed regions. Urbanization has been criticized for leading to problems of breakdown in law and order and being the focus for obvious poverty and decay. Serious problems of local transport and air pollution prevail in many cities. Nevertheless, it is also argued that urban living is a more efficient form of human settlement than rural living and that environmental degradation will be reduced by further urbanization. Well-managed cities — with green spaces, appropriate transport systems, and vigorous programs to renew and upgrade poor quality housing — may be attractive places to live. Thus in many countries policy initiatives are increasingly being directed towards making cities healthier and more environmentally friendly places.

Deforestation is widespread: estimates of the fraction of land transformed or degraded by humanity are between 39 and 50%. In the decade up to 1994 an estimated 154 million hectares of tropical forest were cleared for other use.

Deforestation reduces biodiversity and recent extinction rates are 100–1000 times their prehuman levels. It has direct health effects, such as air pollution from the burning of forests, and indirect effects, such as depriving humanity of potentially important medications. A recent survey of the 150 most frequently prescribed drugs in the USA showed that 57% of them contained compounds derived from or patterned after compounds from other species. Deforestation may also cause changes in the incidence of vector-borne diseases, leading, for example, to increased malaria and leishmaniasis.

Clearly current patterns of global environmental change are unsustainable. The impact of humanity on the environment is related to the size of the population, consumption per capita, and the technologies employed. Halting population growth in the south and unsustainable consumption patterns in the north are key components of any strategy to promote sustainable development. APH

*See also* DEMOGRAPHY; DERMATOLOGY; WATER

**GODS** Chief among the medical gods of the heroic Greeks was ASCLEPIUS (p 710), god of medicine, formally deified in Athens in 420 BC. Asclepius, who had been instructed in the healing art by Chiron, a centaur, was the son of APOLLO (this page) and Koronis, born according to tradition in the mountains above Epidaurus. Machaon and Podalirius were his sons, who accompanied Agamemnon on the expedition to Troy. Homer speaks of Machaeon as 'a doctor worth many men at cutting out arrows and laying on gentle drugs', while Podalirius 'had cunning to find out things impossible and to cure that which healed not'. Of the six daughters of Asclepius, Hygieia, goddess of health, is best known; others were Panacea (the restorer) and Meditrina (the preserver of health). Epigone, wife of Asclepius, was the 'soothing one'.

**GRAND ROUNDS** 'Making rounds' or 'going on rounds' is the term commonly used to describe doctors visiting their patients, in their homes, or more often in the hospital, where the addition of nurses, students, and junior doctors following the chief doctor in procession lends the exercise a certain air of formality. Grand rounds, by extension, are usually held once a week in an auditorium and were the accepted method by which rare or interesting cases were demonstrated to the entire hospital staff. Such a tradition goes back at least to the 19th century, when the great neurologist CHARCOT (p 400) would exhibit his *grandes hysteriques* before the assembled medical establishment of the Salpêtrière; and in American teaching hospitals this format persisted until well into the 1960s. In its most elegant form it would consist of the chief of medicine or his representa-

tive introducing the patient to the audience, explaining that this is a group of doctors interested in his symptoms, and would he mind allowing them to ask him some questions? In most instances the patient would be pleased with the experience and encouraged that so many doctors would hear his case and perhaps make useful suggestions.

By the late 1970s, however, most teaching hospitals had abandoned this format, reflecting concerns about patient privacy and dignity, and also perhaps the decline of bedside teaching in favor of instruction in the classroom and teaching at the blackboard. More often grand rounds now consist of a house officer reading a prepared protocol of a case history, to be used by the expert speaker as a starting point for a canned lecture with slides covering all aspects of a subject. This style of instruction is now much in favor with medical students and junior house officers, who between occasional slumbers and frequent interruptions by strident beepers are satisfied that for once they are really learning medicine — an impression rarely borne out by formal testing several weeks after the event.

The term has so completely lost its original meaning that in many (USA) teaching hospitals nowadays, the timetable of 'Grand Rounds' can be printed and otherwise distributed months in advance, and often includes formal 'presentations' on such subjects as payment methods, health economics, ethical problems, or advances in diagnostic imaging techniques. All are subjects of immediate relevance to clinicians, but their connection to actual patients under treatment is often tenuous. GD

*See also* CLINICOPATHOLOGICAL CONFERENCE; EDUCATION

**GREAT WINDMILL STREET SCHOOL** See BRITAIN

**GREECE** The first medical school (1837) and the Athens Medical Society (1835) were fundamental in the development of medicine in Greece. Many of the new Greek medical graduates continued their studies either in France and Germany (19th century) or in Britain and the USA (20th century). George PAPANICOLAOU (p 740) (Pap test) of Cornell University is one of many examples.

There are today seven medical schools in Greece, which produce more physicians than are needed. This is in addition to those who study medicine abroad either for a better education or because of failing local entry exams. This has now created a crisis. Specialists with unequal degrees of medical skill and experience are unequally distributed, with half of them practicing in the capital, Athens. Despite some recent improvements, medical care

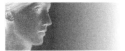

outside the big cities is often appalling. Most Greeks seek medical advice and treatment in the big cities, mainly Athens and Thessaloniki. The crisis of confidence between people and physicians is reflected by the large number of patients who travel abroad, hoping for better management and even cure. This happens despite the availability of some excellent modern and well-equipped hospitals with highly qualified physicians in Greece. Nearly all Greeks have medical insurance, which is usually job-related. The lack of organization of medical care and the influence of factors other than qualifications and efficiency in the appointment of senior medical, academic and administrative staff have a negative influence upon practice and especially upon academic medicine, despite the evident high potential for improvement and devoted physicians. As a compensation, a great number of Greek physicians distinguish themselves abroad in keeping with their tradition, as exemplified by GALEN (p 324), who was born in Pergamos, studied medicine in Alexandria, and became famous in Rome. SGM, CPP

**GREEK MEDICINE** Ancient Greek medicine derived knowledge from many older sources. Greeks, because of their geographical location, were exposed to the influence of Egyptian, Babylonian, Mesopotamian, Phoenician, and Minoan (Cretan) civilizations. They also learned from ancient Jewish medicine.

Pre-Hippocratic medicine was connected with Greek mythology and the temples of Asclepius, chief among the medical GODS.

### The Hippocratic period

The mythological period of Greek medicine was followed by a long, sacerdotal period with priest-physicians. ASCLEPIUS (p 710) left numerous successors, the Asclepiaedes, who continued his work. Their activities were mainly psycho-therapeutic and were practiced in health centers situated near the sea, or near springs in several regions by the Mediterranean Sea.

Along with sacerdotal medicine, a kind of secular medicine also developed, and under the influence of naturalist philosophers — often named 'physiologists' — medicine progressively lost its religious character. Consequently, the Asclepian medicine of the Ionian school in Asia Minor, the Pythagorean school of Croton in Magna Graecia (now southern Italy), and the Empiricism of the school of Cnidos were the precursors of the Hippocratic period.

Hippocratic medicine was founded in the 5th century BC on the basis of Greek physical philosophy. The most important difference between Pre-Hippocratic and Hippocratic physicians was that the former were solely respected craftsmen, the latter both craftsmen and philosopher–physicians.

HIPPOCRATES (p 382) of Cos (born around 460 BC) was the founder of scientific medicine, which flourished in Pericles's 'golden age' of Greece. The following Hippocratic messages are most important and valuable even to current medicine: 'The physician must investigate the entire patient and his environment'; 'The physician must assist nature which is the physician of the diseases'; 'For where there is love of man there is also love for the medical art'; 'The physician must benefit and not harm the patients'; 'The physician must co-operate with the patient, with the patient's attendants and external circumstances'; 'Nothing happens without a natural cause'; and 'Medicine is the most noble of all arts'. Twenty-five centuries later, his teachings are still of great importance, not only in medicine but also in specific aspects referring to the ecology of the environment and atmospheric pollution

### Hellenistic (Alexandrine) period

After Hippocrates' death, his doctrine continued to flourish and also to influence philosophical thinking, as evidenced by the most reliable authorities such as Plato (427–347 BC), ARISTOTLE (384–322 BC) (p 64), and his pupil Theophrastus (372–287 BC).

Alexander the Great, Macedonian King and conqueror (356–323 BC), a pupil of Aristotle, was among his most famous disciples. The Alexandrian school replaced the schools of Cnidos and Cos, for two principal reasons: firstly, Alexandria, with its famous library and its invaluable museum, served as the meeting place of the most eminent scholars of the world, thus becoming a new Athens; secondly, the dissection of human bodies was legalized — old 'taboos' collapsed and Alexandria became the capital of anatomy and physiology.

HEROPHILUS (p 381) and Erasistratus (3rd–4th centuries BC) were among the most celebrated physicians of the Alexandrian school. Herophilus, influenced by the school of COS, was more of an anatomist than a physiologist, while Erasistratus, influenced by the school of Cnidos, was more of a physiologist. Their medical knowledge was not only because of their access to the library of Alexandria, but also because of many years practicing the dissection of human bodies. Although rivals, their remarks and discoveries complemented each other. Both of them, spirited with the ambition that Greek science should embrace the world in its entirety and in unity, tried and successfully imposed their principles on medicine by teaching that 'the only fruitful medical method of thinking is that which views man in his entirety'.

# GOUT

Gout usually presents as an acute arthritis affecting a single joint in the foot. It is caused by an inflammatory response to the deposition of urate or uric acid crystals within or around the affected joint. These urate crystals may precipitate from supersaturated body fluids when the urate concentration, the pH, and the temperature favor this. Such precipitation is particularly likely to occur when the urate concentration is either fluctuating or sufficiently high for long enough. Gout is one of the oldest diseases to be recognized. Its name derives from *gutta*, meaning 'a drop', since the humoral theory of disease suggested that it was caused by a drop of noxious humor falling into the joint. That the condition existed in ancient Egypt is verified by finding tophi (urate deposits) and their characteristic erosions in the bones of mummies. HIPPOCRATES (p 382) distinguished gout from other forms of joint disease and described several of its characteristic features in his Aphorisms, particularly the propensity to affect post-pubertal boys and men and post-menopausal women. This fits with our current knowledge that urate concentrations rise at puberty in the male and after the menopause in women.

## Famous sufferers

Gout is reported to have affected many of the Roman poets, including Virgil, Juvenal, and Ovid. Seneca recognized its familial nature. Indeed, there were efforts to present gout as a noble disease, whose sufferers could trace their ancestry back to Ulysses. Aretaeus the Cappadocian in the 2nd century AD noted the frequency with which the great toe was affected. He also emphasized the completeness of the remissions between the acute attacks and reported an athlete who won a race in the Olympic Games between his acute attacks of gout. GALEN (p 324), also in the 2nd century AD, recognized gout as a distinct entity, emphasizing its hereditary nature in some and its precipitation by 'debauchery and intemperance' in others.

There are few major reports after this until that of SYDENHAM (p 721), who provided the classic English description of gout and emphasized its extreme severity. Writing in 1683, he reported that the part affected 'cannot bear the weight of the bed clothes nor the jar of the person walking in the room'. This distinctive severity was further emphasized by HEBERDEN (p 628) during the 18th century at a time when colchicum (derived from the corm of the meadow saffron) was rediscovered as a beneficial treatment. The active principle of colchicum, colchicine, was isolated in 1814 and its use in acute gout popularized by Scudamore.

Crystals within a tophus were recognized by the inventor of the microscope,

LEEUWENHOEK (p 489), in 1679, but their composition as sodium urate was not known until later. The presence of uric acid in kidney stones was identified by Scheele in 1776 and the composition of tophi as crystals of sodium urate was recorded by Wollaston in 1798. The importance of the pathogenetic role of urate was shown by Garrod in his famous thread test, in which sodium urate crystals were seen to form on a linen fiber suspended in the acidified serum from a gout sufferer. His book on *The nature and treatment of gout and rheumatic gout* (first published in 1859) recognized that the deposition of sodium urate crystals always occurred in an affected joint. He emphasized the importance of the persistent high uric acid concentration and was the first to stress that the factors which predisposed to gout either produced an increased formation of uric acid in the system or led to its retention in the blood. He also wrote 'There is no truth in medicine better established than the fact that the use of fermented liquors is the most powerful of all the predisposing causes of gout', something for which a mechanism is now known. Many of the famous cartoons date from this period. Perhaps the most famous is that by Bunbury entitled 'Origin of the gout', in which the sufferer sits with his foot on a cushion by a table with a decanter of wine, while the devil takes a burning coal from the fire, holds it against the affected bunion, and fans it with his hat.

Gout is well established as having affected many prominent English and European personages, being documented with the English Kings Henry VII and VIII; with Queen Anne and King George IV; and in many of the Bourbons, Medicis, and Hapsburgs. Others said to have been affected include William Cecil, Francis Bacon, William HARVEY (p 363), Oliver Cromwell, John Milton, Isaac NEWTON (p 544), William Pitt, Samuel Johnson, John Wesley, Horatio Nelson, Charles DARWIN

(p 214), Benjamin Franklin, and Martin Luther. Indeed, it is said that it was the incapacity from gout affecting William Pitt which kept him away from the English Parliament when it passed the heavy colonial duty on tea which resulted in the Boston Tea Party and the loss to England of the American colonies.

Modern research has confirmed the correlates of high blood urate concentrations as the associations of plenty. Indeed, the rich and famous have always tended to have a liberal intake of both purine-containing food and alcohol, and these together lead to obesity, which reduces renal elimination of urate. High blood urate concentrations are now recognized as having both inherited and environmental contributions. Those who have inherited such a predisposition, whether because of excessive production of urate or reduced elimination by the kidneys, may be as severely affected as those who have only a small inherited component but who have acquired life-style factors such as obesity, high dietary purine, and/or high alcohol consumption. Thus many races and populations (such as the Maori), in whom gout was once rare, have now acquired a plenteous life-style and are now often troubled by gout.

Landmarks in treating gout have been: (a) the development in the 1950s of the drug, probenecid (which promotes uric acid excretion by the kidney) and its introduction to clinical practice by Talbott; (b) the value of colchicine in acute gout and as a prophylactic agent against gout by Gutman and Yu; and (c) the development by Hitchings and Elion in the 1960s of allopurinol as a xanthine oxidase inhibitor which reduces the production of uric acid and thereby restores a raised urate concentration to normal. Once the urate concentration has been restored to normal for a year or so, further acute attacks of gout become rare.                      BTE

*See also* INBORN ERRORS OF METABOLISM; RHEUMATOLOGY

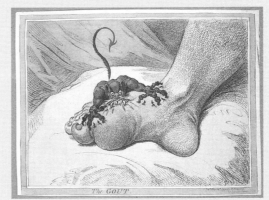

*The gout*, an etching by J. Gillray (1799). (Reproduced courtesy of the Wellcome Institute Library, London.)

The high standards and value of medicine in the Hellenistic period are shown by the fact that anatomy and physiology did not make any significant progress in the 400 years separating Herophilus and Erasistratus from Galen (2nd century AD).

### Greco-Roman (Galenic) period

The Greco-Roman period of medicine is marked by GALEN (Clarissimus Galenus) (p 324), who was born (around AD 129) in Pergamos of Asia Minor and became famous as a physician in Rome in the Emperor's court. His Latin name, Galenus, comes from the Greek 'galenios', which means serene or calm. The so-called 'prince of physicians' was also a prolific writer. He said that 'true medicine is the friend of moderation and the discipline of truth'. He was interested in, and made significant contributions to, many medical disciplines, such as anatomy and physiology (which were inseparable for him), PATHOLOGY, and therapeutics. Galen admired and carefully studied Hippocrates: 'Hippocrates showed the road, but as he was the first who discovered it, he could not go as far as he had wished.' Galen's physiology was greatly influenced by the fashionable Hippocratic theory of the four HUMORS. The work of Hippocrates was more synthetic, whereas that of Galen was more analytical. A fundamental difference was that illness was located in an organ or a system for Galen, while illness was something of a general affliction according to Hippocrates.

Galen's ideas dominated medical thought far into the 16th century and can be considered as precursors of modern experimental medicine.

### Byzantine period

Many historians report that after Galen, medicine experienced a period of decadence and made no progress in the years of the Byzantine Empire.

It is often stated that medicine in this period ceased to be scientific, experimental, or philosophical, and instead became dogmatic under the influence of Christianity, and that there were no famous physicians.

This is not correct, as is illustrated by Oribasius, a native of Galen's birthplace, who studied medicine in Alexandria, discovered many

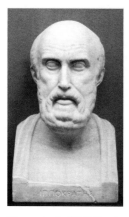

Hippocrates (c 460–357 BCE) (By permission of the International Hippocratic Foundation of Cos.)

new diagnostic and therapeutic medical and surgical methods, was an enemy of empirical medicine, and established himself as an eminent physician of this period.

Byzantine medicine, dominated by the spirit of 'love for one's neighbor', was profoundly humanitarian but also Galenic and Hippocratic in character. It preserved the tradition of Hellenic medicine and passed it on into western Europe. It supported social welfare and the development of hospital medicine. New cures were discovered. Christianity appreciated the importance of human life and started a new period of hope and giving, as summarized by the word 'caritas' (charity).

### Neo-Hellenic period

Modern Greece was officially recognized as a sovereign and independent country in 1830, nine years after the revolution leading to liberation from 400 years of Turkish rule.

Physicians initially were heterogeneous, insufficient, and unequally distributed. They were: physicians who had practiced medicine during the Turkish occupation; foreign physicians, postgraduates mainly of European medical schools, who came to Greece to help with the revolution and stayed after the liberation; Greek national physicians from Europe who returned to Greece; Bavarian physicians and pharmacists serving in the Greek royal court of the Bavarian king; and, finally, empirical physicians who were licensed by the government to practice medicine.

During the Turkish occupation, many talented young Greeks studied medicine in renowned French and Italian universities, with financial support of Greek communities, abroad and philhellenes (friends of Greece). Alexandros Mavrokordatos (17th century), Emmanouil Timonis, and Iakovos Pilarinos (who in the 18th century described a method for the prevention of smallpox) were among the most famous of them.

SGM, CPP

*See also* TEMPLE MEDICINE

**GYNECOLOGY** See OBSTETRICS AND GYNECOLOGY

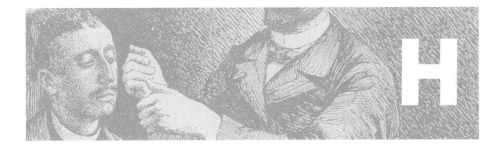

**HARA-KIRI** (sometimes incorrectly called *hari-kari*) is a method of voluntary or obligatory suicide which was prevalent in the Middle Ages among the Japanese samurai class. A samurai might opt for *hara-kiri* rather than capture and disgrace in war, or might be allowed this honorable option in place of public execution of the death penalty.

*Hara-kiri*, or *seppuku*, requires the subject to be clad in a formal white kimono and, using a dagger in his right hand while squatting upright, to open his abdomen from left to right and upwards; he then cuts the carotids or stabs himself in the throat or, if there is a witness present, the suicide must instead be beheaded immediately after the disembowelling.

Self-immolation on the death of one's lord was prohibited by the Tokugawa government in 1668, but *hara-kiri* in other circumstances has continued to be practiced, for example, in the Second World War by Japanese officers facing surrender.

William **HARVEY** (1578–1657). He was born in Folkestone, Kent and received his early education in Canterbury after which he went to Caius College, Cambridge, graduating in 1597. After further study in PADUA (p 447), Harvey returned to London, and in 1609 was appointed physician to St Bartholomew's Hospital. In 1616 he was Lumleian Lecturer on anatomy and surgery where he presented his first ideas on the circulation of the blood. In 1628 he published his classic treatise on that topic, *Exercitatio de motu cordis et sanguinis in animalibus*, challenging the long-held theories of Galen, and provoking condemnation and criticism from the scientific establishment. His practice declined and he retired from St Bartholomew's, remaining in service to the King until 1649. With the subsidence of criticism over the years, in 1651 he published his theories on animal generation and embryology, *Exertationes de generatione animalium*, which was relatively favorably received. He died six years later, aged 79.

**HEALTHCARE SYSTEMS** As access to health services has come to be regarded as a basic human right, governments throughout the world have taken action to implement such access. The earliest such actions were concerned with serious illness, requiring acute care in hospitals after the Renaissance, but, since the beginning of the 20th century, increasing attention has been given to disease prevention, positive health promotion, and provision of diagnosis and treatment to the ambulatory patient.

Every country has a health system that reflects its history, economic development, and dominant political ideology. Its overall characteristics depend on each of the system's component parts.

### Composition

Each system may be analyzed according to five principal components: resources, organization, management, economic support, and delivery of services.

The resources of a health system consist of human resources (personnel), facilities (hospitals, health centers), commodities (drugs, equipment, supplies, etc.), and knowledge. Health programs may be organized under diverse sponsorships, but there is almost always one principal authority of government (at several levels), other governmental agencies with health functions, voluntary health agencies, enterprises, and a private healthcare market. Management includes health planning, administration (supervision, consultation, and coordination), regulation, and legislation. Economic support may come from governmental tax revenues (at different levels), social insurance (statutory), voluntary insurance, charity, and personal households. In economically less developed countries, foreign aid may have a role. The relative proportions among these different forms of support influence many features of a health system. In the industrialized countries, there seems to be a trend toward increasing use of social insurance mechanisms, while in the developing countries, the trend is toward greater use of governmental revenues to finance health services.

Finally, these four component parts lead to the crucial fifth part: the delivery of health services, subdivided into primary healthcare (preventive

**HAMMURABI — CODE OF**

Hammurabi, the founder of the first Babylonian empire, laid down a legal code *c.* 2100 BC, which was discovered at Susa in 1902. Clauses 215–23 relate to medicine, laying down the fees appropriate to various services. Number 221, for example, reads: 'If a physician set a broken bone for a man, or cure his diseased bowels, the patient shall give five shekels to the physician.' The code also set penalties for an unsuccessful outcome: for loss of life or of an eye, the doctor was to have his hands cut off if the patient was a nobleman, or to render value for value if a slave.

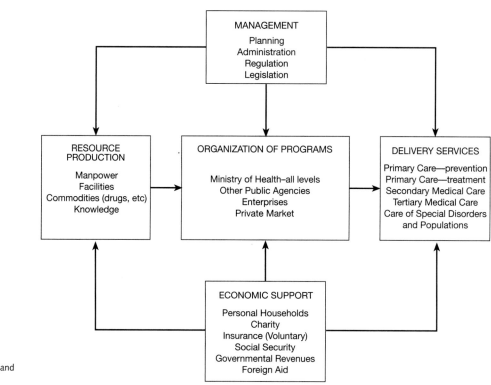

National health system: components, functions, and their inter-dependence.

and curative), secondary care, and tertiary care. The combined characteristics of these five component parts permit the designation of each national health system according to certain types. While history, economic level, and political ideology determine these types, their attributes may be classified according to the degree of market intervention by government. The organization of every health system, it was noted, includes a private healthcare market. The proportions and characteristics of this market depend on the extent of intervention in the market process — supply, demand, competition, and price — by government. This may be measured in different ways, appropriate to each component.

By such analysis, the national health systems in the world's approximately 165 sovereign countries may be scaled into four main types. Going from the least market intervention to the most, these health system types are: entrepreneurial, welfare-oriented, comprehensive, and socialist. This scaling may be applied, furthermore, to countries at high, middle, and low levels of economic development. Health systems, of course, change over time, and this article describes the situation in the late 1980s and 1990.

Analysis of national health systems by economic level and health system type yields a matrix, in the cells of which all countries may be placed. Numerous strategies of financing for healthcare have developed throughout the world. In the industrialized countries, the use of the insurance mechanism was found to achieve stability — as a form of organized self-help, without the reliance on charity or government revenues.

European governments have mobilized financial support to assure people access to medical care since the 1880s. After decades of nongovernmental workers' sickness insurance societies, GERMANY passed a law in 1883 requiring low-wage workers to belong to such societies. This was the birth of social security, and the idea soon spread throughout Europe. In 1888, Austria and in 1891, Hungary adopted similar legislation. In 1911, Britain passed legislation to require low-paid manual workers to have insurance for general practitioner care and drugs, followed soon by the SCANDINAVIAN countries.

Towards the end of World War I, the first social revolution against capitalism occurred, not as expected in Germany but in RUSSIA, where the Bolsheviks took power in 1917. The huge Union of Soviet Socialist Republics started to develop a National Health Service, eventually covering everyone with general revenue financing. By 1937, all the doctors, hospitals, and other resources were taken over by the central government and greatly extended. The Russian Revolution scared the entire capitalist world, goading countries into passing stronger national health insurance legislation. Great Britain debated the DAWSON REPORT (p 131), which laid the foundations for a National Health Service achieved a quarter of a century later.

In the 1920s and 1930s, national health insurance spread throughout Europe. The population coverage and range of benefits in each country were extended. The last European country to adopt compulsory insurance for medical care was France, in 1928.

## Beyond Europe

After World War I, the first non-European country to enact compulsory sickness insurance was Japan, in 1922. It emulated European healthcare patterns, with a free choice of private doctors and fee-for-service payment. When social insurance financing of medical care was first undertaken by a developing country, Chile in 1924, the delivery pattern was finally modified, with the establishment of polyclinics engaging physicians on salary for ambulatory care. Subsequent initiatives in developing countries generally emulated the Chilean pattern. In 1936, Peru was the first country whose social security program constructed a separate facility for insured workers, opening the 'Worker's Hospital' in Lima in 1939. After this, the separate social security hospital — usually much more advanced than the old 'beneficencia' facilities or even the Ministry of Health hospital — became the standard model in Latin America.

## Second World War and the British NHS

With the end of World War II, the post-war planning by the British Beveridge Commission was soon implemented under the Labour Party. Building upon its 1911 doctor's care insurance, its wartime regional hospital scheme, and its long-established local public health authorities, the three-part structure of the British National Health Service was established in 1948. The total population was entitled to service, without any copayment requirements, except for certain drugs. Financial support came 90% from general revenues. In 1974, this complex structure was reorganized into 200 local health districts.

The Nordic countries soon extended their health system coverage in the 1950s to their total populations. Britain had constructed many local health centers, housing general practitioners and others for providing primary healthcare, and this was even more extensive in Norway and its neighbors. Of doctors both in hospitals and health centers, some 90% of Swedish physicians now work on full-time salaries.

## Southern Europe

In the 1970s and 1980s, national health service patterns were adopted in Italy, Greece, and Spain. Each of these countries had long experience with mandatory healthcare insurance. The conversion to national health service arrangements was to be carried out gradually. In ITALY, it started with the 8 northern regions of the 20 into which the country was divided. Each regional authority divided its territory into 'local health units', with populations of 50 000 to 200 000. A general practitioner has a list of about 1000 to 1500 persons, for whom he is paid monthly on a capitation basis. Specialists are employed by the hospitals mainly on full-time salaries, although they may engage in part-time private practice. Hospital beds are abundant and 85% in governmental facilities. GREECE and SPAIN established national health types of health systems in the 1980s. The two major insurance funds — for industrial and for agricultural workers — in Greece were consolidated under the Ministry of Health, which constructed or acquired hundreds of local health centers. Many physicians in private practice were increasingly attracted into salaried public positions in hospitals and health centers.

In Spain, after the death of dictator Franco in 1975, the compulsory sickness insurance was transferred from the Ministry of Labor to the Ministry of Health. Some 93% of the Spanish population is covered through a large network of hospitals and health centers, established by the insurance program, together with facilities operated by the Ministry of Health or even private owners under contract. Hundreds of new health centers were constructed by the Ministry of Health in the 1980s for extending primary healthcare. Progress in population coverage was also made in Portugal.

## Latin America and Cuba

After World War II, social security financing for medical care was extended further in Latin America. Chile — whose leaders were impressed by the British National Health Service — consolidated its several sub-systems to form the Chilean National Health Service in 1952. The social security program, the *beneficencia* hospitals, and the Ministry of Health resources were all coordinated under 12 zones, each directed by a Ministry of Health official. Also, the social revolution in Cuba in 1959 — the first real overthrow of capitalism in the western Hemisphere — generated fear throughout the continent, and gave rise to the US-financed Alliance for Progress. This enabled most Latin American countries to extend the coverage and benefits of their health systems in the 1960s and 1970s.

Soon after its revolution in 1959, Cuba reorganized its health system along socialist lines. Initially all health services were placed under a greatly strengthened Ministry of Public Health. The country's six political provinces were recast into eight health provinces, each subdivided into health regions — 36 in all. Each region had one or more regional hospitals, and the region was subdivided into health areas; by 1968 there were 268 functional health areas. After the revolution, most physicians and pharmacists left the country, and medical education was greatly expanded to replenish the supply. Cuba did not train community health workers or midwives, but insisted on doctors for virtually all medical services. Without midwives, virtually all childbirths were handled by doctors in hospitals. The number of hospital beds was expanded and their distribution equalized between Havana and the rest of the country. The key facilities, however, are some 400 polyclinics, which blanket the country — each serving about 25 000 people. In each polyclinic there are several teams of doctors (for medicine, pediatrics, gynecology, and dental care), serving about 5000 people. Around the polyclinic, since 1984, Cuba has set up small units of a family doctor and a nurse for primary healthcare to about 700 people. Despite the United States' embargo of trade with Cuba, this island of 10 million people has attained the best health record of any country in Latin America.

### Eastern Europe

In spite of its massive losses in World War II, the Soviet Union rebuilt its health system in the post-war 1950s and 1960s. The Soviet health system model was also extended to the other countries of Eastern and Central Europe that came under its control. Replacing the fascist style with socialist health systems in these post-war years was not easy, but the systems worked reasonably well for 50 years, with impressive improvements in measurement of health. Then in the 1970s, when the huge expenditures due to the Cold War caused a serious cutback in health spending, conditions changed. Infant mortality rates began to rise and world-wide attention was drawn to this regression after 50 years of progress. Finally, the communist governments collapsed in 1989, and these health systems are now being slowly rebuilt, with privatization of resources and social security financing (as much as the tax authorities can collect).

### North America

In North America, social insurance for hospital care was finally adopted in one province of Canada, Saskatchewan, soon after the Second World War in 1946. A second province soon followed suit until the federal government took action, extending hospitalization insurance to all of Canada by 1957.

Saskatchewan pioneered again in 1962 with social insurance for doctors' care, with further emulation and extension finally to all of Canada for both hospital and physicians' care by 1971.

Legislation to close the gap of private health insurance for the elderly and the poor was adopted by the United States in 1965. In that year, the Medicare Law applied social security to finance hospital and doctors' care for the elderly, with Medicaid enacted also to use federal and state general revenues for financing healthcare for certain categories of poor people. Health insurance plans linked to salaried doctors in group practices had long been shown to be less costly, by providing incentives for the frugal use of hospital care. Giving this pattern a new name, the health maintenance organization, it was actively promoted by a Republican administration. The Health Maintenance Organization Act of 1973 set federal standards for and subsidized their establishment and promotion; they grew to 12.5 million members in 1983 and to 45.2 million in 1993.

By the 1990s, about 60% of the US population was covered by voluntary health insurance (two-thirds commercial and one-third in the non-profit 'blue' plans), another 12% by Medicare together with 13% by Medicaid. This left 15% of Americans unprotected; these are not the elderly or the poorest, but mainly workers in small shops and their dependents. How to achieve healthcare coverage for these people is the current political issue.

### Communist China

After the communist revolution in 1949, CHINA came very much under Soviet influence in its health system as in everything else. Great progress was made in developing a framework of health services in the 22 provinces, the 2300 counties, and the 27 000 communes. The last, with populations of 20 000–60 000, were further divided into 'production brigades' of 3000 to 5000 each, and these were still further subdivided into 'production teams' of 50 to 500 adults.

Around 1965, under instigation from Chairman Mao Zedong, young Communist Party members or Red Guards mounted a campaign against the Party leadership that became identified as the Great People's Cultural Revolution. For a 10-year period, 1965–75, there was turmoil, in which greater recognition was given to Chinese traditional medicine and many hundred thousands of peasants were trained briefly as barefoot doctors, an idea that became widely accepted in many other parts of the world. After the death of Chairman Mao in 1976, more rigorous training was established for these personnel, qualifying examinations were required, and they became designated as village doctors.

By the 1980s, policies steadily changed toward capitalism and private enterprise. Virtually all services had to be paid for, although various forms of health insurance — covering about 40% of the population — were developed to facilitate these payments. By 1990, with government revenues supporting about 19% of total health expenditures and insurance about 50%, individual families had to bear about 32% of health costs.

The other countries of South-eastern Asia also extended their health systems after World War II. India's Employees State Insurance Corporation continued to reach only about 3.5% of its 800 000 000 people, but the coverage of the general Ministry of Health and Family Welfare was greatly extended through tens of thousands of primary health centers and subcenters. In Vietnam, there is a socialized health system in each of the 40 provinces and 466 health districts; the districts are subdivided into about 8600 communes, each of which has 5 to 10 production brigades. Virtually all households must contribute to the cooperative funds supporting these services. In Thailand, there is a small social security program for regularly employed workers, but most health expenditures come from private sources.

In spite of all the progress in the development of effective national health systems, many problems remain. There is still an inequitable distribution of personnel between urban and rural areas, and within large metropolitan areas, between depressed inner cities and affluent suburbs. The quality of health services is uneven, with inferior quality being common among providers serving the poor. Preventive and health promotional services are deficient in almost all countries. Millions of people, especially in the developing countries, still suffer and die from preventable diseases. In the United States of America, a disgraceful 15% of the population still lacks health insurance.

## World trends

By 1989, some 71 countries throughout the world had developed national legislation for financing healthcare for all or part of their populations. The funds were raised through general revenues or social insurance (social security) or by combinations of the two mechanisms. Under this collective financing, services were provided mainly by either public or private health personnel. The tables indicate the countries that have enacted such legislation, the mechanisms of financing (social insurance and general revenues), and the types of health personnel (private or public) whose services are financed.

Thus the world scene has shown a steadily increasing degree of social support for the costs of health services in virtually all countries. Government has been the main channel through which funds are raised, applying either general revenue mechanisms or social security programs or usually both. At the same time the delivery of services has come to be increasingly through organized frameworks for both inpatient and ambulatory healthcare. The cost–benefit effectiveness of primary healthcare seems to be recognized increasingly in the health policy formulation of virtually all countries. MJR

| ECONOMIC LEVEL (GNP per capita) | HEALTH SYSTEM POLICIES (Market Intervention) | | | |
|---|---|---|---|---|
| | Entrepreneurial & permissive | Welfare-oriented | Universal & comprehensive | Socialist & centrally planned |
| Affluent & industrialized | United States  1 | West Germany Canada Japan  2 | Great Britain New Zealand Norway  3 | Soviet Union Czechoslovakia  4 |
| Developing & transitional | Thailand Philippines South Africa  5 | Brazil Egypt Malaysia  6 | Israel Nicaragua  7 | Cuba North Korea  8 |
| Very poor | Ghana Bangladesh Nepal  9 | India Burma  10 | Sri Lanka Tanzania  11 | China Vietnam  12 |
| Resource-rich | 13 | Libya Gabon  14 | Kuwait Saudi Arabia  15 | 16 |

Types of national health systems: classified by economic level and health system policies.

**HEALTH DEFINITIONS** When we raise our glasses in the toast to 'Good health' what exactly are we honoring?

The word health comes from an Old English word meaning wholeness. The concept covers a person's physical and mental condition, and the general notion of fulfillment. *Good* health implies that degrees of health can be recognized and measured.

A definition with a subjective element is limited because it cannot take into account what the person does not know. For instance, someone may function fully, both physically and mentally, and feel totally at ease, but may be harboring a serious physical disease in its presymptomatic stage. The WHO definition takes for granted the absence of infirmity and disease, declared or latent. Embracing this holistic definition, in 1984 the architects of the

Social security or equivalent protection for healthcare (71 countries) by major type of financing and major mode of service, 1989

| Country coverage 90–100% | Major type of financing | | Major mode of service | |
|---|---|---|---|---|
| | Insurance | Revenue | Private | Public |
| *High income* | | | | |
| Australia | X | | X | |
| Austria | X | | X | |
| Belgium | X | | X | |
| Bulgaria | | X | | X |
| Canada | | X | X | |
| Czechoslovakia | | X | | X |
| Denmark | X | | X | |
| Finland | | X | | X |
| France | X | | X | |
| Germany, Dem. Rep. | | X | | X |
| Germany, Fed. Rep. | X | | X | |
| Greece | | X | | X |
| Hungary | | X | | X |
| Iceland | | X | | X |
| Ireland | X | | X | |
| Israel | X | | | X |
| Italy | | X | | X |
| Japan | X | | X | |
| Kuwait | | X | | X |
| Luxembourg | X | | X | |
| Netherlands | X | | X | |
| New Zealand | | X | | X |
| Norway | | X | | X |
| Poland | | X | | X |
| Romania | | X | | X |
| Spain | | X | | X |
| Sweden | | X | | X |
| Switzerland | X | | X | |
| USSR | | X | | X |
| United Kingdom | | X | | X |
| *Low income* | | | | |
| Costa Rica | X | | | X |
| Cuba | | X | | X |
| Nicaragua | | X | | X |
| Portugal | | X | | X |

| Country coverage 50–89% | Major type of financing | | Major mode of service | |
|---|---|---|---|---|
| | Insurance | Revenue | Private | Public |
| *High income* | | | | |
| Cyprus | X | | X | |
| Libya | | X | | X |
| *Low income* | | | | |
| Argentina | X | | X | |
| Brazil | X | | | X |
| Chile | | X | | X |
| Korea, South | X | | X | |
| Mexico | X | | | X |
| Panama | X | | | X |
| Uruguay | X | | X | |

(*continued opposite*)

(*continued*)

| Country coverage 25–49% | Major type of financing | | Major mode of service | |
|---|---|---|---|---|
| | Insurance | Revenue | Private | Public |
| *High income* | | | | |
| Taiwan | X | | X | |
| *Low income* | | | | |
| Bolivia | X | | | X |
| China | X | | | X |
| Philippines | X | | X | |
| Turkey | X | | | X |
| Venezuela | X | | | X |

| Country coverage under 25% | Major type of financing | | Major mode of service | |
|---|---|---|---|---|
| | Insurance | Revenue | Private | Public |
| *High income* | | | | |
| United States | X | | X | |
| *Low income* | | | | |
| Algeria | X | | | X |
| Burma | X | | | X |
| Colombia | X | | | X |
| Dominican Republic | X | | | X |
| Ecuador | X | | | X |
| Egypt | X | | | X |
| El Salvador | X | | | X |
| Guatemala | X | | | X |
| Guinea | X | | | X |
| Honduras | X | | | X |
| India | X | | | X |
| Indonesia | X | | X | |
| Iran | X | | | X |
| Iraq | X | | | X |
| Lebanon | X | | | X |
| Pakistan | X | | | X |
| Paraguay | X | | | X |
| Peru | X | | | X |
| South Africa | X | | X | |
| Tunisia | X | | | X |

Ottawa Charter for Health Promotion reasoned that to reach the state of total well-being individuals must have, and know how to use, their physical capacities, and personal and social resources. *Well-being*, however, is considered by some to be an aspect of *happiness* rather than health. One's state of health (physical and mental capacities and the ability to use them) is only one of the factors which contribute to happiness or well-being. As the American Constitution puts it, the *pursuit* of happiness is a human right. Consequently, people have a right to the legitimate means of pursuing happiness. This includes an adequate state of health. In this sense an aspiration such as *Health for All* is

credible, but in terms of the World Health Organization (WHO) definition it is not.

Put simply, health is the domain of physical and mental functioning. The *state* of health is then the degree to which these functions are in equilibrium with the physical, biological, and social environment. It is not the same as *fitness*. Fitness is the capacity to do something efficiently; for example, to run one mile in four minutes, using the available oxygen to maximum effect. Not many people who are free of disease and disability can do that, however. It is not the same as *normality*. This denotes the usual state and condition. While it is normal for young people to have

## WHO DEFINITION

In 1948 the WORLD HEALTH ORGANIZATION offered the most comprehensive definition of health: *a state of complete physical, mental, and social well-being and not merely the absence of disease or infirmity*. This defines the perfect state, that is, the *extreme degree* rather than the *domain*, health itself. It does not help us to understand the term *health gain*, which is sometimes used to assess the effect of investment in healthcare.

a full range of physical functions, it is also normal for an octogenarian *not* to be symptom-free.

Health is not *quality of life*, but a definition of health which includes well-being overlaps it. Quality of life depends not only on what an individual can do but also on how he or she perceives the social and material circumstances. The congenital absence of a limb makes it unlikely that an individual is without any kind of infirmity. Nevertheless, that individual may feel entirely fulfilled.

Health, like wealth, is a neutral concept, even though both words have a positive ring. Subjects such as weather or transport *sound* neutral. However, to be useful, they all need to be understood in terms of their components, such as digestion, money, rain, and highways, and these components must be assessed according to some standards.

### Components

For individuals, each component of physical and mental function, such as sight, mobility, mood, can be measured and placed somewhere on a continuum. The individual's position on the scale can be described absolutely, such as having no limit to the range of movements which can be performed, or relatively, according to the movements which most people of that age and gender can manage. A health profile can be constructed from the individual's measured position on each dimension and a judgement made of the overall state of health. For instance, the health of a 55-year-old woman would generally be regarded as good if she were symptom-free, could accomplish, comfortably and unaided, all the activities of daily living, and showed no abnormalities when screened for high blood pressure, high serum cholesterol concentration, cervical cancer, and breast cancer.

The health of a population, too, can be defined in global or specific terms. In Great Britain's General Household Survey, a recurring interviewing survey of about 12 000 households, respondents are asked to rate their health simply as good, fair, or poor. The percentages in these categories are reported. They are also asked about the number of days of restricted activity they experienced in a reference period. In this case *health* means whatever the respondents think it means. In the annual US National Health Interview Survey involving about 45 000 households, some questions probe for specific medical conditions and disabilities as well as for limitations and restrictions of activity. These population surveys describe the health of the population in terms of the proportions who do or do not experience certain types of illness or disability. It also enables changes in the broad state of health

to be noted within and between communities over time.

Other definitions of health are sometimes useful. A definition that attempts to specify what can be identified and measured both in individuals and, with surveys, in populations is:

> Health is a state characterized by anatomical, physiological, and psychological integrity; ability to perform personally valued family, work, and community roles; ability to deal with physical, biological, psychological, and social stress; a feeling of well-being; and freedom from the risk of disease and untimely death.

Health is inconceivable apart from life and, however defined, is compromised by disease or infirmity. Thus, the ultimate, hypothetical example of good health would be a community where all were born intact and survived to an advanced age without any infirmity from disease or injury. The health, or more accurately, health status, of a community is in fact described in terms of death rates, such as the proportion of live-born infants who die before reaching their first birthday, the proportion of middle-aged men who develop coronary thrombosis each year, and similar rates of occurrence of disease.

Summary ways of describing the health of a population are the *average number of years people being born alive now can expect to live*. This is calculated by applying current death and survival rates to the numbers being born. By linking those rates to the proportions known through the relevant surveys to be disabled at various ages, the *average number of disability-free years of life* they can expect to experience from birth or any later age onwards can be calculated.

'Here's to disability-free survival' sounds rather less convivial, however. BW

**HEALTH ECONOMICS** The focus of health economics is about how decision-makers — be they clinicians, nurses, managers, or politicians — make choices about how to allocate scarce resources among competing and alternative technologies to improve the health of the population. While the degree of scarcity varies in different societies (for example, $1 per capita to spend on healthcare in Zambia and over £45 billion to spend on healthcare in Britain), choice is unavoidable. Is it best to spend on healthcare or environmental improvement or education to improve population health? Within the health-care budget, which technologies — screening, diagnostic, and therapeutic — improve the patient's health most at least cost?

To answer such questions, economists deploy their skills to address several interlinked issues, described in the diagram. The issues in box A on the diagram overleaf are concerned with what influences health other than healthcare. Though the correlates among income, education, and other inequalities with inequalities in health are well charted, the causal mechanisms are less well understood. Often it is fashionable to advocate changes in behavior to alter health and, although some such changes have had profound effects (for example, tobacco cessation policies), others remain of questionable efficiency. Nevertheless, marginal investments in interventions other than healthcare may be more efficient than investments in medical care in producing better health. Much economic modeling takes place to evaluate the relative costs and benefits of non-healthcare activities.

The valuation of health (box B) is a topic in which economists have made considerable investments, in part because other disciplines and medical practitioners have been slow to address the issue of the measurement of 'outcomes'. This is a crucial aspect in evaluating the impact of clinical performance on physical, psychological, and social functioning, and utility (patient satisfaction). It is remarkable that the impact of academic research has been so slow to influence the design of trials and public policy.

Why do patients seek healthcare? Their demand for healthcare is mediated by clinicians, who act as their advocates. They demand health and seek assistance from general practitioners and specialists, who demand healthcare on their behalf. Thus it is doctors who create waiting lists, not patients, and it is their referral and treatment thresholds which determine who waits and for how long. Barriers to patient entry into the health system, such as user charges and time costs (such as travel times), influence patient use. However, if it is the doctor who demands healthcare, such barriers to patient access may neither reduce costs, nor increase efficiency nor be equitable. Indeed, in some cases equity may be pursued efficiently by paying patients to consume care (for example, to complete courses of tuberculosis medication in developing countries).

It is also important to understand how provider payment systems influence the performance of hospitals and workers. Another central issue is the issue of substitution — what are the costs and benefits of substituting nurses for doctors? The impact of regulation (such as patent laws and health policies) on the behavior of the pharmaceutical and equipment industries determines not only their prosperity but also the production of health. Health–wealth trade-offs are political and economic issues requiring careful analyses.

Many doctors see economists as working primarily in economic evaluation (box E). With managed care in the USA and market arrangements in Europe, the emphasis is increasingly on cost-effectiveness. This requires that research and development trial designs include outcome measures (quality of life; box B) and cost components. Such evaluative technologies are in their early stages, but already databases provide insights into techniques of evaluating many interventions.

The 'equilibration' between demand and supply of care implies prioritization or rationing of healthcare (box F). There are many financial and non-financial ways of rationing access to care. Rationing denies treatments which give health benefits and which patients desire. It is ubiquitous: even in over-endowed systems as in the USA, where 42 million people have no health insurance. Some of the issues are:

(a) Should rationing be explicit, or implicit (with 'postcode' rationing — that is, according to a person's address)?

(b) If explicit, what should the criteria be? Should they be determined by efficiency or by equity? Societies decide to use scarce resources to treat low birth weight babies inefficiently: how much efficiency should be given up to achieve equity?

The overall evaluation of a healthcare system (box G) involves measuring performance in terms of efficiency, equity, and cost control. Tax funded systems with cash limited budgets appear to facilitate expenditure control, whereas fragmentation in funding (as in the USA) is seen to contribute to cost inflation. Managed care may temporarily alter such trends. Efficiency and equity criteria need to be carefully defined, as do trade-offs, for example, should all patients be treated equally or should there be discrimination in favor of the young and at the expense of the elderly, who have had a 'fair innings'? The principles for such choices need clear articulation, as do the opportunity costs of resultant choices.

The final box (H) integrates knowledge of how healthcare markets work in terms of their incentive structures and in relation to policy targets. This market is characterized by implicit incentives (such as trust and the doctor–patient relationship), which are being questioned because of the frustration of policy makers about medical practice variations, lack of accountability, and the profession's slow progress in establishing guidelines and reaccreditation. Change in 'clinical governance' (particularly if based on cost-effectiveness guidelines) is one way in which performance may be improved.

Thus the scope and potential practice of health economics are very broad. In actual practice, health economics has focused on box E (evaluation) because of funding availability. The need for more investment in the other aspects covered by the subdiscipline is obvious, particularly if public policy is to be better evidence-based.

AKMay

*See also* EVIDENCE-BASED MEDICINE

Herman Ludwig Ferdinand von **HELMHOLTZ** (1821–94). German physiologist and physicist. Helmholtz was a student at the Friedrich-Wilhelms Institut in Berlin which required an undertaking to serve eight years as an army surgeon. A pupil of Müller at the university, with his former fellows Dubois-Reymond and Brücke he founded the 'New Physiology'. In 1847 he published one of the most important scientific

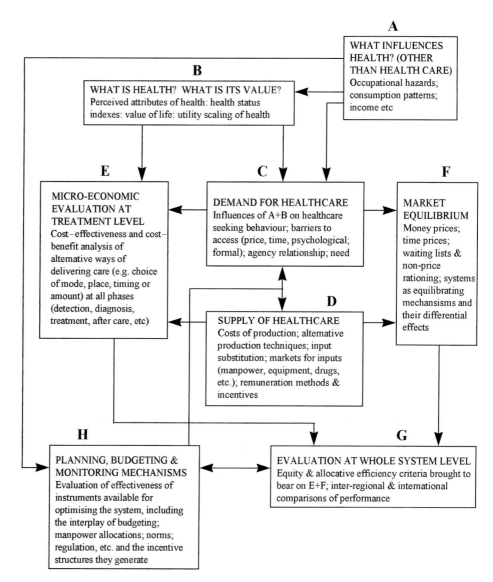

The scope and nature of health economics.

*Source* Williams (1997)

papers of the century. *Über die Erhaltung der Kraft*, which did much to establish the first law of thermodynamics. The next year he was released from the army, becoming professor of physiology successively at Königsberg, Bonn (1855), and Heidelberg (1858). His interests gradually shifted to physics and in 1871 he was appointed to the chair of physics in Berlin, becoming president of the Physikalisch-technische Reichsanstalt in 1885. Although von Helmholtz is remembered for his invention of the ophthalmoscope (1851) he exerted immense influence on science in the 19th century, converting German universities into institutions for organized research. He published a classic handbook of physiological optics (1856–66) and modified 'Young's theory of color vision'. His writings covered a wide range including the physiology of acoustics and music, hydrodynamics, and epistemology.

**HELSINKI — DECLARATION OF** After the Second World War global knowledge of Nazi Germany's outrageous treatment of prisoners, ethnic minorities, and political opponents led to the Nuremberg Trial in 1945–6. Later, in 1948, the judgements formed the basis for a preventive set of rules, the NUREMBERG CODE. Unfortunately the code was so absolute in its wording that it excluded large aspects of health research that were considered very important and ethically acceptable by contemporary democratic societies. Besides, the code was ethically equivocal in stating that 'no experiment should be conducted, unless perhaps physicians themselves take part in the experiment' and that 'the risk involved must never be greater than the importance to mankind of the problem concerned'. Not surprisingly the code's level of abstraction and lack of consistency prevented it from being adopted by doctors in their work with patients in experiments and trials. In one American researcher's words: 'The code was fine for barbarians but did not apply to physician scientists'.

Nevertheless, in the late 1950s and early '60s disquiet resurfaced about the lack of informed consent from participants in published clinical trials. Thus to create a better set of guidelines the World Medical Association published the first Declaration of Helsinki in 1964.

Unfortunately, even this document contained ambiguities that blocked its widespread use in clinical and laboratory experiments in humans. The wording of section 2, paragraph 2, that 'the doctor can combine clinical research with professional care, the objective being the acquisition of more medical knowledge, only to the extent that clinical research is justified by its therapeutic value for the patient' created severe problems. Had the wording been only 'for the patient-group' the unsolvable paradox would have been avoided that original research never knows the answer to a question beforehand, and that a known beneficial treatment should not be tested in order to avoid a multitude of 'me too' studies (repeated for personal gain). This and other differences between ethical principles and the accepted ethics of contemporary biomedical research led to a second attempt by the World Medical Association, which in 1974–75 asked three Nordic doctors to write a new version. The result was the second Declaration of Helsinki from 1995, still valid with a few additions.

The second version retained those paragraphs that had stood the test of time, but replaced paragraphs that had obstructed a general implementation of the Declaration during the preceding decade.

A new paragraph was included on the purpose of biomedical research, not only clinical science, but also understanding the etiology and pathogenesis of disease. There was also an emphasis on the necessary originality of the scientific idea, by specifying that the researcher had an obligation to possess a thorough knowledge of the scientific literature. In this way a quality aspect was introduced in accordance with the axiom that all unoriginal and methodologically invalid research on man is in itself unethical.

The responsibility for participating patients or healthy volunteers was clearly placed on a clinically competent medical person, so that any side effects might be detected at an early stage and immediate interventions applied. Risk assessment was also described in detail, including that of mental hazards.

Another new aspect was the obligation to publish the research results truthfully, this requirement being a forerunner for later initiatives to prevent scientific misconduct. A later addition emphasized children's right to consent when they are old enough to understand.

Probably the most important part of the second version was its statement that 'the design and performance of each experimental procedure involving humans should be clearly formulated in an experimental protocol that should be transmitted for consideration, comment, and guidance to a specially appointed committee, independent of the investigator and the sponsor'. This demand underlines the resulting widespread creation of research ethics committees.

Time has shown that the internationalization of biomedical research, involving many developing countries in collaborative projects, made one of the Declaration's paragraphs too restrictive. Its present wording is that 'every patient — including those of a control group, if any — should be assured of the best proved diagnostic and therapeutic methods'.

# THE TWELVE BASIC PRINCIPLES OF THE HELSINKI DECLARATION

Twelve basic principles are stipulated in the latest version of the Declaration:

- biomedical research must conform to accepted scientific principles
- each protocol should be scrutinized by an ethics committee
- research should be conducted only by qualified persons under the supervision of a clinically competent professional
- the importance of the objective must be in proportion to the risk
- every project should have its risks assessed
- the privacy and the subject's physical and mental integrity must be maintained
- the hazards of the experiment should be predictable, and the study

abandoned if the risks are found to outweigh the potential benefits

- the accuracy of the results must be preserved in any publication, while studies performed not in accordance with the Declaration should not be accepted for publication
- truly informed consent must be obtained from each potential subject
- duress should not occur in obtaining such consent
- in case of legal incompetence, informed consent should be obtained from the subject's legal guardian
- the research protocol should always contain a statement of the ethical considerations involved and should indicate how those stipulated in the Declaration are complied with.

This is still a basic demand within a developed country, but in a developing country it should now be read with the addition 'locally accessible according to national standards'.

For the authors of the second version it was a surprising, but very positive, experience that the principles and the wording were not just applicable to the developed world but were globally applicable. Maybe the explanation can be found in the Declaration's key principle, expressed in the last paragraph: 'In research on man, the interest of science and society should never take precedence over considerations related to the well-being of the subject'. PRii

*See also* BEECHER; BIOETHICS; INFORMED CONSENT; PAPPWORTH

**HEMATOLOGY** The blood or hemopoietic system in humans consists of several interconnected compartments — the peripheral blood, the bone marrow, and the lymphatic system. The circulating blood, about 5 liters in a man, almost 10% less in a woman, comprises a fluid component (the plasma), making up 55% of the total blood volume. The plasma acts as a vehicle for the three basic cell types; the erythrocytes (red cells), the leukocytes (white cells), and the thrombocytes (platelets).

The erythrocytes, or red cells, are largely concerned with oxygen transport; the leukocytes, or white cells, play various parts in defence against infection and tissue injury; while the thrombocytes, or platelets, are immediately involved in maintaining the integrity of blood

vessels and the prevention of blood loss. Although all the red cells appear virtually identical under the microscope, two main types of white cells may readily be distinguished: the granulocytes and the lymphocytes. In the granulocytes the cell cytoplasm is packed with enzyme-containing granules, which are essential for the cells' capacity to kill bacteria. The lymphocytes are members of the immune system and are concerned in defence against infection, particularly viral infection.

Given the large volume of blood which has to be maintained throughout life, the short lifespan of most white cells and platelets (2–5 days), and the survival of red cells (120 days), it is essential that there is a highly efficient factory for production of these cells. This factory is the bone marrow. The compact packaging in nature does not allow wasted spaces and, while embryologically the hemopoietic system is in the liver, the cells which are destined to provide all the blood throughout life migrate to the bone marrow early in fetal life. At birth, because of low oxygen tension in the womb, every bone in the human body contains bone marrow. Thereafter the marrow space begins to contract, although as growth occurs the total amount of marrow increases, such that in an adult man this weighs some 3 kg. A closer look at the bone marrow shows that this is extremely complex, with highly intricate relationships between the various different cell types, which have to mature from a common ancestor to provide the blood cells. It is hardly surprising with such complexity and high turnover that mistakes and problems arise and give rise to a substantial number of blood diseases, both hereditary and acquired.

In conjunction with the peripheral blood and bone marrow, there are also organs normally thought of as part of the immune system (the system of defence against infection, see IMMUNOLOGY). This system consists of the spleen, thymus, and lymph nodes. These lymphoid organs act as sites where lymphocytes (white cells) perform their immune functions and reproduce. The interrelationship between the bone marrow and these lymphoid organs helps to maintain the balance of the cells in the immune system. In addition, the spleen removes from the circulation blood cells that are no longer functioning adequately. The cells are broken down and the products can then be reused.

Hematology is the term given to the discipline of investigation and treatment of blood disorders, to include disorders of the bone marrow, the peripheral blood cells, lymph nodes, and spleen.

## Anemia

Blood is a tissue that has always fascinated man, regarded as the essence of life. The humoral theory of disease was probably based on the ancients' observation of shed blood in various disease states. In the 17th century William HARVEY (p 363) considered that 'Blood acts above all the powers of the elements and is endowed with notable virtues and is also the instrument of the omnipotent creator. No man can sufficiently extol its admirable and divine faculties'. Harvey also felt the blood to be 'The function of life and the seat of the soul'. In 1669 LOWER (p 119) noted that the change from the dark blue of venous to the bright red of arterial blood was due to 'imbibing air in its passage through the lungs'. In 1790 Antoine Laurent LAVOISIER (p 321) discovered oxygen, proving that it was the constituent in air that changed the color of blood. In 1852 von Liebig showed that oxygen combined with a substance in the red cell. Hoppe-Seyler isolated the substance a few years later and named it hemoglobin. Van LEEUWENHOEK (p 489), a draper of Delft, first observed human red cells in 1674, but the detailed analysis of all other blood elements and the development of staining techniques had to wait until the mid-19th century and studies by Paul Ell in 1840 and OSLER (p 602) in 1874. The origin of the cells was debated until 1868, when Neumann showed that they developed from parent cells in the bone marrow.

The 20th century saw a rapid development of understanding and complexity in defining normal and abnormal red cells, white cells, and platelets. Anemia describes a state in which a person has a reduced number of red blood cells in the peripheral blood circulation and hence a reduced amount of the oxygen-carrying pigment, hemoglobin.

***Hereditary anemias*** For red cells to work, all the parts of the proteins that make up the structure have to be in perfect working order. If even one sub-unit is out of place, the function may be distorted. Some of the common blood disorders are hereditary disorders in which one single amino acid may be out of place, and this prevents oxygen being carried accurately. A common example of this is thalassemia, prevalent in many Mediterranean areas. The result of the disorder is that the person cannot maintain the red blood cells at normal levels and if the defect is complete with an abnormal hemoglobin derived from each parent, such persons cannot survive long term. Such hereditary blood disorders may now be treated in a dramatic way with a bone marrow transplant from a family member who is either not affected or is less severely affected. Increasing numbers of such life-saving operations are now carried out. Nevertheless, most people with 'hemoglobinopathy' defects do not have life-threatening problems but remain chronically anemic throughout life. Early diagnosis and genetic counseling are crucial to prevent inappropriate treatment with iron.

### CHLOROSIS

Chlorosis is a term descriptive of the green complexion said to have been characteristic of iron deficiency anemia in young women during the 19th century, but rarely observed today.

***Acquired anemia*** Within developed western countries in the 20th century, the most common cause of anemia relates to deficiency of iron. This may be caused by a decrease of iron in the DIET or, more commonly, by a chronic loss of blood, often from the gastrointestinal tract — for example, due to ulcers — or more commonly, in women, because of heavy menstrual loss. The physician may easily ascertain which mechanism is operative and correct the problem by treating the underlying cause and replacing the deficiency with iron preparations given by mouth. There is, sadly, a widespread view that all anemia must be iron-deficient and it is important to ensure the correct diagnosis before starting long-term iron administration. Iron given for some hereditary causes of anemia may actually cause damage by producing iron overload.

Vitamin $B_{12}$ and folic acid are critical in the development of the nuclear DNA proteins in cells throughout the body. If absent, either singly or together, many tissues suffer the consequences. As the marrow has a continuous turnover of cells, the deficiency of these vitamins may present first as anemia. The predominant cause of vitamin $B_{12}$ deficiency is an inability to absorb the vitamin from the diet because of the lack of a cofactor normally present in the lining of the stomach. This anemia is called pernicious anemia, as before the discovery of $B_{12}$ this was fatal. Currently, treatment of $B_{12}$ deficiency is straightforward, but the vitamin $B_{12}$ needs to be given regularly by subcutaneous or intramuscular injections throughout life. Folic acid deficiency occurs in people who have a poor diet; in people who have bowel problems and malabsorption; or, occasionally, in pregnancy. The pregnant women who are at risk are those who have low folic acid stores before pregnancy and overt deficiency occurs because of the extra demand for the vitamin from the developing baby. Folic acid deficiencies are easily treated with vitamin tablets.

Two other major mechanisms cause anemia. Hemolytic (lysis) anemia — the rapid breakdown of blood cells while still in the circulation — relates to an increased fragility of the red blood

### TWO HEMATOLOGISTS

Gabriel **ANDRAL** (1797–1876). French physician. He succeeded Broussais as professor of general pathology in Paris in 1839 but renounced practice for the study of medical history on account of his wife's illness. Andral was the first French hematologist and recommended gravimetric analysis of the blood in his *Essai d'hématologie pathologique* (1842).

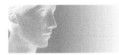

William Bosworth **CASTLE** (1897–1990). American physician. He worked in the Thorndyke Memorial Laboratory, Boston, winning fame for research showing the derangement in pernicious anemia, a condition that had been fatal until Minot and Murphy had shown that patients could be treated with large quantities of raw liver. In 1928 Castle showed that two factors were needed to produce red blood cells: an 'extrinsic' factor in the diet, now known to be cobalamin or vitamin $B_{12}$ (sufficient of which was present in raw liver to reverse the disease), and 'intrinsic factor', secreted by the cells lining the stomach (which were subsequently shown to be destroyed by an autoimmune process in pernicious anemia). Pernicious anemia is now treated with injections of the pure vitamin.

cells. Some red blood cell diseases causing such fragility may be inherited but others are acquired, often when the body produces a protein which attaches to the red cells and shortens their survival. This form of anemia may arise spontaneously or be induced by drugs.

The other main cause of anemia is a large group of disorders in which the bone marrow develops a disease that impairs its function, and there is an imbalance between normal destruction and reduced production. Bone marrow function has to fall below 20% before this becomes a serious clinical problem. Diseases causing such a defect occur predominantly from tumors of the bone marrow such as leukemia or associated disorders.

### Bone marrow and blood cell growth factors

The 1990s has seen the identification and genetic cloning of certain growth factors involved in the intrinsic pathways of blood cell development. Within the pharmaceutical industry, molecular recombinant technology has allowed large-scale production of such growth factors for clinical use. Erythropoietin is the key factor related to red cell production and the product is clinically available for treating some chronic anemias, as in those resulting from kidney disease. Multiple growth factors have been discovered for the development of white blood cells and most important clinically, granulocyte stimulating factor. This product can mature the important white cell component rapidly and is helpful in severe infections where lack of white cells is the main problem. A recent discovery is the additional capacity of this agent, given clinically, to stimulate and mobilize bone marrow stem cells into the peripheral blood in sufficient numbers where they can be harvested and used as an alternative product to bone marrow in transplantation for hematological disorders. This process is called peripheral blood skin cell harvesting.

### Malignant blood disorders

A hematologist or hematological physician will spend a great deal of time dealing with individuals suffering from blood malignancies. In the north of England some 500 new cases per annum occur from a population of 3 million. When people think of blood cancers they automatically think of acute leukemia, and most regard acute leukemia as being commonest in children. In fact, the most common form of blood tumor is lymph-node cancer (Hodgkin's disease and non-Hodgkin's lymphoma), accounting for some 200–250 cases out of a case load of 500. Acute leukemia will account for some 100–120 cases, only one-fifth in children aged under 15. Contrary

to popular opinion, most acute leukemias occur in people aged over 50.

*Childhood leukemia* Four to six per cent of blood cancers occur in children under 15. The most common form of tumor is acute lymphoblastic leukemia, and because this disease arises from a group of cells in the bone marrow, spreading throughout this bone marrow, all the blood cells will be reduced, causing a lack of red cells, normal white cells, and blood platelets. Hence patients develop anemia with a bleeding tendency and predisposition to infection. The past 20 years have seen marvelous improvements in managing childhood leukemia, with the introduction of combination cytotoxic chemotherapy, and in 2001 it is possible to predict that 70% of children will be cured with chemotherapy alone. For individuals in particular poor-risk groups it is also appropriate to carry out marrow transplants, transferring marrow from one person to another early on, and it is hoped that this will improve the outlook. The last five years have seen progress in identifying poor-risk groups, demonstrating specific chromosome abnormalities, and indicating those requiring an early bone marrow transplant.

*Adult leukemia* Once a person is aged over 15, the outlook after conventional treatment with cytotoxic drugs is not so satisfactory. In fact, outcome deteriorates with advancing age. Thus, in patients over 60, accepted conventional cytotoxic chemotherapy will not cure the disease, though it may control it for a while. Even in patients between 15 and 50, the outcome of conventional treatment is unsatisfactory, so that a bone marrow transplant or peripheral blood stem cell transplant (either from a matched family member or using the individual's own recycled tissue) is used to enhance the chance of sustained remission or cure.

### Bone marrow transplantation

During the late 1950s, Donnall E. Thomas, an American physician, began experimenting with allogeneic (transfer of tissue from one individual to another) transplantation in dogs. In the late 1960s and early 1970s he introduced this for treatment of aplastic anemia and leukemia in humans. Forty years since those original experiments, allogeneic transplant using bone marrow or peripheral blood stem cells has become routine and in some diseases very successful. In aplastic anemia (bone marrow failure) with a sibling donor, it is 80% successful. It may be used for treating hereditary anemias (thalassemia) but its main use is for malignant blood disorders. The International Bone Marrow Transplant Registry and its European counterpart compiles detailed information on the outcome for such procedures.

In general, the best results are seen in younger patients who have had a transplant as part of primary treatment within one year of diagnosis. Complications of the procedure continue to hamper progress, and debate continues regarding the validity of outcome versus standard treatment in patients aged over 50.

Donor panels (matched unrelated donor transplants) have become more frequent and complex. The results for such transplants in children are good and continue to improve. Complications of transplants are more of a bar to success in adults but even here patients aged under 40 may have a satisfactory transplant. A recent interest has been the use of cord blood (blood left in the placenta after the birth of a child), as this is remarkably rich in marrow stem cells and provides an alternative source of product for transplants in children.

## Autotransplant — marrow and peripheral blood stem cells

Harvesting and storing 5% of bone marrow, or an equivalent amount of peripheral blood stem cells, allow a patient to undergo an autotransplant (return of the patient's own tissue). Such an approach allows a massive increase in drugs to be given to a patient with a malignant disease (hematological or non-hematological) before return of the marrow. The procedure is the commonest form of transplant world-wide, used for intensification therapy for those who do not have a bone marrow donor. Such an approach is used in acute leukemia, chronic leukemia, Hodgkin's disease, and the other lymphomas. Results of the approach are the subject of great debate and the true place of the procedure has still to be identified. The dash to use this technique in breast cancer, with no evidence to indicate the validity of the approach, is currently a medical and economic concern.

## Lymph node cancer (Hodgkin's disease and non-Hodgkin's lymphoma)

Thomas Hodgkin, born in 1798, described the lymph node disorder which bears his name in 1832. Two hundred years after his birth, it is possible to say that this disease (which arises within cells in the lymph nodes and the spleen) has largely been conquered by radiotherapy and anti-cancer drugs, with many advances over the past 15–20 years. In 1960, only 5–10% of patients would survive five years from the diagnosis. In 1998, even in the most severe form of disease, it is possible to have five years' survival in up to 80% of patients.

Non-Hodgkin's lymphomas are predominantly tumors of B-lymphocytes and a much more heterogeneous group of disorders, whose classification has been a problem to clinicians and pathologists alike. This group of disorders has undergone a 4% increase in incidence throughout the western world during the last 10–15 years, for unknown reasons, and it forms the most common group of hematological cancers. Patients with early stage tumors may be cured with radiotherapy, but even in the most indolent forms of disease it is often very difficult to eradicate, whereas paradoxically in the aggressive forms of disease some 30–40% may be cured with anti-cancer chemotherapy. The role of autotransplantation (transplanting the patient's own bone marrow after high dose chemotherapy) has still to prove that it is an important addition to treatment. Hope for further progress appears to rest on a combination of treatment with cytotoxic drugs, biological response modifiers, and antibodies.

## Bleeding problems

In the 17th century, MALPIGHI (p 37) and Borelli concluded that the dense sponge-work which made up a blood clot was formed from the fluid part of the blood. Not until late in the 18th century did Hewson and John HUNTER (p 398) establish that clots were formed from the 'coagulable lymph'. In 1845 Buchanan showed that the change was brought about by a series of enzymes, and by 1900 the view was accepted that the soluble substance in blood called fibrinogen was converted into the solid-fibrin clot by an enzyme, thrombin. It is now evident that the whole process that causes clotting has to be balanced by an equally complex process in which clotting is prevented, unless a vessel is damaged. These opposing forces of clotting and clot lysis are in a very delicate balance and, once again, may be disturbed if the person inherits a defect of a factor within the clotting cascade or acquires a defect that allows clots to develop.

*Hereditary clotting problems* The classic and well-known hereditary clotting problem is hemophilia, which is split into two types: hemophilia A (classic hemophilia) and hemophilia B (Christmas disease). It was through Queen Victoria that several European royal families came to be affected by hemophilia A (p 329). The first clinical account was written by John Otto from Philadelphia in 1803. Since then we have come to understand the genetic nature of the disorder, in which the defect is passed on via the X (sex) chromosome to male offspring of female carriers (X-linked inheritance). Females rarely suffer from the disease because they are protected by a normal gene copy on the normal X chromosome. There is a 50% chance of male offspring inheriting the abnormal X chromosome and developing the disease. Daughters similarly have a 50% chance of inheriting the abnormal X chromosome and becoming a carrier. The other

50% of males and all females will be normal. The biological defect is absence, or marked reduction, of factor VIII, a particularly important clotting factor in the clotting cascade.

Treatment of the condition is by replacement of factor VIII, which presently has to be obtained from blood products donated by other people. Replacement factors became available from blood plasma in the late 1950s and became much more complex in the 1970s and 1980s, when large amounts of donated plasma from blood transfusion services throughout the world were made into concentrated factor VIII products. This allowed enormous freedom for individuals with the disease. Sadly, much plasma became contaminated with the AIDS virus (HIV), usually when donors were paid to give blood. Once HIV-infected blood had become incorporated in the plasma chain, many hemophiliacs within Britain and the USA became infected. Presently all plasma products obtained through the British blood transfusion service (and similar services elsewhere) are stringently checked for a series of viruses, including HIV, and plasma is treated appropriately to prevent transmission of any form of known virus particle.

It is now possible to produce the normal factor VIII protein by molecular biology, and this product is commercially available. The cost of the product precludes its availability to hemophiliacs in all age groups.                                      SJP

*See also* BLOOD TRANSFUSION; GENEALOGY; GENETICS, HUMAN; ONCOLOGY; TRANSPLANTATION

**HERBAL MEDICINE** Herbal medicine (also known as phytotherapy, phytomedicine, or botanical medicine) is the use of plants or plant parts for medicinal purposes. Such use is the most ancient form of medicine known. Every culture throughout history has evolved an empirical system of using herbs, and herbal medicine forms an essential part of almost all traditional healthcare systems. They play a vital part in traditional Chinese medicine, the traditional medicine of the Indian subcontinent (Ayurveda), Africa, Australia, Polynesia, Indonesia, indigenous American systems of medicine (North and South American), and traditional Arabic systems of medicine (Unani). Herbs form the basis of much modern therapeutics and pharmacology, in which crude herbal extracts were purified to extract the active ingredient. Quinine, atropine, aspirin, and digitalis are some familiar examples; each has a clear and well-documented herbal provenance.

Though many herbal remedies are prescribed empirically, much progress has been achieved through pharmacological and clinical research in substantiating their efficacy. Hypericum for depression, feverfew for migraine, and ginko biloba to improve the circulation in the brain are some of the more widely known examples.

Herbal medicines may have powerful pharmacological effects as well as causing adverse reactions. However, herbalists argue that crude extracts are 'naturally balanced' and thus less likely than purified pharmacological extracts to trigger adverse reactions. Complementary medicine is often seen as safe simply because it is 'natural' as opposed to being produced 'synthetically'. Such blind acceptance should be questioned until we have more information concerning the efficacy, methods of production, potential for adverse reactions, and cross-reactions (particularly with conventional medications) of herbs and indeed all other 'natural' remedies.          GL

*See also* COMPLEMENTARY AND ALTERNATIVE MEDICINE

**HERBAL REMEDIES AND PHYSIC GARDENS**
The very early history of man's use of the plant kingdom is unknown, but the value of plants for shelter, clothing, dyes, implements, and utensils was probably easily established. Their use for food would have been less easy to acquire, such as learning that grass was not nutritious for humans or that tapioca root was poisonous unless cut up and washed or cooked. But to choose plants for medicinal use must have been a difficult task involving many centuries of trial and error (sometimes fatal) because not only had an effective plant to be found, but it had to be matched against a symptom or illness in an era when the nature of disease was not understood.

### Physic gardens

The first knowledge we have of a garden is from China in 2800 BC. It was also there in 100 BC that Emperor Wu Ti originated the idea of a botanical garden, with collectors bringing in plants from far away. The first pictures of gardens are from Egypt in 1400 BC, one of them showing a temple garden at Karnak, where one assumes that priests cultivated the medicinal plants noted in the papyri, such as aloe, caraway, myrrh, and poppy. The concept of botany in the abstract, as a branch of philosophy, was introduced by ARISTOTLE (p 64) in the 4th century BC and he also created one of the first gardens for practical botany.

The establishment of the first Christian monastery at Fayum by St Antony in AD 305 with the ideals of prayers and work — especially gardening — led to the monastic movement which spread to Europe in AD 530 and was the main influence in the establishment of modern botanic gardens.

The plan has survived from the 9th century for a Benedictine monastery at St Gall near Lake Constance, which depicts not only a general garden or *hortus* but also a separate physic garden or *herbularis* next to the infirmary and to the physician's house (the word herb comes from the Latin *herba*, a green crop or grass).

However, it was the Renaissance, with the establishment of universities, that chiefly led to the development of the earlier botanic gardens which began as physic gardens for the education of medical students. The first was in Pisa in 1543, followed by Padua and Florence in 1545. Also established in the 16th century were those at Zürich, Bologna, Leiden, Leipzig, Montpellier, Paris, and Heidelberg.

The idea for the Padua physic garden came from Francesco Bonafede, who had founded the first chair of 'simples' (*lectura simplicium*) in Europe there in 1533 and initially only simples, that is, medicinal plants, were grown. The title simple was used to indicate the single origin of a plant medicine that was later often mixed with others by the APOTHECARY to produce a compound preparation, a '*remedial composita*'. Luca Ghini held the *lectura simplicium* at Pisa, and it was he who had the brilliant idea of drying, mounting, and annotating specimens of plants for study. This invention, the herbarium, was a vital part in the development of botany as a science.

In Great Britain the earliest physic gardens were in private hands. William Turner, the 'father of English botany' (1510–68), had one at Wells, where he was dean of the cathedral. That of the surgeon John Gerard at Holborn was famous for its catalog, the first of its kind ever published and enumerating 1030 plants. Others in London were those of John Parkinson in Long Acre and John Tradescant in Lambeth.

It was the university connection, especially with the faculty of medicine, that led to the foundation of the Oxford Physic Garden in 1621, the name being changed to Botanic Garden in 1840 when the emphasis moved to experimental botany. In Edinburgh, however, it was the need to teach apprentices of the newly allied bodies of surgeons and apothecaries that gave them their first garden in 1656, to be followed in 1670 by the New Physic Garden of the physicians.

In London it was the Society of Apothecaries, not the physicians, who took the lead and in 1673 they founded the Chelsea Physic Garden. Its first gardener, Philip Miller, introduced many new plants from abroad and it became the most richly stocked garden in Europe, sending cotton seed to Georgia to found the American cotton plantations. Carl von Linné (Linnaeus) visited Chelsea in 1733 and taught Miller about his new binomial system for naming plants. Miller's assistant William Aiton went to work in the Royal Garden at Kew House in 1760 and he created Princess Augusta's Physic Garden, which, together with an arboretum, was the origin of The Royal Botanic Gardens, Kew.

A botanical garden has a formally arranged collection of herbaceous plants in Natural Order Beds which are grouped according to families, thus allowing one to compare and contrast the morphological features of related species, for example, in Solanaceae the similarity of the flowers of mandrake and henbane. A physic garden will also have separate collection of medicinal plants. The trees and shrubs, being non-herbaceous woody plants, are often separately placed in an arboretum but, as at Chelsea, they may be interspersed in the order beds, thus pleasantly breaking up the strict geometry. In addition heated glasshouses are essential for tender exotics. A collection of dried specimens constituting a herbarium will be an important feature for the discipline of taxonomy and, naturally, a library is also required. The two essential functions of a botanical garden which separate it from any other garden, however extensive, are those of teaching and research, and facilities for research in the form of special glasshouses and laboratories must be provided.

As knowledge of plants developed there arose an increasing need to replace oral tradition by written records, and these, as we now know, were made in China and Egypt over a thousand years BC. Nevertheless, they had no influence on western medicine and the earliest extant European work dealing with the medicinal plants is the famous *De materia medica* written in the 1st century AD by the Cilician army doctor Pedianos Dioscorides. This described about 500 plants and the influence of this first herbal lasted until the 18th century. It was first illustrated in 512 and with 400 full-page colored paintings of plants it constitutes the *Codex Juliana Anicia*. The invention of printing in 1454 enabled works previously found only in manuscript, together with those newly written, to be quite widely available and the printed herbal (in the sense of a book containing the names and descriptions of medicinal herbs, or of plants in general, with their properties and virtues) became established as an indispensable work. One of the first, von Megenberg's *Das Buch der Natur* of 1475, contains the earliest known botanical wood engraving. The illustrations in all herbals were woodcuts up to 1670 or so but they were themselves copied and recopied until they bore only slight resemblance to the plant they were supposed to depict. Happily there were exceptions, one of the best being Otto Brunfels's *Herbarium vivae eicones* (1530), where the draughtsman and engraver drew from the living plant. Another in this genre was the *De historia stirpium* of Leonhard Fuchs in 1542, although interestingly the text itself was largely a copy of Dioscorides. The figures in Fuchs's work were

## HERBALS

Herbals are treatises intended to enable the user to identify and employ plants for medicinal purposes. Among the earliest manuscript herbals the best-known and the most influential was that of Dioscorides (1st century AD), which was described 1600 years after it was written as 'the foundation and ground-work of all that hath been since delivered'. Thereafter herbals continued to be published (for example, by Pierandrea Mattioli), until the development of printing and wood engraving in the 16th century allowed the reproduction of fine and detailed representation of plants by the great German and Italian botanists. The British contribution was small, resting on such works as that of William Turner (d. 1568) and Gerard's *Herball* (1597). Subsequently herbals became increasingly botanical, moving away from medicine and therapeutic applications.

used by William Turner for the first English herbal in 1551. John Gerard, a London surgeon, produced a very fine herbal in 1597 depicting nearly 1800 plants, which was revised by Tomas Johnson in 1633. It became the standard work on medicinal plants and was influential for many years. Nicholas Culpeper's *The English physician* (1652) was based on astrological herbalism with its strange belief that each disease was caused by a planet and cured by a plant associated with an opposing planet.

As the 17th century progressed the dominant influence of medicine over botany began to wane with the increasing study of plants for their own sake, and gradually herbals were replaced by compendia of drugs such as the *Pharmacopoeia Londoniensis* (1690) on the one hand, and purely botanical works such as Nehemiah Grew's pioneer microscopical work *The anatomy of plants* (1682) on the other. Altogether 79 major herbals were printed in Europe up to 1670, testifying to the great value this type of book had for the physician, apothecary, herbalist, and educated layman, and also for the clergy and monks who helped the common people in time of illness.

### Herbal remedies and drugs

To examine critically the herbal remedies there described in the light of modern knowledge is to realize the difficulties our medical forebears had in grappling with illnesses, the nature of which they did not for the most part understand. Their problem was increased by bizarre hypotheses, such as that of astrological botany, and by the Doctrine of Signatures, to which chemical theories were added by PARACELSUS (p 617). The doctrine held that herbs had physical features which indicated their medicinal use; for example, that those with yellow flowers would cure jaundice.

Furthermore, a good deal of magic and superstition of unknown antiquity crept into the herbals, making with these other factors a final hotchpotch of unproved, useless, and often absurd information. Amazingly, these alleged medicinal properties have been copied right up to now from the printed herbals of the 15th to 17th centuries and they are blandly presented to the present-day public by modern writers on herbalism. Bistort, for example, is exhibited as of proved excellence in diarrhea, dysentery, cholera, and all bowel complaints and in hemorrhages from the lungs and stomach, bleeding from the nose, and mucous discharges, being also considered valuable in diabetes. William WITHERING (p 633), however, presented the scientific approach very well in the introduction to his 1776 work on the British flora:

> Many people will be surprised to find so little said upon the medicinal virtues of plants, but those who are best enabled to judge this matter will perhaps

think that the greater part of that little might well have been omitted. The superstition of former years, operating upon the ignorance of mankind, gave rise to miracles of every denomination … and at length every common plant was esteemed a cure for almost every disease. We shall sooner attain the end proposed if we take up the subject as altogether new, and rejecting the fables of the ancient herbalist, build only upon the basis of accurate and well-considered experiments.

### Modern medicines from plants

Plants are the origin of over 30 important medicines whose value has been proven by scientifically controlled clinical trials. How were these medicines found?

- From folk medicine alone, for example, the opium poppy (*Papaver somniferum*), which contains morphine and codeine.

- Scientific investigation of a folk remedy such as by creating new medicines from the plant compound, as with the synthesis of the heart drug amiodarone and the ASTHMA remedy 'Intal' from khellin (*Ammi visnaga*) used traditionally for kidney stones. Also by discovering a new use for a plant remedy, such as occurred with the Madagascar periwinkle (*Catharanthus roseus*) when the Vinca alkaloids in it were found to be effective against cancer, whilst its folk use against diabetes was disproved.

- Veterinary medicine gave us the oral anti-coagulant drug warfarin when a veterinary surgeon observed that cattle dying of hemorrhage had eaten moldy hay made from sweet clover (*Melilotus officinalis*).

- Organic chemistry led to lignocaine, a local anesthetic discovered from barley (*Hordeum vulgare*) in the course of a purely academic study to find out if genetically different plants were chemically different.

- Observations by patients are valuable. A man found by himself that quinine cured his attacks of palpitation and the related drug quinidine was used for cardiac irregularities.

- Doctors, in the course of their clinical work, found that *Veratrum viride* was effective in pregnancy toxemia and that *Physostigma venenosum* relieved the symptoms of myasthenia gravis.

- Large-scale screening programs have yielded two anti-cancer drugs, paclitaxel (Taxol) from the yew tree (*Taxus brevifolia* and *baccata*) and irinotecan (Campto) from the tree *Camptotheca acuminata*.

Many other remedies are also derived from plants. Foremost among these was the use of the foxglove, *Digitalis purpurea*, for treating heart failure, superbly deduced from an old polypharmacy remedy by William Withering in 1775. The modern heart drug digoxin is obtained by extracting it from the leaves of *Digitalis lanata*. Hyoscine (scopolamine in the USA) used to premedicate a patient for an operation is a constituent of the mandrake plant (*Mandragora officinarum*) and its sedative and anesthetic properties were well known 2000 years ago when it was used for amputation and in the 'death sponge' to relieve the agony of crucifixion. Nowadays it is made synthetically. Atropine, another alkaloid from the same group of plants, the tomato family Solanaceae, is used to correct an abnormally slow heart rate. Formerly it was used in Parkinson's disease, but better synthetic drugs have now replaced it. Colchicine, from the meadow saffron (*Colchicum autumnale*), is used to treat acute GOUT, its value in joint disease stemming from AD 600. Quinine, long of value in MALARIA, comes from the bark of the Peruvian tree *Cinchona ledgeriana*, whose use was found around 1630. Aspirin is the acetyl salt of salicylic acid, a compound first discovered in 1835 in the native British plant the meadowsweet (*Filipendula ulmaria*) then known as a *Spirea*, hence the name of the drug A=acetyl spir=spirea in=a drug termination, as in phenacetin and heroin. The anticancer drug etoposide shows how a medicine can be discovered originally in the community (folk medicine) and then be improved by drug development in a pharmaceutical company. The origin of this drug lies in the finding by the Penobscot native Americans in Maine that an extract of the May Apple (*Podophyllum peltatum*) was useful for growths on the skin. This treatment was extended by physicians to treat genital warts, which are a type of skin cancer. But the extract was too toxic for internal use until Bristol-Myers made the semisynthetic derivative etoposide, which can be given by injection for chemotherapy.

The remedies used in the practice of herbal medicine are quite different from those which have just been described. HERBAL MEDICINE consists of prescribing the whole plant or part of it, and not a pure compound extracted from the plant nor a synthetic medicine. These remedies belong to complementary or ALTERNATIVE MEDICINE, which by definition contains medicines that have never been properly tested. If they had been they would be in the official pharmacopoeia. It tends to be assumed that because a product is natural or has been used for many years, that it is therefore free of toxic effects. This is quite untrue. There are many reports of serious illness and death from herbal preparations. Furthermore it is thought that synthetic drugs ('chemical medicines') are in some way 'different' and more toxic than plant medicines. This approach overlooks the fact that both synthetic and plant medicines are each pure chemical compounds. Assessing drugs by a controlled clinical trial is just as important in revealing untoward side-effects as in demonstrating the beneficial effect of the drug.

The continuing success of plant-derived medicines in combating illness makes it likely that this progress will continue, although it has to be tempered with the knowledge that the discovery of medicinal plants has often been by a lucky incident or by pragmatic trial and error.　AHol

**HEROPHILUS** (*c.*290BC). Born in Chalcedon, he studied medicine under Praxagoras of Cos and was one of the founders of the medical school at Alexandria. One of the founding fathers of anatomy, he advanced medical knowledge by performing human dissections, and even vivisections on executed criminals from the royal jails, and conducting comparative anatomical studies between humans and animals. He described the brain, which he regarded as the center of the nervous system, and among other organs the eyes, liver, salivary glands, pancreas, and sexual organs, and was the first to distinguish between the arteries and the veins. Herophilus also recognized the importance of taking a patient's pulse, trying to assess its rate by using a water-clock. Although none of his works are preserved, it appears he wrote at least 11 treatises, including three on anatomy, one on ophthalmology, and one on midwifery.

Austin Bradford **HILL** (1897–1991). British medical statistician. After developing tuberculosis as a pilot in the First World War, Hill (the son of a professor of physiology), who had wanted to be a doctor, graduated in economics, joining a statisti-

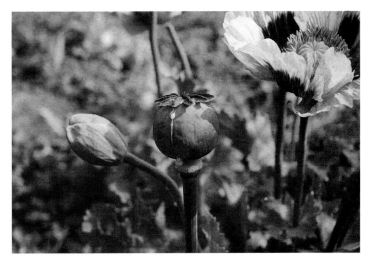

The opium poppy *(papaver somniferum)* showing in the center the incised unripe capsule with the milky juice of opium oozing out. The beautiful flower is on the right.

cal group at the National Institute for Medical Research in 1923. Ten years later he moved to join his friend and mentor, Major GREENWOOD (p 271) at the London School of Hygiene. He went on to become professor of medical statistics, a post which he held until his retirement in 1961, the year in which he received his knighthood. He was also director of the Medical Research Council's Statistical Research Unit. Hill had also been a friend of (Sir) Ronald Fisher, who had introduced randomized controlled trials into agriculture. When after the Second World War the Medical Research Council was allocated a little streptomycin for treating patients with tuberculosis, he persuaded the Council that the only ethical way of allocating the treatment was through such a trial. This was to be the first published RANDOMIZED CONTROLLED TRIAL.

**HIPPOCRATES** (*c*.460–*c*.357 BC), known as the Father of Medicine. Son of a physician, Hippocrates was born on the island of Cos. Little is known of his life but it is thought that, after travelling in Greece and Asia Minor as an itinerant physician, he returned to Cos where he founded a medical school, wrote, practiced, and taught. Of the 72 medical treatises which comprise the *Hippocratic collection,* fewer than 10 are now attributed to Hippocrates (during the same period there were at least 7 other physicians of that name). Whilst acknowledging the humoral theory of disease, the Hippocratic doctrine separated medicine from religion, applying reasoning and observation to medical practice. It focused attention on the patient rather than the disease, and regarded the body as a whole rather than a series of parts. His vivid disease pictures still allow a diagnosis to be made 2000 years after they were written (as in the description of a woman with a five-day course of diphtheria, from which she died). Hippocrates held that health was a balance and illness an upset in the humors (yellow bile, blood, phlegm, and black bile). These humors corresponded to the four qualities (hot, dry, cold, wet), the four seasons, the four ages of man (infancy, youth, adulthood, and old age), the four temperaments (choleric, sanguine, phlegmatic, and melancholic), and the four elements (air, fire, earth, and water),

The highest importance was placed on the honesty and dignity of the physician, and, although the Hippocratic oath is now believed not to be the work of Hippocrates or one of his disciples, it remains eponymous. The writings comprise textbooks, lectures, essays, and case histories from comprehensive clinical observations, recording failure as well as success in diagnosis and treatment; treatises include: *Prognostics; Aphorisms; Epidemics; On airs, waters, and places; Regimen in acute diseases*; and *On fractures.* They were to remain highly influential for many hundreds of years.

**HIPPOCRATIC OATH** See OATHS AND CODES OF CONDUCT

**HIP REPLACEMENT** See ORTHOPEDIC SURGERY (ORTHOPEDICS)

**HISTORIOGRAPHY** Long before professional historians developed an active interest, medicine's past was of critical consequence for medical practitioners and professors alike, eager to recruit the dead to their causes, to commemorate exemplary figures, to inspire their students, and to construct an imposing pedigree for their art. Not least, past heroes long possessed present authority. For the humanist physicians of the 16th and 17th centuries, the treatises of medicine's founding fathers, notably HIPPOCRATES (p 382) and GALEN (p 324), were absolutely canonical; living founts of wisdom, rather than mere objects of antiquarian curiosity.

The first significant attempt to construct a full narrative of medicine's evolution was *Histoire de la médecine d'ou l'on voit l'origine et le progrés de l'art* (1696) by Daniel Leclerc, professor of medicine in Geneva. A derivative English work soon followed: the *History of physick* (1725–26) by the London physician, John Freind. Freind's survey of Greco-Roman and medieval medicine was structured with half an eye to contemporary English debates concerning the medical applications of the Newtonian mechanical philosophy: the past could still settle current controversies.

In the history of medicine, as with political and diplomatic history, the Enlightenment — the age of Edward Gibbon — and, even more so, the 19th century mark the scholarly watershed. Historians began to insist that the past was a different country, truly distinct from the present. Study of long-dead doctors and their august tomes gradually ceased to be definitive of medical thinking itself, and turned into a scholarly passion or pastime in its own right. The first history of medicine in this 'modern' mode was Kurt Sprengel's *Versuch einer pragmatischen Geschichte der Arzneikunde* (1792), which strove to steer a middle course between pedantic antiquarianism and high-flown philosophical interpretations. German scholarship led the field in the 19th century. In his *Lehrbuchder Geschichte der Medizin und der Volkskrankheit* (1845), Heinrich Haeser produced the first professed textbook of medical history — a work that gave consideration to historical EPIDEMIOLOGY as well as to the history of doctors. The first periodical devoted exclusively to medical history, the German language *Janus*, was founded in 1846 — it lasted only two years — and the first chair in the history of medicine was created in Vienna in 1850.

Great attention began to be devoted to furnishing authoritative editions of key texts. Nineteenth-century scholarship produced many of the editions of the classic authors still in use. The works of GALEN (p 324) were edited in Leipzig between 1823 and 1833, while the French philological scholar, Emile Littré, edited Hippocrates between 1839 and 1861. From 1844, the Sydenham Society in England dedicated itself to publishing a renowned series of translations of Greek, Latin, and Arabic medical classics. Alongside the creation of a canon of classical medical texts, book-collecting became a prestigious avocation. Sir William OSLER (b. 1849) (p 602) built up a celebrated personal library, now preserved in Montreal, and, most spectacularly, Sir Henry WELLCOME (b. 1853) (p 316) channeled profits from his pharmaceutical business into the assembling of an enormous collection of medical books, manuscripts, paintings, and artefacts, that was to form the core of the former Wellcome Institute for the History of Medicine in London, now the Wellcome Trust.

Amongst historians of medicine, the pivotal figure is Karl Sudhoff, who was professor of the history of medicine at Leipzig from 1905 to 1925 and director of the first institute of the history of medicine. Sudhoff set particular store by manuscript research. Under his direction, the first enduring journal of the history of medicine was set up (*Sudhoffs Archiv*) and essential reference works were compiled, notably the *Biographisches Lexikon der hervorragenden Ärzte* by August 1884 and Julius Pagel, which began publication in 1884 and took 50 years to complete with its supplements.

Sudhoff's Leipzig institute became the envy of, and model for, medical historians the world over. His successor, the Swiss Henry Sigerist, broadened the intellectual vision of medical history, and, as a committed admirer of the Soviet Union, developed a more socially oriented view of medical history. In 1932 Sigerist was appointed head of the newly founded Institute for the History of Medicine at the JOHNS HOPKINS UNIVERSITY (p 840), Baltimore. From 1933 there appeared, under his guidance, the *Bulletin of the History of Medicine*, and the American Association for the History of Medicine was founded.

Until recently the bulk of writings in the history of medicine have been 'in-house': written by doctors, for doctors, and principally about doctors. This tendency to treat medical history as essentially the contributions of physicians and biomedical scientists to the progress of medical knowledge and practice has come under attack, especially in the present generation. It has been accused of being Whiggish, that is, of judging the past in the light of hindsight. Many historians of medicine nowadays stress the dangers of ana-chronism, and insist, by contrast, that earlier physicians and medical belief-systems must be understood on their own terms, rather than being evaluated in terms of their contribution to modern medicine. They also seek to widen the vision, and pay more attention than heretofore to the history of patients as well as practitioners, to lay wisdom and popular forms of healing, to medical institutions and the paramedical professions, and to the social and political ramifications of medical knowledge. Hopefully a fruitful dialog will develop between the unique medical expertise of 'practitioners' history' and the wider visions of professional historians.          RPor

**HISTORY OF MEDICINE** All societies possess medical beliefs; ideas of life and death, disease and cure, and systems of healing. To speak extremely schematically, the historical development of medicine may be seen in terms of a series of stages. The most elementary belief-systems the world over have attributed sickness to ill-will, to various modes of malevolent spirits, sorcery, witchcraft, and diabolical or divine intervention. Such ways of thinking still pervade the pre-literate tribal communities of Africa, South America, and the Pacific, and were influential in Christian Europe throughout the Middle Ages and the Reformation era. A few radical protestant sects continue to view sickness and recovery largely in providential and supernatural terms; healing shrines such as Lourdes remain popular within the Roman Catholic Church, and faith-healing retains a following.

In Europe from Greco-Roman antiquity onwards, and also amongst the great Asian civilizations, the leading approach to sickness and healing replaced such transcendental explanations by positing a natural basis for disease and healing. Among educated lay people and physicians alike, the body became viewed as integral to a wider cosmic scheme of law-governed elements and regular processes. GREEK MEDICINE in particular underscored the microcosm/macrocosm relationship, the correlations between the healthy human body and the harmonies of external nature. From HIPPOCRATES (p 382) in the 5th century BC through to GALEN (p 324) in the 2nd century AD, 'humoral medicine' emphasized the analogies between the four elements of external nature (earth, air, fire, and water) and the four HUMORS or fluids (blood, phlegm, choler or yellow bile, and black bile), whose balance determined bodily health. The humors found expression in the TEMPERAMENTS and complexions that marked an individual's constitution. The task of hygiene was to maintain a balanced constitution; the role of medicine to restore such balance when disturbed.

The medicine of antiquity, which was transmitted via Islam to the medieval West and remained powerful throughout the Renaissance era, paid great attention to general health maintenance, through regulation of diet, exercise, hygiene, and life-style. In the absence of detailed anatomical and physiological expertise, and without the benefit of a powerful artillery of cures and surgical skills, the ability to advance diagnoses and prognoses was highly valued, and an intimate physician–patient relationship was fostered. The teachings of antiquity, which remained authoritative to the 18th century and still form an undercurrent of medical folklore, were more successful in assisting people to cope with chronic conditions and in soothing lesser ailments than in conquering the life-threatening infections that became endemic and epidemic in the civilized world (LEPROSY, PLAGUE, SMALLPOX, measles, and, later, the 'filth diseases' such as TYPHUS, associated with urban squalor).

This rather personal tradition of bedside medicine long remained popular in the West, as did its equivalents in CHINA and INDIA (Ayurvedic medicine). But in Europe it was gradually supplemented and challenged by the creation of a more 'scientific' mode of medicine, grounded, for the first time, upon precise and systematic anatomical and physiological investigation, epitomized from the 15th century by the dissection techniques that were to become central to medical education. Landmarks in this program include the publication of *De humani corporis fabrica* (1543) by the Paduan professor, Andreas VESALIUS (p 846), the first momentous anatomical atlas and a work that challenged truths received since Galen; and William HARVEY's (p 363) *De motu cordis* (1628), which, by experimentally demonstrating the circulation of the blood and the role of the heart as a pump, put physiological enquiry on the map.

### Further discoveries

Post-Vesalian investigations immeasurably advanced knowledge of the structures and functions of the living organism. Further enquiries saw the unraveling of the lymphatic system and the lacteals (chylous vessels), and the 18th and 19th centuries yielded a finer grasp of the nervous system and the operation of the brain. With the aid of microscopes and the laboratory, 19th century investigators explored the nature of body

A moment in medical history. A direct transfusion of blood by Dr Roussel, Geneva. (Reproduced courtesy of the Mary Evans Picture Library.)

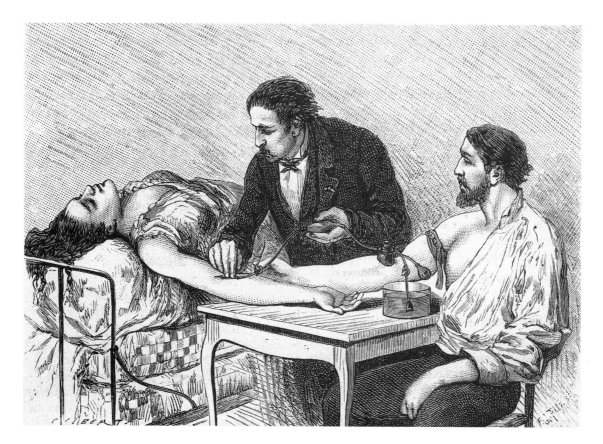

tissues and pioneered CELL BIOLOGY; pathological anatomy came of age. Parallel improvements in organic chemistry led to an understanding of respiration, NUTRITION, the digestive system, and deficiency diseases, and to such specialties as ENDOCRINOLOGY. The 20th century has been the age of GENETICS and MOLECULAR BIOLOGY.

Most spectacularly, 19th century science made enormous leaps forward in the understanding of infectious diseases. For many centuries, rival epidemiological theories had attributed fevers to miasmas (poisons in the air, exuded from rotting animal and vegetable material, the soil, and standing water) or to contagion (person-to-person contact), with little solid evidence to clinch the dispute. From the 1860s, the rise of bacteriology, associated especially with Louis PASTEUR (p 620) in France and Robert KOCH (p 455) in Germany, established the role of micro-organic pathogens. Bacteriology led, in time, to dramatic new cures.

In the short run, however, the anatomically based scientific medicine emerging from Renaissance universities and the Scientific Revolution contributed more to information than to health. Drugs from both the Old and New Worlds, notably opium and Peruvian Bark (quinine), became more widely available, and mineral and metal-based pharmaceutical preparations enjoyed a great if dubious vogue (for example, mercury for SYPHILIS). But it would be tendentious to speak of a true pharmacological revolution before the introduction of sulfonamides and antibiotics in the 20th century, and surgery could make only limited progress before the introduction of anesthetics and antiseptic and aseptic operating-room conditions from the mid-19th century. In short, biomedical understanding long outstripped dramatic breakthroughs in curative medicine, and many would argue that the retreat of the great lethal diseases (DIPHTHERIA, TYPHOID, TUBERCULOSIS, etc.) was due, in the first instance, more to urban improvements, superior nutrition, and PUBLIC HEALTH regulations than to curative medicine. Indeed, the one early striking instance of the conquest of disease — the introduction first of smallpox inoculation and then of vaccination — came not through 'science' at all but through the alert embracing of a tenet of popular medical folklore.

From the Renaissance, medical practitioners increasingly organized themselves professionally, commonly in a hierarchy with physicians at the head, and surgeons and apothecaries nearer the foot, and with other sorts of healers marginalized or vilified (justly or not) as quacks. Practitioners' guilds, corporations, and colleges received royal approval, and medicine gradually became incorporated within the public domain, particularly in the German-speaking parts of Europe, where the notion of 'medical police' (preventive public health) gained official backing from the 18th century. The state inevitably played the leading part in the growth of military and naval medicine and later in TROPICAL MEDICINE. The HOSPITAL sphere, however, long remained largely the responsibility of the Church, especially in Roman Catholic parts of Europe, and of urban philanthropic initiatives. Gradually (some would say, belatedly) the state took responsibility for improving the health of the populations of the emergent industrial societies, through public health regulation and custody of the insane in the 19th century, and through national insurance and national health schemes in the 20th century, although these latter developments often met fierce opposition from a medical profession seeking to preserve its autonomy against encroaching state bureaucracies.

The latter half of the 20th century witnessed the continued phenomenal progress of immensely capital-intensive and specialized scientific medicine. Transplant surgery and biotechnology have captured the public imagination. Alongside, major chronic and psychosomatic disorders persist in the advanced world, and there is little sign that the basic health problems of the developing world are diminishing. This situation exemplifies and perpetuates a key facet and paradox of the history of medicine: the unresolved disequilibrium between the remarkable capacities of an increasingly powerful science-based biomedical tradition and, on the other hand, the wider and unfulfilled health requirements of economically impoverished and politically mismanaged societies.  RPor

**HODGKIN'S DISEASE** See HEMATOLOGY; ONCOLOGY

**HOLISTIC MEDICINE** is a doctrine of preventive and therapeutic medicine which emphasizes the importance of regarding the individual as a whole being integral with his social, cultural, and environmental context rather than as a patient with isolated malfunction of a particular system or organ. Although the term has recently become fashionable, the underlying philosophy is nothing new and has always been inseparable from good medical practice.

**HOLOCAUST** The Holocaust achieved its destructive toll largely because of the active part played by the German medical profession at all levels. The mass destruction produced by the Final Solution arose in medicine and the destructive impact of the Final Solution was magnified by the role of medicine. The crimes of German medicine were not confined to a few evil people working in the isolation of the concentration camps, but involved virtually every element of the German healthcare system, including the German physicians' organization, the public health system, the hospitals, clinics, research centers, and medical schools. It included some of the oldest and most prestigious universities in the world and the foremost scientific research institutions in Germany.

The complicity of the medical profession began with the scientific acceptance of the concept of inherent or biological inferiority. This concept, incorporated within the precepts of eugenics and race hygiene, was promulgated in the German medical profession before Hitler's rise to power. The Nazis found within the culture of German medicine the scientific rationale for legitimizing and fostering of their policies and programs of racial hygiene. The German medical profession and healthcare system became a vehicle for disseminating and implementing Hitler's program of racial selection and destruction.

Members of the German medical profession gave the Nazi party their individual and collective allegiance. Among all occupational groups in Germany, the medical profession had the largest membership in the Nazi party: 45% of German physicians became members, and they tended to join early. Nazi loyalists encompassed country practitioners and the professional élite, including leading professors and scientists. Most university rectors appointed by the Nazis were physicians. Membership in the SS helped ensure an academic appointment. The medical school curriculum included compulsory courses on eugenics and racial hygiene.

The first important programmatic step in the path to genocide was the program of enforced sterilization implemented under a law passed by the *Reichstag* in July 1933. Under this law German citizens who were considered to have, or be potential carriers of, conditions allegedly hereditary were subject to enforced surgical sterilization. The categories included congenital 'weak-mindedness,' schizophrenia, manic-depressive ('circular') insanity, hereditary epilepsy, hereditary chorea minor, hereditary blindness, hereditary deafness, severe hereditary bodily deformities, and severe alcoholism. The sterilization law was drawn up by prominent academicians and researchers, one of the foremost being Professor Ernst Rüdin of the Kaiser-Wilhelm Institute of Psychiatry in Munich. The Munich institute, which was founded by the eminent psychiatrist Emil KRAEPELIN (p 355), played a leading part in the Nazi EUGENICS program.

An estimated 400 000 German citizens were sterilized forcibly. Public health was subsumed by eugenic policy. Patient confidentiality was violated and physicians were required to report patients who might qualify for sterilization. By 1937, 745 eugenic health centers had been established in the Reich. Additional support for state eugenic policies came from the universities, which provided expert advice on eugenic and racial matters through special institutes of genetics and race hygiene. The sterilization program also provided patients used in teaching the compulsory courses on eugenics and race hygiene, as well as for research.

### Racial purification

The program of eugenic purification enacted under the 1933 sterilization law was followed by racial purification under the 1935 Nuremberg racial laws. These laws mandated race as a medical diagnosis requiring a medical examination. The review panel established under these laws included physicians as members.

An architect of the Nuremberg racial laws was a physician, Dr Gerhard Wagner. A Munich general practitioner, Wagner was, until his death in 1938, *Reichsführer* of physicians for the Nazi party. At the 1935 Nuremberg rally, Dr Wagner openly advocated the mass sterilization of Jews and the killing of the mentally and physically handicapped.

While the actual medical killing did not begin formally until after the outbreak of war, the precedents for the program of medical murder had been established earlier, in psychiatric hospitals. Patients in those institutions were considered as 'low life' or 'life without value' or 'useless eaters' and killed by starvation, neglect, or poisoning with medication.

There were four overlapping programs of medical murder: child euthanasia; euthanasia of adult psychiatric patients (known as Aktion T-4); the killing of concentration camp prisoners (designated as Aktion 14f13); and so-called 'wild' euthanasia. The euthanasia programs shared personnel and killing apparatus.

The formal child-killing program began in 1939. It arose from the sterilization program through the Reich Committee for the Scientific Registering of Serious Hereditary and Congenital Illness. This medical expert committee introduced the compulsory registration of all 'malformed' newborn children. Three members comprised an 'expert' subcommittee responsible for deciding which children would die. The doomed children were sent to one of 30 designated killing centers (called 'pediatric clinics'), which had been established in psychiatric asylums throughout the country. Two of these sites, Eglfing-Haar and Brandenburg-Görden, functioned as clinical teaching units for instruction in the killing of children. The preferred method of killing was through starvation and poisoning with overdoses of medication such as phenobarbital.

Some institutions had designated 'hunger houses', where the victims were starved.

Hitler authorized the adult euthanasia program in October 1939. Six killing centers were established. Each had a gas chamber using compressed carbon monoxide and included, in most instances, cremation ovens on the site. The gas chambers, disguised as showers, were developed by a team that included medical experts. The turning-on of the gas was a designated medical act assigned to a physician.

The victims' bodies were exploited for their gold dental work and body parts. The gold taken from the mouths of corpses was used to help finance the killing program. The body parts were sent to academic research institutes.

Over 70 000 people are known to be have been murdered under T-4, which ended in August 1941. The medical killing actually expanded and the number of killing centers increased after this. It extended to occupied Poland and was incorporated into Operation Reinhard for the murder of Jews in the occupied eastern territories.

The children's killing program was expanded to include adolescents and young adults. The killing of adult patients in Germany evolved into a random 'wild' program, which took place in numerous institutions throughout the Reich and continued until virtually the end of the war. Adults murdered in the 'wild' campaign included prisoners and sick foreign laborers.

In 1941, elements of T-4 became Aktion 14f13 for killing concentration camp prisoners. Selected by the medical team, these unfortunates were transported to T-4 gas chambers for execution. The T-4 apparatus provided a transitional killing program until such time as the concentration camps had their own capacity for mass killing. Three of the T-4 killing centers, Sonnenstein, Bernburg, and Hartheim, served as supplemental killing sites for the concentration camps.

In January 1942, less than five months after Hitler's order to terminate formal T-4 activity, fifteen officials met in a Berlin villa on Lake Wannsee to discuss administrative details of the 'Final Solution to the Jewish Problem'. One of the issues considered during that 90-minute Wannsee Conference was the fate of captive Jews who were fit to work and capable of procreation. Serious consideration was given to a program of mass sterilization to prevent both their procreation and the possibility of racial contamination. As a result, horrific medical experiments were performed on inmates of Auschwitz in order to perfect a method of mass sterilization. When mass sterilization was deemed impracticable, the method chosen was death in the gas chamber. The T-4 medical killing program had been a pilot project, a feasibility study, for the largest program of organized mass

murder in the history of humankind. The first commandant of the death camp of Treblinka was a physician who gained his killing experience in the T-4 program at the psychiatric hospital at Brandenburg-Görden, Dr Irmfried Eberl.

## Ghettoization

Death as a result of starvation, privation, and disease was the principal consequence of the Nazi ghettoization policy. The concept of ghettoization — of confining a minority group forcibly into a designated limited area — is centuries old and, although chiefly associated with the repression of Jews, has in fact been much more widely applied. Early in World War II, in occupied Poland in particular, Nazi Germany forced Jews to inhabit ghettos in several cities as well as in smaller locations. The largest ghettos were those in Warsaw and in Lódz.

What seems clear is that no overall policy on the creation or operation of ghettos existed. In Lódz the ghetto was sealed off by April 1940 and was seen initially as a short-term holding measure until the Jews were transported eastwards. Madagascar plan was never seriously considered feasible. In fact, the ghetto survived for some time. In Warsaw, by contrast, it took from autumn 1939, when the first order was issued, until November, 1940, before the ghetto was sealed. In Warsaw, German administrators vacillated between two policies: deliberate extermination by neglect, and use of Jewish skills to provide material useful to the German war effort. In the summer of 1942 this question was settled by the decision to annihilate the survivors at Treblinka.

But before annihilation, the Jewish communities of Nazi-occupied Europe were subject to mass privation, creating an incubator for infections such as TUBERCULOSIS, TYPHUS, and TYPHOID. The Nazi fear of contagion contributed to the policy of ghettoization, which was instituted, in part, as a public health measure to protect the German conquerors from the contagious diseases suffered by the victims of their racial policies.

In Nazi-occupied countries, particularly in Eastern Europe, the health of the conquered population often deteriorated badly and disease and death rates rose. This was especially true of the Jews. In Poland, millions of Jews were forced into ghettos where supplies of food, water, and shelter were grossly inadequate. In Warsaw, the official ration the Germans allowed Jews was 184 calories per day — less than one-tenth of the necessary minimum. Even before the so-called Final Solution began to be implemented, large numbers of Jews were dying of starvation, tuberculosis, typhus, and other disorders.

In Warsaw, which before the war had included in its population almost half a million Jews, these

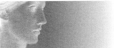

men, women, and children eked out a pinched existence in a primitive part of the old city. Once the ghetto was established in November 1940, almost a third of the city's inhabitants lived precariously in about one twenty-fifth of the area of Warsaw.

Forcible confinement to the ghetto created many problems. Large families lived in a single room. Crowds jammed the streets and sidewalks. Many diseases flourished in such conditions, most notably tuberculosis, which became a major killer.

Overcrowding and lack of sufficient water meant that keeping clean became impossible; lack of cleanliness promoted skin diseases and infestation with lice and fleas. These in turn often carried diseases such as typhus. Sewerage in the Warsaw ghetto was antique and inadequate and outhouses, heavily overused, frequently contaminated wells, a situation followed by various diarrheal diseases, dysentery, and typhoid fever.

Injured and sick Jews had little chance of hospitalization. Before the war, the Jewish Czyste Hospital was arguably the best in Warsaw, a medical haven for non-Jews as well. But that hospital was located outside what became the ghetto and had to be abandoned, along with the bulk of its equipment and supplies. Inside the ghetto, a few small hospitals existed, but the reborn Czyste Hospital had to occupy several buildings, all unsuited to that purpose. The makeshift wards became so crowded that two or three patients occupied the same bed and many lay on the floor and in hallways. Drugs and supplies were almost non-existent and appeals to the Nazis for relief went unheeded.

Although accurate data do not exist, an estimated 80 000 Jews died in the ghetto between November 1940 and the summer of 1942. A Jewish scientist calculated that they all would be dead in five years under the reigning conditions. But, a short time after, the massive deportations to Treblinka began and murder assumed wholesale proportions under the euthanasia-trained physician, Dr Irmfried Eberl.

Many medical scientists considered the racial and killing programs an opportunity to exploit human beings for inhuman experimentation. Scientists regarded the captive, impotent human victims as potential guinea pigs for 'terminal' experiments. Dogs, cats, and horses in Germany were legally protected from experiments performed on human prisoners in SS-controlled concentration camps.

Dr Sigmund Rascher's notorious Dachau hypothermia experiments were performed for the Luftwaffe and the results reported to leading German medical scientists. One scientist linked with the Dachau experiments was Dr Hubertus

Strughold. After the war the American military brought Strughold to the United States, where, in 1961, he became chief scientist of the Aerospace Medical Division of the United States Air Force.

The principal investigator for Dr Josef MENGELE's (p 387) infamous Auschwitz research was the distinguished professor and world authority on genetics and twin studies, Otmar von Verschuer. Verschuer saw Auschwitz as an opportunity to fulfill his research postulate that genetic research required studies on human twins selected at random. In Auschwitz, Mengele functioned as Verschuer's research assistant. Specimens from twin victims murdered in Auschwitz were sent to the Kaiser-Wilhelm Institute of Anthropology in Berlin-Dahlem, headed by Verschuer.

The T-4 euthanasia program was exploited by neuropathologist Julius Hallervorden, then director of the famed Kaiser-Wilhelm Institute of Brain Research in Berlin-Buch. Hallervorden seized the opportunity afforded by the murder of psychiatric patients from Görden who were killed at the euthanasia station in Brandenburg. Specimens from these murdered victims formed part of what was probably the foremost neuropathological collection in the world. After the Soviet occupation of Berlin-Buch, the Kaiser-Wilhelm Institute of Brain Research was moved to Frankfurt. Renamed a Max-Planck institute, the true origins of parts of its neuropathological collection were revealed in Germany only in 1987 and 1988. In 1990, the entire collection from the Hitler period was buried in the Forest Cemetery in Munich. Along with the specimens from the Frankfurt institute were brain specimens from the collection of the Max-Planck Institute of Psychiatry in Munich.

## Anatomy and execution

During the Third Reich, anatomy and execution became inexorably linked, the university institutes of anatomy becoming the benefactors of Nazi terror. The execution chambers of regional jails throughout the Reich became virtual slaughterhouses, with the remains delivered to university institutes of anatomy. Many of the anatomized victims were Polish and Russian slave laborers executed for trivial crimes such as socializing with German women. The German law giving the family the right of reclamation of the body was ignored and eventually suspended. In 1942 the Ministry of Justice prohibited the release of the corpses of executed Poles and Jews for burial by relatives. The approved destination would be a university anatomical institute.

One of those institutes was the Institute of Anatomy of the University of Vienna, which received regular shipments from the execution chamber of the regional court (*Landesgerichte*)

located nearby. The director of the institute, Professor Eduard Pernkopf, was the founding editor of a renowned atlas of human anatomy based on the paintings of subjects anatomized at his institute. The Pernkopf atlas is believed to include paintings of subjects who were victims of Nazi terror. Many of the original paintings included the Nazi symbols, swastikas and SS rune, in the signatures of three of the Pernkopf artists. Pernkopf's loyalty to the Nazi regime was rewarded after the *Anschluss* with his appointment as dean of medicine and subsequently rector of the University of Vienna.

The anatomist Professor Hermann Voss of the Reich's University of Posen exploited the killing programs to develop a nefarious trade in skeletal parts of executed Polish freedom fighters and Jews from a nearby concentration camp. Plaster death masks and busts were prepared from the bodies of the Jews and, together with the victim's skull, sold to the Vienna Museum of Natural History. The masks and skulls of the Jews were displayed in the museum's Race Gallery. In 1991 the masks and skulls of the Jews were turned over to the Vienna Jewish community, but in January 1998 the museum still housed the skulls of the Polish freedom fighters.

Professor Hermann Stieve is known to have used doomed women imprisoned at Ravensbrück concentration camp as subjects for his studies, including the effect of psychic stress (the woman's own impending execution) on menstruation and on the migration of sperm. In the latter case women were impregnated at specific times before their planned execution and their pelvic organs removed upon death to determine the migration of sperm. Stieve published and lectured on his research after the war.

Whereas virtually every medical school in Germany and Austria, and at least two in German-occupied Europe, Strasbourg and Posen, received the cadavers of victims of Nazi terror, only two universities, Tübingen and Vienna, have undertaken a formal investigation into the origins of their collections.

Only a few of the perpetrators of Nazi medical crimes were tried at NUREMBERG. Few of the doctors associated with the euthanasia-killing program were incarcerated for their crimes. Most were permitted to continue to practice with the protection of the Federal Chamber of Physicians (*Bundesärztekammer*). Most of the leaders of the German medical profession during the Hitler regime escaped any accounting for their role. Three of the post-war leaders of the *Bundesärztekammer* (Doctors Karl Haedenkamp, Ernst Fromm, and Hans Sewering) were former members of the SA or SS terror organizations. In 1992, Professor Sewering, who was linked with

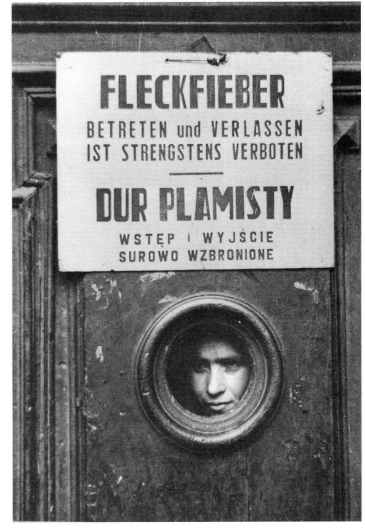

Jew quarantined in the Warsaw ghetto because of typhus in his apartment or building. (Reproduced from *The Warsaw Ghetto in photographs (1984)*, Dover Publications, NY.)

the 1943 killing of a child in the Nazi euthanasia program, was appointed president-elect of the World Medical Association, an international organization responsible for establishing ethical standards in medicine (although he did not serve in this capacity).

Many of the leading scientists associated with Nazi medical crimes continued their academic careers after the war. Mengele's mentor, Verschuer, became the professor of genetics at the University of Münster, where he was responsible for training many of the postwar leaders in genetics in Germany. Professor Stieve was appointed dean of medicine of Humbolt University and a lecture hall at the Berlin Charité Hospital was named in his honor. Hubertus Strughold is known as the father of the American aerospace medicine

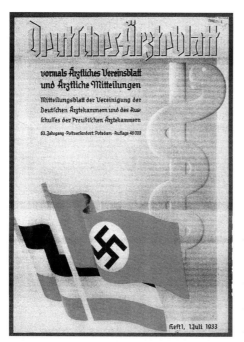

The cover of *Deutsches Ärzteblatt,* July 1933.
(Reproduced with permission from the *Deutsches Ärzteblatt*)

program and the official US Air Force building in San Antonio, Texas, bears his name. Professor Hermann Voss continued his anatomy career and was the co-author, together with his Posen colleague Robert Herrlinger, of a textbook of anatomy, *Taschenbuch der Anatomie,* considered a standard work in the subject. Imprisoned after the war, but never charged with an offence, Eduard Pernkopf was permitted to return to the University of Vienna to work on his anatomy atlas. Pernkopf's *Anatomy* continues to be published under the imprint of the original publisher, Urban and Schwarzenberg.

One war-crimes trial of great importance involved physicians, officially identified as United States of America vs. Karl Brandt *et al,* and usually referred to subsequently as *The Doctors' Trial.* There were twenty-three defendants, almost all German doctors or scientists. The first-named was Karl Brandt, formerly personal physician to Adolf Hitler. Ultimately, seven were convicted and sentenced to be hanged. These included Brandt, Karl Gebhardt (personal physician to Himmler), Joachim Mrugowsky (Chief of the Hygienic Institute of the Waffen SS), Rudolph Brandt (Personal Administrative Officer to Himmler), Wolfram Sievers (non-physician, director of the *Ahnenerbe* Society's Institute for Military Scientific Research), Viktor Brack (non-physician, Chief Administrative Officer in the Chancellory

of the Führer of the NSDAP), and Waldemar Hoven (chief doctor at Buchenwald concentration camp). Eight other defendants were found guilty and received prison sentences, while seven were acquitted.

During the nine-month trial a staggering accumulation of horrific evidence documented the medical atrocities carried out by these persons, evidence presented often by surviving victims. Many of these victims had been prisoners of the Nazis in concentration camps throughout occupied Europe. An unknown but high proportion of these men, women, and children were Jews; others Gypsies and nationals of numerous countries.

Some of the medical 'experiments' included studies of high altitude effects on the human body (Dachau), freezing, malaria, mustard gas (Sachsenhausen and Natzweiler), sulfanilamide (Ravensbrück), bone, muscle, and nerve regeneration (also Ravensbrück), epidemic jaundice, sterilization (Auschwitz and Ravensbrück), typhus (Buchenwald and Natzweiler), poisons, and the destructive human effects of incendiary bombs (Buchenwald).

The guilty verdicts were delivered for charges of murder and crimes against humanity. There was extensive discussion throughout the trial of ethical standards both broadly, in the German medical profession, and specifically in terms of the ethics of human experimentation. One consequence was the enunciation, by the panel of presiding judges on the Military Tribunal, of the NUREMBERG CODE, a 10-point exposition of principles that must hold for human experimentation to be ethically based. Based in natural law, this widely publicized Code has been central to discussions on the ethics of medical experimentation since that time.

Five decades after the Nuremberg Doctors' Trial, which saw the enunciation of the Nuremberg Code on human experimentation, neither the study of medical history during the Third Reich nor medical ethics have become part of the formal curriculum of German medical schools.   WES, CGR

*See also* BIOETHICS; EUGENICS; INFORMED CONSENT

**HOMEOPATHY** Homeopathy is the treatment of illness with very dilute medications derived from plant, animal, and mineral sources. It was founded by Samuel HAHNEMANN (p 391), who noted while translating an English herbal remedy into German that cinchona bark produced the symptoms of malaria, as well as being used to treat it. Hahnemann devised an experimental method that would yield information about individual substances by 'proving', a sort of testing that was applied to many remedies. Hahnemann assembled provers, who took various substances and recorded in great detail any symptoms. The idea was to match the patient's symptoms to a homeopathic drug picture, and give that drug in a very dilute, or 'potentized' form. Clinically this seemed to work and Hahnemann attracted an increasing number of doctors to his ideas, often because they were disenchanted with blood letting, then in vogue.

'Potentization' is believed to result from diluting and shaking the substance and producing a circular motion within the medicine. It is achieved by macerating a plant, such as cinchona (china), and dissolving it in alcohol. One part of this so-called 'mother tincture' is mixed with nine parts (for a 'decimal potency' or D) or 99 parts (for a 'centesimal potency' or C) in 90% alcohol, then shaken vigorously. This process is repeated many times, resulting in very high dilutions. Potencies of 24D or 12C and higher, according to Avogadro's hypothesis, are unlikely to contain even a single molecule of the mother tincture.

Homeopaths claim that the higher potencies (that is, the more dilute potencies) work more powerfully than the lower potencies. With the 'similimum', the name given to the principle of fitting the disease symptoms to the substance which produces similar symptoms, the unusual or uncommon symptoms, which frequently do not fit the condition as described by conventional medicine, are often considered as major pointers to the right remedy. Defining the 'similimum' requires the homeopath to take a detailed and prolonged history so that the drug pictures from the materia medica may be correctly matched to the patient. It often takes several consultations and indeed several remedies for homeopathy to have a long-lasting effect, particularly in chronic illness. Therefore homeopathy is a highly individualized treatment, resulting in different treatments for patients who would receive an identical treatment in conventional medicine.    GL

*See also* COMPLEMENTARY AND ALTERNATIVE MEDICINE.

**HOMOSEXUALITY** The sex instinct usually induces attraction and attachment of men to women. A small minority of people feel an affinity and strong desire for sexual relations with persons of the same sex (homosexuality) or indiscriminate desire for sexual relations with those of either sex (bisexuality).

Homosexuality is observed in some animal species, and is the preferred or only form of sexual activity for an estimated 5% of men and women in modern western society. Many words, mostly derogatory, have been used to allude to male homosexuals. Since the 1960s the most widely used has been gay, which originated in the affected group and is not a derogatory term. Female homosexuals are sometimes also called

gay, but are more commonly called lesbians. Studies of human sexual behavior, for example, those of Kinsey, suggested that as many as a third of all men and about a fifth to a quarter of all women have had at least one homosexual encounter. In single-sex communities where there are no other outlets for sexual behavior, such as prisons, ships on long ocean voyages, and boarding schools, erotic behavior with others of the same sex occurs more commonly than elsewhere.

Attitudes towards homosexuality have varied throughout history. In some cultures homosexual conduct has been accepted and openly practiced. In others it has been punishable by death or imprisonment and in many it has been regarded with disgust, or at a minimum, disdain. In modern western societies, homosexuality has begun to gain acceptance after many centuries in which it was regarded as anything from a capital crime to a form of psychosis. But community standards vary: gay men who are publicly identified still experience stigmatization, victimization, discrimination, or persecution in many places.

### Nature and cause
In a liberal society homosexuality is not regarded as a crime, a mortal sin, or a form of mental illness that requires aggressive psychiatric treatment. Homosexual intercourse (even when it is consensual) is, however, still a criminal offense in many jurisdictions. Homosexual men who have attempted to 'cure' their homosexuality by psychotherapy or by embracing fundamentalist born-again Christianity have a high rate of relapse. Homosexuality appears to be an innate form of behavior, though its precise nature and cause remain obscure. It has been suggested that it may be due to an autosomal recessive gene, though no such gene has been identified. Recent reports have suggested possible neurological anomalies in the configuration of cells in the base of the brain in some homosexual men.

Throughout history, a high proportion of creative and performing artists have been overt or covert homosexuals, sometimes with unhappy consequences, as the story of Oscar Wilde illustrates. At other times their sexual orientation has been accepted or tacitly ignored, as with Noël Coward and those contemporary artists and writers who are known to be homosexual. No hormonal differences between homosexuals and other men have been found.

Unable to cope with rejection by family and society, stigmatization, or their own feelings of guilt about their homoerotic urges, some homosexuals become depressed and suicide may be a tragic consequence. When a popular young man in his late teens or early adult life seemingly inexplicably kills himself, it is perhaps because he has realized that

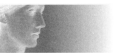

his sexual orientation is irrevocable, and the values of his family and peer group lead him to believe his impulses are so evil he does not deserve to live.

Male homoerotic behavior is usually expressed by mutual masturbation, penetrative anal intercourse, or oral-genital sexual stimulation. Some homosexual men seem to be extremely sexually active and highly promiscuous. When HIV/AIDS first appeared in North America and western Europe in the early 1980s, this combination led to a massive epidemic of AIDS among gay men.

The gay community in several large American and western European cities had begun to 'come out of the closet' in the liberal 1960s. It had organized into an identifiable entity and had become politically active in efforts to assert the rights of gay people to freedom from discrimination, access to employment benefits, and the like. When the HIV/AIDS epidemic struck San Francisco and early epidemiological studies provided some clues about its possible means of spread, the gay community there was able to develop rapidly an effective health education program for safer sexual practices that reduced the risks of transmission, albeit too late for many who had developed AIDS but nevertheless a useful demonstration of how such a sex education campaign should be conducted. The lessons from this have been applied in other American cities and in Scandinavia and Switzerland with some success.

Female homosexuals or lesbians have had a lower profile in most societies throughout history (and Queen Victoria, for instance, refused to believe in lesbianism). Their erotic behavior generally consists of mutual masturbation or oral-genital sexual contact. Lesbian activity has not been criminalized in the same way as male homosexuality and, probably because their sexual activity seldom involves exchange of body fluids, lesbians have been less vulnerable to HIV/AIDS and other SEXUALLY TRANSMITTED DISEASES. JML

**HOSPITALS** After 1500 most European hospitals continued to provide their traditional charitable services that included shelter, food, and spiritual salvation. However, a new ideology of health reflecting social and economic factors associated with the Renaissance expanded their role to encompass the physical recovery of their inmates. With patient populations increasingly composed of younger, unattached workers who sought institutional assistance for their ailments with the hope of returning to their previous occupations, urban hospitals in northern Italy began to function as institutions of first resort for those who became acutely ill. Tuscany, especially the Santa Maria Nuova Hospital in Florence, was at the forefront of this new development. With its 250 beds in the

early 1500s, the patient population consisted mainly of sick townspeople and travelers, especially pilgrims *en route* to Rome. Length of stay was usually brief and mortality low. Previously, barber-surgeons and university-educated physicians had been summoned occasionally as consultants to monastic infirmaries and shelters during medieval times, but their regular presence in the Florentine wards represented a significant shift towards a greater institutional role for medicine and surgery.

Another medicalizing institution was the contemporary 'pox house', first established in several south-west German cities for the care of men and women afflicted by a seemingly novel ailment referred to as '*morbus gallicus*' or French disease by Germans and Italians. The near-epidemic disease — presumably an acute and highly lethal form of venereal SYPHILIS — prompted municipal authorities, private philanthropists, and a new group of specialized physicians to open hospitals for the treatment of the scourge. In 1495, one of the biggest municipal hospitals for pox sufferers in early modern Germany was founded in the city of Augsburg with a capacity of 122 beds. In contrast to older leper- and pesthouses, many of the pox houses were located within the urban walls and featured a permanent medical staff, represented by physicians, barber-surgeons, apothecaries, and empirics responsible for the extensive treatment with mercury.

### Accelerating medicalization

The emergence of modern national states in Europe during the 17th century further accelerated the medicalization of European hospitals. New policies were aimed at increasing the population, necessary for gaining political and economic power as well as military strength. Indeed, European mercantilism considered labor as the key source of wealth, suggesting that productivity was closely linked to the health of citizens. Such considerations were combined with more optimistic notions promoted by Enlightenment thinkers regarding the preservation and rehabilitation of human health. Sickness could, indeed, be controlled, removed, and even prevented through changes in life-style and the employment of several herbal and chemical cures of considerable efficacy. In addition to their traditional efforts at moral redemption, hospitals at this time were also widely viewed as institutions for physical restoration, especially for members of the military and civil labor forces. Such agendas implied a radical reorganization of the hospital from an institution still largely devoted to saving souls to one mending bodies, from simply confining the very young and old suffering from chronic conditions to admitting selected adults afflicted with acute and treatable sickness.

This program, implemented during the 18th century in Europe by the state, local governments, voluntary associations, and corporate professional bodies, allowed the medical profession greater access to vast sectors of the population. Military and naval establishments, such as Britain's Royal Navy Hospital in Plymouth (1762), were among the early models for such care to the sick and wounded, followed by the creation of new institutions for civil use. The first voluntary hospital in Britain to open its doors was the Westminster Infirmary in London in 1720. It was soon followed by a spate of others: Guy's Hospital in London (1726), the Edinburgh Royal Infirmary (1729), London's St George's Hospital (1733), the Winchester Infirmary (1736), the Bristol Infirmary (1737), London Hospital (1740), and Middlesex Hospital, London (1745). All except Guy's resulted from the patronage of 'alliances against misery', composed of civic-minded business men, bankers, lawyers, and teachers, as well as physicians and surgeons.

The last quickly realized the hospital's potential for gaining further knowledge and improving their clinical skills. Most practitioners in private practice continued to be exposed to a series of discontinuous portraits of sickness displayed by those who summoned them for advice. Such fragmentary encounters made it difficult for physicians to assess their diagnostic and therapeutic success. At the same time, shifts in scientific ideology and method promoted the importance of empirical studies and the construction of medical learning based on observation. Hospitals were categorized as 'great nurseries' capable of breeding better healers. By the 1750s, surgeons, especially in France and Britain, had already created programs of institutional apprenticeship designed to promote their professional power and status. Physicians were also keen on studying hospital inmates at the bedside, making diagnoses, observing the evolution of their multiple diseases, and experimenting with new treatments. Although such activities can be traced back to the first wave of medicalization during the 16th century, a more systematic approach emerged at the University of Leiden a century later, leading to the creation of a special twelve-patient teaching ward at Leiden's Caecilia Gasthuis popularized by one of Europe's most famous 18th-century physicians, Herman BOERHAAVE (p 121). Clinical trials and eventually some elementary statistical analyses facilitated the evaluation of traditional remedies and prompted reforms of existing pharmacopoeias. Postmortem dissections performed on former patients provided additional pathological information that could be integrated with the clinical findings to yield clues about etiology and physiopathology.

## Education and research

Indeed, by the 1790s, selected European hospitals, including London's voluntary institutions and the Edinburgh Royal Infirmary in Britain, the ALLGEMEINES KRANKENHAUS in Vienna (p 352), and Paris's Hôtel-Dieu and Berlin's CHARITÉ HOSPITAL (p 354) began to function as sites for comprehensive programs of education and research linked to local universities or medical schools. Here hospital authorities funneled selected patients to special teaching wards, where professors and other attendants, followed by students, made daily rounds, examining and prescribing treatments. Although the learning was essentially passive at Edinburgh and London — students observed what their teachers demonstrated — Vienna and Paris began officially to include senior medical students in supervised diagnostic and therapeutic hands-on activities. Indeed, after the French Revolution, this partnership encouraged the creation of a competitive and hierarchical system of hospital internships meant to furnish postgraduate training. In controlled Parisian ward environments, substantial numbers of poor patients, alive and dead, were selected for systematic study, classification, and dissection. In this quest for medical knowledge and clinical experience, total immersion in hospital life was required. For several years, housestaff and students worked in shifts for long hours, a rite of passage surviving into our own days. France's hospital-based 'medicine of observation' became the main tool for professional medical advancement and improved social status in Europe and America.

## Institutional miasmas

With the hospital firmly established as a medical institution in the 19th century, this new house of recovery was quickly overrun by the sick poor. Overcrowding and lack of institutional hygiene led to deadly cross-infections and postoperative wound complications. A dreaded 'hospitalism' threatened to convert many establishments into 'death traps', shunned even by the sick poor as places of last resort. Administrators blamed a particular institutional miasma or vapor for the problem, a vitiated and dangerous air created by the exhalations of the sick bodies packed into the large wards. The poison seemed to adhere to walls and furnishings, prompting periodic whitewashings and fumigations. Wards were regularly ventilated, and even vacated, furnishings burned and buildings razed. Judging from military experiences, planners were told to build only temporary, disposable wooden structures or barracks. Reformers argued for smaller — 300 bed — cottage-size hospitals, ideally exposed to the prevailing winds for improved ventilation, and single beds for inmates. However, puerperal fever in lying-in institutions suggested that attending physicians also played an important part in the spread of infection. Better nursing practices designed to improve the patients' personal hygiene and ensure a ward's salubrity were also sought. After mid-century, a new design, the pavilion system, became a popular architectural weapon in the war against hospitalism, together with the construction of separate isolation and emergency facilities, surgical amphitheaters, morgues, and outpatient departments.

By the 1870s, new demands for hospitalization were spurred by European and American urbanization and industrialization. As hygienic principles came to dominate the construction and functioning of hospitals, patients once more began flocking to such institutions, attracted in part by the cleansed image rather than the successes of medicine and surgery in both diagnosis and treatment. The new nursing promoted by the Nightingales also promised a disciplined and professional system of care superior to that available in the domestic realm. Stripped of their traditional low status as cleaning women and servants, these informed and trained nurses became true physicians' assistants.

The availability of surgical ANESTHESIA and antisepsis in hospitals progressively enlarged the spectrum of operations to be carried out and promised more recoveries and cures. By the close of the century, therefore, most hospitals were no longer viewed as 'gateways to death' but institutions of first resort operating according to scientific principles. Better organized and cleansed of their deadly miasma, hospitals no longer just catered to the sick poor but now started attracting the growing middle class.

In Europe, but especially in Britain, national governments and municipal authorities became increasingly involved in sponsoring and managing hospitals as part of new responsibilities for unprotected working citizens. Seeking better economic opportunities in a rapidly industrializing society, young people flocked to the cities, where they often lived by themselves, deprived of family or community networks. Upon falling ill, the hospital and its outpatient facilities became their first and often only choice. To prevent a resurgence of institutional contagion, the Public Health Act of 1875 encouraged British municipalities to establish separate isolation hospitals for those suffering from infectious diseases. Moreover, the Poor Law Infirmaries were gradually taken over by local health departments and converted into general hospitals. By 1911, the National Health Insurance Act had eliminated the charitable status of the voluntary British hospitals, placing such institutions within centralized, regional healthcare systems. Public institutions,

however, still tainted by their earlier charitable stigma, were often shunned by well-to-do patients, who sought smaller, privately owned 'clinics' or hospitals for their care.

In the United States, cultural diversity, free enterprise, and bountiful economic resources shaped the hospital's mission from the early 20th century onwards. Religious rivalries and charitable impulses still played an important albeit diminishing part, with private sectarian institutions retaining the notion that the hospital symbolized hope and pious benevolence based on the Scriptures. However, the traditional welfare role was declining as economic, social, and medical considerations gained new importance. Waves of new immigrants created a transient and uprooted population. With their arrival, many religious, ethnic, and national communities sought to protect the new members and provide them with adequate means of care in the event of illness. With Enlightenment ideals about the positive value of health among workers persisting, keeping jobs and productivity frequently required medical intervention, including hospital admission. Thus, a virtual explosion of new voluntary hospital foundations between 1890 and 1920 occurred throughout the land, from ethnic neighborhoods in large urban centers to fledgling suburbs and smaller rural hamlets. Private philanthropy, religious congregations, and industry, with encouragement — at times support — from local governments and universities were instrumental in raising the necessary funds.

## A vast system

Most establishments started as small houses sponsored by networks of prominent and influential citizens. Sectarian Jewish, Catholic, Methodist, Lutheran, and Presbyterian institutions flourished side by side with German and French-speaking ones. By the 1920s, together with private railroad and university establishments and public municipal or state institutions, US hospitals had formed a vast and decentralized system of autonomous corporations spread out across the American landscape, each independently competing for resources and narrowly focused to serve particular constituencies and communities. This phenomenon reflected the nation's democratic ideals, its *laissez-faire* capitalist economy, and a culture based on localism and voluntarism to solve problems. In a most powerful way, US hospitals came to symbolize 'Main Street': community power and pride, and the ability to care for all sectors of the population.

As hospitals shifted their services, earlier charitable and confinement roles were delegated to homeless shelters and soup kitchens, churches and convents, isolation facilities and jails, retirement villages, nursing homes, and hospices. After 1900, upper- and middle-class patients in Europe and America increasingly sought medical care in hospitals, especially for a series of acute medical and surgical conditions. Human experiences such as birth, childhood illnesses, old age, and death also became hospital-bound. Trauma accounted for two-thirds of all surgical admissions. America's growing beliefs in the power and progressivism of science heightened expectations concerning the usefulness of hospitals in making precise diagnoses, reversing disease, and effecting cures. Thus, patients were often hospitalized at early stages in their illness or simply for diagnosis. Hospital-based radiology, electrocardiography, and laboratory tests could reveal the causes of many conditions. Bacteriological studies linked infectious diseases to specific micro-organisms. For treatment, a new generation of chemotherapeutic agents — including Salvarsan for the treatment of syphilis and life-saving sera such as diphtheria antitoxin — improved the odds of success in the battle against specific germs. Fueled by the promise of surgical triumphs based on aseptic methods, new attempts to penetrate bodily cavities such as the chest and abdomen began. Appendectomies, removal of tonsils and adenoids, and later cesarean sections constituted a sizable proportion of hospital admissions well into the 1930s.

New construction methods, greater efficiency, and medical criteria forced significant structural changes on 20th century hospitals. In most urban settings, space had become scarce, suggesting compact, multistoried buildings instead of pavilion-type establishments. The beneficial flow of fresh air could be achieved by mechanical means through central ventilation, heating, and cooling devices, and the new chemical disinfectants kept germs at bay, preventing institutional crossinfections. Vertically expanding to six or more floors, the typical new hospitals placed their kitchens, housekeeping, and storage facilities in basements, while the first floor was reserved for administration, outpatient facilities, and laboratories. In an ascending order, subsequent floors were divided into medical, pediatric, surgical, and obstetric wards. Paying patients demanded private and semi-private rooms, often appealingly furnished to function as home substitutes.

After the Second World War, hospitals consolidated their position as flagships of scientific medicine, and were besieged by a steady demand for more beds and services. Increased specialization and advanced medical technology led the way. Lacking funds, many hospitals in Europe simply retained their antiquated and cramped facilities, monitored by regional or central government agencies that exercised control over location,

finances, and supply of beds. In Britain, implementation of the National Health Service Act of 1946 placed all hospitals under government ownership. Their medical staffs remained closed and decentralized, organized within autonomous divisions. In the USA, a spectacular construction boom added new wings, floors, and buildings to existing facilities and created new ones, all with the help of federal government grants under the Hill-Burton Act of 1946. Generous reimbursement schemes for services from private health insurance schemes and eventually the federally sponsored Medicare and Medicaid programs in the 1960s not only preserved the vast hospital system, but allowed it to expand greatly with steady and generous infusions of capital. Individual voluntary hospitals retained their previous autonomy and medical staffs and remained independent.

## Shift of care

While today hospitals still command the center of medicine's most critical and advanced interventions, the bulk of healthcare delivery is shifting to clinics and patients' homes. Throughout the world, decades of ever-mounting costs of hospitalization have created financial problems in the 1990s for private insurers and governments. Shifts to primary care, health promotion, and disease prevention now often bypass hospitals altogether. Demographics, epidemiology, and current economic conditions are partially to blame for recent attempts to ration hospital care. Aging societies in the developed world are more susceptible to chronic health conditions, best assessed and therapeutically managed in ambulatory settings. When older patients sustain sudden breakdowns of multiple organ systems, the ethics of aggressive and expensive hospital care to prevent dying are increasingly being questioned. Moreover, new and less invasive diagnostic and therapeutic technologies can also be performed without hospitalization. Because of high costs, today's hospitals are becoming intensive care facilities providing acute and highly technical forms of care from the beginnings of life — neonatal nurseries— to complex surgical procedures — emergency trauma and organ transplantation — to medical crises — coronary and intensive care units.

Not surprisingly, the vast network of independent voluntary hospitals in the USA is currently under siege. Restrictive reimbursement schemes instituted by the federal government and private insurers, as well as inefficient, bureaucratized institutions left with low occupancy rates have created this crisis. Smaller community hospitals are closing or merging at a fast rate, while those remaining are purchased by national or regional healthcare corporations, becoming components

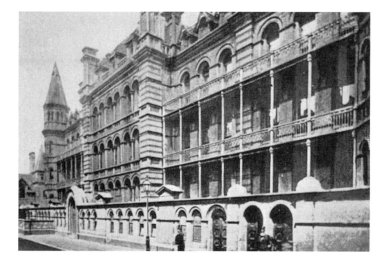

Early view (1850s) of the Hospital for Sick Children, Great Ormond Street, London. (Reproduced courtesy of the Great Ormond Street Hospital.)

of large chains which deliver services for profit. Larger facilities, including academic medical centers, are also merging. This massive restructuring of the American hospital industry has created new and vast markets for capital and has placed hospitals in direct competition with other caregiving institutions, including independent surgical or emergency centers, free-standing diagnostic centers, multispecialty physician practices, and palliative hospices.

At the beginning of a new millennium, hospitals around the world are once more at crossroads. Their ownership, organization, and finances are increasingly subjected to the unfettered forces of a private, largely corporate marketplace with the hope that the new revolution in management will streamline, even ration services and thus save them from extinction. Modern business values and consumerism contribute to these reforms. Although particularly jarring to a decentralized hospital system, such as that in the USA, where hospitals are being transformed into engines of financial gain, this development will also affect other countries with centralized and state-sponsored institutions. The danger is that such business decisions together with the short-term and intensive technological interventions will jeopardize the traditional humanitarianism inherent in hospital care that addresses the emotional and spiritual aspects of illness. Hospitals emerged as communal homes to shelter the needy. As monuments to human empathy and benevolence, they must endure. GBR

*See also* BRITAIN; DISPENSARIES; FRANCE; HEALTHCARE SYSTEMS; MANAGED CARE; USA

**HUMAN EXPERIMENTATION** See BEECHER; CHILDREN – EXPERIMENTATION ON; HELSINKI DECLARATION; HOLOCAUST; INFORMED CONSENT; PAPPWORTH; TUSKEGEE SYPHILIS STUDY

**HUMAN GENOME PROJECT** The first draft of the completed sequence of the human genome marked the beginning of the 21st century, promising to be another landmark in the history of the biomedical sciences. Thus, it took less than a half century between the elucidation of the double helical structure of DNA in 1953 by Watson and Crick, and the sequencing of the entire human genome contained in 23 paired chromosomes, simultaneously by a publicly funded consortium, The Human Genome Organization (HUGO), and the private biotechnology company, Celera Genomics. The biomedical revolution of the 20th century had its genesis in the expansion of knowledge about genetics and the molecules of heredity, DNA and RNA, coupled with an emerging biotechnology, enabling dissection and manipulation of these molecules. The biotechnological advances of the past 30 years have allowed a fantasy of 40 years ago to become a realistic voyage of discovery – namely, the foundation and implementation of the Human Genome Project. This project, initially co-sponsored by the Department of Energy and the National Institutes of Health in the US, began in 1990 (with James Watson, the co-discoverer with Francis Crick of the structure of DNA, as maestro) and a preliminary draft of the human genome was completed early in 2001 and published in back to back issues in February 2001 of the journals, *Science* (**291**:1145–1434, 2001; The Human Genome) and *Nature* (**409**:745–964, 2001: The Human Genome).

In 1993, Francis Collins, a medical geneticist and gene hunter from the University of Michigan, became the Director of the NIH National Institute for Genome Research. At its inception, there was great disagreement within the scientific community as to the value of the Human Genome Project. Many scientists believed the undertaking worthwhile and that much useful knowledge would accrue; others thought that the Human Genome Project would be akin only to stamp collecting and would waste precious resources, both in terms of money and of time. Since then, the Human Genome Project has become worldwide in scope, with efforts by scientists in Britain, France, Italy, Germany, and Japan coordinated through the international body, HUGO. In addition, biotechnology corporations – in particular, Celera Genomics, led by scientist, J. Craig Venter – are competing with the academic and governmental scientific communities in the quest to complete the program. At times, this competitive interaction has become fierce and has led to public acrimony between scientists of the corporate and academic worlds. However, as of late 2000, both the public and private funded initiatives had completed drafts of the human genome which complement one another.

The Human Genome Project's aim is to determine both the location of every gene on each of the 23 pairs of human chromosomes and the precise coding sequences for every gene. Completion of this undertaking will supply a genetic dictionary of inestimable value in understanding the genetic contribution to health and disease.

Each cell, be it human, mouse, fruit fly, worm, or microbe, has a set of chromosomes containing the genetic material, in most cases, DNA (in some viruses one can also find viral RNA, which serves the function of DNA). The DNA contains a double-stranded linear array of subunits, called bases, housed internally within the DNA, which pair with one another to form a structure resembling rungs on a ladder. There are four types of bases contained in nucleotides, adenine (A), guanine (G), cytosine (C), and thymine (T), whose chemical interactions are such that A always pairs with T and G with C. Thus, a linear description of one strand (e.g., ATCG) will define its complementary strand (TAGC). The technology allowing determination of nucleic acid sequences led to a second Nobel Prize for Fred Sanger (UK) and a Nobel Prize for Walter Gilbert (US), who won it jointly in 1980. Genes are discrete sequences of nucleotides that supply the code initially 'transcribed' into a transient RNA, which in turn supplies the information to code for and synthesize proteins ('translation').

Estimates had suggested that the human genome, found in every non-reproductive cell, contains about 3 billion base pairs, coding for about 100 000 genes. An unexpected finding arising from the 'apparent completed human genome data' is that *Homo sapiens* contain about 30 000 genes (a much smaller number of genes than the expected 100 000) contrasted with the worm *C. elegans* (19 099), the fruit fly *Drosophilia melanogaster* (13 061), and the virus, *H. influenzae* (1 740). As of the year 2000, it appears that mouse and human may differ in as little as 300 unique genes. In higher organisms, unlike bacteria and viruses, most of the DNA is non-functional in that it does not code for a gene-product. The function of this 'junk' DNA, corresponding to as much as 85–90% of the total DNA, is not known and is the subject of much speculation.

The major aim of the Human Genome Project, to map the entire genome, requires determining the location and sequences of all the genes on each chromosome. Two types of genetic maps are being constructed: a functional genetic linkage map and a physical map. The genetic linkage map depends upon genetic characteristics and describes the relative location of genes as a function of how frequently they are co-inherited. The closer together two genes are, the greater the chances they will be

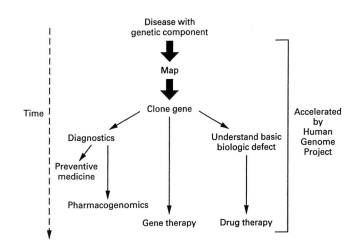

co-inherited. The physical map locates genes relative to actual determined sequences which act as 'landmarks' along the chromosomes. The overall plan involved separating chromosomes and generating both linage and physical maps at lower levels of resolution, which led to maps of greater magnitude of resolution for ultimate deciphering of an entire chromosome. A major challenge to the completion of the project was increasing the automation of sequencing, thereby increasing the rate of sequencing coupled with a decrease in cost for sequencing each base pair. Innovative design and construction of automated equipment and robots by the biotechnology industry made this possible.

## Surprises

The completed human genome revealed a number of surprises: the number of human genes (ca. 30 000) is much lower than expected and does not easily explain the increased biological sophistication of the human being compared with the mouse, the fruit fly, or the worm. The differences between man, primate, and mouse genomes are trivial, suggesting that additional mechanisms that are not solely a function of numbers of genes are necessary to account for the complexity of human beings. The density of genes per chromosome is not uniform, but differs from one chromosome to another. Although we still do not know the function of overwhelming amount of 'non gene-associated DNA', sequence analysis suggests that new gene regulatory mechanisms may lie in these sequences. There is agreement that the first drafts of the human genome have just scratched the surface of our understanding and that the newly spawned disciplines of bioinformatics, genomics, and proteomics will integrate and advance this information such that over the next century we will obtain a detailed understanding of the mechanisms which account for human physiology (the

Steps involved in the genetic revolution in medicine. Uncovering the genetic contributions to an illness is accomplished by cloning the gene for the disease, with the use of the tools of the Human Genome Project. Once the contributing genes and their disease-predisposing variants have been identified, diagnostic tests can be developed to predict future risk — but these tests are most effective when a preventive strategy is available to reduce the risk in persons found to be predisposed to a particular disease. Another rapidly developing application of diagnostics is pharmacogenomics, the prediction of responsiveness to drugs. Ultimately, the real pay-off of genetic research will be the development of new gene therapies and drug therapies, but they will generally require many more years of intensive research. (From *The New England Journal of Medicine* (1999), **341**.)

physiome) and pathophysiology. In contrast to 1990, therefore, few now would doubt the wisdom in undertaking the human genome project.

Completion of the Human Genome Project promises a bounty of riches, particularly in the advance of medicine and the treatment of disease and its prevention. However, as is often common in the path of science (e.g., atomic energy), equally possible is the opening of a Pandora's box, yielding improper use of genetic information. Unique to the design and implementation of the Human Genome Project is that as scientific advances are being made, a great effort fueled by dedicated resources, is simultaneously being carried out to study the ethical, legal, and social implications of human genome research.

Notwithstanding the difficulties of dealing with the implications of being able to read what Sir Walter Bodmer has called 'The Book of Man' (e.g., confidentiality of genetic testing results, the use of genetic information by both the individual and society), it is likely that completion of the human Genome Project and its use will un-alterably change paradigms of medicine. A major paradigm of 20th century medicine was that we are all well until we get sick. In large measure, the role of the physician was to treat sickness. Given a knowledge of one's specific genome and that no individual will be spared some 'bad' genes or genetically documentable risk factors, we are all latently sick. This concept promises to lead to a paradigm shift such that the role of the physician will be to prevent the 'bad' genes from being expressed, a new form of preventive medicine. Thus, as a function of the completion of the Human Genome Project, the 21st century may well become the 'age of preventive medicine'. DAC

*See also* GENETICS; GENE THERAPY

**HUMORS** Humors in medieval times the humors were four fluids supposedly secreted in the body and responsible for a person's character: these were blood, phlegm, choler (yellow bile), and melancholy (black bile). When blood was in preponderance, a man was sanguine or cheerful; phlegm, phlegmatic or calm; choler, choleric or quick-tempered; melancholy, melancholic.

**HUMAN IMMUNODEFICIENCY VIRUS (HIV)**
See AIDS

**HUNGER STRIKE** Wilful self-starvation by prolonged refusal of all food, usually by a prisoner hoping to gain release or as a protest against the conditions of his imprisonment; occasionally by others as a form of protest, generally political.

'Hunger strike' is something of a misnomer, since in total starvation the sensation of hunger disappears after a day or two. Duration of survival

in people totally deprived of food is variable; the average is about four weeks, at which time body weight has been reduced by about half. Impending death is signaled by a marked drop in body temperature. Longer survival times are possible; for example, Terrence MacSwinney, Lord Mayor of Cork, who was arrested in 1920 during the Irish Troubles, fasted for 74 days before dying in coma.

John **HUNTER** (1728–93). British surgeon member of the Surgeons' Corporation (1767). John Hunter was born in Long Calderwood, Lanarkshire. He had little formal schooling and in 1745 moved to Glasgow to lodge with his sister, from whose husband, a cabinet-maker, he acquired considerable mechanical skill. In 1748 he joined his brother William in London, assisting him in his dissections. He showed so much ability that he went to study under Cheselden at the Chelsea Hospital and Pott at St Bartholomew's. He became a master of anatomy in 1753, helping his brother with lectures and carrying out research.

In 1760 he was appointed staff-surgeon to the expedition to Belle Isle, where he studied coagulation of the blood. After serving with the army in Portugal, he returned to London on half-pay in 1763 and started to practice and lecture in Golden Square. Much of his time was spent in the dissection of animals. In 1764 he bought two acres in Earls Court and built a house with facilities for research and keeping animals. In 1767 he was appointed surgeon to St George's Hospital.

In 1771 he married Anne Home and two years later started his lectures on the theory and practice or surgery, the first attempt to give surgery a scientific basis. He was appointed surgeon-extraordinary to George III in 1776. In 1780 he fell out with his brother, who accused him of claiming as his own some observations he had made. He moved from Jermyn Street, where he had been living for some years to Leicester Square in 1788 and continued his researches on experimental pathology.

Appointed deputy surgeon-general to the army in 1786, he was promoted surgeon-general and inspector-general of hospitals four years later. By this time he was recognized as the leading surgeon in London, but as long before as 1773 he had begun to suffer from angina pectoris, which slowly became more troublesome over the years. In 1793 he died suddenly during a wrangle over the allocation of students' fees while attending a meeting at St George's Hospital.

Hunter has been called the father of scientific surgery. He was an indefatigable worker, a brilliant investigator, and an original and stimulating thinker. He was, however, impatient, blunt, and unpolished. His lack of formal education made him a poor lecturer and a worse author. He read little and thus his research depended on his own original observations. He collected a vast range of specimens to illustrate health and disease in man and animals. These form the basis of his museum, which was accepted in 1800 by the Company of Surgeons (now the Royal College of Surgeons of England) with a subvention from the government. Much was lost in an air raid in 1941. Sir Edward HOME (p 719), his executor and brother-in-law, destroyed all Hunter's notebooks and manuscripts in 1823, having published as his own many of the observations recorded in them.

Hunter's publication were numerous. The best-known are: *Natural history of the human teeth* (1771) and *On venereal disease* (1786), in which he claimed, on the strength of self-inoculation, that syphilis and gonorrhea were the same disease: *Observations on certain parts of the animal oeconomy* (1786): *Treatise on the blood, inflammation and gun-shot wounds* (1794, published posthumously and seen through the press by Home)

**HYPERTENSION** is the term that describes a rise of the blood pressure in the arterial circulation. It is a modern disease in the sense that until the invention of the sphygmomanometer by Riva Rocci in 1896 doctors had no way of diagnosing it. During the century that followed, hypertension became the subject of intense study and many great advances were made. It is now known that hypertension is a major cause of stroke, heart failure, renal insufficiency, and accelerated atherosclerosis (narrowing of the arteries by ATHEROMA); that its course can be explosive ('malignant') or more indolent and chronic ('benign'); and that the damage to blood vessels can be assessed during life by examining the fundus of the eye with an ophthalmoscope. In most people the cause of hypertension is not known (so-called 'essential' or primary hypertension), but in about 5% of cases hypertension is secondary to diseases of the kidneys or of the adrenal glands; to narrowing of the renal arteries; to pregnancy; or to drugs such as contraceptives, amphetamine, or cocaine.

Many factors play a part in the causation of hypertension. The output of the heart is sometimes increased, especially early on and in the young. Later, constriction of the peripheral blood vessels (vasoconstriction) is likely to become the dominant feature. Salt plays an important but poorly understood part, and certain groups, particularly Afro-Americans and black Africans, the elderly, and diabetics, may show intense salt sensitivity. Hormones released from the adrenal glands (vasoconstrictor catecholamines and adrenergic sympathetic nervous fibers) play a part, and so does renin, an enzyme secreted by the kidneys that helps to control the synthesis of chemical substances called angiotensin peptides, and thus indirectly causes arterial vasoconstriction and secretion of the adrenal salt retaining hormone, aldosterone. Also involved in hypertension are hormones (produced in the heart and central nervous system) that cause retention of salt by the body, vasoconstrictors such as endothelin, and vasodilators such as prostaglandins, bradykinin, and nitric oxide, whose release or function may be inhibited.

About 5 to 25% of people are classified as hypertensive, depending on what arbitrary level of blood pressure is regarded as abnormal, because blood pressure readings in the general population have a Gaussian distribution. In the United States the desired or optimal cut-off point is now considered to be 120/80 mm Hg. Readings above 130/85 are regarded as 'high normal' and above 140/90 as hypertension. These definitions, based on both systolic and diastolic pressures and not necessarily accepted by experts in other countries, are based on studies showing that blood pressures lower than 120/80 are associated with the least amount of organ damage such as stroke, heart failure, and renal insufficiency. As a result of the massive education, screening, and treatment programs of the past three decades, the incidence of such complications has appreciably decreased. Yet many patients are still unaware of even having high blood pressure, are not receiving treatment, or are not having their blood pressure reduced optimally, so that hypertension remains a common cause of premature illness and death.

As late as 1945 no effective treatment for high blood pressure was available. This is illustrated by the now well-known case history of president Franklin D. Roosevelt, who died in the closing days of World War Two from a brain hemorrhage resulting from untreatable accelerated hypertension. Treatment first became available in the 1950s, with the introduction of the ganglion blocking agents for severe hypertension, succeeded by generations of ever more effective and better tolerated antihypertensive drugs. Yet by 1965 many prominent experts still believed that hypertension represented a 'vascular frailty' that could not be remedied and might even be worsened by lowering blood pressure. It required a whole series of clinical trials conducted between the late 1960s and the 1980s, first on the most severe and later on the mildest forms of hypertension, in young people and in the very old, to show convincingly that treatment at every stage of hypertension could prevent complications and increase life expectancy.

### Effective treatment

In the modern treatment of hypertension it is important that the blood pressure be taken accurately, with the patient relaxed, and that in moderate cases readings should be repeated on several visits before starting treatment. In some

**PIONEERS OF THE SPHYGMOMANOMETER**

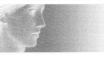

Nikolai Sergeivich **KOROTKOFF** (1874–1920). Russian physician. Korotkoff, a neglected figure in medical history, reported the technique of blood pressure measurement (Korotkoff sounds) in 1905 in less than a page of the *Reports of the Imperial Military Medical Academy* of St Petersburg. After working as a surgeon during the First World War and welcoming the October Revolution, he ended his days as physician-in-chief of the Metchnikoff Hospital in Leningrad. His wife, a RED CROSS nurse who had accompanied him to Manchuria during the Russo-Japanese war of 1904–5, died 21 years later in the Siege of Leningrad in 1941.

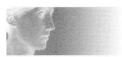

Frederick Henry Horatio Akbar **MAHOMED** (1949–84). English physician. Mahomed was the grandson of the 'shampoo surgeon' to George IV, and son of a proprietor of Turkish baths at Brighton; he qualified in medicine at Guy's Hospital, and modified the sphygmograph to enable arterial blood pressure to be measured. This allowed him to explain the association, noted by Richard BRIGHT (p 522), between contracted kidneys and enlargement of the heart — the connecting link being raised blood pressure. Mahomed entered with notable enthusiasm into the affairs both of his hospital and of the Royal College of Physicians of London; and his death from typhoid fever prevented his giving the Bradshaw Lecture, to which he had been appointed.

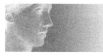

**Jean Martin CHARCOT**
(1825–93). French
neurologist. After a brilliant
career at the Hôpital de la
Pitié, he joined the staff of
the Salpêtrière. Here he
created the greatest
neurological clinic of the day:
he attracted a group of pupils
destined to become leaders in
this specialty; and he set
about the classification of
diseases of the nervous
system. He also described the
Charcot–Leyden crystals of
asthmatic sputum (1853); the
'lightning pains' of tabes
dorsalis (1866); the scanning
speech, the intention tremor,
and nystagmus of multiple
sclerosis (Charcot's triad,
1866); neuropathic
arthropathy (Charcot's joints,
1868); the recurrent fever of
obstructive cholangitis
(Charcot's intermittent
hepatic fever, 1877); and
familial peroneal muscular
atrophy (Charcot–Marie–
Tooth's syndrome, 1886).
Charcot made use of
hypnosis in treating hysterics.
He left a record of his
observations in *Leçons sur les
maladies du système nerveux
faites à la Salpêtrière* (5 vols,
1872–87). He was a
considerable authority on art
as well as being an
accomplished painter himself.

patients the blood pressure recorded in a doctor's office may be atypically high, so-called white-coat hypertension, because of anxiety associated with the encounter. More prolonged observation or home blood pressure monitoring by the patients themselves may be indicated. Proper diet, reduction of obesity, stopping smoking, and regular exercise are the life-style modifications recommended as the initial intervention in mild cases and adjuncts to pharmacological treatment in the more severe cases. Diuretic drugs, which eliminate excess sodium from the body, and beta-blockers, which act predominantly on the heart, are the first line drugs recommended for most patients. Other drugs used are those that dilate blood vessels, either by a direct effect such as calcium channel blockers, or by blocking the sympathetic nervous system (which controls their caliber). Another category of agents, the angiotensin-converting enzyme inhibitors and direct angiotensin-receptor blocking agents, are also widely used and well tolerated. They are especially effective when salt retention and sensitivity are not marked, and specifically useful in treating heart failure, reducing enlargement of the left ventricle of the heart, and slowing the progression of certain renal diseases. Only for a small minority of patients is surgery required, mainly for repair of narrowing of the renal artery, when the obstruction cannot be overcome by inserting a balloon and inflating it, or when this procedure has failed. Future progress resides in better antihypertensive drugs, a greater understanding of the mechanisms causing hypertension, and eventually finding a definitive cure.                                             GD

**HYPNOTISM** The term *neurohypnotism*, or nervous sleep, was coined by James Braid to describe the state, akin to a mesmeric trance, which could be induced by prolonged staring at an object while maintaining a fixation of the attention. (The prefix *neuro* was soon dropped leaving the familiar term *hypnotism*. This word is now more usually applied to the whole topic, whereas *hypnosis* is preferred to describe the state of being hypnotized.) Braid believed that he had found the physiological basis for MESMERISM without the hocus-pocus surrounding that movement. His initial theory was that the paralysis of the eye muscles consequent upon fixed staring led to a peculiar state of the nervous system; further experiments led him to modify the theory and to place more emphasis on mental concentration. Braid completely rejected the concept of a mesmeric fluid, or indeed any other power originating in the operator. One could hypnotize oneself by following his technique; the role of the operator was merely to act as a source of therapeutic suggestion, which was typically much

more effective when the patient was hypnotized than when in the ordinary waking state.

Braid's work greatly influenced the neurologist, Jean-Martin CHARCOT (this page), who introduced hypnotism into the Salpêtrière Hospital in Paris, where he was physician-superintendent. Charcot came too readily to the erroneous conclusion that only hysterical patients could be hypnotized. On the basis of experiments with no more than a dozen hysterical women Charcot attempted to establish the existence of several stages of the hypnotic process brought about by particular physical stimuli.

In Charcot's clinic, hypnotic induction usually began with the visual fixation of a bright light, which produced a state of *catalepsy* marked by rigidity of the limbs; closing the patient's eyes changed this state to one of *lethargy*, with relaxation of the limbs; subsequent pressure on the top of the patient's head normally transformed this second state to that of *somnambulism*, in which the patient would, for the first time since the induction procedure began, become aware of communications from the hypnotist, to which the response would be automatic.

Charcot's clinical reputation and exceptionally dramatic teaching and demonstrating technique led to widespread acceptance of his work, which accorded respectability to hypnotism as a reputable medical procedure. In his demonstrations he was able to mimic, for example, the paralyses and losses of sensation found in traumatized hysterical patients by giving the appropriate suggestions to hypnotized subjects in the somnambulistic state. Thus he believed that he had established an affinity between HYSTERIA and hypnosis, the latter being an experimentally-induced hysteria. Sigmund FREUD (p 321), who attended the Salpêtrière Hospital during this period, described Charcot's work as 'an incomparably fine piece of clinical research'.

However, Charcot's conception of hypnotism soon came under attack from Hippolyte Bernheim, professor of medicine at the University of Nancy. Bernheim had first observed hypnotic induction procedures practiced by Auguste Liébault, a country doctor who treated a wide variety of disorders with simple suggestion. Liébault's technique probably owed as much to the later generation of mesmerists as it did to Braid: he would require his patient to stare into his eyes while repeating emphatically that the patient would go to sleep. Irrespective of the result of this procedure, suggestions were now given to the effect that symptoms would be ameliorated and that the patient would be restored to health. Liébault's success rate was impressive and led to Bernheim's adoption of a similar method in treatment and research.

Among his discoveries, Bernheim found no evidence for the three stages of hypnosis, nor did patients respond to the physical stimuli supposed by Charcot to bring about these stages unless a suggestion to that effect had been implied in one form or another. Charcot had been mistaken in believing that patients were at any time oblivious to their surroundings. Furthermore, hysterical patients were not especially susceptible to hypnosis, most people were more or less hypnotizable, and it was possible to grade the depth of the hypnotic state in terms of the complexity of the suggestions to which they would respond. For the efficacy of therapeutic suggestions, it mattered little where one fell on that continuum; indeed, even in the waking state, many of the phenomena thought to be peculiar to hypnosis could be obtained.

### French controversies

The controversy between the schools of Paris and Nancy was finally resolved with what might be called the triumph of suggestion: it became clear that when people were hypnotized they became very responsive to suggestions emanating from the hypnotist, and their own expectations of what was required of them became crucial. Charcot's research had been riddled with explicit and implicit suggestions. Before he could revise his views, Charcot died; with the loss of its leader, the life also went out of the Paris School, and Bernheim's view prevailed.

At the turn of the century hypnotism became dormant. The reasons for this lack of interest lay partly with the disappointment felt by many physicians that Charcot's work had been discredited. He had, after all, sought a scientific explanation for hypnosis, conceived as a series of states brought about by discrete physical stimuli. The alternative seemed to be the nebulous concept of suggestion, an ill-defined abstraction, which had little appeal. Also, Freud, who had been using hypnotism on the Bernheim model, had by now come to reject it and to adopt the slower, more revealing technique of free association. Succeeding psychoanalysts followed his lead and were rarely to employ hypnotism.

A first revival of interest occurred during the 1914–18 war, when hypnotism was seen as a possible treatment for 'shell-shock' and other consequences of BATTLE NEUROSIS. However, the interest did not last long, as the hypnotic re-living of traumatic events did not seem to have any widespread applicability to the neuroses of the general population. PSYCHOANALYSIS and its derivatives remained the treatments of choice for those who could afford them.

The second revival in hypnotherapy occurred during the Second World War, and has been sustained ever since. Although it again began with the treatment of war casualties, it developed as a series of treatments that could be used with a wide range of disorders in the civilian population.

Tissié hypnotizes his subject Albert in the presence of Dr Azam. From Laurent-Gsell in *Poveau de courmelles, l 'hypnotisme* (c. 1887). (Reproduced courtesy of the Mary Evans Picture Library.)

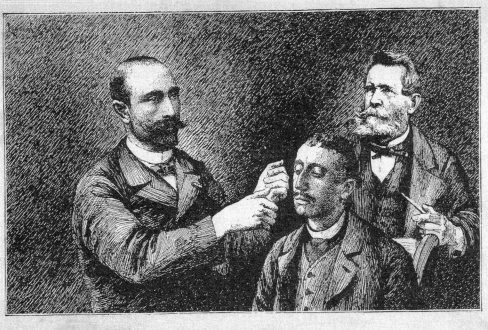

Le Dʳ Ph. Tissié hypnotisant Albert devant le professeur Azam.

These treatments included varieties of relaxation methods, such as autogenic training, the use of guided imagery, and desensitization techniques developed by the behavior therapists.

A list of ailments that are reported to have been cured by hypnotism would be too long to include here. Well-designed studies with control groups are unfortunately not plentiful, and it is impossible to make any very definite statements about the therapeutic efficacy of hypnotism. In general, it seems that the psychosomatic disorders may respond well to hypnotic treatment, a fact which accords with modern understanding of neuro-endocrine and immune system functioning. Psychological influences on what have been generally regarded in the past as purely physical problems are increasingly being demonstrated, and it is no longer surprising when hypnotic intervention leads, for example, to more rapid healing of wounds and burns. Various hypnotic strategies have been adopted to alleviate pain, and research has shown that these can be very effective and are not simply the result of a PLACEBO effect. With conditions such as anxiety neuroses and phobia, there is a good success rate from hypnotic treatment. However, when it comes to changing undesirable habits, such as heavy smoking and drinking, success rates are more modest, and it is clear that extrahypnotic factors, such as the person's motivation, are important in obtaining success with these types of self-inflicted behavior.

The peculiar applicability of hypnotic treatment in cases of multiple personalities disorder has been recognized since the late 19th century. Under hypnosis it is sometimes possible to bring about a fusion of the different personalities or a predominance of one. Sensitive therapeutic management is needed, as it is all too easy to encourage the emergence of further personalities, even in those patients who do not present with this problem. The recent large increase, especially in the USA, in what was once a very rare condition is probably due to the inappropriate use of hypnotic suggestion.

Hypnosis is used occasionally to retrieve forgotten childhood experiences of abuse. However, despite the convictions of patient and hypnotist, it is impossible to distinguish true recall from fantasy, and external validation is always necessary. This caveat also applies in courts of law if any attempt is made with hypnosis to aid the recall by witnesses of previous events.

Many people's knowledge of hypnotism is derived from stage hypnotism. The main dangers in stage performances arise from the carelessness of some hypnotists in ensuring the subsequent well-being of their subjects. Age regression may be upsetting if a 'return' is made to a traumatic past period; people may be required to perform embarrassing posthypnotic suggestions, and sometimes they are not fully awakened after hypnosis. In some countries these negative aspects have been considered sufficiently serious for a ban to be imposed. Hypnotism on the stage is certainly trivialized and a false impression given of its serious applications.

In recent years, much research effort has been directed towards understanding the nature of hypnotism. An experimental approach has been adopted, mainly by psychologists in North America, where expansions in the scope and applications of psychology have been most evident. Thus, it is now commonplace to find controlled studies using scales to assess susceptibility to standardized hypnotic induction, with a variety of control groups of unhypnotized people, or even of people simulating hypnosis, all with careful measurement of numerous variables. Many of the myths surrounding hypnosis have been cleared away, and, in conjunction with advances in neurophysiology and in social psychology, a somewhat clearer picture is beginning to emerge. This work is published in reputable scientific journals, where it has led to the recognition of hypnotism as a serious topic of study, not only because of its various therapeutic applications but also because it can throw light on a variety of psychological processes, especially those of memory and perception, and on the nature of consciousness in general.

However, no overall and generally accepted theory of hypnosis has emerged from contemporary research. A current controversy concerns the notion of the hypnotic trance and whether it is an altered state of consciousness different from normal waking consciousness. Although clinicians generally believe this, much of the experimental and physiological evidence does not support it. It has not proved possible to find a particular brain state associated with the deep trance, and many of the feats achieved by deeply hypnotized subjects can apparently be duplicated by sufficiently motivated control subjects who are not hypnotized. On the other hand, subjectively, hypnotized people report that they feel different when hypnotized. There are great variations in the depths of hypnosis achievable by different people and by one person on different occasions. Laboratory conditions are not usually conducive to achieving deep trances, and it may be more profitable to concentrate research efforts on gifted hypnotic subjects hypnotized by charismatic practitioners in other settings. Hypnosis needs much further research before its psychological and physiological nature can be understood and before its efficacy as a treatment can be assessed.

DWF

Plate 5 The World Food Programme organizes school-feeding (see FAMINE). (Reproduced courtesy of Steven Peters/Tony Stone Images)

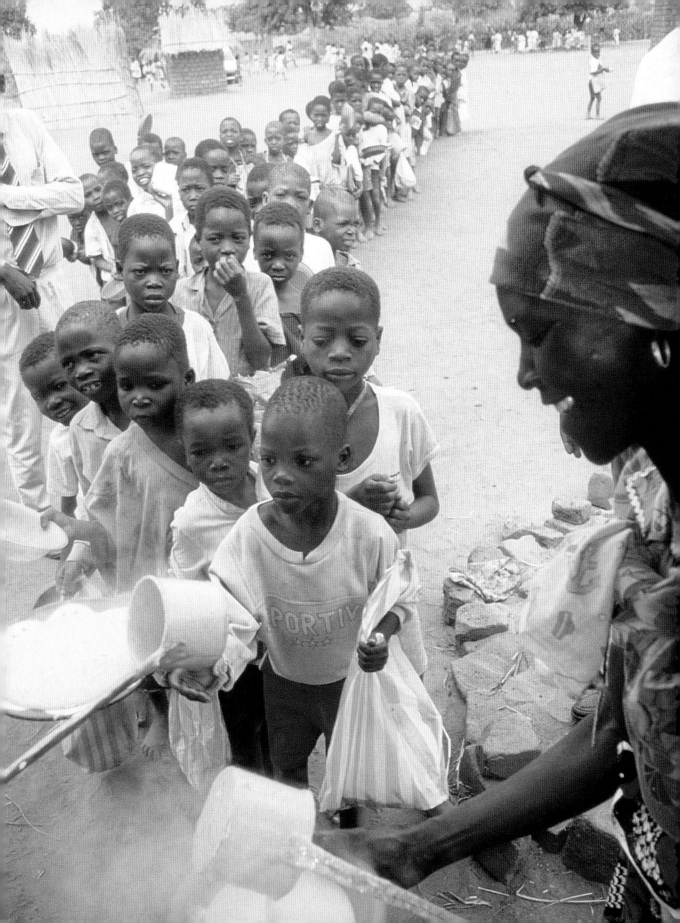

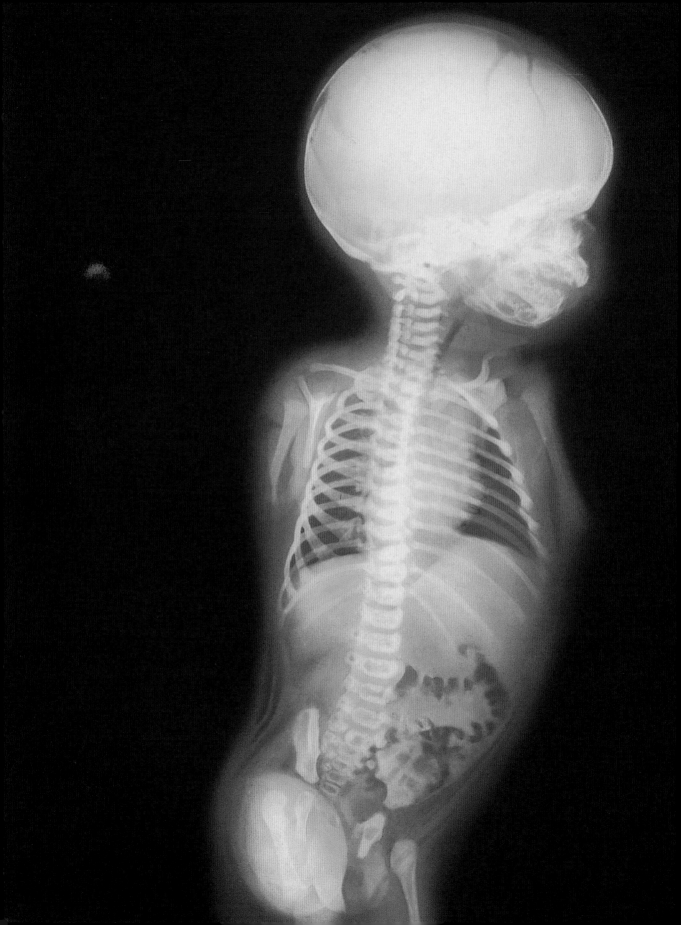

**HYSTERIA** The word 'hysteria' derives from the Greek *hystera* meaning uterus. In classical times, the literally 'displaced uterus' was blamed for many symptoms in women. In the Middle Ages, the concept of 'suffocation of the womb' was still in place, but by the 18th century, although the disorder was still felt mainly to affect women, its origin was thought to reside in the nervous rather than the reproductive system. Hysteria was then characterized by convulsive attacks, pains, the sensation of choking, tics, and paralyses. Undoubtedly, however, many such patients would now receive neurological diagnoses such as epilepsy, multiple sclerosis, or stroke.

By the 19th century, emotional factors were recognized as playing a part, but hysteria was still put down to hereditary weakness and cultural degeneration. Late 19th century work was dominated by CHARCOT (p 400), a neurologist working at La Salpêtrière Hospital in Paris. Charcot was renowned for his theatrical clinics in which patients would demonstrate their hysterical symptoms at his direction in front of eminent, international audiences. Despite his inability to demonstrate a pathological abnormality, he still viewed hysteria as an illness with discernible physical characteristics and believed that some area of the brain must be malfunctioning. He did, however, acknowledge a role for psychological factors in hysteria. FREUD's (p 321) contribution at the turn of the century transformed hysteria from an organic disease causing emotional symp-

A clinical lecture at the Salpêtrière hospital, CHARCOT (p 400) demonstrating with an hysterical patient. Engraving by H. Dochy from the painting by A. Brouillet (1887). (Reproduced courtesy of the Mary Evans Picture Library.)

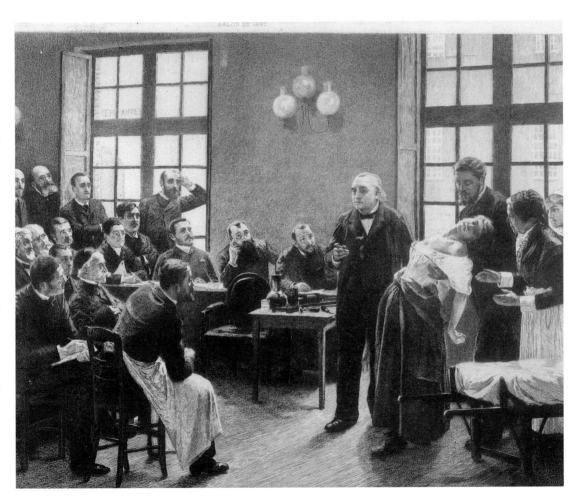

**Plate 6** An X-ray showing the head and body of a child with limb deformities caused by the drug **thalidomide**. (Reproduced courtesy of the Mary Evans Picture Library.)

toms to a psychological disorder causing physical symptoms. He introduced the concept of 'primary gain,' whereby hysterical symptoms performed a symbolic role serving to resolve unconscious, forbidden, primitive urges, particularly of a sexual nature.

### 'Dissociation'

The mainstream view throughout this century has continued to be based on psychodynamic ideas, whereby the patient 'converts' an overwhelming psychic disturbance into physical symptoms. The concept of 'dissociation' is also important and underlies the unconscious nature of the process — the symptoms are neither selected nor fabricated. Hysteria is now generally regarded as a form of somatization, the expression of psychic distress through bodily symptoms. Although the Freudian concept of primary gain is no longer felt to be relevant in most cases, the importance of secondary gain has been increasingly emphasized. This is the potential advantage a patient accrues from continuing illness, such as sympathy, financial benefits, or absolution from normal responsibilities. Other sociological concepts have emphasized the implicit role of the medical profession in encouraging or maintaining symptoms (iatrogenesis).

Although male hysteria was acknowledged even by Charcot, it was generally associated in a negative manner with femininity, delicateness, HOMOSEXUALITY, or 'otherness'. The consequences of the First World War included an epidemic of soldiers returning with paralyses, tics, blindness, and emotional distress. This resulted in a shift in view but, to avoid any of the associations of hysteria, a new socially acceptable model of illness was adopted for the disorder — 'shell shock'. This is an example of the trend, seen in many aspects of PSYCHIATRY, to rename disorders which develop a negative image as a result of their association with underprivileged or undesirable aspects of society.

Whereas initially the term hysteria indicated either a single symptom (such as hysterical paralysis) or, particularly in America, several symptoms (such as somatization disorder — where patients have many chronic medically inexplicable symptoms), the use of the term has since been widened. The label 'hysterical' was allocated to a subgroup of personality disorders characterized by theatricality, egocentricity, and manipulative behavior (now modified to 'histrionic'). In addition, the term 'mass hysteria' has been given to epidemics of unexplained symptoms, transmissible in a way reminiscent of infections through anxiety and modeling. Fatigue syndromes, such as Royal Free disease, chronic fatigue syndrome, and myalgic encephalitis, in which unexplained motor weakness is found in combination with systemic symptoms such as fatigue, fever, and malaise, share many features of mass hysteria.

As a result of this broadening of the use of the term, as well as the pejorative association, formal psychiatric classifications such as the International Classification of Diseases (ICD 10) have now dropped the term hysteria. Its replacement, 'conversion disorder', is now a subheading of the section 'Somatoform disorders'. Despite this, the terminology in day to day use lags behind classificatory systems. Euphemisms such as 'functional', 'psychogenic', 'neurotic', and 'supratentorial' are often used by doctors. In addition, the term has been adopted into everyday language and is used to describe flighty, irrational, or flamboyant behavior, particularly in the context of excessive display of emotion. It is used to describe everything from a touchy film star to a wildly enthusiastic football crowd.

### Somatization

Somatization is the most common presentation of psychological distress and, although narrowly defined somatization disorder is rare, chronic or recurrent somatization is thought to affect as much as 10% of the population. In neurological settings, studies consistently find no organic explanation for physical symptoms in a third to a half of patients. Motor symptoms are most common, such as weakness, incoordination, unsteadiness, and tremor. Hysterical sensory disturbance, blindness, and memory loss are also well described.

The diagnosis of conversion hysteria can sometimes be made on physical examination, especially where inconsistent signs are demonstrated. The mismatch between the severity of a patient's symptoms and their apparent lack of concern, 'belle indifference' is said to bring about a reduction in psychological distress at the expense of physical well-being. It has been said to be a characteristic feature of hysteria, but this view has not held up to scientific investigation. By definition, hysteria works through unconscious processes; however, many still find it difficult to distinguish between it and MUNCHAUSEN'S SYNDROME (where the patient induces or feigns symptoms) or malingering (where the patient is consciously seeking gain from feigning illness). In clinical practice the boundaries are often blurred. A further feature that causes diagnostic problems is that patients with hysteria are more likely to suffer additionally from psychiatric disorders. High rates of depression, anxiety, and personality disorders have been consistently described, but may go unnoticed because of the patient's denial or minimization of psychological symptoms, or because of the doctor's preoccupation with looking for physical disease.

Attempts to study the natural history of hysteria are hampered by the quality of the available studies. The outcome is better, however, when symptoms are of recent onset and co-existent psychiatric disorder such as depression is present. An influential paper from the 1960s by a psychiatrist, Elliot Slater, described the outcome of patients with the diagnosis 'hysteria' admitted to a London neurological hospital. He found that many patients later developed other disorders; he concluded that the diagnosis was invalid and that other underlying diseases should be sought. Recent studies suggest that the rate of misdiagnosis is much lower than previously found.

No controlled treatment studies have been undertaken in hysteria; however, there is good reason to suppose that psychological treatment may be effective as in other areas of somatization. Treating depression and anxiety as well as exploring personal circumstances may help some patients. In others, however — especially those with multiple or long-standing symptoms — avoidance of further deterioration (especially through extensive further investigations) is the main focus of management.          HLC

*See also* BATTLE NEUROSIS

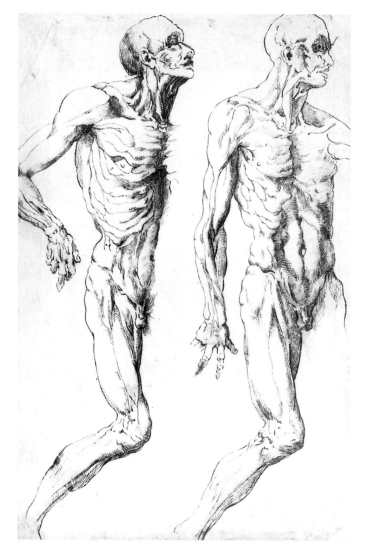

Pen and ink drawings on paper, attributed to the circle of Bartolomeo Passarotti (1529–1592). (Reproduced courtesy of the Wellcome Institute Library, London.)

**ILLUSTRATION AND PHOTOGRAPHY** Since the Renaissance, numerous genres of medical imagery have been invented and developed, some subsequently being abandoned. Most new medical specialties have also been accompanied by their own conventions for representing and understanding the human body. In addition, technological innovations in printing, photography, and imaging techniques, as well as in the means of disseminating images, have all expanded the album of medicine's visual surface. Further still, the sites of medicine (hospitals, pharmacies, laboratories, etc.) have, since the 17th century, increasingly been the subject of pictorial representations, while the twin traditions of picturing medical men (and some women) at work, and of taking their portraits once they have retired, have for centuries been the source of much artistic patronage.

Added together, this accumulation of images amounts to a staggeringly rich visual record (rivaled in no other science). But for too long medical illustrations have simply been used to illustrate medical history. Recently, however, this immense pictorial archive has been examined with great care by some scholars, who increasingly have embraced it not just as an attractive accompaniment to an established story, but rather as a heretofore hidden slice of medical history.

During much of the Middle Ages, the idea that the body was itself the true illustration precluded the development of much medical imagery. To help 'read' the body, books were extensively used, but primarily as vessels to carry verbal descriptions originating from the Greek physician GALEN (p 324).

As Martin Kemp has pointed out, there is 'nothing "obvious" about medical illustration'. The conceit of putting visual depictions of the body at the heart of medical enquiry and instruction was a Renaissance invention. In the same period the conviction grew that knowledge of the body could best be derived from anatomical dissections. The most influential work in the new medical quest for naturalistic representations of body's structure came from ANDREAS VESALIUS (p 846). Disseminated through the printed page, this style of representation gained ever wider audiences, and in time took on a potency of somehow embodying the very touchstone of medical reality.

The body has always simultaneously been a physical reality and a metaphor. In the Renaissance

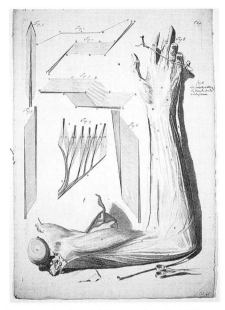

Engraving after Gerard de Lairesse, from Godefridus Bidloo, *Anatomia humani corporis* (Amsterdam, 1685). The main image of the upper arm is accompanied by mechanical diagrams indicating its workings. A handwritten annotation reads 'Geometriques de la disposition.' (Reproduced courtesy of the Wellcome Institute Library, London.)

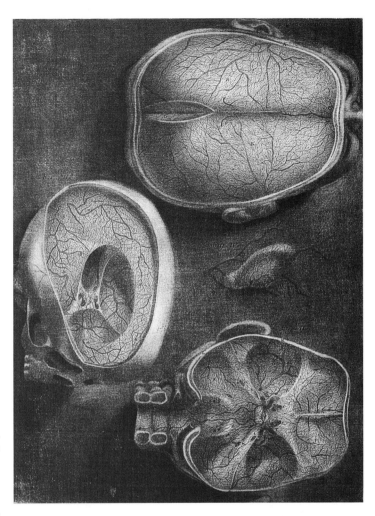

Colored mezzotint by J. F. Gautier d'Agoty, published as a plate in *Anatomie de la tête en tableaux imprimés* (Paris, 1748). (Reproduced courtesy of the Wellcome Institute Library, London.)

the human form was largely envisaged as a world in miniature. Starting in the late 16th century, this concept came to be replaced by mechanical analogies, with mechanisms beginning to figure in representations of the body during the 17th century. And, with the use of the newly invented microscope, some inquirers actually managed to depict these mechanical structures working at a microscopic level.

In the 18th century, the focus of innovative investigations into the body began to focus on less immediately visible body systems such as those of nerves and reproductive organs. In both cases, the findings — treated as two branches of 'natural history' — were recorded and published in well-established representational traditions, though through progressively more elaborate and larger-scale printing techniques.

A new research tradition of pathological anatomy grew up during the 19th century. The concepts of disease already developed by physicians such as Edward JENNER (p 452) were elaborated to lend new significance to the small visual signs of ailment. Earlier holistic notions of disease came to be challenged by a new concentration on discrete pathological changes. The accumulation of pathological analyses was presented within the established naturalistic illustrative tradition, which has ever since remained an essential diagnostic and instructional tool.

Though what was understood by the concept of 'realism' was perpetually under review, it remained the goal of image-making in medicine. Not surprisingly the development of photography in 1839 was almost immediately taken up as a powerful new medical tool. Applied to the inside of the body, however, photographs without color proved of little help. It was instead in mental health that the camera was used with greatest significance, initially by the likes of Hugh Diamond, a superintendent of an asylum outside London, who in the 1850s held that the use of a camera allowed him greatly to improve the systematic typology of mental illnesses, a methodology more famously elaborated by CHARCOT (p 400) at the Hôpital de la Salpêtrière, in Paris. Photography was also used to significant effect in dermatology and later in microscopy.

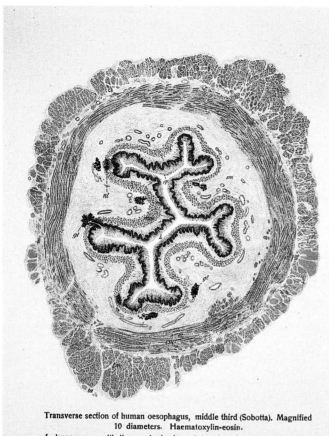

Transverse section of human oesophagus, middle third (Sobotta). Magnified 10 diameters. Haematoxylin-eosin.

*L*, lumen; *ep*, epithelium; *gl*, glands; *nl*, lymph-nodule; *mm*, muscularis mucosae; *sm*, submucosa; *cm*, circular muscle; *lm*, longitudinal muscle; *ta*, tunica adventitia.

Transverse section of human esophagus. Colored plate from B. A. Schaffer's *Textbook of microscopic anatomy* (London, 1912). (Reproduced courtesy of the Wellcome Institute Library, London.)

Photographic portraits of medical professionals also had a lasting impact on the way that medicine has been publicly perceived.

During the 19th century in Germany and France laboratory-based medical science increased, with experiments in organic chemistry and physiology, allowing a variety of the body's activities to be measured systematically. The emblematic instrument in this trend was Carl LUDWIG'S (p 643) kymograph, which enabled the automatic translation of bodily functions into quantitative records. This was a process that symbolized a radically new, nonnaturalistic representation of the body. The visual tradition of graphs and tables it unleashed has continued ever since, throwing up ever new forms of information as well as types of presentation.

Cell theory grew to dominate biomedicine from the mid-19th century, its foundational elements being portrayed pictorially through the use of ever more complex microscopic observations, with their functions being depicted in graphs, tables, and equations. The rise of cell and molecular biology, and the subsequent discovery and investigation of DNA and genes, have led to the fundamental dissolution of the medical vision of the human form. Starting with the application of X-rays, this picture has been further fractured by the development of innumerable instrument-generated visual codes for understanding aspects of the body outside our normal field of vision. However, the more that is learned of cell and gene functions, the more bodily systems are shown to be interdependent. And, while different disciplines have fragmented the once unified study and representation of the body, several influential researchers have recently argued for a return to a more holistic approach to viewing our biological selves.                                                          KA

*See also* ART; IMAGING

**IMAGING** Medical imaging has become integral to all of the clinical and research disciplines of medicine. The images are derived from several different technologies and are based on the emission of different energy wave forms. Those most commonly applied in medical practice are X-rays, gamma rays, positrons, ultrasound waves, and nuclear magnetic resonance.

Few disciplines of medicine can trace their roots to a single instant in time. However, this is the case with medical imaging. On 8 November 1895, Wilhelm Conrad ROENTGEN (p 873) was working in his home laboratory in Würzburg, Germany. Over the previous several months, he had been working with several radiation-emitting tubes. On this particular night, he serendipitously noted that the emissions of his Hittorf tube were causing a barium platinocyanide screen some distance away to fluoresce. He correctly deduced that he was witnessing the effects of a new kind of ray. By 10 January 1896, Roentgen had completed a brilliant set of experiments and published a report that detailed much of what we know about X-rays today, including that: denser materials absorbed more of the rays than less dense materials; that X-rays induced fluorescence in a variety of substances that could serve as receptors for images; and that X-rays were not reflected or refracted or affected by magnetic fields. These discoveries caused an immediate international sensation and led to Roentgen's being awarded the first Nobel prize for physics. They also formed the basis of X-ray imaging. The first medical applications were reported in 1896. The first textbook of medical imaging, *The Roentgen rays in medicine and surgery*, was published by Dr Francis Williams in 1901.

Although X-ray technology has advanced appreciably since Roentgen's time, the basic principles of X-ray emission and absorption still govern X-ray imaging. Within an X-ray tube, high-speed electrons are shot from a cathode to a metal anode. With the rapid deceleration of the electrons, X-rays are emitted. The operator, usually an X-ray technologist, positions the patient so that the relevant body part is exposed to the radiation. During their passage through the body, some of the X-rays are absorbed by tissues, some pass directly through the body onto the cassette holding the X-ray film, and some are scattered by interactions with the molecules in the tissue. The extent to which each of these possibilities occurs depends on the power of the X-rays and the thickness and density of the tissues. Tissue density is the critical feature that allows radiologists to distinguish between types of tissue. For instance, since bones are denser (have a higher average atomic number) than soft tissue, fat, or air, they absorb more X-rays and appear whiter (radiologists say 'more opaque') on radiographs than these other common body elements.

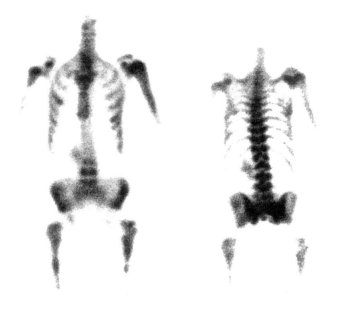

## Radionuclide imaging

The foundations of nuclear medicine — or radionuclide imaging — were established by the reporting of naturally occurring radioactivity from potassium uranyl sulfate by Henri BECQUEREL (p 700) in 1896. He reported emanations similar to X-rays, that had the capacity to blacken film in a darkened place. The elucidation of the physical principles of this radiation by Marie and Pierre CURIE (p 556) (and later by their daughter and son-in-law, the Joliot-Curies) initiated a half century of study that culminated in the human application of radionuclides. Radionuclide imaging has since developed as a method of elucidating both human anatomy and physiology. Unlike X-ray imaging, where the radiation is generated outside the patient, NUCLEAR MEDICINE relies on the administration of a radionuclide by inhalation, ingestion, or injection. The radionuclide is 'tagged' to a molecule designed to be taken up by specific normal or abnormal tissues. As the radionuclide decays, it emits gamma rays, which are transmitted through the body to a crystalline receptor that constructs an image of the target tissue site.

Current single photon emission computed tomography technology has expanded on the capabilities of nuclear medicine by coupling the receptor to a computer and allowing for cross-sectional imaging — images of 'slices' of the target organ — similar to what are viewed on computerized axial tomography (CAT or CT) scans. This has permitted more accurate diagnosis than was previously available by whole organ or 'projectional' images. Attaching radionuclides to an increasing host of molecules has allowed for

the expansion of nuclear medicine imaging to image virtually every organ, and in some cases, to target certain diseases specifically.

A more recent innovation in nuclear medicine is positron emission tomography, or PET scanning. This also depends upon the administration of a radionuclide. However, these radionuclides are of a special type, decaying very rapidly and producing positrons that collide with electrons in the body. Positron 'annihilation' produces paired gamma rays of specific energy, which are emitted in diametrically opposite directions, permitting localization of the point of annihilation in the body by the computerized positron emission tomography system. Tagging positron emitters to molecules participating in cell metabolism has allowed researchers to differentiate normally functioning areas of the brain or heart, for example, from those where metabolism is abnormal. Physicians are also beginning to use positron emission tomography more frequently to distinguish active tumor from slower metabolizing scar tissue or inflammation after cancer treatment.

Amazingly, the name Curie reappears in the history of ultrasound imaging. Pierre and his brother Jacques first described the piezoelectric effect that is the foundation of modern ultrasound imaging. Certain crystals are bipolar, like magnets. Passing an alternating current through the crystal deforms it; once the current is cut off, the crystal seeks to return to its original configuration, and in doing so, emits a high frequency sound, beyond human hearing, whose frequency is dependent on both the nature of the crystal and the electric field. The frequency of ultrasound used for medical imaging ranges from

A bone scan indicating multiple metastatic deposits. (Reproduced from Weatherall, D. J. *et al.* (1996). *The Oxford textbook of medicine*, 3rd edn, OUP.)

## GERMAN PIONEER

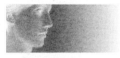

Heinrich Ernst **ALBERS–SCHÖNBERG** (1865–1921). German radiologist. Founder of a private institute for radiology in Hamburg in 1897. He later took charge of the department at St George's Hospital, London, becoming professor in 1907, and the first 'Ordinarius' in this specialty in Germany in 1919. He died as a result of radiation injury. One of the pioneer radiologists, his *Röntgenstechnik* (1903) was the first authoritative textbook; he founded the first German radiological journal as well as the German association of radiologists. He invented the compression diaphragm, showed the harmful effects of X-rays on spermatogenesis, and devised a lead protective screen.

1 to greater than 10 MHz. For some years, the phenomenon discovered by the Curies found few applications in medicine. However, instructed by technologies invented for naval use during the two world wars (largely for detecting enemy submarines), medical ultrasound imaging became practicable in the early 1970s. Modern instruments employ arrays of lead zirconate titanate crystal transducers. Ultrasound is transmitted from the transducer, which is coupled to the body by a thick gel. The sound traverses body tissues at constant speed. Some of the sound waves are reflected by both macrointerfaces (for example, where two major body organs sit adjacent to each other) and microinterfaces (that is, different constituent tissues within organs) and return to the transducer. The ultrasound device uses a computer to place these echoes in space, according to the time elapsed between their transmission and reception, and produces an image accordingly. Ultrasound technology is portable, inexpensive, and avoids the use of potentially damaging ionizing radiation such as X-rays, and produces images in real time — essentially moving pictures that allow for rapid investigation in patients who may have difficulty undergoing other types of examinations. It has become the imaging modality of choice for evaluating fetuses, pregnant women, and critically ill or postoperative patients who cannot be moved, and to guide new, less invasive interventional procedures that can replace surgery for some patients.

## Computerized tomography

Many consider the genesis of computerized tomography scanning to be as revolutionary as the initial discovery of the X-ray. And indeed, as with Roentgen, its progenitors, Cormack and Houndsfield, received a Nobel prize. The computerized tomography scanner takes advantage of a mathematical algorithm called back-projection and the computational power of modern computers to combine fragments of X-ray images exposed from multiple directions into an image that depicts a 'slice' through the body. The resultant images, which can be viewed sequentially to build a comprehensive view of a body part, are far more sensitive to differences in tissue density than ordinary X-rays. Thus, whereas diagnosis on plain X-ray films depends on detecting a departure from the normal in the size or shape of organs, or large density differences, such as finding a soft tissue mass surrounded by the air of the lungs, computerized tomography scanning permits radiologists to detect subtle abnormalities occurring within tissues. This change allows the earlier detection of metabolic diseases, infections, and cancer, and led to a host of new computerized tomography-guided interventional procedures. Using computerized tomography as guidance, radiologists can often replace conventional open surgery by using needles, catheters, and energy-producing instruments to biopsy tumors, drain abscesses, rechannel blocked bile ducts, alleviate pain, and destroy abnormal tissues.

The method used in computerized tomography to combine image 'fragments' also serves as the foundation for subsequent developments in computerized medical imaging, such as magnetic resonance imaging (MRI). This is based on different physical principles to produce a different kind of image. Based on the principles of nuclear magnetic resonance elucidated by Bloch and Purcell (also Nobel prize winners), the details of how images might be generated by magnetic resonance were first propounded by Lauterbur in 1973. Damadian built the first machine capable of human imaging, named it Indomitable, and, after hours of imaging, produced the first human scan in 1977. Since then technical developments and medical applications have proceeded rapidly, spurred by magnetic resonance imaging's unique capabilities to differentiate better among soft tissues without ionizing radiation.

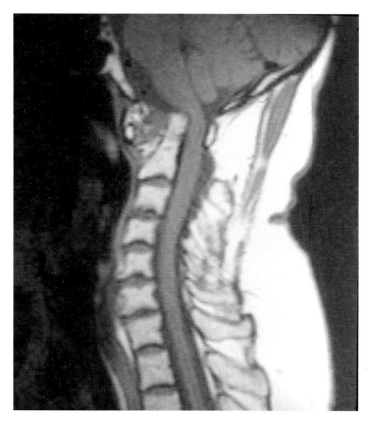

MRI scan of the cervical spine in rheumatoid arthritis. There is atlantoaxial instability; the cervical cord is displaced by the protruding peg. Without MRI, this information would have been obtained by cervical myelography, an unpleasant, time-consuming procedure involving considerable radiation. (Reproduced from Weatherall, D. J. *et al.* (1996). *The Oxford textbook of medicine*, 3rd edn, OUP.)

Magnetic resonance imaging is based on the principle that certain elements occurring in the body are paramagnetic — their nuclei respond to magnetic fields because they have an odd number of protons and neutrons. Fortunately the most common element in the body, hydrogen, is paramagnetic. Placing a patient in an MRI scanner exposes the patient to a strong magnetic field, which aligns the majority of the paramagnetic nuclei along the axis of the scanner. A transducer, or coil, then interrogates the part of interest with a radiofrequency wave, that both flips the nucleus out of alignment with the magnetic field and sets it spinning around its central access (precession). Both the return to alignment and the weakening of precession emit signals that are received by the coil and transmitted to the computer for construction into a cross-sectional image similar to that seen with computerized tomography scans.

The ability of the radiologist to change the sequence of radiofrequency signals permits an almost infinite range of possibilities in how the images will appear, and hence what features of the image can be brought forth to diagnose disease best. Its capacity to depict small differences in soft tissue densities has found particularly important applications in evaluating the brain, spine, bones, joints, and muscles, where it has supplanted more invasive, morbidity-producing procedures and often obviated the need to inject X-ray contrast materials (dye). However, it is still a young technology and new applications, involving all body systems, are being developed constantly. A very recent application is magnetic resonance angiography. In some settings and for some indications, this latter has replaced catheterization and injection of contrast material to diagnose abnormalities of the blood vessels.

During the past quarter century medical imaging has revolutionized medical diagnosis and treatment and has advanced faster than any other aspect of medicine. However, even recent developments are dwarfed by the potential of medical imaging. One may predict the development of less invasive diagnostic and therapeutic procedures; the transformation of medical images from a film to an electronic format; image processing; earlier disease detection for screening and prevention; molecular and functional imaging; and the conflict between the imperative to develop and use improved healthcare technology versus economic constraints. One example is particularly dramatic. Until the introduction of the computerized tomography scanner in the early 1970s enabling examination of deep brain tissues, the brain was imaged by pneumoencephalography — an invasive, frightening, and discomforting procedure. Similarly in the future, virtual colonography using cross-sectional images may replace such more discomforting, invasive procedures as colonoscopy and barium enema.

## New subspecialty

Indeed a whole new subspecialty of medical imaging — interventional radiology — has made its purview MINIMALLY INVASIVE procedures that are replacing more morbidity-producing conventional treatments. This subspecialty uses images to guide the placement of needles, catheters, and other devices as a replacement for open surgery. The effects are that treatment can take place without general anesthesia, often in an outpatient setting, less expensively, with less pain and anxiety, and with more rapid return to normal function. Every part of the body is affected. Surgical breast biopsies for suspected breast cancer have largely been replaced by stereotactic needle biopsies, leading to less disfigurement, fewer complications, and faster recovery. Narrowed or clogged blood vessels and bile ducts can be widened with catheters carrying balloons and held open by stents of plastic or metal. Bits of metal, polymer fragments, balloons, or even glue can be directed into abnormal vessels to block them off before they can bleed and cause damage to the brain or other organs. Life-threatening abdominal abscesses are drained by catheters placed through the skin. Similar new procedures are constantly being devised. Very recently, some researchers have begun to evaluate how such imaging technologies as magnetic resonance imaging can direct even less invasive treatment, using powerful focused sound, heat, or other energies to treat serious ailments with even less damage to surrounding normal tissues.

A second important trend is the movement to electronic imaging. Although the images generated by such technologies as magnetic resonance imaging and computerized tomography are innately electronic, or digital, the conventional mode of transferring, storing, and interpreting them has depended on first printing the images on film. In recent years, picture archiving and communication systems have developed to allow for the acquisition of all medical images, their transmission, storage, and interpretation, by electronic means. Once these systems develop further and mature there will be enormous advantages. Both the current and the past images for a patient will become instantly available to the radiologist who interprets the examinations and the physicians who use them in their treatment. The films will never be lost and will be available to several caregivers, in different locations, at the same time. The huge spaces needed to store films can be reduced to a device the size of a jukebox, at greatly reduced cost. Images can be sent instantly via phone lines or satellite to an expert anywhere on the globe for a second opinion.

## CARDIAC IMAGER

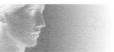

Charles **LAUBRY**
(1872–1941). Parisian cardiologist. Laubry flourished in the 1920s at the Hôpital Broussais. With others he established the technique of injection of radio-opaque substances into the heart and great vessels as a means of studying their anatomy, paving the way for the modern methods of cardiological investigation in the living. In 1939 he published *Radiologie clinique du cœur et des gros vaisseaux*.

Elie **METCHNIKOFF**
(1845–1916). Russian
microbiologist. Metchnikoff
moved to St Petersburg after
teaching biology in Odessa,
but found both uncongenial
and made two attempts to
commit suicide. Finally in
1888 he joined the staff of
the Pasteur Institute in Paris,
where he spent the rest of his
life. He observed
phagocytosis — a word he
coined in 1880 — noted the
macrophage, and believed
that immunity depended
solely on cellular mechanisms.
His views were expressed in
*L'immunité dans les maladies
infectieuses* (1901). He was
awarded the NOBEL PRIZE in
1908.

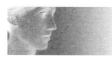

Rodney Robert **PORTER**
(1917–85). British biochemist.
After World War II Porter
developed an interest in
protein chemistry, working in
Cambridge with Frederick
Sanger. As professor of
immunology (the first in
Britain) at St Mary's Hospital,
Porter showed that antibodies
were made up of two heavy
and two light chains, held
together by disulfide bonds.
In 1967 he succeeded Sir
Hans Krebs at Oxford as
professor of biochemistry,
where he remained until his
death in a car crash just three
weeks before he was due to
retire. In 1972, he was
awarded the NOBEL PRIZE for
his research on the chemical
structure of antibodies.

There is also the hope that image processing,
facilitated by images being in electronic format,
will provide greater diagnostic value than is available with film images. Already, radiologists are
using COMPUTERS to achieve this goal. Computer
algorithms facilitate the enhancement of specific
image details for more complete inspection.
Cross-sectional images can be combined into
three-dimensional images and rotated in space to
simulate their appearance during surgery.
Researchers are experimenting with computer-
aided diagnosis — systems that work with the
radiologist to improve his detection of abnormalities and then work with him to decide whether
what has been detected is normal or abnormal,
and if abnormal, what it might be.

### Earlier detection of disease

The continuing development of more sensitive
imaging technologies also portends the possibility of earlier detection of disease. This will allow
the early detection of cancers when they are much
smaller than currently detectable, when changes
are just occurring at the molecular or cellular
level, or when the changes represent premalignant
disease. Medicine is just witnessing the emergence
of imaging agents that respond to genetic
manifestations of early disease by tagging to
molecular receptors indicative of these changes.
The combination of such imaging tests with
more effective non-imaging screening tests may
eventually allow physicians to realize the goal of
decreasing cancer-related mortality.

Ironically, even as imaging technology is poised
to make important new contributions to health, an
even greater revolution is occurring internationally
in how healthcare is organized and financed. These
changes will inevitably influence the extent to
which medical imaging will achieve its potential.
Until the last decade, the emphasis in healthcare
has been on improving technology and applying it
to any situation when it might improve a patient's
health (sometimes referred to as the technologic
imperative). The situation has changed. Now the
emphasis is on value — balancing the benefits for
patients against cost. Since imaging technology
tends to be expensive to develop, acquire, and
operate, such technologies as computerized tomography, magnetic resonance imaging, and positron
emission tomography have often been lightning
rods for this extraordinary paradigmatic change in
healthcare.

Increasingly, decisions about employing medical technology are swinging from patients and
providers to governments and insurers. There is a
greater demand for technology assessment —
decision analysis, Markov modeling, and cost-
effective analysis — and this will have a powerful
influence on whether the full potential of medical
imaging to improve health will be brought to bear
in the future. BJH

*See also* SERENDIPITY

**IMHOTEP** (fl. 2980 BC) Egyptian physician and
sage. Although Imhotep was previously believed
to have been legendary, undoubtedly he was a
historical personage who lived in the third
dynasty during the reign of King Zoser
(2980–2900 BC). He was priest, architect, and
sage, but there is no contemporary evidence of his
being a physician. Under the Ptolemies he
acquired a great reputation for healing and was
deified. Many miracles were wrought at his
temples and he became the God of Medicine. The
Greeks called him Imouthes and identified him
with ASCLEPIUS (p 710).

**IMMUNOLOGY — HISTORY** The science of
immunology originated in the common observation that people recovering from some infectious
diseases are protected from subsequent attacks. A
child who has had measles or mumps, or the
survivor of a SMALLPOX epidemic, is unlikely to
develop the disease a second time. There are three
features of this immune response which make it a
unique biological phenomenon. It is, in the first
place, an acquired response, elicited by the initial
exposure to the disease. Secondly, it persists as an
immunological memory, which may be recalled
and reactivated months or years later. And,
thirdly, there is the extraordinary specificity of the
reaction, as illustrated by the fact that an attack of
smallpox protected against that disease, but not
against yellow fever. The investigation of this
problem has occupied immunologists for over a
century.

In its early years, the science of immunology
was concerned with combating infectious diseases. However, it now encompasses all aspects of
the body's ability to react to foreign or extraneous
substances. Many diseases are associated with
exaggerated or inappropriate immune responses,
commonly known as ALLERGY or hypersensitivity, and a wide range of disorders, autoimmune
diseases, in which the body reacts against itself.
There are also diseases in which the immune
response is not optimally effective, of which AIDS,
due to infection with the human immunodeficiency virus (HIV), is the most striking
example. Immunology has also provided the
rationale and the techniques for such notable
medical advances as blood transfusion and organ
TRANSPLANTATION.

The earliest medical application of immunology was the introduction of VACCINATION
against smallpox by Edward JENNER (p 452).
Jenner was a Gloucestershire physician who
observed that dairymaids who developed cowpox

were protected against smallpox. In 1796, he inoculated a young boy with fluid from a cowpox pustule. A little pustule appeared at the site of injection and then disappeared. Some months later he injected him with material from a human smallpox case and was gratified to observe (as no doubt was the boy) that no disease developed. After some initial resistance, the practice of vaccination (Latin *vacca*, cow) against smallpox became general, although the nature of the protection offered was not understood. Today, vaccination against a plethora of diseases has become common and smallpox has been eradicated. More modern vaccines are being developed, which rely on the ability of DNA purified from microbes to be injected into the body. This microbial DNA produces 'foreign protein', directly triggering the immune system to mount a response to the foreign protein, which mirrors that induced by the invading organism.

In the second half of the 19th century, as a result of the work of PASTEUR (p 620), KOCH (p 455), and others, it became apparent that infectious diseases were due to the invasion of the body by micro-organisms, such as bacteria or viruses. It was also found possible to protect animals from infection by injecting them with altered or attenuated strains of the same organism. This was first observed by Pasteur in 1878, who noted that a culture of chicken cholera, which had been left in the laboratory during a vacation, lost its virulence for chickens, and that animals inoculated with this culture were protected against the virulent strain. He immediately recognized the significance of the observation, and, after confirming the phenomenon in anthrax in animals, applied it to the prevention and treatment of human rabies.

In some diseases it was found that if the animal recovered, its serum protected normal animals from infection. This suggested that immunity was due to a substance — a humoral factor — in the blood. The most striking confirmation of this came from the studies of von Behring on diphtheria and tetanus. In both diseases the damage is done, not by the bacterium itself, but by toxins produced by the organism and circulating in the blood. Von Behring showed that immunization with the toxin was sufficient to protect against the disease, and that this protection could be transferred to normal animals by injecting the serum. He proceeded to treat children with diphtheria by injecting serum from a horse immunized with diphtheria toxin. Von Behring recognized that the protective effect was due to substances circulating in the blood, and coined the term antibody.

The humoral theory was almost immediately challenged by the observations of the Russian biologist Elie METCHNIKOFF (p 412), working in

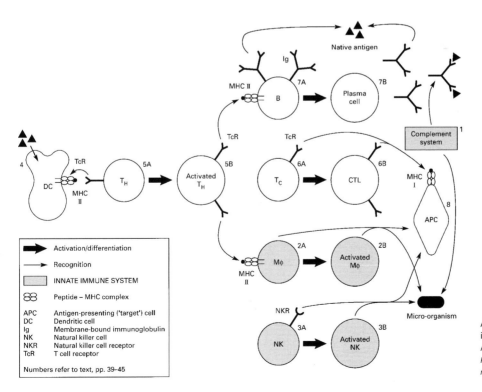

Antigen recognition and cells in the immune system. (From Austyn, J. and Wood, K. (1993). *Principles of cellular and molecular immunology*, OUP.)

Paris. Observing primitive organisms under the microscope, he noted that some cells could take up foreign particles and invading bacteria by a process that he termed phagocytosis. He showed that similar cells capable of engulfing and destroying bacteria were present in the blood of vertebrates and that this process was enhanced in animals recovering from infection. He concluded that these cells were responsible for protective immunity and that the process was a cellular one. The controversy between the proponents of the cellular and humoral theories was a feature of the early years of immunology, but, as often is the case, both groups were correct and immunity comprises both cellular and humoral components.                                  SLei, RLC, DAC

**IMMUNOLOGY** is the study of the protective systems of the body that guard against invasion by foreign organisms and also destroy cells that become abnormal or neoplastic (anti-tumor immunity). Immune-like mechanisms are common to almost all life, beginning with unicellular organisms, extending to both invertebrate and vertebrate multicellular eukaryotes. In humans, immune mechanisms are complex and involve those that are innate to the body (natural or innate immunity) as well as the ability to specifically adapt to meet unforeseen challenges (acquired immunity). Central to all immune mechanisms is the concept of biological specificity, developed at the beginning of the 20th century by Karl LANDSTEINER (p 120) and Lenor Michaelis. The principal advances of immunology have been concerned with explaining in molecular terms how the immune system is activated and how signaling pathways within cells govern immune response (signal transduction). Most importantly, immune cells bear cell-surface molecules or receptors, designed to recognize 'non-self' or foreign molecules termed antigens. The ability of antigens to act as pathologic agents is neutralized by the actions and interactions of immune cells and their products.

### Two types of lymphocytes
The principal cells of the immune system are divided into two main types of lymphocytes (one of the main forms of white blood cells) — T cells (which mediate cellular immunity) and B cells (which are responsible for antibody production) — and monocytes or macrophages (in tissues), whose function is to take up, process, and present antigens to T and B cells. Consequently, macrophages (and specialized types of dendritic cells) are often called antigen-presenting cells or accessory cells. Immune responses fall into two general categories: natural or innate and acquired. The two arms of acquired immunity are cellular immunity

and humoral immunity. In cellular immunity, antigens presented by macrophages activate T cells to release signaling molecules (interleukins and cytokines), which stimulate specific subtypes of T cells, or activate B cells, to differentiate into antibody-producing plasma cells. The two important classes of T cells are the T helper cell and the cytotoxic T lymphocyte. The T helper cell, of which there are two subtypes, regulates immune function through the synthesis and secretion of cytokines, whereas cytotoxic T cells specifically adhere to and destroy abnormal cells. The other arm of acquired immunity, humoral immunity, involves the production of antibodies generated against a specific antigen by differentiated B lymphocytes, plasma cells. Antibodies are released to the blood system and carried 'humorally' to the site of antigen deposition.

In addition to lymphoid organs (for example, spleen, lymph nodes, and tonsils), specialized peripheral immune systems function in the lung, skin, intestine, and nervous system. Interactions have also been documented between the immune system, the nervous system, and the endocrine system, which are giving rise to new insights about immune regulation. These subdisciplines of immunology are variously called neuroimmunology, neuroendocrinology, or neuroimmune endocrinology.

The ability to evoke an immune response is not peculiar to microorganisms. Most foreign substances injected into the body will do so provided they are sufficiently large. The most effective compounds are proteins and polysaccharides. Substances eliciting an immune response are called antigens and the reactive molecules that appear in the serum as a result of immunization are referred to as antibodies. A remarkable feature of the reaction between antigen and antibody is its extraordinary specificity. The chemical nature of this specificity was first demonstrated by Karl Landsteiner. He attached small molecules of known constitution and structure, to large protein antigens and showed that the antibodies produced could distinguish subtle differences in chemical structure. For example, the reaction was not with the whole molecule, but with small parts known as antigenic determinants or epitopes. A protein molecule might elicit a variety of specific antibodies to several different determinants, each capable of reacting with different parts of the molecular surface.

### Antibodies
The antibodies circulating in the serum are extremely diverse, being of several classes. In each class there are antibodies capable of reacting with many different antigenic determinants. The fundamental structure of an antibody is always

the same (Fig. 1). They are protein molecules, called immunoglobulins (Ig), made up of two sets of identical polypeptide chains or sequences of amino acids. There are two heavy (H) chains and two light (L) chains assembled into a Y-shaped structure. The two heavy chains make up the stem of the Y and continue into the arms linked to the two light chains. The latter are of two kinds, kappa and lambda. There are five main classes of immunoglobulin, each with its own characteristic H chain and biological properties. Each immuno-globulin molecule can react with two identical antigenic determinants. The reactive sites are at the ends of the two arms of the Y, and each determinant will, therefore, be in contact with portions of both the heavy and light chains. Each antibody has its own combining site, tailor-made to fit a particular determinant. The number of possible determinants, and therefore the number of different antibodies, is very large.

Antibodies serve various different functions. For example, in bacterial infections antibodies may coat the organisms and facilitate phagocyto-sis, or cause microbes to adhere and agglutinate, immobilizing them. Antibodies may also react with toxins to block their action, as shown by the therapeutic effect of antisera in diseases such as diphtheria. Most importantly, the combination of antibody and antigen may activate the comple-ment system, which enhances many of the protec-tive processes to a large degree.

In addition to the natural role of antibodies in fighting infection, other uses for antibodies have been developed. Purified antibodies may be used as reagents to specifically identify, characterize, and purify the molecules they are directed against. Of great interest in therapeutics is the coupling of antibodies to drugs. The antibody–drug complex can seek out a target and then deliver the drug in high concentrations to the target organ or cell. Two exciting examples of such use are in the treatment of cancer and of blood clots. In the former, anti-cancer drugs are combined with antibodies that can target a specific tumor (by recognizing tumor-specific cell surface molecules). This allows smaller concen-trations of highly toxic drugs to be delivered to a specific tumor site with fewer side-effects than would occur with the same drug in the absence of the antibody. In treating blood clots, antibodies against the fibrin clot are combined with fibrinolytic enzymes and injected into a vein. The antibody targets the fibrin and the enzymes destroy it.

Immunoglobulins are proteins, and as with all proteins their synthesis is under genetic control. If each of the million or more antibodies that the animal can make required a separate gene, it would mean that a very large proportion of the

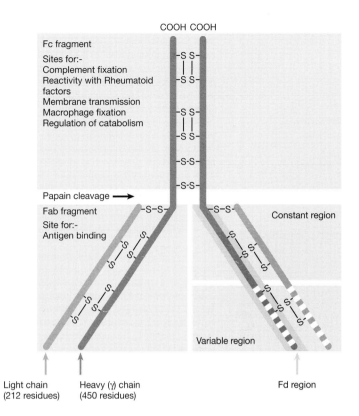

Fig. 1 A diagram of human IgG1. (From McGee, J. O'D., et al. (1992). The Oxford textbook of pathology, OUP.)

genome would have to be taken up with this single task. This is highly improbable, so how is this degree of antigenic variation generated? The answer is that the diversity is not present in the genome of the sperm or ovum, as handed down by the parents, but arises in the lymphocytes of the embryo. In early embryonic development the lymphocytes proliferate at a furious rate. Many die and are eliminated. The vertebrate genome contains several hundred genes devoted to the variable regions of the heavy and light chains of the immunoglobulin molecule. These code for the antigen-combining sites. In the early embryo the lymphocytes have a special propensity for rearranging these genes, producing very many different combinations. There are also special regions of this part of the genome in lympho-cytes, which have a very high mutation rate. These hypervariable regions are an additional source of variation. The combination of the two — gene rearrangement coupled with somatic mutation — appears sufficient to account for the enormous genetic diversity required to produce a million or more different antibodies.

The lymphoid tissues of the body are strate-gically placed to intercept invading organisms (Fig. 2). They guard portals of entry, such as the digestive and respiratory systems, and are located in the draining lymph nodes and blood-filtering organs such as the spleen. In the lymphoid organs the lymphocytes are associated with macrophages, large phagocytic cells which trap and process bacteria and other particulate antigens. These are also antigen-presenting cells, which present the antigenic determinants to the lymphocytes in suitably stimulating form. In tissues throughout the body the macrophages form a network, which is referred to as the reticuloendothelial system. This system may be identified in animals by injecting a suspension of carbon particles into the bloodstream. The particles are rapidly removed from the blood and phagocytosed, staining the lymphoreticular system black.

The recognition of an antigen stimulates the production of immunoglobulins by B cells and specifically activates the appropriate class of T cells. T cells also have receptors on their surfaces analogous to the combining sites of antibodies, which enable them to react with and respond to antigens.

Both B and T cells are lymphocytes which originate in the bone marrow and the thymus gland and migrate to the blood, lymph nodes, and spleen.

They also populate the lymphoid tissues of the digestive system and the lungs. For most of their life cycle they appear as small, featureless cells, 6 μm in diameter, containing small, round nuclei and very little cytoplasm. In this form they function as repositories of genetic information. There are about $10^6$ new lymphoid cells in the human body, and there is a rapid turnover rate, with $10^9$ new lymphocytes being produced daily. They are mobile cells, which circulate between the blood, bone marrow, and lymphoid organs. They enter the tissues from the blood and drain back into the bloodstream through lymphatic channels and lymph nodes. Lymphocytes also filter from the blood into the spleen and bone marrow. Like policemen on the beat, they are constantly on the move, ready to alert the immune defences to any intruder.

During bacterial infections the organisms are trapped in the lymphoreticular tissue, phagocytosed by macrophages, and degraded. The processed antigenic determinants are then presented on the cell surface, in combination with an appropriate class of major histocompatibility cell surface protein, to the lymphocytes by the antigen-presenting cells. The effect is to stimulate specific B or T cells, causing them to divide and multiply. Early in embryonic life each lymphocyte acquires the capacity to respond to a particular determinant. From then on, the cell and all its progeny clones can react with that particular molecular configuration.

There are many potential antigens and the adult animal has cells which can respond to every possible determinant. The number of lymphocytes reacting to any one determinant will, therefore, be small. However, on exposure to antigens these lymphocytes proliferate. Re-exposure to the same antigen, even after a prolonged time, results in a more rapid expansion of lymphocytes capable of generating an efficient immune response (immunological memory). B lymphocytes stimulated by antigens differentiate into plasma cells (Figure on p 412). These large cells, with increased cytoplasm, synthesize and secrete immunoglobulin. Each plasma cell produces an antibody of one specificity, the same for all cells of the clone. Similarly, stimulated T lymphocytes proliferate to give rise to clones of specifically sensitized cells, which can react with the antigen.

There are several classes of T cells, each capable of responding to antigens in a different way. Some can destroy cells invaded by viruses or recognize and kill tumor cells (cytotoxic T cells); others release substances (lymphokines) which stimulate immune and inflammatory cells and may generate a local inflammatory reaction. Episodic inflammatory diseases may have important systemic consequences, resulting in pulmonary disease,

**Fig. 2** Primary and secondary lymphoid tissues. (From Austyn, J. and Wood, K. (1993). *Principles of cellular and molecular immunology*, OUP.)

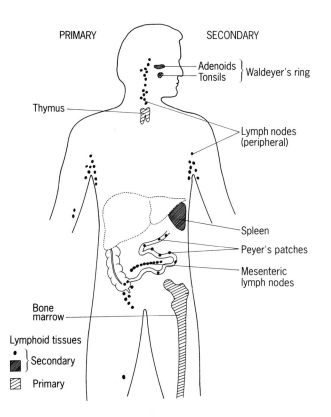

ulcers, periodontal diseases, and even coronary artery disease. In addition to cellular reactions, the T helper cells also help antibody synthesis by providing an additional stimulus to the B cells.

Most infectious agents encountered by the body are prevented from entry by various physical and chemical barriers, which are part of innate immunity. These include the skin and epithelial lining of organs exposed to the exterior, such as the lungs and digestive tract, which synthesize various specially designed protective substances. For example, lysozyme, an enzyme found in many secretions, can break down the cell walls of many bacteria. When micro-organisms penetrate these barriers, they are faced by lymphocytic natural killer cells and the phagocytic cells of the blood and lymphoreticular system.

## Action of phagocytes

The phagocytic macrophages and polymorphonuclear cells engulf and destroy the bacteria using an array of bactericidal mechanisms. Macrophages can secrete powerful cytokines, which have effects on invading organisms as well as stimulating inflammatory responses of other cells. The serum, too, contains a formidable series of biochemical defences, including the complement system. When activated, the latter triggers a complex cascade of enzymatic reactions, the 'complement cascade', which acts to amplify many of the protective devices of innate and acquired immunity. Among other things, components of the complement system recruit polymorphonuclear cells and macrophages to the area, enhance phagocytosis, and combine with antigen–antibody complexes to facilitate the destruction of bacteria and viruses by lysis. All these mechanisms of innate immunity, including phagocytosis and the complement cascade, are an integral part of inflammation — the body's reaction to injury.

Superimposed upon this innate or natural immunity is acquired immunity, which is tailored more precisely to the particular invading organism by producing antibodies and specifically sensitized T cells. Immunity to viruses is largely a T-cell function. This is because, unlike many bacteria, viruses lurk inside living cells out of the reach of antibodies. The cytotoxic T lymphocyte travels through the tissues of the body in an unending search for abnormal cells. Viral infection is signaled by the appearance of foreign antigens at the cell surface. These antigens are recognized by cytotoxic T cells, which attack the infected cell and destroy it, releasing the virus which may then be acted upon by antibodies. Viral infection also induces synthesis of anti-viral proteins, interferons, by other T cells. Interferons are a class of potent cytokines that destroy viruses.

After recovery from an infection the individual retains an immunological memory of the antigens in the form of an expanded clone of B and/or T cells capable of responding to those particular determinants. These memory cells enable the individual to respond to a subsequent infection swiftly and effectively.

The importance of the immune response in combating infection is illustrated by the fact that children born with inherited defects of the immune system succumb to a variety of infectious diseases. For instance, a child born without a thymus gland will fail to develop functional T lymphocytes. The resulting defect renders the infant susceptible to viral and fungal diseases. Children with B-cell defects, who cannot produce immunoglobulins, suffer repeated bacterial infections. In the genetic disease, combined immune deficiency disease, when both T and B cells fail to develop normally, the consequences are even more serious. Often such children have to spend their lives in a sterile environment. Promising investigations suggest that this type of disease may be subject to GENE THERAPY in the near future.

There are also immunodeficiency states which develop as a result of viral infections or from the effects of drugs. The most important of these secondary immunodeficiencies is the acquired immune deficiency syndrome (AIDS), which follows infection with the human immunodeficiency virus. Greater awareness coupled with new drugs directed at the molecular biology of the virus, decreased the death rate from HIV as much as 80% in Europe in 1998, and promising initiatives to develop a 'protective' anti-HIV vaccine are under development.

## Allergy and hypersensitivity

When an immune response occurs in an exaggerated or inappropriate manner and results in tissue injury, this is referred to as allergy or hypersensitivity. The terms were originally meant to describe different phenomena, but time and usage have blurred the distinction and they are now used interchangeably. The discovery that immune reactions can damage the tissues, as well as protect, was made in 1901 by the French physiologists Richet and Poitier when they observed, to their surprise, that the injection of small sublethal doses of toxin did not protect animals from subsequent larger doses, but, on the contrary, rendered them more sensitive. A second injection of a minute and normally innocuous dose caused the animals to collapse and, in some cases, to die. They called this anaphylaxis to distinguish it from phylaxis, or protection.

A mechanism of this kind, known as immediate-type hypersensitivity, underlies many allergic diseases, including such common disorders as hay fever and bronchial ASTHMA. These diseases tend to occur in genetically susceptible individuals and are precipitated by exposure to environmental antigens, which may be inhalants, such as grass pollens or animal dander, or common articles of diet, such as milk or wheat proteins. Immediate-type hypersensitivity is due to a particular class of antibody, immunoglobulin E, which can attach itself to the surface membrane of mast cells in the tissues. The cytoplasm of these cells is closely packed with granules containing potent chemical substances. Antigens entering the tissues combine with antibodies at the surface of the mast cell, triggering the disruption of the cytoplasmic granules. The latter releases pharmacologically active substances which act on small blood vessels, smooth muscle, and mucus-secreting glands. The effect varies with the organ and the species. In man it produces hay fever in the nose and bronchial asthma in the lung. When the antigen is injected, the result may be explosive, inducing acute respiratory or circulatory failure. This so-called anaphylactic shock may lead to collapse and even death in humans, after the injection of an apparently innocuous protein or after a bee sting.

Immediate-type hypersensitivity is but one of several allergic mechanisms. Tissue damage may result from the combination of antibody and antigen to form toxic complexes circulating in the blood. Such complex formation may result in serious disease of the kidneys or the blood vessels, and is not infrequently due to viral antigens. This form of hypersensitivity is known as serum sickness. A related type of injury due to insoluble immune complexes occurs in the tissues and is called the Arthus reaction. There is also the delayed-type hypersensitivity, in which the tissues are injured as a by-product of cell-mediated reactions. This was first discovered by Robert Koch in the 19th century, while he was investigating TUBERCULOSIS. A wide range of human diseases may now be ascribed to reactions of this kind.

### Transplantation, tolerance, and autoimmunity

The immune system responds to foreign antigens and must, therefore, be able to distinguish them from the body's own constituents or self components. The German chemist and pioneer immunologist Paul EHRLICH (p 260) first drew attention to this problem at the end of the 19th century. However, immunologists began to address the matter seriously only after the Second World War, when serious attempts were made to transplant (graft) tissues and organs from one individual (or species) into another. They found that this was not possible, except in identical twins. Transplanted skin, for example, survived perfectly well for a week or so, when it ceased to be viable and was rejected.

The problem was investigated in genetically pure strains of rats and mice, where it was shown that the rejection process was an immune response, mounted against the donor tissue by the recipient. Host lymphocytes become sensitized to antigens in the transplanted tissue, enter the graft, and destroy it. Each individual of a species (apart from sets of identical twins) is genetically unique, and the differences are signaled by a system of antigens known as the major histocompatibility complex. The most important of these, for transplantation, are the class II antigens, which are present on all cells of the body. Elucidation of this problem made it possible to replace diseased organs, such as the kidneys, by transplantation from healthy donors or even cadavers. Donors are now carefully selected to minimize the antigenic differences between the grafted tissues and the host. Administration of immunosuppressive drugs further diminishes the host's rejection response.

In 1953 Sir Peter MEDAWAR (p 819) and his colleagues showed that rejection of skin grafts in mice might be prevented if cells from the donor (or a genetically identical animal) were injected into the prospective recipient while it was still in the womb or shortly after birth. This state of unresponsiveness was called immune tolerance, and we now know that it is maintained by a highly complex mechanism. An important element is that the major histocompatibility complex antigens on cells function as a marker, allowing lymphocytes to recognize 'self' components. An advance in recent years has been the realization that immune tolerance may fail and give rise to diseases in which the body reacts against its own tissues (autoimmunity). These autoimmune diseases — such as rheumatoid arthritis, systemic lupus, and multiple sclerosis — may affect any organ in the body. Many of them occur in genetically susceptible people and some are triggered by viral infections. Although their causes remain largely unknown, treatment of such diseases is often directed at suppression of the immune response by drugs (such as steroids) or even surgically by thymectomy.

The science of immunology has progressed a long way since JENNER (p 452), Pasteur, and Landsteiner. The future of immunological investigation will undoubtedly be bright. Problems that should be amenable to enhanced understanding and ultimate solution include xenotransplantation (transplants between animals), using cells of the immune system to understand the molecular dynamics of signal transduction better, determining the mechanisms of host–microbial interactions, understanding the mechanisms which underlie autoimmune diseases such as diabetes and arthritis, understanding immune components of neoplastic disease, learning more about the complexities of interactions of the immune system with the nervous system and endocrine system that may underlie biological stress, and combining immune specificity with pharmacological efficiency to specifically target drug delivery.

SLei, RLC, DAC

*See also* RHEUMATOLOGY; TRANSPLANTATION

**INBORN ERRORS OF METABOLISM** are a group of over 3000 disorders caused by a mutation in a gene, which is inherited. The term was introduced by Sir Archibald Garrod, a physician who took up the study of urine at the end of the 19th century. In 1897 he first encountered alkaptonuria, a condition which advertises itself most dramatically by the excretion of pitch-black urine. Encountering it in several members of the same family, Garrod was able to explain why some of the members did not develop it after discussing the problem with William Bateson, a botanical friend. They quickly concluded that this disease was inherited according to Mendelian laws but in a recessive fashion. Thus a parent who carried one alkaptonuric gene was unaffected by the disease, but a child who received a gene from each parent developed it.

Inspired by these observations, Garrod studied three other diseases — albinism (the absence of the normal black (melanin) pigment from the skin, hair, and eyes), cystinuria (in which the amino acid cystine is excreted in the urine and may cause kidney stones), and pentosuria (a harmless condition in which a particular form of sugar, xyulose, is excreted in the urine). He used the term inborn errors of metabolism for the first time in his Croonian lectures to the Royal College of Physicians, publishing a second book in 1931, *Inborn factors in disease*, and setting the scene for a biological and medical revolution which has accelerated since that time and which forms the basis of molecular biology today. Garrod suggested that the defect in alkaptonuria was a specific inability to degrade homogentisic acid, the substance that turned urine black. He postulated that this might occur because of the absence of a particular enzyme (a protein catalyst, which accelerates chemical reactions). Nearly 25 years after his death this was shown to be the case, and it has also been demonstrated for many other inborn errors. These include phenylketonuria, a disease in which the enzyme phenylalanine hydroxylase is absent and an excessive amount of the amino acid phenylalanine accumulates in the tissues. Unless the condition is detected very early, giving immediate treatment with a special diet in which phenylaniline is not present, phenylketonuria results in severe mental retardation, accounting for about 1% of cases in the community. Many western countries now carry out routine urine screening tests on every newborn baby.

Other inborn errors include: galactosemia, which affects the metabolism of galactose, a normal constituent of human milk, and if untreated with a special galactose-free diet, may also result in mental deficiency and the formation of cataracts; hypercholesterolemia, one of the most common inherited disorders in humans, in which the body's production of cholesterol is excessive, leading to the extensive formation of ATHEROMA and often death from a heart attack before the age of 25.

Nevertheless, inborn errors of metabolism are not confined to defects in enzymes: they may result from inherited variations of other proteins as well. In sickle cell anemia, for instance, the defect is a single molecular difference between sickle cell hemoglobin and normal hemoglobin (in which the amino acid valine is substituted for the normal glutamic acid at residue number 6 in the beta chain of hemoglobin). The result is that when the blood oxygen concentration becomes lowered the abnormal hemoglobin becomes crystallized and distorts the normal shape, producing a sickle cell appearance. First described by the American physician J. B. Herrick in 1910, sickle cell anemia is marked by periodic attacks of hemolytic anemia (that is, anemia caused by blood destruction) and recurrent severe abdominal and bone pain. Patients with the disease are homozygous for the sickle cell gene, while those who are heterozygous (have inherited only one gene) suffer from a mild form of the disorder. The gene is particularly common in the black population, and the heterozygous trait occurs in about 8% of this group in the USA.

### Types of inheritance

Inborn errors of metabolism may be inherited in one of three ways: *recessively* (in which two genes are present for the condition, one from each parent — for example, cystic fibrosis — *autosomal dominance*, in which a single abnormal gene from one parent will produce the condition — for example, Huntington's disease — or *X-linked*, in which the abnormal gene is carried on the X chromosome (of which there are two in women and one in men) — as in hemophilia or Duchenne muscular dystrophy.

Though many inborn errors of metabolism cause no mental retardation, death, or illness, others do produce serious effects, and in many cases no treatment is available. Much effort has concentrated on early diagnosis in the fetus examining tissue specimens (and particularly DNA) obtained by amniocentesis or chorion villus biopsy and offering early termination of pregnancy if the defect is found. Eventually it is hoped that GENE THERAPY may be the answer to many of the problems raised by these conditions.          AGB

*See also* GENETICS, HUMAN

**INDIA** With its ancient civilization and the invasions and colonialism in recent centuries, one would expect a rich history of medicine and numerous systems of medicine in India. This is so.

## Ancient Indian medicine

The *Atharva Veda*, the last of the four classic treatises handed to man by divinity according to Hindu mythology, embodies information on the maintenance of health and cure of diseases. It has been variously dated from 1600 BC to 600 BC. It mentions fever, consumption, diarrhea, and leprosy among other diseases and contains descriptions of magical practices and herbs for their treatment. The *Atharva Veda* is supplemented by the works left behind by some of the great ancient Indian medical teachers. Chief among them were Caraka, the physician at Taksasila, and Sushruta, the surgeon at Varanasi. The samhitas represent modified versions of their works. Sushruta samhita recommends that a body be placed in a basket and sunk in a river for seven days so as to make it soft and easy for dissection. It describes the existence of 1120 diseases, including smallpox and tuberculosis. Cesarean section, couching of cataracts, removal of vesical calculus, and rhinoplasty were also described. Sushruta described the existence of a thin nerve running by the side of the larynx, the division of which led to hoarseness — a remarkable achievement for those times. He stated that a surgeon needed 20 sharp and 101 blunt instruments and in his *Materia Medica* describes 177 substances of animal origin, 341 of plant origin, and 64 of mineral origin. An oath of initiation is also described.

Ayurveda is the indigenous Indian system of medicine. Prevention of disease is an important aspect with emphasis on hygiene, yoga, and exercise. That hygiene was important to the ancient Indians is obvious from the excellent sanitation systems seen at the excavation sites of the ancient civilizations at Harappa and Mohenjodaro. Similar to the Greek theory of humors, Ayurveda is based on the dosha theory, which maintains that health was dependent on equilibrium among the three doshas — vata (wind), pitta (gall), and kapha (mucus). Vedic India recognized three types of doctors — salya vaidya (surgeons), bhisaks (physicians), and bhisag alharvans (magic doctors).

## The rise of western medicine

As ritual and dogma replaced philosophy in the Hindu religion, and as the caste system took root, the intelligentsia looked down on practices such as anatomical dissections and surgery. The spirit of inquiry was stifled and texts were handed down from generation to generation without any change. Science was replaced by a glib acceptance of ancient theory and practices.

A succession of invasions of northern India further devalued extant medical routines and saw the development of imported variants based on Persian and Arabian practices. Unani was introduced into India around the 11th century AD by the Mughals and Siddha replaced Ayurveda. These, in turn gave way to modern western medicine with the arrival of Europeans to the subcontinent.

The Portuguese were the first to attempt to set up a hospital amid a medical school in Velha Goa. The present Goa Medical College is a continuation of that effort. The first western medical book in India was Garcia d'Orta's *Coloquios dos simples, e drogas de cousas medicinais da India*, published in Goa in 1563. Danish, Dutch, and French settlers made no serious effort at propagating their medical systems. The credit for establishing western medical science on a permanent footing throughout India goes to the British. The INDIAN MEDICAL SERVICE was started in the mid-18th century in Bengal to provide medical care for the soldiers and officers of the East India Company armies, as well as for civilians. Motivated by the need to provide medical attention to their native Indian soldiers and conserve the energies of British physicians to care for their own countrymen who fell victim to tropical diseases, a school for native medical doctors was set up in Calcutta in 1835. A similar school followed in Madras in 1837.

The governor of the Bombay Presidency, Sir Robert Grant, and his able advisor, Dr Charles Morehead, had noted the developments in

## INDIAN MEDICAL SERVICE

The Indian Medical Service (IMS) arose out of the activities of the East India Company, trading in India. The company in its turn came about as a result of a charter granted to the Association of Merchant Adventurers in 1599 by Elizabeth I. By 1614 John Woodall was appointed surgeon-general to the company, and his task was to provide competent surgeons and fit up their chests properly. These surgeons cared for those on shipboard going out east, and also for those employed in India, especially in the trading stations set up there by the company. In 1764 the medical service had military and civil branches, for a navy and army had to be provided to protect the company's interests, especially from the French and Dutch. Hospitals were started and the medical officers were concerned in practice in jails and in mental asylums, as well as with sanitation and public health.

Early in the 19th century acts were passed abolishing the monopoly of the company for trading in India and China. In 1857 there was the Indian Mutiny, after which the British Government took over all the activities of the East India Company. At first the medical services had three establishments in Bombay, Madras, and Bengal, which in 1897 were combined into the general Indian Medical Service, still with military and civil divisions. The Indian Medical Service has a long history of service in many aspects, including medical education. In 1943 an Indian Army Medical Service took away the military branch. In 1947 the Dominions of India and Pakistan were founded and the days of the Indian Medical Service run under British auspices were over.

Calcutta and Madras with considerable interest. They resolved to set up a medical college in Bombay with a difference. Its medical education would produce doctors on a par with those from Britain. The Grant Medical College (and its associated Sir Jamsetjee Jejeebhoy Hospital) was founded in 1845 and it more than fulfilled their expectations, drawing a tribute from the *Lancet* when it eulogized Dr Bhau Daji Lad, one of the first graduates from the college. Dr Morehead was later invited to guide and assist the University of London in improving its own program on medical education. The Government, helped by donations from wealthy Indian merchants, ran all three medical institutes.

HOMEOPATHY made its entry into India when John Martin Honigberger was invited to treat Ranjit Singh, ruler of the Punjab, for paralysis of the vocal cord and edema. The first Homeopathy College was started in 1881 in Calcutta.

## Recent years

In 1944 the Bhore committee, comprising both British and Indian members, and headed by Sir Joseph Bhore, was critical of the British government's role in public health in India. Suggesting that health problems were due to poor living conditions, compounded by the inadequate medical facilities, it called for more medical and paramedical personnel and hospitals to raise healthcare to western levels. The concept of comprehensive healthcare, the primary health center, and that western medicine was appropriate for India were important contributions of the committee.

Since independence the Indian healthcare system has had a definite pattern. The basic units of the system are the primary health centers and their subcenters in the villages and made up of healthcare workers and dais (traditional birth assistants). Secondary care is provided by district hospitals, community health centers, and rural hospitals. At the apex are the tertiary care centers — metropolitan institutions, medical college hospitals, and so on.

Private hospitals and nursing homes are available and account for 70% of healthcare. Health insurance is not common, given that government-run hospitals provide free or inexpensive basic medical care for all. Even advanced treatments, such as bone marrow and cardiac transplants, are available in some of the major medical centers at a fraction of the costs of those in the West. Moreover, drugs are also comparatively inexpensive in India. Non-government organizations are run on a 'not for profit' basis and provide inexpensive generic drugs. Associations of doctors now have crucial roles in furthering public health and preventive medicine, as for example when

pediatricians campaigned to abolish advertisements for breast milk substitutes by powerful multinational companies and championed instead breast-feeding. The development of oral rehydration therapy for diarrhea is another example.

Some institutes that have rendered a yeoman service are the Christian Medical College, Vellore (started by Ida Scudder); the All India Institute of Medical Sciences, New Delhi; the Post Graduate Institute of Medical Education and Research, Chandigarh; the Tata Memorial Centre, Bombay; and the National Institute for Mental Health and Neurosciences, Bangalore.

Ayurveda is still a popular treatment among Hindus, particularly in the rural areas, where most use only this system of medicine. Expense may dictate the form of treatment, especially when the alternative for a villager is expensive allopathic treatment or traveling large distances to visit a modern hospital. Siddha medicine is practiced mainly in Tamil Nadu, being characterized by the importance of the pulse in diagnosis and the therapeutic use of a substance called kuppu and metals such as mercury, iron, and zinc.

Homeopathy flourishes and has overtaken Ayurveda, Unani, and Siddha in popularity. Indeed, some practitioners of modern medicine have either supplemented their practice with homeopathy or have abandoned allopathic medicine in its favor. The reverse is also true, with many graduates of indigenous systems practicing allopathy. However, a 1996 Supreme Court ruling has made such cross-practice illegal. Bone setting, herbal medicine, exorcism, cautery, and branding are all still prevalent in parts of the country.

## Education

There is now a plethora of medical colleges in both the public and private sectors. The Medical Council of India and its counterparts in each of the Indian states serve the same functions as the General Medical Council in Britain. Unfortunately, the comparison ends there, standards in India being far below those in western nations.

Since the 1830s medical education and research have mainly been under the control of the state or central governments. Recently, however, the private sector has made rapid inroads, though the standards leave much to be desired. There are currently about 150 medical schools and 15 000 medical graduates every year in western medicine. Standard western textbooks are used, though Indian textbooks are also popular. The basic degree is the MB, BS, while most institutes offer MD or MS degrees for specialized courses. There are 410 000 allopaths and 510 000 practitioners of Indian systems of medicine in India.

Ayurveda and Unani medical colleges continue to function in India. Today, there are over 150 000

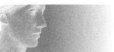
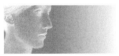

homeopaths and 110 degree colleges with 12 post-graduate colleges in India. There are currently more than a hundred Ayurveda colleges. Medical education in the public sector is inexpensive since the government subsidizes education given its belief that lack of funds should not deter students from pursuing a career in medicine. Many of these students, often the cream, emigrate to the USA, Britain, Australia, or European countries for want of adequate openings and/or facilities to pursue their academic interests.

## Research

The departure of British teachers and administrators in 1947 left a void that is still evident. The many scholarly treatises on a wide range of tropical diseases, epidemiological and other surveys of the whole country, and research conducted at laboratories such as the Haffkine Institute in Bombay, the Institutes for Tropical Medicine and Hygiene at Calcutta, and the Institute at Guindy in Madras remain unequaled models.

In an attempt to encourage medical research, the Government has set up four separate funding agencies — the Indian Council of Medical Research, the Department of Science and Technology, the Department of Biotechnology, and the Council of Scientific and Industrial Research. The first has created 21 institutes and five regional centers for specialized studies, for example, the Institute for Research in Reproduction (currently working on a vaccine against pregnancy) and the Malaria Research Institute in New Delhi.

These funding agencies disburse sums that are large by Indian standards. Critics have pointed to a poor cost–benefit ratio from this largesse, pointing to the paucity of publications that command a high international citation rate, as well as patents and processes transferred to industry. The Indian Council of Medical Research annual budget is Rs 350 million (about US$9 million), some 0.0035% of the country's gross domestic product.

The low priority given to research, along with corruption, bureaucracy, archaic infrastructure, and poor libraries compel many young scientists and physicians to go abroad. That Indians are intelligent and can work hard is evident given that researchers and physicians who migrate to western countries perform well. The Indian-born scientists who have achieved fame abroad include Yellapragada Subba Row, discoverer of aureomycin, and Hargobind Khorana, molecular biologist and winner of the NOBEL PRIZE for physiology or medicine in 1968.

Indian researchers working in India who have contributed to international science include R. J. Vakil, who introduced the anti-hypertensive drug reserpine in 1949; V. R. Khanolkar, who carried out pioneering work on leprosy; Upendra Brahmachari, who discovered the use of urea-stibamine against kala-azar in 1922; S. N. De, who showed the existence of an exotoxin in *Vibrio cholerae* in 1953; V. N. Shirodkar, who introduced cervical cerclage to prevent abortion. European doctors who contributed while working in India include Ronald ROSS (p 481), who, as an IMS officer in 1898, discovered the malarial parasite in the mosquito Anopheles. Waldemar Haffkine, who developed vaccines against cholera and the plague in 1893 and 1896, respectively; and Charles Donovan, who discovered trypanosomes in the splenic pulp while at Madras Medical College in 1903. Sir C. V. Raman, India's only Nobel prize winner in science (physics 1930), also carried out pioneering studies on color and vision.

More recent scientific contributions include A. S. Paintal's research on the J-receptor in the lungs; Noshir Wadia's research on craniovertebral anomalies, tuberculous meningitis, hereditary cerebellar ataxias, epidemic conjunctivitis, atlanto-axial dislocations, and nutritional and parasitic diseases of the nervous system. P. K. Sethi's work on an artificial foot (Jaipur foot), which was made for rural Indian conditions, has found its application in several countries ravaged by LANDMINES. Other important contributions have been made by V. Ramalingaswami on protein-energy malnutrition and goiter, and C. Gopalan on malnutrition; Darab Dastur on central nervous system tumors, tubercular meningitis, and nutritional disease; Dharmendra on leprosy; and R. N. Chopra on medicinal plants in India.

India still lives in its villages and work on community health has been done by Noshir Antia at Mandwa, Mabel, and Rajnikant Arole in Jamkhed in Maharashtra state, and the group SEWA (Self-employed Women's Association) Rural in Gujarat state. Basic research is carried out at the Indian Institute of Science, Bangalore; the Tata Institute of Fundamental Research, Bombay; the Centre for Cellular and Molecular Biology, Hyderabad; the National Institute of Immunology, New Delhi; and the National Institute for Nutrition, Hyderabad. The continual emphasis is to produce much needed life-saving medical and biological devices of international standard at low cost. The artificial heart valve and synthetic bags for blood invented at the Sree Chitra Thirunal Institute, Thiruvananthapuram, as well as the cerebrospinal fluid shunts devised at the All India Institute of Medical Sciences and the Sanjay Gandhi Post-graduate Institute, Lucknow are examples.

The *Transactions of the Medical and Physical Society of Calcutta* was India's first medical journal, established in 1823. There are now about 125 biomedical journals in India, of which about twenty are included in the *Index Medicus*, and three in the *Science Citation Index*. Indian scientists, who form the third largest pool of researchers in the world, publish half the number of articles from the third world. Most of the exceptionally good papers (about 2% of the total) are published in foreign journals. Nevertheless, probably only 5% of doctors read journals.

## Women in medicine

The first woman to become a doctor in India was Anandibai Gopal Joshi, who traveled to the Woman's Medical College of Philadelphia, graduating in the class of 1886. Her thesis was entitled *Obstetrics among the Aryan Hindoos*. Unfortunately she died of pulmonary tuberculosis soon after her return to India.

Women gained entry into Indian medical colleges in the 1880s. Their entry was not as painful or frustrating as that of their counterparts in Britain or the USA. The Grant Medical College, Bombay, for example, opened its doors to women for the medical course in 1888, the first woman to graduate being Freny Cama in 1892. Between 1892 and 1915, 63 Indian women obtained this degree. There are now more women than men in each class in many medical colleges, while women also head many teaching departments.

## Medical ethics

The samhitas are especially noteworthy for their strong ethical, religious, and philosophical principles. Philosophy formed the basis of ethical pronouncements in Ayurveda. Ayur defines the purpose of classical Indian medicine as the prolongation and preservation of life. Veda anchors the science within the Hindu religious tradition. Ayurveda was a secondary science (upanga) linked to the *Atharvar Veda*.

Above all, Ayurveda aimed at the attainment of salvation by which man realizes the identity of the individual soul with the universal consciousness and thus rises above unhappiness, pain, and mortal destruction. The goal of Ayurveda is the cultivation of a sound mind in a healthy body as a means towards ensuring the welfare of the soul and ending the cycle of rebirths. Zimmer summed it up well: 'Ayurveda carefully gathered and sifted the rich inheritance from the preceding generations and interrelated the philosophic background of medicine with religious thought, spiritual life, and ideals'.

The ancient Indian teachers laid down guidelines for the essential qualities of a teacher, who may study medicine, the duties of a teacher and the student, and detailed codes of conduct that continue to command respect.

Despite this heritage from ancient masters, medical ethics remains in the doldrums, with St John's Medical College, Bangalore, being the only teaching institute offering a structured course on the subject. There is but one journal on the subject — *Issues in Medical Ethics* — published quarterly from Bombay.

However, health and education have never been a priority for most Indian politicians. Analysts agree that as long as we fail to give these two portfolios the importance they deserve, many of India's problems are likely to persist.　　SKP

*See also* DEMOGRAPHY; HEALTHCARE SYSTEMS

## INFECTIOUS DISEASES — HISTORY

Infectious diseases are probably the oldest recognized disease of man. Evidence of LEPROSY can be found on corpses from China and mummies from ancient Egypt dating from the 2nd century BC. PLAGUE, a bacterial infection transmitted by rat fleas, often referred to as the BLACK DEATH, is mentioned throughout history. Between 1348 and 1720 there were at least 10 plague pandemics in Europe, which are claimed to have caused the deaths of approximately 25 million people. In the Great Plague of London in 1665 at least 70 000 were infected, many of whom died. SMALLPOX, a lethal virus infection which has now been eradicated from the world, was described in India and China in pre-Christian times. The mummified head of the Pharaoh Rameses V, who died around 1160 BC, had lesions on the skin which were very similar to those left by smallpox. This infection has an additional place in history in that in the eighteenth century the English doctor Edward JENNER (p 452) was the first to demonstrate immunization. He inoculated a boy with fluid taken from lesions on the skin of a milkmaid infected with cowpox (a similar but much milder infection than smallpox). Jenner subsequently proved that the boy was immune to smallpox. This vaccine was eventually responsible for the total eradication of smallpox — the first time that a disease has been wiped out intentionally. However, at the time of writing, two laboratories, one in America and the second in Russia, retain smallpox virus for research purposes and there is concern that other countries might have 'illicit' stocks of the virus for use as potential bioterrorism weapons.

The invention of the microscope by Van LEEUWENHOEK (p 489) in Holland in the 17th century allowed visualization of the larger bacteria for the first time. However, these were not identified and classified until two centuries later. The introduction of the electron microscope in the 20th century allowed the visualization of viruses.

Many factors influence national and international patterns of infectious diseases which are commonly associated with WAR and insurrection. Hepatitis caused serious problems for Allied

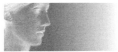

**CAUSE OF SCARLET FEVER**

Gladys **DICK** (1881–1963), with her husband George Dick demonstrated that scarlet fever is caused by hemolytic streptococci (1923) and developed a skin test ('Dick test') for susceptibility to the disease. For this they were nominated for the Nobel prize in 1925, but no prize in physiology or medicine was awarded that year.

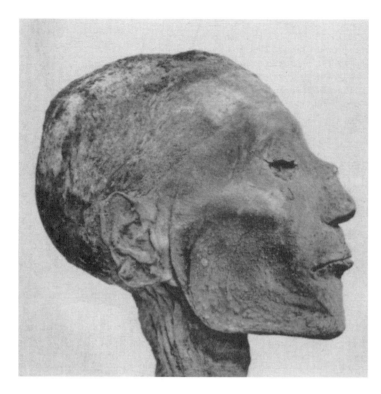

Mummy of Rameses V. The lesions on the face are suggestive of smallpox. (Reproduced, with permission, from Dixon, C. W. (1962). *Smallpox*, J & A Churchill.)

and infections in patients made particularly susceptible by modern medical and surgical techniques such as cancer therapy and organ TRANSPLANTATION. Travel by air has facilitated the importation into countries with temperate climates of infections such as MALARIA normally encountered only in the tropics. The number of travelers each year in the world is over one billion. Approximately 30 million people travel abroad from Britain each year, of whom nearly half a million visit Africa and a quarter of a million visit India. More than 50 000 cases of imported malaria are diagnosed in Europe each year.

The ever-changing spectrum of infectious diseases is illustrated by the fact that, whereas smallpox was eradicated in 1978, several new infections have been recognized. These include food-poisoning caused by bacteria such as *Campylobacter* and *Escherichia coli* 0157, Legionnaires' disease (a type of pneumonia caused by another previously unknown bacterium), and Lyme disease, a bacterial (spirochetal) infection transmitted by ticks from deer to man. The *legionella* bacillus usually originates in the environment (for example, water or air-conditioning systems), while *Campylobacter* and *E. coli* 0157 are acquired by humans from animals, especially cattle, via meat or contact.

The interrelationship between man and animals in the context of infectious disease is remarkably close. Infections contracted directly by man from vertebrate animals are referred to as zoonoses; anthrax, a potentially fatal infection contracted from cattle, and rabies, which is almost invariably fatal, are examples. The acquired immune deficiency syndrome (AIDS), caused by the human immunodeficiency virus (HIV), was first recognized in 1981. The best evidence suggests that HIV is probably a variant of a monkey virus; hence it is also a zoonosis. It was estimated (in 2001) that there are well over 30 million people infected with the virus and 6 million new infections per year. There were 2.3 million deaths attributable to HIV in 1997 alone.

Two zoonoses have been recognized recently. The first, which appeared in the south-west of the United States in the early 1990s, is the hantavirus pulmonary syndrome caused by a virus (hantavirus) transmitted to man from small mammals such as the cotton rat. The infection, a hemorrhagic fever, has a mortality rate of around 30%; there is no effective vaccine against the infection and no cure available. The other newly recognized zoonosis is new variant CREUTZFELDT–JAKOB DISEASE (nvCJD), a rapidly progressive degenerative brain disease which resembles bovine spongiform encephalopathy and is probably contracted by humans by eating beef contaminated with the causative agent of bovine spongiform

troops during the North African campaign in the Second World War. In South-East Asia during the same war there were large outbreaks of dysentery (a diarrheal disease) amongst both Japanese and Allied forces. It is claimed that the availability of sulfonamides (which cured dysentery) to the Allied forces, but not the Japanese, prevented the invasion of Australia. Malnutrition and poverty go hand in hand with infection, leading to a decreased ability to withstand and overcome infection usually exacerbated by a lack of preventive and treatment facilities.

During the 20th century there were many changes in the pattern of infectious disease in developed countries: the traditional contagions such as DIPHTHERIA and POLIOMYELITIS have virtually disappeared, principally as a result of immunization. Indeed, there were hopes that, by 2000, POLIOMYELITIS might have followed smallpox as the second disease to be eradicated. The deadline for this has, however, been deferred as the WORLD HEALTH ORGANIZATION eradication program is behind schedule. Infections caused by bacteria have been controlled by antibiotics. In developed countries many infections have decreased, or even disappeared, while others have become more prominent. Examples of the latter include food poisoning caused by salmonellae, related mainly to the broiler-chicken industry,

encephalopathy, an infectious protein called a prion (*pr* = protein: *i* = infectious). It is probable that cattle acquired the disease by being fed the offal of sheep contaminated with another prion-associated disease called scrapie. Some 104 cases of new variant Creutzfeldt–Jacob disease had been recognized by the end of 2000, 100 in the UK.

AMG

**INFECTIOUS DISEASES** are caused by living organisms. Most are referred to as 'micro-organisms' as they can be visualized only with a microscope: the main groups of micro-organisms are viruses, bacteria, and fungi. There are three other groups, named chlamydiae, rickettsiae, and mycoplasmas, which are intermediate between viruses and bacteria: they cause various infections, the commonest being pneumonia. Whereas chlamydiae, rickettsiae, and mycoplasmas are uni-cellular organisms, viruses are not cells in the true sense — they rely upon the cells of the host (human or animal) for replication and pro-pagation. Some infections are caused by larger multicellular organisms — the helminths or WORMS. The organisms causing infection range in size from tiny viruses, which can be seen only with the aid of an electron microscope, to worms which can be several centimeters long and visible to the naked eye.

Terms synonymous with 'infectious diseases' included contagious diseases and communicable diseases. Not all infections are readily trans-missible — some can originate within an individual's own body.

### Organisms causing infection

Table 1 gives details of the principal micro-organisms causing infection. These are bacteria, viruses, chlamydiae, rickettsiae, mycoplasmas, fungi, and protozoa. The helminths (or worms) include threadworms, roundworms, tapeworms, and worms causing certain tropical diseases such as SCHISTOSOMIASIS. The size of organisms causing infection varies from 0.01 μm (viruses) to many centimeters (worms). Whereas viruses contain either DNA or RNA, the other micro-organisms incorporate both in their structure.

The source of an infectious disease may be another human, an insect, a bird or animal, or an inanimate (non-living) source. Transmission of infection occurs by several routes. Most impor-tant are airborne spread, physical contact, inocu-lation (by needle or insect), or by food and drink. Certain infections such as German measles (rubella) and HIV infection can be contracted through the placenta by the unborn fetus.

Organisms enter the body either by inhalation into the lungs, ingestion (swallowing), or via direct contact (skin or mucous membranes). SEX-UALLY TRANSMITTED DISEASES are transmitted by contact between the mucous membranes of the genital tract. Table 2 illustrates the routes by which various infectious diseases are spread.

The incubation period of an infection is the time between micro-organisms entering the body and symptoms developing. This varies from a few hours, as in certain types of food poisoning, to several or more years, as in HIV infection.

### Pathogenicity of micro-organisms

The term 'pathogenicity' refers to mechanisms whereby micro-organisms cause infection. Certain organisms, such as the common cold viruses, never penetrate below the surface of the mucous membrane (superficial lining) of the nose and throat, while others reach the deep tissues and bloodstream, causing potentially life-threatening septicemia (blood-poisoning). Organisms may produce infection either on their own or via toxins, substances which bacteria release into tissues and bloodstream. Examples of toxin-mediated diseases are diphtheria and tetanus; the bacteria remain at the site of the infection but their toxins circulate in the blood and cause serious effects on the heart and nervous system. The CHOLERA bacterium (*Vibrio cholerae*) causes its effects by producing a toxin that inter-

**Table 1** Micro-organisms

| Type of microbe | Infections caused | Approximate size (μm) | Visible by light microscope |
|---|---|---|---|
| Viruses (e.g. human immunodeficiency virus) | Influenza, colds, measles, rubella, chickenpox, HIV infection, rabies | 0.01–0.3 | No |
| Chlamydia (e.g. *C. pneumoniae*) | Pneumonia Trachoma (cause of blindness) Genital infections | 0.3 | No |
| Rickettsiae (e.g. *R. prowazeki*) | Typhus fever | 0.3 | Sometimes just visible using special stains |
| Mycoplasmas (e.g. *M. pneumoniae*) | Pneumonia | 0.12–0.3 | Sometimes just visible using special stains |
| Bacteria (e.g. *Staphylococcus aureus*) | Wound infections Skin infections Throat infections Pneumonia Endocarditis Septicemia | 0.5–0.8 | Yes |
| Fungi (e.g. *Candida albicans*) | Oral thrush | Larger than bacteria (>5) | Yes |
| Protozoa (e.g. *Plasmodium vivax*; *Giardia lamblia*) | Malaria (plasmodia) Diarrhea (giardia) | Larger than fungi | Yes |

**Table 2** Transmission of infection

| By ingestion (food + drink) | By inhalation | By physical contact |
|---|---|---|
| Food poisoning | Measles, mumps, rubella, influenza | Skin infection (e.g. impetigo) |
| *Salmonella* infection | *Legionella* infection | Sexually transmitted diseases (e.g. |
| Dysentery | Meningococcal meningitis | Gonorrhea, syphilis, and HIV infection) |
| Hepatitis A | | Pneumonia |
| Cholera | | |

| By inoculation | | From birds and other animals | | Transplacental (mother to fetus) |
|---|---|---|---|---|
| By needle: | hepatitis B | Direct: | rabies (dogs) | Rubella (German measles) |
| | HIV infection | | psittacosis (birds) | Toxoplasmosis |
| | | | | *Listeria* infection |
| By insect: | malaria | Indirect: | worms (soil) | Syphilis; cytomegalovirus infection |
| | yellow fever | | toxoplasmosis (cats' feces in soil) | HIV infection |

feres with biochemical mechanisms in the lining of the bowel, leading to the release of large volumes of fluid and electrolytes, causing dehydration and, if untreated, often death.

Certain organisms have a predilection for specific organs or tissue of the body. The pneumococcus causes pneumonia, the meningococcus meningitis, and the gonococcus gonorrhea. The pneumococcus can also cause meningitis.

Infection by one organism may reduce the body's defenses to allow the invasion of another. An example is the influenza virus, which causes severe inflammation of the mucous membrane of the bronchi (tubes leading to the lungs), allowing *Staphylococcus aureus*, a bacterium which resides in the nose or throat of healthy people, to cause pneumonia.

The human body is divided into microbiologically 'clean' and 'dirty' areas. The 'dirty' areas are those that have contact with the outside world such as the skin and bowel. In health, almost all of the other organs and tissues in the body (such as heart, brain, muscles) are sterile (free from microorganisms). Any breakdown in the body's defenses against infection may allow organisms, usually bacteria, from the contaminated parts of the body to penetrate the clean areas. An example is provided by peritonitis secondary to perforation of the large bowel.

Certain micro-organisms, present in the healthy body, seldom cause infection. These are referred to as commensal organisms as opposed to pathogenic organisms, which are the recognized causes of infection. Commensals such as *Staphylococcus epidermidis*, an organism present on the healthy skin, usually causes infection only when the body's defense systems are reduced by disease or treatment. A patient whose resistance to infection is significantly impaired is referred to as being immunocompromised. An example is provided by a sufferer from leukemia who may have no normal white blood cells to combat infection, or a cancer patient being treated with radiotherapy and/or cell-poisoning drugs which depress the immune system. AIDS patients are immunosuppressed because the human immunodeficiency virus (HIV) depresses the immune system (see below).

### The body's response to a micro-organism

The fact that a micro-organism has entered the body does not necessarily mean that a disease process (infection) will result. The organism may be repelled on the surface of the body (skin or mucous membranes) by mechanical barriers or by natural chemical compounds. Should an organism overcome the superficial defenses of the body and pass into the tissues, organs, or bloodstream, it is met by a complex defense mechanism called the immune system (see IMMUNOLOGY). This has two main components — white blood cells (polymorphs, lymphocytes, and macrophages) and various chemical components that interact with these cells. Whether or not an infection results, depends on the capacity of the body's defenses to kill the organism.

Having entered the human body, a micro-organism may:

- be eliminated by the host defenses without stimulating the immune system
- be repelled by the defenses (and, at the same time, cause a reaction by the immune system) without producing symptoms
- cause an infection associated with signs and symptoms and, at the same time, stimulate the immune system

The symptoms of an infection are not caused primarily by the micro-organism but by the reaction of the body's defense system. For example, fever, the most common manifestation of an infectious disease, is produced by the release into

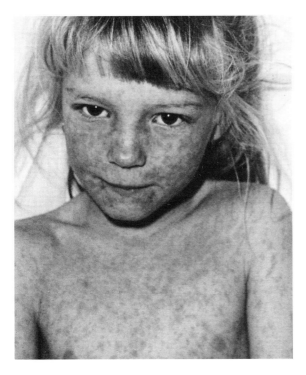

(a)

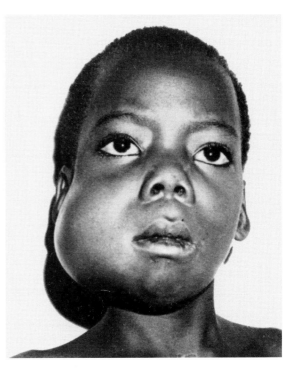

(b)

the body of proteins known as cytokines triggered by the infecting micro-organism. The intravenous injection of these substances can produce symptoms almost identical to those associated with influenza. Viruses stimulate host cells to produce interferons, which have antiviral properties and play a part in overcoming viral infections.

If the body's response to infection is exaggerated as a result of invasion by a particularly virulent organism (for example, the meningococcus), an excessive and uncontrolled reaction may result which can lead to bleeding, shock, and death. If the invading organism has stimulated the body's immune system, with or without symptoms developing, immunity (resistance) to that micro-organism develops. This results from the organism leaving an 'imprint' on the memory of the immune system which repels subsequent challenge by the same organism and thus prevents it from causing an infection. One of the mechanisms employed by the immune system to combat infection is the production of antibodies against specific organisms. These are Y-shaped proteins produced by lymphocytes which bind to micro-organisms and either neutralize them or mark them out for destruction by cells of the immune system. While an immune response with antibody production occurs readily with organisms that invade the body, those that produce only surface

infections, for example, common cold viruses, do not stimulate lasting immunity. Other infections, such as influenza, may stimulate immunity only to one of the many subgroups of an organism and not to other members of the same group. This explains why an attack of influenza (unlike, for example, measles, which has only one strain of the virus which induces lifelong immunity to the infection) does not protect against future attacks by a different strain of the influenza virus. It also explains why the influenza vaccine recommended one year may not protect against strains of the virus causing epidemics in future years.

Although most organisms are eradicated from the body once an infection has been overcome, in some instances they can persist in the body for life. The *Herpes simplex* virus, which causes 'cold sores' around the mouth, and *Toxoplasma gondii* (toxoplasmosis), a protozoal organism transmitted to man by healthy cats and meat, are examples of 'persistent' organisms. Another is the varicella-zoster virus, which causes chickenpox in childhood and may reactivate in later life as shingles. Recovery from TUBERCULOSIS is followed by the development of a dormant state in which the bacterium persists in the body without causing symptoms. It has been estimated that one third of the population of the world has the tuberculosis bacterium in their bodies.

Contemporary manifestations of viral infections: (a) shows a child with measles, and (b) shows a seven-year-old boy with Burkitt's lymphoma involving the right mandible. (From Collier, L. and Oxford, J. (2000). *Human virology,* 2nd edn, OUP.)

Table 3 Vaccines

| Vaccines for childhood | Vaccines for travel | Other vaccines (for occupational or specific uses) |
|---|---|---|
| Measles | Typhoid fever | Hepatitis B |
| Mumps | Hepatitis A | Pneumococcal |
| Rubella | Yellow fever | Influenza |
| Chickenpox* | (Cholera)† | Anthrax |
| Diphtheria | Rabies | |
| Tetanus | Japanese encephalitis | |
| Whooping cough | | |
| Poliomyelitis | | |
| *Hemophilus influenzae* type B | | |
| BCG (tuberculosis) | | |
| Meningococcal ‡ type C | | |

* Not yet available in Britain
† Not recommended as it is relatively ineffective
‡ Not effective against the most common strain (type B) of meningococcus in Britain

Immunosuppression can reactive these persistent or latent pathogens, which are common causes of death in AIDS patients.

### Signs and symptoms of infection

Fever is the cardinal sign of infection. This is commonly associated with non-specific symptoms such as headache and aching in the muscles (myalgia). The signs and symptoms of infection vary according to the nature of the illness and the bodily systems involved. Certain of the common infections of childhood such as measles, are associated with rash; food-poisoning organisms cause diarrhea. If the lungs are involved the patient will have a cough and may be breathless. Meningitis produces headache and sometimes unconsciousness. Skin infection is associated with abscess formation ('boils'); these contain pus — a mixture of bacteria and dead white blood cells.

*Non-specific* treatments for infection include medications such as aspirin which relieve headache or reduce fever. *Specific* therapy, which depends on antimicrobial agents, has revolutionized the treatment of infections caused by bacteria. They have also had a significant effect on fungal and protozoal infections but, as yet, are relatively ineffective against most viral diseases.

### Antimicrobial therapy

Although antibiotics have transformed the treatment of infectious diseases and saved many millions of lives, there are problems associated with their use. These are:

- Although antibiotics are effective against bacteria, fungi, and protozoa, there are relatively few antiviral agents and those that are available, such as acyclovir (used to treat shingles) and zidovudine (also known as AZT or Retrovir, used for HIV infection), do not eradicate viruses from the body but only suppress the disease process. There are no antiviral drugs that are effective against common infections such as measles or a cold.

- Many bacteria, and also certain viruses, fungi, and protozoa, which were previously sensitive to available antibiotics have developed resistance to them. *Staphylococcus aureus*, the first bacterium to become resistant to penicillin (in the 1950s), is now resistant to many other antibiotics. Multi-resistant strains known as methicillin-resistant *Staphylococcus aureus* (MRSA) are causing serious problems, especially in debilitated patients. Other examples of resistant organisms include penicillin-resistant pneumococci (the most common cause of pneumonia), *E. coli* (the most frequent cause of urinary-tract infection), and *Plasmodium falciparum* (the cause of severe and potentially fatal malaria). An alarming prospect is the increase in resistance of *Mycobacterium tuberculosis*, the cause of tuberculosis, to anti-tuberculous drugs. The AIDS virus has developed resistance to zidovudine. To control HIV infection and prevent resistance developing, zidovudine is now given in combination with newer antiviral agents such as lamivudine. Such is the international concern about microbial resistance that the British House of Lords (1998) and the US Congress (1995) have produced reports on this topic.

- No antibiotic is totally free from side-effects, which can range from a mild rash to liver and kidney failure or, rarely, death from anaphylaxis as with penicillin.

- Antibiotics are expensive drugs which contribute a large share to the drug bill in developed countries. In developing countries, because of their cost, many antibiotics are either not available or not readily available.

### Prevention and diagnosis

*Non-specific* Non-specific measures to prevent infection include food hygiene, hand-washing, clean water supplies, and the provision of isolation facilities. In the past, individuals who had been in contact with a serious infection such as diphtheria or smallpox were isolated until the incubation period of the infection had expired. The procedure, known as QUARANTINE, is seldom used today. Health education in the form of advice about sexual health is the basis of AIDS prevention campaigns.

*Specific* Specific measures involve the use of vaccines or, in certain infections, antimicrobial drugs. Antiseptics and disinfectants are also important in the prevention of infection.

There are several types of vaccine (Table 3). One consists of bacteria or viruses which have been inactivated (killed), usually by a chemical process. Whooping cough (pertussis) vaccine is an example. Another, exemplified by poliomyelitis vaccine, contains living micro-organisms, usually viruses, whose virulence has been weakened to enable them to stimulate immunity without causing disease. A third form of vaccine, called a toxoid, contains inactivated toxins, the chemical substances produced by bacteria such as those causing diphtheria or tetanus. Vaccines mimic infections without causing disease and 'trick' the immune system into responding to them, thus producing immunity to the infection.

Unlike the infectious diseases themselves, vaccines usually produce immunity of only limited duration, necessitating repeated doses (boosters). Those that contain inactivated organisms or toxins are generally very safe with few side-effects and can be given to all individuals. 'Live' vaccines, although generally safe, cannot be given during pregnancy as they may theoretically damage the fetus, or to the immunosuppressed, in whom they can cause clinical infection.

Vaccines take several weeks to provide protection against infectious disease, as the immune system has to react and produce antibodies and other protective mechanisms. Immediate protection can be provided by the injection of preformed antibodies obtained from patients recovering from an infection (for example, hepatitis B) or from pooled human blood donations (for example, hepatitis A).

Antimicrobial drugs are employed in selected infections to prevent infection developing. The best-known example is the use of antimalarial drugs to prevent malaria in travellers. Drugs used to prevent infections are called prophylactic agents.

Although some infectious diseases can be diagnosed by the clinician without recourse to ancillary aids, many require the use of a MICROBIOLOGY laboratory for the identification of the infecting organism and the determination (if indicated) of its sensitivity to antimicrobial agents.

It may be possible for the microbiology laboratory to make an immediate diagnosis of the cause of an infection, by collecting a specimen such as pus or sputum and staining it with an appropriate dye (Gram's stain is the most common); the type of organism may be suggested in this way. However, in order to make a definitive diagnosis it is usually necessary for the specimen to be cultured in an incubator to allow the organism to grow; this can take 24 or even 48 hours. For tuberculosis it may be several weeks before the organism can be identified. In most viral infections the diagnosis is made by examining the patient's blood for antibodies to the suspected micro-organism (for example, HIV); these take a week or more to appear. The diagnosis is therefore retrospective.

Various radiological techniques, such as chest X-rays or scans, may be helpful to confirm the diagnosis of infection. They are especially useful in localizing deep pockets of infection, such as abscesses.

## Infection in developing countries

Most developing countries are in the tropics or sub-tropics, where infection is a common cause of illness and death, especially in children. Of particular importance are the classic infectious diseases such as diphtheria, poliomyelitis, measles, and tetanus, which have almost been eradicated from the developed world. Lack of clean water results in the spread of infections contracted from food and water, such as hepatitis and dysentery. Diarrheal diseases and respiratory tract infections are the commonest causes of illness and death in children in the developing world. Tuberculosis is another common cause of death and is often associated with HIV infection. World-wide there are around eight million new cases of tuberculosis and three million deaths each year, the majority in the developing world.

In 2001 it was estimated that between 30 and 40 million people worldwide were infected with the HIV, of whom at least 10 million had developed AIDS. The majority of those infected with HIV live in developing countries. In many sub-Saharan African countries up to 10% of adults are infected with the virus; in Zimbabwe and Botswana this figure is 25%.

Diseases peculiar to the tropics include malaria, leprosy, and worm infestations, such as schistosomiasis (causing liver and bladder disease) and filariasis (a cause of blindness). Malaria occurs in 100 countries and one-half of the population of the world is at risk of contracting it. There are 250 million cases diagnosed every year and 2 million die. The burden of infection in these countries is exacerbated by malnutrition.

## The future

If global warming becomes a reality there could be a significant alteration in the geographical distribution of infection. For example, an increase in environmental temperatures in Europe could result in the migration northwards of insects, such as mosquitoes carrying malaria.

The part that micro-organisms play in the causation of diseases not at present recognized as having a microbial etiology is of increasing interest. The discovery that *Helicobacter pylori* is associated with peptic ulcers has prompted a search for microbial causes for diseases with no known cause such as rheumatoid arthritis and multiple sclerosis. There is a suggestion that coronary artery disease may be associated with *Mycoplasma pneumoniae* infection.

The prospect of bioterrorism — the use of micro-organisms for warfare or acts of terrorism — is a cause for concern. Potential organisms for this purpose include the smallpox virus and the bacteria which cause botulism, anthrax, and plague. AMG

*See also* BIOLOGICAL AND CHEMICAL WARFARE; MICROBIOLOGY

**INFORMED CONSENT** In modern medical practice and research, informed consent is a legal necessity and an ethical imperative, but this was not so until after the middle of the 20th century. Traditionally, the medical profession was paternalist and secretive, upholding an ancient belief that physicians possess special knowledge and skills withheld from all others. While the knowledge and skills were not trade secrets, the mystique attached to them was integral to the healing process, and this justified an authoritarian approach to caring for sick people. Patients and their families were excluded from a decision-making role even in life or death matters. By early in the 20th century, however, the rise of new values in a literate society began to induce a change in the nature of the doctor–patient relationship: patients and their kin began to request, even to demand, a share of decision-making, especially when surgical operations or other invasive interventions were required in the management of their diseases.

Around the mid 20th century, two disciplines, LAW and BIOETHICS, began to bring about a change in the attitude of the medical profession to those who sought help with their ailments. Court cases in which patients or their kin sued doctors when untoward events followed medical interventions they had not understood, produced a growing body of case law that obliged physicians to ensure that all invasive procedures were carried out only with the consent of the patient or responsible person.

The expanding discipline of bioethics provided a foundation of moral theory to underpin the increasing insistence on obtaining formal consent for medical interventions. The evolution of modern concepts of informed consent is discussed in a monograph by Ruth Faden and Tom L. Beauchamp, *A history and theory of informed consent* (1986); this has become an essential reference for lawyers, ethicists, and physicians who have to know and understand the process.

### Cultural variations

There are considerable cultural variations in the extent to which patients and their doctors share in choices and decisions about alternatives in provision of medical care. In the English-speaking world, particularly in the USA, there is far greater insistence on respecting autonomy, the right to make free choices and decisions, than there is among people of comparable educational and socio-economic level in Latin America or southern Europe, where the notion that 'doctor knows best' remains strong. Consequently, medical practice remains more authoritarian and paternalist in those countries than in the USA. Concepts of personal autonomy are foreign to some traditional tribal communities, for example, in parts of Africa

## THE GREAT KILLERS: INFLUENZA

Influenza is an acute viral illness occurring in sporadic epidemic and pandemic outbreaks. Pandemics, affecting many continents, have occurred at intervals varying from 8 to 18 years throughout the 20th century, and probably often before then. Epidemics occur annually in the winter months of temperate zones in many, but not usually the same, communities. Within a community, major cycles usually last 2–4 years. The clinical manifestations of influenza are familiar; although the lining of the respiratory tract is the site of primary infection, systemic symptoms, notably fever, muscle pains, and prostration, are out of proportion to those of local origin. Brief and self-limiting when uncomplicated, the disease can be deadly at the extremes of age and in those with pre-existing cardiorespiratory

disorders because of secondary bacterial invasion of the lung (especially with *Streptococcus pneumoniae*, *Staphylococcus aureus*, and *Haemophilus influenzae*); the pandemic of 1918–19 is thought to have cost 15 million lives. Influenza is caused by three unrelated groups of orthomyxoviruses labeled A, B, and C; pandemics and major epidemics are due to group A. Within the group, however, there appears to be almost infinite antigenic variation, probably as a result of genetic recombination, bedeviling both epidemiology and immunoprophylaxis. Vaccines of attenuated virus of an identified strain confer temporary immunity but are often of little value in a new epidemic.

*See also* INFECTIOUS DISEASES; MICROBIOLOGY

**ENGLISH SWEAT** was a mysterious illness which appeared in 1485 and caused a number of epidemics with a high mortality rate over the next hundred years, after which it seems to have disappeared. It was possibly a form of influenza. The English Sweat either disappeared for no known reason or more probably receded into an illness indistinguishable from 'ordinary influenza'.

and to members of certain religious sects such as the Hutterites. In these communities, tribal elders or religious leaders may make decisions for the collectivity as a whole.

In all orderly societies there are laws or regulations that state the precise ages at which it becomes legal to vote, to buy alcoholic beverages, to get married — and to make medical decisions about such matters as consent to surgical operation, and, more important, the use of contraception and termination of pregnancy. There is much variation among the advanced industrial nations, and even among local districts within some nations, in the legal age of consent — especially in regard to aspects of reproductive care, about which there are strongly held views. In cultures and social groups where religious beliefs about the sanctity of life and the role of parents in the upbringing of their children predominate, young women and men are constrained by local customs (and sometimes law) from making choices for themselves, even perhaps after they are old enough to vote and serve in the armed forces. In some cultures even married women cannot decide for themselves whether or when to use contraceptives: the decision is made for them by their husbands. These matters are determined by laws and customs. For a physician, however, ethics rather than law or custom should be the deciding factor.

## Ethics

The disclosure at the Nuremberg trials of the atrocities perpetrated by the Nazis, including in particular medical experiments that resulted in the death of the individuals upon whom the experiments were carried out, led to the development of the NUREMBERG CODE, governing the principles for ethical conduct of research involving human subjects. The Nuremberg Code established solidly the principle of respect for persons, for human dignity, for the right of persons to make choices for themselves. The Nuremberg Code states without equivocation that the voluntary consent of the human subject of medical research is absolutely essential. This principle, first enunciated in the context of biomedical research, soon came to apply equally to consent to medical treatment — though there are, of course, exceptions and qualifying conditions in some aspects of medical treatment.

Consent to treatment or to take part in a medical research project should be solicited by a senior staff member, not delegated to a junior nurse or medical student.

It is unacceptable to ask patients admitted to hospital, whether in an emergency under stressful conditions or for an elective procedure, to sign a form that grants blanket consent to any and all procedures (some such forms even include granting consent to autopsy in the event of the patient's death).

It is unacceptable to conduct certain tests or procedures without specific consent. In the recent past, it was commonly assumed that the offering of an arm and a vein for the medical attendant to withdraw a sample of blood implied consent to test that blood for anything and everything. The HIV/AIDS epidemic has led to a change in the rules regarding blood tests. The implications of a positive HIV test are so far-reaching that it is unacceptable to conduct the test without the formal consent of the person being tested. (The exception to this rule is anonymous unlinked HIV testing, using samples of neonatal cord blood, for epidemiological surveillance.)

Informed consent is commonly requested in writing, but this is not always necessary. For instance, in telephone surveys, the fact that the respondent answers questions implies consent, and it would in any case not be logistically feasible to obtain formal written consent.

In certain circumstances medical care can be provided without formal consent. An obvious example is an acute medical emergency. A critically ill or injured unconscious person must be given necessary life-saving care without awaiting the niceties of consent procedures that are applicable in routine practice. Another example is when a person suffers from a condition that imposes risk of harm to others. Confidentiality may be violated without the consent of the person if this is essential to protect others from harm. This legal and ethical rule was established by the Tarasoff case, in California in 1976; a psychiatrist did not warn others that a patient he was treating suffered from homicidal paranoid delusions; his patient committed a murder, and in a subsequent civil claim against the psychiatrist's employer, the court ruled that he should have acted without his patient's

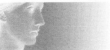
## CONSENT PROCESS

Informed consent has several components:
- The patient or person responsible for the patient, or the subject of a medical research project, must be fully informed of what the physician or other medical attendant is proposing, and what the consequences of this are likely to be. When there are alternatives, each alternative and its advantages and disadvantages must be explained, so the person whose consent is solicited has a clear and fully informed choice among the range of alternatives.

- The right to withhold consent must be communicated, as well as the necessary information to enable informed choice to be made.
- After being fully informed and presented with the range of available choices, the decision must be left to the patient or responsible person. There must be no duress, coercion, extravagant reward, or undue pressure to comply with the request for consent, no penalty for those who choose to withhold consent.

consent in order to protect others. Physicians have a legal duty to prevent patients suffering from conditions that impair consciousness from driving a motor vehicle, even if patients explicitly withhold consent for reporting this fact to motor vehicle licensing authorities.

Patients in a dependent relationship — children and inmates in institutions such as prisons and custodial mental hospitals — cannot legally give consent to treatment. They may, however, provide assent, and whenever possible physicians should explain what they want to do, and seek the agreement of the person to doing it. Children as young as 4 or 5 years can usually comprehend what the physician wants of them, and will cooperate willingly if this is explained and they are asked if the physician can please do it. This simple act of courtesy can lead to harmony in the relationship of child patients to those who are caring for them in hospital; children then willingly, even cheerfully, tolerate discomfort and pain that commonly lead to violent struggles and screaming fits if force rather than common courtesy is applied.                    JML

*See also* BIOETHICS; HELSINKI — DECLARATION OF; TUSKEGEE SYPHILIS STUDY

**INSECTS** There are more species of insects, spiders, mites, and related arthropods than all other living organisms. Insects and related arthropods make up about 90% of the roughly 10 million species estimated to be on the earth. In contrast, mammals and birds comprise only about 0.1% of the species.

Although insects and other arthropods have no single characteristic separating them from all other animals, three features are unique to this group: an exoskeleton (which limits the size of arthropods and keeps them relatively small), a segmented body, and jointed legs. These three characteristics have allowed insects and other arthropods to invade numerous types of habitats and feed on all kinds of plants and animals, including humans, making them some of the most important vectors of disease.

How did insects evolve to feed on humans? Insects first evolved piercing mouth parts so that they could feed on sap and other plant juices. This also made it possible for some species to feed on animals by piercing their skin. Almost everyone has experienced the distressing bite of these plant-feeding bugs — in a manner similar to a mosquito feeding through one's skin.

Since that early development several thousand species of insects and arthropods have further evolved to feed on humans specifically. This has permitted the transmission of various disease micro-organisms from insects and arthropods to humans.

The next step in the evolution of the insect transmission of disease was a change in disease micro-organisms. At first, human blood on the mouth parts of insects provided only a limited capacity for moving microbes from an infected human to an uninfected one. The time between feedings was long, the blood on the insect's mouth parts would dry, and the microbes mostly perished. But over time some microbes learned how to multiply and persist in the body cavity of insects, enabling them to be passed from human to human. Thus the insect became an effective vector of disease. For example, the malarial protozoan parasite may multiply both in humans and mosquitoes, greatly increasing its chances for transmission.

### Mosquitoes

Numerous mosquito species can transmit microbes and are thus associated with serious diseases such as MALARIA, filariasis, YELLOW FEVER, dengue, and encephalitis.

*Malaria* All mosquitoes, including the *Anopheles* mosquitoes that transmit the protozoan pathogen that causes malaria, require water for their larvae to feed and grow. Anopheline mosquitoes, depending on the species, prefer pool or stream water for raising larvae, which feed on living and dead organic matter in the aquatic ecosystem.

The female adult anopheline mosquitoes require a blood meal to produce viable eggs. Although some species prefer humans, others prefer different mammals or birds. Some of the anopheline mosquitoes feed on both humans and animals. Anopheline female mosquitoes may be attracted to feed on humans wearing perfume or aftershave lotion. In contrast, males of all mosquito species do not bite humans and other animals, but feed on the nectar from flowers.

After a full blood meal, females fly off, usually to the wall of a building, to rest and digest their recent meal. The observation of this resting behavior led to the control program of treating the walls of buildings with insecticides to kill the female mosquito. This successfully controlled malaria, until the mosquitoes evolved resistance to the insecticides. Currently, such resistance in mosquitoes is a serious world-wide problem.

Malaria infects over 500 million people each year, killing some 2.7 million of those infected. About 90% of all malaria cases, as well as 90–95% of the world's malaria-related deaths, occur in Africa. Between 1970 and 1990, in the African countries of Rwanda, Zambia, and Togo, the malaria incidence increased from 4-fold to more than 150-fold, and continues to rise.

Fortunately, in some regions of Asia and South America, the incidence of malaria decreased from 1950 to 1980. Yet even in these regions the malaria rate has remained fairly stable at about 5 million cases per year since 1980. In other regions, malaria is still on the rise. For example, in 1991, Peru recorded about 34 000 cases; by 1992 that number had nearly doubled to about 55 000 cases. Likewise in Bangladesh the incidence of malaria increased from about 33 000 cases in 1988, to 64 000 cases in 1991, to 125 000 cases in 1993.

Many changes in the natural environment have fostered the rising incidence of malaria. In parts of Africa deforestation exposes land to sunlight and produces temporary pools of water, where the human-biting malaria-transmitting mosquito, *Anopheles gambiae*, may breed. In African areas where human populations are doubling almost every twenty years, more people are living in close proximity to the water ecosystems where mosquitoes breed. The mosquito vectors also continue to evolve resistance to insecticides, while the protozoan pathogens are evolving resistance to antimalarial drugs. Together these changes are making control efforts less effective than in the past, so that malaria is now a serious problem in many parts of the world.

*Filariasis* The filariasis parasite, *Filariasis bancrofti*, develops in humans and is transmitted by a wide range of mosquitoes. Many years passed before scientists understood the complex relationship between the filariasis parasite and its two hosts, humans and the mosquito. After a mosquito bites an infected human, the parasite moves into the thoracic muscles of the insect and there develops into an adult. The adult worms move down to the tip of the proboscis of the mosquito, ready to emerge when the mosquito bites to feed. In this way the adult parasite is transferred to the human host to multiply and continue the cycle of infections.

The major vector of filariasis is the common house mosquito, *Culex quinquefasciatus*, which breeds in pools of water, even in water caught in tin cans and old tires. Many of the female culecine mosquitoes rest in houses, ready to feed on humans; some even roost under sinks and toilet rims. Depending on the region, filariasis also can be transmitted by other anopheline mosquitoes, such as *Anopheles hycanus*, *A. gambiae*, and *A.*

*funestus*. In contrast to the widespread incidence of malaria, however, filariasis is generally restricted to tropical countries.

The human infection rate in areas such as Kilgare, Kenya, may be as high as 24%. Although filariasis has declined in several areas of Africa, it has increased in the Nile delta of Egypt from a previous low 1% to a staggering 20% of the population in 1991.

*Yellow fever* The yellow fever virus is spread by the urban mosquito, *Aedes aegypti*, after it becomes infected by feeding on infected humans. The virus multiplies in the mosquito and, after developing for about two weeks in its tiny host, may be transmitted by the mosquito as it bites uninfected humans. *A. aegypti* is known as the urban mosquito because it can breed and reproduce in towns and cities. It uses the water that often accumulates in flower pots, old tires, tin cans, and similar water holding vessels. Relatively little water can support large populations of mosquitoes.

Yellow fever is a serious disease, endemic to Africa and other tropical areas; it probably originated in Africa, where it spread from monkeys to humans. Monkey populations harbor the virus, and mosquitoes that bite monkeys pass it across species to humans.

When first recognized, yellow fever did not seem as serious in Africa as in the Americas, where the human populations were quite dense. In large cities, yellow fever spreads rapidly. However, as the African population continues to expand and urban areas increase in size and density, the incidence of yellow fever is expected to rise there as well.

Yellow fever infections in infants frequently result in immunity if the infant survives. In adults, however, yellow fever is more deadly than malaria. Fortunately, the number of human cases of yellow fever in the world is generally low. In a recent epidemic of yellow fever in Maranhao State, Brazil, the incidence was reported to be 3.5 per 1000, with the number of deaths per case at 16.4%.

*Dengue* The dengue virus is also spread by the urban mosquito, *Aedes aegypti*. Recently, the incidence of dengue has been rising, probably

## MEDICAL ENTOMOLOGISTS

René-Antoine Ferchault **RÉAUMUR** (1683–1757). French scientist, naturalist, entomologist, and physician, Réaumur wrote a monumental work on insects, the six-volume *Mémoires pour servir à l'histoire des insectes* (1734–42), and discovered regeneration of lost limbs in Crustacea. He made technical improvements in the iron and steel industries. He is mainly remembered for his thermometric scale, now obsolete, which took the freezing point of water as zero but the boiling point as 80°.

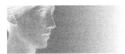

Howard Taylor **RICKETTS** (1871–1910). American microbiologist and epidemiologist. He carried out important field studies of Rocky Mountain spotted fever, succeeding in transmitting the disease from man to laboratory animals, and demonstrating the causative organism, which was subsequently named for him: *Rickettsia*. He showed that this organism is carried by ticks and transmitted to man by their bites.

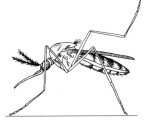
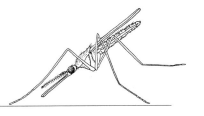

Resting positions of mosquitos: *Culex* (left); *Anopheles* (right). The latter can be recognized by their characteristic posture. (From Dawood, R, (ed.) (1994). *Travellers' health: how to stay healthy abroad*, 3rd edn, OUP.)

owing mainly to increasing population densities in cities. Each year an estimated 80 million people in the world become infected with dengue. Most of the serious infections occur in large urban cities.

Recently, a new mosquito called the tiger mosquito or *Aedes albopictus*, has been introduced into the United States and can transmit dengue and various other diseases.

Indeed, the problem of new species being introduced into new regions is becoming a world-wide problem, as the human population grows and trade between disease areas increases.

### Tsetse flies

*Sleeping sickness* Sleeping sickness, caused by the protozoans *Trypanosome gaminess* and *T. rhodesiese*, is transmitted between humans and other mammals by tsetse flies, *Glossina palpalis* and *G. tachinoides*. The adult flies produce fully grown larvae, which they deposit in protected locations of dense vegetation until they emerge as adults. Adult tsetse flies are found near water, where they easily infect humans when people collect water, bathe, or merely live close to a river or similar aquatic ecosystem.

Sleeping sickness is serious in humans on the African continent. For example, in south-eastern Uganda, the number of cases increased from 50 in 1970 to 4496 cases in 1979, though it has leveled off at about 1266 more recently. In addition to *Trypanosome gaminess* and *T. rhodesiese*, strains of the protozoan are also found in the blood of wild game animals, including *T. vivax*, *T. congolense*, and *T. brucei*.

Western strains of cattle are extremely susceptible to the trypanosomes transmitted from wild game by the tsetse fly. Indeed, the presence of the fly and the parasite in humans and cattle has prevented enormous areas of Africa from being inhabited by humans and their livestock. Attempts to control the fly using DDT and dieldrin have been partially effective, but this had adverse environmental effects.

### Houseflies

World-wide, the housefly, *Musca domestica*, is one of the most common insects in the world living in close proximity with humans. Its larvae live in human and animal wastes and an adult housefly easily produces 500 offspring in about two weeks under favorable conditions. This enormous number of eggs and the short generation time have led some biologists to calculate that houseflies theoretically could cover the earth 3 to 4 feet deep in about four months, provided abundant food for larvae and adults was available. Because adult flies emerge from human and animal wastes, they are heavily contaminated with

bacteria, viruses, and other microbes. The adult flies become further contaminated when they walk on and feed on human and animal wastes and then contact food eaten by humans. Houseflies spread disease by contact, not by biting.

*Enteric diseases* Houseflies and other non-biting flies, as well as several other insects such as cockroaches, help transmit enteric diseases such as diarrhea, typhoid, salmonellosis, and diseases caused by *Staphylococcus* and *Streptococcus*. They do this by either walking on or by eating contaminated food, feces, or vomit. The contaminated flies then either walk on or defecate on uncontaminated food, depositing infectious bacteria and other pathogens.

Houseflies also breed in human and animal feces and also in other wastes such as garbage and dead animals. Without adequate waste treatment facilities, the number of contaminated houseflies may be enormous. In dairy barns and pit privies, there may be literally clouds of flies.

The number of infections caused by houseflies each year is unknown. However, the number of humans infected by diarrhea, typhoid, and diseases caused by *Salmonella*, *Staphylococcus*, and *Streptococcus*, is about 4 billion per year, causing over 15 million deaths each year. Houseflies have a significant role in contaminating food and water with these pathogens.

### Blow flies

The larvae of most blow fly species, *Phaencia spp.*, live in decaying flesh of animals and can transmit several enteric diseases. In emerging from decayed flesh, the flies easily become contaminated with various microbes, some pathogenic. The adult blow flies also visit and feed on dead animal bodies, becoming further contaminated. They visit human foods, especially unprotected meats, thus contaminating the foods humans consume.

In the past blow fly larvae were used to clean out dead flesh from human and animal wounds. One or two species of blow flies attack contaminated areas of sheep and related animals; in some circumstances, the flies end up literally eating the sheep alive.

### Blackflies

Blackfly larvae, *Simulium spp.*, live in streams, attached to rocks and other objects in the water, where they capture minute particles of organic matter drifting in the stream water for their food. Blackfly larvae are found in fast flowing, well-oxygenated streams. Control of the fly larvae is easy by treating streams with pesticides. Yet these pesticides often have detrimental impacts on aquatic fauna and flora. Not only are blackflies a

**Plate 7** A false-colour transmission electron micrograph of *Salmonella typhi*, the causative agent of **typhoid** fever in humans. (Reproduced courtesy of Science Photo Library.)

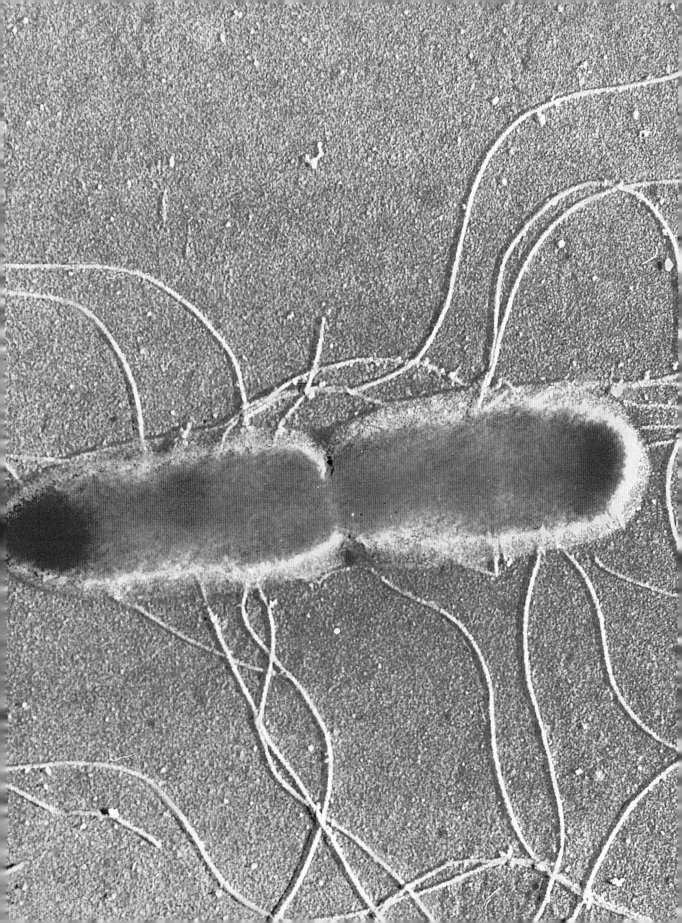

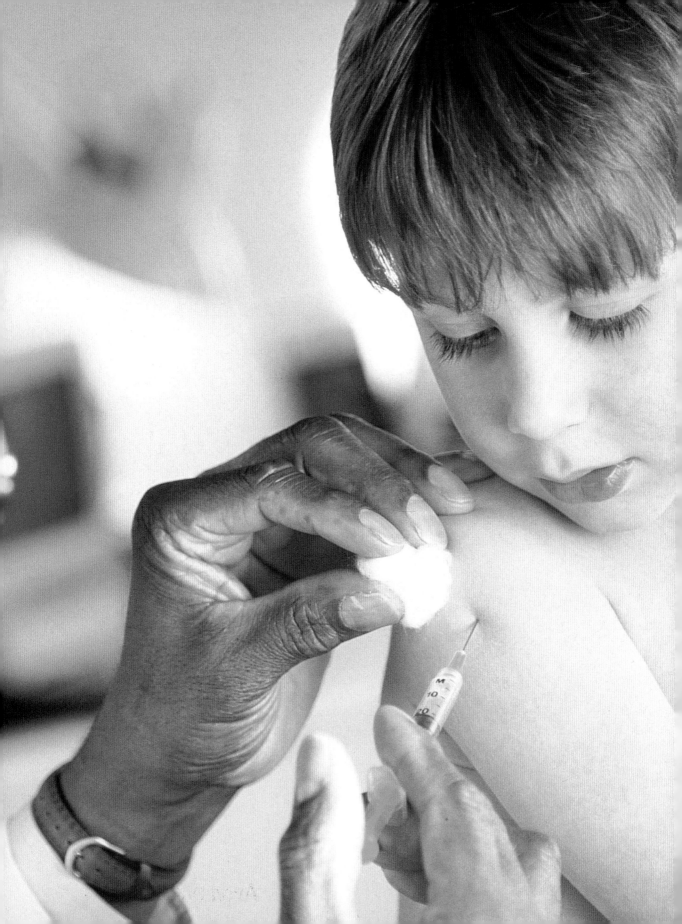

nuisance to sportsmen and gardeners because of their painful bites, but they are vectors of diseases such as river blindness.

***Onchocerciasis (river blindness)*** River blindness is caused by a microfilial worm, *Onchocera volvulus*. The microfilariae are picked up by blackflies, *Simulium damnosum*, from infected humans and then survive in the gut of these blackflies. The microfilariae migrate to the thoracic muscles and then to the proboscis of the flies. Later the fly feeds on uninfected humans and spreads the disease.

Onchocerciasis resembles sleeping sickness because it develops very slowly in humans. Its delayed symptoms and lack of overt signs of infection frequently make treatment difficult. Eventually, many people become blind because the flies migrate into their eyes. An estimated 38 million people are now blind and 110 million people have impaired vision because of onchocerciasis in Africa and other tropical regions.

## Fleas and plague

Adults of the common flea species *Xenopsylla cheopis* feed on the blood of many mammals. The adult fleas deposit their eggs on their hosts; these eggs roll off the host and drop to the nests or dwelling floor. The larvae live on the organic matter found in the nest, rugs, or cracks in floors. When the larvae mature, and the adult flies emerge, they seek out dogs, cats, and other mammals, including humans, as hosts. They feed on the blood of their new host by piercing their skin and have been effective vectors of plague.

At present, human PLAGUE, transmitted by fleas, is on the rise. The plague-bacteria parasite, *Yersinia pestis*, is transmitted by human contacts and the bites of fleas associated with rodents.

Rodents, such as the European rat (*Rattus rattus*) and Asiatic rat (*Rattus nrvegicus*), become infected with the plague bacillus and eventually die, but the plague organism survives. The flea abandons its dead host and looks for new hosts, including humans. The plague bacilli often multiply in the flea's foregut and sometimes the gut becomes blocked by a mass of bacilli. When the flea tries to feed, packets of bacilli are dislodged into the wound of the new host, thus infecting him.

The European rat and Asiatic rat have invaded most ecosystems in the world, living in close contact with humans. Other native rat species may also serve as hosts for both the plague and flea vectors. Different flea species can also transmit plague, including *X. astia* in Asia and *X. brazilliensis* in South America. *X. cheopis* originated in the Nile Valley in Africa and from there probably invaded Europe.

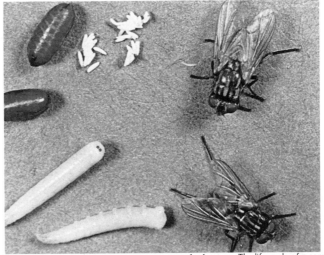

The life-cycle of a common housefly: egg, larva (maggot), imago (adult).

In the 1980s there were 1327 reported plague cases in the world; in 1993, there were 2194; and by 1994, 2935. During the 1990s, nearly 60% of the reported cases occurred in Africa.

## Lice and typhus

Human lice, *Pediculus humanus*, in contrast to fleas, spend their entire life cycle on their host. The eggs of the louse are glued to the hairs of the human host. Both the immature lice and adults feed on the host, creating much discomfort and itching, which can break the skin and help spread disease.

The typhus pathogen, *Bacillus typhi exanthematicum*, is picked up by lice, and the pathogen passes through the gut of the louse without affecting it. During feeding, the contaminated lice defecate, and humans scratching the bite enable the pathogen from the lice feces to enter their blood stream. Typhus is another disease associated with high densities of people and poor hygiene, often occurring in army barracks and jails. Crowding facilitates the spread of lice (*Pediculus humanus*) among troops and jail inmates.

Typhus may also be transmitted to humans by direct contact with infected mucous membranes or by inhalation of the pathogen from an infected person. While many insect-borne diseases (such as malaria and yellow fever) are found mainly in the tropics, typhus may occur everywhere.

## Blood-sucking bugs

Bed-bugs (*Cimex lectularis*) and triatomids (*Panstrongylus megistus*) are referred to as true bugs and have piercing, sucking mouthparts with which they feed on the blood of humans. They lay their eggs in beds and other areas of houses,

435

where both the immature and adult bugs feed on humans at night. Bed-bugs usually remain in the cracks and crevices of the mattresses. The thatch used in huts in many parts of the world provides an ideal place for the triatomid bugs to hide during the day. The triatomids are often larger than bed-bugs and can travel longer distances to feed on human hosts.

***Chagas's disease*** Chagas's disease is a type of sleeping sickness caused by *Trypanosoma cruzi*. This is transmitted by several biting bugs, including bed-bugs, *Cimex lectularis*, and triatomids, *Panstrongylus megistus*. Once these bugs bite an infected person, the pathogen develops in the bugs. The infection spreads when the infected bug feces are scratched into a wound by humans as with typhus. People may also be infected by ingesting or inhaling the pathogen. Since *P. megistus* typically feeds on the face, near the mouth, the probability of human infections is increased. This feeding behavior of these bugs earned them the popular name 'kissing bugs'.

Control of Chagas's disease focuses on reducing the cracks and crevices where the bugs can hide and using a residual insecticide. Such control efforts have reduced the incidence of the disease. For example, in Brazil, where intervention programs have been carried out during the past ten years, Chagas's disease infections have declined by 30% in some communities.

### Ticks

Ticks are not insects but are their relatives, belonging to the group known as acari that includes ticks and mites. Many ticks have complex life cycles, such as those in which the larvae feed on one host and the adult feeds on another.

A bedbug, resting on human skin.

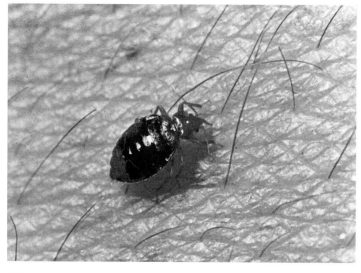

For example, adult deer-ticks *Ixodes dammini* (or *I. scapularlius*) feed on deer but their larvae on rodents. Both stages will feed on humans. The eggs of ticks are laid on the host and drop off the host to the ground when the eggs hatch; the young larvae climb to the top of grasses and similar vegetation and attach to their new host as it brushes against the vegetation. Both larvae and adult ticks have several pairs of legs that facilitate their reaching out to attach to a host when it passes.

***Lyme disease*** Lyme disease, caused by *Borrelia burgdorferi*, is the most common vector-borne disease in the USA, having been reported in 47 states. It is caused by a spirochete similar to the one causing syphilis. It is thought to have existed naturally in the United States without incident, until major ecological changes occurred in the 20th century. Then suburban areas expanded at the same time as the white-tailed deer population increased from 2000 in 1945 to 9500 in 1990 in Massachusetts. The coexistence of abundant rodent *Peromyscus leucopus* and deer-tick *Ixodes dammini* (or *I. scapularius*) populations allowed the Lyme-disease organism to spread rapidly. Dramatically expanding since the initial description of the disease in 1976, Lyme disease now infects nearly 12 700 people in the United States each year. It is also becoming a problem in Europe and Asia, more than 30 000 cases having been recently reported in Germany.

***Relapsing fever*** African tick-borne relapsing fever is also caused by a spirochete, *Borrelia crocidurae*. The vector is the tick, *Ornithodoros moubata*. Different species of the spirochete and species of ticks exist in the North African and Mediterranean region; eastern Mediterranean, Middle East, and China region; central and western United States, and Mexico region; and Central and South American region.

After feeding on an infected person, the spirochetes pass through the tick's gut in a manner specific to the strain of the pathogen and species of tick. The spirochetes invade most organs of the tick, including the salivary glands, which aid in the transmission of the pathogen when a new host is bitten. The spirochetes may be also passed from an adult tick to its eggs via transoval transmission. The ticks' ability to live for a year and continue transmitting the spirochetes to humans contributes to the widespread incidence of this disease in adults. Fortunately, however, the incidence of relapsing fever is low, only 0.9% in West Africa.

***Rocky mountain spotted fever*** Upon first study, the spotted fever organism neither appeared to be a virus nor a bacterium; thus, the organism was called a 'rickettsia' and named *Dermo-centroxenus rickettsi*. However, the infective organism is closer to a virus than a bacterium, because it infects the nucleus of a cell. Like the spirochete for relapsing fever, it may also be transmitted by trans-oval means from the adult tick to its eggs, thus furthering the spread of the disease.

The infective agent is transmitted by several tick species. In the United States, the primary vector is the wood tick (*Dermacentor andersoni*) in the west and the dog tick (*D. variabilis*) in the east. In Mexico and other South American regions, the transmission of the pathogen is by another tick, *Amblyomma cajennse*. Between 1981 and 1992, 9223 human cases of spotted fever were reported in the United States, but with effective control the incidence of the disease appears to be declining.

### Bees

Honey bees and other bees provide the essential service of pollinating about one-third of the world's crops and its natural vegetation. Without bees food production would be severely reduced and many natural species of plants would become extinct.

On the negative side, the sting of honey bees and the new Africanized bee or 'killer bee' may cause deaths in the United States as well as in other parts of the world. In the United States, more people die from the allergic reactions to bee stings than from bites by poisonous snakes.

Although a few species of arthropods are pests and some are vectors of deadly diseases, most arthropods are beneficial and essential to the functioning of the natural ecosystem. Without the millions of species of arthropods that exist on earth, the natural aquatic and terrestrial ecosystems could not function effectively and the quality of the environment would suffer. Arthropods are vital for degrading and recycling wastes, pollinating crops and native vegetation, controlling pests attacking crops, and providing food for birds, fishes, and wildlife. DPim

*See also* MALARIA; RHEUMATOLOGY; TYPHUS; YELLOW FEVER

## INSURANCE: LIFE AND OTHER TYPES

Within the ambit of life insurance come not only products (contracts) which depend upon death or survival to a certain date in the future (for example, whole life, endowment, term insurance), but also other policies insuring against disability, (income protection; total and permanent disability benefit, long-term care, elderly care) and the diagnosis of major disorders (critical illness insurance). The common defining factor in all these contracts is that they are for long-term coverage and the insurer cannot refuse to renew throughout the duration of the policy. Thus the assessment of the medical risk at the inception of the contract takes on added significance because the underwriter and his medical advisor cannot subsequently amend the terms of acceptance, even in the event of a significant change in the health of the policyholder, or the experience of a group of risks in total.

Premium rates are developed from mortality tables based on the experience of insured lives rather than the population as a whole; by eliminating the majority of lives with terminal and

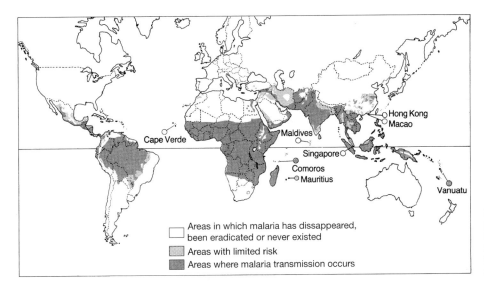

Geographical distribution of malaria (1991). Note, however, that the exact distribution varies somewhat from time to time. (Reproduced courtesy of WHO.)

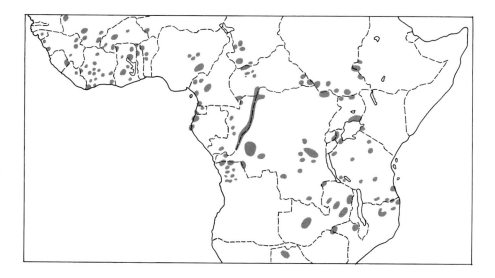

Geographical distribution of yellow fever and of mosquitoes capable of spreading the disease. (Reproduced courtesy of Dawood, R. (ed.) (1994). *Travellers' health: how to stay healthy abroad*, 3rd edn, OUP.)

very high-risk conditions the actuary can make assumptions about the mortality of insurance applicants that are markedly lower than would be the case if life insurance were granted without the selection process.

Most life assurance written in Britain is underwritten purely on the disclosures by the client made in the application form. It is in the insurers' interests to minimize acquisition costs and therefore in the main it will require only formal reports because of material disclosure, the age of the individual, or the level of the sum insured.

In Britain, most personal medical attendants are familiar with completing such reports from patient's records and often the insurer will ask for details of specific illness(es) mentioned in the application. It is commonplace for personal medical attendants to enclose copies of any relevant hospital reports. Personal medical attendants' reports provide a detailed outline of significant medical disorders allowing more accurate assessment by the insurer.

### Medical examination

Traditionally, examinations were performed by independent physicians on behalf of life companies but in recent times more personal medical attendants are being asked to examine their own patients. Increasingly, examinations are being carried out by a paramedic (usually a registered nurse), who will record height, weight, blood pressure along with urinalysis for protein, glucose, and blood. In addition, the paramedic will ask questions about medical history, family history, and social and life-style habits, such as alcohol, smoking, exercise. In the USA the paramedic examination often includes the collec-

tion of blood and urine samples for laboratory analyses.

For large sums insured or where there are relevant medical histories other tests may be performed; electrocardiograms, particularly treadmill ECG stress tests, may be requested routinely for multi-million pound policies but also for lesser amounts when there are co-existing coronary risk factors such as hyperlipidemia, hypertension, and smoking. Other tests include blood biochemistry, lipids, HIV, microscopic urinalysis, and cotinine (to check non-smoker status).

### Clinical, population, and insured lives studies

The availability and analysis of major impairment studies have demystified the underwriting process, which until after the Second World War was more often based on the opinions (and prejudices/idiosyncrasies) of individual consulting medical officers rather than any scientific data. Today, when challenged, most life offices can muster sound evidence for many of the more common impairments for which ratings may be imposed; these will include hypertension, obesity, asthma, diabetes, vascular disease, kidney and bowel disorders, and cancer. A considerable volume of material relating to the mortality of these disorders has been analyzed mainly by the Society of Actuaries and American Academy of Insurance Medicine in the USA and their findings have been published at regular intervals.

The average physician's understanding of medical aspects of life insurance is naturally limited. While most doctors recognize that the prime concern is assessing the effects of current medical status on future mortality, many seem unaware that the underlying mortality assumptions are based on insured lives rather than the general population at large. This means in practice that the latter group's mortality is around 60% of the former. In addition the medical profession generally takes a short-term view — perhaps five, maybe ten years — of most conditions, whereas life insurers are often concerned about the effects of medical conditions over significantly longer periods, often twenty to thirty years or more. Bearing both these points in mind it is instructive to consider how the various clinical and insured lives mortality studies are interpreted and why misunderstandings can arise.

If one takes as an example ulcerative colitis, several clinical studies paint a favorable picture of the prognosis with long-term mortality only marginally higher than the general population. However, the main insured lives study on inflammatory bowel disease showed a moderate increase in mortality when analyzed against the mortality assumptions used in the basic premium rates.

In terms of insurability the excess mortality associated with virtually all significant conditions is assessable via mortality studies of clinical populations and insured lives. However, not all serious conditions will necessarily be insurable; for example, the high risk of recurrence in the early years after treatment for most aggressive cancers rules out quoting commercially viable premiums until the initial extra mortality has dropped to affordable levels, usually after two to five years. Large cancer studies, particularly the SEER programs in the USA, now chart the risks associated with the major cancers at durations over twenty years from treatment, highlighting those tumors where excess mortality continues to be a feature despite the fact that a 'cure' has seemingly been achieved.

## The rating of substandard lives

With the development of insured lives studies starting at the beginning of the 20th century in the USA, the underwriting of substandard lives was put on a more scientific basis. During the period between the world wars a numerical system of rating was established which is still used today. The principle of the system assumes the average risk is 100% mortality and each factor influencing mortality is expressed numerically in terms of percentage extra/reduced mortality. Debits and credits are allocated in multiples of five depending upon whether there is a favorable or unfavorable influence. For example, a 40-year-old man whose blood pressure averages 175/100 would probably merit rating of an additional 100 percentage points for his hypertension but his loading might well be reduced if there were positive features such as a

normal lipid profile, good family history, or satisfactory treadmill ECG. Evidence of sustained normotensive blood pressure control by medication may be commensurate with ordinary standard rate premiums.

## Disability

Life underwriters assess a variety of products based on disability, defined as either the inability to work at one's normal occupation or the occurrence of a specific illness or event such as a stroke, heart attack, or cancer (so-called critical illness or 'dread disease' insurance). Estimation of future morbidity — particularly if it is a work-related disability — is no easy task especially when attitudes to incapacity have a high degree of subjectivity and the 'will to work' is difficult to gauge. The insurer's ability to assess such morbidity risks is not made any more simple by the fact that many doctors in their reports tend to gloss over or ignore non-life-threatening conditions such as 'stress', mild anxiety/depression, and musculoskeletal disorders which are major causes of recurrent incapacity.

Compared to mortality risk assessment, underwriting disability risks tends to be much more conservative. Often there is a lack of objective information relating to future morbidity and the medical reports from the patient's own personal medical advisor or general practitioner may not have sufficient detail. Given that the results for most disability insurers have been generally poor, it is not surprising that the underwriters and actuaries have taken a cautious line when quoting terms, particularly on lives with impaired health.

Rating disability coverage is either based on extra premium loading or on the use of exclusions. By way of example the risks associated with hypertension or marked obesity are manifold and do not lend themselves to exclusion; thus premium loading is usually applied. On the other hand, the risk associated with back or other musculoskeletal disorders because of their recurrent nature is not easily quantifiable in cash terms and thus most insurers will apply specific exclusions.

The main problems that arise are usually linked to the doctor–patient relationship. There will be times when information about a patient's medical history is passed to an insurance company (only after signed consent by the patient, who is also protected under the Access to Medical Reports Act) which will be of a nature that will need sensitive handling (for example, the true nature and extent of a cancer resection may not be known by the patient but an insurer's special terms of declinature may be unwittingly revealing).

Rather more frequently patients are strongly reassured by specialists about the significance (or lack thereof) of their medical condition or the results of investigations. It is common practice for medical professionals to play down the negative aspects of a condition, but underwriters and their medical advisers must take a long-term view. Interpretation of ECG variations is often a case in point; equivocal abnormalities tend to be glossed over in order to avoid worrying the patient but in the absence of more conclusive investigations cannot be ignored in the underwriting process.

Several countries have passed laws covering the rights of the disabled to goods and services. While there are naturally variations in practical terms, the approach on insurance is broadly similar, namely, insurers are able to adjust the terms they quote on disabled applicants as long as there are supportive and relevant data to justify such discrimination. In Britain the Act has generated a number of challenges and on occasion underwriters have been forced to amend adverse decisions where there proved to be no statistical justification. In most cases however, there has been a compromise solution that usually has satisfied both parties.

### Genetics

The development of the HUMAN GENOME PROJECT that ultimately will map the one hundred thousand pairs of genes that make up the human genome has given rise to much debate about the social, ethical, and legal consequences such knowledge will bring. Life and health insurance have been the focus for discussion especially in countries like the USA where healthcare cover (medical expenses insurance) is primarily provided by commercial insurers.

In Britain more attention has been put on life insurance which is seen — quite erroneously — to be a vital requirement in effecting a private house mortgage. Despite the logic that insurers have employed in attempting to reassure customers that genetic testing will have little or no effect on their insurability, many pressure groups have not been convinced that private insurance companies can be trusted to handle and interpret the emerging genetic data in a responsible fashion.

The Human Genetics Advisory Commission was established in December 1996 as a non-statutory advisory body to report to the UK health and industry ministers on issues arising from developments on human genetics. They issued a report in December 1997 at the same time as the Association of British Insurers issued its code of practice on genetic testing. The code, openly available on the internet, sets out in detail all aspects relating to genetic testing emphasizing the continued importance of consent to disclosure, confidentiality, privacy, and appeal mechanisms. The government has welcomed these detailed reports and is promoting an independent evaluation system to review the scientific and actuarial evidence result-

ing from a genetic test that might contribute to decisions used by insurance companies in the underwriting process.

Although the above overview is written from the perspective of the British insurance industry, the basic principles of life assurance and selection of risks are similar world-wide. A recurring theme in the global insurance industry in the 1990s has been the increased government interest in the life/health insurance industry.

Many countries recognize the escalating economic pressures (aging populations, cost of services, etc.) that will be put upon their social security and national health insurance systems in the first quarter of the 21st century. Although most will wish to maintain the main principles of the welfare state and universal healthcare, it seems inevitable that the funding and administration of such schemes will increasingly involve the private sector in partnership with the state.

## THE AIDS RISK FOR LIFE INSURANCE

The 1980s saw the possibility of an epidemic that might have threatened the financial status of the life insurance industry. In order to protect the funds of millions of policyholders, companies were forced to assess the amount of extra reserves necessary to cover the 'expected' claims. Various projections about the impact of AIDS were made and insurers introduced HIV tests for all those who were considered to be in high-risk groups and for applicants applying for substantial levels of cover.

Mainly owing to governments' education programs most predictions were wide of the mark and at the time of writing the spread of the disease has not penetrated as widely into the general population as was expected. There was criticism of the insurance industry's response to the situation and, although with hindsight certain aspects could have been handled better, it would have been imprudent in the late 1980s not to have taken swift action using the conservative projections.

Today insurers run into very few problems on the question of HIV tests. The test is frequently based on saliva analysis, which for the average applicant is more user-friendly than a blood test. The sensitivity and specificity of saliva tests are broadly in line with blood with very few equivocal or false-positive results.

At the same time, if the private sector takes an increasing role in healthcare provision, this will fuel the arguments of many powerful lobby groups who in promoting their members' interests effectively propound the view that everyone has a right to insurance. Changes in societal attitudes have brought about legislation on disability discrimination and medical data protection. It is possible that additional constraints will be proposed that will further diminish the insurers' ability to underwrite and base their terms on the degree of risk each person brings to the total fund. In this environment of change and challenge to the *status quo*, medical risk assessment will need to adapt but as long as life and health insurance remains a voluntary undertaking, insurers will continue to insist upon the right to select the business they write based upon the assumptions made in the underlying mortality and morbidity rates. RCro, PBC

**INTERNAL MEDICINE — USA** Internal medicine in the United States had a vague beginning. The term is probably based on its German forebear, *Innere Medizin*. The discipline was based initially on clinical observations of several American physicians, among whom William OSLER (p 602) was the most notable. Several physicians of Osler's generation formed the Association of American Physicians in 1886. The Association comprised physicians (some also noted pathologists) and was based partly on the close relationship of basic science (in those days, mainly pathology, microbiology, and physiology) with clinical medicine and the importance of clinical investigation to patient care. It eschewed the politics and the democratization of the AMA (American Medical Association), which bitterly opposed it.

Internal medicine was also born in the early reformed medical schools, of which JOHNS HOPKINS (p 840) was the prototype. Other early schools included Columbia, Cornell, Washington University, Chicago, Iowa, and Michigan. These schools pioneered full-time departments of internal medicine, consisting of a professor and a small group of associates who were full time in the medical school. They could devote most of their efforts to teaching and research and were not dependent on private practice for their livelihood. These 'academic' departments of medicine, with Johns Hopkins leading the way, also introduced internship and residency training.

As internal medicine gained its identity, its practitioners were identified primarily with diagnosis and prognosis. Early diagnostic tools included the X-ray, electrocardiogram, and smears and cultures, as well as analysis of the chemical composition of blood, urine, and other secretions. History taking and physical diagnosis were the internist's primary stock in trade, and hospital wards were the laboratory. During World War II, internists served as medical consultants for the armed forces and carried out important research on blood replacement, traumatic shock, and, with the discovery of sulfonamides, treatment of infections. After the war, academic departments of internal medicine came into their

own primarily because of the ready availability of research grants from the federal government, which in turn led to a sharp increase in the faculty. Many of these faculty members were engaged primarily in clinical (and in recent years) basic research. Early figures are not available; but in the late 1940s, departments of medicine had on average between six and ten faculty members. In 1996, there were over 20 000 department of medicine faculty members in 125 allopathic US medical schools. The increase in the size of the educational and research establishments was accompanied by a considerable increase in trainees in internal medicine, many of whom became practicing internists, mostly subspecialists.

During the past twenty years, internists expanded their interests to encompass important new technology, particularly in cardiology, gastroenterology, pulmonary disease, and nephrology. The internist became primarily a therapeutician rather than a diagnostician. Many diseases formerly under the aegis of surgeons or not treatable at all (such as peptic ulcer, tuberculosis, most cancers, and malignant hypertension) became under the purview of internal medicine and its subspecialties.

### Organization

The largest internal medicine organization in the USA is the American College of Physicians. Founded in 1916, mainly by physicians from New York, the college moved its headquarters to Philadelphia in 1926, where it has been located ever since. By 1996, it had over 100 000 members divided into four categories; masters (349), fellows (24 145), members (52 044), and associates (24 675). It also included 15 174 medical student members and 171 honorary fellows. The American College of Physicians is governed by a board of regents, who are elected nationally, and a board of governors, who are elected by regions (states). For many years, its mission was continuing education. It introduced a self-assessment examination (now in its twelfth iteration), constructed an in-training examination for residents, and publishes a widely circulated journal, the *Annals of Internal Medicine*. In 1956, a group of internists formed the American Society of Internal Medicine, concerned with the socioeconomic welfare of internists and their patients. As American medicine became more politicized and regulated, the college also felt that it had to address social, economic, and public policy concerns. Because of the overlap between the college's and Society of Internal Medicine's public policy agenda, several attempts to merge the two organizations occurred but failed. However, influenced by the increasingly complex and difficult environment in which American internists are now forced to practice, the leadership of both organizations felt that internal medicine must speak with a single voice; and on 1 July 1998, they merged into one organization — the American College of Physicians–American Society of Internal Medicine. While this is the most important organization in US internal medicine, others are configured into the Federated Council for Internal Medicine, whose members include the Association of Program Directors of Internal Medicine, the Association of Professors [Chairs] of Medicine, the American Board of Internal Medicine, the Society of General Internal Medicine, and the Association of Subspecialty Professors. The federated council is primarily an organization that exchanges information and has little policy-making power. There are also many subspecialty societies in internal medicine.

## American Board of Internal Medicine and subspecialty medicine

The American Board was organized by the American Medical Association and American College of Physicians in 1936 to develop and promulgate standards for clinical training in internal medicine. Board certification is voluntary and was conceived initially as an accolade to recognize an élite cadre of physicians. The board's purpose is to assure the public that certified internists have the requisite knowledge, skills, and attitudes necessary to provide excellent medical care. A private, non-profit organization based in Philadelphia, the board administers written examinations and evaluates the clinical competence of the 22 000 residents and fellows being trained in the 408 internal medicine and 1472 subspecialty programs.

In the beginning, interest in 'having boards' was limited mostly to academics (fewer than 5000 were certified after the board's first ten years). This changed with the explosive growth of internal medicine after World War II. Thirty years after its founding, the board was certifying over 1000 internists annually; and by 1997, this number had reached nearly 8000. By setting and maintaining high standards of clinical performance, board certification has gained broad acceptance as the most important marker of clinical competence in internal medicine. It has become a virtual requirement for employment in academic institutions and for many healthcare systems. Some 97% of internal medicine trainees voluntarily seek this credential; and more than 90% are successful in being certified. Because of the importance of certification, the board has played an important part in shaping internal medicine in the USA. Its decision in 1990 to limit all certificates to ten years will further extend its influence in clinical practice as recertification becomes mandatory

for future generations of internists and medical subspecialists. The board took this step to assure the public that its diplomates remain competent and up-to-date over their professional lifetimes.

Internal medicine is the largest medical specialty in the USA, comprising almost a quarter of all trainees and clinicians. The number of certified internists exceeds that of the next two largest specialties, pediatrics and family practice, combined. Heightened interest in careers in internal medicine has been stimulated by four decades of generous federal funding for training, by advances in biomedical research (especially in the subspecialties), and by the influence of large and talented departmental faculties on graduate medical education.

The growth of internal medicine is due to interest in the medical subspecialties. Cardiology, gastroenterology, and pulmonary medicine were formally recognized by the American Board as early as 1940. Presently, one-half (77 000) of all physicians certified in internal medicine also hold certificates in at least one of the 11 major subspecialties, which, in descending order by size, are cardiology, gastroenterology, pulmonary medicine, oncology, critical care medicine, geriatrics, nephrology, hematology, infectious diseases, endocrinology, and rheumatology. Interest in subspecialty careers reached a peak in the early 1980s, when nearly 80% of internal medicine residents opted to continue training in one of these disciplines. In the 1990s, however, interest in subspecialization declined, a response to changes in federal funding stemming from an oversupply of subspecialists; a perceived shortage of primary care physicians; and the acceptance of MANAGED CARE, which seeks to make healthcare more efficient and less costly. The trend away from subspecialization is evident in board annual tracking data, which indicate that fewer than half of 1997 internal medicine graduates had entered subspecialty training. However, this contraction has not reduced the overall size of the specialty since it has been offset by a renewed interest in ambulatory and hospital-based generalism. This latter group of practitioners are referred to as 'hospitalists', and their function is similar to the hospital-based internal medicine consultant in Britain. General internists are also becoming more numerous again in academia, where they are responsible for much of the medical student teaching, serve as resident role models, and are leaders in health services and clinical outcomes research.

## Current issues

*Primary care in general internal medicine* In the USA, the practice of internal medicine includes a generous amount of preventive and primary care. Primary care — defined as first contact, continuing, and coordinated care — has always been a part of internal medicine, although this role has become more important with the advent of comprehensive subspecialty medicine. The traditional role of the general internist as a diagnostician and consultant has declined steeply, and probably exists now only in isolated regions that are not well represented by medical subspecialists. Most internists spend less of their time in hospitals, and many are wholly based in office practice. At the other extreme, some internists ('hospitals') now spend all of their time managing the general medical problems of hospitalized patients.

In recognition of these trends, the American Board is promoting the concept of the general internist as 'Doctors for Adults', to make a distinction from activities of family practitioners. In general, family practitioners concentrate on families, children, and pregnant women, while general internists focus more narrowly on older adults with complex problems and those who are chronically ill. Constructive relationships exist between the generalist specialties (internal medicine, family practice, and pediatrics), which have collaborated to develop some combined training programs leading to dual certification with as little as a single year of additional training. Primary care in the USA, therefore, is characterized by its diversity of generalist physicians, a system that is well established and understood by the profession and most patients.

Increasingly, physicians are organizing across specialty lines to form primary care groups consisting of general internists, family practitioners, and pediatricians rather than vertical single specialty organizations consisting of internists and medical subspecialists. These newly configured groups are usually well positioned to negotiate with various health plans to provide cost-effective, comprehensive care for defined patient populations.

*Medical subspecialties* Although subspecialists provide some general care to patients, most limit their professional activities to patients with specific illnesses. In this capacity, they offer specialized consultative services; provide advanced and highly technical care (such as interventional cardiology); or function as physician-scientists and educators in university medical centers. Subspecialty clinicians are more oriented towards hospital care than generalists; but on occasion, they also provide 'principal care', a special category of primary care in which a subspecialist may provide all, or almost all, the medical services for patients whose complex chronic conditions are dominated by a single

illness. Examples of 'principal care' include patients with end-stage renal disease or organ transplantation.

Unlike surgery, internal medicine and its subspecialties have stayed together in large part because departments of medicine and board certification have been strong stabilizing forces for the cohesive integration of the specialty. Similar to the situation in Britain, medical subspecialists must first be fully trained in internal medicine. To look ahead, it seems likely that the medical subspecialties will continue to differentiate to include new disciplines as they evolve. Some of these will be recognized by board certification.

*Internal medicine workforce* At present, the physician workforce is in a state of flux, being heavily influenced by inconsistent market forces emanating from large healthcare systems, small group practices, and academic medical centers. Failure to enact comprehensive federal healthcare reform legislation in the mid-1990s fueled the influence of market forces in the health sector. Consequently, a patchwork of federal and state policies has been enacted to protect patients from the worst effects of a purely market-driven healthcare system. Most health policy analysts believe that the supply of physicians (including internists) is in serious excess in the USA. The leading internal medicine organizations have publicly supported limiting federal funds for training programs to create incentives that will provide better alignment between the total number of trainees and the number of graduating US medical students. At present, the total number of residency positions is roughly 150% of the number of US medical graduates. An influx of international medical graduates fill many training slots in internal medicine and most continue to practice in the USA permanently. Controversial legislative initiatives are being considered to reduce federal funding to this group of trainees as a mechanism to control physician supply.

An analysis of staffing patterns in managed care organizations indicates there may soon be up to a 50% excess of medical subspecialists. Additional evidence suggests that there may soon be an oversupply of primary care physicians, including internists. The impact of these realities, combined with enacted and proposed changes in federal funding for residency training, appears to have contributed to the recent decline in interest in the subspecialties (the most definite decline, over 30%, has occurred in gastroenterology, infectious disease, and rheumatology). Many thoughtful observers conclude that it is time to develop a better system for determining the physician workforce than simply leaving it to the vagaries of the medical marketplace and the whim of incremental government action.

## The future

With the changes in the US healthcare system, internal medicine and its subspecialties face a time of uncertainty for several reasons. The first is the surfeit of subspecialists and generalists. The second is whether general internal medicine will retain its franchise to provide primary care. The third is whether the medical schools and teaching hospitals will continue to maintain the size of their faculties or whether fiscal considerations will force them to downsize. The answers to these questions are not yet at hand. Those who see the glass as half empty will argue that internal medicine in the USA is too large and needs to get leaner and meaner. Those who argue that the glass is half full will posit that internal medicine must be the intellectual leader and the harbingers of quality care. The answer is probably somewhere in between.                                         RGP

**INTERNET** The internet is a network of computers that can exchange information by communicating with one another via cable, telephone lines, or satellites using radio waves. It began in the 1960s at the height of the Cold War as a closed circuit linkage of COMPUTERS in the US Department of Defense, intended to ensure secure communication in the event of hostilities with the Soviet Union. It soon spread to other US government departments, then to academia and to business, commerce, and private individuals. By the late 1990s the internet had been adopted as an efficient and inexpensive means of communication in many professions, including medicine. Also by the late 1990s almost a third of private households in the USA and smaller but rapidly rising proportions in other nations had at least one computer, and a high proportion of these computers are linked actually or potentially to other computers all over the world. Mass production of microprocessors and other components has led to rapid reduction in price and an even more rapid increase in the capacity and speed of information transfer within and between computers.

The World Wide Web is a related computer-based information system that was developed at CERN (Conseil Européan pour la Recherche Nucléaire), the European laboratory for particle physics. This uses computer technology and software programs to transmit 'hypertext', a system for the transfer among computers of pictures and large documents such as medical journals, even entire books, that can be opened and viewed on computer screens at the receiving end.

The principal uses of the internet and the World Wide Web in medicine are for communica-

tion of clinical and administrative information, and for education — undergraduate, graduate, and especially continuing medical education.

## Communication

With suitable safeguards to ensure confidentiality, patients' records can be transmitted over the internet from one doctor's consulting room to another, or between a tertiary care hospital and distant peripheral clinics, or to the members of an internet discussion group, any of whom can provide opinions and advice about the diagnosis and management of difficult or puzzling cases. Internet discussion groups have become a widely used means of communication among doctors in professional colleges and societies in many parts of the world, used mainly for continuing medical education and dissemination of notices about matters of professional interest. Doctors working all over the world can take part in some specialized internet discussion groups, for example, in cardiothoracic and orthopedic surgery.

The internet is a valuable means of instantaneous world-wide notification of outbreaks of dangerous contagious diseases of high public health importance such as viral hemorrhagic fever and epidemic influenza. It is routinely used by the WORLD HEALTH ORGANIZATION, the US Centers for Disease Control and Prevention, and similar information clearing-houses, to post weekly updates of notified cases of communicable diseases. The serial publications of these organizations, CDC's *Morbidity and Mortality Weekly Reports* (*MMWR*) and WHO's *Weekly Epidemiological Record* (*WER*), circulate more widely, and of course far more rapidly, over the internet than they ever did in print format. These publications are in the public domain, so anyone can use their internet connections to open them; to read *Morbidity and Mortality Weekly Reports*, visit http://www.cdc.gov/epo/mmwr/mmwr.html and to read *Weekly Epidemiological Record*, visit http://www.who.int/pub/wer.html.

As well as internet discussion groups and World Wide Web sites for professional use, there are huge numbers intended for the lay public. Many offer advice and suggestions about health and disease in general, and many others are disease or body system specific. These vary from reliable, informative, and truthful information and advice to outright quackery and deceit, and there is little guidance for uninitiated web-surfers, who must attempt to discriminate truth from lies. There are internet discussion groups and web sites for concerned patients, and parents of patients, with every imaginable medical disorder: obesity, anorexia, asthma, arthritis, psoriasis, chronic fatigue syndrome, fibromyalgia, insomnia, incontinence, multiple sclerosis, and innumerable others.

Distance education can be offered to students and to health professionals over a wide region, perhaps transcending national borders, using interactive internet discussions in which teachers offer a formal course of instruction, usually expecting students to answer questions and solve problems. This is particularly useful in countries such as South Africa, Australia, and Canada where distances are large and educational resources are limited, rather thinly spread, and mainly confined to big cities. The Maintenance of Competence program of the Royal College of Physicians and Surgeons of Canada, and the Maintenance of Professional Standards program of the Royal Australasian College of Physicians are among several that provide objective information as part of systems for recertification of specialists.

Internet-based distance education has several advantages over traditional correspondence courses. There is little need for paper to flow frequently, or indeed at all, between teacher and learners. It can be far more interactive than paper-based correspondence courses, allowing frequent and profuse questions and problem-solving exercises and feedback to students of the teacher's opinion of students' answers. Apart from the capital cost of computers and development of course material, the internet is cheaper than paper-based correspondence courses, eliminating the cost of paper and postage.

Several sets of more sophisticated lectures have been developed, for example, the 'Epidemiology super-course' which is based at the University of Pittsburgh, and is accessible at **http://www.pitt.edu/~super1/**. This offers lectures on special topics in epidemiology, all of which have been extensively peer-reviewed and are frequently updated.

All the leading, widely circulating journals of medicine and the sciences have 'home pages' on the World Wide Web, and some, for instance, the *British Medical Journal*, post their entire weekly contents electronically as well as by mail to subscribers. The *British Medical Journal*, and several other widely circulating medical and science journals, are accessible to anyone who has an internet connection (the *BMJ* is at **http://www.bmj.com**). Many other journals post their table of contents, abstracts, and selected other editorial content. Some journals are accessible by password only to users who must pay a subscription fee. Some, like their paper equivalents, support the cost of maintaining a web site in part by carrying advertisements, though these are seldom obtrusive.

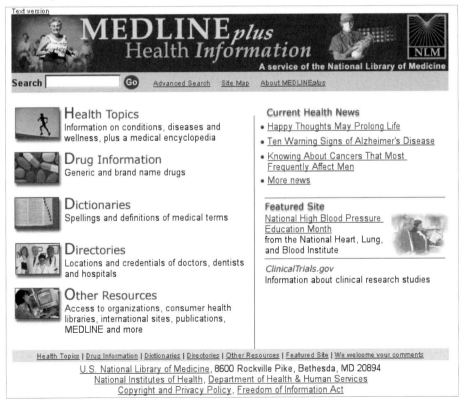

## EARLY AND RECENT

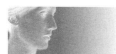

Guilielmo **SALICETTI**
(Guilielmus di Saliceto)
(c. 1210–77). Italian surgeon.
Salicetti was professor of
surgery in Bologna (c. 1268):
he moved to Verona in 1276.
The leading Italian surgeon of
the 13th century, his *Cyrurgia*
(first printed 1476) was a
widely consulted textbook for
many years. He reintroduced
the knife in place of the
cautery favored by the Arabs
and regarded suppuration,
inevitable after use of the
cautery, as undesirable. He
recorded crepitus as a sign of
fracture, distinguished
between arterial and venous
bleeding, noted contralateral
paralysis in skull wounds, and
appreciated the venereal
origin of chancres and bubos.

Maria **MONTESSORI**
(1870–1952). Italian
educationalist. Montessori
was the originator of the
well-known system of
teaching which bears her
name and was the first
woman in Italy to graduate in
medicine, from the University
of Rome in 1894. Her
methods were originally
devised for educating
backward children and
proved so successful that
she developed them for
application to normal children
of lower age groups.

There is an ongoing debate about the relative
merits of electronic versus paper communication
of original articles and information about recent
advances in the medical sciences. Proponents of
traditional journals assert that journal archives
must be paper-based and that convenience and
portability make paper journals the method of
choice for many purposes. Advocates of electronic
journals proclaim the merits of instant world-
wide transmission, avoidance of waste paper, and
the potential for additional sensory input such as
sound and moving pictures to illustrate clinical
features of medical conditions. The reality is that
each has its merits and uses, and its disadvantages.

Between the early and the late 1990s, that is,
within the space of about five years, the internet
and the World Wide Web have probably at least
doubled the volume of information that flows
from source to destination in the health sciences
as well as greatly increasing the speed with which
the information is transferred.

It remains to be seen whether the human mind,
even the mind of the most dedicated doctor, can
keep pace with this profuse flow of information,
and retain the capacity to discriminate what is
really important from what is trivial and
ephemeral.                                    JML

*See also* EDUCATION; JOURNALS; TELE-
MEDICINE

**ITALY** The words choler, melancholia, and
phlegm are still in use today. Pythagoras introduced them in the 6th century BC, while teaching
at his famous medical school in Crotone — at
that time Magna Graecia — on the HUMORS that
influence human behavior. Among the followers
of Pythagoras, Empedocles from Agrigento, an
anatomist, embryologist, and physician, was possibly the most illustrious, his reputation surviving
well into the Middle Ages.

Besides its impact on the Magna Graecia
medical culture, Greek influence was also predominant in Roman medicine, as CELSUS (p 806)
points out in his *De re medica* (c. AD 30), a historical appraisal and a summary of medical and
surgical knowledge of his time, that was highly
considered as a textbook up to Renaissance times.
GALEN (p 324), who worked in Rome in the 2nd
century AD, was of Greek origin. Few men have
influenced the progress of medical sciences as
Galen did.

It is hard to separate history from legend in
assessing the evidence of medical achievements in
the Middle Ages. Most important was the spread
of Christianity, which emphasized giving help and
relief to sufferers. Benedictine monks were particularly active: hospices and hospitals were built
along the main routes in the early Middle Ages, to
assist travelers and pilgrims. Some still exist, while

traces of others can still be found in place names
today. The Crusades prompted the institution of
the Knights Hospitalers' Orders, devoted to assist
merchants, soldiers, and pilgrims. The Order of
the Knights of Jerusalem, then of the Knights
of Malta, founded by Amalfi merchants, still
operates today.

Greek and Arabian medical traditions merged
in the first medical school in Italy, established in
SALERNO (p 448), around the turn of the
10th century AD, initially supported by the
Benedictines of Monte Cassino. It was the first
and only European institution where a degree in
medicine could be obtained, and it attracted
medical scholars from the whole of Europe.
Graduates of the school worked in Italy, France,
Germany, and England. In England, the court
physician at the time of Edward the Confessor
was a Salerno graduate.

From Salerno stemmed the medical school
at the University of BOLOGNA (p 447), founded
in the 12th century. Bologna was possibly the first
university fitting the modern idea of such an
institution. A century later, professors and
students overflowed from Bologna to PADUA
(p 447). Bologna and Padua became the most
important centers of medical studies in Italy. For
several centuries, the use of Latin as the language
of science fostered a great mobility of teachers
and students among the universities of Europe,
such as Paris and Montpellier in France, and
Oxford and Cambridge in Britain (a distinguished example being William HARVEY (p 363)).

Later, universities were founded in Naples
(1225), Siena (1241), Perugia (1266) (where, for the
first time, the denomination *Universitas studii* was
used), Florence (1320), Pisa (1338), and Pavia
(1361).

Several Renaissance painters and sculptors
were keen students of anatomy. Among them,
LEONARDO da Vinci (p 40) has a place of outstanding importance for his drawings and descriptions. The career of Leonardo da Vinci marked a
turning point in medical research and started the
quest for instruments of investigation. Galileo
Galilei built a THERMOMETER and a microscope.
Marcello MALPIGHI (p 37), professor at Bologna
and a corresponding member of the Royal Society,
published a treatise on macroscopic and microscopic pulmonary anatomy in 1661.

Rather than '*Anatomicorum princeps*' — he has
been considered by some — the Bologna
professor Giovanni Battista MORGAGNI (p 621)
was a pathologist, a pathophysiologist, and a clinician. His *De sedibus et causis morborum per
anatomen indagatis* represents a landmark in
medical knowledge. His interests encompassed all
topics in medicine, and several diseases still bear
his name. The spread of medical knowledge later

gave rise to medical schools of distinction and renown all over the world, in France, England, Spain, Germany, and America.

It is not possible to discuss here all the achievements of Italian medicine in modern times. Nevertheless, not to mention the name of Camillo Golgi would be a serious omission. A histologist who worked at Pavia, his name is linked with the study of the nervous system and of subcellular organelles. Working in Rome with Giovanni Battista Grassi and Ettore Marchiafava, Golgi also made a contribution to studies on MALARIA, then a major health problem in Italy.

## Organization of healthcare today

In 1978, Law no. 833/78 replaced the previous system of health insurance with the Sistema Sanitario Nazionale (national health system), which provides health assistance for every citizen. The organization of the system depends on the state and, at peripheral levels, on the regional and local council and Uniti Sanitarie Locali (local health units).

The Decrees 502 and 517 (1993) modified in part the organization. The number of local units has been drastically reduced, so that now each of them supervises the health problems of a territory corresponding to the geographical limits of a province. Greater internal management autonomy was granted, on commercial lines, to the new local health enterprises.

Hospitals have been divided into local hospitals directly managed by local health enterprises, and hospital enterprises, with a management of their own. The latter are defined as 'hospitals of national importance and/or highly specialized hospitals'. University hospitals take part in the National Health System in two ways. Eight university hospitals are managed directly by the universities (for example, in Naples and in Rome) and have special agreements; they fall under the supervision of regional authorities. All other university hospitals are part of the hospital enterprises having special agreements with the regional authorities. The participation of a university in a hospital makes the latter a health enterprise by definition, since university units are considered 'highly specialized' ones.

About 400 000 beds are still available under the National Health Service, less than one fifth being privately owned and bound to the service by agreements. Such a number is provisional, since the current trend is to decrease this number drastically.

Employees, nurses, and physicians are hired by the National Health System, the local health enterprises, and the hospital enterprises according to their qualifications, on the basis of civil service personnel collective contracts. So far, university teaching personnel engaged in the public health service have become automatically part of the personnel of the hospital enterprises, though maintaining their academic status. Modifications to this regimen are in progress, but not yet defined by law.

In medical practice, national collective agreements determine the optimum patient/physician ratio, terms of employment, limitations in private practice, and conditions governing the work of specialists. Citizens are free to choose their doctor, within the limited list size given to every physician. At a doctor's request, a patient may be admitted to hospital, emergencies being dealt with by the hospitals' emergency and admission departments. Local health enterprises authorize laboratory and instrumental investigations requested by the doctors, for which in some instances the patient must pay, as they must for non-essential drugs. Exemptions can be granted for those on low income and for diseases requiring continuous treatment.

Private practice is open to all physicians belonging to the College of Physicians who are not employed by the National Health System. They are also allowed hospital privileges.

The National Health Fund is made up of contributions paid by citizens, social contributions, and state funds.

Medical personnel working for the National Health Service in local hospitals are paid by the local health enterprises. Local health enterprises pay their own doctors; university physicians receive their salary from the university. An integration of the pay is provided when the salary is less than the one received by a National Health Service physician in the same position.

## Medical education

All medical schools in Italy are controled by the state, through the Ministry of University and Technological Research, and confer a legally recognized degree. The Ministry approves the statutes of the universities, publishes details of, and controls the competitive examinations for, academic posts, ratifying the consequent nominations made by the faculties.

Italy has many medical schools. Some universities have established branches in neighboring cities, where courses are also held.

Since 1986 medical degree curricula have undergone profound changes, also in connection with the European Union regulations. Despite each university having some autonomy in organizing its own curriculum, a common core allows students to transfer from one university to another without serious problems. Subjects are distributed over six years, for a total of 5500 hours. Each year is divided into two periods, at

## SALERNO

Salerno, on the west coast of Italy, just south of Naples, is famous in medical history for housing the first medical school of real pretensions in Europe, flourishing in the 11th and 12th centuries. It would be pleasing to think that it was here that Arabic medicine met the Christian medicine of the Benedictines of nearby Monte Cassino, but there is no firm evidence. It is certain that southern Italy and especially Sicily were much influenced both by Greek and Islamic cultures, as they moved along the Mediterranean. Several medical books were published from Salerno, and of especial interest is that there were female physicians and students. The practice of medicine came under the jurisdiction of the Emperor Frederick II, who in 1221 decreed that doctors would have to pass examinations set by the masters in Salerno. Moreover, no one was allowed to start an education in medicine until the age of 21, the previous three years being spent in the study of logic; the medical course lasted five years. This sort of pattern has therefore persisted for about 800 years.

the end of which the student faces the examinations in the subjects taught in that period. Preclinical medicine is taught in the first three years and includes chemistry, physics, anatomy, physiology, biochemistry, and general pathology. In the last term of the third year the student may choose to spend 150 hours either in a laboratory or on a ward. Clinical medicine, preventive, and social medicine are taught in the following three years, with courses in subjects such as pharmacology, pathology, internal medicine, general surgery, obstetrics and gynecology, pediatrics, neurology, psychiatry, medical and surgical specialties, legal medicine, hygiene, to mention the main ones.

Since 1987, medical faculties have determined each year the maximum number of places for new students, who are admitted after a placement test to the first year. The degree in medicine is conferred after all curricular requirements have been completed and a thesis discussed. Graduates work for six months in university clinics or in selected hospitals rotating in internal medicine, general surgery, obstetrics and gynecology, and emergency units, before taking their board examination. Postgraduate specialization schools are established in every faculty. Their organization and curricula depend on European Union regulations, under the control of the Ministry.

Graduates may apply for doctoral courses (*dottorato di ricerca*) organized by the universities in various subjects of biomedical research. Each doctorate has its own curriculum, which includes the various research activities. The candidate chooses the topic of the research to be performed and works under the supervision of a tutor. Research may be carried out in a university or qualified research institution in Italy or abroad. Once the curriculum has been completed, a national committee evaluates the research, the published papers, and the thesis, which is discussed. At any institution, a doctorate was once considered as the means of obtaining an academic position. However, shortage of funding has lately prevented the establishment of an adequate number of courses.

Most universities have undergraduate schools aimed at training personnel to work in the

National Health System and in the universities as nurses, technicians, or administrators.

## Physicians

The number of physicians in Italy was 332 588 at the 1996 census, in a population of 57 268 598. This huge number is because in 1971, as a result of the 1968 revolution, access to university was opened to young people licensed from high schools of every kind and no longer limited to those graduating from upper secondary schools (*liceo*). In those years the medical profession was an appealing career chosen by many young people. In the academic year 1976–7 medical students made up 13.3% of all first year students in Italian universities, compared with an average of 7.5 in pre-1968 years.

Thus in 1977 there was a dramatic increase in graduates from medical school which continued for ten years. By 1987, faculties were allowed to program enrolments, reducing the number of graduates slightly in subsequent years. Most Italian doctors range in age between 36–45 and the decrement trend is apparent when looking at the group aged 26–30. The situation causes the dramatic problem of medical un- or underemployment, since younger doctors are prevented from entering into the active profession by the 'wall' — the number of active colleagues aged 36–45.

## Allied health workers

In Italy there are three distinct groups of ancillaries and nurses. Registered nurses are employed both in hospitals and in community care services and have a variety of roles, ranging from ordinary ward services to surgical assistance, geriatric care, and outpatient services.

The role of health visitors has recently expanded, also as a consequence of the recent reduction of long-term hospital wards. Such patients are now taken care of in various recently established institutions within the community. Some health visitors are also employed by local or municipal authorities.

Pediatricians work mainly in pediatric hospital nurseries, but may be employed by local health authorities. Some also work in the community.

APol MVG

William **JAMES** (1842–1910). American psychologist. William James was born in New York, the brother of Henry James the novelist. He started his study of medicine at Harvard, but broke off to explore the Amazon with Louis Agassiz; subsequently he went to Europe to study with HELMHOLTZ (p 372), VIRCHOW (p 853), and BERNARD (p 102). He took his MD from Harvard in 1869 but never practiced. Indeed, his studies seem to have induced a neurosis and he remained at home for some time as a semi-invalid. For just over a year in 1872 he taught physiology at Harvard, but then moved on to what was then physiological psychology. By 1890 he published *The principles of psychology*, which helped establish the subject as a science on a par with biology. He then entered a religious phase, applying psychology to religious experience, and these studies with his later works in philosophy started furious arguments. In philosophy he was a pragmatist, judging ideas by their consequences. This remarkable man made important contributions to psychology, religion, and philosophy and became world-renowned and much esteemed. He was empirical and not fanatical so that he has left no school to follow him, and one suspects that he would not have wished to.

**JAPAN** Until the Second World War, Japan was considered to be one of the most civilized nations in the Orient, as there was much interest and concern about public health in both the private and public sectors alike. The general state of health, however, was unsatisfactory. TUBERCULOSIS and other acute infectious diseases ranked high among the causes of death, and the infant death rate was also high. The average life expectancy in 1935 was under 50 years (46.9 for men and 49.6 for women).

After the war, American influence and the advent of antibiotics greatly improved healthcare in Japan. Birth control guidance, improvement of environmental hygiene, mass examination for tuberculosis, and increased opportunities for regular health check-ups for the early detection of adult chronic diseases such as HYPERTENSION, malignancy,

cardiac disease, and DIABETES became possible. Through increased health education and public awareness about the prevention of chronic disease, the life-span of the Japanese began to extend steadily. By 1998 the average life expectancy of the Japanese had reached 77.16 years for men (compared with 73.8 years for the Caucasian male population of the USA, in 1996) and 84.01 years for women (79.6 for American Caucasian females). Thus, Japanese men ranked second in the world in terms of longevity, next to Iceland. Moreover, the average life expectancy for women was the highest in the world. The consequence of this achievement, however, was a rapidly aging population structure. Some of the reasons underlying this notable change were: a drastic decrease in deaths from tuberculosis and other infectious diseases; a marked decline in the infant death rate; and the homogeneity, lack of poverty, and lack of disadvantaged groups in Japanese society.

The high infant death rate in the past has been partly due to the fecundity of Japanese women, and partly to infant deaths from infectious diseases and malnutrition. In children less than 12 months old, the death rate in 1925 was 150 per 1000 live births. By 1940 it had fallen to 90 per 1000. The decline continued steadily after the Second World War; in 1960 it was 30.7 per 1000, and in 1997, 3.7 per 1000. Such a rapid decline was not seen elsewhere in the world, and today Japan ranks among the nations with the lowest infant death rate.

The adult death rate in the population was 14.6 in 1947, two years after the Second World War, but had fallen to 7.3 in 1997 (compared with 9.4 in the USA in 1994). The notable decline in general and infant death rate mentioned above, reflects the striking improvements achieved in general health conditions during these periods.

### Changes in the causes of death

Until around 1950 tuberculosis, pneumonia, and other infectious diseases were the principal causes of death of the Japanese. After that, deaths from cerebrovascular disease increased rapidly, and in 1951 this became the most common cause of death, cancer ranked second, and cardiovascular

## TWO JAPANESE MICROBIOLOGISTS

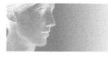

Baron Shibasaburo **KITASATO** (1852–1931). Japanese bacteriologist. He was the first to obtain a pure culture of *Clostridium tetani* and worked on immunization against tetanus and diphtheria (1890). He isolated tetanus toxin and proved it could be used to immunize against tetanus. He used killed bacterial cultures for vaccination and isolated *Pasteurella pestis* in the Hong Kong epidemic of plague independently of Yersin (1894).

Kiyoshi **SHIGA** (1870–1957). Japanese microbiologist. After graduation Shiga became an assistant to Kitasato. From 1901–3 he worked with EHRLICH (p 260), returning to take charge of a department of the Kitasato Institute. In 1919 he was made professor at Keijo, Chosan. He carried out valuable work on plague and tetanus, but his name was made by isolating the dysentery bacillus now known as *Shigella*.

diseases third. In 1981 cancer ranked first, followed by cerebrovascular and cardiac diseases.

What reasons underlay the rapid decrease of cerebrovascular deaths in the 1970s, which had long been the principal cause of death in Japan? First, the dietary habits changed, particularly the high salt intake (average 15 g/day); the intake gradually decreased to 12 g/day through extensive health education. Secondly, regular health examinations focusing on blood pressure measurement, which became widely available, to the general public from 1955, allowed the early detection and treatment of hypertension, thus reducing deaths from cerebrovascular disease, and extending the average life expectancy of the Japanese. Cardiac disease is now the second most important cause of death in Japan; however, it is very low compared with the USA.

Among malignant diseases, lung cancer ranks highest, followed by stomach cancer, which is diagnosed at an early stage, as gastrointestinal X-rays and gastroendoscopy screening are readily accessible to the general public. Early cases of stomach cancer are successfully managed by surgery. Also, the decrease in salt intake, and westernization of dietary habits, are assumed to be contributory factors tending towards a gradual decrease in cases of stomach cancer; but colon cancer cases are steadily increasing.

## Medical problems

Japanese medical care costs much less than in the USA and other western countries. Japan had a per capita annual healthcare expenditure in 1996 of US$1741 (¥182 805) compared with the American figure of US$3925. Surgical operation rates and their costs in Japan were about one-quarter of those in the USA. This is because the Ministry of Health and Welfare controls medical fees and all other charges in Japanese medicine. However, annual medical expenditure has gradually increased up to US$276 billion (¥29 000 billion) in 1997, and the costs of medical care of the elderly over the age of 65 reached 31.5% of the total annual medical expenditure in Japan (US$ = ¥105).

The number of hospital beds in Japan per capita is the highest in the world. The average length of hospital stay in Japan was as long as 22.0 days in 1998, and cost per inpatient per day US$223 (= ¥24 557), given the longer hospital stay when compared with the USA; the cost of one outpatient attendance was US$76 (= ¥8028).

Japanese patients stay in hospital for an unusually long time when admitted because of illness; however, this may be offset against their total vacation time. The Japanese are seen much more often by doctors in primary care or hospital outpatients than in other western countries. They visit their doctors on average 17.9 times yearly. In 1996 there were about 240 908 doctors serving a population of 126 million in Japan; however, there were only about 928 896 nurses, including both registered and 'practical' nurses. They have to work hard and to carry a heavy physical load because of a chronic shortage of hospital nurses. Many graduate nurses do not stay long in their posts and many big hospitals have had to close some of their wards.

There is a universal health insurance system controlled by the Japanese government, allowing anyone to be seen in the outpatient department of most hospitals or dispensaries at any time. However, they often have to wait two or three hours for 3 minutes' consultation with doctors as there are so many outpatients. A doctor's income (the fees payable for outpatient consultations) is calculated according to the number of consultations and not by the length of time required for each consultation. The Japanese healthcare insurance system is very much appreciated by the elderly, as virtually all their medical costs are paid.

Today, Japan faces a growing problem of how to provide medical and welfare care for an aging population. The administrative measures needed to cope with this situation are lagging behind the need. Although the proportion of people over 65 in the whole of Japan is still just 15.3% (1997), in some remote rural areas where there is a population drift to the cities, villages may have over 20%.

As the elderly population increases, so do medical costs. The entire population is at present covered by one of several health insurance organizations, and medical costs are paid to the hospitals and physicians on a fee for item of service basis. This method is under review by a joint commission comprising representatives from health insurance organizations, hospital authorities, the Japan Medical Association, and learned societies.

## Expenditure

In 1997, 7.4% of the Japanese gross national product was spent on medical care, but it is becoming increasingly difficult even to maintain this level. A rise is considered to be inevitable by most doctors. The Japanese government, however, is trying to keep expenditure below 7%. An amendment of the Health and Medical Services Law for the Aged and an increase in the number of intermediate nursing homes are some of the principal measures proposed to contain rising costs, as is a redistribution of medical expenditure. Japan has twice as many hospital beds per unit population as the USA, and too many elderly people are long-stay residents in hospital. It is intended to reduce hospital admissions and to shorten lengths of stay by the provision of intermediate nursing homes and improved community care with visiting nurses. The government will be asked to provide adequate financial assistance to the private sector, to build and run these intermediate nursing homes. The qualified registered nurses who gave up working after marriage will be encouraged to offer home-care nursing, assisted by trained helpers, publicly subsidized; voluntary workers will also be encouraged to help.

The social security budget in Japan is much smaller than that of many western nations; if increases in medical expenditure can be rationally and effectively curtailed, it should be possible to increase the budget for social security benefits, including community care.

It is also essential to improve housing conditions. In an urban environment, high-rise apartments should be planned in order to secure extra living space. More elderly people live with their children in Japan when compared with most western nations. If this is to continue, larger family homes will be needed as well as trained helpers subsidized by public funds, to assist the relatives caring for the elderly. Housewives and elderly people who are healthy enough to work could be recruited for this purpose.

As the age of retirement in Japan has been increased from 55 to 60 in recent years and may soon rise to 65, it will be increasingly important to create a social structure offering opportunities for work, social activities, and learning for the elderly. The new intermediate nursing homes may have to be provided in urban environments so that the elderly in these homes can be in touch with their younger relatives; elderly people of experience and ability may be able to help in youth educational programs. These social activities will give the elderly people a chance to find a meaning in life and at the same time help them to stay mentally young.

## Medical education

Contemporary Japanese medical education is based on western medicine; yet, until 120 years ago, medicine in Japan was predominantly of Chinese origin. Chinese medicine was brought to Japan in AD 554, but medicine did not develop extensively before 1550. From 1641 on, with the arrival of Dutch physicians, Dutch medicine was introduced and spread in Japan, centering on Kyushu Islands in the south. This, in turn, led to the founding of private medical schools. In 1849, SMALLPOX vaccine was imported into Japan, and was eventually used throughout the country.

In 1870, shortly after the ascension of Emperor Meiji, the Japanese government decreed the adoption of German medicine. The first medical school specializing in German medicine was founded in 1877 in Tokyo (the predecessor of the Faculty of Medicine, Tokyo Imperial University), with professors of medicine recruited from Germany. Subsequently, national medical schools were built in cities such as Kyoto, Sendai, Sapporo, and Fukuoka.

By 1939, there were 13 medical schools in Japan. During the Second World War the number of medical schools was increased to 34, to train military doctors. As the war progressed, the number of Japanese medical schools further increased to 51. After the war, the system was changed under the guidance of the Allied Occupation Forces, being rapidly replaced by the Anglo–American style. Under this system, a student enters medical school after graduation from high school, undertakes two years of a pre-medical school curriculum, out of a total of six years of medical education.

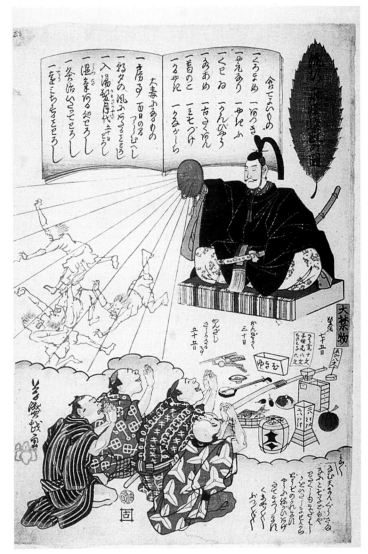

Paying homage to the deity who banished measles. (Reproduced courtesy of the National Library of Medicine, Bethesda, MD.)

Before the Second World War a license to practice medicine was conferred automatically on all graduating students of medical schools. A change took place after the war, so that only those who completed a year of rotating internship after graduation became qualified to take the medical licensing board examination and obtain a license.

In 1963, the internship program was abolished as the result of opposition by the interns, who saw their year of training as working without pay. Now students take the national medical licensing board examination immediately after graduation; those who qualify receive a stipend while training in university hospitals or other public or private teaching hospitals.

By 1969, there were 46 medical schools in Japan. But a shortage of doctors became apparent in rural areas, so that a government policy was implemented to allocate at least one medical school to each prefecture. Between 1970 and 1979, the number of medical schools was increased to 80 (including 51 national or prefectural medical schools, and 29 private ones, a system which continues today).

The enrollment of students increased proportionally, reaching 8360 in 1981. The government considered this to be a surplus, and advised schools to cut back on admissions, resulting in a decrease in the number of medical students to 7695 in 1998. The teacher–student ratio in medical schools is 1 to 2.0. Currently there are 19.1 doctors per 10 000 population, fewer than in Britain and the USA.

Pre-war Japanese medical schools tended to value basic medical science. This was a characteristic of German medical education, resulting to some extent in a lack of bedside training. During the postwar era, many medical personnel came to Japan from the USA to advise Japanese schools on their development. Medical textbooks and journals published in Britain and the USA were imported, and exposure to such literature seems to have increased the regard for clinical medicine. However, the staff's dedication to teaching clinical medicine is still lacking, particularly when compared with the specialist training programs in the USA. This is attributed to the attitude of the medical school professors, who over-encourage young students to pursue basic medical research rather than to acquire clinical skills from an early stage in their training.

Most drugs prescribed in Japan are pharmaceutical products of western origin. But Chinese herbal medicine, as well as moxibustion and acupuncture, have been covered by health insurance since 1976. Thus the application of both western and Oriental style medical treatment is gradually gaining ground in present-day Japan.

### Nursing education

In Japan there are three different routes to become licensed as a registered nurse: a three-year course of nursing school attached to the hospital; a three-year course at junior college of nursing; or four-year course at a college of nursing. Only ten colleges of nursing offered the last type of course in 1988, but during the past 11 years, the number has increased to 76 in 1999 and 40 of them have graduate courses. Hence the level of academic nursing in Japan has been improving in clinical competence, and nurses can now assume a major role in healthcare in Japan.                SH

*See also* HEALTHCARE SYSTEMS

**JEHOVAH'S WITNESSES** See RELIGIOUS SECTS

Edward **JENNER** (1749–1823). British physician. Son of a vicar, Jenner was born in Berkeley, Gloucestershire, and after receiving his early education locally, and an apprenticeship to a country doctor, he went to St George's Hospital, London, in 1770, to study anatomy and surgery under John HUNTER (p 398). Three years later he returned to Berkeley, where he established a practice and remained there until his death. Jenner is remembered for his proof that cowpox gave immunity to smallpox and the development of the smallpox vaccine. The practice of smallpox inoculation had been introduced into England in 1721 by Lady Mary Wortley Montagu, wife of the British Ambassador to Turkey. It was frequently fatal; over the course of 25 years, Jenner realized that milkmaids who had been infected with cowpox were unaffected by the smallpox inoculation. He reported the results of his experimental observations of 23 cases to the Royal Society, but the subject was considered too unsubstantiated to be published. Jenner therefore published *An inquiry into the causes and effects of the variolae vaccinae* privately in 1898. Despite the skepticism of a large proportion of the medical profession, within a few years the technique of vaccination was widespread and mortality from smallpox had decreased dramatically. As a naturalist, Jenner wrote several works describing his observations of birds in the English countryside. His work was recognized more outside than within Britain.

**JOHNS HOPKINS HOSPITAL** See USA

**JOURNALS** Medical research is incomplete unless it can be communicated, which is best done by publication (as one scientist told his students, 'think, work, publish'). Not only does this present the findings, but it enables research findings to be disseminated widely, can give these in the detail that fellow experts need, and can record them in permanent form.

Scientific journals were not introduced until 200 years after the invention of printing; they arose in the mid 1600s with the formation of the new scientific societies such as the French Academy and the Royal Society of London. Although there were a few journals specifically devoted to medicine, these were fleeting and medical men published mainly in general scientific rather than medical journals. The 19th century saw the beginnings of the specifically medical journal. Moreover, during this century there was a large expansion in the number of journals published, particularly in Germany, as well as two important trends and an evanescent one: respectively, the establishment of the general medical journal, the beginnings of the specialist journal, and the publication of the 'one-man' journal. The general journal is aimed at all doctors, the specialist journal deals only with a single specialty (such as cardiology), and the one-man journal is written and edited by an individual.

### Establishment of the general journal

In the 19th century two prominent editors of general journals, Thomas WAKLEY (this page) of the *Lancet* and Ernest HART (this page) of the *British Medical Journal*, used their journals to fight against privilege and nepotism and to campaign against social evils, such as poor medical care in WORKHOUSES and the armed forces, air pollution, and the adulteration of food. Wakley, the more prominent of the two, was able to carry his campaigns even further by being elected a member of parliament in Britain, and by the time he died in 1862 had laid secure foundations for the general journal. The latter aimed at informing, instructing, commenting, and amusing — providing a mixture of original papers about medical research with up-to-date comment and current news. Though the *Lancet* had been established in 1823 and the *British Medical Journal* in 1828, another general journal, now called the *New England Journal of Medicine*, had started even earlier in Boston, USA, in 1812. Nevertheless, for its first 150 years of publication it did not have a major impact, either nationally or internationally, and the national medical journals in other countries, such as France, Austria, Australia, and The Netherlands, followed the pattern established by the *Lancet* and the *British Medical Journal*. One notable feature of 19th century journals was their failure rate: a large proportion of those founded ceased publication within a few years, particularly in Germany. Editors often found themselves short of material to print and resorted to copying articles printed in other journals, with or without permission or attribution.

Another positive feature was the launching of the specialist journal: by the end of the First World War virtually every specialty had at least one journal devoted to it (often published by the

society concerned) and as new specialties were started so journals were started to serve them. During the 1930s and after the Second World War the pace of subdividing medicine into specialties continued and was reflected in the number and character of the specialist journals. Other countries besides the USA and Britain began to publish specialist journals, notably Scandinavia. The character of some of the new specialist journals also changed: they became 'super-specialist' or even 'super-super-specialist'. At the same time, reflecting the need for doctors to cover the field adequately, several new types of journal were introduced — including the abstract journal, the review journal, and the medical newspaper.

Before the beginning of the Second World War it became apparent that the number of scientific journals was increasing both regularly and rapidly — by 6–7% a year, thus doubling every 10–15 years and rising ten-fold every 35–50 years. Before the 20th century the total number had been modest because of the failure rate of so many new journals. Thereafter, journals continued to be published, but survived, probably for several reasons: their guaranteed circulations due to their association with specialist societies; the enormous rise in research and library budgets (together with the great expansion of the latter); and innumerable new findings from the vastly increased amount of research.

### Total numbers

Today estimates vary of the number of journals, because not all are included in the list maintained by the US National Library of Medicine. It seems likely that there are at least 24 000 medico-scientific journals, and there is little sign of a slow down in the appearance of new ones. The popular view was that such an increase in the number and complexity of journals has been a sign of the scientific community's folly and self-agrandizement. Others, however, argued against such a simplistic view. Professor Derek de Solla Price, of Yale University, showed that scholars have read and written at much the same rate over the past three centuries, and for similar reasons: communication and assessment of the results and the prestige of the individual or the research group. New journals are started not only to cover new subjects but also because the disciplines of many readers cross fixed boundaries, and, for instance, molecular biologists need to know what is going on outside their own particular subspecialty. The number of scientists working in research may well add up to the total number there has been throughout the past, with a roughly constant proportion of scientists per journal. History has shown, moreover, that faced with information overload, scientists have always managed to cope. Initially information

## NOTABLE EDITORS

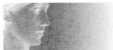

Thomas **WAKLEY** (1795–1862). British physician, reformer, and editor. Wakley was a friend of William Cobbett and well aware of the jobbery and nepotism in the medical profession. He founded the *Lancet* in 1823, publishing reports of hospital lectures and operations and attacking hospital administration and the Royal College of Surgeons. Coroner for West Middlesex from 1839 until his death he sat as Member of Parliament for Finsbury from 1835–52. He obtained a pardon for the Tolpuddle Martyrs. Clauses from his Private Member's Bill were adopted in the Medical Act 1858. He reduced adulteration by publishing analyses of foods in the *Lancet* (1851).

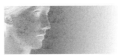

Ernest **HART** (1836–98). English medical editor and publicist. Hart entered ophthalmic surgery in St Mary's Hospital, becoming dean from 1863–9. He also worked for the *Lancet*, but in 1866 he became editor of the *British Medical Journal*, a post which he retained until shortly before his death in January 1898 — the second volume for 1897 still has him as editor. He gradually gave up practice, but turned his attention to public issues — the improvement of poor law hospitals, diseases carried by water and milk, smoke abatement, the medical education of women, and medical life insurance.

*(continued overleaf)*

(continued)

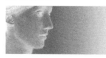

Franz Joseph
**INGELFINGER** (1910–80).
American physician and
medical editor. Ingelfinger
was born in Germany and his
family moved to the USA in
1922. He trained in the new
specialty of gastroenterology
at the University of
Pennsylvania, and returned to
Boston as chief of the section
of gastroenterology at the
Boston City Hospital. There,
between 1942–67 he trained
a remarkably successful group
of young physicians. In 1967
Ingelfinger embarked on a
new career — as editor of the
*New England Journal of
Medicine*. He promulgated
what became known as 'the
Ingelfinger rule', that is,
refusing to publish
information that had been
prereleased to the Press. This
caused some resentment and
anxiety among science
writers, but has generally
been accepted and followed
by other editors.

was synthesized in encyclopedias, then in abstracting and review journals, and most recently in computer databases. The last in particular has proved useful for 'literature searches' — finding out what has been published on a topic, and where, and how much this has been quoted in subsequent publications ('citation'). The US National Library of Medicine produces the *Index Medicus*, and a growing variety of electronically accessible catalogs of medical, scientific, and related information. These can be used to read on computer screens, and to download and print, all the indexed articles on a specified subject, their abstracts, in some cases even the full text. This is among several popular uses of the INTERNET.

### Weighing in the balance

From the beginnings of scientific publication editors have tried to ensure that their journals acted as filters rather than as sponges, which absorb everything submitted for publication. Such filtration was by 'peer review' — the evaluation of submissions by experts. Initially, this was done by members of the editorial board, but with the increasing complexity of research most editors now also have a further team of expert advisers, or 'referees'. These reviewers answer questions about the newness, credibility, and importance of the new work, and play an important part in the ultimate decision about its suitability for publication. Given that the rejection rates of the principal general medical journals now approach 90%, and those for the specialty journals 60% — and that publication in a major journal has an important, and often crucial, role in any assessment of an individual or a department for further research grants, tenure, promotion, and prestige — such peer review clearly has a pivotal role in science, and until recently little has been done to study either its process or outcome. Recently, editors and others have started to study these and to report their findings at international conferences devoted specifically to peer review.

Not only has the price of journals risen inexorably, but for some time the medical community has been concerned about delay in publication and difficulties in distribution, especially to the developing world. Hence it was natural to turn to the electronic media to help solve some of these problems. The initial experiments were with on-line services, not only for retrieving references, but also for transmitting the contents of a journal coincidentally with its publication in conventional form. The enormous expansion of the INTERNET has now enabled journals to achieve electronic dissemination much more simply than before, and most of the principal ones now have their own website. Not only can this medium give

the full text and illustrations for an article, but it can also speed up peer review and print comments or changes, or both, to the published article. Again, some have suggested that research findings that have not undergone formal peer review should be posted on the internet to allow expert comment — a system similar to preprints that already exist in most scientific disciplines. Although some senior members of the scientific community frown on such an extension of publication — fearing its lack of scientific rigor and the potential for harm by publicizing scary results that have not been validated by peer review — it seems likely that such a system will creep into practice, very much as unreviewed work is currently reported to colleagues around the coffee table. If so, no doubt some way will be found of introducing rigor into the electronic presentation, given that some sort of peer review has been a part of publication ever since the *Journal de Sçavans* and the *Philosophical Transactions of the Royal Society* were first published in 1665.                                    SPL

**JUDAISM** is the oldest of the monotheist religions. Jews claim descent from Abraham, the son of Terah, so the historical roots of the Jewish faith can be traced back about 3,000 years. Since the rise of Christendom, Jews have been frequent victims of persecution, massacred in large numbers in pogroms, segregated in ghettos, and in those parts of Europe controlled briefly by the Nazis, systematically exterminated in the HOLOCAUST. Jewish customs include ritual CIRCUMCISION of newborn boys. This custom is said, probably correctly, to promote sexual hygiene. There are several major groups of Jews, notably Ashkenazi and Sephardim, and orthodox and reform synagogues. Judaism has remained relatively free of deviant sects. A central feature of the Jewish culture is a great respect for scholarly activities and the arts; Jews are therefore strongly represented in such professions, including medicine. Among some communities of orthodox Jews, many generations of consanguinous marriages, a consequence of living in segregated ghettoes rather than part of their faith, has led to a high prevalence of genetic disorders such as Tay–Sachs disease. Compared with non-Jews of similar socioeconomic background, Jews have low incidence rates of certain kinds of cancer, for instance, cervical cancer, but high prevalence rates of metabolic diseases such as DIABETES.

Jews adhere to some important dietary customs that may have originated in empirical observations of adverse consequences of eating and/or drinking certain food items. Thus, they do not eat pork or partake of meat and milk or milk products together.

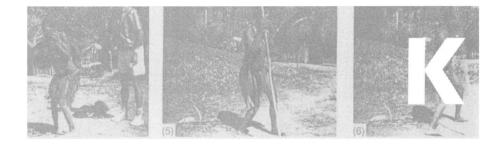

**KALA-AZAR** (Hindi for 'black fever') is a serious chronic infection with the protozoan parasite *Leishmania donovani*. Without treatment it carries a mortality rate which may be as high as 90%. It is usually a zoonosis, that is, a disease of animals which can be transmitted to man. The animals are mostly wild and domestic canines and rodents, and transmission occurs via biting sandflies of various *Phlebotomus* species. The disease is prevalent in the Mediterranean littoral, East and West Africa, Asia Minor, southern Arabia, India, China, and South America. Also known as visceral leishmaniasis, kala-azar is predominantly an infection of the reticuloendothelial system; the cardinal features are fever, wasting, anemia, and enlargement of lymph nodes, liver, and spleen, the spleen in particular often reaching a great size. Hyperpigmentation of the skin of the hands, feet, face, and abdomen is common, accounting for the name 'kala-azar'. Death is usually the result of intercurrent infection, but when diagnosis is made early and treatment (antimony preparations are the first choice but other compounds are effective in resistant cases) is quickly introduced, almost all patients recover.

*See also* INSECTS; LEISHMANIASIS

**KEYHOLE SURGERY** See MINIMALLY INVASIVE SURGERY; SURGERY, GENERAL – HISTORY

Heinrich Hermann Robert **KOCH** (1843–1910). German bacteriologist. After service as a medical officer in the Franco-Prussian war, in 1872, Koch was appointed district physician (*Kreisphysicus*) in Wollstein, a small town in Posen. Here he established his own laboratory, culturing *Bacillus anthracis*, the organism of anthrax (1876), studying sporulation, and developing photomicrography of bacteria. In 1880 he was appointed to a vacancy in the Department of Health and con-

cerned himself with the bacteriology of wound infection and with improving technical methods. He isolated *Mycobacterium tuberculosis* in 1882 and in the same year enunciated the four postulates (Koch's postulates) to be satisfied before accepting an organism as the cause of a specific disease. In 1883 he visited Egypt and India, where he identified the *Vibrio cholerae* as the cause of cholera and the Koch-Weeks bacillus as responsible for a conjunctivitis which was common locally. He noted the presence of amebae in those dying with dysentery. On a later visit to Africa he showed that relapsing fever was due to a spirochete carried by a tick. *Ornithodorus moubata*. His latter years were occupied by controversies over tuberculin, which he had prepared in 1891. At first he claimed it as a cure for tuberculosis but he was later forced to recant. He denied that the bovine *M. tuberculosis* was pathogenic to man. He was awarded the NOBEL PRIZE in 1905.

**KURU** is a uniformly fatal (within months rather than years) degeneration of the brain characterized clinically by incoordination and mental changes, and pathologically by spongy changes in the brain. The disease occurs only among a small group of primitive people in central New Guinea, and is now rapidly on the decline. It is transmissible to subhuman primates by inoculation of brain material; the agent has not been precisely identified but is clearly a slow virus bearing a close resemblance to the agent which causes scrapie in sheep and CREUTZFELDT-JAKOB DISEASE in man. What is known of the epidemiology is consistent with human-to-human transmission by the ritual cannibalistic practice of eating the brains of dead relatives. Like the disease itself, this custom is now almost extinct, largely as a result of its discouragement by missionaries.

*See also* CREUTZFELDT–JAKOB DISEASE

A series of pictures taken from a 16-mm movie sequence of a patient with kuru. Midline postural instability and the inability to stand still are shown as the patient gets up and stands. As she walks she shows a wide-based, ataxic gait. Turning, even with the aid of a stick, leads to severe unsteadiness and loss of balance. (From Weatherall, D. J. et al. (1996). *The Oxford textbook of medicine*, 3rd edn, OUP.)

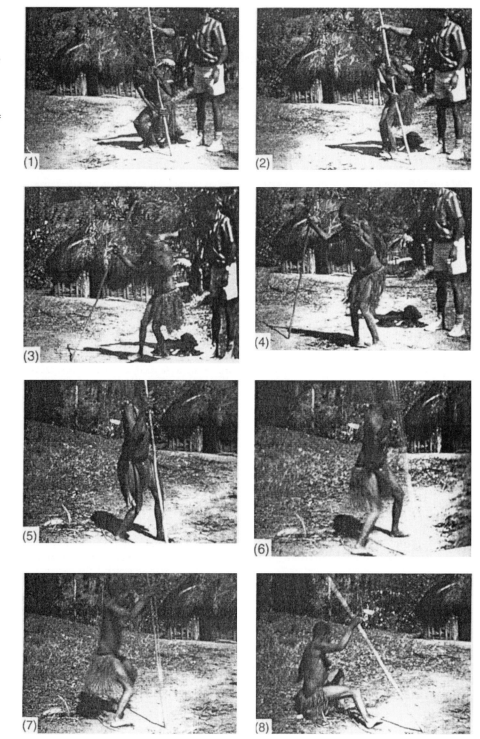

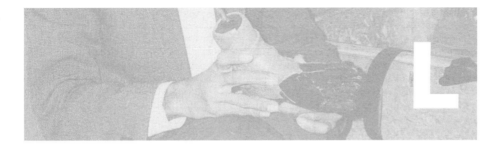

**LABORATORY MEDICINE** comprises experimental research and its practical application in patient and population management and the transmission of its findings in medical education. It merits notice, cognitively, because of its production of new and routine medical knowledge at a special site away from the bedside and socially, because of its place in the massive industry of modern western medicine. In the past century, laboratory research has been increasingly institutionalized in universities and industry and also in government and philanthropically funded institutions. The laboratory is involved in two main aspects of routine medical practice: for populations, in laboratories dealing with public health matters; and for individual patient management, in hospital laboratories. In these two situations, diagnostic and other routine testing often goes hand in hand with epidemiological or clinical research. Research and routine laboratory medicine are inextricably linked.

Elements of laboratory medicine may be traced to antiquity and indeed the name is derived from the Latin root which also gives us 'labor' and is related to the alchemists' 'elaboratory'. None the less the scale of laboratory medicine today, and the degree of authority invested in it, distinguish it as uniquely modern. Laboratory medicine arose in the 19th century when there was an increasing recognition by individuals, professions, industry, educational authorities, and governments that experimental science was, for all sorts of reasons, a valuable activity. The modern laboratory scientist, the creation of this outlook, had appeared in Europe and North America by the end of the 19th century, but historians agree that Germany was the source of many of the important features of this new sort of worker. German universities, and more particularly their specialized *institutes* with their powerful professorial chiefs, were the model for laboratory science for the rest of the world. In particular, at the Institute of Chemistry at the University of Giessen in the 1840s, the chemist Justus von LIEBIG (this page) built the first modern scientific research school, training students who published in specialist journals and went on to head their own departments.

Physiology, along with chemistry, was the science on which reformers endeavored to build a new practice of medicine. At the University of Berlin, a contemporary of Liebig's, Johannes Müller, built a research school that aspired to study physiology by integrating animal experiment, comparative anatomy, embryology, and histology. Simultaneously in France a few men, notably François Magendie, were trying to make physiology a pure science based almost entirely on animal experiment. However, the power of the French hospitals and the CLINICOPATHOLOGICAL tradition, ensured there was very little institutional support for the subject. In Britain, particularly in England, the commitment to laboratory science was even less pronounced, notably because of the dominance of the great clinical teachers and a descriptive or natural historical approach to body form and function.

### German influence

By the second half of the 19th century the new basic sciences had become sufficiently prominent in Germany for foreign students, including North Americans, to flock there. Equally important, the first changes in medical practice consequent on the introduction of these sciences to the bedside appeared. At a new physiological institute at Heidelberg, Hermann von HELMHOLTZ (p 372), explicitly studying animal function in physical and chemical terms, devised the ophthalmoscope. At his major Institute of Physiology in Leipzig, Karl LUDWIG (p 643) produced the kymograph for graphically recording body function. Conceptually this device was the basis of clinical instruments, such as the sphygmograph and the sphygmomanometer, that were introduced into bedside medicine by physiologically minded physicians in the late 19th and early 20th century. The use of these devices was not simply the isolated application of laboratory medicine to practice; rather it involved a fundamental reconceptualization of the body in laboratory terms. The meaning of blood pressure, for example, ultimately referred to animal experiments carried out a long way from the ward. One of the most

**EARLY BIOCHEMIST**

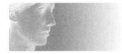

Justus von **LIEBIG**, Baron (1803–73). German chemist. After working with Gay-Lussac in Paris, Liebig was appointed professor at Giessen in 1824, where his teaching of chemistry was based upon laboratory instruction. He succeeded to the chair of chemistry in Munich in 1852. Liebig was one of the early biochemists and founder of agricultural chemistry. He discovered chloroform and chloral (1831), hippuric acid (1829), and tyrosine (1829). He showed that carbohydrates and fats were oxidized in the tissues. He was unwilling to accept the role of bacteria in putrefaction and is now generally remembered for his meat extract.

striking programmatic arguments, that clinical medicine could and should eventually be based almost entirely on physiological research, was developed by France's most famous physiologist, Claude BERNARD (p 102), who set it out in his acclaimed and still widely read *An introduction to the study of experimental medicine* of 1865. The *Introduction*, nevertheless, is a 19th century text, based on secular, optimistic, and positivist assumptions about the nature of science that accord well with those Victorian ideals that deified the view that the progress of western society was inevitable and uncomplicated. In this respect it is notable that many Victorian clinicians who, in general, embraced science in medicine, were concerned about the damaging effects of the laboratory on a traditional *art* devoted to healing. Such suspicion, of course, was not limited to the 19th century, for the debate continues today.

### Clinic to bench

If the laboratory was moving into the ward, other developments in Germany made it possible to move the work of the clinic to the bench. Cell theory was largely the creation of the pupils of Müller and by mid-century it was converted into a comprehensive theory of disease. Rudolph VIRCHOW (p 853), after 1856 director of a pathological institute in Berlin, whose *Cellularpathologie* appeared in 1858, was a major architect of the theory. To agree that cells were the basis of disease was to establish two new authorities in medicine: the microscope and its user. The diagnosis of disease could now be made by taking away parts of the body or its products — biopsy specimens, blood, sputum, urine, etc. — to a distant laboratory site, where cells could be examined for abnormalities in their number and conformation. Many standard hematological investigations, such as red cell counts and hemoglobin estimations, date from this period.

Physiology was the locus of the relatively backward professionalization in the medical sciences in Britain. At Cambridge, after 1870, Michael Foster established a research school that, along with its progeny, eventually equaled any in Germany. The foundations of new clinical approaches were built by many of Foster's students. The work of W. H. Gaskell on the heart's rhythmicity was used in the first two decades of the 20th century by Thomas LEWIS (p 188) at University College Hospital, London, in his fundamental work with the electrocardiograph (a device conceptually dependent on the kymograph). Across the road (Gower Street), the physiological researches of William Bayliss and Ernest Starling in University College formed the backbone of a new clinical discipline — ENDOCRINOLOGY.

Thus admiration for the laboratory changed the structure of practice. One of the most striking features of the growth of medicine during the 20th century was the increase in medical specialization. Specialization is often construed as a natural process, a passive response to a quantitative growth of medical knowledge. The reverse, however, is much nearer the case. Medical specialties were deliberately created by transforming the shape of medical knowledge. Clinical investigations did not simply pile up facts about disease at random, quite the opposite. New ideas about disease based on laboratory research shaped the salient facts about what constituted a disorder. Atrial fibrillation (uncoordinated contraction of muscle-fibers in the heart), for example, was literally inconceivable without Gaskell's work.

Experimental physiology was largely introduced into clinical medicine by enthusiasts and teachers at famous institutions and only slowly were its new concepts and attendant practices adopted by the medical profession as a whole. This situation contrasts markedly with the adoption of the ideas and techniques of another laboratory science: bacteriology. That 'germs' of some sort might be the cause of disease was an idea widely discussed in the mid 19th century. However, in the 1880s a finely-honed theory describing specific bacteria as the causes of febrile illness was produced in Germany, notably by Robert KOCH (p 455). The rapid incorporation of this theory into medicine depended in part on the rigorous laboratory techniques such as microscopy, animal inoculation, culture of bacteria, etc. that formed its basis. Between 1880 and 1890 many of the bacteria of the common infectious diseases had been identified — those of TYPHOID, TUBERCULOSIS, CHOLERA, DIPHTHERIA, and tetanus having been described within the first four years of the decade. Like the other laboratory sciences, what was significant about bacteriology was its transfer of authority from the ward to the laboratory. From the late 19th century onwards, whenever a clinician, anywhere, diagnosed a disease such as diphtheria, he or she was ultimately invoking laboratory criteria, even if a laboratory test was not used on any particular occasion.

### Revolutionizing therapeutics

Bacteriology tied bedside and basic science together in another way — by revolutionizing therapeutics. That diseases might be prevented by injecting a weak dose of their presumed causative agent was an ancient view enshrined in SMALLPOX inoculation and vaccination. It had been the basis of many of the experimental studies of Louis PASTEUR (p 620) in Paris. In the early 1890s, two of Koch's assistants claimed that small doses of the newly discovered diphtheria toxin could be injected in animals to produce active therapeutic antisera. Trials were started on sick children using sera raised in animals. Controversy over the serum's efficacy raged at the time and does to this day. There were, however, three important longer-term outcomes of this approach to treatment. First, the early 20th century saw an explosion of 'vaccine' treatments for infectious diseases. Thus the medical profession and public alike saw medicine as finally becoming 'scientific' in the sense of being laboratory based. Second, prophylactic vaccinations — for instance, for diphtheria — were established in large-scale public health programs. Again, however, the efficacy of some of these vaccines has been contested. Third, diphtheria antiserum was the foundation of the growth of research and development in what were to become multinational drug companies such as Hoechst, Merck, and Glaxo-Wellcome-SmithKline Beecham.

## Salvarsan

Laboratory research for specific therapeutic agents transformed early 20th-century therapeutics. In 1909 Paul EHRLICH (p 260), working in Frankfurt, announced the discovery of salvarsan as a cure for SYPHILIS. Salvarsan was the outcome of animal experimentation and the most up-to-date possibilities of chemical synthesis. Around this time, too, the medical press was deluged with claims (accredited and discredited) from physiology laboratories for the isolation of the active principles of endocrine glands. Thyroxine, for instance, was isolated in 1914. Reputable pharmaceutical companies produced these agents in large quantities and, along with disreputable ones, flooded the market with putative extracts from every known gland for relieving every conceivable ailment.

Besides being the site of original research in the 19th century, laboratories were institutions where routine tests on clinical samples and specimens were performed. Successful doctors might even have a laboratory in their home. Even modest practitioners testing a patient's urine or examining blood through the microscope in their own consulting rooms were practicing laboratory medicine. Provision of clinical laboratories for diagnostic investigations varied by country at the beginning of the 20th century. The great European centers of medical study at Freiburg, Bern, and Munich were among the most admired by advocates of laboratory medicine. In these places, laboratories were attached to wards and were under the direction of the physicians in charge, who also therefore had facilities for clinical research. In Britain and most of North America, things were rather different. By the end of the century most large hospitals had a laboratory where bacteriological tests were carried out, but nearly all urine testing and hematological examinations would have been performed by juniors in 'side rooms' attached to wards. Although, in a very few places, a medical career as a pathologist was a possibility, specialization in any of the clinical laboratory sciences, such as bacteriology, was not conceivable. Funding for any sort of laboratory-related clinical research was virtually non-existent.

The other discipline in which the laboratory became visible at the end of the 19th century was public health. The pattern of laboratory establishment varied. In Britain, for example, public health work was usually carried out by hospital or university laboratories. This often served to establish university medicine at the apex of the local hierarchy. In the United States, public health laboratories were set up by local and state departments to diagnose and track communicable diseases and to produce sera and vaccines. Relatedly laboratory medicine was an important arm of imperialism. The description of the natural history of the parasites implicated in many of the major tropical diseases — MALARIA, sleeping sickness, SCHISTOSOMIASIS, amebic dysentery, filariasis — was followed by the introduction of more or less effective preventative and curative measures for the colonials and later, in some cases, for the indigenous populations. At home and abroad, laboratories were crucial to the personalizing of public health services. Though not necessitating it, laboratory medicine allowed a focus on the individual as the site for the study of the detection and prevention of disease, to the neglect, some have argued, of the broader economic and social causes of sickness.

Conceptually, laboratory medicine was a 19th and early 20th century creation. The history of it in the later 20th century is largely one of massive elaboration dependent on commercial, philanthropic, and government investment. But the growth of laboratory medicine in the 20th century was not a simple quantitative increase. Rather it was part of a wholesale reorganization of medicine in which university academic departments and their associated hospitals were established as the apex of a hierarchy of laboratory-based medical services. Such restructuring has involved a fundamental reorganization of medical work leading to an increased integration and division of medical labor. This restructuring, which began at the turn of the century, was not peculiar to medicine. It was carried out in many institutions — for example, those of industry and education — in conformity with the dictates of 'scientific management'.

### Philanthropy in the USA

The story of laboratory medicine shifts westward, to the United States, in the 20th century. Here philanthropy was one of the prime movers in changing traditional approaches to the study and treatment of sickness. The change in medical work, however, was simply one aspect of the reorientation of American higher education, which was procured by capitalist finance. During the Progressive Era, new engineering and technical schools were established and the wealthiest men and women in the country founded universities, for example, Johns Hopkins, Vanderbilt, Stanford, and Cornell. Reformers who targeted medicine admired the German model and aimed at making medical schools and hospitals into university-based centers of research and seats of scientific education. The flagship of the new medicine was the JOHNS HOPKINS (p 840) medical school and its hospital in Baltimore. Here an array of talented figures created an institution which was widely admired and adopted as a model for reform elsewhere. Philanthropic money eventually ensured the establishment of a full-time or nearly full-time professorial system at American medical schools, especially after the famous and damning report by Abraham FLEXNER (p 258) on American medical education of 1910. Flexner came out firmly in favor of medical students being rigorously trained in the laboratory sciences.

Philanthropic money also funded specialized research institutes centered on the laboratory. There were European precedents for these, notably the Koch Institute in Berlin and the Pasteur Institute in Paris. In 1906 the Rockefeller Institute Laboratories were dedicated in New York, and in 1910 a hospital devoted to clinical research was opened alongside them. Rufus Cole, former director of the biological laboratory at Johns Hopkins, developed the Rockefeller hospital as a center that trained a generation of European and American clinical researchers in combined bedside and laboratory study. Such specialized research fostered the growth of laboratory-based specialism in medical practice, for example, hematology.

By the 1920s, clinical research involving the laboratory drew increasingly on biochemistry, which displaced bacteriology as queen of the medical laboratory sciences. For example, the isolation of insulin by Frederick BANTING (p 236) and Charles BEST (p 236) in 1921 relied on blood tests for glucose as well as on animal and clinical experiments. Besides being the basis for research, blood biochemistry was gradually introduced in everyday clinical practice at this time. In the 1920s, simple tests for metabolites became available and large hospitals established biochemical or clinical pathology laboratories. A new specialism, clinical biochemistry, appeared and doctors began to think of traditional clinical entities, such as DIABETES, as metabolic disorders.

Western governments had become convinced that laboratory research might improve a nation's health and its prestige. In Britain, for example, the Medical Research Committee (later Council) was

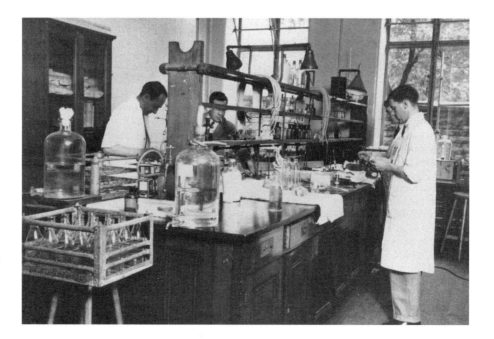

The biochemistry laboratory of the Royal Infirmary of Edinburgh in the 1930s. (Reproduced courtesy of the Lothian Health Services Archive, Edinburgh University Library.)

formed to administer funds, raised under the 1911 National Insurance Act, for the study of tuberculosis. It was soon steered by its managing committee towards funding various medical research projects based in the laboratory. Walter Morley Fletcher, its first secretary, was a Cambridge-trained physiologist who endeavored to control the funding of all medical research in Britain, taking the view that research in the basic sciences laid the foundations for the understanding of disease. At the other extreme from Fletcher were clinicians (usually associated with the Royal Colleges) and public health officials who saw too much energy wasted on the laboratory sciences, considering that investment in bedside observation or epidemiology would be more productive.

The years immediately after the Second World War saw the expansion of academic medicine and the flourishing of the laboratory in every aspect. One reason for this was the optimism which medical professionals, politicians, and the public invested in medicine. Insulin therapy, penicillin, and the decline of the major infectious diseases were all used as evidence that, through medicine, social progress could most rapidly be facilitated. In creating the National Institutes of Health (the American equivalent of the Medical Research Council), which now has a massive research complex at Bethesda, Maryland, the United States federal government committed itself to supporting medical research, especially laboratory-based research. Foundations as well as governments poured money into medicine. Pharmaceutical companies invested unprecedented amounts in drug development. Academic clinical departments expanded and proliferated. Increasingly, research became expensive and multidisciplinary, being carried out by teams of clinicians, basic scientists, and technicians. Frictions over leadership and salaries developed. Inter-war antagonisms over funding priorities — basic science or clinical medicine — persisted. On the ward, laboratory tests that had once been optional extras became mandatory parts of diagnosis and treatment.

MOLECULAR BIOLOGY, IMMUNOLOGY, and GENETICS have now displaced biochemistry as the basic sciences which shaped much clinical research, although as an ancillary to patient management the biochemical laboratory has made itself indispensable. The relations between laboratory research and the ward are well illustrated by work on the structure of proteins. These were widely studied from the late 1950s and hundreds of variants of hemoglobin were described, some differing from the normal by only a single amino acid. Some of these abnormal hemoglobins were associated with manifest diseases, which were investigated clinically and experimentally as genetic disorders. The genes considered at fault in such disorders were mapped on chromosomes in the laboratory using techniques such as cell culture.

Everyday clinical work, especially in hospital, has been transformed since the Second World War by laboratory studies and technological developments. Such developments, coupled with routine laboratory analysis, have been the basis of the management of many life-threatening conditions often by intensive care, and surgery. Some contest that this is the best approach to these conditions and argue that there has been a disproportionate distribution of resources into laboratory medicine while the social problems caused by chronic degenerative disorders, let alone poverty, accrue. At the bedside, too, clinicians and others question the value of the innumerable laboratory tests performed on the sick yet, not least from fear of litigation, numbers continue to rise. Whether laboratory medicine has succeeded as the agent of social progress it promised to be is an open question.                                        CL

*See also* EDUCATION; FOUNDATIONS; RESEARCH INSTITUTES; SPECIALIZATION

Théophile René Hyacynthe **LAËNNEC** (1781–1826). French physician. As a boy during the Revolution Laënnec worked in the hospitals at Nantes, becoming third surgeon at the Hôpital de la Paix in 1795. In 1799 he moved to Paris, becoming physician to the Hôpital Beaujour (1806), to the Hôpital Necker (1816), and professor and lecturer at the Collège de France (1822). He devised the stethoscope and published *De l'auscultation médiate* (1819). In this book he analyzed and described the sounds audible in diseases of the lungs and of the heart, firmly establishing the value of auscultation. His terminology is still in use today. Laënnec was the leading clinician of his day in France, but a poor lecturer and unpopular because of his royalist views. He died from pulmonary tuberculosis, a disease of which he had made a profound study.

**LANCETS** The lancet, a razor-sharp blade 5–7.6 cm long, has been a symbol of medicine since ancient times. It is still the most commonly found object among medical antiques and modern instruments. In 1474 Caxton wrote: 'he did his vysage to be kutte with a knyf and lancettis', which was probably the first reference to a lancet in English. By the 18th century lancets had become important symbols of the doctor's growing status. By then they had become elaborate and elegant in folding guards of ivory, tortoiseshell, or mother of pearl, carried in the waistcoat pocket.

Lancets were used for bloodletting, opening abscesses, circumcision, and other minor operations, most commonly cutting babies' gums in the belief that this hastened teething, which was thought to be dangerous. As infant mortality was high, and most of these deaths occurred between the ages of 6 months and 2 years, the age of cutting teeth, it was widely believed that teething was a cause. In 1839, 5016 deaths in England and Wales were attributed to teething: in 1910, the figure was 1600.

The custom of lancing babies' gums probably originated with the French surgeon, Ambroise PARÉ (p 320), who introduced it as a humane alternative to even more violent treatments such as blistering, bleeding, placing leeches on the gums, and applying the cautery to the back of the head. Paré described how he got the idea from an autopsy on a baby.

> When we … diligently sought for the cause of his death, we could impute it to nothing else than to the contumacious hardness of the gums … When we cut his gums with a knife we found all his teeth appearing … if it had been done when he lived, doubtless he might have been preserved.

The idea that failing to lance gums contributed to infant death rate recurred frequently in the literature of the next four centuries.

The custom increased during the next 300 years. Joseph Hurlock, who wrote a book on teething, advocated gum lancing in every disease or ailment, whether the tooth was evident or not. One of the few medical men who regarded teething as natural was William Cadogan, and he was much criticized for this.

Lancing the gums became common practice. John HUNTER (p 398) would lance a baby's gums up to ten times. J. Marion Sims treated his first patient, a baby 18 months old: 'as soon as I saw some swelling of the gums, I at once took out my lancet and cut the gums down to the teeth'. The physician Marshall Hall wrote that he would rather lance a child's gums 199 times unnecessarily than omit it once if necessary and he instructed his students to do it before, during, and after the teeth appeared, sometimes twice a day. In 1846 the Scottish physician, Andrew Combe, recalled that when he began practice 'the lancet was in great vigour and a well-employed medical man almost lived in a stream of blood. *Vigorous practice* was the order of the day'.

By the mid-19th century abscesses still needed to be opened, but the lancet was used less often on babies because it was becoming clear to some that teething was not a cause of serious disease in infants and that bloodletting was a dangerous, rather than a therapeutic, procedure. Opinions about both were increasingly divided and ambivalent. Typically, Charles WEST (p 175), founder of the Hospital for Sick Children, Great Ormond Street, London, wrote that dentition was 'a perfectly natural process', yet he continued to advocate gum-lancing, advising, '[I]t may be necessary to repeat your scarification several times with the same object …'.

By 1867 the American physician Samuel Gross complained that young doctors no longer used their lancets. Yet in 1883 distinguished physicians still insisted that dentition is 'a powerful predisposing cause of diarrhea and enteritis'. The different views engendered anger and competition. The Liverpool physician Boyd Joll roused his critics to anger by advising students to leave the 'lancet in your waist-coat-pocket'. He was expressing increasingly humanitarian attitudes, new ideas about childhood, about blood, along with increasing dissatisfaction with violent treatments and greater belief in the reparative powers of nature in acute diseases. Thus the practices of lancing the gums and of bloodletting declined at a time when other forms of surgical interference (for example, tonsillectomy, tenotomy (cutting a tendon) for clubfoot, and surgery for cleft palate) were increasing. Also, the development of antisepsis and asepsis in surgery discouraged 'pocket-knife surgery' because elaborate knives and showy lancet-cases were revealed as potentially dangerous.

Lancing gums and bleeding were increasingly criticized and both continued to decline. By 1896 some observers were 'even going so far as to say that the growth of teeth causes no more symptoms than the growth of hair'. Others criticized bleeding. In 1898 in New York the pioneer pediatrician Abraham Jacobi pronounced, 'Lancing the gums has lost most of its charms'.

Child health was improving and the infant death rate was falling but some, especially dentists and pathologists, still regarded teething as potentially pathological and advocated lancing. Between the world wars there were still pediatricians who asserted that 'teething can give rise to serious symptoms', including 'diarrhea, vomiting, eczema, bronchial catarrh, and convulsions, as well as screaming fits and strabismus'. Medical texts, especially those on dentistry, still advocated gum-lancing. This common view among dentists and pathologists may have been related to their striving for professional advancement and recognition.

Today no one lances gums or bleeds patients, but lancets (now usually called scalpels) became increasingly important as modern surgery developed. Today they lie in profusion on the operating tray, streamlined, sterile, and with disposable blades. We may now have substitutes for cutting, but it will be a long time before lancets are totally displaced from medical procedures.               AD

**LAND MINES** have been described by the US Department of State as the most toxic and widespread pollution facing mankind. The statistics bear out this grim assessment. The epidemic of mutilation by anti-personnel mines has now spread to more than 80 countries, constituting what is recognized as a global health crisis. Some 400 million land mines have been dispersed since World War II; many millions remain undetonated in some of the world's poorest countries; another 100 million mines are held in stockpiles ready for dispersal; two million mines are laid for every 100 000 removed; 500 people are killed or maimed every week by land mines; in Angola one in 334 citizens is an amputee. And we could go on and on with these statistics, but they ring hollow in the affluent societies which have never heard a mine detonating, and they fail to depict the anguish and suffering of the victims, often children, maimed for life, and destined to eke out an existence on crutches or hobble in pain on rudimentary prostheses.

Land mines are vicious weapons and their makers have no hesitation in incorporating the latest technology to improve them so as to inflict even greater mutilation and suffering on their victims. There are blast mines, fragmentation mines, butterfly mines, bounding mines, mines with anti-handling devices to kill those who try to defuse them, and smart mines which can be pre-programmed to self-detonate (but as many as half fail to do so, leaving the need for conventional mine clearance). Mines can be laid by hand or by remote delivery; they can be scattered over wide areas from artillery or rocket warheads, aircraft or helicopters, which can disperse as many as 2000 mines in a few minutes.

So what is being done to control this epidemic of mutilation? Until recently, the answer might have been a despairing chronicle of well-intentioned but failed efforts by numerous international bodies and individuals. Then the remarkable happened. The International Campaign to Ban Landmines (ICBL), an organization coordinating the voices and efforts of over 1300 organizations in over 75 countries (which was awarded the Nobel peace prize in 1997), met in Dublin Castle in September 1998, and the little-known nation, Burkina Faso, became the 40th country to ratify the Ottawa Treaty, thereby ensuring that the Convention on the prohibition of the use, stockpiling, production and transfer of anti-personnel mines and on their destruction would come into force on 1 March 1999.

An internationally binding ban on land mines is in reality only the beginning of the solution. It ensures that when one mine is removed, twenty are not being laid elsewhere, as is the case at present. Nevertheless, the populations of mined countries must continue to live amongst the mines, to work their mined farmlands, to suffer maiming and death and see their children hobble

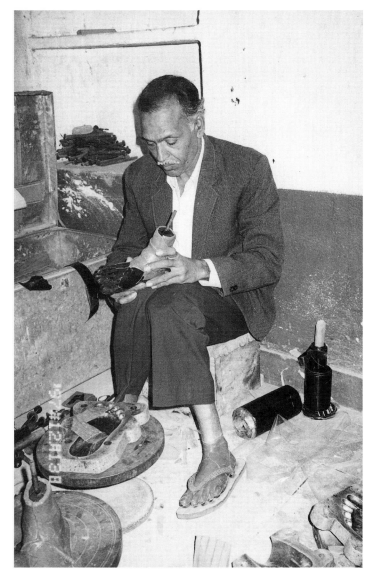

on stumps, while their political leaders see already impoverished economies drained by the toll of mine casualties and the loss of arable land — until their region is cleared of mines and the people can once again walk in safety.

One of the urgent imperatives, therefore, in the campaign against land mines is to reduce the risks of injury from mines among the indigenous population through mine-awareness programs, which have the objective of educating civilians as to how mines work, how they may be detected and cleared, how mined areas may be identified, and how to give primary first aid to victims of land mines. Such programs are now a standard part of the overall strategy in mine-infested countries,

An amputee making a Jaipur foot.

463

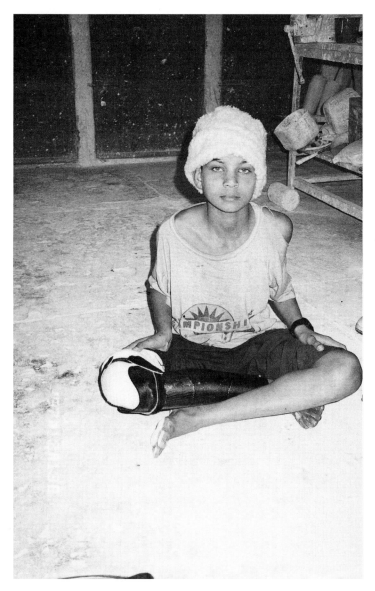

A young amputee from India.

expectedly from the Sawai Man Singh Hospital in Jaipur, where the 'Jaipur foot', a simple but ingenious prosthesis costing less than US$30, was developed for Indian amputees, whose injuries usually result from falling from trains. But now the Jaipur foot is in demand in many mined countries, where its low price and simplicity of production (often by trained local amputees) and its durability make it suited to the circumstances of developing countries where the people often go barefooted and work in damp rugged conditions.

Following enforcement of an effective ban on the production of land mines, and assuming their illegal dispersion can be controlled, global energies can now be directed towards the daunting task of clearing the world of mines. This will be the challenge for this new century. The technology can be developed but it will be costly, and much more than the annual £10 million per year pledged by the EU and USA will be required if the stated objective of clearing the mines by 2010 is to be achieved. Using contemporary methods for clearing mines, which basically consist of probing the ground inch by inch, is slow (one deminer can clear about 50 square meters in a day), dangerous (for every 5000 mines cleared, one deminer is killed and two are injured), and expensive (to remove a mine costing between $3 and $30 may cost from $300 to $1000). The UN has estimated that to clear the world of the mines that have been laid would cost $33 billion, and that at the present rate of clearance it would take a thousand years even if no new mines were laid.

Scientific and technological developments will undoubtedly revolutionize the present very primitive methods of clearing land mines, but as it has taken the nations of the world to come together to prevent further destruction of the planet, so too, it will take another major international initiative to allow the unfortunate people of mine-ridden countries to walk again in peace.

Disparate mankind, sundered by national boundaries, bemused by cultural, ethnic, and religious characteristics, can overcome its differences and prejudices to unite in the cause of protecting our planet, and, though the issue here is the eradication of land mines, perhaps it is not too much to hope for a greater gain, that by applying the land mine solution to other issues threatening our future existence, we may strive for that which should be the inherent gift of being endowed with intelligence, namely, that a collective harmony of thought and expression may permit us to take an evolutionary step in the furtherance of civilization.                                   EO

*See also* WAR

but they must be developed so as to be effective among often poorly educated people, and they must be intensified in the areas where they are needed.

Mine awareness may reduce casualties, but unfortunately does not stop them. For those surviving a land mine detonation there is the inevitability of coping with life as an amputee. For most victims living in the poorest countries of the world the prospect of being able to walk again depends on a cheap and durable prosthesis being available. A major contribution to the amputee victims of land mines has come un-

## LANGUAGE

'Gold were as good as twenty orators'
*William Shakespeare*
'Racks, gibbets and halters were their arguments'
*John Oldham*

Language, or the formulation and communication of meanings, takes many forms: body language, the language of gesture and mime, the language of music and dance, computer language, the language of military signals and artillery fire. Here, however, we are concerned only with verbal language, the language of words.

Words are signs, encoded with meaning. They may be heard, seen, or even touched. To be understood, the words must be decoded by those who know the code used (for example, English, Spanish, Arabic, Russian). A code here indicates a system of words with agreed arbitrary meanings.

Saussure, 'the father of modern linguistics', likened language use to a game of chess. He thought the state of a set of chessmen corresponded closely to the state of a language. The respective value of the pieces depends on their position on the chessboard, as linguistic terms derive value from their relation to other terms. The positions and relationships change continually according to established rules. And, finally, to pass from one state to the next, only one chess piece has to be moved: there is no general rearrangement. Similarly, in language use we only add one word at a time, however rapidly we do this. Further to these points of Saussure, we might also say that, with a finite number of different chess pieces, each with limited types of move, limitless numbers of combinations and sequences are possible. And in verbal language, with a finite number of different vocal sounds or letters of an alphabet, limitless numbers of combinations and sequences are possible.

Saussure also introduced into linguistics the terms 'the signifier' (*le signifiant*) and 'the thing signified' (*le signifié*). In the 1920s, Ogden and Richards similarly distinguished 'a word' from its 'referent' (what the word refers to). The 'act of reference' involves thought. For clear thinking with words such terms must be kept in mind.

### Form and matter

As with any other medium of human expression, spoken and written language involves form and matter. Form relates to the grammar of language, that is, to the rules of syntax (word connections) and accidence (word inflexions). Form also concerns the morphology of words, spoken and written, and so includes phonology and graphology. Matter relates to the meaning or semantic content of the language expressed. Semantics is the study of meanings.

Chomsky in 1985 concluded that grammar is autonomous and independent of meaning. This may certainly be the case. As an example he gave a nonsensical sentence of five words:

'Colorless green ideas sleep furiously'.

The sentence, though grammatical, is self-contradictory and transmits no meaning. If language involves the formulation and communication of meanings, is Chomsky's sentence still language? On the contrary, I walked into a small shop and said five words, in telegram fashion:

'Bread — milk — girl — sick — please'.

Though grammar was lacking, this was language in action, for the shopkeeper handed me the bread and the milk with an expression of sympathy. We can lack grammar and still communicate, but we cannot communicate without semantics. In most language use, however, the form relates to the matter, the grammar to the semantics.

The term 'semantics' was not widely used until the 20th century, but there is an early reference to what was much later to become semantics:

'Who is this that darkeneth counsel by words without knowledge?' *Book of Job* (? *c.* 1600 BC ? *c.* 500 BC)

And Robert Browning gave us a relevant satirical line from the 19th century:

'He said true things but called them by wrong names'.

Naming is at the root of semantics and language use.

The semantic content of spoken and written language may be examined in various ways. For instance, the 'density of the thought' may be gauged by the number of expressed simple ideas divided by the number of words employed (suggested by Henri Morier).

### Structuralist grammar

Following the work of Chomsky, linguists have given much attention to the surface structure and deep structure of sentences and phrases (structuralist grammar as distinct from traditional grammar). 'Bill dropped the book' and 'The book was dropped by Bill' are syntactically different sentences as regards surface structure. Semantic interpretation at a deeper level indicates that the deep structure or meaning of the two sentences is virtually the same.

In contrast, the surface structure of the sentence 'She pushed the boy with a book' is ambiguous. The deep structure could be either a sentence such as 'With a book she pushed the boy' or one such as 'She pushed the boy who had a book with him'. Chomsky called the analysis into surface and deep structure 'Phrase structure grammar'. It has been convenient to use labeled 'tree diagrams' for showing different levels of this type of analysis.

Transformational grammar formulates rules for mapping out possible surface structures from the deep structures. For example, stating rules for the transformation of sentences from active to passive voice, and *vice versa*, or rules for placing adverbs relative to verbs.

In speaking and writing we need never have heard or read of phrase structure grammar and transformational grammar. But perhaps related processes are involved in unconscious mechanisms underlying language use. Chomsky thought that there are computational processes underlying language activity which are not accessible to consciousness.

Most of us use the language tool without thinking of the tool itself, and without consciously knowing exactly how we do it (as we swallow our food without knowing exactly how we do it). Yule has commented that any individual speaker has a more comprehensive 'unconscious' knowledge of how language works than any linguist has yet been able to describe.

## Abstractions

Abstractions are easy to form with the tool of language. My pillow is soft. This ripe plum is soft. So is this tomato. From these objects we can abstract or take away the general notion or concept of softness. But there is no objective referent for the word 'softness' itself; there are only objects that are soft. Isolated or pure softness, the concept of softness, is an abstraction and is nowhere to be found. Similarly in clinical medicine, there are no diseases, only sick people. Diseases, such as influenza and scurvy, are abstractions or concepts.

Abstractions are useful but deceitful. Ogden and Richards referred to them as bogus entities or linguistic fictions. Yet abstractions can effect great economy in our thinking. They allow us to manipulate notions of whole groups of similar things, processes, and qualities in a condensed or synoptic form. We can make propositions about properties and relations of whole classes of things and processes, where a single class may entail large numbers of particular items. Abstractions may also be invented to solve problems. When we don't really know why we do something we sometimes say it is 'our will'. Or we may alleviate despair with words like 'immortality' and 'salvation'.

Having no objective referents but referring rather to general notions or concepts inside human heads, abstractions may be very flexible, sometimes dangerously so. Abstractions may be very subjective and people may argue about them (freedom, justice, honor, etc.), for one person's abstractions are seldom quite the same as another's. 'Licence they mean when they cry liberty', wrote John Milton. 'They fight among themselves for so-called freedom', wrote Goethe, 'but looked at closely, they are slaves against slaves'.

Yet we continue to abstract. We separate a certain quality of a thing from its other qualities and consider it in isolation as if it were a real thing. We may even give it personality. 'Honour pricks me on', says Shakespeare's Falstaff (*Henry IV Part 1*), and then goes on cynically, 'Yea, but how if honour pricks me off when I come on? How then? Can honour set to a leg? No ... Or take away the grief of a wound? No ... What is honour? A word. What is that word, honour? Air'.

## Emotive and propositional speech

Speakers and writers are disciplined by their medium of expression, grammar and semantics, but feeling, emotion, and mood may have great influence on what words and ideas come to mind at any given time.

Hughlings Jackson distinguished propositional speech from emotive speech. He thought that to speak is not simply to utter words, it is to utter propositions. The words relate to each other. One word is not merely added to another. On the other hand, strong emotion may lead to a more automatic, interjectional type of speech, tending to or towards inferior speech. Cries of alarm ('Fire! Fire!'), and distress ('Help!'), and swearing in anger ('Goddamn it!') are examples. Another neurologist, Henry HEAD (p 745), observed that even the longest of such exclamatory or automatic phrases does not convey a complete logical statement of some propositional act of thought.

In the clinical disaster of aphasia (loss of speech, see next page), emotional speech is less affected than propositional speech. A patient bereft completely of all propositional speech may still be able to use words to express emotion, as in cries of alarm, distress, and anger. In less severely affected aphasic patients, emotion may still allow utterance of words otherwise inaccessible. One of Alajouanine's patients, accompanied by his son, was asked: 'What is the name of your son?' The patient could not say the name, became distressed and agitated, then turned to his son and cried 'Help me, Raymond!'. With the outburst of emotion he was able to retrieve the name of his son.

For centuries, and in different ways, poets and writers have told us that art merely makes verse, that great thoughts come from the heart, that only the heart is poet. So the findings in aphasia are here of some interest. There is abundant clinical evidence in aphasia that surges of emotion can make words and ideas come to mind when they are otherwise inaccessible.

## Channels of verbal communication

'A mighty maze but not without a plan'

Alexander Pope

# APHASIA

In aphasia there is impaired or lost capacity to formulate and/or understand words as signs with meaning. It is caused by focal damage to the dominant (usually left) cerebral hemisphere (the upper part of the brain), most often because of head injury or stroke. Spoken and/or written language may be affected.

In Broca's aphasia there is damage to part of the frontal lobe of the brain and the aphasia is mainly expressive. Speech output is greatly reduced and may be restricted to a very few words. The words uttered are pronounced slowly, hesitantly, often with much apparent effort, and the sounds may be mispronounced. Sentences are typically ungrammatical, with frequent word omissions. Emotive speech is usually less affected than propositional speech. Writing is similarly affected. Writing difficulties are usually compounded by an accompanying hemiplegia (weakness of one side of the body), so that the patient has to learn to write with the non-dominant hand.

The patients can demonstrate by gestures and actions that they understand what they hear and read. The patients are usually aware of their errors in speaking and writing and may make great efforts to try to correct them.

In Wernicke's aphasia there is damage to part of the temporal lobe (the side part of the brain surface) and the aphasia is primarily receptive. There is impaired understanding of spoken and written words, including words that the patients themselves have uttered. Thus their word output is secondarily affected because the monitoring effect of understanding their own words is disabled. The patients cannot show by gestures or actions that they understand what they hear and read. They speak freely, fluently, even volubly, but their speech lacks meaning. The sentences may be reasonably grammatical, but give little information.

Words used are often inappropriate or may be meaningless. One word may be substituted for another because of a similar sound or because of belonging to a similar class. Non-existent words may be coined and speech may be reduced to an unintelligible jargon. Writing is affected comparably to speaking. Usually the patients do not recognize that their speech and writing are abnormal.

There may be mixed forms of aphasia, such as a combination of Broca's and Wernicke's aphasias to form global aphasia, as well as isolated or partial forms such as pure word dumbness (without affecting writing) or pure word deafness or pure word blindness.

Classification of the types of aphasia in any detailed way is difficult. Many such classifications have been offered but there is no general agreement. In a particular patient, it is probably best to describe the form of the aphasia empirically, according to the disturbances of language function produced.

Classification of the causes of aphasia is less difficult, and is linked to general medicine. The principal causes are head injury; stroke (vascular damage due to blood clotting, bleeding, or blockage by a clot that has come from elsewhere); inflammation (including abscess); and innocent or malignant tumors. After treatment for the underlying medical or surgical condition, a program of speech re-education should be considered.

Classification of aphasia according to the severity of the communication handicap is of great importance for the patients, their families, and their relationships and responsibilities. A tentative classification here might be:

Group 1: those who cannot make their daily needs known to family, friends, or nursing staff.

Group 2: those who can make their daily needs known but cannot perform any gainful employment because of the communication handicap.

Group 3: those who can carry out some gainful employment if in a protected environment.

Group 4: those who can independently earn a living, though substantially below their pre-aphasia level.

Group 5: those who can return to their pre-aphasia occupation.

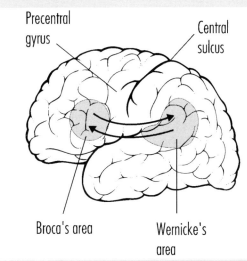

Broca's and Wernicke's areas. In Broca's aphasia, patients are often unable to speak, although they are capable of normal tongue movement and sometimes of habitual expressions such as 'thank you'. In Wernicke's dysphasia, the patient's speech may be fluent, but it is meaningless because the words are wrong or jumbled up, and the patient cannot understand relatively simple commands.

Verbal communication within a language involves four primary channels of encoded information:

Input: auditory comprehension of words, reading comprehension

Output: oral expression, writing.

To be understood, this encoded information needs to be decoded by a person knowing the language code in question.

There are also four related channels of non-encoded (non-verbal) communication such as:

Input: auditory perception of non-verbal sounds, visual perception of objects and movements

Output: gesture, actions.

There are thus at least four possible channels of input and four possible channels of output. Some of these combinations are much more important than others. The most important combination would be oral expression $\rightleftharpoons$ auditory comprehension for ordinary conversation, as one person encodes ideas into words, another decodes and understands the message, then encodes to reply and so on.

Linguists may use an almost algebraic system of combinations of the various communication channels, with repeated encoding and decoding, to test, analyze, and understand a subject's speech. For example: to follow verbal instructions by appropriate action (auditory comprehension → action, or reading comprehension → action); to designate or point to objects named (auditory or reading comprehension and visual perception → gesture); to name objects or movements (visual perception → oral expression or writing); to name non-verbal sounds (auditory perception → oral expression or writing); to read aloud (reading → oral expression); to write to dictation (auditory comprehension → writing); to be involved in written correspondence or examinations, or filling in official forms (reading → writing).

These channels of communication can be kept in mind as a preliminary synoptic framework for exploring and localizing problems of language function. This is useful for analyzing language difficulties in people learning a foreign language, in patients with APHASIA (p 467), and in children with learning problems such as dyslexia (disordered reading, usually associated with difficulties in writing). If indicated, standardized language tests may follow the preliminary survey.

## Dyslexia in children (developmental dyslexia)

In 1970 the World Federation of Neurology defined dyslexia as 'a disorder manifested by difficulty in learning to read despite conventional instruction, adequate intelligence, and sociocultural opportunity'.

A typical dyslexic child appears to be of normal or above average intelligence before entering school, and learns to speak at about the usual age. But during the first two or three years at school, the child does not learn to read normally. The disability may not be discovered until about the age of 8 or 9 years. Then, while spoken language skills may seem to be normal, written language skills may be at about the level of a 5 or 6 year old. Reading, writing, and spelling are affected and the dyslexic child may fail continually in these skills and in subjects depending on them.

As the children find themselves falling behind their peers in their written work they may become frustrated and unhappy, often feeling stupid and inferior. This may undermine their self-confidence and discourage them from further learning. They may be regarded as unintelligent or lazy or both. Crystal referred to 'the blighted school career of such children, when no one recognizes their handicap'.

The incidence of developmental dyslexia has been variously estimated as between 5 and 10% of the child population, boys being affected 3–5 times more frequently than girls. More than one member of a family may be affected. The causes of the dyslexia are not well understood.

Clinically, the children seem to have difficulty in dividing their spoken words into the component sounds, and correlating these with the letters and syllables of written words. This may obviously lead to problems with written words, since the latter are derived and codified from the sounds of spoken words.

On reading aloud from a text, dyslexic children may omit words, phrases, or even sentences. They may make substitutions ('all' for 'some') or change words ('sifters' for 'suffers'). They may invert words (saying 'on' for 'no', 'saw' for 'was'). They may interpolate letters or words of their own. All this handicaps the child from understanding the text clearly. Spontaneous writing, including written answers to questions and writing to dictation, may be comparably affected. Severely impaired scores for verbal tests compared to performance tests are of key importance in the diagnosis of developmental dyslexia.

When treating children with dyslexia it is essential to have a caring and sympathetic teacher who will help them achieve or regain self-confidence and a wish to learn. Patient but intense individual teaching is desirable and progress should be gradual from simple tasks to complex ones.

The teacher must ensure that each letter of the alphabet is perceived correctly, checking for any confusion between letters, such as b and d, or p and q. An analytic method is valuable. Printed words causing difficulty are analyzed into individual letters or sounds corresponding to those of the spoken word. For instance, 'exit' may be analyzed, the sounds separated, and the word pronounced e — x — i — t, rather than the word being perceived and pronounced only as a whole. The children should be taught to recognize and analyze their errors when reading aloud from a text (omissions, substitutions, inversions, changing letters in words, their own interpolations).

The sequencing of the individual sounds of spoken syllables or words may be linked to the sequencing of visual signs, for example, colored blocks, as well as to printed letters. Visual and auditory sense learning may be supplemented by touch and kinesthetic (muscle and joint sense) learning. The children may feel the outlines of plastic, embossed, or engraved letters and words, and trace their outlines with the fingers as well as say them aloud and write them.

Play therapy is important. This may include children trying to recognize plastic letters by touch while keeping their eyes closed, as well as the use of toys and games involving letters and words.

### Conclusion

Words are perceptible signs but they are not the message. They are only the means of conveying the message. One person may say 'I have a headache'. Others may convey exactly the same message by saying '*Ho mal di testa*', '*Tengo dolor de cabeza*', or '*Ich habe Kopfschmerz*', according to the language code used (Italian, Spanish, or German).

It is hard to better the view of Thomas Hobbes: 'For words are wise men's counters, they do but reckon by them: but they are the mony of fooles'. JHT

*See also* NEUROLOGY

**LAW** The earliest contacts between law and medicine may have occurred because courts required medical evidence to help them settle disputes or liability involving wounding, rape, concealment of birth, virginity, paternity, and violent and unnatural deaths. But the primitive beliefs held by both disciplines were such that both the medical evidence concerned, and the use to which it was put by the courts, bore little resemblance to what happens today. It was not until the 13th century that it became recognized in England that the purpose of a trial is to determine by a process of reasoning the truth as to the facts at issue. Instead, innocence, guilt, or liability was determined by primitive procedures and tests, of which the most well known was trial by ordeal.

European medicine was strongly influenced by the classical Greek masters and their interpreters, and this continued to be the case in Britain — with which much of this article is concerned — until the 17th century. HIPPOCRATES (p 360) thought that the function of the brain was to attract the vapors from the body, and ARISTOTLE (p 64) believed that the heart was the seat of the intellect. In one famous legal case GALEN (p 324) was able to convince a Greek court of the legitimacy of a child born to a woman 11 months after her husband's departure on foreign military service by pointing out that, although the child bore no resemblance to her husband, it did resemble closely a man at whose portrait she had been gazing during her confinement.

### Expert medical evidence and the courts

The prohibition by the Lateran Council in 1215 of the clergy from officiating at trials by ordeal meant that the courts had to find other methods of proof. Most European countries resorted to Roman law by introducing an inquisitorial (civil law) system of justice, under which expert medical evidence was tightly controlled and restricted to experts who were recognized by the courts as competent, and this remains the position in those countries today. But the English courts were unwilling to introduce a system of justice based on Roman law, with which few English lawyers were familiar. Left to their own devices the royal courts introduced an accusatorial (common law) system which, unlike the inquisitorial system, made no provision for expert medical evidence.

Medico–legal AUTOPSIES were rarely carried out in England till the 19th century, whereas they had been carried in both Italy and North Germany as early as the 13th century, mainly in cases of suspected poisoning. Here they anteceded by several years the introduction of anatomical dissection for teaching and research. When John HUNTER (p 398), William Hunter's (p 88) even more famous brother, appeared as an expert witness in John Donellan's trial for murder in 1781, and was asked by the judge whether the victim's death had been caused by poisoning, Hunter replied 'I should rather suspect it to be apoplexy, and I wish the head had been opened, as it might have removed all doubts'.

This infuriated the judge, who strongly criticized Hunter for refusing to commit himself. But Hunter was fully justified in refusing, as an incomplete autopsy had been carried out by a surgeon who had failed to observe the requirement established on the continent during the previous century that all the cavities of the body must be opened at autopsy. In fact, the first book on FORENSIC MEDICINE in the English language, a translation of one of the standard European works on the subject, was not published until 1797, and no provision was made for coroners to order autopsies and toxicological analyses in cases of suspected violent or unnatural death until 1836.

Introduced in Britain in 1858, medical registration facilitated the identification of medical practitioners who had been properly trained. In due course laws were passed, mainly several in PUBLIC HEALTH, conferring various privileges and responsibilities on registered medical practitioners, including certification of deaths and stillbirths, and for cremation, prescribing of controlled drugs, notification of infectious diseases, and compulsory orders for detention of mentally ill persons. Unlike other countries it is not an offence in England for an unregistered (or unlicensed) person to practice medicine, although it is an offence for unregistered persons 'willfully' to misrepresent themselves as registered medical practitioners. But the requirement that the misrepresentation must be 'willful' makes it very difficult to obtain a conviction, and hence few prosecutions have been brought. However, unregistered persons may be prosecuted for carrying out certain activities that are restricted to registered medical practitioners and registration is a condition of appointment to certain posts.

## Police authorities

The replacement of the parish constable by an organized police force greatly improved law enforcement and opened up possibilities for medical and other scientific evidence to assist in detecting crime. As a result, police authorities in the larger metropolitan areas started to call on the services of local doctors to help them collect and interpret evidence of crimes such as homicides, wounding, and rapes. Later, the motor vehicle led to an increase in alcohol-related road traffic accidents, and medical evidence was required to establish whether the drivers concerned were impaired by alcohol. Accordingly, police authorities in many parts of Britain began to pay retaining fees in return for which local doctors undertook to be available to examine the drivers concerned. The introduction in 1967 of a statutory blood alcohol concentration above which any driver could be convicted of an offence resulted in a large increase in cases and nearly all police authorities appointed police surgeons.

It was realized that the basic professional training of doctors in forensic medicine was inappropriate and a postgraduate diploma of medical jurisprudence was introduced by the Society of APOTHECARIES to encourage a higher quality of medical evidence. The diploma rapidly became recognized as a requirement for appointment as a police surgeon. In this, as in many other aspects where medical expertise can enhance law enforcement, Britain was far behind the rest of Europe. Police surgeons had been appointed in Italy as early as the 13th century, and attendance at a course held by the Vienna Medico–Legal Institute had been recognized since the end of the 18th century as an essential qualification for appointment as a police surgeon in almost all European countries.

It might have been expected that the greatly increased exposure of doctors to legal processes would have resulted in student instruction in the legal and ethical basis of medical practice. But there is very little evidence of this. Moreover, career opportunities in forensic pathology in Britain cannot begin to compare with those provided by the university medicolegal institutes in Europe. The specialty is not part of the National Health Service, and universities see no reason to fund forensic medicine departments adequately to provide a free service for the courts.

## Expert medical evidence

The provision of expert medical evidence for the courts illustrates one of the most striking and controversial differences between the accusatorial (common law) and inquisitorial (civil law) systems of justice. Under the latter, medical evidence can be given only by experts recognized by the court and the objective is to settle disagreements over the medical evidence before a case comes to court. The so-called 'battle of the experts', as may occur in open court under the accusatorial system, is regarded as contrary to the interests of justice. Expert medical opinion is given to the court mainly in written form as part of the 'dossier' and full disclosure of all relevant evidence is mandatory.

Under the accusatorial system, medical evidence is confrontational. Advantage can be, and often is, obtained by counsel for the one side attempting to discredit evidence given by expert witnesses called by the other side, who may be taken by surprise by the late disclosure of facts of which they were unaware.

In one well-known case, counsel told a pathologist he was calling as an expert witness that on no account was he to discuss the case with a colleague working in the same department who was to be called as an expert by the other side. Foreign lawyers find it incomprehensible that this should be allowed to happen and question whether the purpose of the accusatorial system of justice is to arrive at the truth, as opposed to scoring the most points. Hence their reference to the 'English sporting theory of justice'.

The confrontational environment engendered by the accusatorial system is unsuited to providing the courts with expert medical opinion. By exposing expert witnesses to cross-examination aimed at discrediting their evidence, it fails to take account of the difficulties experienced in expressing an unequivocal opinion on what are, in effect, biological issues. As such they are bound to involve uncertainties, not least those resulting from the wide variation that exists between individuals, and in the same individual at different times. This is recognized under the inquisitorial system, for example, in France, where only the judge is allowed to question expert witnesses.

The position of the expert witness is particularly difficult in medical negligence cases, where liability often depends upon whether the procedure that caused the damage is recognized by a competent body of medical opinion as 'reasonable' in the circumstances. Surgeons may often have to take split-second decisions when encountering unexpected operative situations. If damage results, those decisions are subjected in retrospect under the accusatorial system to long-drawn-out confrontational legal proceedings to determine whether the surgeon acted reasonably. Few other professions are at such risk of legal proceeding as a result of having to take instant decisions.

Although the independence and integrity of forensic medical and scientific expert witnesses are rarely ever questioned, in several recent cases convictions have had to be quashed on appeal because experts have not disclosed evidence that might have assisted the other side. This is an inevitable consequence of a system under which expert witnesses are retained (and paid) to produce evidence in support of the side that calls them. An expert can hardly be expected to 'score an own goal' by volunteering such information in court and might well not be given the opportunity to do so unless asked a directly relevant question. In some of these cases, notably those involving suspected (Irish Republican Army) terrorist activities, the persons concerned had been in prison for several years before their convictions were quashed.

### The impact of law on medical practice

The professional conduct of doctors is subject to various laws, judicial decisions, and regulations relating to the interventions they carry out. These include specific legislation such as that dealing with the prescription of controlled drugs, termination of pregnancy, notification of infectious diseases, certification of deaths, and cremation as well as more general law such as that relating to the requirement to obtain informed consent and to comply with the duty of care. The most controversial topic is the uncertainty of the law dealing with medical decisions affecting life and death, such as those arising out of the introduction of new medical technologies, such as assisted conception, artificial prolongation of life, and, even more recently, cloning.

On the other hand, in the absence of any contractual requirements, there is no obligation on doctors at English law to offer assistance in situations where life is in immediate danger. England is probably unique in that a doctor (or indeed any citizen) can stand idly by and watch a child drown in three feet of water without incurring any legal consequences. Furthermore, doctors who do intervene are at risk of being sued in negligence if they fail to show the requisite duty of care. As a result, several common law countries have introduced 'good Samaritan' legislation to offer some protection to doctors who stop at road accidents to render assistance. Even so, a study carried out

by the American Medical Association in states that have such legislation revealed that less than half the doctors surveyed would stop at an accident because of the risk of being sued.

The legal constraints on the professional conduct of doctors are supplemented by the ethical principles with which doctors are required to comply, unless there are strong reasons to the contrary. These are based mainly on respect for the integrity of patients and the best interests of their health. Nevertheless, they may conflict with the law — in some countries the law requires doctors to assist, or otherwise to become involved in, brutal, inhuman, and degrading practices such as judicial amputations, flogging, and executions.

The most controversial source of conflict is the failure of English law to protect the ethical principle of confidentiality. Unless sensitive medical information is treated confidentially, sick or injured persons will be reluctant to consult doctors and unwilling to make full disclosure of relevant aspects of their medical history. This is well recognized in civil law countries, where doctors who fail to respect the 'medical secret' may be severely punished under the penal code. However, damages for the English common law offence of breach of confidence can be awarded only if it has resulted in pecuniary damage, which is rarely ever the case. In 1981 the Law Commission strongly criticized the inadequate protection afforded by English law to confidential medical communications, and drafted a bill to protect them.

England is one of the few countries where confidential medical information is not given protection (privilege) against disclosure in court proceedings. Doctors may be compelled by subpoena to attend court; disclose their patients' confidential medical records; and answer questions about them. Judges are usually willing to listen to reasons given by a doctor why the notes should not be produced, but they have absolute discretion to compel disclosure, and are known to be reluctant to comply. Personal medical records often contain sensitive medical information that is irrelevant to the case including information about other members of the patient's family.  JH

*See also* NO-FAULT COMPENSATION; PROFESSIONAL REGULATION

**LAZARETTES** 'Lazarette' and 'lazaret' are variants of 'lazaretto', meaning lazar-house, that is, a house or hospital for poor and diseased persons, particularly those with unpleasant conditions. 'Lazaretto' has also been used to describe a place of QUARANTINE. The derivation is of course from Lazarus (*Luke 16*), the beggar full of sores, who was laid at the rich man's gate but who achieved ultimate salvation in Abraham's bosom.

# LEPROSY

Leprosy is a chronic communicable infection (also designated Hansen's disease) of humans caused by the bacterium *Mycobacterium leprae* (an organism similar to that causing tuberculosis); skin eruptions and damage to superficial nerves (leading to loss of sensation) are classic features, but the eyes, testicles, and mucous membranes of the nose and throat may also be affected.

The disease has a long and colorful history. Numerous references to it exist in the Bible, but Hebrew and Greek terminologies were used as terms for a wide variety of skin conditions which remain important in the differential diagnosis. Excellent (skeletal) evidence exists that the infection was widespread in medieval Europe; studies in Danish graveyards (and elsewhere) by V. Møller–Christensen have produced much information. Incontrovertible evidence exists (also from skeletal evidence) that Robert the Bruce (1274–1329) had leprosy. The term was first used in the English language in 1535. Today the infection has largely disappeared from temperate areas, but throughout the world (most in tropical and subtropical regions) at least one million people suffer from leprosy; the number infected may be much more. Several problems exist about the precise numbers affected; however, in 1988 the WORLD HEALTH ORGANIZATION Expert Committee on Leprosy recommended that a case should be defined as one either 'requiring or under treatment'; this has eliminated many inactive cases, which formerly remained on registers.

The infection exists world-wide and usually possesses a male preponderance — often in a ratio of 2:1. Two principal forms of the infection exist: *lepromatous*, in which very many organisms are present, and there is widespread chronic inflammation of subcutaneous tissue, and the mucous membranes of the upper respiratory tract, face, and testes — with sterility and enlargement of the breasts in men; and *tuberculoid*, characterized by skin eruptions, which initially have raised, reddish borders, and are anesthetic, and thickened nerves. Untreated, the lepromatous variety has a bad prognosis, whereas tuberculoid may improve spontaneously with disappearance of the disease followed by complete recovery. Intermediate forms are also recognized on clinical/histological grounds.

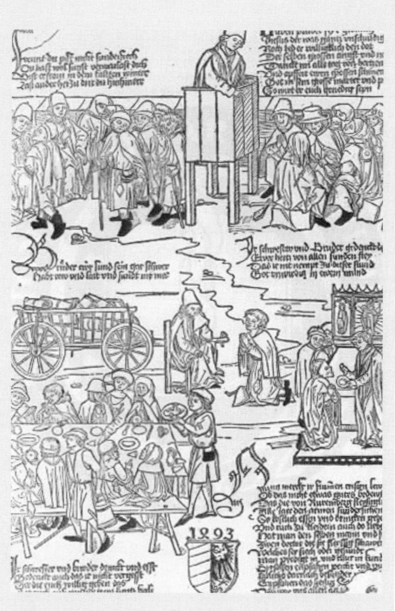

A 15th century broadsheet on the care and treatment of leprosy patients. (From Tollet C. (1892). *Les edifices hospitaliers depuis leur origine jusqu'a nos jours,* Paris. Reproduced courtesy of the National Library of Medicine, Bethesda, MD.)

(*continued opposite*)

*(continued)*

The incubation period of leprosy is usually long, frequently 20 years or more (although it may be as short as a few weeks). Probably most infections begin in childhood or early adult life, sometimes associated with immunological 'stress', for example, puberty, pregnancy or menopause.

The causative organism *M. leprae* was first demonstrated by the Norwegian G. A. HANSEN (p 431) in 1873; it had previously been considered that the disease was 'inherited'. Both genetic and environmental factors are involved in the 'host response' to infection. Immunological factors account very largely for the varied clinical picture.

The mode of infection is unclear. Nevertheless, prolonged physical contact with an infected person seems important in most cases. The organism may be found in large numbers in nasal secretions, probably an important factor in person-to-person transmission. Skin disease is also a focus of bacteria. Accidental infection (through inadequately sterilized needles used for injections or tattooing) results occasionally. The importance of an animal reservoir of infection is unclear.

Diagnosis depends ultimately on the characteristic changes in a specimen under the microscope; however, the lepromin skin test indicates the presence of some resistance to *M. leprae* (the causative organism) and may be of value in cases difficult to diagnose clinically.

Patients are treated with chemotherapy using long-term sulfones, and more recently newer antibacterial agents such as rifampicin or clofazimine. These have reduced the world incidence substantially in the last two decades. The progress of the infection is arrested by dapsone — which rapidly renders an individual non-infectious. An important problem relates to the side-effects of the more effective agents. Sometimes these produce an exacerbation of symptoms associated with leprosy itself. A further problem lies in a world-wide increase in resistance to dapsone (the first and most widely used agent). Multiple agents have been advocated to counteract this problem.

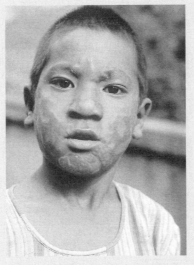

The lesions resulting from leprosy can clearly be seen on the face of this man. (National Library of Medicine/WHO.)

Prevention depends on identifying proved (bacteriologically positive) cases with subsequent isolation and treatment. In the long term, physiotherapy, reconstructive surgery, and vocational training are of great importance — but only when the progress of active infection has been arrested. The objects of leprosy control are: the interruption of transmission of infection; cure (and rehabilitation); and the prevention of associated (usually long-term) deformities.

Provided correct measures and the wise use of chemotherapy are implemented, there seems no reason why the infection should not eventually be totally eliminated from the world. There is also a move to avoid stigmatization, abolishing the term leprosy, substituting Hansen's disease.

GCC00

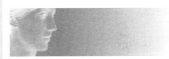

Joseph **BANCROFT** (1836–94). English-Australian physician. Born in Manchester he emigrated to Brisbane in 1864. He recognized LEPROSY in Queensland, and discovered the WORM which causes filariasis, later named *Wuchereria bancrofti*. He also studied the culture and diseases of plants, and invented a process for drying meat which yielded pemmican. He was a reluctant member of a Royal Commission set up to study the rabbit problem in Australia, which experimented unsuccessfully with fowl cholera. He also practiced medicine.

---

**LEISHMANIASIS** is infection with a protozoan parasite belonging to the genus *Leishmania*. It occurs in various cutaneous forms, and in the visceral form known as KALA-AZAR.

**LEUKEMIA** See HEMATOLOGY

Joseph **LISTER** (1827–1912). Born in London of Quaker family, Lister studied medicine at University College, London graduating in 1852. He then moved to Edinburgh, as assistant to the professor of surgery, and his future father-in-law, James Syme. In 1860 Lister was appointed regius professor of surgery at the University of Glasgow and 9 years later returned to Edinburgh as professor of surgery and surgeon to the Royal Infirmary. In 1877 he took up the chair of surgery at King's College, London. In 1891 he became chairman of the newly created British Institute of Preventive Medicine, which he had strived to establish (later named the Lister Institute), and between 1895 and 1900 he was president of the Royal Society. He retired from practice in 1896.

**LITERATURE** Doctors appear in so many novels and plays that a short account must be selective and personal, limited in this case largely to European classics. They seldom play a major part, except for the occasional hero or villain. Singling them out for special attention does not mean that they are in any way unique; a medical qualification may in fact be irrelevant. Nevertheless, their portrayal in fiction does provide an opportunity to learn how lay people view doctors; naïve medical readers will no doubt be shocked by the amount of ill-feeling.

PHYSICIAN-WRITERS

**John ARBUTHNOT**
(1667–1735). British
physician and writer. A wit
and a friend of Pope, Gay,
and Swift, he contributed to
*The memoirs of Martinus
Scriblerus* (1714) and wrote
*The history of John Bull*
(1712), being the first to use
this name for the archetypal
Englishman.

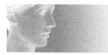

William Somerset
**MAUGHAM** (1874–1965).
British physician and writer.
He never practiced medicine,
publishing his first novel *Liza
of Lambeth* the year he
qualified as a doctor. His most
celebrated work was *Of
human bondage* (1915),
which was said to have sold
10 million copies. In addition
to novels and short stories he
wrote many successful plays.

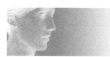

Osborne Henry **MAVOR**
(1888–1951). British
physician and playwright.
After being professor of
medicine at Anderson
College, Glasgow, for a short
time, he devoted his time to
writing plays under the
pseudonym of James Bridie.
Of his more than 40 plays the
best known are *Tobias and
the Angel* (1930), *The
Anatomist* (1931), and
*Daphne Laureola* (1949).

(*continued opposite*)

Through the ages the behavior of doctors has
been imaginatively dissected — and on the whole
found wanting. This is perhaps hardly surprising
given that medieval 'doctors' were often quacks
and of lowly standing, but as late as the 18th
century they were feared, largely because their
remedies were so unpleasant. Their standing
improved somewhat towards the end of the 19th
century, when technology began to provide them
with new skills, but debate about their character
and behavior continues.

## Professionalism

Fictional works by medically qualified writers,
however partisan, might be expected to give some
idea of life and work as a doctor. Medical and surgical practice in the 18th century, for example, is
documented with coarse realism by Tobias
Smollett, surgeon's mate and unsuccessful physician, in *The adventures of Roderick Random* (1748)
and *The expedition of Humphry Clinker* (1771).
There are many doctors in his books, not always
sympathetically drawn.

Sir Arthur Conan DOYLE (p 114), who took high
professional standards for granted, collected 15
stories of medical life in *Round the red lamp* (1894),
'to make doctors something more than mari-
onettes'. One of his strongly held beliefs was in the
importance of the healing touch, 'that magnetic
thing which defies explanation or analysis'. He compared the energetic and up-to-date young doctor
unfavorably with the wise old physician (not for the
last time in fiction): 'I thought of his cold, critical
attitude, of his endless questions, of his tests and his
tappings. I wanted something more soothing' — a
sentiment many patients would heartily endorse today.

A romantic, black-and-white view of medical
practice can be found in Francis Brett Young's *The
young physician* (1919) and *My brother Jonathan*
(1928), in *Arrowsmith* (1925) by the Nobel prize
winner, Sinclair Lewis, who came from a medical
family, and in A. J. Cronin's *The citadel* (1937).
Their books were best sellers but the appeal has
not lasted, perhaps because they are too self-
consciously of their time. More substantial is *The
Pasquier chronicles* (1933–41) by another doctor,
Georges Duhamel. The hero in the epic is a
doctor and biologist (scientist) who is involved in
the social and philosophical issues of a society in
crisis, and not surprisingly reflects the increasing
rift between science and humanism.

Of the few uncomplicatedly sympathetic
portraits of doctors by non-medical writers,
Dr Tertius LYDGATE (p 477) in George Eliot's
*Middlemarch* (1871–2) provides the best known
stereotype of the traditional English physician. He
'was convinced that the medical profession
offered the most direct alliance between intellec-

tual conquest and social good. He cared not only
for "cases" but for each individual' — sentiments
that have a modern ring. He was a good man, idealistic and ambitious, but emotional entangle-
ments led to his downfall, condemning (*sic*) him
to successful and fashionable practice instead of
an independent life of research, which he so much
desired.

Many doctors, all except one totally dedicated,
grace the various tales known collectively as the
*Comédie humaine* of Honoré de Balzac; the most
sympathetic is the 'beloved' Dr Bénassis in *The
country doctor* (1833). Walter Scott's Dr Adam
Hartly in *The surgeon's daughter* (1828) is decent,
competent, and incorruptible, as upright as his
teacher, Gideon Gray ('there is no harder worker
in all Scotland and none more poorly requited').
Dr Edward Hope in Harriet Martineau's
*Deerbrook* (1839) is selfless and uncomplaining
about the calls made on him. One of Émile Zola's
last novels, *Dr Pascal* (1893), provides an idealized
image of the humane, hard-working, broad-
minded physician, who is not interested in
making money.

An excellent opportunity to show the doctor in
a good light arises when he is confronted by disaster. Young and much traveled Dr Thurnall in *Two
years ago* (1857), the last of Charles Kingsley's
social novels, at first upsets the local villagers by
his prediction of a cholera outbreak, but when the
epidemic strikes, he is rapidly accepted because of
his courage and dedication. By contrast, though,
Dr Stockman in Ibsen's *An enemy of the people*
(1882) is reviled and ostracized by the community
for attributing an epidemic to deficiencies in the
water supply. Dr Rieux in Albert Camus's celebrated novel *The plague* (1947), sometimes
inhuman and ruthless in the eyes of his patients,
is a dedicated and concerned doctor, capable of
facing up to his powerlessness and frustration in
the face of the epidemic. An arrogant exterior
may hide the humility and compassion of the best
doctors.

## Mixed views

Ambivalent attitudes towards doctors are displayed by Shakespeare and Dickens. Shakespeare's
views have to be considered in the context of their
time, when much treatment was undertaken by
quacks, such as the contemptible Dr Pinch (*The
comedy of errors*, 1594). On the whole, proper
doctors are treated with respect: the physician
who treated Lear (*King Lear*, 1608) is humane and
considerate; the Scottish doctor called to the
unhinged Lady Macbeth (*Macbeth*, 1606) admits
that the illness is beyond his competence, and is
thought none the worse for saying so.

The dedicated physician Lord Cerimon
(*Pericles*, 1609) is repeatedly praised:

'Your honour has through Ephesus pour'd forth/ Your charity, and hundreds call themselves/ Your creatures who by you have been restor'd; and "Reverend Sir, /The Gods can have no mortal officer/ More like a God than you".'

But he is responsible for restoring Pericles's wife, Thaisa, to life, and so might be considered a special case.

Less certainty exists about more conventional doctoring. The French Dr Caius (*The merry wives of Windsor*, 1602), 'that calls himself doctor of physic' (a remark made by his sworn enemy, Sir Hugh Evans, who could be biased), is nevertheless described as a fool and a physician by his maid-servant, Mistress Quickly. Pericles complains 'Thou speak'st like a physician, Helicanus/ who minister'st a potion unto me/ That would'st tremble to receive thyself'. And there is the well-known sentiment in *Timon of Athens* (1623 Folio): 'Trust not the physician,/ His antidotes are poison, and he slays/ More than you rob, takes wealth and lives together.'

Compared with the unflattering way in which Dickens treated lawyers, doctors come off lightly. Although numerous, none plays a major part in his novels. They are often gently ridiculed; none is learned or high-principled. Sir Parker Peps (*Dombey and son*, 1848) is 'one of the Court physicians, and a man of immense reputation in assisting at the increase of great families'. Mr Jobling (*Martin Chuzzlewit*, 1843) is an unscrupulous knave, 'who had a habit of sucking his lips and saying "Ah"… which inspired great confidence'. Dr Slammer (*Pickwick Papers*, 1837–9) is small, fat, and irascible. Others exhibit more admirable qualities. Dr Jeddler (*The battle of life*, 1844) 'looked on the world as a gigantic joke', although he was kind and generous. Dr Bayham Badger (*Bleak House*, 1852–3), a fashionable and ambitious general practitioner, is rather a fool but generally sound, and Dr Alan Woodcourt, the young ship's surgeon in the same novel, is tender-hearted but sensible. Mr Chillip (*David Copperfield*, 1849–50) is a kind and amiable village practitioner.

None of Dickens's doctors is particularly memorable, in stark contrast to the hilarious descriptions of the medical students in *Pickwick Papers*: Benjamin Allen, 'he presented a rather mildewy appearance', Bob Sawyer, and others. And his graphic exposure of the dangerous activities of Sairey Gamp and Betsy Prig (*Martin Chuzzlewit*) alerted society to the scandal of untrained nurses.

### The sins of doctors

Doctors are accused of every sin, including murder (Herman Melville, *White-jacket*, 1850; Frank Danby, *Dr Phillips, A Maida Vale idyll*, 1887; Hjalmar Söderberg, *Dr Glas*, 1900). The prize for

the most decadent goes to the central character, Dr Bardamu, in L.-F. Céline's astonishing first novel, *Journey to the end of the night* (1932). He is a seedy and ignorant individual who shares the degradation of the society in which he works. Any high-mindedness is destroyed by the nightmare of the city and its denizens. Céline had been an idealistic doctor (as was CHEKHOV) (p 84), and, arguably, by denigrating the medical profession he was reflecting his own disillusionment. But the greatness of the novel lies in its profound despair at the sordidness of the human condition, from which no one — least of all doctors — can escape.

The three doctors in Anton Chekhov's plays (*The seagull*, 1895; *Uncle Vanya*, 1900; and *Three sisters*, 1901) share all the worst characteristics: cynicism, indecision, incompetence, and little knowledge of medicine; two of them are alcoholic. Dr Astrov in *Uncle Vanya* 'knows as much about medicine as I know about astronomy.' Chekhov ('I look upon medicine as my lawful wife …') seems to be warning that the basic human instincts are a constant threat to the passionate involvement of the dedicated physician. Dr Plarr in Graham Greene's *The honorary consul* (1973) is profoundly cynical (as are so many of Greene's characters), but is redeemed by his devotion to medicine.

Scarcely concealed contempt for the arrogant pride, pedantry, and certainty of doctors is widespread. 'There are worse occupations in this world than feeling a woman's pulse' (Laurence Sterne, *A sentimental journey*, 1768). Dr SLOP (this page) in *The life and origins of Tristram Shandy* (1760), by the same author, is a figure of fun, perhaps in order to exorcise the unpleasantness of medical treatment at the time. Love of money has been a popular theme since Chaucer's doctor of physic in *The Canterbury tales* (c. 1387) — a man of importance, serious, sober, and moral, 'who knew the cause of every malady' and appreciated gold 'in special', not for the money, of course, but for its use as a cordial in therapy. 'Be a physician, Faustus', says the Devil in Christopher Marlowe's *Dr Faustus* (1604), 'heap up gold/ And be eternized for some wondrous cure.'

Amusing descriptions of the sleight of hand with which doctors receive and dispose of their fee are given by Ivan Turgenev in *The district doctor* (1852) and by Marcel Proust in *A la recherche du temps perdu* (1913–26). Anthony Trollope's *Dr Thorne* (1858), who scandalizes his colleagues by offering change when paid for consultations, is firmly put in his place. 'The true physician should hardly be aware that the last friendly grasp of the hand had been made more precious by the touch of gold.' Perhaps financial transactions removed the awe and fear by reducing the doctor to the status of tradesman, or

(continued)

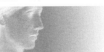

Axel Martin Fredrik **MUNTHE** (1857–1949). Swedish doctor and psychiatrist. Born in Oskarshamm, Sweden, Munthe studied at Uppsala University and with CHARCOT (p 400) in Paris, becoming the youngest MD ever to be created in France. He practiced in Rome and in Capri and is remembered especially for his book of reminiscences called *The story of San Michele* (1929), the place being the name of his villa on the isle of Capri. The book is sensitive and delicate, with a charming and charmed view of life and death as a doctor sees it.

### DOCTORS IN FICTION

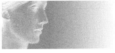

Dr **SLOP** is the irascible, clumsy, and bigoted Catholic doctor in Laurence Sterne's novel *The life and opinions of Tristram Shandy* (1760–7). In his eagerness to demonstrate a new type of obstetrical forceps, Slop, a 'little squat, uncourtly figure', inflicts permanent deformity on the hero's nose.

(continued on p 477)

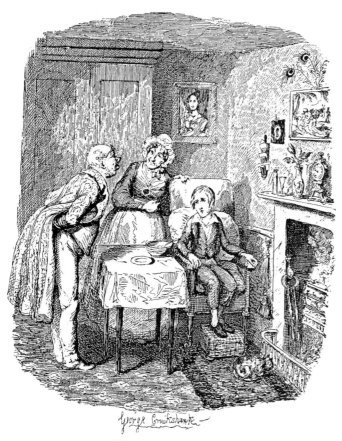

*Oliver recovering from Fever*

Oliver recovering from fever. From *Oliver Twist* by Charles Dickens.

based on his acquaintance with the important medical men of the day. *The doctor's dilemma* (1906), though not one of his best, is particularly harsh on the undignified behavior of doctors. The polemical preface is a comprehensive criticism of the medical establishment: 'The tragedy of illness at present is that it delivers you helplessly into the hands of a profession which you deeply distrust'. 'Let no one suppose that the words doctor and patient can disguise from the parties that they are employer and employee.' 'It is simply unscientific to allege or believe that doctors do not under existing circumstances perform unnecessary operations and manufacture and prolong lucrative diseases.'

Proust, too, suffered at the hands of doctors, who could do little for his ASTHMA; one of them is said to have nearly killed him through too aggressive treatment. He was naturally skeptical:

> 'The mistakes made by doctors are innumerable'. In *A la recherche du temps perdu* he writes, 'For each ailment that doctors cure with medications (as I am told they occasionally succeed in doing) they produce ten others in healthy individuals by inoculating them with that pathogenic agent a thousand times more virulent than all the microbes — the idea that they are ill'. An excuse for his own hypochondria, perhaps?

He dissected his physicians with the same intensity as he did his other characters, and found them wanting: autocratic (Dr Dieulafoy), arrogant (Dr du Boulbon), narrow-minded and consumed by self-interest, unconcerned with any deeper meaning to life other than the physical ills they could not cure. The renowned specialist, Dr Cottard, is self-important and ineffectual, 'an imbecile'. And yet, fear of illness forced Proust in the end to concede: 'To believe in medicine would be supreme madness, if not to believe in it were not an even greater one, for from this heaping of mistakes have come out in the long run some verities'.

Doctors, particularly specialists, as portrayed in *The doctor's dilemma* and in the ridiculous figure of Sir Roderick Glossop, brain surgeon in P. G. Wodehouse's novels, are arrogant, snobbish, and patronizing. General practitioners are little better: Dr Raste in Arnold Bennett's *Riceyman steps* (1923) had 'the pompous solemnity of a little man conscious of rectitude'; 'often spoke more loudly than he need — the result of imposing himself on the resistant stupidity of the proletariat'; and 'had a general preference for not being quite sure; he liked to postpone judgement'.

Despotic, callous, and unsympathetic attitudes are displayed by Dr Tyrell in Somerset MAUGHAM's (p 474) *Of human bondage* (1915), by the hard working but ultimately bribable medical

worse: 'We are angels when we come to cure, devils when we ask for payment' (Walter Scott, *The abbott*, 1831). That people might feel better for paying is not considered.

Some of the more scathing opinions of doctors have come from writers who suffered from chronic ill-health. Molière, who repeatedly coughed up blood from TUBERCULOSIS while acting, wrote six plays in which doctors, 'who know nothing about curing', are pilloried. He complained in *Le malade imaginaire* (1673), 'Why does he need four doctors — is not one enough to kill a patient?', and berated the medical profession,

> 'Your best knowledge is pure nonsense/ Vain and impudent doctors/ With your fine Latin words you cannot cure/ The suffering that is driving me to despair.'

Bernard Shaw's well-known contempt for doctors was also based on his own experience. Pompous doctors with names to match like Sir Ralph Bloomfield Bonnington, Cutler Walpole, and Sir Colenso Ridgeon crowd his plays, many

superintendent, Hofrat Behrens in Thomas Mann's *The magic mountain* (1924), and by the boorish medical hierarchy in A. E. Ellis's *The rack* (1958). The last two are powerful descriptions of the physical and mental claustrophobia suffered by the victims of tuberculosis SANITARIUMS, and are highly recommended for the many examples of patient–doctor non-communication.

A recurrent complaint is that doctors have no time to talk to patients: they 'never tell you anything outright' and 'no one stops for a few moments to say a few words' (Alexander Solzhenitsyn, *Cancer ward*, 1970). It is only fair to add that in this case the staff themselves recognize their failure. Bedside manners, too, leave much to be desired: doctors are insensitive and insincere, they have 'a healthy man's jovial condescension' (*Of human bondage*) towards ill people, and are poorly equipped to deal with serious illness and dying. Leo Tolstoy's harrowing novella *The death of Ivan Ilyich* (1884) is an indictment of the confusion and false optimism of doctors faced with an illness they cannot diagnose: 'the doctors couldn't say what was the matter — at least they could, but each said something different.'

Rivalries among doctors do little for their image. Examples can be found in *Middlemarch* between Dr Lydgate and the general practitioners; in *The doctor's dilemma*; in Virginia Woolf's *Mrs Dalloway* between Sir William Bradshaw and Dr Holmes; in *My brother Jonathan*, with its two brothers — one dedicated and the other worldly-wise and bored; and in *The rack*, where doctors squabble over private patients. Anthony Trollope's *Dr Thorne* brings down the wrath of the self-elected leader of the profession (appropriately called Dr Fillgrave) for doing his own prescribing and collecting money. William Thackeray in *The adventures of Philip* (1861–2) contrasts Dr Firmin ('among the meanest scoundrels of fiction' — Squire Sprigge, a famous editor of the *Lancet*) who, although 'only a doctor', becomes a consultant through the help of fashionable friends and a good marriage, with the kindly and professional Dr Goodenough, believed to be based on John Elliotson, professor of medicine at University College Hospital, London, to whom he dedicated *The history of Pendennis* (1848–50). Dr Raste (*Riceyman steps*) is made to voice the age-old professional antagonism: 'I'm not a specialist. He uttered the phrase with a peculiar intonation, not entirely condemning specialists, putting them in their place, regarding them very critically and rather condescendingly, as befitting one whose field of work and knowledge was the whole boundless realm of human pathology.'

AP

*See also* AUTHORS; POETRY; TRUANTS – DOCTORS IN OTHER WALKS OF LIFE

Otto **LOEWI** (1873–1961). German pharmacologist. After graduating in 1896, he devoted himself to physiology and pharmacology, working first at the Physiological Institute in Marburg; during this period he spent some months at University College London under E. H. Starling. He then spent four years (1905–9) as associate professor in Vienna, before becoming professor of pharmacology in Graz, Austria, where he spent most of his career (1909–38). After the Nazi occupation, he emigrated to the USA in 1940 to be research professor at the College of Medicine of New York University. His main discovery concerned the appearance of a chemical substance in the perfusate of a frog's heart following stimulation of its nerve supply that was able to inhibit the action of a second heart receiving the perfused fluid (1921–6); this substance was later identified as acetylcholine, which had been isolated by Sir Henry Dale in 1914. Dale and Loewi were jointly awarded the 1936 NOBEL PRIZE for this work.

**LUNG CANCER** See CHEST MEDICINE

**LYING-IN HOSPITALS** Two events in the first half of the 18th century shaped the future of maternal care. From about 1740 medical practitioners for the first time became regularly involved in both normal and abnormal childbirth; in other words, midwifery joined physic, surgery, and pharmacy as part of the medical curriculum. The second event was the rapid growth of HOSPITALS. Because these were judged to be a success, it was natural to establish lying-in hospitals on the same model. By the end of the 18th century several lying-in hospitals had been established, funded in Britain by voluntary subscriptions and staffed by MIDWIVES and honorary (unpaid) medical men. On the European Continent, lying-in hospitals, which came into being at the same time, were generally funded by the state or local government, and the medical staff was salaried.

Lying-in hospitals varied in size. Most were smaller than the general hospitals, the exception being the ALLGEMEINES KRANKENHAUS in Vienna (p 352). Its maternity hospital — the hospital with which Ignaz SEMMELWEISS (p 479) was associated — was, by the 1840s, providing obstetric care for 5000 women a year. The only then British hospital of equivalent size was the Rotunda in Dublin. Other British lying-in hospitals in the mid-19th century usually delivered around 100 to 200 babies a year.

It was fortunate that lying-in hospitals were fewer and smaller than general hospitals, because they were extremely dangerous places to have a baby. Although a lying-in hospital might continue

(continued)

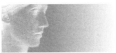

**DR LYDGATE** Dr Tertius Lydgate is a character in *Middlemarch* (1871–2) by George Eliot (Mary Ann Evans), a work saluted by Virginia Woolf as 'one of the few English novels written for adult people'. In it George Eliot delineates the detail of life in an English provincial town on a spacious and well-lit canvas. Her analysis of the developing medical profession has been praised. Lydgate represented a new type doctor emerging from the surgeon apothecary (one with diplomas from both the College of Surgeons and the Society of APOTHECARIES), the forerunner of the enlightened general practitioner of today. He was motivated by the prospects of scientific advance and medical reform; his use of the stethoscope and his wish to conduct AUTOPSIES placed him in the *avant-garde* of his profession.

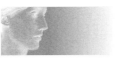

Dr **JEKYLL** is the antihero of Robert Louis Stevenson's *The strange case of Dr. Jekyll and Mr. Hyde* (1866). Dr Jekyll is a philanthropic and well-liked physician who develops an interest in the dualism of personality. Experimenting with drugs, he succeeds in separating the good and evil sides of his own nature, the latter being intermittently personified as Mr Hyde. The book recounts how Mr Hyde gradually gains the upper hand, culminating in the doctor's self-destruction.

## Queen Charlotte's Hospital

### A. Maternal mortality from all causes

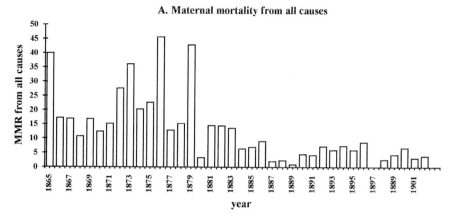

### B. Maternal mortality from sepsis only

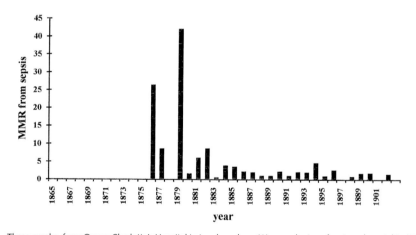

These graphs, from Queen Charlotte's Hospital in London, show (A) annual rates of maternal mortality (MMR) from all causes (1865–1902) and (B) from sepsis only (1876–1902). Antisepsis was introduced in 1880. (Source: Williams, W. (1904). *Deaths in childbed.* Royal College of Physicians, London.)

for a while with few maternal deaths, sooner or later all of them suffered horrifying epidemics of puerperal fever. There are records from the 18th century of whole wards of lying-in women being 'swept away' and the dead buried two in a coffin in an attempt to hide the awful mortality from the public. Even in less ferocious epidemics, most patients were infected and the fatality rate could be 50% or higher. The hospital authorities did not know what to do.

Obstetricians knew that the risk of death in a hospital delivery was ten or more times higher than that of a home delivery with unskilled assistance in the meanest of slums. At the height of an epidemic of puerperal fever in Paris in the 1850s, an obstetrician at the famous Maternité hospital is said to have intercepted a woman in labor as she climbed the steps to the hospital and implored her to turn round and go home if she valued her life. Although a few obstetricians in the 1830s advised the closure of these deplorable institutions, most protested that their hospitals provided a service for the poor and were essential for teaching. Throughout the mid-19th century maternal mortality remained as high as ever. Then a sudden unanticipated revolution occurred: the introduction of Listerian antisepsis.

## Introduction of asepsis

Joseph (later first Baron) LISTER (p 473) introduced antisepsis into surgical practice in 1865, publishing his results in 1867. In 1868 a Swiss obstetrician visited Lister in Glasgow and was so impressed that he went straight home and introduced a similar antiseptic technique in his lying-in hospital in Basel. The result was dramatic. Maternal mortality rapidly fell from 50–60 maternal deaths per 1000 deliveries to five per 1000. A Danish obstetrician followed suit in 1870, and by the 1880s obstetric antisepsis was established in most lying-in hospitals in western countries, with a startling reduction in mortality.

By 1888, a British obstetrician was able to say that lying-in hospitals were no longer 'hotbeds of death and disease in which no woman could be confined without serious risk, hardly less grave than that of a capital surgical operation'. Reports from all over the world, he said, had shown that lying-in hospitals were now places where 'a woman is as safe if not safer than if she was confined in a large and luxurious house with nurse, physician, and all that money can now procure'. This transformation was due to the discoveries of Lister, based on the work of Louis PASTEUR (p 620). Contrary to received opinion, Semmelweis's work in 1847 had almost no effect on reducing maternal mortality, except locally in Vienna and later in a few German

hospitals. Lister had never heard of Semmelweiss until the 1890s; nor had most British obstetricians until Listerian antisepsis was established and a group of surgeons and obstetricians suddenly 'discovered' Semmelweiss as the pioneer of antisepsis. In a series of later biographies, Semmelweiss was portrayed (incorrectly) as the conqueror of puerperal fever, and as a tragic hero and martyr, unjustly neglected by past generations. There are few more striking examples of medical hagiography.

Until the 1880s, the best that could be said about the lying-in hospitals is that they provided poor mothers with a warm bed, ample food, rest, and the rare luxury of being waited on, which explains why they were so popular with patients. But they did so at the cost of a horrific mortality rate. After 1880s, antisepsis, asepsis, safe CESAREAN SECTION, and new methods of ANESTHESIA and analgesia, led to lying-in hospitals becoming specialist centers that were increasingly popular with all classes of women. By the 1980s, home deliveries had virtually disappeared in all but a few western countries, and the offspring of the old lying-in hospitals, the modern maternity hospitals, and maternity departments of general hospitals had become the normal and usually the safest place for women to have their babies.                          IL

*See also* OBSTETRICS AND GYNECOLOGY

**LYME DISEASE** See INSECTS; RHEUMATOLOGY

**LYMPHOMA** See HEMATOLOGY

**A DISAPPOINTED MAN**

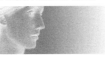

Ignaz Philipp
**SEMMELWEISS**
(1818–65). Hungarian obstetrician. In 1846 when working at the Allgemeines Krankenhaus in Vienna, Semmelweiss noted that the maternal mortality in the ward attended by students was far higher than in that staffed by nurses. He suspected the difference was due to the students coming directly from the dissection room and infecting the parturient women they examined. When he enforced their thorough washing, the maternal mortality fell from 9.9% to 1.3%. His views were not acceptable to his superiors and he left Vienna for Budapest, where he became professor of obstetrics in 1855. In 1861 he set out his findings in *Die Aetiologie der Begriff und die Prophylaxis des Kindbettfiebers*. It was badly received and in 1865 he suffered a mental breakdown and died, ironically from septicemia from a wound infection.

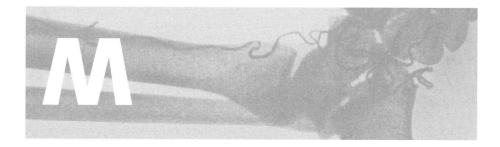

# THE GREAT KILLERS: MALARIA

**MALARIA** is caused by a plasmodium, a single-celled parasitic organism transmitted by anophalene mosquitoes to mammals including humans. Plasmodia are highly species-specific: only specific vertebrates and mosquito species are parasitized by specific varieties of plasmodia. Four main varieties of plasmodia affect humans; two of these, falciparum and tertian, are the most common. Many other varieties of malaria exist, some specific to other mammals such as monkeys, some affecting only birds. These do not infect humans, but have been useful to research workers seeking to develop vaccines that could protect humans against malaria.

Malaria, like TUBERCULOSIS, could be called 'Captain of the men of death'. In Africa it kills over a million people a year; worldwide it affects 200–300 million people, causing chronic debility in many. Prevalent in tropical and subtropical countries, it may occur wherever mosquitoes that carry the malaria parasite occur and conditions allow the parasite to flourish and reproduce. In the past, and potentially in the future, this has

included many temperate zones. Indigenous malaria occurred in England and parts of western Europe in the 1920s, and cases may have occurred in Kent as recently as the 1960s. In the 1820s malaria was common in the southern USA, the Mississippi Valley, and New England; cases occurred even as far north as Ottawa, Canada, despite the harsh winters. Occasional cases arising from bites by local mosquitoes have occurred near airports in New York and Toronto in the 1990s.

Malaria is among the diseases that have shaped the course of history. The marshes near Rome were a breeding ground for mosquitoes, and the decline of the Roman Empire may have been accelerated when the drainage systems the Romans built fell into disrepair, allowing the mosquitoes to breed and the disease to return. The Mayans in the Yucatan Peninsula of what is now Mexico, the temple builders in Cambodia, among others, may have fallen victim to malaria.

Only female anophalene mosquitoes require a blood meal, and therefore carry the malaria parasite. Anophalenes are smaller than the culecine mosquitoes which we see and hear on hot summer evenings. When they are feeding, their head, thorax, and abdomen form a straight line at an oblique angle to the skin, unlike culecine mosquitoes, which have a hump-backed appearance. But they are so small and inconspicuous that they escaped notice until Ronald ROSS (p 481) who worked in the south of India in the late 19th century, identified them as the villain responsible for carrying the malaria parasite.

Ross's investigations, including microdissection to show the stages of parasite development in the female anophalene mosquito's stomach and salivary glands, led to his being awarded the NOBEL PRIZE for Medicine in 1902. Previously, Alphonse LAVERAN (this page) had discovered malaria parasites in human blood. He too received the Nobel prize, in 1907.

Until the connection was made between mosquitoes and malaria many hot, wet,

humid, and swampy regions in temperate as well as tropical and subtropical regions were made virtually unfit for human occupation by the presence of mosquitoes and malaria parasites. The names given to the disease — malaria means bad air, and another name was swamp fever — were clues to its environmental origins, but it was long thought to be a perfect illustration of the miasma theory of disease — that is, one spread by foul and poisonous emanations from rotting flesh or vegetation.

Control of malaria requires understanding of the life cycle of the malaria parasite, the plasmodium. When a female anophalene mosquito takes a blood meal, she ingests plasmodia that begin the sexual phase of their reproductive cycle; they form cysts in the mosquito's stomach, which rupture to disgorge the next phase of the life cycle, microscopic organisms called sporozoites that migrate to the mosquito's salivary glands, where they are released and injected directly into the blood stream next time the mosquito takes a blood meal. The time required for all these developmental phases to occur in the mosquito is temperature-sensitive: it takes less time in hot weather than in cool. This explains the higher prevalence of malaria in the tropics than in temperate zones.

### Epidemiology

Ronald ROSS (p 481) not only discovered the link between malaria and anophalene mosquitoes, he also developed mathematical models that explain the EPIDEMIOLOGY. He was a pioneer in the art of developing mathematical models to fit the empirical observations of epidemic spread of disease. When malaria parasites are injected into the blood stream, they disappear for about ten days from the peripheral blood for a period of development in the liver; at the end of this latent period, huge numbers of plasmodia invade the peripheral blood stream, all attacking red blood cells simultaneously, devouring and destroying them, releasing

Charles Louis Alphonse **LAVERAN** (1845–1922). French physician. After service in the war of 1870 Laveran was appointed associate professor in the military École Val de Grâce. Posted to Algeria in 1878, he undertook research on malaria and in Constantine on 6 November 1880 found the parasite responsible. From 1884–94 he was professor of military hygiene at Val de Grâce, but left the army in 1896 to work at the Pasteur Institute. He was awarded the NOBEL PRIZE in 1907 for his work on protozoa.

*(continued opposite)*

*(continued)*

new generations of parasites that repeat the process of attacking and destroying red blood cells. The periodicity of this repeated invasion of red blood cells by new generations of parasites every two or three days causes the characteristic regular peaks of high fever and drenching sweats that debilitate victims of malaria. Some parasites either remain dormant in the liver or subsequent generations return to the liver to be released at some later time. This causes the recurrences or relapses characteristic of the disease. Destruction of massive quantities of red blood cells causes anemia and a characteristic sallow appearance in people who do not have heavily pigmented skin. It may cause jaundice, as well as liver damage, brain damage, and enlargement of the spleen.

Mosquito control was the key to successful development of many tropical regions, for example, the central American isthmus of Panama — where YELLOW FEVER, carried by the other principal variety of mosquito, culecines, was a more deadly hazard even than malaria.

Malaria has been treated with quinine for centuries. During and since the Second World War, other antimalarial drugs, the first of which was atebrine, have been developed. Antimalarial drugs work by killing plasmodia or inhibiting their reproduction, but drug resistance is a perennial problem. Likewise, mosquitoes soon become resistant to insecticides such as DDT and more powerful (but also more toxic) second and third generation insecticides such as parathion.

Malaria control therefore relies increasingly on other tactics: bednets impregnated with insecticides protect people, especially children, in regions where mosquitoes are nocturnal feeders. Other control measures include the use of larvicides to kill mosquito larvae; seeding ponds with fish or amphibia that feed on the larvae; and, where feasible, draining or covering water to deprive mosquitoes of breeding sites.

It is important for all who may be exposed to malaria to know the habits and the habitat of the mosquitoes in the locality where they are at risk of being bitten: some mosquitoes breed only in deep shade in stagnant water; others breed in sunlight in fast flowing streams; some take their blood meal only at dusk or dawn, others are indiscriminate feeders. It is wise always to expose the minimum area of skin to the risk of bites by wearing long-sleeved shirts and long trousers rather than shorts, to use insect repellent on exposed skin surfaces, and to take particular care at times of the day when the local variety of mosquitoes look for their blood meal.

For over twenty years the World Bank and other UN agencies and non-governmental organizations have invested heavily in a program of tropical diseases research, in which development of a vaccine against the malaria parasite has been a priority. However, despite the investment of much money and many years of diligent effort by some of the world's best research workers, there is little so far to show for this. There are many problems, some related to the difficulty of

identifying effective ways to enhance the natural immunity that many people seem to develop in endemic regions, others due to the problems of growing malaria parasites in artificial media. Some 'natural' immunity is associated with a genetically determined abnormality of red blood cells, the sickle-cell trait. Over the millennia, exposure to malaria has led to a high prevalence of this trait among certain ethnic groups of African origin, and, while they may be less prone to malaria in malarial regions, they may experience other severe medical problems in environments where they are not exposed to malaria.

Malaria is resurgent in many regions where for some years it was so well controlled that many people believed it had been eradicated. For example, in the late 1970s Sri Lanka and much of India were free of malaria for a few years. But by the early 1980s cases were occurring again in ever larger numbers every year, and by the late 1990s the incidence of malaria had risen again to levels not seen since before World War II. Now, however, the malaria parasites are often resistant to antimalarial drugs and the mosquitoes are often resistant to insecticides.

As the world's average ambient temperature increases in these days of global warming, malaria remains a terrible threat to the health of humans in a widening belt of the world's subtropical waist. By 2050, over half the human race will live in regions at risk of malaria.                                                JML

*See also* INSECTS; TROPICAL MEDICINE; WORLD HEALTH ORGANIZATION

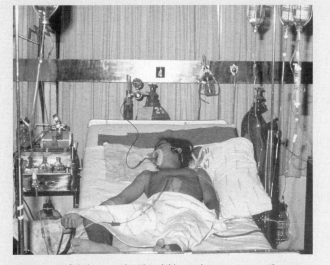

Intensive care failed to save this Thai child, seen here in a coma with severe falciparum malaria. (Courtesy of Professor D. A. Warrell.)

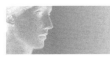

Ronald **ROSS** (1857–1932). British medical scientist, entomologist, and epidemiologist. Following suggestions of his mentor Patrick Manson, he searched for the link between mosquitoes and MALARIA, eventually finding that only the small, inconspicuous anophalene mosquitoes carried the malaria parasite. He did micro-dissections to show the development of the parasite in the female mosquito's stomach and its migration to the salivary glands. He received the NOBEL PRIZE in 1902 for this work. Ross also worked out the first mathematical models of malaria epidemiology, and in his spare time, wrote poetry.

A MILITARY
MALARIOLOGIST

Neil Hamilton **FAIRLEY**
(1891–1966). Australian
physician. Immediately after
graduating in Melbourne in
1915, Fairley joined the
Australian Army Medical
Corps and carried out work
on schistosomiasis
(bilharziasis), for the
diagnosis of which he devised
an antigen which was used
for decades. His work on
intravascular hemolysis and
on the anemia of malaria
won him the Fellowship of
the Royal Society in 1942.
Joining the Australian
Medical Corps at the
outbreak of the Second
World War, his work on the
protection of troops serving
in heavily malarious areas,
first with mepacrine and then
with proguanil, was critical in
the success of the Pacific and
Burmese campaigns.

**MALARIA AND WAR** Sir Ronald ROSS (p 481), discoverer of the mosquito vector of MALARIA, once mused that the history of malaria and war might almost be taken to be the history of war itself, so closely were the two intertwined. Ross can be forgiven a little exaggeration here, but certainly the conditions of war favor the dissemination of malaria. Population movement — whether of troops or refugees — may introduce exotic parasites to new areas, just as non-immune populations are exposed to infection if they move into areas in which the disease is endemic. Damage inflicted during war to drainage and irrigation systems may also extend the breeding places of malaria-bearing mosquitoes. At the same time, malaria has often had a dramatic impact upon military campaigns and, in recent times, it has even been used as weapon of war.

The most deadly form of malaria is that caused by the *Plasmodium falciparum* group of parasites, once thought to be a single species, but now known to be at least five subspecies. Probably originating in West Africa — where it is still the most common form of malaria — *falciparum* is now distributed widely throughout the tropical world. Another species of malaria parasite common in Africa is the less fatal *P. malariae*, but perhaps the most important militarily is the rarely fatal but debilitating *P. vivax*. While probably of Mediterranean origin, *vivax* is now common in Asia and in parts of central and eastern Africa. Until the mid-20th century, it was also found in many low-lying areas of Europe, including Britain and the Netherlands. It is the type of malaria probably responsible for most of the casualties from fever in Roman and Grecian campaigns, and, more recently, in the Salonika and Sicilian campaigns of the First and Second World Wars. Malaria is spread by the *Anopheles* mosquito, whose larvae grow in slow-moving or stagnant water, including collections as small as a human footprint.

Much of what we now call malaria was previously termed 'ague', marsh fever, or 'intermittent' and 'remittent' fever, so we can never be certain of the extent to which malaria affected military campaigns. Nevertheless, taking into account the symptoms described by eye-witnesses and their descriptions of the environment in which military campaigns were conducted, we can make a reasonable guess as to the prevalence of malaria. Among those who may have fallen prey to malaria is Alexander the Great, who was stricken by fever when returning through Asia Minor after years of campaigning in the East. Fever of a seemingly malarious kind also appears to have been responsible for much of the sickness during the Crusades (along with dysentery) and in armies fighting in Mughal India. With the systematic collection of mortality statistics from the 18th century we are on firmer ground. Malaria was certainly chief among the diseases which struck the ill-fated British expedition to Walcheren, The Netherlands, in April 1809. The area in which troops were deployed was a disease-ridden marsh and, by September, only 4000 of the original force of 39 000 were fit for duty. When the army was finally withdrawn in February 1810, 4000 had died from disease and 11 000 were still in hospital.

Malaria was also prominent among diseases encountered by Europeans in tropical campaigns. If not the chief cause of mortality, malaria was usually the principal cause of sickness (along with SEXUALLY TRANSMITTED DISEASES). The worst effects of the disease were controlled from the 1820s by quinine — the active ingredient of cinchona bark — given prophylactically as well as in the treatment of hospital cases. As a result, malaria deaths began to fall rapidly from mid-century, and there was some success in controlling the incidence of malaria on tropical campaigns, such as the Magdala and Kumasi campaigns in Africa, in 1867–8 and 1873–4, respectively. However, the low incidence of malaria on these occasions may have been the result more of luck than judgement and, outside their barracks, European troops continued to be vulnerable to the disease. This was shown dramatically during the First World War in several theaters, but most notably Macedonia, Mesopotamia, and East Africa. During 1918, for example, around 90% of British and French units serving in Macedonia had contracted malaria, despite attempts to enforce quinine prophylaxis, while, in East Africa, the predominantly Indian British-led expeditionary force suffered as many as 38 000 admissions to hospital (chiefly from malaria) within the first four months of 1917. Such high casualty rates led military medical officers to conclude that quinine prophylaxis was of little use. Many soldiers feared that the drug caused sexual impotence and they were reluctant to take it. Even when taken regularly, it seemed not to confer adequate protection.

At the outbreak of the Second World War, most medical officers thought that quinine could, at best, only suppress rather than prevent infection, and commanders were advised not to rely too heavily upon it. In any case, in the Allied armies, the supply of quinine had been greatly reduced by the Japanese invasion of the Dutch East Indies, where most cinchona trees were cultivated. As a result, the Allies began to turn to synthetic substitutes, most notably the drug mepacrine (Atebrin), which had been synthesized by German chemists in the 1930s. Experimental trials in Queensland, Australia, showed that mepacrine could confer a high degree of protection, and this was further shown in the field in New Guinea, where the malaria rate among Australian troops declined from 740 per 1000 in December 1943 to only 20 per 1000 by November 1944. In other theaters of the war, however, it took much longer to establish the use of mepacrine as a regular feature of military life, as the Allied armies learned to their cost during the invasion of Sicily in 1943 and, later, on the Italian mainland. In Burma, however, strict anti-malaria discipline paid dividends and General William Slim's threat to sack commanders who neglected the health of their men succeeded in reducing the malaria rate in the British-led 14th Army from a high of 60% of total strength in 1942 to around 10% in 1945.

The control of malaria was also aided greatly, from 1944, by the use of the insecticide DDT, which was sprayed from the air and on the ground. DDT provided much needed protection for troops operating in intensely malarious areas such as the Kabaw Valley (Valley of Death) in Burma and in the Pontine marshes and other low-lying areas of Italy, parts of which had been deliberately flooded by the Germans to hinder the Allied advance and to engender an epidemic of malaria. However, in almost all circumstances in which malaria was encountered, Allied forces had the upper hand in controlling the disease in the last years of the war. The official medical historian of the British Army in Burma has gone so far as to declare that the differences in malaria rates were 'one of the most important reasons why the Japanese were defeated'. However, as Slim acknowledged, only during the last phase of his campaign did his army enjoy a higher standard of health than the Japanese. He also acknowledged that this was due as much to the rapid return of malaria casualties to duty as a result of forward treatment facilities as to prevention itself. Starved of supplies and dispirited in retreat, it is little wonder that the Axis powers had less success in controlling malaria during the final years of the war.                                    MH

*See also* INSECTS; TROPICAL MEDICINE; WAR

**MANAGED CARE** is any attempt to influence the access and delivery of healthcare by financing and management strategies. With this definition, all healthcare has been and will be managed. Managed care is often considered an outgrowth of the healthcare reform movement of the 1990s. This is not true — managed care has been around a long time. For example, employers of railway workers in the 1800s developed a managed care plan to cover traumatic injuries. In fact, fee-for-service is managed care. However, new models of managed care have emerged. The debate about these new models is not about managed care, *per se*. Instead, it is about *how* care is managed and *how* these new models may change access and delivery of care.

These new models of care refer to managed care organizations. These managed care organizations are a business approach to healthcare delivery.

## CLASSIFICATION OF MANAGED CARE ORGANIZATIONS

Managed care organizations can be classified according to the following five characteristics:

- How physicians are paid for primary care services (salary, capitation, or fee-for-service).
- Whether health maintenance organization physicians see only their own organization's patients.
- The nature of the health maintenance organization's financial arrangements with other businesses that provide services to patients enrolled in their plan.
- The risk and reward structure for participating physicians.
- The size of the 'risk pool' (patient populations and their disease characteristics) used to share the risk or rewards.

Four main categories emanate from these characteristics: health maintenance organizations, provider-sponsored organizations, preferred provider organizations, and point of service plans. Health maintenance organizations cover care only when patients go to physicians and hospitals within the network. Provider-sponsored organizations are similar to health maintenance organizations except that they are owned and operated by independent physicians and hospitals rather than an insurance entity. Preferred provider organizations allow patients to choose from a larger network of physicians and do not require primary physician referrals to see specialists. Point of service plans are even more flexible in that they pay for out of plan care, but they usually require higher co-payments. Point of service plans have grown at the fastest rate. Managed care organizations may offer plans from each of these categories and, therefore, may be organizationally complex.

The United States spends more on healthcare per person than any other country — nearly $2500; 14% of the gross national product. A strong voice decrying the current spending level is the business community. Prepaid healthcare is the solution being proposed by employers to control costs and managed care organizations are the vehicles of change. The percentage of patients enrolled in managed care

*(continued overleaf)*

*(continued)*

organizations has grown from 14% in 1987 to 75% of all Americans with private insurance in 1998. Of Medicare beneficiaries in 1997, 15% — 5.6 million people — were enrolled in managed care plans. The number of plans has increased four-fold in the last few years to total 409. Clearly, this business approach to healthcare delivery is being touted by employers and, in terms of Medicare, by government as well.

Any mechanism to constrain costs of healthcare delivery, whether by national plans with fixed budgets or by managed care plans, will affect the access to and delivery of healthcare. Some effects will be good, some bad. Which are good or bad will depend on the perspective of the stakeholder in the healthcare delivery chain. Physicians are concerned about not being able to deliver care that they think is the best. They also see a shift in profits and note that leaders of some managed care organizations have large salaries that siphon off dollars from delivering care, while physicians may be 'deselected' when they care for the more ill patients. Patients are concerned about being able to choose their doctor, and access to care by specialists. They are also concerned about a new financial incentive for their providers — when a fixed budget profit is maximized by reducing services (such as length of stay in a hospital after delivering a baby). Employers, on the other hand, see variation in treatment decisions by providers and believe improved financial arrangements could modify incentives to assure more appropriate care.

These diverse perspectives, along with examples of abuses from each, have reached Congress. New legislation is being proposed to protect patients. Examining these proposed changes tells a great deal about how managed care organizations have changed access and delivery of healthcare. One proposal calls for health maintenance organizations to pay for emergency room visits if a 'prudent' person has reason to believe they face an emergency (and not just if they truly have one in retrospect). Another provision will require health maintenance organizations to set up affordable, accessible processes to appeal a decision to deny care. Some legislation will make it easier to sue managed care organizations for malpractice, and prohibit 'gag' rules that forbid physicians from discussing treatments the health maintenance organization will not cover. One provision will require health maintenance organizations to provide detailed information about the drugs covered in their plan.

A growing aspect of emphasis for managed care organizations is quality of care. Organizations have survived by reducing costs to employers. However, as profit margins for managed care organizations decline through reduced spending on healthcare prompted by competition and improved management, many believe that quality of care will be the deciding factor for choosing among plans. Published evidence is scanty, but it suggests that care under managed care is as good, and may be better, than care with fee-for-service.

Managed care is a reality, but how care will be managed continues to evolve. Hopefully, this evolution will assure that access is guaranteed for those who derive benefit, compassionately dissuade access for care that is not beneficial, and foster a desire to know the difference. EE

*See also* HEALTHCARE SYSTEMS; USA

---

**MARTYRS** There are not many instances of medical thinkers and scientists who have gone to their deaths on account of their beliefs, although there have undoubtedly been some. For example, SERVETUS (this page), a Spaniard who had studied medicine in France, was condemned to death by the Protestant leader John Calvin for proposing (correctly as it turned out) the theory of the lesser or pulmonary circulation of blood, contradicting the teaching of GALEN (p 324); he was burned alive in Geneva on 27 October 1553.

*See also* SAINTS

## MASSACHUSETTS GENERAL HOSPITAL
See USA

Henry **MAUDSLEY** (1835–1918). British psychiatrist. As a student at University College, London, he won ten gold medals, and after qualification considered a career in the Indian Medical Service. For this, he had to have experience in mental illness, and, after two short appointments in asylums, he decided to devote himself to this specialty, a decision which must have been reinforced when he married the daughter of the psychiatrist, John Conolly. After serving as the medical superintendent of a Manchester lunatic hospital he moved to London, becoming editor of *Mental Science*, and subsequently being appointed professor of medical jurisprudence at University College. His writings were influential, particularly a textbook on mental illness, and increasingly favored the concept of heredity and degeneracy as important causes of mental illness. Pessimistic about the value of asylums in treatment, he nevertheless gave the London County Council a large sum of money to build the research institute and teaching center associated with the mental hospital now named after him, though this was not to open before his death.

**MAYO CLINIC** See USA

**McGILL UNIVERSITY** See CANADA

**MEDIA** Coverage of health matters by the mass media has grown dramatically over the past fifty years. Nowadays most newspapers have at least

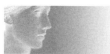

one health correspondent; and regularly they devote a section specifically to health matters. The broadcast media also give much time to health matters, and some countries have TV channels devoted to health. Hospitals and doctors' consulting rooms are also regularly the setting of soap operas and dramas.

The World Wide Web offers thousands of health related sites, and increasingly members of the public can access information on health as easily as doctors. This is one factor contributing to what many see as a fundamental change in the relationship between doctors and patients, with the relationship becoming much more egalitarian.

The news media cover all health issues, but there is a bias towards the new and the dramatic. Thus new and risky surgical operations receive a great deal of coverage, whereas the more mundane — for instance, mental illness and the problems of aging — receive much less. 'Lifestyle' issues — such as smoking, drinking, diet, and exercise — are widely covered on news and feature pages.

The tone of media coverage of health matters is changing. Thirty, even ten, years ago, doctors tended to be treated uncritically, and the media concentrated on promoting 'a doctor's view of health'. Increasingly, however, such views are being questioned by the media. 'Exposures' of doctors and their practices have become common, and the mass media will often promote complementary medicine. These changes reflect broader social changes, and it's impossible to know how much the media are leading public opinion and how much simply reflecting it. Probably both.

Many of the news stories are derived from medical journals, particularly the weekly general medical journals, but an increasing number of organizations — professional associations, research institutions, and pharmaceutical companies — are keen to use the media to promote issues that are important to them and to raise their own profile. These organizations increasingly employ public relations consultants to spread their messages, and the media are regularly manipulated. Wise consumers of the mass media are constantly alert for subtext and ask themselves 'Who is trying to sell what to whom?'

What is the effect of this increasing media coverage of health matters? The usual answer is that people are better informed about health, more able to take charge of their own health, and more likely to be discerning and critical consumers of healthcare services. This may be true, but scientifically sound studies of the effects of increased health coverage are scarce. Indeed, it has been argued that the mass of published material may actually reduce understanding of health issues — partly because of

the way it is selected and partly because of the inevitable tension between the scientific complexities that underlie medical stories and the need for short, clear, and exciting stories. Certainly the result of using the mass media for health education has been disappointing. For instance, doctors thought that once the evidence was gathered on the harmful effects of smoking some powerful messages through the media would solve the problem. But this was not the case, and research has shown that simply transmitting messages through the media — either through advertising or editorial coverage — is not enough on its own to change behavior.

Although it is hard to be sure about the overall effects of health coverage in the media, there have been some examples of where the media have had important effects on particular issues. It was a television program that first suggested that children around nuclear installations may be at increased risk of leukemia and some solid cancers. Doctors and others might have complained that the program was sensational and scary, but its central proposition turned out to be true. Unfortunately television programs are not good at conveying the size of a risk, and pictures of young children dying of cancer inevitably have an impact that dull statistics cannot match. The media are regularly accused by doctors and health authorities of creating 'scares'. These 'scares', which may now receive world-wide coverage, include: the contraceptive pill and breast cancer and thromboembolic disease; vaccines causing autism or brain damage; 'flesh-eating bugs' (necrotizing fasciitis); vitamin K and childhood cancer; breast implants causing autoimmune disease; mobile phones causing brain tumors; and bovine spongiform encephalopathy spreading to man and causing CREUTZFELDT–JAKOB DISEASE.

There is a tendency to blame the media for these 'scares'. However, most of those listed above have their origin in reports in the scientific media. One exception is the 'flesh-eating bug,' a good example of a media-created scare. Necrotizing fasciitis is a well known but rare condition. The media identified some cases and attached the sobriquet 'flesh-eating bug.' Other media, excited by the idea, searched backwards in time and over a large geographical area for cases — and of course found them. They reported them, and a huge amount of publicity and a scare was created. Many medical journalists understood what was happening, and tried to hold the stories. But editors insisted on running them: they could not be the only newspaper or news program to 'miss' such an important story.

Scare stories arise because of problems in understanding and describing risk and uncertainty. The risk to humans of bovine spongiform encephalopathy (BSE) is unknown. It may prove to be huge; it may be trivial. In such circumstances, it's hard for the media to get the message 'right.' In contrast, the risk of third-generation contraception pills causing more deep vein thromboses than second-generation pills is well known. The relative risk is something close to a twofold increase: the new pills cause twice as many deep vein thromboses as the old. But the absolute risk is 10 more cases a year among a million women — up from about 10 for the old pills to 20 for the new. Ideally, the mass media — and medical journals — would give both figures: people make different decisions depending on the way the information is presented. Unfortunately, the media, driven by regulatory authorities, gave only the relative risk and caused unnecessary panic.

### Leaks to the press

One particular conflict between doctors and journalists has been over the publication of studies reported in medical journals. The editors of journals make journalists wait until the studies are published in their journals — arguing that the peer review process aims at ensuring the study is sound and that doctors will be better able to understand the study if they have the full scientific paper rather than a few paragraphs in a newspaper or on television. Journalists claim that studies of importance to the public should be reported immediately and not have to wait for the peer review process. Some journals have refused to publish papers that are leaked to the press, but a system has now been devised by the International Committee of Medical Editors for allowing publicity before publication in restricted circumstances.

Ironically, one of the few circumstances where a scientifically sound study has shown a positive effect of the media has to do with the reporting of stories from medical journals in the media. Researchers showed that studies selected from the *New England Journal of Medicine* for reporting in the *New York Times* were more likely to be cited in scientific journals than articles not selected. And it wasn't that the journalists were simply selecting the most important studies because those selected but not reported — at a time when the *New York Times* was on strike — were not better cited.

The influence of the media on health and healthcare is considerable, even if not clearly defined. That influence is likely to grow as the World Wide Web develops into a medium that can be easily accessed by everybody (probably through their televisions) and as the media become increasingly global, with people all over the world having access to the same television channels.                                    RS

*See also* JOURNALS

Gregor Johann **MENDEL** (1822–84). Austrian monk. Born in the Moravian village of Heizendorf, Mendel was educated locally and at the Philosophical Institute of Olmütz. At the age of 21, hampered by poverty, he entered an Augustinian monastery in Brünn (now Brno) as a means of security. After studying theology, Greek, and Hebrew at Brünn Theological College, he was ordained as a priest in 1847 and went to teach in a local school. In 1850 he attempted unsuccessfully to pass an examination to gain the teaching license required by the authorities, and he was thus sent by his Abbot to study at the University of Vienna for two years. It was there that he was introduced to the sciences, plant biology and hybridization and on his return to Brünn in 1853 he resumed teaching and carried out plant experiments in the monastery gardens. He bred and crossbred the edible pea and formulated the laws of segregation and independent assortment of characters, which are now recognized as basic laws of heredity. He reported his findings in a paper read at a meeting of the Brünn Society for the Study of Natural Science in 1865; it was published in the society's *Transactions* but it made little impact. In 1868 Mendel was elected Abbot of the monastery, leaving him little time for further scientific work. He died in 1884, sixteen years before his work on heredity was rediscovered and independently confirmed by three scientists.

**MESMERISM** takes its name from Anton MESMER (p 487), whose medical thesis argued that the course of a disease was determined by gravitational influences from the sun and moon. He subsequently thought that it might be possible to mimic these invisible forces by using magnets, whose force also operated at a distance. The first patient on whom he tried this treatment was a woman suffering from various manifestations of HYSTERIA; Mesmer found that he could remove her symptoms by placing variously shaped magnets on her body and stroking her with them. Further experiments showed that the therapeutic effect could be transferred from a magnet to non-magnetic objects, such as paper or bone, which were equally effective. In the light of these experiments, he was led to postulate the existence of a new force, different from terrestrial magnetism, which he termed *animal magnetism*. He subsequently found that his own hand or even his gaze could communicate this energy to the patient. Thus, he argued that an ill person had a deficiency of animal magnetism, which could be supplemented by a therapist, especially one such as himself endowed with a great amount of magnetism.

The new treatment caught on, resulted in opposition from the Viennese medical establish-

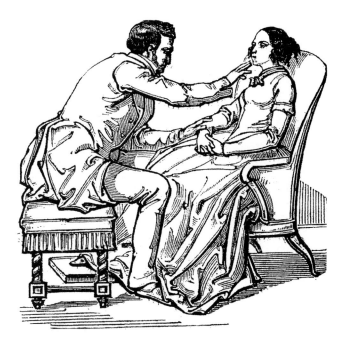

A mesmerizer at work.
(From Dupotet, C. (1862). *L'art du magnétiseur*, Paris.)

ment, and led to Mesmer moving to Paris, where he developed the *baquet* for group treatment. This consisted of a shallow wooden tub filled with bottles of water and iron filings, which Mesmer 'magnetized'; iron bars conducted the animal magnetic fluid to the patients, who sat around holding the bars and applying them to the site of their pain. Under these conditions many patients suffered 'crises', faints, seizures, and other physical effects, which Mesmer had come to consider were an essential preliminary to cure.

Royal commissions were established to investigate the many reported cures and to pronounce on the supposed existence of animal magnetism. Their largely negative findings helped to discredit Mesmer, although, lacking any clear alternative, the magnetic theory remained a durable explanation for the undeniable changes observed in some patients.

As well as opponents, Mesmer had attracted many followers. Among them was the Marquis de Puységur (1751–1825), who was responsible for a new approach to treatment. Puységur's first patient did not show any dramatic crisis in response to Puységur's magnetic stroking; instead, he went into a passive trance-like state. Puységur found that he could talk to the patient, make him behave in various ways, affect his memory and his perceptions. His patient also appeared to be more intelligent than in his waking state and to be capable of performing various paranormal feats, such as telepathy and clairvoyance. Not only was

the patient curable through mesmerism: in the mesmerized state he could diagnose and suggest cures for others. Puységur called this sleep-like state *somnambulism* and began to use *somnambulists* as assistant physicians.

Many cures were reported by Puységur, whose theory now came to differ from the purely physical theory of Mesmer in that he believed that the magnetic fluid was transmitted to the patient by the exercise of will-power on the part of the operator. In spite of the fact that Puységur's work rid mesmerism of its orgiastic element, his uncritical approach led to the association of somnambulism with paranormal powers, an association which was an anathema to medical and scientific orthodoxy, and which led to mesmerism being considered the concern of charlatans.

Nevertheless, some reputable and idealistic people concerned themselves with mesmerism, especially in Germany and later in Britain. The best-known British practitioner was John Elliotson, professor of medicine at the University of London, who was renowned as an innovative and highly skilled physician and free-thinker. Elliotson was forced to resign his academic and hospital appointments after controversy with more orthodox medical colleagues over his demonstrations with the Okey sisters, two young women who were a considerable spectacle when deeply mesmerized. Thomas WAKLEY (p 453), the editor of the *Lancet*, considered them to be impostors and became an implacable opponent of mesmerism.

### FOUNDER OF MESMERISM

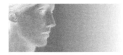

Franz Anton **MESMER** (1734–1815). Swiss physician. Mesmer, who practiced in Vienna, was inspired by Mead's book on the influence of the planets on the body. He used magnets to draw out the 'animal gravitation', which he later called 'animal magnetism'. Finally his hands took the place of the magnet and with them he claimed to infuse 'mesmeric fluid' (the origin of the term 'mesmerism'). Expelled from Vienna in 1778, he established a clinic in Paris which attracted a large following, including Marie Antoinette. The Revolution and the disapproval of orthodox practitioners forced him to leave France for Switzerland.

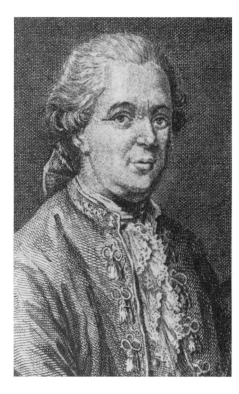

Portrait of Anton Mesmer, from an engraving by Dupin after a drawing by Desrais. (Reproduced courtesy of the Royal College of Physicians of London.)

mediumistic trance as somnambulists learnt to induce trance states in themselves and to communicate with 'the spirits'. The spread of spiritualism to Europe helped to push mesmerism as such into the background, but there were further reasons for its slow decline. At the time of its initial formulation, mesmeric theory had been a reasonable attempt at a scientific explanation of the psychological effects one person might have upon another. But during the 19th century the theory became untenable in the light of advances in neurophysiology and electromagnetism. And towards the end of that century, when HYPNOTISM seemed to have encompassed mesmeric phenomena and to have adopted psychological explanations for its effects, there was clearly no need to postulate the transmission of nervous energy from one person to another.

Although mesmerism itself is no longer taken seriously by scientists and physicians, the techniques of the mesmerizers may have produced a somewhat different physiological state from that involved in hypnosis, where touch is rarely involved, and to that extent the subject may still be open to research. 	DWF

*See also* CULTS AND QUACKERY

The *Lancet*'s ban on mesmeric writings extended to other medical periodicals, and Elliotson responded by publishing his own journal, *The Zoist*. In *The Zoist* the extraordinary reports of mesmerically-induced anesthesia first became widely disseminated. These originated mainly from James Esdaile, a surgeon in India, who carried out many major operations under mesmerism. Mesmeric infirmaries were established in London and in a few other cities, where treatment of a wide variety of complaints, including surgery under mesmeric anesthesia, became available. The infirmaries ran into financial difficulties and were short-lived; above all, the advent of chemical anesthesia killed off for surgical purposes the use of the less reliable mesmerism. This discovery proved a major set-back for the mesmerists, as anesthesia was a genuine effect which had served as a demonstration of the reality of the mesmeric influence on a patient; otherwise the critics could maintain with Wakley that all was trickery. With the demise of the *Zoist* in 1864 and the death of Elliotson, the mesmeric movement lost its impetus in Britain.

In the USA, mesmerism and public exhibitions of somnambulism had achieved some popularity by the 1840s. During that decade a new religious movement, spiritualism, began to sweep the country and altered the nature of mesmerism. What had been a mesmeric trance now became a

**MICROBIOLOGY** Micro-organisms are life forms that are so small that they cannot be seen with the naked eye. They include bacteria, viruses, fungi, algae, and protozoa. Our world teems with these tiny creatures, and, even now, less than 10% of the micro-organisms on earth have been characterized. The microbial biosphere is one of the most exciting biological frontiers left to explore. Microbiology encompasses the study of micro-organisms in all of their environmental niches, from deep sea vents, to arctic ice caps, in oceans, in the soil, and inside our bodies. Life as we know it without micro-organisms would be catastrophic. For example, we would be without food, since micro-organisms transform nitrogen from the atmosphere into forms that plants can use as food. Animals, such as sheep and cattle, depend on micro-organisms to digest food. In humans, harmless micro-organisms in our guts provide essential vitamin nutrients and compete against potential disease-causing microbes. Micro-organisms are essential for decomposing plants, animals, and other wastes in the biosphere so that nutrients are recycled and reused for renewed growth. Micro-organisms help destroy toxic compounds in the biosphere and they are an essential part of aquatic food chains. Micro-organisms are important for the production of beer and wine and many foods including yogurt, bread, and cheese.

Since their first isolation in the 19th century, micro-organisms have been exploited for their ability to produce antibiotics; clean up oil spills and other types of toxic chemicals released into the environment; produce various chemicals for industry; clean up sewage; and extract minerals such as copper and uranium. More recently, micro-organisms have been modified by the biotechnology industry through genetic engineering to produce insulin and other pharmaceutical and chemical products.

Despite the many beneficial, underappreciated roles of micro-organisms, the word microorganism is often associated with disease and is often used synonymously with 'germ'. The inference of 'germs' is that they are bad for us, and our collective historical memory contains many examples of how this came about. The plagues of past centuries, such as the BLACK DEATH, smallpox, and LEPROSY continue to horrify and fascinate. These ancient scourges take on new meaning as we encounter new afflictions such as AIDS, Ebola virus outbreaks, and Legionnaire's disease. Diseases that we once considered tamed, if not eradicated, such as TUBERCULOSIS, are reappearing and our modern antibiotic arsenal against many disease-causing micro-organisms (that is, pathogens) is endangered as microorganisms develop an array of mechanisms to resist antimicrobial agents.

The first micro-organisms were observed by an amateur lens grinder from Delft in 1674, Anthony van LEEUWENHOEK (this page). He took specimens from common sources — water droplets, his mouth, foods — looked at them under his homemade lens, and observed a hitherto unseen world of tiny organisms of different shapes and sizes ('animalcules'). He reported his results to the Royal Society of London, where they were discussed. These discoveries led to a heated debate, which lasted for several centuries, on the origin of such creatures. Long before Leeuwenhoek, the Greek philosopher ARISTOTLE (p 64) had taught that mice emerged from moist soils or that worms developed from slime. Following this line of thought, various scientists from the 17th to the 19th century proposed that living organisms, including micro-organisms and maggots, detected in spoiled foods or drinks, arose from non-living materials. This was the theory of spontaneous generation. Others, using tenets of a new approach known as the scientific method, proposed that living organisms could arise only from other living organisms and that contaminated materials must have arisen because they contained unseen organisms that multiplied. The debate was unequivocally resolved in 1861 through the elegant experiments of Louis PASTEUR (p 620), a brilliant pioneer microbiologist, who determined that the agents responsible for spoiling broths were microorganisms. Pasteur made other important dis-

coveries in microbiology. Besides discrediting the theory of spontaneous generation, he and associated researchers developed methods to decrease micro-organisms in foods by gentle heating, a process now known as pasteurization still used today to eliminate harmful micro-organisms from milk and other products.

Pasteur's first microbiological investigations were grounded in industrial microbiology with the discovery of the microbial origins of wine and beer souring. After first applying microbiological knowledge to improve industrial processes, Pasteur and others, such as his insightful contemporary, Robert KOCH (p 455) and his co-workers, then turned their attention to microorganisms that caused human diseases. The key to the characterization of these micro-organisms was the development of staining methods that allowed the better visualization of bacteria under the light microscope and the isolation of microorganisms as separate species, called pure cultures. By inoculating and growing bacteria on solidified culture media and distinguishing between species through various morphological and biochemical criteria, disease-causing organisms were purified and identified. Coupled with the development by Koch of criteria, known as Koch's postulates, for showing that a specific micro-organism was the source of a specific disease, the end of the 19th century was distinguished by the discovery and characterization of micro-organisms causing anthrax, tuberculosis, PLAGUE, meningitis, gonorrhea, TYPHOID fever, tetanus, DIPHTHERIA, dysentery, and pneumonia, to name a few.

At the same time that the microbial causes of infectious diseases were being elucidated, Pasteur and others discovered that bacteria could change into harmless variants under different cultural conditions and treatments and that these harmless variants could then be used as vaccines. Pasteur first developed vaccines to control chicken cholera and anthrax in sheep and finally he vaccinated a human against rabies. Even without the knowledge that micro-organisms cause disease, it had been long appreciated that humans could develop immunity to disease. Centuries ago, the Chinese had noted that persons who survived a SMALLPOX outbreak were immune to subsequent attacks. They used this knowledge to inoculate people by having them inhale dried scabs from infected victims in the hope that they would be protected. Edward JENNER (p 452), in Britain, observed that milkmaids, who had been first exposed to cowpox, were immune to smallpox infection. He produced the first vaccine by inoculating patients with material from cowpox lesions and showing that they were protected from smallpox.

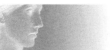
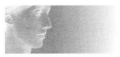

John Franklin **ENDERS** (1897–1985). American microbiologist. Studying and working at Harvard, Enders carried out research on immunology and viruses until 1946, when he set up a laboratory to research infectious diseases at the Children's Medical Center in Boston. In 1954 he was jointly awarded the NOBEL PRIZE for physiology or medicine for research on the growth of the polio virus in cultures of various types of tissue. This work led directly to development of the first polio vaccine by Jonas SALK (p 664).

## Vaccine development

The development of vaccines against infectious diseases is a cornerstone of public health initiatives. Modern techniques have permitted the development of several methods for vaccine production including the inactivation of microbial toxins, the use of components of microbial cells, the use of live non-disease-causing microbial varients, and even the injection of naked DNA. During the 20th century, the development of vaccines to control diseases such as tetanus, diphtheria, polio, whooping cough, measles, hepatitis B, smallpox, and other important diseases helped to contribute to the post-modern impression that infectious diseases are no longer a threat. In fact, vaccination against smallpox was so successful that the world was declared smallpox-free by the WORLD HEALTH ORGANIZATION in 1980. It is of concern that a renewed smallpox threat, to a largely unvaccinated population, has recently been discussed in the context of biological warfare.

The investigations of Pasteur, Koch, and many others associated with the so-called golden age of microbiology (1850s to 1930s) were focused on the isolation and identification of specific micro-organisms, primarily bacteria causing disease, and the development of effective vaccines against them. More recently, the development of technologies such as the electron microscope has allowed scientists to identify even smaller micro-organisms, such as viruses, than those seen with the light microscope, and also permitted the analysis of the contents of microbial cells. Coupled with the powerful methods of molecular genetics, molecular biology, and biotechnology, more complex questions about how micro-organisms cause disease (mechanisms of pathogenicity) and new ways to identify micro-organisms, even if they cannot be grown using traditional culture methods, have been and continue to be investigated. Methods of molecular biology have also been applied to discover the very nature of the nucleic acid (DNA or RNA) sequences of bacterial and viral genomes. Thus, no genome will be secret in the future and the potential discovery of the function and interactions of every protein from a micro-organism will revolutionize diagnosis and disease prevention.

## Bacteria

Bacteria are generally single cell creatures displaying the properties of all living cells: the transfer of genetic information from one generation to the next; a cellular physiology which includes a membrane surrounding the inner contents of the cell; a capacity to find or breakdown nutrients to feed themselves; and a capacity to change by mutation and other genetic alterations. The average length of a bacterial cell is 2 μm and the diameter 0.5 μm. Based on observations under the microscope, the bacterial world consists of differently shaped cells which mostly fall into the categories of rods (bacilli), spheres (cocci), and spirals. Some disease-causing bacteria with these shapes include those causing pneumocccal pneumonia and boils (cocci); gonorrhea (diplococci); salmonella food poisoning and botulism (rods); cholera (curved rods); and syphilis and Lyme disease (spirals).

With the development of methods of electron microscopy, bacterial genetics, and molecular biology, especially during the second half of the 20th century, many of the secrets of the bacterial cell have been exposed. Bacterial cells have simple organization and lack the complexity of plant and animal cells, which contain membrane-bound compartments (organelles), such as mitochondria or chloroplasts. As with all cells, the interior of a bacterium is enclosed by a cell membrane that regulates the passage of materials in and out of the cell and, in bacteria, is associated with molecules involved in energy production. The interior of the cell contains the genetic material, a single bacterial chromosome, in a region called the nucleoid. The size of the chromosome varies in different bacterial species. Reproduction of bacterial cells requires the replication of the bacterial chromosomes so that each new cell receives one complete copy of the chromosome. Therefore, cell division, the process in which the bacterial cell divides to produce two daughter cells of equal size, in a process called binary fission is closely synchronized with chromosome replication.

***Plasmids*** Some bacteria also contain additional genetic material, called plasmids, which consist of small self-replicating circular pieces of DNA. Plasmids are usually not essential for cell survival, but may carry genes, such as those which make the bacterium resistant to various antibiotics or which code for harmful toxins. Plasmids may be transferred between micro-organisms and they have played a large part in spreading some genes throughout the bacterial world. Their properties have been exploited for genetic engineering methods which permit cloning genes such as that for insulin into modified plasmids.

The interior of bacterial cells, known as the cytoplasm, also contains enzymes and chemicals required for the cell to grow and reproduce, molecules such as ribonucleic acid (RNA), which are involved in protein synthesis, and thousands of structures, called ribosomes, where protein synthesis occurs. Bacterial ribosomes are different from the ribosomes in human cells and these differences are exploited for developing antimicrobial agents which are toxic for bacteria but not for human cells. The bacterial cytoplasm may also contain granules, called inclusion bodies, used to store various chemical nutrients.

The part of bacteria outside the cytoplasmic membrane is unique to bacteria and is called the cell wall or peptidoglycan. The latter prevents the bacteria from bursting and also establishes their shape. This structure differs chemically in different bacteria and is the basis for distinguishing two major classes called Gram-positive, or Gram-negative bacteria, based on their staining properties with two different dyes. This staining procedure was developed by a Danish physician, Hans Christian Gram in 1888 and remains important for distinguishing bacteria even today. A gram stain is still the basis of the diagnosis of infectious diseases such as gonorrhea. The cell wall is also the site of action for many antibiotics, especially penicillins. Because bacteria are the only living organisms with a peptidoglycan cell wall, antibiotics which are specific for this type of cell wall are selectively toxic for bacteria.

## Projections

Many bacteria carry structures that protrude from or are external to the cell wall. Many carry long protein projections (flagella) that extend outward from the cytoplasmic membrane to the exterior of the cell and are involved in cell motility. These structures spin like propellers, allowing bacteria to respond to chemicals in their environment by either moving closer or further away from them. Bacterial cell surfaces may also be covered with short, thin hairlike projections, largely composed of protein, called pili. Pili are sometimes concerned in the specific attachment of bacterial cells to host cells. Other bacteria may be surrounded by a thick structure, generally composed of sugar molecules, called a capsule or slime layer. The capsule is implicated in the attachment of bacteria to various surfaces. An interesting example of this are the bacteria which cause periodontal disease; they attach to the surface of the tooth by their capsules forming a dense microbial biofilm called plaque. In some cases, capsules protect bacteria against natural ingestion by cells in our bodies, called phagocytes. Finally, some bacteria can produce spores which enable them to survive in unfriendly environmental conditions, including extreme heat and dryness. Some spore-forming bacteria produce some of the most deadly toxins known, for example, tetanus and botulinum toxins.

One of the more exciting recent developments in bacteriology has been applying molecular and genetic methods to determine how bacteria cause disease, to identify the genes involved, and to investigate their regulation. Each bacterium has an array of strategies to produce disease and the challenge of medical microbiology today is to discover, for each disease-causing bacterium, what these tactics are. Thus, for each pathogen, investigators are determining the ways in which bacteria adhere to cells or tissues, penetrate, spread, and multiply in the body. The many strategies used by bacteria to interfere with or escape our bodily defenses, which include the immune system, are also a matter of intensive research. The processes by which bacteria cause damage to the host — for example, through the production of toxins (cholera, diphtheria) or through stimulation of immune responses (toxic shock syndrome) — have been especially important aspects of investigation. Information derived from these studies has led to new strategies for controlling diseases, including ways to stimulate our immune systems and vaccines. Many of the ecological factors (temperature, availability of oxygen, nutrient availability, for example) which contribute to disease are also being studied. These new aspects of research will provide information on the factors which regulate whether disease-causing genes are functional when grown in different host sites.

## Viruses

The term virus was used by the Romans to mean poison. Their presence was first appreciated in the late 1880s when investigators learned that some disease agents might pass through filters that held back the smallest bacteria. Cell-free filtrates were implicated in diseases such as yellow fever and foot and mouth disease. Unlike many bacteria, viruses require living cells in which to grow and cannot be propagated on artificial laboratory media. Methods to grow viruses in the laboratory using tissue or cell culture methods (growth of living cells in a Petri dish) were initiated during the 1920s, but these cultures tended to be heavily contaminated with bacteria and other agents. In the 1930s, Ernest Goodpasture and his colleagues determined that viruses might be grown in embryonated hen's eggs and after this discovery, several viruses could be grown in the laboratory environment and studied. With the discovery of antibiotics that inhibit bacterial and fungal growth, improved methods of cell culture were developed. The search for improved methods of culturing viruses continues. The use of cell culture to grow viruses was the breakthrough required to grow viruses in sufficient numbers to produce vaccines against them. Methods of electron microsopy to visualize viruses, coupled with molecular biology and genetics, are now used to dissect viral genomes and to study their proteins and determine how they cause disease.

Viruses are part of the microbial world but differ from bacteria in their structure and are much smaller. They are not composed of cells, but contain genetic material which is either DNA or RNA and which is surrounded by a protein coat known as a capsid. The capsid may be either helical or icosahedral (20 plane faces) and may contain a single or many different proteins. Some viruses are surrounded by membranes which are acquired as they emerge from the host cell or nucleus. Viruses cannot replicate outside their host cells. Some viruses, known as bacteriophage, infect only bacterial cells, while others infect various other animal cell types (for example, papilloma virus, which causes warts, and herpes virus replicate in epithelial cells; hepatitis A virus replicates in the liver). Viruses are considered to be molecular parasites because they use the metabolic machinery of the host cell to replicate. The basic steps of the replication cycle of viruses include attachment to the cell surface; penetration of either the entire virus or just its nucleic acid into the cell; removal of the protein coat if required (some viruses inject only their genomes into the cell interior); synthesis of proteins required for viral replication; replication of the viral nucleic acid (for which different strategies are used depending on whether the viral genome is RNA or DNA, single stranded or double stranded), synthesis of viral coat proteins; assembly of viral particles; and release from the cell.

When a virus is released from its host, it may or may not kill the host cell, depending on the mechanisms by which it is released. Viruses may produce unwanted effects in host cells including cell death and various detrimental morphological changes, as well as altering the properties of cells, such as causing them to behave like tumors (a process called transformation). Some viruses remain in cells as silent genetic material and emerge later to replicate only under conditions of stress. Viruses using these strategies include the human immunodeficiency virus (HIV) and the virus causing herpes.

## Prions

The recent outbreaks of bovine spongiform encephalitis have focused attention on some of the least understood micro-organisms, called prions. Prions are simpler in structure than viruses and are considered to be infectious proteins. Their mechanisms of reproduction and transmission are being intensively studied. Prions have been implicated in diseases which have very slow onsets and cause chronic progressive central nervous system degeneration including KURU, a degenerative neurological disease associated with cannibalistic rituals in New Guinea, and CREUTZFELDT–JAKOB disease.

## Protozoa and fungi

Protozoa and fungi have a cell structure that is more similar to human than bacterial cells (i.e. eukaryotic). Protozoa are generally single-celled micro-organisms and include several different groups, for example, amebae and trypanosomes. Their life cycles may be complex, with many morphological forms and developmental stages. Often protozoan parasites have a life cycle which includes survival in the environment and one or more hosts of different species, such as mosquitoes and humans. Protozoan or parasitic diseases cause some very serious diseases in tropical countries, malaria being among the most prevalent. Water supplies in many communities are infested with protozoan organisms and have been the source of enormous diarrheal disease epidemics including cryptosporidium, giardiasis, and amebic dysentery. Along with algae, fungi are an important group of micro-organisms and play a significant part in recycling nutrients in the environment. Fungi include yeasts (so important to the food and drink industry), molds, and mushrooms. Some fungi cause human diseases, often infections of the skin and hair (e.g. athlete's foot), and are collectively called mycoses. Sometimes fungi which do not normally infect healthy people cause opportunistic infections in persons severely weakened by diseases such as AIDS and some cancers.

## Emerging infections

The 20th century was remarkable for the discovery of the specific agents causing infectious disease and for developing methods to eliminate or control them. This has led to significant reductions in deaths from infectious disease in industrialized countries. It is easy to forget that infectious diseases remain the leading cause of deaths world-wide with significant disparity in the amount of illness and death due to them in industrialized and non-industrialized countries. In many developed countries, the perception of the last few decades has been that microbial diseases are tamed, if not eradicated. Many were unprepared for the emergence of seemingly new or newly recognized diseases such as hemorrhagic fevers caused by the Ebola and other viruses, AIDS, hemolytic uremic syndrome, and Legionnaire's disease. Nor were they prepared for the resurgence of diseases, such as tuberculosis and cholera, that were previously considered well under control and decreasing in occurrence. The panacea presented with the discovery and use of antibiotics for treating bacterial infections is now threatened because of the development of microbial resistance to the many antibimicrobials which were once effective, and by deteriorating living conditions that favor epidemic spread.

Causes for the emergence of these new or renewed microbial threats include the increased awareness or recognition of certain micro-organisms as pathogens; the detection and identification of previously unrecognized microbial pathogens; the evolution of more virulent or antibiotic-resistant micro-organisms; and the intrusion of humans into previously untouched environments. In some cases, genetic rearrangements and exchanges ('mutations') may have created a micro-organism with entirely new properties enabling it to cause disease (influenza virus, for example). However, these changes are not only brought about by the micro-organisms, but also by environmental, economic, and behavioral factors. For example, immunosuppressed people (such as those having treatment for cancer, or with AIDS) are more susceptible to various infections which might be successfully counteracted if the immune system was intact. The ever-increasing proximity between animal habitats and human settlements has made it more likely that micro-organisms normally found only in animals now cause disease in humans (PLAGUE is a well-known historical example of this; however, more modern examples might include HIV and the lethal hemorrhagic hantavirus infection). International travel ensures that all infectious diseases have the potential to be spread world-wide. Modern methods of animal husbandry and handling, which include the extensive use of antibiotics to control disease or promote growth in animals, may promote the spread of antibiotic-resistant micro-organisms in animals used for food.

All these threats can be controlled only if they are detected and understood. Basic research is required to develop knowledge of how to identify new micro-organisms and to uncover their strategies in causing disease. This information must then be applied to developing new vaccines, diagnostic agents, and antimicrobial drugs. In this way, an international and effective response to high-risk communicable disease outbreaks may be mounted. Over the past century and a half of medical microbiology, we have learned that infectious diseases will remain a continuing and ever-changing challenge. These renewed challenges remind one of the comment made by the microbiologist, Hans Zinsser in 1935: 'Infectious disease is one of the few genuine adventures left in the world'.                                            J-ARD

**MIDWIFERY** 'It is hardly too much to say that midwives must have begun nine months after there were two women and one man on earth' (*Sir Francis Champneys, Presidential address to the obstetrical society, 1895*).

As long as there have been recorded accounts of childbirth, women in countries across the world have chosen midwives to attend them. The word 'midwife' originates from the Anglo-Saxon *mid wyf*, meaning 'with woman'. In many other languages, 'midwife' has a similar meaning and it may also translate to mean 'wise woman', as in the French *sage femme*.

In the developed countries, midwifery has remained a predominantly female occupation, but in the last century it has become a regulated profession. Most births now take place in hospital and, for many women, birth has become a medicalized event. However, midwives continue to see themselves as the specialists in the normal 'life event' of childbirth, concerned with the emotional, spiritual, physical, and social well-being of women, their babies, and families. Throughout the western world there is a move towards setting up and maintaining publicly funded services where the same midwives provide continuity of care to women and their families during pregnancy, labor, and the early weeks after birth. Midwives work in the community as well as in hospitals and call on the skills of doctors only when complications arise. This trend is supported by the WORLD HEALTH ORGANIZATION: 'The midwife is the most appropriate and cost-effective type of health care provider to be assigned the care of normal pregnancy and normal birth, including risk assessment and the recognition of complications.'

By comparison, in traditional societies, each community will identify local women who are seen to have particular expertise of being with women who are giving birth. Although they may have had no formal training, usually these women are respected elders who have had children themselves. Knowledge of HERBAL REMEDIES and massage techniques may be part of the skills that have been handed down throughout the centuries. Sometimes, these women will also be called to attend the sick and dying. They may be involved in rituals around the laying out and DISPOSAL OF THE DEAD; hence the oft-quoted notion of the person who 'sees you into the world and sees you out the other end'. In western society, these women no longer exist but historically they were known as 'midwives'. Western society refers to such women in developing countries as 'traditional birth attendants', but the title given to them by their own communities will often translate to mean 'with woman' or 'wise woman'. It should be remembered that in these countries, the infant and maternal death and illness rates are appallingly high as a result of all aspects of poverty. The World Health Organization sees midwifery education and development as a proved strategy to improve this.

Some of the earliest references to midwives may be found in the art and papyri of ancient Egypt. In

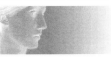
**CHAMBERLEN**. The Chamberlen family made up a dynasty of obstetricians founded by a French protestant emigré William Chamberlen who settled in Southampton, England, in 1569. His son Peter Chamberlen the Elder (d. 1631) trained in Paris and was probably the first to use the short obstetrical forceps zealously guarded as a family secret for over a hundred years. He moved to London in 1596, and became a barber-surgeon and accoucheur to the queens of James I and Charles I. He was prosecuted by the Royal College of Physicians of London for prescribing, escaping imprisonment only through the intercession of the Archbishop of Canterbury with the president.

Peter the Elder's brother, Peter Chamberlen the Younger (1572–1626), was a barber-surgeon and licensed by the Bishop of London to practice midwifery.

Peter the Younger's son, also Peter Chamberlen (1601–83), trained at Cambridge and Padua. He lectured on anatomy to the barber-surgeons and became physician to the King. Arguments with the Royal College of Physicians over the incorporation of midwives under his presidency led to his being deprived of his fellowship in 1649.

Peter's eldest son, Hugh Chamberlen the Elder (?1632–?), trained under Mauriceau in Paris and translated his textbook. He was appointed physician to the King in 1673 and elected a fellow of the Royal Society in 1681. It is thought that he sold the family secret to the Dutch obstetrician, Hendrik van Roonhuysen, in 1692. *(continued overleaf)*

(continued)

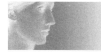

**CHAMBERLEN**. Hugh's brother, Paul Chamberlen (1635–1717), practiced as a midwife, but was better known for his anodyne necklace.

Hugh Chamberlen the Younger (1664–1728), son of Hugh Chamberlen the Elder, studied at Leiden, graduated from Cambridge in 1689, and practiced with success as an obstetrician in London.

A man-midwife. The instruments and bottles behind the man-midwife contained potions which, it is alleged, he used to stimulate carnal desire in his patients. (From Fores, S. W. (1793). *Man-midwifery dissected*, London. Reproduced courtesy of the Wellcome Institute Library, London.)

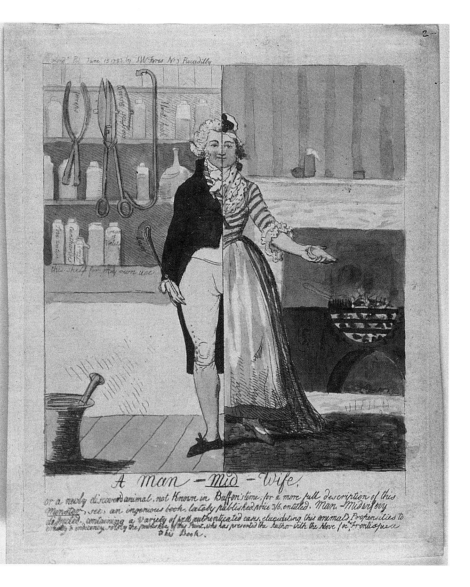

the EBERS PAPYRUS we learn that in ancient Egypt, midwifery was a female occupation. Midwives attended normal childbirth, including royal births. Similar references to midwives as the skilled practitioners of childbirth can be found in other ancient texts such as the *Old Testament*, the *Talmud*, and the *Tao Te Ching*.

Records from ancient Greece and Rome show that midwives were an honored class. In these civilizations, midwives were divided into two categories: those who assisted at normal births, and those of superior skill, who were consulted in the case of difficult labors. This role division within midwifery was to continue in European countries until doctors established themselves as the specialists in the complications of childbirth.

Little is written about midwives in Europe after the fall of the Roman Empire until the medieval period, by which time Christian religion had assumed authority and opposed both formal medicine and secular education in its drive to eradicate paganism. The church set up systems of jurisdiction in a wide range of human affairs, including the licensing and regulation of midwifery. Midwives were among the thousands who were persecuted and executed in the 'witch hunts' that swept across Europe in the 14th and 15th century. Towards the end of this period, European cities began to implement structures for the regulation of midwifery and gradually, over the centuries, the Church relinquished its role to municipal and state authorities.

From the 16th century until the middle of the 19th century, most midwives remained uneducated and, as women, they were denied access to the increasing body of medical knowledge that was developed in universities. An exception was to be found at the Hôtel Dieu in Paris, a charitable monastic institution, founded in the 16th century in order to provide free birthing services to the poor as well as instruction for midwives. By the 18th century this school was renowned throughout Europe. One of the Hôtel Dieu's earliest scholars was Louise Bourgeois, who educated midwives and became famous as the official royal midwife and writer of three midwifery books. Louise Bourgeois first attended the queen, Marie de Medici, in 1601 at Fontainbleau. Two hundred people were present at the long and difficult birth of this, the queen's first baby.

Louise Bourgeois was married to a surgeon. Other educated women, interested in the prospect of earning an honorable livelihood, were able to gain access to medical knowledge through their contacts with surgeons. Women such as Hester Shaw, a prominent London midwife in the 17th century, were thus able to develop their midwifery skills and earn a considerable income by attending wealthy women. Increasingly, though, their role was being taken over by male physicians. Known originally as the 'man midwife', the male birth attendant would eventually assume the title 'obstetrician', meaning 'to stand before'. The beginning of the fashion to employ a man-midwife is attributed to Louis XIV of France, who employed a court physician, Boucher, to attend his favorite mistress, Louise de la Vallière, in 1663 and, again, Jules Clement to attend the Dauphine when she gave birth in 1682. However, it was a female midwife,

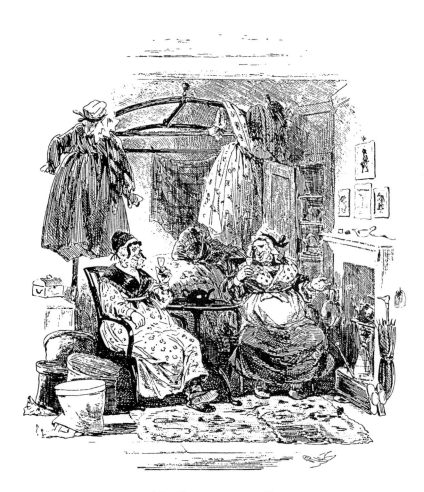

*Mrs. Gamp proposes a Toast*

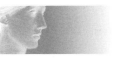

### DICKENS'S MIDWIFE

Sairey **GAMP**. Mrs Gamp, a character in Dickens's novel *Martin Chuzzlewit* (1843–4) was a disreputable, grasping, and alcoholic nurse of wide professional range, equally at home at 'lying-in or laying-out'. She would adjure her employers to 'leave the bottle on the chimley-piece, and don't ask me to take none, but let me put my lips to it when I am so dispoged' (Ch. 19). To 19th c. readers, Sarah Gamp, together with her friend and colleague Betsey Prig, provided a popular and not inaccurate caricature of the nursing profession. Her name also became synonymous with the large cotton umbrella she invariably carried.

Her character formed in Dickens's mind during walks in the 'deep lanes' of Finchley, where he had taken a cottage in the early summer of 1843 (after serialization of the novel had already begun). It was acknowledged that she was drawn from life. Dickens's own later comment was:

Mrs. Sarah Gramp was, four-and-twenty years ago, a fair representation of the hired attendant on the poor in sickness. The Hospitals of London were, in many respects, noble Institutions; in others, very defective. I think it not least among the instances of their mismanagement, that Mrs. Betsey Prig was a fair specimen of a Hospital Nurse; and that the Hospitals, with their means and funds, should have left it to private humanity and enterprise to enter on an attempt to improve that class of person— since, greatly improved through the agency of good women.

Sairey Gamp, the notorious midwife from Charles Dickens's *Martin Chuzzlewit*.

Sir Robert
**MANNINGHAM**
(1690–1759). British man-
midwife. The son of a bishop
and first destined for the law,
Manningham changed to
medicine and became the
leading man-midwife in
London. In 1739 he
established the first wards for
parturient women in Britain in
the parochial infirmary of
St James, Westminster. He was
ordered by the King in 1726
to investigate the case of Mary
Toft of Godalming, who
claimed to have given birth to
several rabbits.

**EARLY PRACTITIONER**

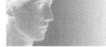

**TROTULA** (11th century).
Italian physician. The existence
of Trotula is uncertain. Some
authorities held that she was a
teacher at Salerno and wife of
Johannes Platerius, others that
'Trotula' was nickname for all
Saliternan midwives. Extensive
writings, especially on
gynecology and midwifery, are
attributed to her.

Madam de Coudray, who was appointed as 'the Official French Midwife' by Louis XV with a brief to lower the infant and maternal mortality rates of 18th century France. Madam de Coudray proceeded to teach the art and science of midwifery to 10 000 students in over forty cities.

The lucrative nature of attending the wealthy in childbirth attracted an increasing number of men into midwifery throughout 17th and 18th century Europe. The fashionable status symbol of employing men-midwives was boosted significantly by the invention of the obstetric forceps and the gradual establishment of birth as a medical science. Men-midwives promoted the use of forceps to shorten labor and save lives. Since instruments could be used only by surgeons, and only men could be surgeons, such practices presented a severe threat to women who were employed as midwives. Educated midwives decried the use of forceps by medical men. Jane Sharp, who lived in the 17th century and was the first English midwife to write a midwifery text-book, quoted the Scriptures in defending mid-wifery as a female occupation, 'there being not so much as one word concerning men midwives mentioned there that we can find'.

### Women activists

Elizabeth Cellier was an English political mid-wifery activist, whose claim to fame includes a spell in the stocks. In 1688, she tried (unsuccess-fully) to persuade doctors to join her in a pro-posal to set up charity hospitals that would incorporate a midwives college, similar to the Hôtel Dieu.

A century later, Elizabeth Nihell, a midwife who had trained at the Hôtel Dieu and who prac-ticed in the Haymarket, London, with her surgeon-apothecary husband, described men-midwives as 'a band of mercenaries who palm themselves off upon pregnant women under cover of their crochets, knives, scissors, spoons, fillets, speculum matrices, all of which and espe-cially their forceps …are totally useless'. Elizabeth Nihell's vehement protestations about men-mid-wives included venemous personal attacks on William Smellie, the greatest 18th century practi-tioner and teacher of midwifery. She alluded to his large hands as, 'the delicate fist of a great horse-godmother of a he-midwife'. There were also some doctors who expressed the view that the need for men-midwives was being exagger-ated, as were the complaints about incompetent and dangerous female midwives.

Other early midwives, who have a place in history became of their attentive recording of their work, include Justine Siegemundin, who was midwife to the Court of Prussia in the 17th century, and whose name is still used to describe a standard method of managing an arm presenta-tion; Catherine Schrader, who was called to com-plicated births in Holland in the early 18th century; Sarah Stone, who practiced in the West Country in Britain in the 18th century; and Martha Moore Ballard, who kept a diary record-ing the 996 women she attended in America between 1778 and 1812.

Unfortunately, perhaps the most famous mid-wife of all is to be found in Charles Dickens's fictional caricature of the drunken, slovenly Sairey GAMP — whose name would be used to describe and discredit local, working class midwives in Britain around the turn of the 19th century (p 495). A successful campaign to eradicate the practice of the untrained midwife and to develop a regulated midwifery profession was spearheaded by socially influential, aristocratic, and middle class women. Midwifery offered the possibility of responsible work with practitioner status, in a discipline where there was no competition from men, since all com-plicated cases would be handed over to doctors. Campaigners such as Alice Gregory, daughter of the Dean of St Paul's, and Rosalind Paget, saw them-selves as saviors of the poor and asserted that pro-fessional midwifery would reduce the rate of infant and maternal deaths. Eventually, in 1902, the First Midwives Act saw the start of legislation that would formulate restrictive practice requirements, a pow-erful supervisory apparatus, and a plenary system designed to make it impossible for uneducated, working class midwives to continue to practice. As in other European countries, legislation would also ensure that the regulation of midwifery practice and education would support the development of a respected profession.

### Defining its role

Throughout the world in the 20th century, mid-wifery had to continue to define its role in rela-tion to the medical profession, but it also had to be clear about where it sat in relation to another emerging professional group. The profession of nursing arose as a necessary workforce when medicine established its dominance within hospi-tal structures. As normal childbirth moved into hospitals under the domain of obstetricians, mid-wifery began to be seen as a specialization of nursing in Britain and in previous British juris-dictions. In many countries the role of the midwife as a practitioner in her own right became eroded into that of an 'obstetric nurse', subordi-nate to the obstetrician. Today, there is an effort to address this. In particular, in Britain, New Zealand, and Canada, midwifery courses are now predominantly for people who do not have a nursing qualification and who undertake a minimum of three years' education in order to become a practitioner of midwifery.

In the Netherlands, midwifery has never been seen as a specialization of nursing. Midwifery has benefited from government-funded education and regulation since the mid-18th century. Competition between obstetricians and midwives has rarely been an issue, since self-employed midwives are the only practitioners funded by the state to provide total care for all women undergoing normal childbirth. General practitioners can claim government funding for maternity services only if there are no practicing midwives in their geographical area. Thus the role of the midwife as the practitioner of normal childbirth is protected by the state. Where complications are identified, the midwife hands over care to the obstetrician. State funding for obstetricians is limited to covering only those women who are referred by the midwives as having complications. The obstetrician depends on the midwife for referrals, and this competition encourages what Dutch midwives refer to as a 'woman friendly' approach from obstetricians. Midwives can attend women who choose to give birth in hospital but roughly one third of all births occur safely at home, with the midwife as the sole practitioner.

In most other western countries, midwives are developing a role where, unlike in Holland, they continue to be involved in the care of the women whom they refer to obstetricians, thus enabling continuity of midwifery care. Collaboration between midwives and obstetricians and respect for their separate but complementary roles is seen as being in the best interests of childbearing women. Within this context, midwifery care is increasingly occurring in the community, with referral to doctors only when the midwife identifies a need. Women are asking to be cared for in labor by the same midwives who provided their antenatal care; thus many midwives now work in both the community and hospital setting. Midwifery is developing its own academic base within universities. An evidence-based approach to organization and practice has seen an ever-growing number of midwives involved in relevant research.

Although in western societies most women still choose to give birth in hospital, home birth with midwives is increasingly being shown by research to be a safe option for women considered to be at low risk. This depends on supportive hospital services near at hand — in particular, an efficient ambulance service staffed by paramedics for the rare occasions when transfer from home is needed in an emergency. In Britain, where the home birth rate fell from about 50% to 1% in the last 50 years, since government reports acknowledged the safety of home birth for most women, there is a steadily increasing demand for this service. In some areas, between 4–15% of births now occur at home, with community midwives employed by the National Health Service in attendance. In New Zealand and Ontario, Canada, where in recent years government legislation has endorsed public health service funding for self-employed midwives, home birth is also increasing, with excellent documented outcomes and high levels of maternal satisfaction.

For women who give birth in hospital in western society, the trend is towards the mother and baby returning home within hours or a couple of days if there are no complications. Midwives then visit women at home to make sure that all is well for both the new mother and the baby and to give support and advice, particularly about breastfeeding.

To provide continuity of care that is centered on the individual needs of women, midwives are increasingly working in small teams or group practices. For both self-employed midwives and those employed within public health services there is a trend towards 'caseload practice', where individual midwives are paid to take responsibility for coordinating the total care of a defined number of named women. They work when the needs of the women dictate and are therefore not responsible for staffing the hospital wards, a task which is carried out by a core staff of midwives who choose to work shifts. These midwives are experts at providing care for women who need to be in hospital because of complications. It is generally recognized that with increased responsibility and autonomy for midwives comes the need to develop structures that address accountability and support as well as regulation that ensures appropriate standards of midwifery education and practice.

The midwifery profession has moved into the 21st century with a mandate from women to work with them during their experience of childbirth. This mandate is based on the understanding that childbirth is more than the physiological process of growing a baby, giving birth, and nurturing a new infant. It is a complex life event, one that for many women is a rite of passage involving significant ritual and personal development. Women throughout the world are turning to midwives, whom they see as the practitioners who are most able to respond to their individual needs, even when there are complications, in a way that addresses the physical, emotional, social, and spiritual aspects of childbirth. In the words of Caroline Flint, a well-known, contemporary British midwife:

'To be a midwife is to be "with woman" (the meaning of the Anglo-Saxon word) — sharing their travail, their joys and their delights. To be a midwife is to engage in a close and intimate relationship which often lasts only as long as the pregnancy, birth and puerperium, but the effect

**MINERAL SPRINGS** supply natural water containing appreciable concentrations of salts and gases dissolved from the rocks and soil through which it has flowed. The discovery of such springs and their supposed medicinal qualities dates from earliest history; HIPPOCRATES (p 382) in 400 BC described contemporary watering places in his work *Airs, waters, and places*, and Pliny in 77 AD wrote about the mineral springs of Europe. Many of the springs discovered by the Romans are still well known, for example, those at Aachen (Aix-la-Chapelle) and Baden-Baden in West Germany, at Spa in Belgium, and at Bath in Britain. Others whose waters have achieved world renown include Harrogate, Vichy, Dax, Selzer, Bad Pyrmont, Ems, Wiesbaden, Baden (Switzerland), and Carlsbad (Czech Republic).

In the USA, mineral springs have not been exploited to the same extent. Of about 8800 which exist, only some 400 have been used commercially. A few are well known, for example, Saratoga Springs, New York, and White Sulfur Springs, West Virginia.

of which travels down through the centuries in the image women have of themselves and their abilities and worth…Midwives and women are intertwined, whatever affects women affects midwives and vice versa — we are interrelated and interwoven.'                                          NL

*See also* LYING-IN HOSPITALS; NURSING – AS A PROFESSION

**MIGRAINE** See NEUROLOGY

**MINIMALLY INVASIVE SURGERY** A new and general concept of 'minimal invasiveness' in surgery was first proposed by Wickham in 1986 because of the radical changes in the treatment of kidney stones between 1979 and 1983. During this time the serious and traumatic operation of surgical removal of stones was at first replaced by their telescopic extraction through tiny 1 cm tracks made from the body surface into the kidney, and later by the advent of extracorporeal shockwave lithotripsy. With this latter method stones within the kidney were fragmented by the application of a focused shockwave from outside the body. This shockwave was passed from the generator, either electrical or acoustic, though the soft tissues of the body to impinge on the target stone and to fragment it. Particles of stone then passed through the natural urinary passages to the exterior. With the latest machines of this type, called lithotripters, no anesthetic is needed; the patient's body is not invaded; and the whole procedure has become a walk in/walk out event like going to the dentist. Nevertheless, it is fully effective in treating the patient's stone disease.

Thus a dramatic change occurred in the treatment of kidney stones. Major trauma had been avoided but the same therapeutic effect had been produced. The results of treatment by open surgery, telescopic surgery, or lithotripsy were compared in 1986, showing an enormous diminution in mortality and complications if these new procedures were used. Patients were suffering from the same conditions but the reduction in trauma was achieved because open access surgery had been replaced by 'minimal access' procedures or 'keyhole surgery' dependent upon the introduction of far more advanced instruments.

Meanwhile, similar changes were taking place in other specialties. For example, gynecologists were beginning to control bleeding from the uterus by coagulation of its lining rather than by removing the whole uterus. Orthopedic surgeons were using a telescopic technique to remove knee cartilages without the need for open operation. Medical gastroenterologists were removing gallstones from the bile ducts with flexible telescopes and retrieval baskets passed through the stomach and duodenum into the bile duct.

By 1986 it seemed possible to predict the way in which interventional therapy was destined to develop in the next decade and at the beginning of a new century many common interventional procedures have already been converted into 'minimally invasive' techniques because the resultant reduction in morbidity has become so obvious.

Although a simple telescope had first been used to inspect the abdominal contents in 1901, it was Palmer (in France) and Semm (in Germany) in the 1960s and 1970s who initiated the use of ancillary instruments passed through small secondary tubes inserted through the abdominal wall to carry out operative procedures on the female reproductive organs. Why this technique was not seized on by general surgeons at this time is a mystery. So far as the upper abdomen was concerned, it was left to the medical gastroenterologists and radiologists in the 1970s to remove gallstones from the bile duct telescopically through the normal gastrointestinal passages. This was followed by direct puncture of the gall bladder with endoscopic stone removal in 1986. Only in 1987, when the removal of the whole gall bladder was carried out by Mauret in France, was the full potential of this technique appreciated. The method was rapidly taken up by general surgeons and the term 'keyhole surgery' coined, although this was only one operation out of many that had been developing in other specialties over the preceding 10–15 years. The surgeon now had no need to grope inside the abdomen with his hands, but could observe and carry out his operation remotely and less traumatically by watching a television monitor.

Telescopic removal of the gall bladder is a simple operation and is a further example of the much greater general concept of minimal invasiveness now permeating all aspects of interventional therapy. Although a considerable part of minimally invasive treatment may be classified as keyhole surgery — using a telescope passed into the abdominal cavity — many more complex operative techniques have been pioneered in other specialties with the same aim of reducing open surgical trauma. The very delicate operations carried out in the middle ear by ear, nose, and throat surgeons using operating microscopes are an example, as is the endoscopic removal of the prostate, which dates back as far as 1927.

## Future development

In intestinal surgery for tumors the surgeon can now remove the whole of the esophagus by endoscope. Segments of stomach and bowel may be removed telescopically and joined up again entirely within the abdominal cavity. Rectal tumors may be removed telescopically through the anus, thus in many cases averting the need for colostomy or other types of bowel diversion. Diseases of the biliary tract are almost completely accessible to the endoscopist or interventional radiologist.

In the chest, the lungs, or portions of them, may be removed telescopically, and various forms of heart surgery can be carried out through catheters introduced into peripheral vessels by the radiologist. Through these catheters balloon dilatation or laser disobliteration of the coronary arteries can be performed without the gross invasion of the chest cavity as is now required for bypass surgery, which is rapidly being replaced by radiology and endoscopic techniques. A blockage in a peripheral artery of the body is now being treated by the introduction of dilating balloons followed by the insertion of hollow metallic splints to maintain the newly dilated artery in an open position to allow blood flow to resume. Hence the need for open surgical intervention on these vessels, including even the abdominal aorta, will gradually be phased out.

In gynecology, removal of the lining of the uterus by diathermy or laser coagulation is rapidly removing the need for hysterectomy, which even if required, may be carried out telescopically through the abdominal cavity and the mobilized organ removed by way of the vagina.

In orthopedics, telescopic examination of the knee and removal of a damaged cartilage are common, but similar techniques are being extended to other joints in the body. Quite probably the extensive open operations for the replacement of the hip joint will gradually be replaced by the endoscopic refashioning and relining of joint surfaces with artificial materials or even cartilage grafts.

Ear, nose, and throat, and eye doctors are increasingly using the operating microscope and telescope for their work. Open traumatic procedures for removing the larynx and large portions of the face for treatment of cancer are rapidly being superseded by internal endoscopic examination and laser dissection or coagulation and a new specialty called 'base of skull surgery' is in evolution. Neurosurgeons may now remove prolapsed intervertebral discs using mini telescopes and micro techniques on a day case basis under local anesthesia and, ultimately, very accurate intracranial brain surgery will be increasingly managed by the endoscope and robot. This catalog of changes is almost endless and serves to highlight the general concept of minimal invasiveness coupled with instrumental technical advances.

## Secondary effects of techniques

The rapidity of recovery and passage of patients through the treatment sequence is soon going to render the large, hotel type of hospital obsolete. As much as 70 or 80% of this form of intervention can be carried out on a day case basis in smaller, stand alone units with good transport access. The emphasis on inpatient nursing care will be less in the ward but more demanding in the interventional suite, and will become more community based, day case surgery becoming the norm, with patients being visited postoperatively in their homes. Patients will benefit further as they will be able to decide more easily the timing of their treatment and, with a very short convalescence period, will be able to return to normal activity much more rapidly, with obvious economic benefit.

The type of doctor will also change. Patients may find that their treatment is carried out by a radiologist or even a technician rather than by the conventional open operative surgeon. Surgeons will need to be trained and retrained as primary microendoscopists or bioengineers rather than as anatomical carpenters as at present.

The specialty boundaries may become obscured. For example, skilled endoscopists may be able to remove a knee cartilage or a kidney stone as competently as they remove a rectal tumor or a uterus. A new breed of organ-related diagnostic physician may emerge, while the active interconventional treatment may be carried out by a non-organ-oriented endoscopist. Pre- and postoperative care will be supervised by anesthetists and intensive care physicians and not by surgeons.

Healthcare funding will need to undergo an appreciable shift from the support of hospital hotel services to the purchase and maintenance of high technology equipment, such as lasers, robots, videos, and camera systems, coupled with complicated X-ray and scanning machines. The health economists will need to become accustomed to this necessary relocation of equity from one discipline to another, and also to promote the introduction of new technologies more rapidly into the system.

### Conclusion

A revolution in interventional medical treatment has occurred in the past decade fueled by the desire of the doctor to obtain a satisfactory cure if possible without a mutilating operation, and actively aided by the spectacular developments in instrumental technology. Undoubtedly what makes patients ill during an open operative intervention is the damage caused by the surgeon in achieving his target object. By reducing this surgical trauma, morbidity and mortality are vastly reduced. Many procedures are now carried out through small apertures by telescope and may be categorized as 'keyhole surgery'. Nevertheless, this title should not be allowed to trivialize and obscure the vast change in attitudes to interventional therapy that may be as significant as the introduction of the first general anesthetic in 1846.

It used to be said that a surgeon should have 'the eye of an eagle, the hand of a woman, and the heart of a lion'. Perhaps a better description at the millennium should be that the eye of the eagle has been replaced by a magnified telescopic image, the hand of the woman by an increasing instrumental delicacy, and the heart of a lion by a rather more judicious use of the human cerebrum.　　JEAW

*See also* ARTHROSCOPY; ENT; NEPHROLOGY; ORTHOPEDICS; SPECIALIZATION; SURGERY

**MISNOMERS — EPONYMOUS** Eponymy is generally considered to mean affixing the name of the scientist to all or part of what he has found; however, in practice, as Stephen Stigler writes, 'No scientific discovery is named after its original discoverer'. Indeed, Mark Ravitch adds that they are often named after people who have misunderstood the eponymous lesion or have even been misquoted. An extreme case is the statement that 'every scientific discovery is named after the last individual too ungenerous to give credit to his predecessor'.

Commonly, the eponym derives from the person who popularized something, rather than the one who first described it. This is partly because often the relevance of an entity becomes clear long after it has been documented. Also, with the vast body of medical literature, it may be difficult to discover a previously undescribed or a

## MISADVENTURES

**MISADVENTURES** are often due to the well-meaning application of new methods and procedures that subsequent observations and experience show to be harmful, and to events caused by contamination of blood, blood products, vaccines, etc., that evaded detection in time to avert disaster.

Striving to cure or prevent disease, doctors eagerly — and sometimes uncritically — embrace innovations for which success has been claimed, commonly by eminent professional leaders whose opinions are unsupported by scientific evidence. This has led to the choice of some strange weapons in the quest for better health. Misguided theories and unproved hypotheses may be blamed for much needless suffering. These account for a considerable share of the disease, disability, and premature death attributable to the actions of the medical profession.

Such misguided ideas go back centuries: one only has to think of the emphasis on blood letting, enemas, and purgation to realize that the richer the person the more they were at risk from enthusiastic doctors, whose fees bore no relation to their successes. In modern times a variety of treatments have been introduced and then withdrawn. Thus hemicolectomy for

'autointoxication'; lobotomy for assorted mental and emotional disorders; irradiation of the thymus to prevent the mythical condition of status thymolymphaticus; prevention of threatened miscarriage by using diethylstilbestrol that caused cancer of the vagina in daughters born to these women — all are examples of 20th century medical mistakes that we look back on now with a mixture of horror, sorrow, and anger. Other tragedies were unavoidable because of the limitations of medical science at the time they occurred; because vaccines and human blood products, for example, were contaminated with previously unknown or undetected lethal pathogens (such as HIV); or because of failure to consider the possibility of delayed adverse effects of diagnostic or therapeutic methods and procedures. Some well-known examples appear in the Table.

Many similar episodes could be listed, some that amount to disasters, some of them true accidents, others aggravated by blind obstinacy or stupidity on the part of the attending doctors. Much ink has been spilt describing and lamenting these events, and in increasingly litigious times much money changes hands among doctors,

malpractice insurers, lawyers, and occasionally even the unfortunate victims of these medical misadventures and mistakes.

There are signs of improvement. The rise of EVIDENCE-BASED MEDICINE, insisting on demonstration of efficacy and safety of new drugs, together with close scrutiny of doctors' and other health professional workers' actions by routine peer review and medical AUDIT, all help to reduce risks of harm to patients.

But there are countervailing forces, too. One is the complexity of modern medical practice, where as many as a hundred or more specialists and technicians may be directly involved in providing care for a patient with a serious, life-threatening illness. This leads to many problems of communication, may delay transmission of early warning signals to the responsible attending physician, and may blur the boundaries to such an extent that no one is unmistakably in charge. Some drug companies have knowingly put the interests of their stockholders ahead of the interests of patients, who have taken drugs after evidence of harmful adverse effects has been deliberately withheld or suppressed. Some diagnostic and therapeutic procedures which are beneficial at the time have delayed adverse effects that may

*(continued opposite)*

*(continued)*

**Some 20th-century medical misadventures**

| Agent | Year(s) | Consequences |
| --- | --- | --- |
| **Contaminated vaccines, blood products, etc.** | | |
| BCG vaccine | 1930 | 207 of 251 newborn babies developed tuberculosis in Lübeck, Germany; 72 died |
| Yellow fever vaccine | 1942 | 28 000 cases of hepatitis among US servicemen, 62 deaths |
| Polio vaccine | 1955 | 125 cases of paralytic POLIOMYELITIS |
| Human growth hormone | 1980 | CREUTZFELDT-JAKOB DISEASE, several hundred cases world-wide |
| Blood transfusion | c.1980–86 | HIV/AIDS, Hepatitis C, many thousands in France, Canada, USA, Japan, etc. |
| **Adverse drug reactions** | | |
| Mercurial teething powder | 1890–1951 | 'PINK DISEASE' (chronic mercury poisoning) affected many thousands of infants, some fatally |
| Chloramphenicol | 1946–c. 1960 | Aplastic anemia; 200 cases in 1952 in USA, many thousands world-wide, especially in developing countries |
| Thalidomide | 1956–61 | 9000–10 000 reduction deformities of limbs, over 8000 in W. Germany |
| Phenothiazines | 1953–c. 1975 | Tardive dyskinesia—that is, disfiguring body tics; many thousands of cases |
| Estrogens | c. 1946–71 | Vaginal cancer, genital tract dysplasia among daughters exposed *in utero*; estimated 10 000 affected in USA |
| Oral contraceptives | 1958–present | Thromboembolic disorders, estimated 500 deaths/year in USA |
| Supplementary oxygen | 1930–50 | Retrolental fibroplasia (blindness) in immature and low birthweight infants |
| **Diagnostic procedures** | | |
| X-rays | c. 1920–75 | Cancer, leukemia; even low-dose diagnostic X-rays can cause cancer after exposure of early developing fetus |

not declare themselves for many years, perhaps not until the next generation. One example is the exposure of an early developing fetus to very small diagnostic doses of X-rays, which can cause harm to adult offspring a generation later.

**Record linkage**
One essential requirement to detect harm as soon as possible and so minimize the risks, is an efficient health information system with comprehensive record linkage so that facts about present health, occurrence of cancer, cause of death may be unequivocally linked to past encounters with healthcare systems, past use of drugs, exposure to diagnostic doses of X-rays. This is feasible in nations and societies that have comprehensive publicly supported health services. But guardians of privacy and advocates for restricting access to past medical records (or, worse, deliberate destruction of these records) impede the efficacy of these safeguards. Public education and advocacy by members of the health professions, especially by eminent physicians, is the best way to tackle this problem. In the same way, improved approaches to the education of doctors and members of other health professions can sensitize all who care for patients to the hazards of medical care. Problem-based learning, the concept of lifelong medical education, and emphasis on a critical, skeptical attitude towards all forms of diagnostic and therapeutic regimens and procedures may go a long way towards minimizing the kind of medical mistakes — perhaps better described as disasters — that are listed in the Table.　　　JML

*See also* ADVERSE DRUG EFFECTS; BLOOD TRANSFUSION; ERRORS; THALIDOMIDE

new entity. For instance, although the Valsalva maneuver (1704) had been described earlier by Ambroise PARÉ (1634) (p 320) and even earlier by Leonard of Bertapagglia (1497), it was Antonio VALSALVA (p 252) who popularized it and put it to use in practical situations.

Another such example is that of the eponym that undoubtedly has caused more heartache and outpouring in the medical literature — Crohn's disease. It is currently accepted that Leon Ginzburg and Gordon Oppenheimer were conducting an investigation into the nature of non-specific granulomatous disease involving the ileum, under the guidance of the surgeon, A. A. Berg. When Burrill Crohn came across two such patients, he collected Ginzburg's material, added his own cases, and planned to present it at a conference, as the sole author. It was then suggested by Berg that Ginzburg and Oppenheimer be (in alphabetical order) co-authors on the paper. Berg himself declined to be a co-author because he did not wish to append his name to a paper that he had himself not written — else it may well have been called Berg's disease today. However, although Crohn put this disease on the map, it is now known that Thomas Kennedy Dalziel gave the first complete description of the lesion as early as 1913. With national pride playing an important part in the development of eponyms, the Scottish still like to call the disease Dalziel's disease.

Some have received eponymous immortality through sheer error. The Plummer–Vinson syndrome, consisting of dysphagia (difficulty with swallowing), upper esophageal web, glossitis (inflammation of the tongue), and anemia was actually described by Adam Brown Kelly and Donald Paterson in 1919. What Vinson described in 1922 were patients with dysphagia and anemia, but no glossitis, while together they wrote a paper on lower esophageal spasm. Plummer, remarkably, did not ever publish a paper on the subject. This inaccuracy stemmed from an article by Sir Arthur Hurst in 1925. Similarly, the ampulla formed at the junction of the common bile duct and the duct of Wirsung, termed the ampulla of Vater, was actually described by Giovanni Santorini. The anatomic lesion that Abraham Vater had described was a periampullary diverticulum. Unfortunately, this fact was misunderstood by Claude BERNARD (p 102) and in his landmark book *Mémoire sur le pancréas*, he referred to ampulla of Water (probably the printer's devil) and this led to the eponym.

Jean-Nicolas Marjolin, in 1828, referred to *ulceres cancroides* of the skin, probably referring to cancer-like ulcers. Marjolin did not associate them with trauma nor did he state that they were malignant. However, when Robert William Smith, in 1850, saw patients with cancer developing in burns ulcers on the skin, he labeled them Marjolin's ulcers because of the similarity in appearance between his cases and those of Marjolin. When John Chalmers Da Costa in 1903 and John Addison Fordyce in 1914 used the term again, the eponym stuck. Ironically, burns ulcer cancers were first described by his teacher and nemesis, Baron Dupuytren (1839). In what appears to be poetic justice, the palmar contracture termed Dupuytren's contracture was itself first described by Sir Astley Cooper.

Paradoxical misnomers also exist. Krukenberg tumors (Friedrich Krukenberg, 1896) were initially believed to be primary ovarian tumors, but were discovered by F. Schlagenhaufer in 1902 to be metastatic carcinomas. Likewise, the sign of Leser–Trelat consists of a sudden appearance of seborrheic keratoses (warts) in association with an internal malignancy. Later investigations showed that what Edmund Leser and Ulysse Trelat described in 1890 were actually senile angiomas; Hollander was the first author to make the correct association, in 1900.

Bureaucracy is an important contributory factor. Salmonellae are named after Daniel Elmer Salmon, who was Director of the Bureau of Animal Industry of the US Department of Agriculture when Theobald Smith, his subordinate, discovered the pathogenic bacteria 'salmonellae'. Smith had to settle for second place in authorship, behind his superior, thus resulting in this misnomer.

An unusual way to be an eponym is exemplified by Klinefelter's syndrome. H. F. Klinefelter states that the syndrome named after him was the result of unselfish action by Dr Fuller ALBRIGHT (p 265), who after they jointly described the syndrome, allowed Klinefelter to put his name first on the list of authors.

The ideal eponym, one that honors both the discoverer and the person who established its importance, would be lengthy and unwieldy. A case in point is J. F. Fielding's suggestion that Crohn's disease be a term to describe the narrow concept of terminal ileitis and Dalziel's syndrome be used to document the broad concept. Unfortunately, it is impossible to replace established eponyms. The tradition of creating eponyms, including misnomers, is likely to continue in the future. It may only be appropriate since medicine is, after all, an imperfect science.                     SAP

## MISSIONARIES — MEDICAL AND MISSION HOSPITALS

Western standards of social welfare and medical care embody Christian values. Christ showed compassion for the poor, the disabled, and the outcasts of society. He healed the sick, and taught his disciples to do likewise. Early Christians became the first medical missionaries. During an outbreak of bubonic PLAGUE in Alexandria in 256 AD, when most citizens fled the city, only the Christians stayed to care for the victims, and many lost their own lives. By the 4th century they had established community *nosokomita*, places for care of the sick. The modern hospital developed from medieval monastic institutions. During the Reformation, as Trevelyan said, 'the disendowment of hospitals was more injurious to the poor than the disendowment of monasteries'. When

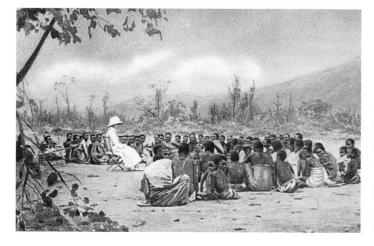

Yao tribespersons attend a 'hearers' instruction class in Christian teaching at Mangoche, Nyasaland in the early part of the 20th century. (Reproduced courtesy of the Mary Evans Picture Library.)

Christian missionaries went to the 'Third World', they found appalling medical need; by the beginning of this century most missionary societies had medical departments.

Before the 19th century western medicine had little to offer. But the advent of scientific medicine coincided with the Industrial Revolution, expanding trade, geographical exploration, and increased world awareness by the West. One of the first missionary doctors was Dr John Thomas, who accompanied the Baptist William Carey to India in 1792. The Edinburgh Medical Missionary Society, founded in 1841, was the first such medical society in Britain. The Church Missionary Society, established in 1799, let nearly a century pass before developing a medical outreach, which subsequently became very extensive.

Some individuals of true greatness devoted their lives in service abroad and became an inspiration to others. David LIVINGSTONE (this page) is remembered as an explorer of Central Africa and the Zambezi, sponsored by the Royal Geographical Society from 1856. Initially based at mission stations, his early journeys were undertaken to discover locations where further healthy bases might be established, many missionaries having died from MALARIA. He crossed Africa from coast to coast, revealed to the world the routes to its interior, and showed that, with the use of quinine, Europeans could live there. He is also remembered as a pioneer in the fight against slavery, for his epic endurance to the end, then for the story of how devoted Africans carried his embalmed body 1500 miles through unfriendly territory to the coast: his final resting place is in Westminster Abbey.

Albert SCHWEITZER (p 504) was a doctor of philosophy and of theology, a famous organist and authority on Bach, when, at the age of 30, he decided to become a medical student and devote the rest of his life to service in AFRICA. He reached Gabon in 1913, built a hospital at the remote location of Lambaréné, described in his book *On the edge of the primeval forest*, and died there in 1965, aged nearly 90. A truly Olympian character, awarded the Nobel peace prize, his personal philosophy was contained in three simple words — 'reverence for life'.

Sir Wilfred GRENFELL (p 299) was a pioneer physician to the fishing villages of Newfoundland's Labrador coast. Known as 'Grenfell of Labrador', his missionary work there attracted hundreds of Canadian, American, and British doctors, nurses, and medical students.

Mission hospitals had a significant role in medical education. Of necessity, many nursing schools were established. Dr Peter Parker founded the Ophthalmic Hospital in Canton in 1834: of him, it was said 'he opened the gates of China with a lancet, when European cannon could not

heave a single bar'. Medical schools developed in CHINA at Canton (1866), Tientsin (1881), Mukden (1884), and Soochow (1894): the first Chinese to graduate (1892) (in Hong Kong) was SUN YAT-SEN (p 178) who became the founder of the Chinese Republic. The Peking Union Medical College (1906) established very high standards. Women of India had often been denied medical attention because of *purdah*. Recognizing their plight, women missionaries founded two medical schools for training women doctors, at Ludhiana (1894) by Dame Edith Brown and at Vellore (1918) by an American doctor, Ida Scudder. The Vellore hospital became the Christian College of South India of international repute.

Most mission hospitals remained small and located in rural areas. The influence of medical missionaries is often remarkable and out of all proportion to their numerical strength. By western standards the staffing ratio of doctors is very low in relation to clinical demand. The better the hospital, the greater is the demand, patients often traveling great distances. A problem of developing countries is that, though the central government provides hospitals in the capital and main provincial towns, rural areas are poorly served. The further from the main towns, the more pressing are the medical needs, and it is here that most medical mission hospitals are sited. Many have outlying dispensaries and maternity centers or mobile clinics; roads are often poor, transport is scarce and expensive, so basic medical help needs to be reasonably close to hand.

### Pioneering role in leprosy

LEPROSY is one disease in which medical missions have played an important and often pioneering part. This was so even before specific treatment was available, and isolation in leper colonies was usual: the name of Father Damien is remembered in this context. In India the Mission of Lepers, established in 1873, became the Leprosy Mission in 1966: many pioneers in treating leprosy during that period were missionaries. In recent years Paul Brand in Vellore has been a leading figure in reconstructive surgery, physiotherapy, and rehabilitation of deformed victims of leprosy. Mother Teresa's name is associated with leprosy, and with rescue of abandoned babies and those dying in destitution on the streets of Calcutta. The Salvation Army's world-wide care for the poor and deprived is well known.

Another topic of great concern has been child welfare. The synergy of poverty, malnutrition, and endemic disease leads to very high mortality for the 'under-fives'. Experience with static and mobile child welfare clinics has shown that much of this is preventable. David Morley's book *Paediatric priorities in the developing world* has

**TWO BRITISH MISSIONARIES**

David **LIVINGSTONE** (1813–73). British physician, missionary, and explorer. From the age of 10 Livingstone supported himself by working in a cotton factory and eventually paid his way through medical school. In 1840 he traveled to South Africa for the London Missionary Society and thereafter undertook many journeys into the interior, especially in what were then called Bechuanaland and Nyasaland. Later he became obsessed with a desire to find the source of the Nile; after one journey in 1871 he had been almost given up for lost when he was found by the American journalist, J.M. Stanley.

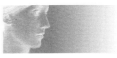

Sir Albert **COOK** (1870–1951). English surgeon. After graduating in 1895, Cook left for Uganda to serve under the Church Missionary Society, and within three months of starting work he had opened the Mengo Hospital in Kampala. His brother, Jack, later joined him, and together they enlarged the hospital and established a clinical laboratory and library. During his work he proved that hookworm infestation could cause severe anemia and, with his brother, was the first to describe sleeping sickness in East Africa. He is the founder of modern medicine in Uganda.

Albert **SCHWEITZER**
(1875–1965). German-French
philosopher, theologian, and
physician. After appointment
as principal of the theological
faculty in Strasbourg,
Schweitzer decided that his
duty lay in the medical care
of the sick poor in Africa and
trained in medicine. He
settled in Lambaréné, Gabon,
French Equatorial Africa, in
1913, built a hospital with his
own hands, and maintained
it. Interned briefly in 1914 as
a German subject, he
returned to Africa to work in
his hospital in 1925. In 1952
he was awarded the Nobel
peace prize.

been influential in governmental organization of health planning.

Where medical cover is limited, conditions requiring surgery often present at an advanced stage, for example, hernias, uterine fibroids, and thyroid tumors may be massive. Cataract is common in tropical countries; Sir Henry Holland performed 60 000 cataract operations in India. The Commonwealth Society for the Blind provides clinics in some mission hospitals. In the pioneer days it was often the dramatic successes of surgery that made western medicine, and particularly preventive measures, acceptable to other cultures.

Despite the pressure of heavy work loads, there have been outstanding contributions to research. DAVID LIVINGSTONE (p 503) described symptoms and signs of anthrax, blackwater fever, bilharzia, tropical ulcers, maggot fly boils, relapsing fever due to tick bite, eye infection by an 'insect' moving in the aqueous chamber (a filarial worm causing river blindness, onchocerciasis), and animal trypanosomiasis caused by the tsetse fly. Without realizing its profound significance, he wrote, 'myriads of mosquitoes showed, as they probably always do, the presence of malaria': he strongly advocated the use of quinine. It is worth noting that when he qualified, bacteriology did not exist, insect transmission of infective organisms was unknown, and tropical diseases were almost unexplored. Sir Patrick Manson, to many 'the father of tropical medicine', went to China in 1865, aged 21, to help an overworked missionary, studied filariasis, and discovered that a mosquito carries the causative parasite. In the early 1920s Sir Clement Chesterman was a pioneer in the use of tryparsamide for the cure of sleeping sickness in the Congo. In 1958 Denis Burkitt in Uganda described the malignant tumor which now bears his name: from an academic post he traveled 10 000 miles across Africa tracing the locations and cause of this condition. There have been many other contributions to medical literature.

The extent and nature of medical problems (and inherent personal dangers) facing missionary doctors and nursing sisters have often been daunting, particularly in the early days, when understanding of tropical diseases and their treatment was poor. By 1977 a WORLD HEALTH ORGANIZATION campaign eliminated SMALLPOX worldwide. Modern treatment has greatly reduced the incidence of conditions such as sleeping sickness and yaws. Diseases such as leprosy, bilharzia, filariasis, and amebic and bacillary dysentery can now be cured. Thus great medical advances have taken place in the 20th century, but new serious problems have arisen.

During recent years many developing societies have been devastated by the spread of AIDS and tuberculosis. The World Health Organization records that 'in 1995 about one third of the 17 million HIV infected people world-wide were also co-infected with tuberculosis. Of these, 70% live in sub-Saharan Africa, 20% in Asia, and 8% in Latin America and the Caribbean'. By 1997 30.6 million were infected with HIV/AIDS. The Global Report on the HIV/AIDS epidemic by the United Nations shows that in 1997, 5.8 million people were newly infected, that 90% were in developing countries, and two thirds of the total world number were in sub-Saharan Africa; over 50% were in 15–24 year olds. Affecting young workers, these diseases imperil national economic productivity. Most do not know that they are infected by HIV and treatment is very expensive. Uganda is one of the first African countries to make a concerted effort to prevent the spread of the virus, and the proportion of infected adults has now dropped. Unsterile needles, infected blood transfusions, and drug-resistant malaria are problems which may affect visitors or expatriate aid workers.

Political instability in some African countries has worsened their fragile medical cover. For example, during insurrections in Sierra Leone all rural hospitals, governmental or missionary, were partly or completely destroyed, the staff sometimes massacred. The hospital where I had worked was maintained with great difficulty: treatment concentrated on malnutrition, TUBERCULOSIS, and war wounds; community health teams worked in refugee camps. The hospital was attacked on Christmas Day 1992, a senior nurse killed. In February 1998 retreating rebel Guinean troops looted the hospital and beat the nursing staff; despite these trials its work continues. A Catholic hospital 35 miles away came under threat: as they tried to flee to safety, the car of a doctor and his family was machine gunned and all were killed. Civilian government was restored to the country by Nigerian forces in April 1998. Angola, Burundi, Congo (Zaire), Liberia, Rwanda, Mozambique, Somalia, and Sudan have all suffered from civil wars. In Africa much death and brutality comes from the man-made 'Kalashnikov epidemic'. Those who sow discord and supply arms usher in new dark ages. It is hoped that the new century will see resolution of tribal and other conflicts and growth of political unity within the new nations.

### Drought and civil war

Medical needs of developing countries have always been great, but of recent years the tragic exacerbation by the twin horrors of drought and civil war has led to catastrophic levels of malnutrition and suffering. This can be met only through massive international assistance by the Red Cross,

UNICEF, American government, anti-famine agencies such as Oxfam, the French and German equivalents, and emergency organizations such as Médecins sans Frontières. Among mission hospitals there is greater coordination of resources, such as the bulk purchase of drugs by local inter-denominational Christian Health Associations, helped by organizations such as Equipment for Charity Hospitals Overseas (UK), aid in staffing by volunteer organizations, financial assistance by Christian Aid and the Government Department of International Development.

The pioneering days of medical missionaries may have passed, but their work goes on, with increased emphasis on preventive medicine. In Africa there are still 1000 mission hospitals, often short-staffed, though the need for expatriate help has lessened as skilled indigenous medical staff have become available. Teaching hospitals are now usually managed by central government. Some hospitals in Nigeria are jointly run by church and state. The Christian College at Vellore, with over 1000 beds and 350 doctors, is still supported by the Church of South India. There is a general devolution of responsibility from western missionary societies to overseas churches. But in poorer developing countries the medical needs of rural areas are still very great. Other religions also run medical services in some of the world's poorest countries and regions; for example, there are Islamic, Buddhist, and Hindu mission hospitals.

Early in the 20th century, mission hospitals were in the vanguard of recognizing, meeting, and raising awareness of medical problems in developing countries. Increased media coverage has very literally 'brought this home' to everyone: meeting those needs has become a shared responsibility. JLWil

*See also* WORLD HEALTH ORGANIZATION

**MOLECULAR BIOLOGY** The origin of the molecular biological revolution is usually attributed to the observation by Griffith in 1928 that it is possible to 'transform' a 'rough' strain of a bacterium — the pneumococcus — (which lacks a capsule and is not harmful to mice) into a 'smooth' strain (which has a capsule and kills mice) by injecting living rough organisms with dead smooth organisms into a mouse. This phenomenon is an example of what is now called genetic engineering. It is worth pointing out to those who are worried that genetic engineering is new and man-invented that bacteria have long used this 'technique'.

A group at the Rockefeller Institute for Medical Research led by Oswald Avery repeated these experiments. They showed that similar transformations would occur in the test tube and that detergent extracts of the smooth organisms were effective at producing it. They went on to demonstrate — to their own surprise and the even greater surprise of the scientific community — that the active principle in the extracts of the smooth bacteria was DNA, a material previously believed to have only a structural function. This single experiment convinced the scientific community that DNA was the material of which genes were composed and gave rise to an intense interest in the chemistry and structure of this class of nucleic acid. This led to the elucidation in 1953 of the double helix structure by Watson and Crick, based on the crystallographic studies of Rosalind Franklin and Maurice Wilkins. Because this structure carried with it the mechanism by which DNA could replicate and maintain its specific sequence, it had an enormous influence and rapidly led to the decipherment of the genetic code and the mechanism of protein synthesis. This revolution of the 1950s and '60s was concerned with the analysis of DNA and enabled scientists for the first time to determine the structure of genes. It led eventually to the rapid techniques for sequencing DNA by Gilbert and by Sanger, and opened the way to the sequencing of whole genomes. Several smaller genomes, from viruses, bacteria, yeasts, and nematodes, have already been completed and the preliminary aspects of the HUMAN GENOME PROJECT were completed in 2001.

In the 1970s a second revolution occurred allowing the manipulation of genes. It arose from the discovery of plasmids — spontaneously occurring pieces of bacterial DNA which transmit, among other things, antibiotic resistance from one organism to another; the discovery of 'restriction' enzymes, which bacteria use to destroy DNA foreign to them, cutting the DNA at specific sequences which they do not have in their own DNA; and from the discovery of the enzyme 'reverse transcriptase'. This enzyme transcribes RNA into DNA, which is the opposite direction of the usual sequence in protein synthesis and is a trick used by a family of viruses (including the virus causing AIDS). The discovery of plasmids, of restriction endonucleases, and of reverse transcriptase made it possible to manipulate genes at will. The consequences of this 'genetic engineering' have given rise to the biotechnology industry. The discovery by Mullis and his colleagues (1986) of the polymerase chain reaction, that allows genes to be amplified without having to clone them in bacteria, was a further striking advance in our ability to analyze and manipulate genes and has had a profound effect on the practice of biology and medicine.

### Large-scale production of natural products

Many potent biological molecules made by plants or animals were discovered because of their bio-

**Examples of therapeutic uses of cytokines**

| | |
|---|---|
| IFN-α | Hepatitis B antigen positive carriers |
| | Hepatitis C |
| | Hairy cell leukemia |
| IFN-β | Multiple sclerosis |
| IFN-γ | Chronic granulomatous disease |
| IL-2 | Cancer therapy — generation of LAK cells |
| TNF-α | Cancer therapy |
| | Infections with pneumocystis and toxoplasma (mice) |
| CSFs | Marrow stimulation after chemotherapy |
| | Therapeutic uses for antibodies to cytokines and for cytokine inhibitors |
| Anti-TNF-α | Rheumatoid arthritis and Crohn's disease; and for septic shock (in mice) |

There were more than 100 new biopharmaceuticals in autumn '98 undergoing clinical development.

logical activity but occur *in vivo* at such low concentrations that purification by conventional techniques was extremely difficult and production in pharmaceutical amounts impossible or extraordinarily expensive. Important groups of such molecules are hormones, cytokines, and growth factors.

Although some major protein hormones had been purified before the advent of biotechnology and one, insulin, was in common use as a drug, many others were first made in substantial amounts by biotechnology. One good example is erythropoietin, a hormone made in the kidney which enhances blood production and which has had great success as a drug for treating the anemia of chronic renal disease. Growth hormone, used for treating dwarfism in children, can also be made by genetic engineering, which is cheaper than extracting it from large numbers of human pituitary glands and also free of the danger of having been contaminated with the prions that cause CREUTZFELDT–JAKOB DISEASE that tragically occurred in the past.

Cytokines are also intercellular messengers but unlike hormones are not secreted into the general circulation but act locally. They tend to be produced in even smaller amounts, and until the advent of molecular biology most of them were unknown. A growing number of these biological compounds have been produced including (at a minimum) three interferons, originally described as anti-viral agents but having major actions on cell function; thirteen interleukins; various 'colony-stimulating factors' and other growth factors; the two species of 'tumor necrosis factor' and three members of the 'transforming growth factor β' family. Together these are responsible for many aspects of cell differentiation and activation.

The initial attempt to use cytokines for treatment was disappointing. It turned out that they were quite capable of producing severe toxic reactions. For example, one of the early discoveries from the purification of alpha interferon was that the symptoms one suffers from with virus infections are not due to the virus itself but to the high concentration of interferon produced. While it may be reassuring to patients with virus infections to know that they feel ill because their host response to the virus is vigorous, it does limit the use of larger doses of these materials for therapeutic purposes. Furthermore, at high doses the biological activities of cytokines are multiple and overlap and it is difficult to find compounds that have a single effect. Nevertheless, increasing experience has produced therapeutic uses for the cytokines and perhaps particularly for the inhibitors of their action. Interleukin 2 has found a use in tumor treatment, as has tumor necrosis factor. However, perhaps more striking is the use of antibodies to tumor necrosis factor in the treatment of septic shock in experimental animals and there is evidence of its efficacy in rheumatoid arthritis. A few examples of the pharmaceutical uses of the common cytokines are shown in the Table. Many of the more recently described factors await evaluation in treatment; this is a time-consuming step-by-step procedure.

### New ways of making antibodies

A quite separate revolution in the 1970s arose from the original work by Köhler and Milstein, which led to the development of 'monoclonal' antibodies — individual antibodies that can be produced in substantial amounts. The original techniques were 'cell biological' and the antibodies were made from mouse tumor cells after fusion with individual antibody forming cells. Although the technique enables a wide range of antibodies to be made it is restricted to antibodies that mice can make. This excludes some antibodies, which may be wanted in man, for example, antibodies to the rhesus blood groups. Moreover, the antibodies made are murine and are recognized as foreign by humans, so that their use as therapeutic agents in man is limited. Molecular biological techniques have largely overcome these problems and it is now possible to make chimeric antibodies of which the great majority is human and only small regions in the 'business end' come from the mouse. Such chimeric antibodies are proving extremely useful for treatment and are likely to become increasingly widely used in several diseases.

However, even more substantial innovations are at hand. It is now possible by genetic manipulation to introduce the genes coding for a particular human antibody into the germ line of an animal of a different species or into a plant.

Human antibody can then be harvested from the blood or the milk of the animal or from the plant for human use. Pursuing a quite different strategy, Winter and his colleagues have devised methods of making antibodies that circumvent immunization altogether, by constructing enormous phage libraries displaying random associations of amino acids within the binding regions of antibodies displayed on bacteriophage. It is possible to select with antigens those immunoglobulins that react specifically and at high affinity with the antigens involved. Having selected the binding site fragment, this can then be engineered into antibody molecules containing Fc regions with effector properties of one's choice. Eventually, these techniques for obtaining antibodies will be more powerful, quicker, and cheaper than current techniques and allow us to foresee the generation of virtually unlimited arrays of antibody molecules directed against any chosen antigenic pattern. Since antibodies can inactivate many biological molecules; and antibodies to hormone and cytokine receptors can also act as 'agonists' (drugs that produce the same effects as biologically active molecules), the therapeutic implications of these new technologies are immense. A whole branch of the biotechnology industry devoted to the use of antibodies is developing.

## New vaccines

So far the greatest contribution made by medical intervention to human health has been the introduction of active immunization against infectious disease. Starting with SMALLPOX VACCINATION in the 18th century, many lethal diseases have been substantially eliminated, including smallpox, YELLOW FEVER, POLIOMYELITIS, DIPHTHERIA, and more recently measles and hepatitis A and B. Where these diseases persist it is because vaccination is not effectively used for social and environmental reasons. Traditionally vaccines have either been living attenuated organisms (smallpox, yellow fever, polio, and measles), inactivated organisms (polio), or (more or less) purified proteins such as the toxins of diphtheria and tetanus suitably modified, or the hepatitis B surface antigen. Many infectious diseases have not so far yielded to vaccination. These include some virus infections, the most notable perhaps being the lentivirus infection with HIV that gives rise to AIDS and many diseases due to parasites, both protozoal and metozoal, which are of enormous importance, particularly in the developing world. These include MALARIA, LEISHMANIASIS, and SCHISTOSOMIASIS. Probably new approaches to vaccination are required to produce effective vaccines and molecular biology has allowed several highly ingenious approaches.

In the first place, the attenuation of organisms to make them incapable of producing disease while still giving rise to immunity can now be approached in much more scientific ways by the deletion or modification of particular genes. It is also possible to incorporate antigenic portions of one parasite into another organism, which can then be used to introduce it into its host. There has been widespread experimentation with the vaccinia virus used for immunizing against smallpox to introduce into it antigens that can immunize against other diseases and to remove from the vaccinia those genes which cause it, in a few cases, to give rise to complications such as encephalomyelitis. While no such vaccines are in use in man, a successful engineered vaccinia vaccine incorporating portions of the rabies virus is used as infected bait to control rabies in the wild population of animals in continental Europe.

It is also possible to make, by the techniques of molecular biology, isolated proteins which can be used as immunogens to protect against disease. This has proved highly successful with hepatitis B and the widespread immunization of populations is certain to be the first successful intervention in preventing human cancer. Primary hepatoma, which is common in the Far East and in Africa, depends for its development on the liver cells having been infected with hepatitis B or hepatitis C virus. If hepatitis B or C can be eliminated from the population many hepatomas would not occur.

One problem with much of the new technology is that it is expensive and therefore will be difficult to apply to the developing world; it also requires cold storage of the vaccines for their delivery. The technique of DNA immunization can overcome these difficulties. This involves incorporating the DNA coding for immunizing antigens into plasmids (which normally grow only in bacteria) and injecting these into animal muscle. Muscle is made up of interconnecting cells, so that injections into muscle always end up with the material being inside the cell. In these circumstances plasmids express the introduced antigens at least for some time and thereby immunize the host. Plasmids, being pieces of bacterial DNA, are cheaply and rapidly grown in bacteria, and being solely DNA do not require refrigeration. The technology is being improved, particularly by adding adjuvants to make them more powerful antigens. If DNA vaccination can be safe and effective in humans, it will represent an important advance, introducing vaccines on a massive scale without enormous economic cost.

The development of antibiotics has been based for the last half century on the observations by DUBOS (p 247) on the competition among bacteria and fungi living in soil, where organisms secrete compounds that inhibit their competitors' growth. This approach has been immensely fruitful, as the repertoire of antibiotics shows. However, the rapid increase in antibiotic resistance among pathogens has led to the situation where new classes of antimicrobial drugs are urgently needed. To meet this need, new targets in the micro-organism need to be identified. This is being achieved by taking advantage of 'bacterial genomics', where sequencing the whole genome of an organism allows the pattern of gene expression *in vivo* as well as *in vitro* to be studied. Genes can be identified whose expression is essential to the establishment of infection *in vivo*, and drugs developed to inhibit the action of these gene products. The first drugs developed in this way are likely to be available for clinical use within the next five years.

A related approach is to search bacterial genomes for products that subvert the host immune response. Many micro-organisms have learnt to synthesize the same types of protective molecules — complement control proteins, Fc receptors, MHC molecules, and protease inhibitors — that mammalian cells use for their own protection. Such molecules are also attractive candidates as targets for antimicrobial therapy.

### DNA fingerprinting

The work of Alec Jeffreys created an entirely new way of uniquely identifying human beings. This technique, known as DNA fingerprinting, relies on the fact that we all contain within our genomes, multiple, and highly variable, repeats of small sequences of DNA whose real function *in vivo* is unknown and which are relatively unstable so that an individual's pattern of these constitutes a 'fingerprint'. Jeffreys has developed several ingenious techniques by which such fingerprints may be created, and in doing so has produced a true revolution in FORENSIC MEDICINE. It is now possible to match human tissue (and this includes semen) accurately to a particular individual; to perform rigorous tests for genetic relationships such as paternity; and, potentially, to identify an individual from a single cell, be it a hair, a drop of saliva, or a piece of dandruff. These techniques have already proved valuable in investigations of crime; but have many other uses in the identification of individuals or the establishment of relationships between them.

### Genetic manipulation of cells and animals — gene therapy

The new techniques of gene manipulation make it possible to alter the genetic composition of a living cell with capacity for growth and therefore to introduce genes that will function into the tissues of living animals and humans. This carries with it the promise of being able to treat single-gene genetic disease. Indeed, the first experiments testing an immune disease due to the deficiency of a particular enzyme — adenine deaminase — and the treatment of cystic fibrosis by introducing into lung cells the normal form of the gene that is deficient in this disease, are already being undertaken. Although there are formidable practical difficulties in targeting genes in humans, the notion of being able to treat serious life-endangering diseases such as muscular dystrophy and the hemoglobinopathies is promising and exciting. Although some disquiet about genetic manipulation of somatic cells has in the past been expressed, there is now a wide consensus in favor among doctors and bioethicists. There is similar agreement that trying to modify the germ line of humans, that is, to create by genetic manipulation individuals with 'desirable' traits, is, for the foreseeable future, not permissible. On the other hand, genetic manipulation of the germ line in both plants and animals is being widely undertaken. Many purposes for which transgenic organisms are used are agricultural, but the preparation in this way of biopharmaceuticals is a real prospect as mentioned above for human antibodies.

There is also growing interest in genetically modifying farm animals, particularly pigs, whose organs can be used for transplantation into humans. The reasons why pig kidneys and pig hearts cannot be transplanted into humans are now moderately well understood and it is at least potentially feasible that relatively few genetic manipulations will make such organs suitable for transplantation. Primarily these are likely to concern the introduction of the human pattern of complement control proteins into the pig, and the modification of certain transglycosidases to produce a human pattern of heterophile (carbohydrate) antigens. As the supply of human organs is inadequate and will become even more so, there is a growing need for such a form of treatment.

### Tumor suppressor genes

Molecular biology has led to the discovery and analysis of genes that have a role in the induction or prevention of cancer: oncogenes and tumor suppressor genes. Oncogenes were first recognized in viruses that can give rise to tumors in animals, where it became apparent that these viruses contained in their own genome homologs of host cellular genes which in their own host presumably have functions other than giving rise to cancer. A systematic analysis of the phenomena has shown, perhaps disappointingly, that there are very many such genes and they all seem concerned with various aspects of the regulation and control of the growth of normal cells. Several genes are enzymes that phosphorylate a particular amino acid, tyrosine, in other proteins. This is a common and important mechanism of controlling the activation of proteins. From such work much has been learnt about the control of cell activation and about genetic predisposition to individual tumors.

A related class of genes exists whose products hinder tumor induction and whose malfunction predisposes to tumor formation. The nuclear protein is a particularly striking example of a tumor suppressor and abnormal forms are common in many forms of human cancer. In the foreseeable future it may be possible to detect people at increased risk of developing a particular tumor and to keep them under close medical surveillance. It may also become possible to intervene in the formation of individual tumors.   PJL

**MONTPELLIER** See FRANCE

**MULTIPLE SCLEROSIS** See NEUROLOGY

**MUMMIES** During the early part of the 19th century it had become common practice for European travelers to return home from their winter vacation with an Egyptian mummy. Many of these were unwrapped, or 'unrolled', at social events in private houses and, although much scientific information could have been gathered from these investigations, they were, in general, not carried out by persons with a medical or scientific background and inevitably little important information was gathered. There were, however, notable exceptions, among which were those carried out in London by the Saville Row surgeon Thomas Joseph Pettigrew (1791–1865) and Augustus Bozzi Granville (1783–1872). The latter described ovarian dropsy in an Egyptian mummy from the Persian Period. The organs from this mummy were discovered recently in the British Museum and the authors have been fortunate to

# MOUNTAINEERING

The mountain environment is hostile and physically dangerous. Mountaineering, particularly at high altitude, requires physical ability and stamina. Although rock-climbing and alpine mountaineering up to 4000 m carry risks of injury and death comparable with many contact sports, climbing the world's highest peaks involves extreme risks: the death rate for members of expeditions to peaks over 7000 m high is around 4%. The causes of this mortality are a combination of mountain accidents (avalanche, stonefall, and the effects of storms), cold, and the lack of oxygen, causing medical conditions that are specific to high-altitude mountaineering.

The amount of oxygen diminishes with increasing altitude. Around 4000 m, the available oxygen is around one half that at sea level; on the summit of Mount Everest (8848 m) this falls to less than one third, just sufficient to sustain life for some hours. Acclimatization is the process by which man adapts to the lack of oxygen at altitude involving an increase in hemoglobin production, and changes in respiration and cellular enzyme systems. Acclimatization of a visitor from sea level to 4000–5500 m takes several weeks. Above 5500 m climbers can continue to acclimatize and reach altitudes higher than 8000 m without bottled oxygen — if they are fit, determined, lucky with the weather, and have the technical ability. Permanent habitation much above 5500 m is impossible. Above this altitude, deterioration, working against acclimatization, sets in. A gradual decline in exercise tolerance, loss of

appetite, and loss of weight take place over months, weeks, or days depending on the altitude. A stay of some months is possible at 6000 m, whereas above 8000 m climbers deteriorate rapidly within several days.

## Medical problems caused by lack of oxygen

**Acute mountain sickness**. It has been recognized since ancient times that travelers from sea level to 3500 m or above develop headaches, lassitude, nausea, and sometimes vomiting. This is called acute mountain sickness. It is self-limiting and usually lasts several days. The headaches are treated with simple pain killers. Some prevention is possible by taking acetazolamide, a drug which is a diuretic and an inhibitor of the enzyme carbonic anhydrase, before reaching 3500 m. Acetazolamide is now little used, first because the symptoms of acute mountain sickness are transient, and also because the drug sometimes has unwanted effects (tingling fingers, occasional confusion, and, rarely, allergic reactions). Gradual ascent is the best way to prevent acute mountain sickness.

**Pulmonary and cerebral edema** are severe forms of acute mountain sickness, with the accumulation of fluid in the lungs and the brain. Recognized in 1960, pulmonary edema is uncommon below 3500 m but occurs in 2% of trekkers to 5000 m. Usually, the patient seems to have acute mountain sickness that fails to improve and becomes severely breathless at rest. Crackly breath sounds

become audible. This is a medical emergency. The treatment is with oxygen, with descent, with mask or pressure bag, or with nifedipine, a drug which blocks calcium channels. Breathlessness improves, sometimes dramatically with treatment.

In cerebral edema, fluid accumulates in the brain. The pressure within the skull rises and the brain becomes swollen, causing headache, confusion, drowsiness, and unsteadiness, sometimes with double vision. Swelling of the optic disc (papilledema) may be seen with an ophthalmoscope. Occasionally a stroke-like episode occurs — sudden weakness or numbness of one side of the body. Like pulmonary edema, cerebral edema is serious and potentially fatal. Treatment is with oxygen by mask, descent, or pressure bag, and the potent steroid drug, dexamethasone.

Early pulmonary and cerebral edema respond well to treatment. If the conditions are untreated, or the patient continues to ascend, both usually worsen over the course of several hours. Pressure bags have been used for these conditions since the early 1980s. The patient is inserted into a specially designed body-bag, which is inflated by a footpump. A simulated descent of up to 1000 m can be achieved.

**Other problems** Noticeable fluid retention occurs commonly above 3500 m; puffiness of the face and hands is often apparent and is self-limiting. Above 5000 m, small hemorrhages within the retina occur in about

*(continued overleaf)*

(continued)

A hyperbaric chamber in use in central Tibet. (Photo: Chris Bonnington, 1998. Reproduced with permission.)

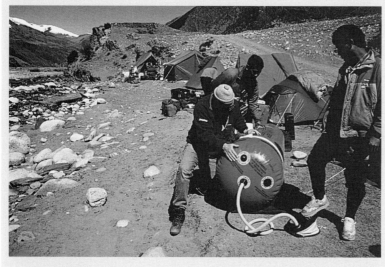

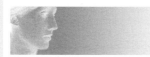

John Scott **HALDANE** (1860–1936). British physiologist. He was the leading respiratory physiologist of his time and carried out practical research into the causes of explosions and death in mines (1906), war gases (1914–18), and deep-sea diving. In 1911 he led an expedition to Pike's Peak, Colorado, to study the effects of atmosphere on breathing. He published an important work, *Respiration*, in 1922.

a third of subjects. They almost never cause symptoms and resolve spontaneously; very occasionally massive retinal hemorrhages cause loss of vision.

Strokes are more common at altitude than at sea level. They are caused by the increased viscosity of the blood, dehydration at altitude, and changes in blood clotting. Early treatment is with oxygen, descent, and aspirin. Many high altitude strokes are mild and resolve completely.

**Cold and ultraviolet radiation**

Hypothermia, that is, a fall in core temperature below 35°C, occurs at subzero temperatures and with frostbite is especially common at high altitude. In hypothermia there is shivering, exhaustion, and confusion leading to coma. Emergency treatment on a mountain is by gradual rewarming — space blankets, huddling, warm drinks, or a warmed sleeping bag. Frostbite occurs when flesh freezes. Fingers and toes (or face, ears, and nose) become doughy and white, and then hard, like meat in a deep freeze. Several days after thawing massive blisters develop. Early treatment of frostbite is by gradual warming — for example, in hand-hot water. Wound hygiene is essential. Antibiotics may be needed. Amputation is carried out in severe cases, but remarkable improvement may take place over several months and often makes surgery unnecessary.

Excess ultraviolet B radiation causes severe sunburn at high altitude, especially on snow. Protection with clothing is essential. Sunscreens are of limited value. Treatment of severe altitude sunburn is with soothing lotions such as calamine, and if necessary steroid creams. There is a risk of skin cancer after prolonged exposure to high-altitude ultraviolet A and B radiation.

Snow-blindness is an intensely painful inflammation of the conjunctiva and cornea which occurs some hours after exposure to ultraviolet light on snow. The eyes feel as if they have been blasted with sand. Treatment is with painkillers and steroid eye-drops. Prevention (goggles/glasses, or in an emergency any eye covering) is mandatory whenever traveling over snow.     CC

*See also* ALTITUDE SICKNESS; EXTREME ENVIRONMENTS

be allowed to examine them histologically. This work has shown that the condition described by Granville was almost certainly a tumor called a cystadenoma of the ovary.

The unwrapping of Natsef-Amun in Leeds by members of the Leeds Literary and Philosophical Society also took place at about this time (1828). This is another mummy which has been reinvestigated more recently by the Manchester Mummy Team. Microscopic examination of tissue from the groin of this mummy showed evidence of filarial WORMS. There is no direct evidence that Natsef-Amun suffered from elephantiasis (swelling of the legs, one of the complications of infestation with this worm) but there was separation of the skin from the underlying tissues of the feet which would be consistent with extensive fluid in this region being removed during mummification. Other evidence of filariasis in ancient Egypt has been suggested from representations in tombs of enlarged male external sex organs and from the swelling of the legs and abdomen seen in depictions of the Queen of Punt at Hatshepsut's Temple at Deir el Bahri. One of the nerves supplying the eyeball from Natsef-Amun showed microscopical changes suggestive of peripheral neuritis. Many poisonous substances, including antimony and lead, were used therapeutically in ancient Egypt and possibly the peripheral neuritis is the result of the treatment of filariasis and hence an early example of doctor-induced (iatrogenic) disease.

After this work in the 1820s, the enthusiasm for the investigation of mummies appears to have waned, and it was some 80 years later (in 1910) when a more scientifically based investigation took place in Manchester led by Dr Margaret Murray, who was then the assistant keeper in Egyptology at Manchester Museum. She was limited by the lack of radiological and adequate microscopical techniques at that time, but fortunately material from Nekht-Ankh and Khnum-Nakht, the 'two brothers' examined by Margaret Murray, were retained and consequently available for further re-examination by the authors in the early 1970s. The material was supplemented by fragments of liver, intestine, and lung from the canopic jars of the mummies. Microscopic examination of the lungs showed extensive scar tissue associated with fine particles of sand, a condition very similar to silicosis. This condition has been seen in several other mummies since that time, and it would appear to have been a widespread disease in ancient Egypt. Although, given the amount of building in stone carried out in ancient Egypt, the condition might be occupational, it is far more likely that most cases were due to the inhalation of fine particles of sand, particularly during sand storms — which were probably a problem in ancient Egypt as they are in the present day. The same condition has been described in the lungs of desert dwellers from the Sahara and the Negev.

Another landmark in the study of ancient Egyptian mummies was also taking place in the early part of the century in Cairo. Mark Armand Ruffer, who was professor of bacteriology there, was the first person to apply modern microscopical techniques to examining tissues from mummies. Most noticeably these studies revealed the presence of the parasite responsible for bilharzia, or SCHISTOSOMIASIS (*Bilharzia haematobium*) in the kidneys of a mummy. More recently the widespread distribution of schistosomiasis in ancient Egypt has been shown using serological techniques. In addition, Ruffer described naked-eye evidence of disease, including a smallpox-like eruption in the skin of a mummy and changes caused by disease in the bones of Egyptian mummies.

Interest in the microscopical examination of mummified tissue was renewed some 50 years later by A. T. Sandison, working in Glasgow, but the main impetus to the study came with the unwrapping and post mortem examination of mummies in

Members of the Manchester Museum team unwrapping Mummy 1770.

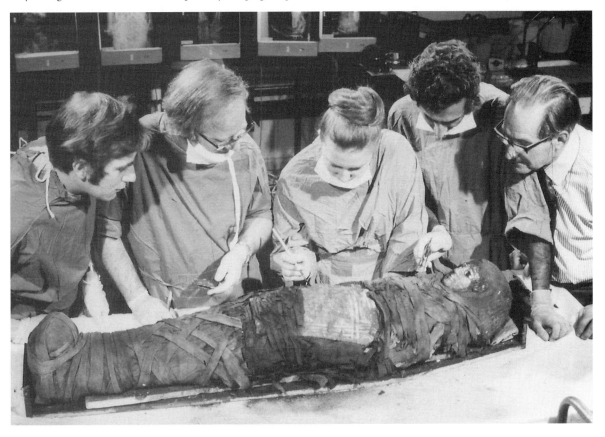

America and in Manchester. This work showed the widespread nature of parasitic infestations in ancient Egypt. The roundworm Ascaris was found in Pum II, unwrapped at the Pennsylvania University Museum in 1974, while Nakht, who was examined in Toronto in 1977, was found to have been suffering from bilharzia and whipworm (Trichinella) infestation. Eggs of a tapeworm (Taenia) species were also found in his intestine. The finding of the latter two parasites is particularly interesting given that they are associated with eating meat, and Trichinella in particular with pork. This finding indicates that the ancient Egyptians were not strictly vegetarian and that in some periods of the year they must have eaten pork. One suggestion is that the pig was associated with Seth and the Legend of Osiris, and it may be that it was eaten only on the anniversary of his birthday. The religious prohibition of pork, then, probably goes back to ancient Egyptian times, and originally may have been based on good hygiene, although, of course, the ancient Egyptians had no way of recognizing the association between Trichinella infestation and pork.

**Parasitic infestation**

The unwrapping of Mummy 1770 in Manchester produced further evidence of parasitic infestation. During preliminary radiographs of the mummy a radio-opaque nodule had been seen in the front of the abdominal wall and after the removal of this nodule, microradiography showed that it contained a calcified guinea worm. The legs of this mummy had been amputated, but it was not possible to determine whether this had been carried out before or after death. If the former, then the lack of healing at the ends of the bones indicate that Mummy 1770 did not live for more than week or two after surgery. The calcified worm found in the abdominal wall was, of course, the male, which dies after copulation. The female migrates to the legs, where it may cause ulceration and (as it was in some more remote parts of the world until very recently) was probably treated by carefully pulling the worm out through the ulcer and winding it on to a stick. If the worm broke, then complications ensued, which may well have required amputation. People become infested with guinea worms when they drink water containing immature forms, and clearly this would be a constant problem where sanitation was inadequate and where there was a total lack of appreciation as to the cause of such a disease.

Yet further evidence of parasitic infestation was found in the intestine of the mummy Asru. This mummy had been unwrapped but not submitted to autopsy in the early part of this century in Manchester and a package containing her intestines had been found lying between her legs. Examination showed immature forms of the parasite Strongyloides in the wall of the intestines. Like schistosomiasis, this infestation was acquired if immature forms penetrated the feet when people came into contact with contaminated water. In ancient Egypt the only opportunity the people had to sow their crops was at the time of the inundation and under these circumstances they would be particularly susceptible to such infestations.

Whilst undoubtedly much information may be gained about disease in Ancient Egypt from autopsies of mummies, Egyptian mummies are valuable antiquities and, since the importation of further specimens has been banned by the Egyptian authorities, museum authorities quite properly are loath to allow investigations that might damage them. Consequently other methods have been sought whereby specimens can be obtained for microscopical examination. In Manchester initially attempts were made to obtain cores of tissues using bone trephines, but in general 'soft tissue' from mummies is too brittle to be taken this way. Much more success has been gained by using endoscopes (fine telescopes that can be passed into the body). Fortunately, during the mummification process the ancient Egyptians removed the brain after breaking through the roof of the nose with an iron hook. This has provided a route whereby the endoscope can be introduced into the skull and specimens taken without causing further damage. In addition, the left lung, stomach, liver, and intestines were also removed during mummification, usually through a vertical incision in the left side of the abdomen. This created a space into which an endoscope can be introduced through the chest or abdominal wall, and the technique has been particularly valuable in obtaining samples of residual lung. A cyst of a hydatid (a worm that infests dogs, sheep, and humans) was identified by this method in the lung of Asru. Further evidence of hydatid disease was found in an isolated head from the Manchester Museum, and clearly the dog tapeworm was a problem in ancient Egypt.

Conversely to all these findings, the more common diseases of modern populations appear to have been rare in ancient Egypt. Thus evidence of disease of the blood vessels is scanty; earlier reports dealt largely with calcification in blood vessels rather than atherosclerosis, although one researcher found evidence of both ATHEROMA and calcification of the blood vessels, while another team also described the microscopic appearance of atherosclerosis in three peripheral arteries from different mummies.

The early death of ancient Egyptians, together with dietary and environmental factors, may also have been important factors in the low frequency of cancer in Ancient Egypt. In particular, very few malignant tumors of the soft tissues have been found, and radiologically there is a striking absence of secondary tumors in the bones of ancient Egyptians. ET, PT

**MUNCHAUSEN'S SYNDROME** Hieronymus Karl Friedrich, Freiherr von Münchhausen (1720–97) was a younger son in the noble house of Rinteln-Bodenwerder in Brunswick. After a distinguished career as a cavalry officer in the Brunswick regiment, he retired to his estate to live the life of a country gentleman. Among his friends he acquired a reputation for telling tall tales based on his travels and on his military and sporting exploits, but much exaggerated and embellished by the inventions of his vivid imagination. Without the knowledge of Baron von Münchhausen, Rudolf Eric Raspe (1734–94), while a refugee in England from his native Germany, wrote *Baron Munchausen's narrative of his marvellous travels and campaigns in Russia*, a slender volume dated 1785 and published anonymously in Oxford in 1786. Raspe wrote the book in English, anglicizing the spelling of the baron's surname to Munchausen. In subsequent editions, other anonymous authors added tales of fiction and fantasy, often with satirical allusions to contemporary events. The popular appeal of the book continued and during the past two centuries many of the fantastic exploits of the fictional baron have attracted the talents of some of the best book illustrators. The tales have also been made into films. Raspe, the author of the original *Adventures of Baron Munchausen*, though a man of sharp intellect and wide interests, had a complex and flawed personality, so that much of his life was spent as a fugitive from the consequences of his deceits.

In 1951, Richard Asher, a physician in London, wrote an article, published in the *Lancet*, under the heading *Munchausen's syndrome*. 'Here is described a common syndrome which most doctors have seen, but about which little has been written. Like the famous Baron von Münchhausen, the persons affected have always travelled widely; and their stories, like those attributed to him, are both dramatic and untruthful. Accordingly, the syndrome is respectfully dedicated to the baron, and named after him.' Munchausen's syndrome was soon accepted as a particularly apt name for a type of factitious disorder.

Persons who manifest Munchausen's syndrome seek urgent medical attention and often gain hospital admission by simulating illnesses with dramatic but untruthful complaints. The psychopathology underlying such a pattern of symptoms, which includes masquerading of disease, pathological lying, and wandering, is poorly understood, though it is thought to be a form of psychological defence mechanism. As the source of his inspiration for the name, Asher cited a particular edition of the *Singular travels, campaigns and adventures of Baron Munchausen* by R. E. Raspe and others, edited and with an introduction by John Carswell, illustrated by Leslie Wood, and published by the Cresset Press in 1948. There have been periodic suggestions that the eponymous nomenclature involving Baron Münchausen should be dropped, in favor of such terms as 'peregrinating problem patients' or 'hospital addiction'; not surprisingly, all have failed.

In 1977, a bizarre form of child abuse was named 'Munchausen's syndrome by proxy' by Sir Roy Meadow, an English pediatrician, who described mothers who not only invented stories of illness suffered by their children, but who also sometimes substantiated the stories by fabricating false physical signs. Child victims of mothers manifesting Munchausen's syndrome by proxy have themselves been designated as suffering from the 'Polle syndrome', named after the infant whose father may have been Baron Hieronymus Karl Frederich von Münchhausen. In 1744 the baron married Jacobine von Dunten, who died without issue in 1790. At an advanced age Baron von Münchhausen married a 17-year old girl, Bernhardine Brun, who gave birth to a daughter,

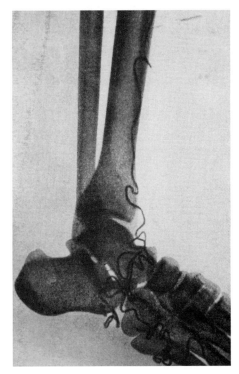

An X-ray of Mummy 1770 showing a guinea worm in the leg.

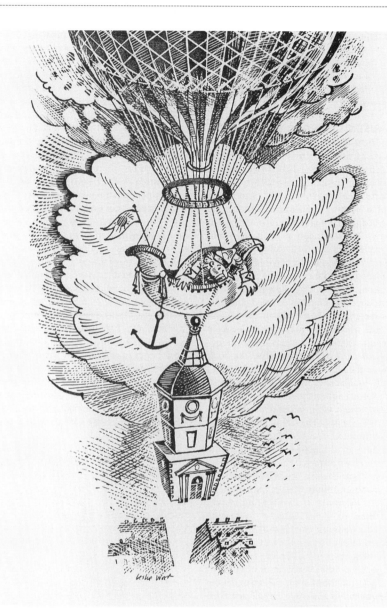

The raising of the Royal College of Physicians of London and its suspension from a balloon for three months is included among Baron Münchausen's later surprising adventures.
(Drawing by Leslie Wood, 1988.)

**MURDER** Very few doctors or nurses have committed murder, and, apart from the dreadful circumstances of the HOLOCAUST, most of the incidents have been in a domestic setting. In January 2001, however, a former single-handed doctor in Manchester, UK, was convicted of murdering fifteen of his elderly women patients (and forging the will of one of them). He had given them injections of heroin, mostly on afternoon house calls, and research after the trial suggested that the total of murdered patients might have been much higher, possibly another 256 cases. Harold Shipman had been present at the death of 20% of all his patients who died (compared with less than 1% for the average family doctor), and probably half of all the death certificates he signed were related to murder. This episode will lead to increased monitoring of family doctors' practices in Britain (especially of single-handed practitioners), with the aim of improving inadequate standards rather than detecting murder. An open full public inquiry into the Shipman case conducted by a High Court judge started in June 2001. *See also* FORENSIC MEDICINE; PROFESSIONAL REGULATION.

Polle, in 1795; Polle died when she was a year old. Thus, Baron von Münchausen (albeit with an anglicized version of his name) and his family have contributed three names to eponymous medical nomenclature. It was, however, Raspe who deceitfully used the name of the baron for his own tales of fantasy, and it was these tall tales which led Asher to use the term Munchausen's syndrome.                    DDG

**MUSIC** The practice of medicine and music have often gone hand in hand. Many doctors have also been musicians. The first five professors of music at Oxford were all physicians, and over the years the roll of medico-musical practitioners includes, among others, Lepold AUENBRUGGER (p 165), Caspar Bartholin, Theodor BILLROTH (p 518), Herman BOERHAAVE (p 121), Robert BOYLE (p 125), Thomas Campion, Sir Francis Champneys, Leopold Damrosch, George Ethridge, Christian Fenger, Oliver Goldsmith, Henry Harington, John Hemmeter, Florient Kist, William Kitchner, Peter Lichtenthal, James Naylor, William Pitts, Albert SCHWEITZER (p 504), Richard Shuckbugh, Harold Sternlicht, Alan Tyson, Herman von HELMHOLTZ (p 372), William Wallace, and T. J. Walsh (founder of the Wexford Festival).

Doctors' orchestras have been founded in many cities, including London, New York, and Vienna. There are numerous flourishing, and highly competent, hospital choirs.

To balance this practitioner roll, there is an equally impressive history of medico-musical traditions: the lore on proportions, concordance, dissonance, and balance as developed by the Pythagoreans; the different types of shaman (witch-doctor or priest) and their drums; the role of mantric sound-syllables and rhythms for inducing healing through altered states of consciousness. In many cultures, medicine and music are combined in ceremony (the priest-doctors of ancient Egypt or the medicine men of the American Indians) often under the aegis of one particular god in a pantheon: Apollo in Greece; Saraswati in southern India. Contemporary sound-healers, such as Jonathan Goldman or Jill Purce, draw on ancient traditions in their chanting of overtones to integrate the chakras, involving a spiritual aspect.

### Underlying issues

What are some of the issues behind this medico-musical association?

An underlying principle of medicine concerns the relation between normal and abnormal. Doctors' knowledge of the normal arises from a study of the anatomy, physiology, and psychology of the human body and mind (the psyche-soma). This knowledge provides an essential base for understanding what can go wrong in the psyche-soma. Equally, their study of what goes wrong, the abnormal, often provides doctors with unexpected insights into the normal.

One of the more direct contributions that doctors can make to musicology is the painstaking archaeological sleuth work involved in diagnosing what exactly a famous musician suffered from and how his illness affected his life and work. What was the exact nature and effect of Beethoven's deafness? Of the extraordinary flexibility of Paganini's hands? Did Marfan's syndrome lie behind the size of Rachmaninov's hands that stretched those wide-spaced chords, a new pianistic sound, at the start of the second piano concerto? What part did Schumann's psychiatric illness play in the spine-chilling effects of alienation and twilight states he instilled into his setting of the Eichendorff Liederkreis? How far was Smetana confronting symptoms of tertiary SYPHILIS (tinnitus and paranoid auditory hallucinations) in his two string quartets? Or Mahler, a childhood psychological trauma in his first symphony?

Time and again, such medical studies show how a musician resorted to his art to overcome what might otherwise have been an insuperable handicap. Through music, their illnesses became creative experiences. Chopin, according to Liszt, used his art to reflect the tragedy of his life (with TUBERCULOSIS). In reflecting their tragedies, musicians somehow transcend them. There are some lessons here for the debate on the quality of life, for music therapy, and for the healing professions generally.

When applied to music, this relation in medicine between the normal and abnormal works in various ways. The core of music has to do with sounds, which we perceive primarily through our ears and our faculty of hearing. Our understanding of the anatomy and physiology of hearing, and of those occasions when hearing is disturbed (as in the medical specialty of audiology), can contribute directly to this core.

A key fact about our hearing and balance is that their anatomical apparatus, the stato-acoustic system, is already well developed by the 28th week of fetal life, considerably in advance of other sensory channels, such as vision or touch. This suggests that our primary sensory patterns are auditory and that our earliest experiences and model of the world are sound based. The intrauterine world is full of sounds coming from inside and outside the mother's body, including her voice and the pulsations of her uterine arteries. By 5 weeks, the fetal circulation is established, the fetal heart contracting. So when we start to hear, we pick up a counterpoint of two regular heart-rhythms with variation in pace, stress, and grouping (into 2s, 3s, 4s etc.). We begin to experience interactive rhythms with entrainment (the pull of one rhythm on another) and synchrony. Our sense of time in the womb is *kairos* (entrained to the person as a whole organism) as well as *chronos* (entrained to an external clock).

This priority of auditory sensation means that in communicating as Rousseau and Darwin intuited, we sing and dance before we speak. As babies, we respond to the intonations of another's voice (and subsequently interpret central features of music according to where we learnt our first words). In our later language, pitch and rhythm

**PHYSIOLOGIST-MUSICIAN**

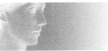

Boris Petrovitch **BABKIN** (1877–1950). Gastroenterologist and neurophysiologist. After being awarded a research fellowship with PAVLOV (p 729) he held the professorship of physiology at Nova Alexandria's College of Agriculture, and later at the University of Odessa. Despite his close association with the great Pavlov, Babkin was sentenced to imprisonment in 1922 by the Soviet authorities, with whose recently introduced policies he disagreed. On release from prison he joined Professor Ernest Starling in London for two years. He was appointed to the chair of physiology at Dalhousie University in Halifax, Nova Scotia, in 1924 and four years later was given a research chair at McGill. Babkin was a talented musician and composer; his earliest composition at the age of 15 was, appropriately enough for a physiologist, 'The Pussy Cat Gavotte'.

(prosody) underpin syntax. What ultimately tells in what we or others say is often the music behind the words. Think of the wartime speeches of Hitler and Churchill. Think, too, of the significant roles assigned to birds and dolphins (mermaids) in our various mythologies, and of the fascination with birdsong shown by composers from Janequin to Messiaen.

Our two ears combine to provide us with a single hearing field (our binaural hearing). This has important consequences for the localization of sounds in space, a problem which has inspired many musicians including Gabrieli, Berlioz, and Stockhausen. Birds often use song to establish territorial boundaries. According to Bruce Chatwin, Australian aboriginals may do the same, drawing on an ancestor's song to define these boundaries, and aligning the contour of a melody with the contour of the chosen piece of land. Music, an aboriginal told Chatwin, is a memory bank for finding our way about the world.

The simultaneous presentation, that started in the womb, of more than one stream of sound has, in polyphony, provided a bedrock for many types of music. The exercise of separating these two streams of sound and feeding one into the left ear and the other into the right (so-called dichotic listening) throws light on how we create our aural 'reality', how we may override the location of sound by the need to form coherent contrapuntal lines, and how we integrate the different functions of the right and left sides of our brain.

## Hearing

From medicine we learn that a complex faculty such as hearing entails connections with many other systems in the psyche-soma: the 'triune' brain of cortex, limbic system, and brain stem; the systems which underlie our capacity to move, dance, and sing; and the systems whereby we experience and express emotions or understand and articulate speech. Just as the material of music draws deeply on expansions such as silence, noise, repetition (rhythm), contrast (variation), so our medical understanding of what is happening when we are making or listening to music draws on these experiences and expands that of 'pure' hearing.

One example of this inter-connectedness may be seen in the phenomenon of synesthesia, that capacity to combine sensory modalities, to hear sounds in color or as tactile textures. Recent brain studies show that hearing music stimulates the occipital cortex (the area in the back of the brain surface associated with vision) even when our eyes are closed. Synesthesia has intrigued musicians, from Josquin and his Renaissance experiments in word painting to Scriabin and Messiaen. It has an important role in song writing, where

the aim is clearly to bridge the two languages of poetry and music. Studies on synesthesia illuminate our understanding of our earliest steps in symbolizing and in integrating our verbal self with those other selves (like the musical one) which predate our use of words. The obverse side of synesthesia may be seen in a musical 'savant', whose focus of expression may be confined to music, compensating for other skills that are unfulfilled because of blindness, for example, or autism.

Other approaches to the connection between the language of music and words have been pursued by laryngologists and neurologists. The first are engaged, with singers, on such issues as phonation, the neuromuscular basis of vocal mechanics, the adaptation of the voice to the ever-expanding demands put on it; and with pediatricians and child psychiatrists, on the analysis and synthesis of voice sounds, the formation of everyone's idiosyncratic cry, which, in certain instances, can help in the diagnosis of a particular disease.

Neurologists have explored certain abnormalities of musical experience (the 'amusias') along lines similar to those undertaken into the abnormalities of speech (the 'aphasias'). The distinctions they outline point to various often clearly defined problematic areas: vocal amusia, the loss of the ability to sing; instrumental musical or receptive amnesia, the loss of the ability to play an instrument, to recognize a familiar tune, or to discriminate melodic patterns; musical alexia and musical agraphia, the loss of the ability to read or write down a series of notes; basic disorders of rhythm entailing a failure to reproduce rhythmic patterns or to distinguish between them; tone deafness, which may have a genetic origin. Through such distinctions, one can begin to appreciate why at least ten systems of the brain may be required to recognize 'Happy Birthday' just by the tune.

Besides the amusias, another abnormalities which may throw light on the neural basis to music are those rare types of epilepsy that are triggered by music and may be accompanied by auditory hallucinations (and hence lie on the boundary of physiology and psychology). These are associated with disturbances in brain rhythms in either temporal lobe (the sides of the brain surface).

Further insights into this neural basis for our musical experiences and for the way our hearing and listening link with other systems are coming from increasingly detailed studies on how the normal and abnormal brain functions. These studies entail observing, through positron emission tomography scans, the blood flow (and hence the activity) of different sites in the brain

| Energy centers (CHAKRAS) | Much variation possible | | |
| | Selected notes from harmonic series | Vowel-sounds | Colors |
|---|---|---|---|
| Cosmic center PURE CONSCIOUSNESS — SAHASRARA | | ee | silver |
| Mental center AUM Cognition MIND — AJUNA | | eh | cerulean |
| Throat center HAM Knowledge-teaching Listening-hearing ETHER — VISHUDDHA | | eye | blue |
| Heart center YAM Love Touch-skin AIR — ANAHATA | | ah | green |
| Navel center RAM Power-expansion Sight FIRE — MANIPURA | | oh | yellow |
| Genital center VAM Contraction Tongue-taste WATER — SVADISHTHANA | | oo | orange |
| Root center LAM Cohesion Nose-smell EARTH — MULADHARA | | ur | red |

Integrating the Chakras through overtone chanting: suggested connections between centers of energy (chakras), notes selected from the harmonic series, vowel sounds, and colors. Considerable variation is possible. (After Golman, J. (1992). *Healing sounds*, Element Books, Dorset.)

when different mental activities are undertaken — such as listening to pitches and tone color of individual notes; to combinations of notes; to sequential patterns of notes; to a piece of music; or to music in our head when we are composing music.

An overall impression from any of these studies is the variety of networks involved and the speed at which they operate. Among more specific findings are that different aspects of playing music activate different areas in the brain. Playing scales on their own, for example, involves different areas from the playing of scales when part of a musical composition. Concordant pitch combinations prompt symmetrical neurone firing patterns of electrical impulses in the nerve cells. Discordant pitch combination prompt erratic firing patterns. And we are

PERIPHERAL

Two EARS. each with:

Outer: Pinna
Passage to drum

Middle: Ossicles
Transmission of
(sound) vibrations

Inner:

Cochlea;
Analysis of
sounds for
pitch and
timbre

Semi-circular
canals;
Balance and
orientation in
space

Cochlear
nerve

Vestibular
nerve

Auditory nerve
(VIII)

CENTRAL BRAIN

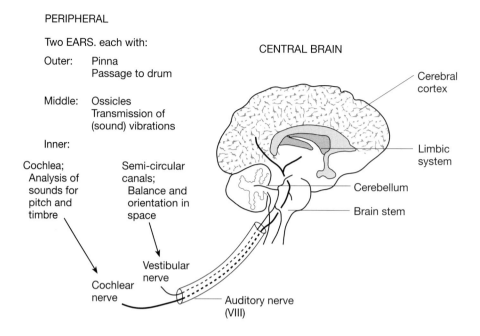

Cerebral
cortex

Limbic
system

Cerebellum

Brain stem

Neural pathway of hearing

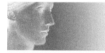
remarkably sensitive to differences of tone color. This heightened discrimination of tone colors, coupled with the direct association of auditory input and emotion/memory in certain brain areas (temporal lobe, corpus callosum, and limbic system), is one reason why a mother can single out her infant's cry from a ward full of others.

Music is inseparable from dance, and, though we may take it through our ears, we respond to it through our whole body. As a result of the entrainment experienced in the womb, our biological rhythms may be modulated by rhythmic events going on around us. Musicians, along with dancers and competitive athletes, describe the near instantaneous interactive rhythms that become established in the course of their work. Lullabies, marches, work songs, sea shanties; the intimacy of a string quartet or a jazz group; or just the audience response to an entrancing performance, all illustrate these rhythmic empathies which have medico-musical applications. For example, setting up an entrainment system by inserting appropriate sound-filters in the biofeedback between voice and ear improves the quality of a singer's voice, or a linguist's pronunciation, and may be used to repair sound-spectrum deficits in stutterers and dyslexics.

The varied body parts used in playing different instruments determine the many occupational hazards to which musicians are prone. Indeed, the list of these hazards reads like a medical textbook, and a course in how to avoid them (including techniques for planning body movements, correct posture, and expansion/relaxation as in the Alexander or Thiberge methods) has now become part of a musician's training.

The musician's use of the doctor's skills is complemented by the doctor's use of the musician's art. Music has been called upon for pain relief; as a general environmental sedative, especially in centers for disturbed children and adults; in critical care as a means of reaching a comatose patient; in geriatric wards to engender some contact for those with Alzheimer's disease or senile dementia; in the obstetric wards through simulated heart beat sounds or other 'lullabies' for babies before and after delivery; and in anesthesia to counter tension, during an operation, such as for cataract under local anesthesia.

Music has found a place in treating those with cardiovascular and inflammatory bowel diseases. For the blind, musical scales have been used in electronic travel aids to display distances between objects. For children suffering from developmental delay, and others similarly challenged, music has proved valuable in enhancing communication and learning. As rhythm, music may enter the treatment of stuttering or, as melodic intonation, that of aphasia. Associated with play, music may provide a channel of access to autistic or withdrawn children.

Along with other art therapies, music can serve as a means of creating a shared 'potential space', in which patients can feel safe enough to find and tell their own stories. In this space, the therapist offers, through music, a resonating chamber, where these stories can be heard and understood.

Through music it is claimed that, from our earliest years, we can expand our embodied self; enhance our capacity to feel; and develop our acquisition of social and intellectual skills. The task of consolidating such claims by logical and statistical techniques that would satisfy a traditional scientist is formidable. But under the spur of EVIDENCE-BASED MEDICINE, and an enlightened critique of conventional research methods, music therapists are moving from a position of empiricism ('we've tried this here and it works') to scrutinizing closely what they are doing, and describing their results in terms that ensure comparability with others. They are setting up a cycle of research, based on the creative principle: I do, therefore I am.

In this cycle, therapists address two central questions: what is it in music that heals? What are the grounds for music therapy in medical practice? With colleagues in medicine and the basic sciences, and working particularly with well-controlled single case studies, they analyze in detail the situations they face, the context in which they face them, the changes they expect and observe, the means at their disposal (including an impressive range of improvisatory skills in music and beyond), and the appropriate research plans to measure outcomes, biases, confounding variables, and the play of chance. In aiming to combine rigor with imagination, they are shifting the underlying perspective from man as a machine to man as a musical composition; from man as a patient with so many deficits, to man with untold possibilities of biological/musical form. A list of sources is given in the 2nd edition of this book. Further publications include Aldridge, D, *Music therapy* (1996); O'Shea, J, *Music and medicine* (1990); and Storr, A, *Music and the mind* (1992). *See also* DANCE; OPERA

RH

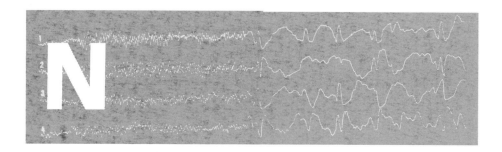

**NATURAL CHILDBIRTH** In the early 20th century, diseases such as rickets were common among the urban poor in Britain. Medical intervention in childbirth was also common, often in the form of general anesthesia and forceps delivery. Still maternal death rates remained high. The 'natural childbirth' movement developed as a reaction to these conditions, just before the maternal death rate in Britain began its long overdue fall from 1935 onwards.

*Natural childbirth* was the title of a book published in 1933 by an English doctor, Grantly Dick-Read. As a boy in Norfolk, he had wondered why

A mother gives birth in a birthing pool, attended by her midwife. (Photo: Sheila Kitzinger, reproduced with permission.)

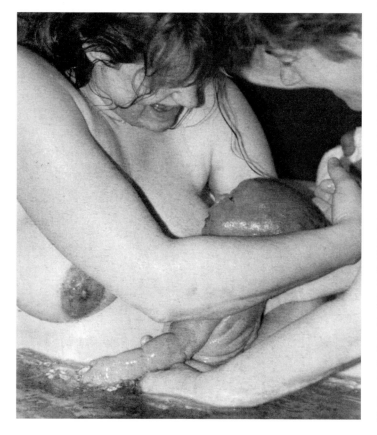

women suffer pain in childbirth while animals apparently do not. He was introduced to the technique of relaxation during the First World War while a medical officer in the Indian Cavalry Corps. He spent a year in hospital obstetrics before entering general practice in southern Britain. In 1934 he entered private obstetric practice. When the National Health Service was introduced he moved to Johannesburg, but returned in 1953, after which he lectured and wrote.

In *Childbirth without fear* (1944), Dick-Read argued that the vicious circle of the 'fear-tension-pain syndrome' was responsible for the pain of labor, and that 'in 90–95% of cases, severe pain can be avoided or overcome by the elimination of fear and tension'. He believed that prenatal instruction was essential for pain relief, that emotional factors during labor are also important, that obstetrics and surgical gynecology are incompatible disciplines, and that obstetricians paid insufficient attention to normal pregnancy compared with the abnormal.

Many of his ideas are now accepted, but some were overstated, and Dick-Read remained at odds with the British obstetric establishment. In 1947 he was invited to lecture in the USA, but his radical approach did not gain favor there and the growing American natural childbirth movement turned instead to 'psychoprophylaxis'.

Psychoprophylaxis, which had been developed in the Soviet Union, was based on Pavlovian conditioning. It argued that the fear and pain were learned responses to uterine contractions and could be unlearned using, for example, breathing techniques. Ferdinand Lamaze (1890–1957), a French obstetrician, introduced psychoprophylaxis in Paris after visiting Russia in 1951 with his colleague Pierre Vellay. An American, Marjorie Karmel, gave birth in Paris and on returning to the USA she published, in 1959, a book called *Thank you Dr Lamaze: a mother's experience in painless childbirth.* Soon afterwards she founded the American Society for Psychoprophylaxis in Obstetrics.

'Prepared childbirth' became popular in the USA as the American Society for Psychoprophylaxis in Obstetrics, working alongside obstetricians without trying to challenge their authority, encouraged antenatal education. Another movement that began in the USA in the 1950s was the La Leche League, which provided support groups, counseling, and role models for women who wanted to breast-feed. Within a few years the League had over 3000 groups throughout America and in many other countries.

More recently other French obstetricians have become well known for their views on natural childbirth. Frederick Leboyer, author of *Birth without violence* (1974), suggested that birth is a traumatic experience for the baby and should be as gentle as possible. He advocated avoiding bright lights and, after delivery, symbolic bathing of the baby by the woman's partner. In the 1980s Michel Odent extended the use of water, saying that bathing reduced labor pain and that delivery itself could take place under water. His views generated controversy, but many British hospitals installed 'birthing pools'. Subsequent research concluded that underwater birth may carry some risk to the baby.

Underlying the natural childbirth movement since the 1930s has been the desire for women to be in charge of childbirth. Their regaining control has paralleled women's increasing independence in society. Some tension between women's autonomy and obstetricians' expertise is inevitable, but doctors have recognized the disadvantages of overmedicalizing childbirth. Interventions are being rigorously appraised, leading to the abandonment of unnecessary procedures such as pubic shaving and routine enemas, and reduction in the rates of forceps delivery. General anesthesia is now infrequently used, though epidural anesthesia is common. The aim of keeping childbirth natural is now the norm. In future, the debate will be the extent to which women can choose unnatural childbirth, particularly CESAREAN delivery.                    JOD

*See also* OBSTETRICS AND GYNECOLOGY

**NATUROPATHY** See COMPLEMENTARY AND ALTERNATIVE MEDICINE

**NEAR-DEATH EXPERIENCES** Since the earliest of times those who have been (or who have believed themselves to be) near to death have reported profound or unusual experiences. Although such near-death experiences may be unrelated to the nearness of actual death, certain elements have persisted across cultures and time. These elements may possibly have been shaped by having heard, earlier in life, of others having had such experiences. Despite this, the ubiquity of such reports across time and place is striking. Persistent themes have included: an experience of peace, well-being, and absence of pain; a sense of

detachment from the physical body, progressing to an out-of-body experience; an entering of darkness, ended by a tunnel experience with panoramic memory and warm feelings; an experience of a warm attractive light, which is entered and in which others are met.

It is not known how common near-death experiences are since surveys tend to provide a self-selecting sample. Both sexes seem equally subject to them, and there appears to be nothing demographically distinct about those who have had a near-death experience save that they are more interested in spiritual matters. This might well be a consequence rather than a cause, because great spiritual and religious changes have been noted as a consequence.

The form that a near-death experience takes seems to depend on the cultural background of the person experiencing it. A Hindu might encounter Yamjaj but never Jesus; the reverse would be true for a Christian. It might, however, be argued that it is the individuals reporting the experiences who are culture-bound rather than the experiences themselves, the same experience being reported differently according to culture.

Some have suggested that these experiences are an epiphenomenon of terminal deprivation of the oxygen supply to the brain. This may produce some of the changes in perception and attitude, but many of those who report them had no oxygen deprivation, and some had only the belief that they were about to die rather than an actual risk of so doing.

The type of threatened death seems to have some effect on the form or extent of experience. Visual images and meeting people seem commoner in those threatened with death by terminal illness or drowning, but are rare in falls or accidents without head injury. Panoramic memory seems rare in uncompleted suicide and near-death experiences seem to be uncommon when near-death has been caused by sedative drug overdoses.

People who have had near-death experiences seem to show less materialism and preoccupation with social success than those who have not.

---

**WHAT IS NATURAL CHILDBIRTH?**

Natural childbirth is difficult to define. Many people have a vague feeling that human reproduction was straightforward before modern life interfered with it. For example, seventy years ago a book about Kalahari bushmen described childbirth as 'a simple affair. If the family is on the move and the pains of labor come on, the woman retires behind a convenient bush and, unhelped by anyone, unless there be another woman in the party, she fulfils this duty of nature. She may be detained an hour or two, but the discomfort is over practically as soon as the baby is born'. Studies have shown, however, that the risk of death in childbirth is much higher in rural Africa than in developed countries.

---

## DEATH, ALMOST, BY DROWNING

A good example of a near-death experience was given by a Scottish doctor, James Lowson in the *Edinburgh Medical Journal* (quoted in *The perfect storm*, by Sebastian Junger). Bound for Sri Lanka in 1892, he was in a ship that sank in a typhoon: 'many years ago my old teacher used to describe how painless and easy a death by drowning was — "like falling about in a green field in early summer"— and this flashed across my brain at the time. I appeared to be in a pleasant dream, although I had enough willpower to think of friends at home and the sight of the Grampians, familiar to me as a boy, that was brought into my view. Before losing consciousness the chest pains had completely disappeared and the sensation was actually pleasant'.

Some, like President Reagan, feel that they have been spared to complete their mission and that their plans have been vindicated. Others report an enduring sense of cosmic unity and the unimportance of previously unmet worldly goals, preferring thenceforth to care for and help others. Although interest in spiritual matters seems to increase after such an experience, denominational allegiance seems to decrease and tolerance of differences grows. These changes have been said to resemble the changes induced by lengthy PSYCHOANALYSIS.

It remains unclear why some return from a real or perceived close call with death bearing a vivid account of an extraordinary experience whilst others report nothing whatever.                    JB

**NEPHROLOGY** is the study of the structure and function of the kidneys in health and disease, from fetal development to the atrophy of old age. The subspecialty of kidney medicine is commonly called nephrology.

### History

From HIPPOCRATES (p 382) onwards, the study of urine was practiced as an indication of bodily well-being. GALEN (p 324) first recognized that urine is produced by kidneys. In the classic 7th century treatise *De Urinis*, Theophilus recognized that urine was made by percolation of blood by the kidneys. MALPIGHI (p 37) described the filtration apparatus of the kidneys, the glomeruli, in 1661, but better understanding of kidney function had to await developments in microscopy in the early 19th century and chemistry in the early 20th century.

Cotugno, in SALERNO (p 448), first described albumin (protein) in the urine of patients with the nephrotic syndrome, but did not understand its significance. In Britain, the Exeter physician John Blackall in 1818 published a book on dropsy and coagulable urine, but it was the physician Richard BRIGHT (this page) at Guy's Hospital, London, who made the connection between this and kidney disease. Applying the then revolutionary approach of correlating clinical findings with morbid anatomy, Bright published the first of his famous reports on renal disease in 1827. He showed that albumin in the urine correlated with diseased kidneys. Producing remarkably accurate descriptions of kidney diseases, he showed that the excretion of urea was depressed in disease and that it accumulated in the blood. He demonstrated that low blood protein was associated with urine protein leak. In the 1850s he opened the first specialist renal ward. For the next century nephritis was to bear the eponym 'Bright's disease'.

The fundamental concept that urine is formed by filtration of the blood by the renal glomeruli, and then modified by the renal tubules, was first enunciated in his thesis by the German physiologist Carl LUDWIG (p 643) in 1842. Further understanding of this filtration/reabsorption theory of urine formation was enhanced by the introduction of renal tubular puncture techniques and the study of living nephrons in the 1920s and '30s, led by the physiologist Alfred Richards at the University of Pennsylvania. Over the same period, Homer Smith at the New York University School of Medicine developed concepts for measurement of renal clearance of urea and other solutes which are the foundation of modern practice.

Renal biopsy (taking a small sample of living kidney tissue by needle for histological study) was introduced by Iversen and Brun in Denmark in 1951. This made possible the study of renal disease at all stages of illness.

It is now recognized that many different diseases can damage the kidneys and cause renal failure. Such damage to the renal filtration apparatus, the glomerulus, is often mediated by deranged immunological responses. Despite our growing understanding of these disorders, disappointingly few are responsive to treatment. Many of the clinical developments in nephrology in the last 50 years have been in the amelioration of the effects of renal failure, or in the replacement of renal function by hemodialysis or transplantation.

Hemodialysis was the first treatment to replace the many functions of a complex organ. It was perhaps prophetic that in the first description of the physicochemical process of dialysis in 1862, Thomas Graham used the example of the dialysis of urea out of urine. The prototype artificial kidney was constructed in 1913 by Abel, Rowntree, and Turner, who removed toxins from dogs' blood by dialysis of blood through collodion tubing. Application of this technique to humans had to await the development of anticoagulant drugs and manufactured membranes, the first of which was cellophane used for sausage skins. Not until 1943 did Willem Kolff design an artificial kidney with an adequate area of membrane to carry out the first successful hemodialysis on a patient. Long-term dialysis became possible when Scribner and Quinton in Seattle in 1960 designed an artificial arteriovenous shunt which allowed permanent access to the blood circulation.

The first attempts at renal TRANSPLANTATION in humans were by Mathieu Jaboulay, who attempted two pig-to-human transplants in Lyon in 1906. The very severe rejection of animal kidneys transplanted into man has not been overcome. The use of 'humanized pig kidneys' (kidneys from pigs carrying inserted human genes) may prove a solution, but has been held up by fear of transferring pig viruses to humans.

## EARLY NEPHROLOGISTS

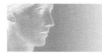

John **BOSTOCK** (1773–1846). English physician. The son of a Liverpool physician, he practiced in Liverpool, but moved to London in 1817. There he lectured on chemistry at Guy's Hospital, where he shone in the reflected glory of collaboration with Richard BRIGHT. His particular contribution was in demonstrating that in patients with renal disease the serum contained an excess of urea and was deficient in albumin, while the urine was of low specific gravity. Bostock also gave a complete description of hay fever, drawing on his own experience as a sufferer.

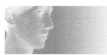

Richard **BRIGHT** (1789–1858). British physician. He traveled widely between 1810 and 1818. In 1820 he was elected to the staff at Guy's Hospital and in 1837 became physician-extraordinary to Queen Victoria. Bright was an unimpressive lecturer; his genius lay in correlating clinical observations with post-mortem appearances. In his *Reports of medical cases* (1827) he established the association of edema and albuminuria with nephritis (Bright's disease).

The first transplants between humans, performed in the USSR in 1933, failed. Success was first achieved in the Peter Brent Brigham Hospital in Boston. From 1947, transplants were used to provide temporary renal function for patients with reversible renal failure, but rejection prevented long-term graft function, first achieved in a transplant between identical twins in 1954, earning the surgeon, Joseph Murray, a NOBEL PRIZE.

In the late 1950s, total body irradiation was used as immunosuppression and some successful living related donor transplants were undertaken, notably in Paris. The development of immunosuppressive drugs, first used by Sir Roy Calne in 1960, enabled successful unrelated cadaver transplantation, which by the early 1970s had become a routine operation.

## Functions of the kidneys

The kidneys excrete waste products and toxins, and control salt, water, and the mineral balance in the body. It is these functions that are largely replaced by dialysis treatment. The hormonal functions of the kidney are less well known, but are vitally important and much of the drug treatment of renal failure is aimed at replacing these functions.

Renin is a circulating hormone produced by the kidney. It is secreted in excess when the renal arteries are narrowed, and in many chronic renal diseases. This stimulates overproduction of angiotensin II in the circulation, which causes high blood pressure. The development of drugs which either block the formation of angiotensin II, or the receptors to it, has been an important advance in treating high blood pressure.

A role for the kidney in stimulating the formation of red blood cells was first proposed in 1906, but erythropoietin, the hormone produced by the kidneys to stimulate the bone marrow, was only isolated and characterized, and its site of secretion in the cells lining the kidney tubules identified, in the last 30 years. The cloning of its gene, and its insertion into cultured monkey kidney cells so that they produce human erythropoietin, have made available a treatment which corrects the anemia of renal failure, and has greatly improved the quality of life of patients with renal failure.

Inability to control blood calcium concentrations with consequent bone disease has been recognized in renal failure since the 1930s. In 1970 Fraser and Kodicek showed that the kidney converts vitamin D to its active form, calcitriol: without this, the serum calcium concentration falls, and the bones are softened. The availability of calcitriol and closely related alfacalcidol as therapeutic drugs in renal failure has prevented much of renal bone disease.

## Disorders

Cystitis, infection of the urine in the bladder, is the most common of all urinary tract diseases. It is particularly common in women, is painful, but seldom causes structural damage in the absence of DIABETES or urinary tract abnormalities, and is rarely life-threatening. It usually responds rapidly to ANTIBIOTIC treatment.

Scarring of the kidneys by infection is most frequently seen in reflux nephropathy, which occasionally leads to renal failure. This process starts in infancy or even *in utero*, and runs in families. It results from delayed development of the valve at the lower end of the ureter (the tube leading from the kidney) where it enters the bladder: when the bladder contracts to express urine, some urine refluxes to the kidneys. If infection is present abscesses form in the kidneys, and can lead to scarring. Scrupulous prevention of infection during childhood, while the valves mature, usually prevents damage. Operative intervention is now rarely necessary and has only minor effects on the natural history of the illness.

*Glomerulonephritis (nephritis)* This term describes the diseases, formerly known as Bright's disease, in which the glomeruli are damaged by inflammation and scarring. Several types of glomerulonephritis have been identified by renal biopsy; they respond in different ways to treatments. Many of them are caused by abnormal immunological responses. An abnormal immune response to streptococcal infection was responsible for many cases of glomerulonephritis, especially in children, until the 1950s, when the advent of penicillin, the first effective treatment of streptococcal infection, greatly reduced its frequency in developed countries.

Another lesion responsive to treatment is minimal change disease, in which the abnormalities in the glomeruli are shown only by electron microscopy. It affects mainly children. Massive loss of protein in the urine causes low blood albumin concentrations and edema (waterlogging of the tissues), susceptibility to infection, and increased tendency to blood clotting. These features occur whenever there is heavy proteinuria (protein in the urine) and are known as the nephrotic syndrome. Minimal change was disabling and often fatal until the introduction of corticosteroids in 1950, to which it responds rapidly, although periodic relapse is common. It does not lead to kidney failure.

Some of the most aggressive forms of glomerulonephritis can be reversed by heavy immunosuppressive treatment. However, most of the common, slowly progressive forms of glomerulonephritis are currently unresponsive to such treatment and possible benefits are outweighed by side-effects.

*Drug-induced disease* Most drugs or their metabolites are excreted through the kidneys, and some are concentrated there. Some very valuable antibiotics, anti-cancer drugs, and immunosuppressants damage the kidneys when used at high dose or for prolonged periods. Many drugs, particularly anti-inflammatory analgesics and some antibacterials, can cause a rare inflammatory reaction in the kidney called acute interstitial nephritis. There have been a few outbreaks of renal failure in Europe due to herbal medicines containing germanium or Chinese herbs, and similar side-effects of folk remedies are common in Africa (bush teas) and Hong Kong (carp gallbladder).

In 1953 Spühler and Zollinger in Switzerland noticed a high frequency of fatal kidney failure in people consuming large quantities of painkillers, a practice common among watchmakers. Epidemics of this 'analgesic nephropathy' were described from many countries, especially Australia, Scandinavia, Belgium, and Germany: it was the most common cause of renal failure in some areas. Improved education, the withdrawal of phenacetin (believed to be one of the toxic ingredients), and the use of single analgesics rather than mixtures, have been followed by a gradual decline of this disease, which is now relatively rare in most countries.

*Genetic diseases* Over 100 dominant or recessive diseases and chromosome disorders affecting the kidney are known. However, polycystic kidney disease (where the substance of the kidney becomes destroyed by slowly enlarging cysts), the most common genetic disease to cause renal failure, presents in adult life. It accounts for 8% of cases of renal failure in Britain. It is caused by mutations in one of at least two genes, on chromosome 16 and chromosome 4, which code for similar proteins in the cell membrane. The genetic abnormalities in many other renal diseases have now been identified. This has not yet resulted in major changes in treatment, but genetic counseling and prenatal diagnosis are rapidly improving.

*Urinary obstruction* Obstruction to the outflow of urine from the kidneys causes renal dysfunction, which may be irreversible if obstruction is long lasting. In younger people congenital abnormalities and renal stones are the common causes. In the elderly it is predominantly a disease of men with an enlarged prostate gland causing obstruction of the bladder outflow.

*Acute renal failure* Acute renal failure is renal failure of rapid onset, and the phrase commonly implies reversibility. In 1941 during the London Blitz, Bywaters and Beale described this condition caused by crush injury. Other causes include septic abortion, accidents of childbirth, blood loss, fluid depletion, infections, snakebite, acute obstruction, and drug side-effects. Both hemodialysis and peritoneal dialysis were used in the 1940s but success was limited. Artificial kidneys of improved design made hemodialysis a routine procedure by the late 1950s and peritoneal dialysis became an acceptable alternative for some patients from the early 1960s. With the use of these techniques patients rarely die of acute renal failure, although many still die from the severe illness that caused it.

*Chronic renal failure* Chronic renal failure is long lasting, irreversible kidney failure. The most common causes are diabetes, glomerulonephritis, polycystic kidney disease, hypertension, urinary obstruction, and genetic disorders. The frequency rises steeply with age; in the USA it is particularly common in black people and in Britain it is more frequent in immigrants from countries such as Africa, the Caribbean, and the Indian subcontinent than in Caucasians. In some countries diabetes accounts for over 35% of patients starting renal replacement therapy. Tighter control of diabetes and hypertension could substantially reduce the incidence of end-stage renal failure but demand commitment to long-term meticulous care from both patient and doctor.

During chronic renal failure excretory function fails, causing accumulation of toxic substances from the diet or metabolism: fine control of fluid and electrolyte balance is also lost. Sodium and water are usually retained, causing high blood pressure. Endocrine functions are deranged — calcitriol and erythropoietin under-produced, and renin sometimes over-produced.

Once renal function falls below 30% of normal, deterioration often progresses even if the disease that caused it is quiescent. This progression was attributed by Brenner in 1982 to the surviving glomeruli being subjected to excessive pressure (glomerular hypertension), causing excessive protein to leak through the filter with progressive scarring of the glomeruli (focal glomerulosclerosis). The process can be slowed by tight control of blood pressure and avoidance of excessive protein intake. A very low protein diet may help but the evidence is equivocal and there is a risk of malnutrition.

## Treatment

*Renal replacement therapy* Renal transplantation is the gold standard, but, with the increasing numbers of elderly and diabetic patients accepted for treatment, a third of patients are unsuitable for such surgery. Even among those suitable for transplantation, the supply is limited by the shortage of donor organs and in most countries few patients over 65 receive transplants.

Since 1960 long-term hemodialysis has been the mainstay. Long-term peritoneal dialysis developed at about the same time, but its widespread use dates from the introduction of continuous ambulatory peritoneal dialysis in the late 1970s. Sodium and water retention remain a problem in most dialysis patients, leading to problems of control of HYPERTENSION.

*Hemodialysis* Blood is taken from a suitably modified blood vessel and passed over a semipermeable membrane which allows small molecules and toxins that accumulate in renal failure to pass through it. Blood cells and larger molecules such as proteins are retained. The other side of the membrane is perfused by a fluid which carries away the waste products. Some substances removed by dialysis such as amino acids and vitamins may need to be replaced by appropriate diet or supplements.

Dialysis is a two-way process so the dialysis fluid must be purified, and its content carefully controlled, especially with regard to solutes such as sodium, calcium, potassium, and dextrose. Many of the early problems of long-term dialysis were due to impurities entering the patient from the tap water used to produce dialysis fluid. Of particular importance was aluminium poisoning, which caused dementia, bone disease, and anemia. Zinc, copper, and chloramines used in water disinfection, caused hemolytic anemia. Febrile reactions from bacterial growth were common. Production of ultra-pure water by successive filtering, softening, and reverse osmosis eliminated many of these complications of dialysis therapy.

The 30 m of sausage skin in Kolff's first artificial kidney has been replaced by a dialyzer containing thousands of hollow fibers, which enable 80 ml of blood to be spread over a surface area of more than 1 m$^2$ to allow solute exchange. The process is monitored by pressure sensors on the inflow and return lines to detect obstruction to flow; a monitor detecting air or froth in the venous bubble trap to prevent air embolism; sensors which monitor the temperature and ionic concentration of the dialysis fluid; and gauges which measure the pressures on both sides of the membrane. A computer, programmed by the nurse, controls the rate of fluid removal, displays all measurements on screen and sounds alarms.

Patients in chronic renal failure usually require dialysis three times a week for at least four hours. Between treatments patients must restrict their intake of water, salt, potassium, and phosphate and take their prescribed protein. A serious problem in hemodialysis is securing access to blood flow from the patient at an adequate rate. This is not possible from peripheral veins. The plastic arteriovenous shunt devised by Scribner and Quinton in 1960 was the mainstay for six years, but was plagued by recurrent clotting and infection. It was replaced by the Cimino-Brescia fistula, a subcutaneous connection between an artery and a vein which stimulates the vein to grow and maintain a high blood flow.

Cellulose dialysis membranes are poorly biocompatible, and stimulate many inflammatory reactions as blood passes over them. This does not allow the passage of molecules bigger than 12 000 molecular weight, and many important toxins are thought to be in the range of 12 000–30 000 molecular weight. One such substance is beta II microglobulin, a product of inflammation, which is deposited as amyloid around bones and joints causing pain and fractures in many patients after five years of hemodialysis. Newer synthetics more biocompatible and more permeable dialysis membranes may perhaps alleviate such problems but are also expensive.

*Hemofiltration* With high permeability membranes it is possible to operate a circuit similar to dialysis but with no dialysis fluid. 'Ultrafiltrate' is filtered from the blood and discarded. It is replaced by an electrolyte solution. This is more expensive than hemodialysis but removes large molecular weight substances better and may have some clinical advantages. It may be used to treat acute renal failure because the system can be run slowly throughout the illness. This allows high volume intravenous feeding in patients unable to eat or drink, and good control of blood pressure. Hemofiltration can be combined with hemodialysis (diafiltration) to increase removal of toxins.

*Continuous ambulatory peritoneal dialysis* The peritoneum is a natural membrane through which solute exchange can take place between blood in the capillaries under the peritoneum and fluid introduced into the peritoneal cavity. In peritoneal dialysis carefully controlled solute solutions are introduced into the peritoneal cavity. In continuous ambulatory peritoneal dialysis these solutions are left *in situ* for six hours and then exchanged. Waste products are washed out at each exchange. Fluid control is potentially difficult as the high urea content of the blood in renal failure creates an osmotic pull such that fluid is transferred into the patient. To prevent this and allow fluid removal from the patient, dextrose is added to the fluid as an osmotic agent. Dextrose is cheap and effective but slowly absorbed, blunting appetite and causing obesity. After long periods of peritoneal dialysis, particularly if infection has intervened, the dextrose may be absorbed rapidly and lose its osmotic effect. Newer osmotic agents are being sought. They must be very slowly absorbed from the peritoneum and non-toxic. Icodextrin, a glucose polymer of high molecular weight, is a promising agent.

The main complication of continuous ambulatory peritoneal dialysis is peritonitis. The silastic catheter which remains in the abdomen is readily colonized by bacteria from the skin, which evade the body's defences by forming a protective layer of slime. The use of peritoneal dialysis is limited by its efficiency. It is a very valuable treatment, allowing considerable freedom of life-style, in the early stages of renal failure. However, when the kidneys are completely destroyed peritoneal dialysis may not provide adequate replacement of renal function.

## Conclusion

One of the great successes of medicine in the last fifty years has been the development of effective renal replacement therapy. It is surprising that a process as crude as dialysis can adequately replace the excretory function of the kidneys and maintain life over twenty years or more. The judicious use of peritoneal dialysis, the advent of new hemodialysis membranes, and the availability of hormones to replace the hormonal functions of the kidney have greatly improved the quality of life of patients on dialysis. Transplantation is now a routine highly effective treatment: over 50% of transplants still work after ten years.

There has been less success in devising treatments to prevent renal failure. Better treatment of diabetes and hypertension would substantially alter the situation. New understandings of immunology offer hope that some immunological renal disorders will become amenable to treatment.                          TGF, DK

*See also* MOLECULAR BIOLOGY; IMMUNOLOGY

**NESTORIAN MEDICINE** The Nestorian Christians were followers of Nestorius, Patriarch of Constantinople, who in AD 431 was denounced by the Council of Ephesus for his heresy (that Christ had two distinct natures, divine and human). The doctrine, however, continued to flourish in Syria and the East, and the Nestorians, debarred from eminence in Church and State, turned to medicine. The medical school and hospitals at Edessa (Urfa, the 'Athens of Syria') were taken over, and a school was established, which for a time rivaled that of Alexandria. Despite the success of Nestorian practitioners, they were expelled from the empire in 489 by Emperor Zaro at the instigation of the orthodox Bishop Cyril. The Nestorians then moved to Persia, where they established further medical schools, the most famous being that at Jundisha-pur. Here the most liberal-minded Christians

came together with advocates of Greek free thought and the ancient knowledge of the East — Hindu physicians were to be found among the professors. For two centuries the Nestorians translated Greek medical texts into Arabic, thus contributing to the flowering of Arabian medicine in the 7th century and long afterwards.

*See also* GREEK MEDICINE

**NEUROLOGY—HISTORY** In 1681, Thomas Willis coined the term 'neurology', based upon his 'doctrine of the nerves'. Subsequently this discipline was generally taken to embrace that aspect of human biology dealing with the structure and function of the central and peripheral nervous systems, including the neuromuscular system. More recently, however, a distinction has been drawn between neuroscience, the study of structure and function, and clinical neurology. The latter is the practice of a physician concerned with the diagnosis and treatment of disorders of the nervous and neuromuscular systems. Plainly, there is some overlap with PSYCHIATRY, which is primarily concerned with disorders of the mind.

Many organic nervous diseases studied by neurologists, such as dementia, profoundly affect mental function; and assessment of defects of memory and cognition is undertaken by neuropsychologists. There is growing evidence that several disorders falling primarily into the realm of psychiatry, such as depression and schizophrenia, may be associated with specific biochemical disturbances and are thus, in one sense, organic. In the 19th century, especially in continental Europe, many doctors practiced neuropsychiatry, embracing both organic and mental disorders, but the increasing demands of the two specialties have meant that in the last 50 years neurology and psychiatry have been practiced as distinct disciplines.

### Neuroscience infrastructure

ARISTOTLE (p 64) regarded the brain as a structure whose purpose was to cool the blood; however, in the Middle Ages the widely-held view was that its fluid-containing cavities or ventricles had a secretory function. Gradually, it was realized that the brain was concerned with mental function, and particularly with cognition, memory, and 'common sense'. In the 18th century Franz Josef GALL (p 641) and Johann Gaspar Spurzheim were among the first to postulate a doctrine of cerebral localization relating individual parts of the brain to different intellectual, physical, and mental functions. This led to their espousing the discipline of PHRENOLOGY, which for some years had a considerable vogue.

Much effort was devoted to attempts to correlate different external contours of the skull to the function of underlying areas of the brain, specifically in relation to human behavior and physical activity. As interest in this pseudoscience waned, information derived from the study of pathological changes in the brain gradually emerged; for example, Paul Broca postulated that an area in the inferior part of the left frontal lobe might impair the production of speech. It soon became apparent that not just speech but other so-called higher cerebral functions were un-equally divided between the two cerebral hemi-spheres and that the frontal, parietal, temporal, and occipital lobes of the brain differed in func-tion. For example, Wernicke showed that the recognition and understanding of speech are controlled by part of the left temporal lobe in right-handed individuals. Sometimes the right temporal lobe controls this function in those who are left-handed. It was also realized that the occip-ital lobes are concerned with recording visual information, and that a part of each temporal lobe is concerned with hearing.

Earlier views suggested that the multiple outfold-ings of the cortex of the brain (the gyri, separated by sulci) were random. These were soon replaced by the recognition of a consistent pattern and by neuroanatomical and microscopical studies confirming that the cells in the cerebral cortex (the grey matter) are organized in discrete layers, which vary in different cortical areas. Indeed, Brodmann constructed a mosaic-like brain map comprising 50 areas, each numerically demarcated, and postulated that each might have a specific function. Although that view was later shown not to be strictly correct, knowledge of specialization in structure and func-tion continued to emerge. Ramon y Cajal devel-oped his neuronal theory suggesting that nerve cells and the axons (fibers) or dendrites (small processes) to which they gave rise controlled activ-ity in the nervous system. The Russian anatomist, V. A. Betz, described the giant nerve cells in the motor cortex. Some of the principal nerve fibers and tracts concerned with voluntary movement (motor activ-ity) originate from these and pass down through the white matter of the brain and spinal cord.

In the second half of the 19th century, the school of localizationalists held sway; among its leaders were Hughlings Jackson, von Monakow, Pierre Marie, and Henry HEAD (p 745). With the aid of skilled neuropathologists, who increasingly began to relate abnormalities of structure and function to pathological changes in the nervous system and to their clinical consequences, a new discipline of pathophysiology emerged. Neuro-physiology had, in parallel, begun to define the principles of conduction in nerve pathways and, through the work of SHERRINGTON (p 646) and others, reflex action was recognized and defined.

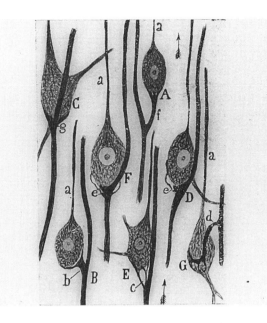

This led to the discovery of the synapses (points at which two nerve fibers come into con-junction). Gradually, it emerged that transmission of nerve impulses across synapses usually requires the secretion of a neurotransmitter substance, such as acetylcholine or dopamine, which reacts with receptors on the target cell or nerve fiber. As the years passed, many more neurotransmitters were identified, enhancing the development of neurochemistry and neuropharmacology.

Studies of neuronal behavior defined the prop-erties of excitability, excitation, and response, and the all-or-none theory of nervous transmission. This was followed by the recognition that, while some neurones are excitatory, others are inhibitory, and that integration or the control of a response in a target neurone or organ innervated by such a neurone depends upon the regulated control of excitation and inhibition.

Just as evidence of the specialized function of different parts of the cerebral cortex was recog-nized, the function of the cerebellum in modulat-ing voluntary motor activity was gradually defined. So too was the crucial role of the brain stem and its reticular substance in controlling sleeping, wakening, and consciousness, coupled with the recognition that certain brain-stem centers have a vital role in cardiorespiratory function. Gross damage to the brain stem may seriously impair these vital functions and so 'BRAIN-STEM DEATH' came to be equated with brain death.

### Foundation of clinical neurology

As such knowledge developed, it inevitably influenced neurological diagnosis, as it became

Detail of neural connections, from Ramon y Cajal's *Recuerdos de mi vida*, Madrid 1923. (From the National Library of Medicine, Bethesda, MD.)

**GERMAN NEUROLOGIST**

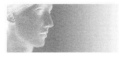

Paul Julius **MÖBIUS** (1853–1907). German neurologist. He described ophthalmoplegic migraine, the Leyden–Möbius type of muscular dystrophy (1879), weakness of convergence in thyrotoxicosis (Möbius's sign, 1886), and also congenital absence or aplasia of facial, bulbar, and other muscles (Möbius syndrome).

possible, through examining a patient, to define such phenomena as weakness, paralysis, involuntary movement, loss of sensory function (whether involving the special senses or somatic sensation), and reflex change. Abnormalities such as heightened reflexes in paralysed limbs due to dysfunction of the 'pyramidal' or corticospinal tract, or an extensor plantar response (first recognized and described by Babinski), confirming such an abnormality, added to the precision of diagnosis.

These and other physical signs made it possible to localize a lesion or pathological process within the nervous systems, while expert history taking to define the nature and speed of onset of the resulting symptoms helped to define its nature. Thus, symptoms resulting from a stroke (hemorrhage into, or loss of blood supply to, a part of the nervous system causing infarction), usually develop suddenly, while those due to infection or inflammation, whether caused by micro organisms or a disorder of immune function, arise over hours or days, and those due to a degenerative process or to tumor formation in the brain or spinal canal tend to evolve over weeks or months. At best, however, despite the skill and experience of many notable neurologists of the late 19th and early 20th centuries ancillary diagnostic techniques became of increasing importance in many countries.

### Aids to diagnosis

Among the first important diagnostic aids was ophthalmoscopy. Examination of the optic fundus could reveal information about the state of the arteries and veins and could also indicate, through the presence or absence of papilledema (swelling of the optic disc), whether or not the pressure inside the skull was raised. In 1885, Corning introduced lumbar puncture for examination of the cerebrospinal fluid; this became a vital procedure in diagnosing meningitis and some other inflammatory brain disorders. While it carried significant risks if a brain tumor was present, examination of the cerebrospinal fluid for bacteriological, cellular, and biochemical abnormalities contributed fundamentally to neurological diagnosis for over half a century and still has a limited role today.

Expanding neurophysiological knowledge led in the 1930s to the introduction of electroencephalography (the study of brain waves through the intact skull) through the work of Berger, Adrian, and others; electromyography (electrical examination of the function of the muscles) soon followed, as did measurement of nerve conduction velocity; these techniques have made a notable contribution to the understanding of neuromuscular disease. More complex techniques of measuring sensory-evoked potentials recorded from the brain or over the spinal cord during somatic, visual, and auditory stimulation followed; these techniques, too, have been valuable aids to diagnosis.

However, the introduction of neuroradiology gave the greatest impetus to neurological diagnostic accuracy. X-rays of the skull and spinal column are still useful, but contrast methods introduced to facilitate imaging of the brain and spinal cord, such as myelography, carotid and vertebral angiography, ventriculography, and air (or pneumo-) encephalography played an increasingly important part in the 1930s and for 30–40 years subsequently, despite the discomfort, potential risks, and inconvenience involved with each.

Nevertheless, the localization of tumors of the brain and spinal cord depended crucially upon such methods until the painless and harmless techniques of computerized axial tomography (the CT or CAT scan) came along, to be followed rapidly by nuclear magnetic resonance (NMR), with its improved resolution and its ability to recognize and define not only strokes, neoplasms, aneurysms, and many other lesions readily recognized by older techniques, but also the plaques of multiple sclerosis, for example. Ultrasonic methods, including the Doppler technique of studying blood flow in the extracranial blood vessels, have been invaluable in defining some causes of stroke, especially those resulting from narrowing of the carotid arteries in the neck. Studies using radioactive substances, including single proton emission computerized tomography and the much more expensive and elaborate positron emission tomography (PET scanning), have given useful morphological information but more importantly functional information relating to metabolic changes in the brain in health and disease.

Neuropathology has enabled the recognition at post-mortem of the disease responsible for the patient's symptoms.

Furthermore, biopsy techniques of muscle and to a lesser extent of nerve, and occasionally of the brain itself, have proved increasingly useful in diagnosis.

The skills of the neuropsychologist in assessing faculties such as thinking, learning, memory, communication, calculation, spatial conception, time sense, the notion of the body image, and other aspects of cognition also make an important contribution. Studies of abnormalities of these functions consequent upon brain disease in the borderland between neurology and psychiatry may be invaluable. Moreover, assessments by speech and language therapists, and occasionally by academic linguists, have helped to define abnormalities of speech and language consequent upon brain disease. Thus has emerged the discipline of psycholinguistics.

Important, too, are other contributions. The neuro-otologist studies abnormalities of hearing and of balance; the neuroimmunologist autoimmune diseases of the nervous and neuromuscular systems; and the human geneticist and molecular biologist inherited diseases of the nervous system, and conditions in which genetic susceptibility is important. To quote but one example in multiple sclerosis, there is now clear evidence of genetic susceptibility; against that, background environmental factors (commonly viral) may precipitate an autoimmune reaction in the nervous system, producing demyelination in the optic nerves, brain, and spinal cord.

## Treatment

For many years it was conventional criticism that neurology was often powerless to alleviate or cure. The contribution of neurosurgery in managing tumors of the nervous system and of aneurysmal subarachnoid hemorrhage has long been acknowledged, and in recent years the vascular surgeon has made a major contribution to stroke prevention by using endarterectomy to remove areas of narrowing in the carotid arteries. The conquest of many formerly fatal diseases such as tuberculosis and other forms of meningitis is largely history, though the recent emergence of multidrug-resistance tuberculosis in many parts of the world, and of antibiotic-resistant pneumococci, for instance, is a cause for concern. HIV infection and AIDS, with their profound effect upon the central nervous and neuromuscular systems, have presented doctors with another challenge. Intensive care has saved many patients who would formerly have died from head injury, stroke, or acute paralysing disorders such as the Guillain-Barré syndrome or transverse myelitis. The techniques of relieving intractable pain, whether with increasingly effective drugs, peripheral nerve stimulation, surgery, or even acupuncture, have also transformed pain management. Increasing emphasis upon rehabilitation has greatly improved the lot of many patients suffering weakness, paralysis, or other dysfunction due to various neurological disorders. Thus although many neurologic diseases remain incurable, there are none whose effects cannot be modified by pharmacological, physical, surgical, or psychological means.

The increasingly effective drugs now available for treating epilepsy, such as the glutamate antagonists; the introduction of serotonin antagonists for migraine attacks; and the introduction of levodopa and its analogues for Parkinson's disease, are just a few examples. Neurochemistry, which has elucidated specific enzyme defects in some nervous disorders such as Wilson's disease and Refsum's disease, has led to effective treatment.

Perhaps our greatest hopes now relate to discoveries in human genetics and molecular biology, as the genes responsible for more and more progressive disorders of the nervous and neuromuscular systems are being increasingly identified. In some, the missing gene product has been identified, bringing in prospect gene therapy using an appropriate vector to carry the missing protein back into the damaged cells. In some dominantly inherited disorders, such as Huntington's disease and myotonic dystrophy, abnormal amino-acid repeats have been identified, and methods are now being explored to try to mitigate the effects of these abnormalities.　　　　JW

*See also* GENETICS, HUMAN; IMAGING; MOLECULAR BIOLOGY; NUCLEAR MEDICINE; PAIN; PHARMACOLOGY, CLINICAL PHARMACOLOGY, AND THERAPEUTICS

**NEUROLOGY** Clinically, neurology is concerned with diseases affecting the brain, spinal cord, peripheral nerves, and muscles. Disorders of thought processes and emotion are considered to lie within the realms of PSYCHIATRY, although the two specialties overlap, particularly for ALZHEIMER'S DISEASE or psychosomatic symptoms. Modern neurologists work closely with specialists in related disciplines: with neurosurgeons in treating tumors and subarachnoid hemorrhage; with neuroradiologists, who image structural disease of the brain and spinal cord; and with neurophysiologists, who use electroencephalography to investigate blackouts and use nerve conduction studies and electromyography to classify the diseases of peripheral nerves and muscles.

Diagnosing neurological diseases is founded on clinical principles, and pays close attention to the patient's history and to careful physical examination. The advent of non-invasive investigations, such as computed tomography and magnetic resonance imaging of the brain and spine, means that most neurological diagnoses can be made in outpatients. The most common conditions seen by neurologists in the clinic are: headache and facial pain; blackouts and epilepsy; peripheral and cranial nerve disease; spinal nerve root disorders; stroke and transient ischemic attacks; multiple sclerosis; Parkinsonism and other movement disorders; dementia; and giddiness. Together, these account for about three-quarters of consultations. Fortunately, most patients with neurological symptoms do not have a disabling or fatal illness. Bodily symptoms, such as headache, tingling, or clumsiness, are often a result of stress or other psychological disorders, such as depression.

Modern neurology presents doctors and medical researchers with richly varied challenges to improve diagnosis and treatment of neurological diseases. Refined clinical skills are essential for accurate diagnosis in the clinic. Everyday clinical practice confronts complex ethical issues. Effective treatments are increasingly available for disabling disorders, such as multiple sclerosis, motor neurone disease, and peripheral neuropathy, all previously considered untreatable. Ingenious APPLIANCES developed by medical engineering can minimize disability. Neurobiological and neurogenetic research is revolutionizing our understanding of neurological diseases and prompting the design of new treatments.

Some common varieties of neurological problems include the following.

### Blackouts and epilepsy

Attacks of unconsciousness present a common diagnostic problem. Common causes include epilepsy, irregular heart rhythms, and simple faints. Epilepsy results from storms of uncoordinated electrical discharges in the brain. Sudden loss of consciousness results from generalized epileptic discharges throughout the whole brain. These may either involve momentary 'absence' or 'petit mal' attacks, in which the patient becomes blank and inaccessible for a few seconds, or typical 'grand mal seizures', with falling and violent limb shaking often associated with tongue biting and urinary incontinence. In contrast, focal epileptic discharges produce different types of symptoms depending upon where they arise in the brain. These range from repetitive twitchings of the limbs, to episodes of automatic behavior or stereotyped hallucinations.

Diagnosing epilepsy generally depends upon a characteristic description of attacks provided by the patient or a witness. Seizure discharges can be detected by electroencephalography, although the results are often normal when recorded between attacks. An underlying cause of a patient's epilepsy is usually not identifiable; only occasionally is it genetic, but sometimes it results from structural brain damage after severe head injuries or from brain tumors detectable by magnetic resonance imaging.

Anti-epileptic drugs, principally phenytoin, carbamazepine, and sodium valproate, either abolish or diminish seizures in most patients. Newly developed drugs, such as lamotrigine, vigabatrin, and gabapentin, are often helpful in epilepsy resistant to these conventional drugs. A few patients are unresponsive to any drug treatment and may be considered for neurosurgical treatment to remove the focus from which the epileptic discharges are arising in the brain —

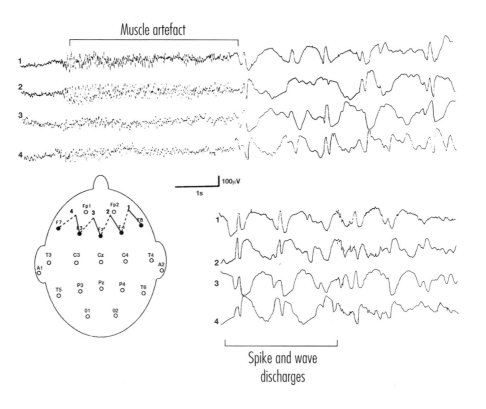

Electroencephalogram in grand mal epilepsy. This shows irregular spikes and waves preceded by a few seconds of high-frequency muscle artefact as the convulsion began.
(From Donaghy, M. (1997). Neurology, OUP.)

particularly if their attacks arise within the temporal lobes.

Modern treatment of epilepsy usually permits patients to follow a normal life-style, allaying the old stigma that epilepsy represents a form of insanity. In most countries, patients with epilepsy are barred from driving until free of seizures for one year; for many this constitutes the main disability caused by their epilepsy.

## Headache and migraine

Headache and facial pain are two of the most common symptoms encountered in everyday neurological practice. Most headaches do not signal medically serious disease, although they may cause considerable disability by intruding on everyday life, and distress because they raise thoughts of serious underlying disease, such as a brain tumor. The most common headaches are migraine and muscle tension headache.

*Simple migraine* causes discrete bouts of intense throbbing headache, lasting between three hours and three days. These are generally associated with nausea or vomiting and dislike of loud noises or bright lights. The headache is usually one-sided, at least at the onset. In **classic migraine** the same type of headache is preceded by a temporary visual disturbance lasting 15–30 minutes, manifesting as patches of lost vision, tunnel vision, brightly colored spots (photopsia), or zig-zag lines (fortification spectra). Occasionally this 'aura' causes temporary speech loss, pins and needles, or limb weakness. Migraine tends to run in families. Attacks may be precipitated by menstrual periods, cheese, chocolate, or wine. Drugs to treat individual attacks include simple pain killers, ergotamine, and recently introduced 5-hydroxytryptamine-agonist drugs such as sumatriptan. Patients disabled by frequent severe attacks should eliminate any identified precipitating factors from their diet if possible. They may prevent regular and disabling attacks by taking daily prophylactic medications such as propranolol or pizotifen.

Tension headache consists of a tight band or pressure sensation encircling the head; brief bouts of this will be familiar to most people. When chronic, it is present in varying severity on most days, and tends to worsen as the day goes by. The cause of tension headache is not clear, but sustained contraction of scalp muscles is often blamed. It may occur in depressive illness or anxiety states, but is usually encountered in hard-working yet otherwise well-balanced individuals. Treatment may include advice about reducing stress, undertaking regular physical exercise or relaxation, and low dosage antidepressant drugs such as amitriptyline.

*Medically sinister headache* Only occasionally does headache signify serious disease requiring investigation with brain imaging or lumbar puncture. Headache of abrupt onset, often during physical exertion, occurs in subarachnoid hemorrhage. Gradually worsening daily headache, worse on awakening, occurs when raised pressure within the skull results from brain tumors, abscesses, hydrocephalus, or benign intracranial hypertension. Meningitis causes headache associated with stiffness of the neck and dislike of bright lights. In elderly patients, inflammation of blood vessels called giant cell arteritis causes severe scalp tenderness; prompt treatment with steroids is essential to prevent blindness due to involvement of the eye's arteries.

## Stroke

Strokes are sudden neurologic disturbances due to diseased brain blood vessels. Those resulting from blocked brain arteries are termed 'ischemic strokes'. If brain arteries burst, blood clots form either within the brain, 'intracerebral hematoma', or within the meningeal membranes which surround the brain, 'subarachnoid hemorrhage'. These ischemic and hemorrhagic forms of stroke are clearly distinguishable by brain scans, which show whether bleeding has occurred. Stroke is a common cause of severe disability and death, particularly in the elderly. For reasons not wholly clear (but related in part to improved blood pressure control), stroke is becoming less common in western countries.

*Ischemic strokes* cause loss of normal neurological function in the part of the brain deprived of its blood supply. Most commonly, strokes cause weakness of one side of the body (hemiplegia) or difficulty with speech (aphasia) when the blockage affects the middle cerebral artery, or loss of half of the field of vision (hemianopia) if a posterior cerebral artery is blocked. Small blood clots, called emboli, are the usual cause of blocked brain arteries. Emboli usually come from a heart with diseased valves or an irregular rhythm, or from narrowed carotid arteries in the neck. Once an embolus has lodged in a small artery, the surrounding area of brain dies, permanently losing its function. No treatment can prevent permanent brain damage once an embolus has firmly lodged for an hour or two, but recent evidence shows that very early administration of 'clot-busting' drugs (or thrombolytics) can reduce this damage. Fortunately, emboli sometimes break up and pass onward, restoring blood flow. If this occurs within the first few hours, complete recovery of neurological function quickly follows. If complete recovery occurs within 24 hours, such attacks are termed 'transient cerebral ischemic attacks (TIAs)'. These signal an increased risk of permanent stroke in the future. Prompt assessment is required to identify any reversible risk factors. If the emboli arise from a severely narrowed internal carotid artery, surgical reboring (carotid endarterectomy) may reduce the risk of further attacks or future stroke. Patients can reduce their risk of further strokes by taking daily low-dose aspirin (50 mg a day), which beneficially affects blood coagulation and the tendency to form emboli.

*Subarachnoid hemorrhage* is the most usual form of hemorrhagic stroke, and occurs when weakened arteries rupture into the meningeal membrane coverings around the brain. It causes an abrupt severe headache, and sometimes instantaneous death. Brain imaging may visualize the hemorrhage, or lumbar puncture detects blood in the spinal fluid. The source of the bleeding is pinpointed by X-rays of brain blood vessels (angiogram). Most usually it arises from a distended weakened artery wall or aneurysm. This can be repaired neurosurgically to prevent recurrence. Recently neuroradiologists have started obliterating aneurysms from within blood vessels, thereby eliminating the need for a neurosurgical operation in some patients.

Less frequently the hemorrhage comes from a tangle of blood vessels present from birth, an arteriovenous malformation. Some patients have a normal angiogram test, often smokers or oral contraceptive consumers, and they have a better long-term outlook. Subarachnoid hemorrhage is a serious condition, and permanent brain damage may occur even in those who survive the initial hemorrhage. This is because the continued presence of blood in the meningeal coverings of the brain can induce spasm of other brain arteries many days later, resulting in secondary ischemic strokes.

### Multiple sclerosis

Multiple sclerosis is due to attacks of damage to patches of myelin (the lining of the nerve fibers) in the white matter pathways of the brain or spinal cord. This demyelination blocks the transmission of nervous messages along the nerve fibers within the affected pathway. The underlying cause of multiple sclerosis is not known, but the leading contenders are an autoimmune attack by the body upon its own myelin or the effects of a viral infection. It is particularly common in temperate countries. Multiple sclerosis usually causes a succession of attacks affecting different parts of the nervous system. Particularly vulnerable are the optic nerves, which transmit messages from the eyes to the brain, with loss of vision; the spinal cord, causing limb weakness and impaired urinary control; and the brain stem, causing

double vision and loss of balance and coordination. Partial recovery occurs after each attack, and this may be speeded up by short treatments with corticosteroids. A diagnosis of multiple sclerosis is based on a history of relapsing and remitting symptoms — that is, symptoms affecting at least two separate areas of the brain or spinal cord at different times. Investigations may support this clinical diagnosis; delayed visual evoked responses may reveal slowed transmission along optic nerves affected by a previous silent attack. Magnetic resonance brain scans show widespread plaques of demyelination within the white matter (myelin) of the brain.

The clinical course and severity of multiple sclerosis are unpredictable for any individual patient. At the mildest extreme, a patient may only ever experience two attacks representing episodes of demyelination. At the other extreme, severe disability may result from progressive accumulation of widespread plaques of demyelination. Such patients often become wheelchair bound, and clumsiness may limit the use of their hands. Most patients with multiple sclerosis fall between these two extremes. These range from those who have a few attacks during their lifetime but no appreciable residual disability, to those in whom numerous attacks have caused a degree of permanent disability but who remain reasonably independent. No treatment can prevent further attacks of multiple sclerosis or enhance the degree of eventual recovery from each attack. However, regular administration of β-interferon does reduce the frequency of attacks and may reduce the amount of long-term disability which results. There is no clear evidence that dietary manipulations are effective, though supplementation of polyunsaturated fatty acids has been popular with some. For those who are cruelly disabled by multiple sclerosis, often as young adults, skilled rehabilitation can minimize the degree of disability.

### Neurodegenerative diseases

Certain disabling neurological diseases result from progressive and premature death of specific groups of nerve cells in the brain or spinal cord. These neurodegenerative diseases are particularly common in the elderly. They include the memory loss of ALZHEIMER'S DISEASE, the movement disorder of Parkinson's disease, and the muscle weakness of motor neurone disease. They are usually of unknown cause and inherited forms account for less than 10%.

*Alzheimer's disease* is the most common cause of dementia. To begin with, the symptoms are minor and may be attributed to absent-mindedness. Then errors of judgement are noted and alarm is generated eventually when the names of family members can't be remembered and there is loss of interest in hobbies and recreations. Memory is lost along with other cognitive abilities, such as calculation, reasoning, and insight. Ultimately the personality disintegrates: 'He is not the same man that I married'. After death, it is found that nerve cells have been lost from the cerebral cortex and other parts of the brain and microscopy reveals the characteristic 'neurofibrillary tangles' originally described by ALZHEIMER (p 39). Although Alzheimer's disease itself is not treatable or preventable, brain scans may reveal alternative causes for dementia, such as multiple small strokes, or a hydrocephalus which may improve after neurosurgical shunting to drain the cerebral ventricles.

**Parkinson's disease** involves a 'pill-rolling' tremor of the hands, 'lead-pipe' rigidity of the limbs, and slowed movements causing reduced facial expression and blinking, small handwriting, poor manipulation, and a slow shuffling gait. It results from loss of the nerve cells in the substantia nigra of the brain stem which normally secrete the neurotransmitter dopamine. After death, microscopic inspection of surviving nerve cells shows characteristic Lewy body inclusions. Parkinsonian symptoms improve substantially with L-dopa medication, which supplements this deficiency of dopamine. Later in the disease, L-dopa becomes less effective, and patients' responses may fluctuate dramatically. Similar Parkinsonian syndromes may also be a side-effect of major tranquilizer drugs used in psychiatry which block dopamine's actions.

**In motor neurone disease** (amyotrophic lateral sclerosis) the muscles waste away and weaken. This is a result of death of those lower motor neurones (nerve cells) which directly supply the muscles and also of the upper motor neurones in the brain which control them. The disease starts either in a limb with weakness, or in the muscles of the mouth and throat, causing difficulty in speech production, eating, swallowing, or breathing. It does not affect skin sensation, or the control of urination or sexual function. Mental faculties are preserved, highlighting the distress of patients, who are fully conscious of becoming prisoners within bodies they can no longer move. No cure is known for motor neurone disease, and no way is known of arresting the inevitable deterioration. Recently the drug riluzole has been shown to prolong survival slightly in motor neurone disease, although it is not clear that it preserves muscular functions.

### Infections

**Meningitis** is an infection of the meningeal membranes covering the brain. It may be caused by bacteria, viruses, or fungi. The range of infections has widened now that many patients have impaired immune defences due to organ transplantation or AIDS. Bacterial meningitis is a serious disease causing permanent brain damage or death unless diagnosed promptly and treated with antibiotics. Initial symptoms of headache, fever, neck stiffness, and intolerance of light may progress to coma within hours. Diagnosis is by lumbar puncture yielding cerebrospinal fluid containing copious inflammatory cells and bacteria; hemophilus, neisseria, pneumococcus, and TUBERCULOSIS are the species of bacteria most commonly encountered.

**Encephalitis** is an inflammation within the substance of the brain, either due to invasion by viruses (such as *Herpes simplex*, the 'cold sore' virus) or as a remote effect of viral infections elsewhere in the body (such as measles). Headache, fever, and seizures develop, often with speech difficulties, confusion, or coma. The exact virus responsible for acute encephalitis is commonly not identifiable. The antiviral drug acyclovir treats the *Herpes simplex* form; nowadays most patients with encephalitis receive this drug pending accurate virological diagnosis. Without treatment, encephalitis may cause death, or leave residual memory disturbances, epilepsy, or Parkinsonism. Fortunately, many patients now recover from encephalitis.

The brain may be affected by some slowly progressive infections. CREUTZFELDT-JAKOB DISEASE (similar to mad-cow disease or bovine spongiform encephalopathy) is due to a subviral particle called a prion and causes dementia accompanied by sudden ('myoclonic') limb jerkings. Sub-acute sclerosing panecephalitis is due to latent measles virus infection of the brain, also causing myoclonic jerking and intellectual decline; it is becoming extremely rare now that children are routinely immunized against measles. HIV infection can cause a slowly progressive dementia. Slowly progressive leg weakness (tropical spastic paraplegia) results from infection with another retrovirus, human T-cell lymphocytotrophic virus.                    MD

*See also* INFECTIOUS DISEASES; LANGUAGE

**NEUROMUSCULAR DISEASES** involve either the muscles or their nerve supply causing muscle weakness, paralysis, and sometimes muscle wasting. Diagnosis depends on analysis of the clinical and family history, examination to detect weakness or wasting of individual muscles, estimating the blood levels of enzymes such as creatine kinase, using electrophysiological measurements of activity in muscles or nerves, or removing by needle or surgical biopsy a sample of muscle for microscopical or biochemical study.

## Motor neurone disease

Motor neurone disease (amyotrophic lateral sclerosis or Lou Gehrig's disease — after a famous baseball player) is a degenerative disorder usually of middle or late life. (See NEUROLOGY)

## Spinal muscular atrophies

The spinal muscular atrophies are conditions affecting the anterior horn cells of the spinal cord but not the upper motor neurones. Sometimes the cranial nerves are also affected, giving rise to difficulty with speech and swallowing, less often impaired eye movements or facial weakness. Most types are inherited in a recessive manner due to a gene located on chromosome 5. A severe infantile form (Werdnig–Hoffmann disease) causes diffuse muscular weakness, floppiness of the muscles, progressive paralysis, respiratory insufficiency, and usually death in the first year of life. Milder varieties cause localized, restricted, or more diffuse weakness of limb and trunk muscles.

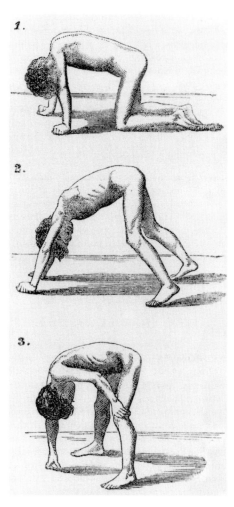

Gowers's sign or maneuver from the book *Pseudohypertrophic muscular paralysis*, published 1879. (From Emery, A. (1994). *Muscular dystrophy: the facts*, OUP.)

## Neuropathies

Neuropathies are disorders of the peripheral nerves. Localized neuropathies may be due to physical injury or compression due to disease. The ulnar nerve may be irritated behind the inner side of the elbow (funny bone) giving rise to tingling and pins and needles in the little and ring fingers, and sometimes wasting of the small hand muscles. The carpal tunnel syndrome is caused by compression of the median nerve at the wrist due to swelling of flexor tendon sheaths resulting from overuse; it may produce pins and needles in the fingers and thumb, which often waken the patient from sleep. Blockage of the arteries to peripheral nerves may be due to diabetes, or inflammation of the arteries as in polyarteritis nodosa or leprosy.

Diffuse disease of the peripheral nerves (polyneuropathies) may be due to vitamin B1 deficiency (nutritional or due to chronic alcoholism), heavy metal poisons (lead, arsenic, gold, etc.), diabetes, malignant disease, drugs such as isoniazid, leprosy, or vitamin B12 deficiency in pernicious anemia. In the Guillain–Barré syndrome patients develop weakness rapidly at first in muscles of the shoulders, upper arm, hips, and thighs with occasional tingling and pins and needles in the fingers and toes over a few days, sometimes leading to paralysis of all four limbs and even of the respiratory muscles, requiring assisted respiration. If serious complications such as respiratory weakness can be prevented or controlled, patients ultimately recover completely. Steroid drugs are of no value but plasma exchange (plasmapheresis) may help. There are also many hereditary or genetically determined forms of polyneuropathy, including Charcot– Marie–Tooth disease, in which muscular weakness and wasting are usually limited to muscles below the knees and those of the hands.

## Muscular dystrophies

Muscular dystrophies are inherited muscle degenerative diseases. The Duchenne type, being X-linked, affects virtually only boys. Some do not walk until 18–20 months; all have difficulty in walking by about three years, with frequent falling, clumsy running, difficulty in climbing stairs, and getting up from the floor. The calf muscles are often enlarged, but the upper and lower limb muscles are weak and wasted. Most patients are confined to a wheelchair by the age of 10 and few survive beyond the age of 25. Death is due to respiratory infection or disease of the heart muscle. The culpable gene was characterized in 1987 by Kunkel and his colleagues at Boston Children's Hospital, leading later to the discovery that dystrophin, a protein, is totally absent in boys with Duchenne dystrophy and greatly reduced in the Becker type and in many female carriers of the Duchenne gene, some of whom show variable degrees of muscular weakness (manifesting carriers). An immunochemical method of staining for dystrophin has added precision to diagnosis by muscle biopsy. Isolation of the gene allows the accurate identification of female carriers (especially among the sisters of dystrophic boys). Prenatal diagnosis in pregnant carriers is now possible using chorionic cell biopsy, feasible earlier in pregnancy than amniocentesis, thus making possible selective abortion of affected males.

Other types of muscular dystrophy, such as the Becker, or the limb-girdle varieties, begin later. They tend to run a more benign course, and may affect specific and facioscapulohumeral groups of muscles.

## Myotonic disorders

Myotonia is a form of delayed muscular relaxation: after the patient is asked to relax, there is an after-contraction which can be recorded electrically. A patient being asked to open a hand after gripping an object is unable to do so quickly and the fingers uncoil slowly. A tap on the tongue or on a limb muscle produces a dimple, which slowly disappears. Myotonia congenita is generalized from birth, but no other disability develops. The outlook is excellent, but the myotonia, worse in cold weather, restricts movement. In some families myotonia congenita is dominantly inherited (Thomsen's disease). A recessively inherited variety beginning late in childhood is also benign. Myotonia may be relieved by drugs such as quinine, procainamide, or phenytoin, but the response is variable.

In dystrophia myotonica (Steinert's disease), on the other hand, myotonia is often limited at first to the hands, and may be clinically unobtrusive or detectable only by electromyography. Facial weakness, cataracts, weakness of sternomastoid muscles, and distal wasting and weakness of limb muscles develop usually in adolescence or early adult life. The condition, due to a gene on chromosome 19, is progressive and disabling, most patients dying before the normal age. Infants of mothers with myotonic dystrophy may be very 'floppy' or hypotonic at birth, and often show marked developmental delay before developing typical myotonic dystrophy in adolescence.

## Inflammatory myopathy

Polymyositis is an autoimmune disease in which one type of white blood cells, the lymphocytes, become sensitized against the muscles and invade and damage them. There is often, but not always, muscle pain and tenderness with diffuse, non-

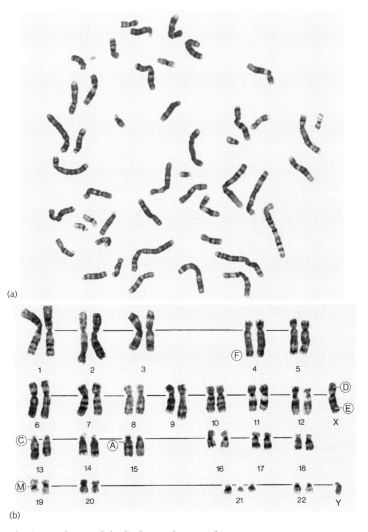

(a)

(b)

selective weakness of the limb muscles near the trunk. Sometimes there is difficulty in swallowing and inflammation of the skin, when the condition is called dermatomyositis. This condition may occur at any age, but in middle or late life it often complicates malignant disease in the lung or elsewhere. Treatment with drugs such as prednisone and immunosuppressive agents such as azathioprine is usually successful, except when the disease is associated with cancer.

Viral diseases of muscle include influenzal inflammation (myositis) and Bornholm disease (an acute myositis with fever, causing difficulty in breathing and pain in the chest wall and diaphragm for a few days and due to Coxsackie A3 virus). Bacterial inflammation may be due to *Staphylococcus aureus,* while infestation with the parasite *Trichinella spiralis* (trichinosis or trichiniasis), acquired through eating undercooked contaminated pork, may mimic polymyositis.

Chromosomes stained to show banding patterns by which each can be identified. (a) Shows a chromosome spread. (b) The karyotype derived from the chromosome spread. Indicated are the positions of the genes for various dystrophies: Duchenne and Becker (D); Emery-Dreifuss (E); limb girdle of childhood (C) and (A); facioscapulohumeral (F); and mytonic dystrophy (M). (From Emery, A. (1994). *Muscular dystrophy: the facts,* OUP.)

Polymyalgia rheumatica, a disease of the elderly, gives diffuse muscle pain which restricts movement but produces no weakness; the response to treatment with steroids is immediate.

## Myasthenia gravis

Myasthenia gravis is another autoimmune disease; circulating antibodies form against the acetylcholine receptor (specialized nerve ending) on the surface of muscle fibers with which acetylcholine (released at the end of nerve fibers when they activate muscles) combines. This antibody coats the receptors so that acetylcholine cannot have its full effect; the muscles become weak and fatigable; repeated contraction causes increasing weakness. Typically the condition, more common in women and beginning at any age, affects external ocular muscles, with drooping of the eyelids towards the end of the day, with or without double vision. Often the patient finds it difficult to speak, swallow, and chew (difficulty in chewing which increases during a meal is almost diagnostic). Variable weakness of limb muscles without wasting is also common, always accentuated by exercise. The diagnosis is confirmed by estimating circulating antibodies and clinically by injecting intravenously edrophonium chloride (Tensilon); this reverses the weakness, if only for a few seconds or minutes. This drug inhibits cholinesterase, the enzyme which breaks down acetylcholine. Sustained benefit may be produced by longer-acting drugs such as pyridostigmine. In the long term, it is more effective to remove surgically the thymus gland producing the T lymphocytes, which by interacting with B lymphocytes help to produce the antibodies. Steroids and immunosuppressants are also helpful. In an acute emergency, plasmapheresis may be of temporary benefit.

## Other muscle disorders

The so-called floppy infant syndrome includes many benign congenital myopathies of variable severity and rate of progression associated with specific structural abnormalities in the muscle fibers. In some metabolic and endocrine myopathies patients develop weakness of the muscles in the upper arm and legs. This is often seen in patients with thyrotoxicosis, whereas the reverse (hypothyroidism) may cause slowness of muscular contraction and relaxation, with muscular enlargement.

In the so-called familial periodic paralyses of dominant inheritance patients have episodes of diffuse muscular weakness, precipitated by exertion or by a heavy carbohydrate meal. In some, the attacks are accompanied by a rise in serum potassium (hyperkalemic type), in others by a fall (hypokalemic type). Several other muscle disorders are associated with abnormalities of fat metabolism. JW

**FOUNDER FIGURES**

Pedro Manuel de
**ALMEIDA LIMA**
(1903–83). Portuguese neurosurgeon. Almeida Lima was born in Lisbon and educated at the university there, where his father was professor of physics and university President; he abandoned an early interest in geology (he was briefly in charge of the seismology section of the Lisbon Geological Observatory) in favor of the medical sciences. Lima's well-known collaboration with Egas Moniz began almost immediately. With the support of Moniz he was enabled to develop his experience and skill at the London Hospital under Sir Hugh Cairns, whose neurosurgical unit there had been established in 1932. Among his contributions, the development of cerebral angiography is of great importance. In collaboration with Moniz he established, in 1926, the feasibility of visualizing the blood vessels of the brain by the radiographic contrast method, working first with dogs and cadavers and later with patients. Lima was also responsible, with Moniz, for the introduction of psychosurgery in 1935 by performing the first frontal leucotomy for treatment of an organic psychosis.

(*continued opposite*)

## NEUROSURGERY — HISTORY

While neurosurgery in its current form is a modern development, medical practitioners have been attempting to treat intracranial disease with surgery since neolithic times. Trepanned skulls are found in the relics of many primitive cultures. The purpose of these operations remains obscure, but the pathological evidence indicates that many patients survived these operations, whatever their object. Trepanning was widely practiced in pre-Columbian America and was observed in Africa well into this century.

Neurosurgery as a specialty is less than a century old. The pioneering efforts of the great European general surgeons to operate on the brain became possible because of the development of ANESTHESIA in 1846 and the introduction of antiseptic surgery by LISTER (p 473). Enormous gains in understanding clinical neurophysiology and neurological localization in the brain came just before modern neurosurgery was born and were extremely important to the development of rational surgery. Sir William Macewen was the first to describe successful removal of intracranial tumors, mostly meningiomas arising from the lining of the brain, identified because of their protrusion through the skull. Godlee is generally credited with having been the first to operate upon an intrinsic brain tumor in a modern hospital setting. Sir Victor Horsley was the first surgeon to devote a substantial part of his practice to neurological diseases. He established neurosurgery as a surgical discipline, but it remained for Harvey CUSHING (p 537) to make it a specialty.

In 1901 Harvey CUSHING (p 537) returned to JOHNS HOPKINS HOSPITAL (p 840), where he had received his general surgical training, after a year of research with Kocher in Bern. Against the advice of his chief, William HALSTED (p 746), he elected to limit his practice to neurological diseases early in his career. During the succeeding 12 years in Baltimore, he applied the meticulous anatomical surgical techniques of Halsted to the nervous system and reduced the enormous morbidity and mortality of neurosurgical procedures to levels which rival those today. It is less appreciated that Cushing, with his mentors, Halsted and OSLER (p 602), founded the Hunterian Surgical Laboratory at Johns Hopkins and originated the concept of the trained clinician/scientist in academic medicine. Pusepp was Harvey Cushing's counterpart in Europe. He also specialized in neurosurgery and built a neurosurgery center in the Baltic similar to the one Cushing began in Boston. Unfortunately, the political events in Russia and the Baltic in the early part of the century destroyed his contribution, which is now largely forgotten.

In 1912 Cushing went to Boston to the Peter Bent Brigham Hospital, where he continued his innovations. The use of suction in surgery and of electrocautery for stopping bleeding both came from his operating rooms. Cushing and his colleagues published extensively on the pituitary and its disorders. His book, *The pituitary body* (1912), founded surgical ENDOCRINOLOGY. His surgical experience led to a classification of malignant tumors of the brain (gliomas), a detailed description of acoustic neuromas, and clarification of meningiomas. Through his efforts a school of surgery developed which soon became worldwide. Cushing drew students from many countries and they in turn spread the Cushing concept that neurological patients required dedicated surgeons and special departments for their care.

### Early operations

The first general surgeons who undertook neurosurgical operations concentrated on visible tumors and infections. As the discipline developed, a limited number of other neurological diseases amenable to treatment were added. Operations for trigeminal neuralgia (tic douloureux) were common and Cushing's interest in the pituitary led many of his followers to concentrate upon these rare tumors. Some meningiomas located in favorable areas could be totally removed, and others were at least partially removable. Gliomas were usually treated by lobectomy if possible, by internal decompression, or by simple cranial bony decompression when a deep-seated tumor could not be found. Acoustic tumors were operated upon by subtotal intracapsular removal. Neurosurgeons treated trauma to the nervous system and some blood clots (hematomas) were successfully removed. The mortality of these early efforts was enormous and rarely improved on the natural history of the disease.

### Change from palliation to cure

Walter DANDY (this page), a pupil of Cushing and his successor at Johns Hopkins, was responsible for the philosophical changes that moved neurosurgery from a PALLIATIVE discipline to its modern concepts of accurate localization of disease and surgery for cure. In 1918 Dandy introduced the new technique of ventriculography, which for the first time allowed the accurate preoperative localization that was mandatory for success. Dandy added the concept that the goal of every operation should be the cure of the offending lesion. He was successful in the total removal of acoustic tumors. He was the first to operate upon arteriovenous malformations and the first to clip intracranial aneurysms. Through his operations for tinnitus and vertigo, Dandy established the concept of functional neurosurgery, in which

symptoms of neurological disease are treated by operations upon the nervous system. Dandy also performed an equally remarkable laboratory investigation, which established the causes of hydrocephalus and is fundamental to our understanding of the circulation of the cerebrospinal fluid.

Before Walter Dandy's time, all cerebral localization was carried out by assessing the neurological history and determining the attendant signs. This was a fallible technique in the best of hands, and many of Cushing's operations were simple decompressions when the tumor could not be found. Abnormalities seen on plain radiographs of the skull followed. Dandy's ventriculography allowed accurate localization of intracranial lesions and remained a standard technique until the 1970s. In 1931 Egas MONIZ (p 538) and ALMEIDA LIMA (p 536) introduced cerebral angiography (X-rays of blood vessels), which demonstrated all kinds of vascular lesions and, after refinement, assessment of the cerebral circulation. Myelography (X-ray examination) with positive contrast (radio-opaque) agents was introduced by Siccard and Forrestiere. This technique allowed localization of spinal lesions.

The first functional technique for cerebral localization was radioactive brain scanning. The accumulation of a radioactive material after intravenous injection could be imaged to provide additional information about intrinsic abnormalities which might be difficult to demonstrate because of a paucity of anatomical distortion.

Early angiographic studies were limited by the contrast agents available, and the need for direct puncture of the blood vessels. Development of safe contrast agents was paralleled by the use of intravascular catheters. Simple catheter techniques were soon replaced by flexible catheters, which could be manipulated into individual brain vessels from a distant source, such as the femoral artery in the groin. Angiography became safe, much less painful, and highly specific. These dramatic advances prepared the way for the endovascular therapeutics of today.

Similar advances occurred in myelography. The first agents were unsatisfactory, but the introduction of iodized oil (pantopaque) made myelography practicable and safe. However, these oils were poorly absorbed by the body. They have been replaced by water-soluble agents, which are readily excreted. Each new agent has fewer problems than those it replaced, and myelography has become less and less complicated.

Until the early 1970s air studies, angiography, and myelography were the standard diagnostic techniques on which neurological localization and neurosurgery depended. In the early 1970s computerized axial tomography was introduced

(continued)

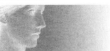

Harvey Williams **CUSHING** (1869–1939). American neurosurgeon and physiologist. He began his academic career at JOHNS HOPKINS (p 840). In 1912, he became first chief of surgery at the Peter Bent Brigham Hospital. He carried out many craniotomies to remove brain tumors, usually under local anaesthesia. He observed changes in body appearance associated with pituitary tumors (Cushing's syndrome), and also noted that removal of the pituitary led to atrophy of the genitals. As author of the classic biography of William OSLER (p 602), he shared Osler's interest in medical history.

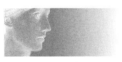

Walter Edward **DANDY** (1886–1946). American neurosurgeon. Dandy became head of neurological surgery at the JOHNS HOPKINS Hospital, where he introduced many technical procedures and trained younger associates. He developed diagnostic methods for localizing tumors by injection of air into the cerebral ventricles or into the spinal subarachnoid space (pneumoencephalography). He was among the first to localize and remove prolapsed intervertebral discs.

(continued overleaf)

(continued)

Antonio Caetano de Egas **MONIZ** (1874–1955). Portuguese neurosurgeon. Moniz was the foundation professor of neurology in Lisbon in 1911 and the first to carry out cerebral angiography (1927) and frontal leucotomy (1935). A man of many and varied talents, he wrote an operetta and was a distinguished historian and literary critic. He was elected to Parliament in 1908, and became Foreign Minister in 1918. A political quarrel in 1919 led to a duel and his retirement from politics. He was awarded the NOBEL PRIZE for medicine in 1949.

and a revolution in imaging began. This scan uses a computer to capture and display the large amount of information generated by X-rays passing through the body which cannot be displayed on conventional film. The capture of these images and the techniques for their display were the work of Hounsfield, although advances have occurred widely since his original monumental contribution. The computerized tomography scan revolutionized intracranial and spinal imaging. For the first time the intracranial tumor and all of its effects upon the brain could be seen. Spinal cord tumors were seen less well, but the combination of computerized tomography imaging with water-soluble myelography provided superb visualization of intraspinal structures. The accuracy of scanning was remarkable — the brain and spinal cord could be seen with a test that was generally safe and painless. The impact upon neurosurgery was enormous — neurosurgeons could assess: the results of trauma accurately; the location of tumors and their effects on the rest of the brain; the presence of blood and the location of hematomas; the degree of hydrocephalus; and the source of spinal fluid obstructions, congenital abnormalities of the brain, and, of equal importance, the postoperative status of the brain of patients who were not doing well after surgery. The accuracy of scanning changed the focus of neurology and neurosurgery from diagnosis to treatment.

The addition of magnetic resonance imaging (MRI) was equally revolutionary. Not only were intracranial abnormalities seen with detail unimagined before, but the normal structures of the brain were visualized with great accuracy. Functional abnormalities, such as the plaques of multiple sclerosis, or small lesions, such as those of subclinical strokes, leave changes which can be seen. Furthermore, exposure to radiation is avoided by the use of magnetic fields. The current techniques of magnetic resonance imaging provide the anatomical standard by which all other localizing studies are judged. The neurosurgeon may now rely upon precise diagnosis and accurate localization so that the surgical incisions can be minimized, important surrounding structures are identified in advance, and a rapid postoperative assessment of patients with problems is available.

In the late 1980s the concept of three-dimensional reconstruction using both types of images was developed. The computer programs to carry out these reconstructions now allow anatomically accurate reconstruction of images of the head, skull, brain, and its appendages with virtual anatomical accuracy.

Refinements in the physical characteristics of MRI continually improve resolution and have led to the new technique called 'functional imaging'.

The original techniques allowed anatomical imaging only. Advances have led to images which assess function and dysfunction of the brain. These allow researchers to examine localization of specific functions in the brain such as speech in individual patients. Dysfunctions such as the epileptic seizure focus or the sequels of head injury can be identified. We are still in the very early phases of using MRI to study function of the normal brain and to examine the effects of diseases upon those normal functions.          DML

**NEUROSURGERY** Between the end of the Second World War until the mid-1970s, neurosurgery matured, and remarkable advances were made throughout the world. The techniques were largely those of Harvey CUSHING (p 537) and Walter DANDY (p 537) modified by outstanding surgeons in many countries. Surgery for trigeminal neuralgia, operations on pituitary tumors, removal of intracranial and spinal tumors, and the treatment of trauma were all important aspects of neurosurgery. TRAUMA, in particular, was studied extensively during and after the Second World War and in the lesser wars that followed. However, a number of new topics were added or developed from earlier beginnings.

In 1934, Mixter and Barr described operations for the removal of the ruptured intervertebral disc which had herniated into the spinal canal. The recognition of the herniated disc as a frequent cause of disabling lumbago and sciatica received immediate surgical attention throughout the world. The herniated lumbar, and subsequently the cervical disc, became a principal focus for neurosurgeons, particularly in North America. Surgery for these disc protrusions remains an important part of neurosurgical practice today.

Egas MONIZ (this page) and ALMEIDA LIMA (p 536) introduced frontal leucotomy for treating psychiatric disease in 1935. Surgery on the frontal and temporal lobes and the thalamus was explored broadly in the 1940s and 1950s. While the techniques were of great value for many patients, psychosurgery has virtually disappeared, for pharmacological, social, and political reasons. There is now a modest interest in re-examining the concept of psychosurgery for some psychiatric and psychological dysfunctions based on the greatly improved understanding of the brain and its functions.

Stereotactic localization of subcortical structures had been in laboratory use since the time of Horsley and Clarke. Through the 1940s and 1950s, several surgeons developed instruments that allowed the destruction of deep brain targets for the treatment of tremors and other forms of abnormal movement and for pain and epilepsy. The techniques were most widely employed for the tremor or Parkinsonism, and thousands of patients world-wide were treated. The development of effective medication virtually eliminated stereotaxis by the mid-1970s.

In the past five years there has been an enormous increase in the use of stereotactic surgery for Parkinson's syndrome and other disorders of movement. Research into the organization of the human motor system has led to an improved understanding, which in turn allows surgery to be much more precise. The relief of symptoms is substantially better than with older operations and the risks to patients are reduced.

### Epilepsy and pain

Convulsive seizures are among the oldest afflictions of recorded history and certainly one of the most dramatic. Epilepsy was a major study of early neurologists and Horsley attempted to treat epilepsy in the earliest days of neurosurgery. However, it remained for Wilder PENFIELD (p 138) and many colleagues at the Montreal Neurological Institute to make the study and treatment of epilepsy a serious surgical venture. Penfield made great contributions by establishing the first extensive cerebral localizing maps for man, categorizing the epilepsies, and providing relief for many afflicted patients. The rise in epilepsy surgery was paralleled by the development of more effective anticonvulsant drugs, and the need for epilepsy surgery diminished somewhat. Nevertheless, temporal lobectomy, hemispherectomy, and removal of isolated abnormal areas of cortex for the control of epilepsy all became standard neurosurgical procedures.

Treatment of trigeminal neuralgia was one of the first operations to interest neurosurgeons. Foerster described the effects of dividing spinal nerves for the relief of PAIN. Spiller suggested division of the anterolateral quadrant of the spinal cord and neurosurgeons prided themselves on their skill in doing this operation (cordotomy) for the relief of pain, usually the pain of cancer. Mullan suggested performing the operation with a needle inserted through the skin into the spinothalamic tract. This operation became so popular that it supplanted the open operation. More recently, the development of long-acting narcotics for cancer pain has reduced the need for cordotomy.

Neurosurgical interest in trigeminal neuralgia continues. Rather than the open operations used by earlier surgeons, Sweet devised a technique of insertion of a fine needle carrying a radiofrequency current behind the Gasserian ganglion through a foramen at the base of the skull. The technique has been modified by the injection of noxious agents, and in one form or another the

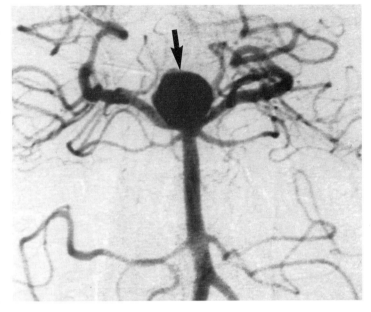

percutaneous procedure has virtually eliminated trigeminal surgery.

An alternative development has been microvascular decompression by Jannetta. He theorized that trigeminal neuralgia often results because abnormal blood vessels compress or irritate the trigeminal nerve in the posterior fossa. Jannetta has devised ways of moving these nerves using microsurgical techniques through a limited exposure. Undoubtedly the operation is successful and carries no risk of facial sensory loss, which may attend the other techniques.

Neurosurgeons have also pioneered the use of pain-relieving procedures which attempt to alter nervous system function by electrical stimulation. Various devices, to be placed around

Arteriogram showing a basilar apex aneurysm. The large globular aneurysm is seen nestled between the two posterior cerebral arteries at the apex of the trunk of the basilar artery.

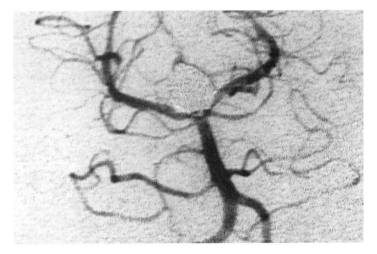

Endovascular coils have been placed in the aneurysm, obliterating it completely, with preservation of all normal vessels.

peripheral nerves, over the spinal cord, or within the brain, are available and have been in use for over 20 years. They remain helpful in a limited number of patients, but are the province of a few experts.

### Diversion of the cerebrospinal fluid

Hydrocephalus was understood after the pioneering work of Dandy, and many neurosurgeons attempted to relieve the problem. Cushing and Dandy used open craniotomy to puncture the lamina terminalis, thus opening the ventricles into the subarachnoid space. A variety of techniques to divert the spinal fluid into some other body cavity were proposed, but none were effective until the development of valved systems that allowed the controlled delivery of excess spinal fluid into the vascular system or abdomen. There are now several of these shunts available. All share the basic concept of a valve that regulates pressure or flow, thus controlling the flow of fluid from the ventricle into a body cavity where it can be absorbed. Because of the reduced number of complications, the peritoneum is now the most common site of diversion. Hydrocephalus has been changed from a uniformly fatal or disabling disease into one in which a child may be restored to relatively normal function.

The development of small fiberoptic scopes allows the inspection of the interior of the ventricular system of the brain. With these magnifying devices, which allow the ventricles to be carefully explored, it is possible to perform the operation of third ventriculostomy originally devised by Cushing and Dandy through a single burr hole and a very small incision. This MINIMALLY INVASIVE SURGERY relieves hydrocephalus (swelling of the brain through obstructed drainage) in many patients and avoids the use of any of the shunting devices.

### Congenital anomalies

The successful treatment of other forms of congenital anomalies of the nervous system has been equally dramatic. While nervous system function cannot be restored, it is possible to prevent complications, treat the other anomalies, and allow these children to live a worthwhile life by repair of the spinal defect. Craniosynostosis, the premature closure of skull sutures which produces marked skull deformities, can be repaired as well. These children, who previously would have been relegated to the life of a freak, are made to look acceptable.

Surgery in the neck on the blood vessels supplying the brain has been in common use for over 40 years. Operations on the vertebral system are usually limited to unusual abnormalities and are the province of a few highly specialized vascular surgeons. By contrast, stenotic disease at the carotid bifurcation (the point where the carotid artery divides) has been treated by general surgeons, vascular surgeons, and neurosurgeons throughout this time. In the recent past, extensive studies have demonstrated the validity of endarterectomy for patients with over 70% narrowing of the carotid artery. Additional studies are under way to investigate the question of whether restoration of blood flow will be beneficial in patients with less than 70% narrowing who have ischemic symptoms.

Walter Dandy first demonstrated the feasibility of surgery to occlude cerebral aneurysms and remove arteriovenous malformations. The focus of neurosurgery in the 1950s and 1960s was largely on these two abnormalities, and many of the most famous surgeons of the time were vascular surgeons. The early operations were often complicated and mortality was high. Ligation of carotid and vertebral arteries in the neck was used as an alternative to try to reduce the pressure within the aneurysm and thus reduce the risk of hemorrhage. Other surgeons attempted to wrap the intracranial aneurysms after exposure because of the lack of adequate metal clips for their occlusion. McKenzie, Olivecrona, and Norlen all introduced new clips, which improved the surgeon's chance for aneurysmal obliteration. Scoville developed the concept of the spring-loaded clip, and now many other prominent surgeons have produced individual clips and entire systems of clips for use in aneurysm surgery. Improvement in anesthetic techniques, use of hypothermia, the new clips, and the reduced risk of angiography all allowed successful treatment of aneurysms and arteriovenous malformations during this period.

### Magnification, microscopic anatomy, and the development of modern neurosurgery

By the early 1960s, several neurosurgeons had suggested that magnification with an operating microscope would be advantageous in many procedures. William House introduced the operating microscope to neurosurgeons through his treatment of acoustic tumors. Yasargil, after a year of study in Vermont with Donaghy, returned to Zürich, where he began to apply microsurgical techniques in all kinds of neurosurgical operations. His results in aneurysm and acoustic surgery showed such an advantage over existing surgical techniques that microsurgery soon became the standard and formed the basis for the enormous improvement in the treatment of neurosurgical diseases which has occurred in the past 20 years.

#### Aneurysms and arteriovenous malformations

During the early history of aneurysm surgery it was not clear that operation resulted in an advantage over the natural history of the disease. The long-lasting study of subarachnoid hemorrhage, aneurysms, and their treatment sponsored by the National Institutes of Health, showed the advantage of surgery if done with a small resultant morbidity and mortality. The microsurgical techniques and the surgical skills pioneered by Yasargil produced a morbidity and mortality of under 10% and allowed most competent neurosurgeons to carry out these operations, which had been the province of only a few master surgeons before.

The principal cause of mortality in those patients who survive the first subarachnoid hemorrhage is rebleeding. Study of the natural history, coupled with improvements in management techniques, has allowed aneurysms to be treated on an urgent basis, thus eliminating the rebleeding risk. The second major problem is vasospasm, which produces ischemic stroke. Allen introduced calcium-channel-blocking agents for the prevention of these ischemic effects, providing the first reasonable treatment for this dreaded complication.

The same microsurgical techniques that allowed the precise identification and obliteration of aneurysms, have helped in treating arteriovenous malformations. Individual blood vessels can be identified and controlled, and the treatment of these vascular anomalies in the brain is now feasible. Previously surgery was sometimes carried out but most published studies did not clearly improve on the natural history of the disease. Now endovascular obliteration of feeding vessels, direct surgery, and focused radiation are combined to improve outcomes.

*Tumors of the cerebellopontine angle* Tumors of the acoustic nerve have been a neurosurgical challenge since the days of Harvey Cushing, who treated them with subtotal removal, but preserved and improved cranial nerve function. Walter Dandy showed that total removal and cure was possible, but at the expense of facial paralysis. This remained the standard until the microsurgical era, when total removal became routine, and the surgeon could focus on preservation of cranial nerves. Modern microsurgeons save the facial nerve routinely, cure is expected, and mortality has almost disappeared. Increasingly, surgeons report salvage of residual hearing or restoration of hearing in patients with small tumors in whom functional hearing is preserved.

*Tumors of the skull base* The broad variety of tumors at the base of the skull were treated ineffectually until the recent past. Many of these are benign, but eventually cause death of the patient by inexorable progression of loss of cranial nerve and, finally, brain-stem function. Neurosurgeons and otorhinolaryngologists have combined to develop a variety of new surgical techniques which are quite different from traditional neurosurgical operations. Some require operating through the mouth, dividing both the upper and lower jaw, operating through the face or sinuses, or surgical exposures around the eye, and are combined with extensive dissections in the neck. These radical operations now allow successful surgery on tumors that were considered inoperable a decade ago.

*Intramedullary spinal cord tumors* Enhanced magnetic resonance imaging has revolutionized the surgeon's ability to diagnose and understand tumors in the spinal cord. The nature of the tumor may be guessed with accuracy and its extent measured with certainty. Microsurgical techniques, coupled with spinal cord monitoring, allow delicate dissection of the tumor with continuous assessment of spinal cord function. The favorable tumors that are encapsulated can usually be removed with only a limited risk of paralysis. Gliomas which infiltrate the core are generally not curable, but palliation with preservation of function is possible.

*Brain and spinal cord trauma* One of the greatest advances in neurosurgery has been in treating trauma to the nervous system. These advances have not come from technical surgical achievements, but are based upon clinical research, which has greatly increased our understanding of the pathophysiology of injury to the nervous system.

The pathological consequences of injury to the spinal cord have been studied in great detail and are now well understood, although nothing can be done to restore function in most cases. Collins and his associates have shown a beneficial effect of steroids administered in very high doses immediately after the injury, the first demonstration that any treatment is of benefit in severe spinal cord injury.

Even more progress has been made in brain injury. While a seriously damaged brain will not recover and regeneration is not possible, the secondary effects of brain injury are now much better understood and can be treated. This is because some neurosurgeons have led the way by studying and understanding the complex relationships between increased pressure within the skull secondary to injury, its effects upon blood flow, and its mechanical effects upon the brain. These studies have led to techniques for ameliorating the damaging effects of all these factors upon potentially recoverable brain cells. Hence, there has been a dramatic improvement in the mortality and morbidity of serious head injury.

*The management of gliomas and chemotherapy* Much effort has been expended on gliomas, but these intrinsic brain tumors remain an unresolved problem. The immediate effects of tumor growth can be palliated by surgery. There is some evidence that radiation therapy is beneficial for slow-growing gliomas, and it is certainly beneficial in the short term in more malignant tumors. Many chemotherapeutic agents have been tried, but the only tumors commonly cured by chemotherapy are medulloblastomas in children. Such treatment continues to be under intense study. Nevertheless, the malignant gliomas remain among the most devastating of all known tumors.

### Developing aspects of neurosurgery

*Endovascular therapy* Catheter manipulation within arteries supplying the nervous system has greatly improved the treatment of many kinds of vascular abnormality and some tumors. Spinal cord arteriovenous malformations may often be treated by obliteration of nutrient vessels, rather than by open surgery. A combination of surgery and endovascular obliteration is sometimes required, but reduction of blood flow generally makes surgery much safer. Equal success has occurred in treating cerebral arteriovenous malformations. It is now common for these blood vessel abnormalities to be treated by a combination of endovascular obliteration produced by the injection of sclerosing agents, with techniques to occlude feeding vessels. Focused radiation techniques for small areas of residual malformation can then be added. Such combined methods have greatly reduced mortality and morbidity.

The endovascular treatment of aneurysms was introduced at about the same time that treatment of arteriovenous malformation was begun, but progress has been slower. The original techniques included balloon occlusion of aneurysms or their parent vessels and the injection of adhesives. Current focus is principally on the use of minute metal coils, which are released into the aneurysm and induce electrothrombosis. The treatment of specific aneurysms such as those of the basilar apex is predominantly by this method now.

*Repair of peripheral nerves* The use of the operating microscope and microsuturing techniques has allowed much more precise repair of severed or injured peripheral nerves. This aspect of surgery is no longer restricted to neurosurgeons. Neurosurgeons have added the possibility of re-innervation of paralyzed arms by repair of brachial plexus injuries through the use of intact nerves in the vicinity and in the treatment of painful peripheral nerve injuries.

*Stereotaxy and stereotactic radiosurgery* There has been a dramatic increase in the treatment of movement disorders with stereotactic techniques. The source of the abnormal movements in Parkinson's syndrome and related diseases may be identified with microelectrode recordings in the thalamus and small, precisely made lesions in the brain will eliminate the abnormalities of movement. Similar improvements in understanding of the pain pathways in the human thalamus have led to a rebirth of the use of stimulating devices for the treatment of intractable pain.

Stereotactic biopsy is now routine and many tumors are identified so that more rational decisions about treatment can be made. Open surgery can be avoided, particularly with the use of stereotactic radiosurgery. Stereotactic craniotomy has been developed well now. Tumors are localized by these stereotactic techniques and approached through limited exposures. This adds a margin of safety for the patient and allows precise removal of the tumor without injury of the surrounding brain.

Stereotactic radiosurgery is an old technique which was introduced by Lars Leksell in the late 1960s. The original device focused the radiation from a cobalt source to a small area, avoiding the side-effects of widespread radiation of the brain. Linear accelerators now have been developed to do the same thing. The goal is intense radiation of a small area with total destruction of the tumor while sparing radiation of the surrounding brain. Stereotactic radiosurgery is now being widely used for secondary tumors and some benign tumors such as meningioma or acoustic neuroma. The procedures are safe and effective for many patients.

*Epilepsy and the study of brain function* Epilepsy surgery is an important expansion in neurosurgery. Monitoring techniques have been developed which allow a longitudinal evaluation of brain activity and abnormalities. Grids of electrodes can be inserted surgically over the brain's surface to localize areas of brain dysfunction precisely. Patients can be monitored for several weeks by this technique. Functional imaging allows areas of brain abnormality to be visualized with improved localization of the implanted grids or other electrical monitoring techniques. The studies have led to improved understanding of the localization of language and memory function and are being expanded to other functional studies in the brain.

*Neurological intensive care* Patients with intracranial and spinal disease require intensive support if they are to recover fully from their disease and its treatment. A new specialty of neurological intensive care has developed in the past decade. These intensive care specialists come from many medical disciplines, but focus their interests upon the nervous system. Improved monitoring techniques allow careful study of brain electrical activity, brain blood flow, and brain function. Spinal cord monitoring techniques are less advanced. The goals of neurological intensive care are to provide the best environment for the recovery of function and to prevent additional injuries that might come through lack of oxygen, blood flow, or from increased intracranial pressure.

*Spinal reconstruction* For many years spinal surgery consisted of removing herniated discs, the treatment of trauma, the removal of tumors, and correction of a few congenital or acquired anomalies. In the past five years, new methods of reconstruction of the spine have been developed. There are now many metal systems of screws, plates, rods, wires, nuts, and bolts which allow the spinal surgeon to fix the unstable spine to correct anatomical abnormalities. Because of improved methods of fixation, decompressive techniques have grown more radical. There has been a broad emphasis in neurosurgery and in orthopedics upon spinal reconstruction after surgery for trauma and tumors. There has also been a dramatic increase in the ability to deal with the consequence of degenerative spinal disease.

There is emphasis now upon disc replacement and the development of an artificial disc. None are on the market as yet, but several versions are in clinical trials. An alternative to disc replacement is the use of various artificial devices which replace the disc, but also fuse the spine.

## Monitoring techniques

One advance of the past 10 years has been the development of electrical techniques that allow continuous assessment of the function of the spinal cord, the visual and auditory systems, the brain-stem, and the peripheral and cranial nerves. Surgeons can now carry out operations with increased safety because the transmission of electrical signs can be recorded continuously.

*Three-dimensional imaging* The three-dimensional techniques in computerized tomography scanning have improved dramatically the imaging of the nervous system and its surrounding bony structures. The accuracy is so great that the surgeon can have an exact understanding of the location of tumors. Furthermore, this system can be used in the operating room to demonstrate exactly where a tumor is located, thus guiding the surgical exposure. Three-dimensional imaging has also proved invaluable for such long-standing spinal problems as assessment of the continuity of fusion, bone, or the size of a neural foramen.

## Developing topics of greatest interest

A rapidly developing aspect of neurosurgery concerns the treatment of all kinds of brain tumors. The first significant increases in longevity of patients who had had surgery for malignant brain tumors followed the use of time-release local chemotherapy around the tumor bed. GENE

THERAPY has also reached the clinical trial stage. The modification of genes which can specifically target brain tumors has occurred in the laboratory and some patients have been treated. The delivery of specific toxins to poison tumor cells is also at the clinical trials stage and may be available soon.

Spinal reconstructive surgery continues to develop and is maturing as a specialty for both orthopedics and neurosurgery. The artificial disc may soon become a reality.

The identification of several growth factors and neural transmitters offer hope for Alzheimer's disease and stroke. Most would require the continuous infusion of the factors involved, so time-release polymers and programmable infusion pumps are also under investigation. In the laboratory nitric oxide has proved to be important in the injury that follows stroke and the development of drugs to counteract such noxious agents is of prime importance. Recent clinical trials have already shown the value of existing thrombolytic agents for stroke. Minimally invasive surgical techniques continue to develop, and the surgeon can expose tumors through smaller and smaller incisions.

There is considerable interest in the amalgamation of imaging techniques and operating room requirements into an advanced operating room system which will allow imaging control of surgery, verification of surgical result, and functional study of the brain in the course of an operation. Robotic control of neurosurgical instruments is likely to become important. Ultrasound will assume greater and greater use for imaging during operations. Functional imaging will be routine and will help understand the effects of diseases upon the brain and the effects of therapy of these diseases.

## Conclusion

Neurosurgery is barely 100 years old and has been a mature specialty for less than 50 years. Modern neurosurgery began with the advent of magnification techniques and is less than 30 years old. The early years of the specialty were devoted to clinical diagnosis, categorization of the diseases to be treated, and palliative surgery which prolonged life and function. Dandy introduced the concept of localization by imaging the nervous system and curative surgery which dominated the specialty until the 1960s. The addition of magnification to the neurosurgical operating room brought new emphasis on maintenance of functional integrity of the nervous system, particularly cranial nerves, and has reduced mortality and morbidity to levels that seemed unattainable only a few years earlier. New imaging techniques have revolutionized diagnosis. Most patients are now seen early in the course of their disease when symptoms are minimal and when satisfactory treatment is more likely.

Recent developments changed the discipline yet again. Endovascular therapies are revolutionizing the treatment of vascular disease. Stereotactic radiation may replace some of the most demanding operations. Minimally invasive surgery reduces the surgical consequences for the patient, but often demands more technical skill from the surgeon. Spinal reconstruction is maturing rapidly and opens an extremely common human condition (the prolapsed disc) for neurosurgical treatment. Functional imaging is revolutionizing our understanding of the pathophysiological effects of neurosurgical diseases and the consequences of their treatment.

Neurosurgery has changed from a discipline characterized by uncertain diagnosis and treatment, with very high mortality and morbidity, to one of precise diagnosis and localization with mortality and complication rates which are lower than those of many much simpler specialties. It has redefined itself every 25–30 years. The new era will emphasize minimally invasive techniques to preserve, restore, and improve lost or impaired neurological function.                    DML

*See also* SPECIALIZATION

Isaac **NEWTON** (1642–1727). British scientist and mathematician. Born in Woolsthorpe, Lincolnshire, Newton was educated at Grantham and in 1661 went to Trinity College, Cambridge. After graduation he spent a year in seclusion in Woolsthorpe on account of the plague at Cambridge, during which time he laid the foundations of much of his work. He returned to Cambridge, became a fellow of Trinity College in 1667, and the following year became Lucasian professor of mathematics. He remained at Cambridge for nearly thirty years, often studying alone but with frequent correspondence with other scientists and the Royal Society, of which he became a fellow in 1672. He published his *Philosophae naturalis principia mathematica* in 1687, in which he described his laws of motion and the law of gravitation. In 1689 he became Member of Parliament for the university, a position which he held until the dissolution the following year; he was re-elected in 1701 but took little part in politics. After a period of depression, Newton was appointed Warden of the London Mint, and became Master in 1699. Shortly afterwards he resigned his fellowship and professorship at Cambridge and moved to London. In 1703 he was elected president of the Royal Society, an office which he held until his death, and in 1704 he published his work on light and the effects that light produces, *Opticks*. He was knighted in 1705 and his later years were spent revising his *Principia*; a second edition was published in 1713 and a third edition in 1726. Newton died in March 1727 and was given a state funeral and burial in Westminster Abbey. As well as his writings on physics and mathematics, Newton also wrote on chemistry, alchemy, ancient chronology, prophecy, and theology. One of the greatest scientists of all time, Newton's work epitomizes the revolutionizing of science in the 17th century. In medicine his work was to be built on by BOERHAAVE (p 121), an influential Dutch physician and teacher who promoted mechanistic explanations of disease in medicine.

**NEW ZEALAND** New Zealand is in the southwest Pacific Ocean, and similar in size to the British Isles. The north–south orientation produces climates ranging from cool temperate in the south to subtropical in the far north. Alps, volcanoes, rugged coasts, fiords, sandy beaches, and rich pastoral countryside make this one of the most beautiful countries on earth. The Maori, a Polynesian race of people, settled the land 800–900 years ago. In 1770, the English explorer James Cook charted much of the coastline. European sealers and whalers began to arrive soon afterwards. Formal settlements were established by colonists from the British Isles in the North and South Islands in the 1840s, at what have since become the cities of Auckland, Wellington, New Plymouth, Nelson, Christchurch, and Dunedin. In 1996, these and other cities and large towns held about 80% of the population of 3.68 million; the remaining 20% lived in scattered and often rather isolated rural communities that present difficulties in providing medical services.

When the European settlements were established there were about 90 000 Maori people living mainly around the coast in small tribal groups. Many thousands were killed in tribal warfare after the acquisition of firearms or died from infectious diseases introduced by the European sealers and whalers. The Treaty of Waitangi, which was signed in 1840 by Maori tribes and the British Crown, established a partnership between the two races. At this time the Maori population was only 70 000 and reached a nadir in 1896, when the numbers had declined to 42 000. In the last 100 years the Maori population has increased dramatically to 523 371, constituting in the 1996 census 15% of the population. In addition, 5% of the total population are Polynesian from the Pacific Islands, 2% Chinese, 1% Indian, and 77% of European descent. Immigration in recent years has increased the cultural diversity of the population.

### Medical services

*Public hospitals* Governor Sir George Grey established public hospitals in each settlement in the first decade after the settlers arrived. These hospitals were for both Maoris and Europeans in financial need. Provincial councils were responsible for running local hospitals until they were dissolved in 1876.

By the time the first Hospital Act of 1885 established regulations for the management of hospitals, there were 28 hospital districts. The hospitals were funded a third each by local rates, central government, and donations and patient fees. The Social Security Act in 1938 ensured that all citizens were provided with free hospital care, and in 1957 central government assumed full responsibility from local authorities for funding hospital services.

In 1996 public hospitals provided 19 637 general beds; a ratio of 7.3/1000 population, with a total of 507 258 admissions in that year. The average length of stay was 6.5 days.

*Private hospitals* A private hospital system with emphasis on elective surgery has for many years operated in competition with publicly funded hospitals. In recent years, with the availability of health insurance, more operations have been performed in private hospitals. Most life-threatening conditions continue to be treated in the public hospitals, although open-heart surgery is performed in three private hospitals. There are 1261 private surgical beds.

Private health insurance, held by one third of the population, is used to meet in whole or in part the cost of surgical operations or other medical treatment.

*Medical practitioners* The first doctor, Dr Joseph Crocome, arrived in 1838 to serve the whalers and sealers around the coast of the South Island. Several medical practitioners came with each settlement in the 1840s. Medical registration by government officials was started in 1867, when 133 doctors were serving 228 000 people. In 1924 the medical profession assumed responsibility for both registration and discipline after the establishment of the New Zealand Medical Council.

By 1997 there were 8738 medical practitioners, of whom 30% were women. The proportion of doctors from each ethnic group was European 84%, Chinese 4.3%, Indian 3.9%, Maori 2.5%, and others 5.3%.

The low number of Maori doctors remains despite both medical schools having offered preferential entry for Maori applicants for over a decade. Overseas trained doctors constituted 34% of the workforce. Doctors in training constituted 24% of the total workforce. The median age for women doctors was 36, and for men 42. In 1996 there were 254 doctors per 100 000 population, but general practitioners remain unevenly distributed throughout the country.

*Medical schools* In 1870, the University of Otago in Dunedin was established and by 1885 provided a full medical course to enable students to complete their clinical training in New Zealand. The first woman to graduate was Emily Siedeberg in 1896; she spent the next 30 years managing and providing obstetric services in a maternity hospital, St Helens, in Dunedin. In 1937 the medical class size was increased to 120, with students completing their final year of clinical training in Auckland, Wellington, Christchurch, and Dunedin.

A second school of medicine was established in Auckland in 1968. This has grown and diversified to meet the needs of Auckland, which has one third of the population of New Zealand. Clinical schools have since been established in Wellington and Christchurch, each providing three years' clinical training for 60 students a year from the University of Otago. Overall, about 250 medical students graduate each year. Appreciable proportions of medical graduates are lost by emigration, mainly to Australia, but those lost are replaced by immigrants from Britain, India, Sri Lanka, and other countries.

*Medical research* The Otago Medical School was firmly based on the tradition of the Edinburgh School and from early times there has been a focus on inquiry and research. In 1937 Sir Charles Hercus, then dean of the Otago Medical School, established the Medical Research Council, responsible primarily for funding biomedical research. In 1990 the Health Research Council replaced the Medical Research Council with a broader responsibility to cover research into public health, social sciences, and Maori health as well as biomedical research.

*Health and Disability Commissioner* The position of Commissioner was established in 1994 'to promote and protect the rights of health and disability consumers'. A Code of Rights for Consumers has been developed for all public and private hospitals. The post of Commissioner was created after a major public debate about the ethical responsibility of health professionals to inform patients about the risks and potential benefits of any proposed treatment or research procedure. The Commissioner has a staff of patient advocates, one in each public hospital to advise patients and negotiate with health professionals.

*Voluntary societies* The Plunket Society was established by Sir Truby King in 1907 to improve the health of women and children. The society has provided training for Plunket nurses to care for babies and children in the first years of life. Several Karitane Hospitals, which emphasized the importance of diet, were established to help mothers and babies with feeding difficulties and to provide training facilities for Karitane nurses. Infant mortality rate (in those aged under 1 year) fell rapidly from 40/1000 in 1907 to 6.7/1000 in 1995.

Many voluntary groups provide support for patients and their families including the Cancer Society, the National Heart Foundation, the Epilepsy Society, and the Alzheimer's Association, to name but a few.

## Health of New Zealanders

***Life expectancy*** Life expectancy in 1996 for non-Maori New Zealand males was 73.7 years and for females 79.1 years. In comparison, both male and female Maoris have a reduced life expectancy of 68.3 and 72.9, respectively.

***Causes of death*** New Zealand uses the 9th revision of the International Classification of Diseases based on the death certificate supported by other sources of information. About 10% of deaths are subject to a post-mortem examination.

Death rates from cancer have increased slightly in the past decade. Major cancer sites causing death are for men, lung 23%, large bowel 15%, and prostate 13%, and, for women, breast 20%, large bowel 15%, and lung 15%.

Death rates from ischemic heart disease (heart attacks) have halved in the last 30 years and continued to fall from 1989 to 1994 by 20% for men and 15% for women.

***Patterns of illness*** The main causes of hospital admission in infancy are premature birth and the effects of birth anoxia; in childhood, respiratory infections; and in young adults trauma from motor vehicle crashes. Ischemic heart disease is the commonest cause of admission from middle age onwards.

Diabetes, a serious health problem, is increasing in prevalence and associated with obesity in adult Maoris and Pacific Islanders. The incidence of selected communicable diseases is comparable with that in the USA. Acute rheumatic fever and meningococcal meningitis remain important illnesses, particularly for Maori and Pacific Island children.

***Maternity and women's health*** Since the 1960s there has been an increased focus on women's health. General practitioners, independent midwives, and obstetricians provide maternity care. Most women (98%) have their babies in hospital. Breast-feeding is strongly encouraged. In a 1991 survey 94% of mothers initiated breast-feeding, and 79% and 62% of mothers maintained breast-feeding at eight and twelve weeks, respectively. These figures are high compared with most western countries. Maternity care is free in New Zealand.

***Infant and child health*** The infant mortality rate in 1995 was 6.7/1000 live births. This has been falling, but is still high compared with many northern European countries. Unexplained sudden infant death is a cause of concern, at a rate of 1.4/1000 live births and treble this rate in Maoris.

***Care of the elderly*** Care of the frail elderly and patients with disabilities is undertaken in private hospitals and rest homes. Few elderly people are cared for long term in public hospitals. Most patients receive a government subsidy to cover costs, although this is subject to a means test. Assessment by a geriatrician is required before admission to a rest home, and serious efforts are made to encourage people to remain with support in their own home.

***Mental healthcare*** The first asylum was established in Wellington in 1853 and other hospitals were opened in each province. One of the first mental hospitals in which patients were all accommodated in villas was opened in Wellington in 1907. In 1993, 4372 patients were first admitted to mental hospitals, most being voluntary admissions. In the last 15 years many large mental hospitals have been closed and most patients placed in community homes or discharged from care into the community.

***Maori health*** The life expectancy of Maoris, both male and female, is six years less than for non-Maoris. Like many other colonized people, some Maoris lose their cultural roots and become marginalized second-class citizens with high prevalence rates of alcohol and substance abuse and high suicide rates.

Maori infant death rate is twice that of non-Maoris, most being attributed to SUDDEN INFANT DEATH SYNDROME. Hearing impairment from inadequate treatment of middle ear infections occurs in up to one-quarter of children. This has a serious effect on future learning and employment. A high level of smoking, particularly amongst Maori women, has resulted in a lung cancer rate twice that of non-Maori women. Maori rates of admission to mental hospitals are three times that of non-Maoris. A higher prevalence of cancer of the cervix, diabetes, chronic lung disease, and obesity also contributes to the lowered life expectancy.

Some Maoris still consider western medicine to be a method of control rather than help. Historically the Maori people did not distinguish between life and health: how one dealt with illness contributed to one's life experience and wisdom. To encourage western medical practice and to reduce the influence of tohunga (indigenous healers), a Suppression of Tohunga Act was passed late in the 19th century. At the turn of the century two distinguished Maori doctors, Maui Pomare and Sir Peter Buck, made great efforts to improve health by introducing a Maori health nursing scheme. This scheme, however, was soon absorbed into the Public Health Department, and Europeans within the department assumed responsibility for Maori health services, replacing the Maori nurses.

Until the 1970s, Maori aspirations were largely ignored, and the past process of assimilation continued. In 1984, the Labor government made a strong commitment to support biculturalism and to recognize the Maoris as the indigenous people of 'Aotearoa' (New Zealand). The government also allowed Maori Treaty of Waitangi grievances from 1840 to be reviewed and the Crown has since made compensatory payments for land confiscated after the Land Wars in the 1860s.

With the health reforms in 1993, the Maori people have taken greater responsibility for planning and providing health services for themselves, but the government decided not to create a separate Maori Health Authority. Tohunga (traditional healers) are again encouraged, but receive no public funding. Maoris trained in western medicine, according to Professor Eru Pomare, can complement but not replace tohunga without inflicting substantial harm to Maori culture.

***Accident compensation*** Since 1974 a no-fault accident compensation scheme has operated in New Zealand for everyone including tourists from overseas. All injuries, whether or not work-related, are covered. The emphasis is on rehabilitation to encourage an early return to work. People in general can no longer sue for compensation. In 1995 there were 1.4 million claims, of which 10% were for moderate or severe injuries; a further 126 000 claimants received continued support for injuries of previous years. Injured people receive 80% of their pre-injury wage.

An analysis in 1994 of 77 000 injuries showed that 13% were transport related, 20% due to accidental falls, and 17% due to medical or surgical complications. Over the years the levies to fund the scheme have become more focused, with high-risk industries (such as forestry and meat packers) paying much higher levies. Motor vehicle license fees meet the cost of traffic accidents.

## Health administration

***Health administration and expenditure*** In the 19th century the focus of public health was on the control of infectious disease by QUARANTINE, VACCINATION, and improved sanitation. Hospitals were under the control of local authorities, while the government Department of Health operated separately through district health officers.

The Social Security Act, passed by the first Labor Government in 1938, provided health benefit subsidies from general taxation. New Zealand was the first free market economy to introduce these universal benefits, including free pharmaceuticals, laboratory tests, and public hospital care. In 1983 the 25 hospital boards were replaced by 14 area health boards, responsible for all public funding of health services including health promotion, disease prevention, personal treatment, and caring services for a defined population.

Total expenditure on health has increased steadily, from NZ$4.7 billion in 1986 to NZ$6.8 billion in 1996, but at 7.6% of gross domestic product remains low compared with other Organization for Economic Cooperation and Development countries. Since 1989 the government has been trying to transfer more health costs to private funds (including health insurance). This now accounts for 24% of expenditure on health.

Publicly funded real expenditure has increased in the last 10 years, from NZ$4.2 to 5.2 billion at a rate of 1.3% per year, while privately funded expenditure rose from NZ$0.6 to $1.6 billion at a rate of 6.7% per year. The government believes that it cannot continue to meet the total cost of universal healthcare and is targeting people in the lower income groups while encouraging others to take private health insurance.

***Health reforms*** In 1993 the Health and Disabilities Service Act radically reshaped the healthcare system and separated purchaser from provider functions. Four regional health authorities funded on a population-based formula acted as purchasers of integrated health services from both public and private providers in their region. Public hospitals as the principal providers were accountable for performing a defined number of each operative procedure.

'Pharmac', a subsidiary company of the regional health authorities, has aggressively forced international pharmaceutical companies to reduce the price of all drugs in a class to that of the cheapest drug or cease to receive a government subsidy.

General practitioner services remain on a fee for service basis, with targeted assistance for lower income groups by using a community services card. The government wishes to develop capitation-based funding for general practitioner services. The doctors have responded by forming independent practitioner associations to develop MANAGED-CARE schemes.

Greater equity of access to free elective surgery in public hospitals is being attempted, with the development of national guidelines for all people on waiting lists for surgery throughout the country. Waiting lists will be replaced by a booking system using waiting times. Patients in lesser need are to be referred back to their general practitioner.

A redistribution of surgical services to metropolitan hospitals is continuing despite vigorous local opposition to the closure of several rural hospitals. These small hospitals have been costly to run and cannot provide the surgical experience required to maintain surgical competence.

Overall New Zealand health services provide people with a high standard of comprehensive care, including advanced technical procedures such as kidney, heart, and liver transplants.   DN

*See also* HEALTHCARE SYSTEMS; NO-FAULT COMPENSATION; THEORIES OF ILLNESS

Florence **NIGHTINGALE** (1820–1910). British nurse. Nightingale received her early education at her home in Derbyshire, then went to the Institute of Protestant Deaconesses at Kaiserswerth in Germany for nursing training. She returned to England in 1853 and was appointed superintendent of the Hospital for Invalid Gentlewomen in London. On the outbreak of the Crimean War the following year, through her friendship with the secretary of war, Sidney Herbert, she was invited to travel to the Crimea with a small group of nurses under her direction, to establish a nursing service for the British army there. Stationed at SCUTARI, where (as reports in *The Times* had shown) conditions of hygiene, sanitation, treatment of the 5000 wounded and sick, and lack of food were deplorable, she transformed the barracks into a military hospital with clean wards, a laundry, and efficient administration and nursing, reducing the mortality dramatically. In February 1855 the death rate of soldiers admitted to the hospital was 42%; by June of that year it had fallen to 2%. She returned to England in 1856, a national heroine, and a fund of £50 000 was raised by public subscription, which she used for the training of civilian nurses. In 1859 the Nightingale School and Home for Nurses was established at St Thomas's Hospital, London, providing accommodation and a training center for pupils. She also continued her attempts to reform the army medical services, producing a document, *Notes on matters affecting the health and efficiency and hospital administration of the British army*. A royal commission was established in 1859 and many of her recommendations, such as the establishment of an army medical school, the reform of sanitary facilities in barracks, and hospital regulations, were implemented in the following years. Thereafter she took no part in public life, seldom leaving her sickroom, from which, nevertheless, there issued a stream of reports and recommendations. The best known of these, *Notes on nursing, what it is and what it is not*, was published in 1859.

**NOBEL PRIZE** Selecting candidates for a Nobel prize in physiology or medicine — 'The domain of physiology or medicine' according to the testament of Alfred Nobel — is complicated and time consuming. Nobel stipulated in his testament that the prizes should be distributed to those who 'during the preceding year shall have conferred the greatest benefit to mankind' and that they should 'be awarded for physics and chemistry, respectively, by the Swedish Academy of Sciences; that for physiology or medical works by the Karolinska Institute in Stockholm; that for literature by the Academy in Stockholm; and that for champions of peace by a committee of five persons to be elected by the Norwegian Storting [Parliament]'. These institutions work separately and totally independently and may follow slightly different procedures for their work, but there is a common timetable — for example, invitations for proposals for prize candidates for next year are sent out during September, the final date for acceptance of proposals for the current year's prize awards is January 31.

For medicine the Faculty of the Karolinska Institute (then consisting only of full professors), was the body responsible for awarding the prize. During the 1970s as Swedish law was altered, making all written documents from the Karolinska Institute public property, secrecy could no longer be upheld for the Nobel proceedings. Accordingly a new body had to be created. The new Nobel assembly at the Karolinska Institute is private and thus able to uphold total secrecy. Like all the prize awarding bodies, the Karolinska Institute also has a Nobel committee.

Written proposals regarding prize candidates by qualified people mentioned in the Nobel statutes should be sent to the Nobel committee. The following bodies, by statute, have the right to submit proposals for the award of prizes: members of the Nobel assembly at the Karolinska Institute; Swedish and foreign members of the medical department of the Royal Swedish Academy of Sciences; Nobel laureates in physiology or medicine; members of the Nobel committee at the Karolinska Institute; full professors of the medical faculties in Sweden and corresponding medical faculty members in corresponding colleges in Denmark, Finland, Iceland, and Norway; members of corresponding posts in at least six other medical faculties elected according to a suitable system for the distribution among the different countries and their seats of learning; and other scientists from

Nobel prizes for physiology and medicine, 1901–2000

| 1901 | Emil von Bebring (Germany) | Diphtheria antiserum |
|------|----------------------------|----------------------|
| 1902 | Ronald Ross (UK) | Mosquito and malaria |
| 1903 | Niels Ryberg Finsen (Denmark) | Ultraviolet light in lupus vulgaris |
| 1904 | Ivan Petrovich Pavlov (Russia) | Conditioned reflex |
| 1905 | Robert Koch (Germany) | Tuberculosis |
| 1906 | Camillo Golgi (Italy) and Santiago Ramon y Cajal (Spain) | Structure of nervous tissue |
| 1907 | Charles Louis Alphonse Laveran (France) | Malarial parasite |
| 1908 | Paul Ehrlich (Germany) Elie Metchnikoff (France) | Immunity Phagocytosis |
| 1909 | Theodor Kocher (Switzerland) | Thyroid disease |
| 1910 | Albrecht Kossel (Germany) | Bases of nucleic acid |
| 1911 | Allvar Gullstrand (Sweden) | Physical properties of lens |
| 1912 | Alexis Carrel (USA) | Vascular suture |
| 1913 | Charles Richet (France) | Anaphylaxis |
| 1914 | Robert Bárány (Austria) | Vestibular apparatus |
| 1915 | No award | |
| 1916 | No award | |
| 1917 | No award | |
| 1918 | No award | |
| 1919 | Jules Bordet (Belgium) | Lysis by complement |
| 1920 | August Krogh (Denmark) | Contractility of capillaries |
| 1921 | No award | |
| 1922 | Archibald Vivian Hill (UK) Otto Meyerhof (Germany) | Production of heat in muscles Lactic acid metabolism |
| 1923 | Frederick Grant Banting and John James Richard Macleod (Canada) | Insulin |
| 1924 | Willem Einthoven (Netherlands) | Electrocardiography |
| 1925 | No award | |
| 1926 | Johannes Fibiger (Denmark) | Discovery of the *Spiroptera* carcinoma |
| 1927 | Julius Wagner-Jauregg (Austria) | Malaria treatment of dementia paralytica |
| 1928 | Charles Nicolle (France) | Transmission of typhus fever by the louse |
| 1929 | Christiaan Eijkman (Netherlands) Frederick Gowland Hopkins (UK) | Discovery of the antineuritic vitamin Discovery of growth-stimulating vitamins |
| 1930 | Karl Landsteiner (Austria) | Human blood groups |
| 1931 | Otto Warburg (Germany) | Intracellular respiration |
| 1932 | Charles Sherrington and Edgar Douglas Adrian (UK) | Function of neurones |
| 1933 | Thomas Hunt Morgan (USA) | Function of chromosomes |
| 1934 | George Hoyt Whipple, George Richards Minot, and William Parry Murphy (USA) | Liver treatment of pernicious anemia |
| 1935 | Hans Spemann (Germany) | Embryonic development |
| 1936 | Henry Dale (UK) and Otto Loewi (Austria) | Chemical transmission of nerve impulses |
| 1937 | Albert Szent-Györgyi (Hungary) | Studies on vitamin C |
| 1938 | Corneille Heymans (Belgium) | Respiratory reflexes |
| 1939 | Gerhard Domagk (Germany) | Antibacterial action of sulfonamide |
| 1940 | No award | |
| 1941 | No award | |
| 1942 | No award | |
| 1943 | Henrik Dam (Denmark) Edward A. Doisy (USA) | Discovery of vitamin K Chemical structure of vitamin K |
| 1944 | Joseph Erlanger and Herbert Spencer Gasser (USA) | Studies of single nerve fibers |
| 1945 | Alexander Fleming, Ernst Boris Chain, and Howard Walter Florey (UK) | Antibacterial action of penicillin |

*(continued overleaf)*

Nobel prizes  (*continued*)

| | | |
|---|---|---|
| 1946 | Hermann Joseph Müller (USA) | X-ray induced mutations |
| 1947 | Bernardo Alberto Houssay (Argentina) | Role of anterior pituitary in carbohydrate metabolism |
| | Carl F. Cori and Gerty T. Cori (USA) | Carbohydrate metabolism |
| 1948 | Paul Müller (Switzerland) | DDT as an arthropod poison |
| 1949 | Walter Rudolf Hess (Switzerland) | Hypothalamus and autonomic function |
| | Antonio Egas Moniz (Portugal) | Prefrontal lobotomy |
| 1950 | Edward Calvin Kendall, Philip Showalter Hench (USA), and Tadeus Reichstein (Switzerland) | Adrenal hormones |
| 1951 | Max Theiler (USA) | Yellow fever vaccine |
| 1952 | Selman Abraham Waksman (USA) | Discovery of streptomycin for tuberculosis |
| 1953 | Hans Adolf Krebs (UK) | Citric acid cycle |
| | Fritz Albert Lipmann (USA) | Coenzyme A in intermediary metabolism |
| 1954 | John F. Enders, Frederick C. Robbins, and Thomas H. Weller (USA) | Poliovirus in tissue culture |
| 1955 | Hugo Theorell (Sweden) | Oxidizing enzymes |
| 1956 | André Fédéric Cournand, Dickinson Woodruff Richards (USA), and Werner Forssmann (Germany) | Cardiac catheterization |
| 1957 | Daniel Bovet (Italy) | Synthetic vasoactive drugs |
| 1958 | George Wells Beadle and Edward Lawrie Tatum (USA) | One gene-one enzyme concept |
| | Joshua Lederberg (USA) | Bacterial genetics |
| 1959 | Severo Ochoa and Arthur Kornberg (USA) | Biological synthesis of the nucleic acids |
| 1960 | Frank Macfarlane Burnet (Australia) and Peter Brian Medawar (UK) | Acquired immunological tolerance |
| 1961 | Georg von Békésy (USA) | Physiology of the cochlea |
| 1962 | Francis Harry Compton Crick, Maurice Hugh Frederick Wilkins, and James Dewey Watson (UK) | Molecular structure of DNA |
| 1963 | John Carew Eccles (Australia), Alan Lloyd Hodgkin, and Andrew Fielding Huxley (UK) | Ionic mechanisms affecting nerve cell membrane |
| 1964 | Konrad E. Bloch (USA) and Feodor Lynen (Germany) | Metabolism of cholesterol and fatty acids |
| 1965 | Francois Jacob, André Lwoff, and Jacques Monod (France) | Genetic control of synthesis of viruses and enzymes |
| 1966 | Francis Peyton Rous (USA) | Cancer-producing virus |
| | Charles B. Huggins (USA) | Hormonal treatment of cancer |
| 1967 | Ragnar Granit (Sweden), H. Keffer Hartline, and George Wald (USA) | Chemical and physiological processes in the eye |
| 1968 | Robert W. Holley, H. Gobind Khorana, and Marshall W. Nirenberg (USA) | How genes control cell function |
| 1969 | Max Delbrück, Alfred Hershey, and Salvador Luria (USA) | Use of phage in studies of inheritance |
| 1970 | Julius Axelrod (USA), Bernard Katz (UK), and Ulf von Euler (Sweden) | Chemical mediators of nerve transmission |
| 1971 | Earl W. Sutherland, Jr (USA) | Mechanism of hormone action: cyclic AMP |
| 1972 | Gerald M. Edelman (USA) and Rodney R. Porter (UK) | Structure of immunoglobulins |
| 1973 | Nikolas Tinbergen (UK), Konrad Z. Lorenz, and Karl von Frisch (Germany) | Studies of animal behavior, instinct |
| 1974 | Christian de Duve (Belgium), Albert Claude, and George E. Palade (USA) | Cell biology |
| 1975 | David Baltimore, Renato Dulbecco, and Howard M. Temin (USA) | Interaction of tumor viruses and nucleic acids in cells |
| 1976 | Baruch S. Blumberg (USA) | Discovery of hepatitis B virus |
| | D. Carlton Gajdusek (USA) | Slow-acting viruses |
| 1977 | Rosalyn Yalow (USA) | Radioimmunoassay |
| | Roger Guillemin and Andrew Schally (USA) | Isolation of hypophyseal peptides |
| 1978 | Werner Arber (Switzerland), Hamilton Smith, and Daniel Nathans (USA) | Restriction endonucleases |

(*continued opposite*)

Nobel prizes *(continued)*

| Year | Recipients | Field |
|------|-----------|-------|
| 1979 | Allan MacLeod Cormack (USA) and Godfrey Newbold Hounsfield (UK) | Computer-assisted tomography |
| 1980 | George Snell, Baruj Benacerraf (USA), and Jean Dausset (France) | Immunogenetics: the histocompatibility complex |
| 1981 | Roger Sperry (USA)<br>David Hubel and Torsten Wiesel (USA) | Cerebral hemispheric function<br>Mechanisms of vision |
| 1982 | Sune Bergström, Bengt Samuelsson (Sweden), and John Vane (UK) | Prostaglandins and biologically related substances |
| 1983 | Barbara McClintock (USA) | Mobile genetic elements |
| 1984 | Niels Jerne (Switzerland)<br>Cesar Milstein and Georges Koehler (UK) | Concept of the 'network theory' of the immune system<br>Production of monoclonal antibodies |
| 1985 | Michael Stuart Brown and Joseph Leonard Goldstein (USA) | Cholesterol metabolism |
| 1986 | Stanley Cohen (USA) and Rita Levi-Montalcini (Italy) | Mechanisms regulating cell growth |
| 1987 | Susumu Tonegawa (Japan) | Genetics of antibody diversity |
| 1988 | Sir James Black (UK),<br><br>Gertrude Belle, and George Herbert (USA) | Design of new therapeutic compounds<br>Design of new drug treatments |
| 1989 | John Michael Bishop and Harold Eliot Varmus (USA) | Derivation of oncogenes |
| 1990 | Joseph E. Murray and Thomas Edward Donnall (USA) | Organ transplantation |
| 1991 | E. Neher and B. Sakmann (Germany) | Ion detection in cell membranes |
| 1992 | Edwin Krebs and Edmond Fisher (USA) | Protein enzymes |
| 1993 | Richard Roberts and Philip Sharp (USA) | Genes, DNA, and introns |
| 1994 | Alfred G. Gilman and Martin Rodbell (USA) | G-proteins |
| 1995 | Edward B. Lewis (USA), Christiane Nüsslein-Volhard (Germany), and Eric F. Wieschaus (USA) | Early embryonic development |
| 1996 | Peter C. Doherty (USA) and Rolf M. Zinkernagel (Switzerland) | Immune defence |
| 1997 | Stanley B. Prusiner (USA) | Prions |
| 1998 | Robert F. Furchgott, Louis J. Ignarro, and Ferid Murad (USA) | Nitric oxide in the cardiovascular system |
| 1999 | Günter Blobel (USA) | Mechanisms of organelles |
| 2000 | Arvid Carlsson (Sweden), Paul Greengard (USA), and Eric Kandel (USA) | Signal transduction in the nervous system |

*Note:* The nation listed refers to the site of the prize-winning work, not the birthplace of the scientist.

whom the assembly may see fit to invite proposals. There is an official statement saying that 'personal applications for an award shall not be taken into consideration'.

These regulations enable several outstanding and well-known universities to have a permanent invitation to submit proposals for candidates. Other less well-known universities are invited according to a rotating schedule.

## Evaluation

All submitted proposals are handled by the Nobel committee, consisting of five ordinary and ten co-opted members, all on an equal footing.

The first task of the committee is to determine whether the proposed candidates are prizeworthy. With knowledge of previous Nobel awards, and the list of candidates already evaluated and proved worthy, the committee then decides which proposals will be dealt with further.

The final evaluation is divided into several steps. The first is a written evaluation by one or more scientific specialists, ending in a recommendation either to continue the evaluation into a second stage or to reject the proposal. The decision on this level lies with the Nobel committee.

The second and final step is a very thorough process, often extended over years, during which Swedish and international experts make their studies, investigations, and evaluations of the work carried out by the candidate. This step includes the often difficult task of determining what has been done by the candidate him/herself and what by his/her associates and collaborators — or by other researchers or groups of researchers.

When the complete material has been assembled, the full Nobel committee has to make its final decision: is the candidate worthy or not worthy? When the Nobel committee has decided that the proposed candidate is worthy, its investigations and final decision are submitted to the Nobel assembly at the Karolinska Institute. The final decision is taken by the Nobel assembly at the Karolinska Institute in a plenary meeting of all fifty members. The decision is made public not later than November 15. Generally it is made public during the first half of October. The decisions are final and without appeal, while the deliberations as well as the votes are kept secret.

Self-evidently there are many prizeworthy candidates within physiology or medicine and some kind of unofficial waiting list must exist for an individual to reach the top and be selected for a specific year. It is very seldom that the stipulations of the Nobel testament can be followed with regard to the words during 'the preceding year' shall have conferred the greatest benefit on mankind. Hence the evaluation whether a candidate is prizeworthy or not may take several years. Moreover, there are well-known examples of men who received their prizes several decades after their original discovery, given that the greatness of the work was not previously understood, or that recent results have proved the work to be correct, and so on.　　　　　LEB

*See also* FOUNDATIONS

**NO-FAULT COMPENSATION** describes alternatives to traditional litigation which grant compensation to personal injury victims without the requirement that such victims prove their injuries were caused by someone else's fault. No-fault compensation schemes have grown up as a consequence of the criticism that the elusive search for fault wastes resources and leaves a high proportion of accident victims uncompensated.

### No-fault schemes
No-fault schemes first appeared in workers' compensation plans at the turn of the century, and have spread to almost every endeavor in which human activity can cause personal injuries. The workings of such plans vary widely, depending on the types of compensation offered (medical expenses, loss of earnings, etc.); the prerequisites to a successful claim (for example, Israel and many North American regimes cover only motor vehicle accidents); the seriousness of injuries covered (many North American automobile plans leave the most serious injuries to the traditional tort (law) system); and whether the plan is compulsory for all potential victims. A crucial distinguishing factor, and the focal point of the controversy regarding no-fault compensation, is the extent to which a no-fault plan takes away the right to sue.

The accident compensation system which came into force in NEW ZEALAND in 1974 merits scrutiny as representative of many common features of no-fault plans. This legislated scheme purports to provide compensation for *all* personal injuries caused by accident occurring in New Zealand or suffered by New Zealand residents traveling overseas. The present level of compensation is not high, being reduced from that offered by the scheme before its 1992 revision, and in no way matching that of a common law award of damages. Compensation will be given for medical treatment, vocational retraining, and additional matters such as home help and childcare costs. The extent of payments is governed by a host of regulations, and victims are increasingly being required to make up the difference between their actual costs of treatment and the sums provided by the scheme.

The largest source of compensation under the New Zealand scheme is for loss of earnings. A successful claimant will receive 80% of earnings lost as a result of his or her injuries, such compensation potentially continuing to the age of qualification for national superannuation. Various limitations on the entitlement exist. There is a prescribed maximum amount payable. At periodic intervals there will be a medical assessment of the claimant's capacity for work. If that capacity is 85% or more, loss of earnings compensation shall cease, regardless of the lack of any opportunities for employment. In the case of a fatal accident, where loss of earnings compensation would have been payable to the victim, it will be paid to the victim's surviving spouse and dependants for a limited time. All benefits are indexed to accommodate inflation. Additional benefits payable in the event of a death arising from a personal injury are a funeral grant of NZ$3145 and sums of NZ$4500 to a surviving spouse and NZ$2252 to each surviving child (NZ$3 = £1, US$1.55).

Although the scheme formerly provided for lump-sum payments of up to NZ$27 000 for 'non-economic' losses (such as pain and suffering and loss of enjoyment of life), this type of compensation has now been abolished. In its place is a periodic payment known as an 'independence allowance', which is available to claimants who have suffered a disability of 10% or more of their 'whole body' function. The amount payable is small, being a percentage of the maximum of NZ$61.88 per week (for 80% disability or more), depending on the degree of disability.

### The no-fault debate
Two substantial criticisms of New Zealand's scheme likewise challenge many less comprehensive versions of no-fault compensation plans in place in other jurisdictions. The first is the legislated exclusion of claims for personal injury 'caused wholly or substantially by gradual

process, *disease*, or infection' except in the case where such injury has arisen in the course of employment, a 'medical misadventure', or is 'a consequence of personal injury or treatment for personal injury'. This exclusion of disease claims from New Zealand's scheme is indefensible on any ground other than that of the scheme's limited resources. Why should the cancer sufferer be forced to accept the meager assistance of a social welfare benefit, while the drunken daredevil injured by his or her foolishness receives the greater compensation offered by the no-fault scheme?

The unfairness of the disease exclusion influenced court decisions on the scope of the scheme before its 1992 reworking, resulting in some surprising rulings in favor of claimants who sought cover for 'personal injuries by accident', which the lay person might suspect were no more than the effect of disease. Thus compensation was granted to a woman with a history of back trouble who suffered pain upon bending down to pick up milk bottles; to a child who suffered an apneic attack (cessation of breathing) due to unknown causes; to the woman who did not give her informed consent to a novel form of treatment for cancer; and to the woman who suffered a 'nervous breakdown' in the middle of a grueling management course.

The 1992 legislative reworking of the scheme attempted to exclude such veiled disease claims by introducing more restrictive definitions of 'accident' (… the application of force or resistance external to the human body … but not any gradual process … ), 'medical misadventure' (in addition to medical negligence, a medical mishap will be covered only if its consequence is both severe and rare, occurring in 1% or less of cases of similar treatment), and 'personal injuries' (which, as to mental injuries, include only those suffered as a consequence of actual physical injuries *to the claimant*). Undoubtedly, however, the unfairness of the disease exclusion continues to be one of several factors blurring the dividing line between cover under the scheme and the lack thereof.

The second major criticism of the New Zealand scheme focuses on the legislated bar to litigation for damages 'arising directly or indirectly out of personal injury covered by this Act'. Serious questions have been raised about the desirability of a system of no-fault compensation such as that in place in New Zealand, where the victims of rape or other assaults, gross medical negligence, or automobile collisions involving alcohol cannot sue for full compensation. Such results appear particularly incongruous in a legal system which unhesitatingly accepts the propriety of the civil lawsuit for property damage (such as damage to the *automobiles* involved in a collision) and a host of other interests protected by the law.

New Zealand personal injury lawyers are continually seeking avenues to circumvent the legislated bar on litigation. Lawsuits based on mental suffering resulting from the personal injury suffered by *another person* are becoming more common (for example, witnessing an automobile accident involving one's spouse). In 1982 the Court of Appeal ruled that the prohibition on personal injury litigation did not extend to claims for punitive (exemplary) damages, which are designed to punish rather than compensate. This door to the courthouse was widened when a single High Court Judge later ruled that punitive damages could be awarded in a case where negligence, as opposed to intentional conduct, was alleged against the defendant.

### Unique scope

Despite over 25 years of operation of the New Zealand scheme and its intense study by other jurisdictions, it remains unique in its scope of operation and the extent of its bar on litigation. Although the 1974 Report of the Australian National Committee of Inquiry, chaired by Mr Justice Woodhouse (who likewise chaired the 1967 New Zealand Royal Commission which preceded the New Zealand scheme), recommended a full no-fault system for Australia, including compensation for disease, its recommendations were not acted upon. The exhaustive inquiry into compensation for personal injury conducted by the English Royal Commission, chaired by Lord Pearson, rejected the New Zealand approach in its 1978 Report. Despite the fact that the British Medical Association and the British medical Royal Colleges support introducing of a no-fault scheme, this proposal is, to date, opposed by the British government, if only on the grounds of cost.

The most positive aspect of the New Zealand scheme is its relatively low cost, which is not merely a function of the modest benefits payable. By largely doing away with the need to determine fault, administration costs are low — generally amounting to 6% of expenditure. This is a substantially lower percentage than that found in compensation systems requiring proof of fault.

### Sweden's insurance regime

In contrast to New Zealand's extreme form of no-fault compensation, Sweden employs a multilayered system of accident insurance to achieve many of the same goals, as several writers have stated (such as P. M. Danzon in the International *Review of Law and Economics*, 1994; 14: 4537). At the primary level is a universal social insurance providing generous cover for losses caused by disease, accident, or death. Because it compensates without reference to fault, there is no incentive to sue for many minor personal injuries.

This universal social insurance is supplemented by four further insurance schemes, which aim at compensating personal injury victims at a level comparable with that achieved through a tort action, largely without the necessary of proving fault (although certain types of claim are essentially fault based). The cover provided by these supplemental schemes is aimed at work-related injuries and disease, traffic accidents, medical and dental treatment injuries, and injuries caused by any manufactured drug. Although only traffic accident insurance is compulsory, the influence of the other schemes is wide as most individuals claim under the schemes which are negotiated on their behalf through collective agreements (work injuries); their county council (medical injuries); or the agreement reached between the drug manufacturers and a consortium of insurance companies (pharmaceutical injuries).

Tort law survives in Sweden to compensate the accident victim who can prove fault in the few aspects falling outside the focus of the no-fault insurance schemes. Differing rules govern the right to sue of a participant in each of the four schemes. The worker covered by a scheme forming part of a collective agreement is precluded from suing his or her employer, but the victim of a medical injury does not forego the chance to sue, although such suits are now rare, given the liberal amounts awarded under the scheme. In general, claims available under the insurance schemes are deducted from any award in tort.

Although the Swedish version of no-fault compensation may be criticized for favoring some particular sorts of injuries, thereby raising the predictable problems of demarcation of cover, it may appear to some a more realistic form of no-fault compensation than that in place in New

## NOISE

Noise is a loud sound, generally unpleasant. Most pervasive in urban, overcrowded, and industrialized areas, it has also been called 'unwanted sound', 'superfluous sound', 'sound without value', 'pathogen', or 'noise pollution'. Sensitivity to noise varies considerably, educated professionals and intellectuals being the most averse to it. One British study found 20% of people to be 'supersensitive' and 25% 'imperturbable'.

The intensity of sound waves is measured in decibels (dB). It is expressed on a logarithmic scale, so that a small numerical change reflects a large increase in sound. On this scale a whispered sound would be 20 dB; the ambience of a public library 35 dB; an average home 50 dB; a quiet residential neighborhood 55 dB; normal speech 60; a vacuum cleaner 70; a busy office 80; heavy city traffic 90; and a garbage truck, pneumatic hammer, rock concert, or noisy bar, or loud thunder 110–120 dB. A loud automobile horn would emit a sound of 115 dB; an air-raid siren 140, and being close to a jet engine 160 dB. Special devices are available to measure ambient noise, and the result indicates the potential of effects, physical or psychological, on the subject exposed to it.

Most clearly defined are the effects of noise on hearing. Damage to the inner ear (the organ of Corti) has been variously postulated to be due to constriction of the blood vessels supplying the inner ear, direct trauma, or metabolic changes, with secondary scarring. A single exposure to a sound over 140 dB may permanently damage hearing. According to a 1990 National Institutes of Health consensus report, a sound environment up to 75 dB is safe, but exposure above 85 dB for eight

hours a day for many years may eventually induce deafness. There is considerable variation in susceptibility to noise-induced damage to hearing, concomitant use of agents such as aminoglycoside antibiotics being a notable exacerbating factor. About 20 million Americans are regularly exposed to sound levels dangerous to hearing; 28 million have impaired hearing; and, of these, some 10 - million cases are at least in part attributable to loud sounds. Hearing loss tends to affect first the high frequencies but may be generalized. It interferes particularly with the comprehension of speech and may be accompanied by tinnitus. Even young infants' hearing may be damaged by noise; and the popularity of rock music and portable transistor radios with headsets clearly constitutes an appreciable risk to young people.

Other physical effects of exposure to noise are less well defined. Acutely, noise induces a flight and fight reaction, releases adrenaline and similar agents, and causes the blood vessels to contract (vasoconstriction). It may cause acute hypertension. In animal experiments, exposure to continuous noise has been found to cause chronic hypertension. In man, noise has been considered to be a possible contributing factor in the pathogenesis of chronic hypertension. Noise has also been claimed to contribute to enlargement of the left ventricle of the heart, raised blood cholesterol concentrations, and even atherosclerosis. In rats, noise has been found to damage the embryo and cause reduced fertility. In one study, a noisy environment has been claimed to prolong hospital stay, perhaps as a result of delayed healing.

Many studies on the effects of noise have

identified psychological changes, including sleep deprivation and behavioral changes. People working in noisy environments tend to make more errors, wrong decisions, become more aggressive, irritable, aloof, non-involved, impersonal, prone to burnout, less caring, less altruistic, and less helpful. Noise may cause a narrowed focus of attention, a perception of loss of control over the environment, feelings of helplessness, or depression.

Noise is a problem in hospitals, once areas of quiet, now often having noise levels of 50–70 dB night and day, reaching occasional intensities of 110 dB. It is also a problem in operating rooms. In several studies some 20–50% of hospital patients have complained of noise. It originates largely from telephones, loudspeakers, monitors, therapeutic devices, and people shouting instead of speaking softly. In hospitals, as elsewhere, ambient noise may be controlled by changing architectural designs, providing quiet rooms, using simple methods such as rubber bumpers, and pads on various equipment, and moderating the unpleasant impact of monitors, phones, and pagers. At work sites ear plugs and muffs may be required. Noise cancellation technology has been made possible by the development of new techniques such as head sets with batteries that cancel out undesirable frequencies. In some areas communities have been active in reducing noise by restricting times for building and constructions, putting limits on radios, loudspeakers, steam whistles, leaf blowers, drums, or shouting peddlers, or by making it illegal to make a noise that can be heard at more than 200, 300, or 600 feet away, and educating people about the danger which excessive noise poses to hearing. GD

Zealand. Its administrative costs are comparably low. The no-fault systems of both countries aim to achieve the laudable goal of an equitable system of loss-spreading, whereby society undertakes to compensate its members for *all* those personal injuries which are an inevitable part of daily life in our modern world.

Variations on the theme of no-fault insurance exist in several other countries as well as New Zealand and Sweden, primarily to protect physicians and public health authorities from the risk of legal claims in the event of idiosyncratic reactions to routine preventive vaccinations.     RMah

*See also* LAW; MISADVENTURES

**NORDIC COUNTRIES** See SCANDINAVIA

**NUCLEAR MEDICINE** The patient lay stretched out on a comfortable table. Standing alongside a technologist prepared an injection and explained that the syringe contained a solution of radioactive molecules designed to attach to one or other tissue in the body. When injected these would be carried by the bloodstream to that tissue — perhaps a cancer. A device called a camera, but one recording the radiation from radioactive atoms rather than light, was then placed over the patient to image the sites of disease. This would help the radiologist make a diagnosis or help the patient's physician provide care.

That person is an imaginary patient in a nuclear medicine service — most often found within a department of radiology. The images produced need skill to be interpreted, by a nuclear medicine physician or radiologist, who may have as colleagues technologists, radiopharmacists, and medical physicists. If necessary, the same drug, when bound to a source of more damaging radiation, might be injected later to treat and eradicate the cancer or other disease.

## Beginnings

Radiology and nuclear medicine are perhaps the only specialties that trace their origins to a specific month, if not a day. Both are children of the very end of the 19th century; matured in the 20th century; and owe their origins to chance. But chance is not always an orphan. The individuals concerned — ROENTGEN (p 873) and BECQUEREL (p 700) — were careful experimental scientists.

Roentgen, a German physicist, was experimenting in the small Bavarian university town of Würzburg. In November 1895, while working with cathode-ray tubes in a darkened room he noticed by chance fluorescence at a distance. He went on to discover that the fluorescence was caused by penetrating but hitherto undiscovered radiations from the cathode-ray tubes. These

radiations he called X-rays, using the algebraic symbol *x* for an unknown. Before the end of that year, Roentgen had used the new rays to image the internal structure of the body — the bones of his wife's hand.

In February 1896 while working in France and prompted by this awareness of radiation, Becquerel discovered radioactivity. The story has it that he placed lumps of pitchblende on sealed photographic film in the sunlight, intent on finding out if the rays of the sun induced any penetrating fluorescence in the mineral. On developing the film after a cloudy day, he was surprised to find as much blackening of the photographic emulsion as had occurred in bright sunlight. He realized that the pitchblende itself was a source of the energetic rays. We now recognize that these rays result from natural radioactivity.

Later, Mme (Dr) Marie and Dr Pierre CURIE (p 556) described natural radioactivity and discovered radium. Subsequently, Mme Eve Curie observed the artificial induction of radioactivity. Rutherford, a British-educated, New Zealand physicist working at McGill University in Montreal, Canada, went on to discover the structure of the atom. All won NOBEL PRIZES — Becquerel and Marie Curie jointly.

Another insight, crucial to the development of nuclear medicine, came when the Hungarian scientist, Georg von Hevesy (a former student of Rutherford) first used the tracer principle. He experimented with a plant having its roots in a water bath containing a radioactive isotope of lead. Hevesy followed the rate of passage of the tracer through the stem of the plant with an instrument able to detect radioactivity. This use of radioactive atoms, present in minute amounts but acting as a marker of other, non-radioactive atoms — the tracer principle — was an important link in the evolution of nuclear medicine. It required only that Hevesy's insight was applied to living humans instead of plants, and for the tracer to be administered by injection.

## Subsequent developments

Despite these insights, the only radioactive materials available before 1940 were isotopes of such elements as lead, radon, radium, and uranium. Few of these play a part in the normal functions of our bodies. And then came WAR, where cyclotrons and nuclear reactors led to the ghastly horrors of Hiroshima and Nagasaki. And yet war resulted in the availability of a range of radioactive elements produced from these same cyclotrons and reactors. The radioactive elements, or isotopes, permitted understanding of the function of the thyroid gland in health and disease and the development of a range of tools to

## HUSBAND AND WIFE

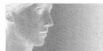

Marie Sklodowska **CURIE** (1867–1934). Franco-Polish physicist. She was forced to leave Warsaw for political reasons and in 1891 joined her sister in Paris to study at the Sorbonne. In 1895 she married Pierre CURIE the physicist. She and her husband, together with Henri BECQUEREL (p 700), were awarded the Nobel prize for physics in 1903 for discovering radioactivity. In 1893 they had isolated two new elements from pitchblende, radium and polonium. For this she received the Nobel prize for chemistry in 1911.

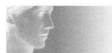

Pierre **CURIE** (1859–1906). French physicist. Curie married Marie in 1895, and with her and BECQUEREL (p 700) won the Nobel prize for physics in 1903 for their discovery of radioactivity. He discovered piezo-electricity and made contributions to magnetism and other physics. He described the three radioactive emanations of radium, later designated as α, β, and γ, that is alpha, beta, and gamma particles and rays. In 1906 he was run over by a dray in Paris and killed. His daughter, Iréne, born in 1897, married Frédéric Joliot, and together these two carried on and advanced the work begun by her parents.

examine the human body, its functions, and its fluids.

With the availability of radioactive tracers to inject into the body, early developments focused on measuring the amount of radioactivity wherever it localized. It quickly became apparent that much more would be gained from making images of the distribution of radioactivity in organs or in the body as a whole. Yet the gamma rays from radioisotopes are not susceptible to optical bending as occurs in an optical lens. Benedict Cassen solved this by using a moving detector which traversed the body, or organ, in a stepwise manner and recorded the pattern of activity only immediately below the detector. The image that resulted was called a scan.

Later Hal Anger developed the gamma camera. This uses electronics rather than mechanics to act as a lens for gamma rays. In converting the gamma rays, first into an electronic signal and then into an image, the information becomes digital and can be measured easily and the image processed mathematically.

The resulting techniques permit examination of virtually every bodily organ and system. It was soon found that a radioactive version of the element technetium (technetium-99m) had ideal physical properties for detection by a gamma camera. Moreover, it causes only a little radiation exposure to the patient. It could also be delivered to hospitals and clinics in a weekly supply of a radioactive parent — molybdenum-99 — in a generator from which the technetium-99m may be obtained daily. Ironically, technetium no longer occurs naturally on earth (having all decayed away from among the primordial star matter which makes up our planet). It certainly has no role in natural bodily processes. Nevertheless, because of the physical properties of technetium-99m, much human ingenuity has gone into preparing compounds of this nuclide now used to examine many parts of the body.

Instrumental in the development of nuclear medicine, physicists continue to have an important role in its evolution. Complex machines need careful selection, testing, calibration, and quality control. These tasks are carried out by technologists and medical physicists. Such physicists in larger facilities contribute to educational programs as well as carrying out research into new techniques or ways of displaying and analyzing images.

### Nuclear pharmacy

Only a few naturally occurring elements are used by the body. For example, iodine (as iodide) is selectively concentrated in the thyroid gland, as are calcium salts in bone. Both of these facts have

been used in nuclear medicine. However, the range of techniques which characterize modern nuclear medicine are possible only because nuclear pharmacists have learned how to combine a radioactive atom with a carrier molecule creating a radiopharmaceutical. The carrier molecule determines how that radiopharmaceutical behaves in the body, while the radioactive atom allows for its external tracking. An analogy is the cowbell. The bell itself (the radioactive tracer) is of no intrinsic interest to the herdsman, but its signal reveals the whereabouts of the cow (the carrier molecule).

Radiopharmaceuticals are made by radiopharmacists either in a hospital or at a commercial manufacturing facility. In larger hospitals, particularly teaching hospitals, the radiopharmacist is usually part of the staff, contributes to educational programs, and does research into the development of new compounds.

The radionuclide used in 90% or more of clinical nuclear medicine tests is technetium-99m.

### Modern nuclear medicine

As a result of these developments nuclear medicine now has a place in the day-to-day practice of medicine. Typical applications of nuclear medicine include:

***Detecting tumor spread in bone*** Calcium phosphates concentrate in bone. Bis- or di-phosphonates localize in bone when used in treating such bone disorders as Paget's disease and osteoporosis. Similarly, technetium-99m-methylene di-phosphonate concentrates in sites of increased bone turnover, such as sites of tumor spread (metastases). Because this tracer is detectable at such sites very early in the disease, technetium-99m-methylene di-phosphonate is used for its early diagnosis. Sites of increased uptake of the radiotracer are found when radiographs (X-rays) of bone show no abnormal finding. Furthermore, unlike other imaging methods, nuclear medical images may be made of the whole body, allowing for a survey of all or most of the skeleton — an important step when there may be no symptoms to alert the physician to a particular site to examine (Fig. 1, p 558).

### Early diagnosis of osteomyelitis

Technetium-99m-methylene di-phosphonate also localizes in sites of bone infection, called osteomyelitis. When this disease is suspected, both early and late images are made. On the early images when the radioactive compound is still mostly in the blood, there is an area of more general increased activity. On delayed images this is seen in particular to be in bone. The use of such 'two-phase' imaging makes nuclear medicine tests more specific — anyone who has had an infection such as a boil knows that at such sites the blood flow is increased, with a characteristic throbbing pain in tune with the heart beat. Such abnormalities are apparent on gamma ray scans much earlier than on radiographs, permitting prompt treatment and less progression of the disease.

*Diagnosing reduced blood flow to the heart* Technetium-99m methoxy isobutyl isonitrile is a radioactive tracer localizing in heart muscle that has a normal blood supply. A patient with chest pain of uncertain cause might have a test using this material. After injection sectional images are made and may show reduced blood flow, which indicates (depending on the extent and severity of the abnormality) partial or complete obstruction of the (coronary) blood vessels supplying the heart (Fig. 2). The test is used to select those who need further testing by heart catheterization.

*Seeking sites of postoperative infection* Infections are associated with an increase in the white blood cells and the local migration of these cells into the infection — the pus that may accumulate in a boil is an example. However, not all infections are as readily located. Postoperatively a patient may become increasingly feverish without any obvious site of infection. Blood may be taken from the patient, the white cells separated, and labeled with a tracer which enters cells such as indium-111 hydroxyquinoline. When reinjected some of these cells will localize in the infection, if present. Images of the radioactive label then help the diagnostician to locate the site of infection.

*Mapping tumor spread* A patient with thyroid cancer returns to the clinic for follow-up. She has an I-131 sodium iodide scan which shows abnormal localization in the chest despite a normal lung radiograph. This finding is typical of small sites of tumor spread throughout the lungs. A much larger dose of the same tracer is then injected for treatment and on subsequent follow-up the disease is found to have been eradicated.

Such techniques of nuclear medicine are not confined to people. Veterinary schools also have diagnostic services using radioactive tracers. Typical applications are the use of technetium-99m-methylene di-phosphonate bone scans to elucidate the nature of injuries to the limbs of racehorses, or I-131 sodium iodide to treat cancer of the thyroid in dogs — a species in which this disease is common.

## Tomography

In all early radiological methods a disadvantage was that two-dimensional images were made of a three-dimensional object — the human body. The result was a superimposition of structures. This often limited the detection of disease or the clarity of the images. All radiological methods have, therefore, progressed to use sectional imaging to increase the detectability of disease. Such sectional images are made mechanically or electronically. The technique is called tomography (Greek *tomos* meaning slice), and contiguous slices reveal structure just as sliced bread reveals the inner structure of a loaf.

*Positron emission tomography* Though great ingenuity has made it possible to trace many biological processes using compounds of technetium-99m, the purist may object that such methods are playing fast and loose with Hevesy's tracer principle in that technetium-99m is neither naturally occurring nor metabolized. Positron emission tomography has evolved in part to address this.

The most common elements in our body are hydrogen, carbon (C), nitrogen (N), and oxygen (O) with smaller amounts of calcium, iodine, iron, and other trace metals. It so happens that there are isotopes of C, N, and O, all of which share some unusual characteristics. All three have very short half-lives (20, 10, and 2 minutes, respectively) and all decay by converting a nuclear proton to a neutron by emitting a positron. Readers of science fiction will recognize this as a positive electron — anti-matter. Very soon the positron encounters an ordinary electron, and with matter and anti-matter the result is mutual destruction — the stuff of science fiction. However, the conservation of mass-energy requires that the mass of these particles is converted to gamma ray energy, according to Einstein's famous equation ($e = mc^2$). For equally complex reasons (related to conserving angular momentum), the gamma rays are paired at 180° to each other. These rays may be imaged very readily since detecting the pair helps in locating the original positron event — and thus the site in the body of the original compound labeled with radioactive C, N, or O.

Because these radioactive tracers have such brief half-lives they cannot easily be distributed from a central facility but are best made in a small cyclotron at the hospital. In addition to C-11, N-13, and O-15, tracers such as fluorine-18 (which substitutes for hydroxy groups in biological molecules) or rubidium (acting like potassium in localizing in healthy heart and other muscle) may also be made.

In the past, the cost of the cyclotron and positron detector or camera has often limited positron emission tomography to research uses. However, of late it has increasingly come to be applied to routine clinical care, particularly for detecting tumor spread or blood flow in damaged heart muscle. Thus unnecessary cancer surgery

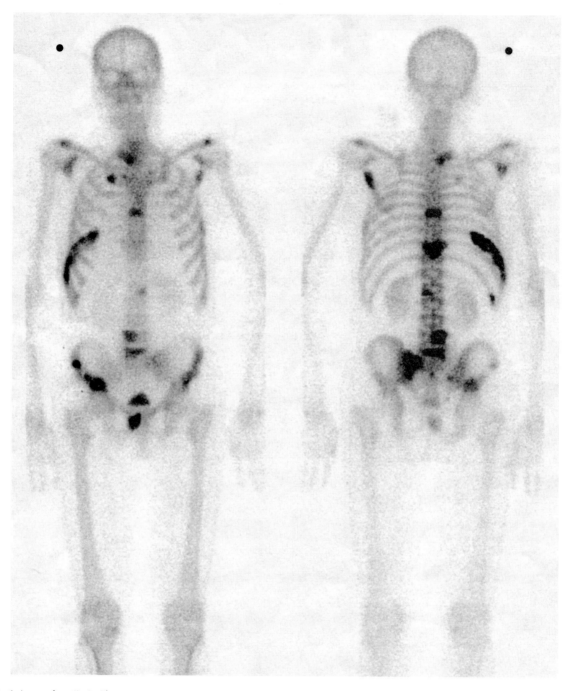

**Fig. 1** A scan of a patient with prostate cancer made after injecting technetium-99m-methylene di-phosphonate. Radiographs had been negative, but the multiple sites of increased uptake of tracer indicate that the cancer has spread into bone.

may be avoided, or patients selected who will benefit from surgery to improve the blood supply to the heart.

### Treatment with radioactive tracers
Radioactive atoms of different kinds produce several types of radiation. Gamma-rays, such as X-rays and light, are part of the electromagnetic spectrum and are very energetic so that they readily penetrate tissues and may be imaged. Alpha and beta radiations are particles (helium nuclei and electrons, respectively), and being larger do not easily penetrate tissues. Their energy may be used as a destructive force.

Molecules labeled with radioactive atoms that emit alpha and beta radiations may be used to treat disease. For example, iodine-131 emits both gamma and beta radiations. As sodium iodide, it has been used to image the thyroid gland and remains in widespread use for treating overactive glands (Graves's disease) as well as cancer of the thyroid gland which has spread. Indeed, thyroid cancer is one of the few cancers which may be cured after it has migrated to other organs, such as the lung.

Palliative treatments for cancers that have spread to bone (using strontium-89 citrate) and the abdominal cavity (using a phosphorus-32 colloid) have been used to relieve pain and other symptoms. More recently, antibodies against cancer cells and labeled with iodine-131 or similar radionuclides have been used successfully in late stage cancers, such as lymphoma, for which no other treatment is available. Such methods require many caregivers, besides admission to special hospital beds with adequate measures to ensure the safety of patient and staff in the presence of large doses of radiation. For example, when iodine-131 was used for diagnosis a typical dose might be 0.37 megabecquerels (10 microcuries), whereas for treatment, doses of 7.4 gigabecquerels (200 millicuries) or more might be used. The extent to which such methods will become widely available is uncertain.

### The future

The medical diagnostic applications of radiation began with studies of the human skeleton when Roentgen first took what would be called a radiograph of his wife's hand. The early years of imaging the body focused on examinations of its structure, and this was partly true of nuclear medicine in early techniques such as liver scanning. However, the second century of all of the radiological sciences is witnessing an increasing emphasis on examining function. The reason is not hard to seek as, trauma aside, most diseases begin as disordered function and, when death results, it is usually because one or more organs cease to work properly. The strength of nuclear medicine lies in applications to examine organ function, recalling its origins in Hevesy's tracer principle.

Simplistically it is possible to see in nuclear medicine two undesirable traits. The first is the dehumanizing influence of machines, with their potential to deconstruct the compassionate, caring context of medical practice. The second is the fear that high-technology medical practice, which by its nature is expensive, will make the care of the sick potentially unaffordable for those not insured against such needs.

The provision of care in any aspect of medical practice requires a balance between compassion and ensuring that the best possible care is provided. That sometimes requires technology-intensive tools. The challenge is not to ignore technology but temper its use with humanity.

Diagnosis and treatment with nuclear medicine are often much less complex and expensive than with alternative methods. Thus, in reducing stays in hospital and facilitating early and accurate diagnosis, technology is proving to be part of the solution to the problem of providing high standards of care without further increases in its cost.

BL

*See also* IMAGING; ONCOLOGY; X-RAYS

**NUREMBERG CODE** The Nuremberg Code was the first internationally recognized set of guidelines dealing specifically with non-therapeutic human experimentation. It originated under the special circumstances of the Nuremberg Medical Trial of 1946–7, where 23 defendants stood accused of participating in horrific experiments in Nazi concentration camps. Throughout the

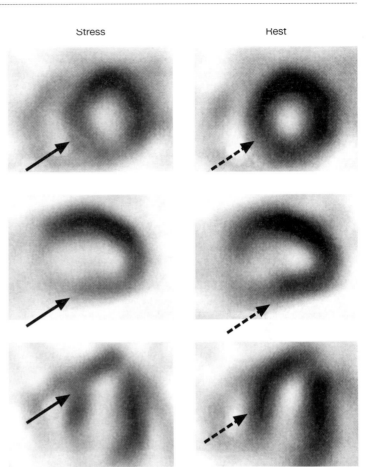

Stress        Rest

**Fig. 2** Selected tomographic sectional scans of the chest in planes at right angles to each other made after injecting technetium-99m methoxy isobutyl isonitrile while the patient's heart was stressed. Sites of decreased blood flow to heart muscle (arrows), indicating obstruction of blood vessels, are apparent. Comparable images made at rest show some recovery, indicating that the vessel obstruction is not complete.

trial the judges tried to establish historical standards relating to human experimentation, which they found through multiple sources but principally through the testimony of two American physicians, Andrew Ivy and Leo Alexander.

The code stipulates several major provisions: the voluntary consent of the subjects is essential (and they should be competent to give it — not children, the mentally ill, or captive populations such as prisoners, where coercion might be used); the experiment must yield fruitful results for the good of society unprocurable by other means; the study should be based on the results of animal experiments; the experiment must be conducted to avoid all unnecessary physical and mental suffering; no experiment should be conducted if there are good reasons for supposing that death or disabling injury will occur; the degree of risk should never exceed the humanitarian importance of the question; proper protective precautions should be taken; the experiment should be conducted only by scientifically qualified personnel; the subject should have the right to end the experiment, and the physician ought to end it if continuation is likely to cause injury or death.

The judges based the code on what were perceived to be customary principles in medical science — what Ivy described as rules 'in force by common understanding and practice'. Yet there were never any clear guidelines governing research in the major Allied countries before Nuremberg, although frequent references from the prosecution to the Hippocratic OATH made it seem so. HIPPOCRATES (p 382) emphasized the obligation to benefit the patient but was silent on human research ethics. Other historical authorities who wrote on medical ethics also devoted very little space to experimentation procedures. Thomas PERCIVAL'S (p 629) *Medical ethics* (1803) mentioned only the importance of competent research and in 1865 Claude BERNARD (p 102) cautioned against harming the subject but approved experimentation on prisoners condemned to death. The critical principle of informed, voluntary, and competent consent was absent or vaguely worded in the writings of subsequent authorities and dealt solely with therapeutic experiments. Only the 19th-century physician, William Beaumont, mentioned the need for voluntary and informed consent in the context of non-therapeutic experiments.

The absence of any formal or even coherent guidelines meant that ethical questions were left to the discretion of individual researchers, and vulnerable populations such as institutionalized children, prisoners, soldiers, the moribund, and the intellectually disabled were over-represented as subjects of research. In the USA, use of prisoners in experiments was often justified in the name

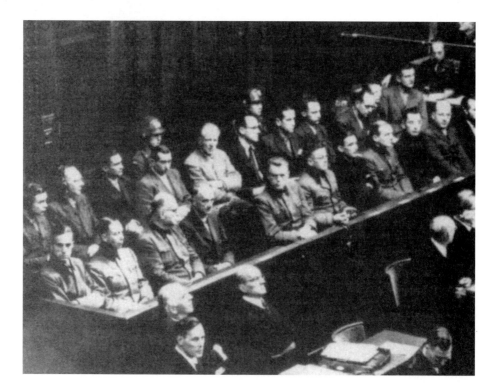

The 'Dock' of defendant physicians at the 'Doctor's Trial', November 1946. (Reproduced courtesy of UPI/Bettman Newsphotos.)

of social redemption and, under the imperatives of World War Two, the Medical Research Council in Britain felt justified in asking conscientious objectors to volunteer for risky experiments with hepatitis and malaria as their contribution to 'war work'.

Orphans were used extensively in American experiments. In 1911–16 there were 68 reports of experiments on children in one pediatric journal. Physicians rarely mentioned parental consent and frequently referred to the children as 'material'. However, such experiments were less easy to justify publicly, and in 1911 Dr. Hideyo NOGUCHI (p 874) of the Rockefeller Institute found himself at the center of a public storm over his use of orphans as experimental subjects in a diagnostic test for syphilis.

Ironically, it was in pre-war Germany where public controversy first led to government action. Here, the research effort was unrivaled and accompanied by vigorous public comment. In 1900, after a public scandal about experiments on minors with serum infected with syphilis, the government issued a directive that demanded the procurement of voluntary and informed consent and prohibited non-therapeutic experiments on children and incompetents. The Reich government issued further guidelines in 1931 after the death of 75 children in Lübeck during experiments with TUBERCULOSIS vaccinations. These guidelines contained most of the points included in the Nuremberg Code; some have argued they were more inclusive since they covered therapeutic as well as non-therapeutic experiments. At the medical trial there was much controversy over the legal status of the Reich circular, but regardless of its legal status it undoubtedly represented a more detailed and advanced guide for investigators than any that existed at the time in the rest of Europe or America.

The Nuremberg Code is the most famous document issuing from the medical trial and is generally recognized as a watershed in the history of human experimentation. Nevertheless, subsequent research practices have not always lived up to its high standards. In 1962, Dr Maurice PAPPWORTH (p 616), a freelance teacher for the higher medical diploma in London, claimed that morally unacceptable experiments on human beings had been carried out on a large scale in teaching hospitals throughout Britain over the previous 20 years. Pappworth's allegations followed three years after those of the respected anesthesiologist and Harvard professor, Henry BEECHER (p 94), who made similar comments about research practices in the USA.

In view of the apparent ineffectiveness of the Nuremberg Code and the narrowness of its scope, the World Medical Association drafted the

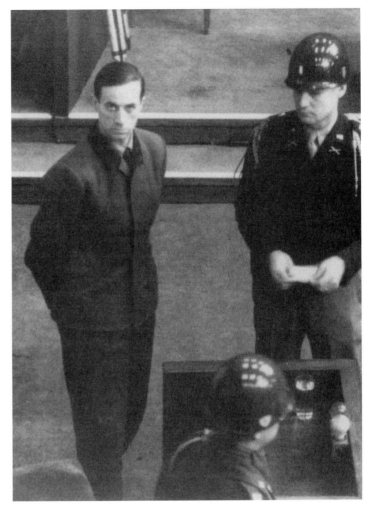

Declaration of HELSINKI (1964), which was designed for professional use and distinguished between therapeutic and non-therapeutic research. (This code waived the requirement to gain consent if the patient was unable to give it and research was therapeutic.) Nevertheless, the Nuremberg Code remains one of the most important documents in the history of human experimentation. It has served as an authoritative reference point for general debate and for critics of human experimentation. Successive codes and legal mechanisms have referred implicitly or explicitly to Nuremberg when setting guidelines and limits to acceptable experimentation. As many historians have noted, the code's enduring value lies in the judges' vision that 'certain basic principles must be observed in order to satisfy moral, ethical and legal concepts'. JHaz

*See also* BIOETHICS; HOLOCAUST; INFORMED CONSENT

Karl Brandt, personal physician to Adolf Hitler and Reich Commissioner for Health and Sanitation, sentenced to death by hanging. (US Army Photo, Ray D'Addario.)

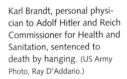

**NURSING — AS A PROFESSION** Throughout its history nursing has been something of an institutional orphan in the hospital but also in the community, constantly casting around for political space and reference points within which to build a coherent identity and power base. Nursing has also played an important social part as mediator between groups of differential status as a conduit into care. That role has been shaped by pressure on all sides: medicine, managers, policymakers, professions allied to medicine, and patients. The in- and go-between nature of nursing has rendered it both functionally critical to, and yet often invisible within, the healthcare division of labor.

Significantly, it was Sairey GAMP (p 495), the notorious character in Charles Dickens's novel *Martin Chuzzlewit* (1844), who has often been perceived as the spark plug for nursing reform during the 19th century. A 'female functionary, a nurse and watcher, and performer of nameless offices about the persons of the dead', Mrs Gamp quickly became synonymous with the 'old' order of healthcare. Superstition, corruption, coarseness, age, prejudice, presumption, dirt, and drunkenness contrasted deeply with that of the 'new' nurse. The 'new' nurse embodied the ideal attributes of the emerging order of healthcare: enlightenment, rationality, science, Christian purity, innocence, virtue, youth, freshness, gentleness, hygiene, sobriety, gentility, and intelligent obedience. Sairey Gamp and her counterpart, the 'new nurse', soon came to symbolize the discrepancy between the 'old' and the 'new' order in healthcare.

Interestingly, the nurse reformers, keen to promote professionalization, looked to the

doctors for inspiration. In doing so, they adopted the rhetoric that doctors had deployed some 50 years earlier against quacks or irregular practitioners. Sairey Gamp was to quackery what the new nurse was to gentlemanly practice in the respective registration campaigns. Unlike her unruly counterpart, Sairey Gamp, the 'new' nurse was to be inculcated with the rationalist ethos and values of scientific medicine, facilitating her compliance with medical orders. Training provided the ideal means of institutionalizing a stable, hierarchical social order in the evolving institutions at the turn of the century. The 'new' medicine, sound and scientific, required new regimes of nursing to be applied assiduously and accurately. Within this new symbolic and scientific structure Florence NIGHTINGALE (p 548) came to epitomize the clinical and cultural counterpoint to Sairey Gamp. In her hands 'character' became short-hand for skilled observation, obedient compliance with medical orders and vigilance, the touchstones of skill in the rhetorical armory of reformed nursing.

Although skilled nursing was not unknown before Florence Nightingale, it is she who is often credited with disciplining and deepening its basis. The domiciliary nurse, in the guise of Sairey Gamp, had been demonized, but it was the home and not the hospital that was the dominant locus of care. Nursing became a key constituent in the reform of the hospital, as the care of sickness began to shift from the home into hospital.

The hospital provided a valve for recruitment, career routes, and training standards for doctors and nurses. It was the site around which the politics of state registration segregated. The pursuit of registration by nurses was part of a wider, international movement and support network of nursing leaders sharing a common set of values and vision. Their political ethos involved commitment to improving the economic and social status of nurses and women through state registration and nationally-determined standards of nursing education. Together these defined what it meant to be a trained nurse.

For nurses in Britain, the reference points for reform therefore borrowed from medicine and nursing in the USA and resulted in the passing of the Nurses' Registration Act in 1919 and the establishment of the General Nursing Council (GNC) in 1919 as its educational and regulatory body. One issue that remained vexatious, however, was the place of specialist groups within the 'new' profession created by registration. A caste system divided MIDWIVES, mental, male, fever, and children's nurses from general nurses, who were situated at the apex of the occupational pyramid. Echoing earlier medical maligning of specialists,

Nuns, nurses, and patients — some of them sharing beds — as depicted in a 15th century illustration of the Hôtel Dieu, Paris. (Reproduced courtesy of the Mary Evans Picture Library.)

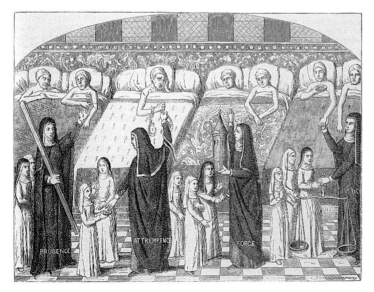

they were regarded as inferior owing to their (in some cases) shorter and more limited scope in training. One of the chief arguments against separate and specialist qualifications for nurses was that they provided a 'back door' of entry into the profession for 'inferior' practitioners. So, although a semblance of unity was created by registration, its substance was more precarious still.

In the 1960s and 1970s, the failure to contain expenditure by rationalizing nursing work led policy makers in Britain to look to management for other ways of engineering efficiency. They proposed that nurses take their place within the management fashion of the day, consensus management. Peaking in popularity in the 1970s, the tide of opinion subsequently changed from consortia working towards agreed objectives to one which favored giving people what they want rather than what the producers provided. Under the new public management, professional expertise (and expenditure, it hoped) was to be pinned down by quality assurance, clinical audit, and performance indicators.

Research was the next strategy recruited in service to rationalization. From the 1940s onwards, nursing came under increasing scrutiny from social scientists keen to explore the psychosocial dynamics of nursing in terms of outcomes such as productivity, patient recovery, staff turnover, and morale. It resulted in Britain importing models of care organization from the USA. American ideas and methods were also evident through the Rockefeller Foundation, which provided the initial seed-corn and fellowship funding for university development.

Higher education for nurses shifted seismically in Britain only when the government's own policy in higher education moved towards 'massification' in the late 1980s. Nursing became both a beneficiary of and contributor to the expansion of higher education, especially for women. How sustainable such development might be in the face of cost-containment pressures, workforce re-engineering and redesign initiatives, and the 'intensification' of care remains to be seen.

Nursing's nomadic status, at times, aligning itself with medicine or the state, and occasionally with feminism and radical political movements, means that it is more often an anomaly rather than an analog in relation to other groups. Perhaps it is time to reinvoke the early nurse historians, Adelaide Nutting and Lavinia Dock, who, drawing upon the work of Russian zoologist and anarchist, Petr Kropotkin, used an ethological model of behavior to endorse the 'biological' basis of altruism and hence nursing. They argued that the species most capable of survival are those who have co-operated with each other in 'mutual aid'. Accordingly, symbiosis might ensure that reci-

procity, recognition, and reward regulate relations between patients and practitioners in the future.

AMR

**NURSING IN BRITAIN** Historically, the women in a household cared for the sick of their family, just as they fed and clothed them in health. The care of the indigent and homeless sick devolved mostly on religious communities until the Reformation.

In the 19th century the Industrial Revolution saw the rise of a prosperous middle class of manufacturers who began to seek professional advancement for their children. Medicine attracted many applicants, all able to pay for hospital experience, and doctors soon needed to divide beds among themselves for teaching purposes. In the first half of the 19th century, hospitals in London and the big provincial cities had so many medical students that there was no need of nurses, except as unskilled attendants. One effect of this surge of medical training was that acute medicine and surgery provided all the 'interesting' cases and 'good teaching material', and the chronic sick, the enfeebled aged, and the psychiatrically ill were not wanted in the voluntary hospitals. This had far-reaching effects on the development of the nursing profession.

There were two important facts that made nursing women's work. First, nursing was always seen as part of domestic household work; secondly, there were 2.5 million women, mostly spinsters and widows, seeking means of support through work. Working-class women might hope to find employment in factories, where, although badly paid and overworked, they met outside their homes, and learned the facts of industrial life. Middle-class women could be governesses, often working only for their keep, or clerks working a 60-hour week for 12 shillings. When, during the Crimean War (1854–56), Florence NIGHTINGALE (p 548) showed that there was work that intelligent women could do in hospital, so enthusiastic was the response that by the 1890s more women wanted to nurse than could be trained. Thus for nearly three-quarters of a century nursing in Britain was fashioned by a great pioneer and by the social trends of Victorian England. Nurses were to be women, and dedicated to their work; they were thus doubly vulnerable to economic exploitation, and remained so until the middle of the 20th century.

Our feelings and ideas about pre-Nightingale nursing derive from two sources. One is fiction; how powerful is the image of Sairey GAMP (p 495), and of the women whom Scrooge saw quarreling over his clothes after his 'death'. The other is fact. St Bartholomew's Hospital, London, has continuous records from 1549; from the accounts of the governors' meetings one may picture the work of the sisters (charge-nurse), who lived in a room off their wards, gave simple care, fetched the patient's food from the buttery, washed their ward linen, and spent their 'spare' time in spinning. Much unpretentious care was given, often with heroism in times of plague and pestilence.

Miss Nightingale's new recruits were, not unnaturally, rather disdainful and disapproving about those whom they were replacing. Their predecessors might have been forgiven for some of the ways in which they maintained fortitude in days before anesthetics and antiseptics. A sister wrote in 1902 about what she saw on entering the first school at St Bartholomew's Hospital in 1877:

Drunkenness was very common among the staff nurses, who were chiefly of the charwoman type, frequently of bad character, with little or no education, and few of them with even an elementary knowledge of nursing … One woman I remember who came some little time after I did, and under whom I worked, had been a lady's maid, and had never done a day's nursing. She was, however, of a decidedly superior class to any of the others … Nursing, as you understand it now, was utterly unknown. Patients were not nursed, they were attended to, more or less … The work was very hard — lockers, locker boards and tables of course to scrub every day. No, we did not as a rule scrub the floors, though I have scrubbed the front ward of Matthew on a special occasion before 6 a.m. … The patients had their beds made once a day, the bad ones had their sheets drawn at night … then you thought nothing of having fourteen or fifteen poultices to change. All wounds of course suppurated, and required poulticing two or

three times a day … the thermometers in use then were very much longer than those in use now, and had to be read while in position, as they ran down at once when removed from the mouth or armpit. They cost 12/6d each. The sisters and nurses never used a thermometer, the dressers and clerks took the temperatures when required.

This was the nursing scene in 1877. Infection, both medical and surgical, was rife. The nurse worked long hours at hard work with little reward. Light was, however, breaking on the hospital scene. Anesthesia had arrived to relieve the lot of the patients and of surgeons; the nature of infections such as TYPHOID and CHOLERA began to be understood. Doctors were now able to cure. The nurse stopped scrubbing the floor, and began her role by taking over duties delegated from the doctor.

### End of 19th century

Nursing in the 1880s and 1890s involved physical and mental stress. Infectious diseases abounded and could be fatal. Yet by the end of the 19th century the new nurse of Florence Nightingale's ideals had displaced the pre-Crimean one. Hospitals and their matrons (nurses in charge of hospitals) were much concerned with the length of nurses' training, which successively rose from one to two and then to three or four years. In the closed world of hospital wards and nurses' homes, nurses still retained the dual aspect of domestic work and personal care. The following account was written by a woman who began to train in 1916, and who later headed Lady Minto's Indian Nursing Service. She says of her probationer days:

---

**NURSE-EDUCATOR**

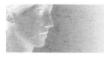

Dame Mary Rosalind **PAGET** (1855–1948). British nurse and midwife. Trained as a nurse, Paget worked at the Westminster Hospital, the London Hospital, and the British Lying-in Hospital before returning to the London Hospital, where she remained for many years. Having realized the need for better education in midwifery, in 1881 with a small group of women, she founded the Midwives' Institute, which later became the Royal College of Midwives. She was also one of the founders of what was to become the Chartered Society of Physiotherapy and founded and edited *Nursing Notes* for many years.

---

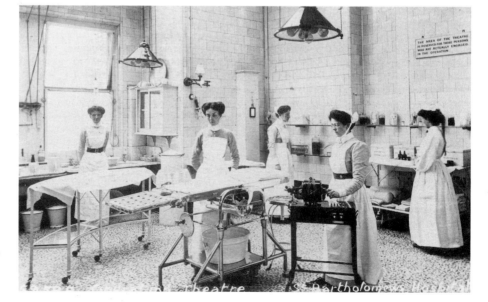

The coming of anesthetics and asepsis began the emergence of a technical role for the nurse at the turn of the 19th century, as shown in this photograph of an operating room at St Bartholomew's Hospital.
(Reproduced by permission of the Medical Illustration Department, St Bartholomew's Hospital, London.)

Life was hard. Cleaning and washing patients, making beds, giving bedpans, and then cleaning again … lockers, brasses, mackintoshes, spittoons. Very seldom were we probationers allowed contact with anything interesting or instructive. Many fell by the way, as often as not because of the ward sisters' stinging sarcasm. Medical students suffered in the same way but they were in the wards each day for a short time only.

With our long hours on duty, one particular patient depended so much on the personal touch of the individual nurse. We really did see them through their illness, which I think made our job so absorbingly interesting. We were at their bedside each day for ten to thirteen hours … and for twelve hours on night duty … we became part and parcel of their sufferings.

Treatments included saline infusions, bread, linseed and kaolin poultices, and mustard plasters. I have seen cupping done to relieve congestion and have myself applied leeches.

In the wards probationers (student nurses) worked under continual blame and criticism. It was as if training had to be made as rigorous as possible, so that only the strongest survived. It is sometimes said that this was the result of rule by elderly spinsters, but this is a simplistic view. Medical students were managed in much the same way by the consultants: ward rounds were often painful occasions, when learners were held up to ridicule in front of their patients.

The effect of the First World War on nursing was tremendous. There were 2 million casualties on the Western Front alone, mostly adult men, so that there were many spinsters and widows who would have to earn a living after the war.

The College of Nursing was founded in 1916 to further nursing interests, and now survives as the Royal College of Nursing, the main professional body concerned with educational policy, ethical standards, and conditions of service. In 1920 a General Nursing Council was established to supervise instruction and examinations, and to compile a register of trained nurses. Yet in the 1930s nurses still worked long hours at low pay. By then the nursing role was well established: it was to give comfort; the patient always came first. Nurses did not run unless there was a fire or hemorrhage. Such axioms were not thought of as clichés, but as truths to be followed.

It was accepted that 'good nursing' might still save lives when no medical cure existed. Diabetes was treated by insulin, but lobar pneumonia patients still suffered a long dangerous illness culminating in a crisis, through which nurses hoped to bring them. Healthy young men who had a hernia operation stayed in bed until the stitches were removed. A drug called prontosil had been discovered which could cure infections. Blood transfusion was becoming common, so

surgical shock was retreating. Lung surgery was becoming safer, and heart surgery was on the horizon.

**World War II**

During World War II women won advancement in many fields, while sharing the hardships of the battlefield and the prisoner-of-war camps. Many new forms of work were opened up to women. Nursing had lost its old appeal as the major area of work available to women. It was now seen as a job of low pay with hard work in Victorian premises, and many women were no longer eager to tolerate such conditions. In an endeavor to fill vacancies, more auxiliaries and students were recruited, so that the ratio of untrained and trained staff altered for the worse. The age of entry was lowered in the hope that there were many young people who went elsewhere because they were too young to nurse. Headmistresses now saw nursing as an occupation for the undereducated and were unwilling to help intelligent candidates to nurse.

The inauguration of the NHS in 1948 should have been a time of hope. A free health service was to be one basis of the new caring society, but nurses and doctors were depressed and anxious. Assistant nurses were now a statutory grade, working for enrollment with the General Nursing Council. One-year 'crash' courses for people with wartime nursing experience abounded. 'Cadet' schemes for children leaving school were legion, in the hope that bridging the gap between school and hospital would keep up numbers. All these increased the imbalance between untrained and trained staff. Those who qualified and remained in nursing were promoted early and without training to posts of responsibility. In some areas the number of patients awaiting admission was high and the staff meager.

A change came, too, in the traditional role of the nurse. Antibiotics and renal dialysis and other technical procedures were being introduced. Cure became more common, and the quality of nursing care of less obvious importance to the outcome of an illness, if not to the well-being of the patient during it.

Suggestions and proposals for the ailments of the nursing profession were not lacking. Many thought that more money for staff would solve all problems, others that harsh prevailing attitudes must be cured. Some wanted the training lengthened, some shortened. All wanted the syllabus reorganized, but not all in the same direction. Everyone agreed that many students were unequal academically to the demands of the syllabus; their eventual failure was traumatic and discouraged recruitment, but if they were not recruited, there was no one to do the work. Matrons went on recruiting missions to Africa, the West Indies, and Asia seeking potential students, pupils, and auxiliaries, and tutors found that they must teach English as well as nursing. By the 1960s 35% of the nursing force came from overseas. Wastage in 1961 was 39% overall, and many registered nurses went to the USA, Canada, and Australia, where conditions were better and salaries higher. This further increased the imbalance between trained staff and learners. Yet the great advances in medicine and science that occurred in the second half of the 20th century gave nurses marvelous opportunities in care. The student nurse must today have experience not only in her training hospital, but also in elements of psychiatric nursing, midwifery, community service, and the care of the elderly. She can specialize in a variety of disciplines, not only in hospital, but also with the armed services, in occupational health, with a primary-care team, the prison service, overseas nursing, or in the community. If she chooses the last, she can be a health visitor, a district nurse, a midwife, or work in a family planning clinic.

The work of the district (community) nurse has changed in content and method. People live longer, to suffer more degenerative diseases; in many areas there are large immigrant populations with pressing problems, especially among women. Some diseases disappear, some make sporadic reappearances; some problems, like CHILD ABUSE, come increasingly to attention. Nurses increasingly work as a part of a team with general practitioners and health visitors, with unrivaled opportunities to give total care. She sees the patient's life-style, his social problems, and those of his family and relatives. A great deal of the nursing in Britain is done by relatives in the home, many of whom need the support of the nurse over technical procedures, and advice and teaching on how to cope with problems.

In hospital, the ward is the center where nurses learn most of their art and science, and where the general public most often meets them. The ward sister was traditionally the linchpin in this important setting, and until the Second World War stayed in the post for years, often living in a bedsitting room attached to the ward, and devoting her life to it. Consultants depended on her clinical judgement; she was the stable element on the ward team, often at great personal sacrifice. She had no nursing superior but Matron, until 1966, when the structure of the hospital service was reorganized. Sisters became nursing officers of both sexes, nursing officers managed a group of wards, senior nursing officers co-ordinated their work and were responsible to a principal nursing officer. In many ways the results were painful. Those who liked bedside nursing saw that pay and pension prospects demanded that they move up the promotion ladder. Matrons disappeared: unit officers took on management positions without formal training. Senior nurses had to reapply for their own re-named positions, and sometimes found themselves rejected after years of performing their duties apparently to everyone's satisfaction. Thus the 1970s became a time of crumbling attitudes and beliefs, and awakening of economic awareness. Hospitals had assumed that there would always be a supply of low-paid workers to move goods by hand, and of student nurses to do most of the nursing. Now everyone was working shorter hours, earning bonuses and overtime pay, and union activity in hospitals was increasing. At the basic clinical level it was possible to perceive an air of hope and professional self-awareness of the immense changes in all aspects of medical and surgical care, and techniques such as renal dialysis, positive pressure ventilation, and cardiac monitoring became available. Nurses became essential members of teams that became increasingly specialized. As they gained insight into the uniqueness of their role, they also refined the method of registration, examination, and evaluating their professional competence. On-going assessment of practical skills in giving and planning individual care, knowledge of responsibilities for drug therapy, ability to plan for a group of patients, and for the nurses who give that care, has taken the place of classroom tests.

### Academic education

As academic entry standards for nurses have risen, so it seemed increasingly inappropriate that intelligent women should have to choose between

Nursing as a vocation. The nursing sister in the early 20th century divided her life between the patients in her ward and her sitting room which led off it.
(Reproduced by permission of the Medical Illustration Department, St Bartholomew's Hospital, London.)

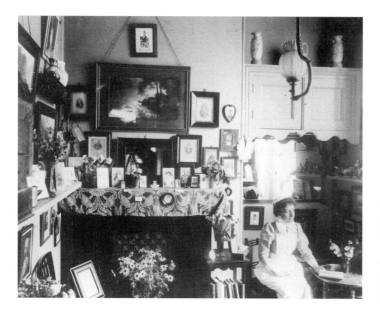

an academic education and work which they had a deep desire to undertake. Courses shared between a university and a school of nursing, which would lead to a degree and to state registration as a nurse, were approved. Apart from the number of courses based in schools of nursing, there are professors of nursing in several universities in England, Scotland, and Wales. There are now also opportunities to take a master's degree or a doctorate in many universities. Some of these are taught degrees that offer clinical nursing as a specialty. Under Project 2000, proposed by the United Kingdom Central Council (successor to the General Nursing Council) and approved by government, all nurses in training will have become students rather than workers, and it seems likely that nursing will soon become an all-graduate profession.

How is the trained nurse seen today by the public and by her peers? In the 19th century the qualified nurse's tradition had three historical strands — domestic, military, and religious. Today the domestic element has largely disappeared; caps and aprons are rarely seen. 'Officer' as a title with its connotations of rank, is used only by the armed forces. The religious component is largely confined to hospice care, where it still makes an important but ecumenical contribution.

Hospital schools of nursing have joined to form colleges, most affiliated to, or part of, a university or college of further education. Most student nurses still pursue the traditional three-year syllabus, but there are many university courses leading to a degree. Under Project 2000, programs are offered by approved colleges under which students take a three-year course, of which the first year is common ground, while the next two years are devoted to general, psychiatric, and mental handicap experience.

Provision of hygienic care, and those tasks which were the sole work of the nurse up to the 19th century, have been largely delegated to healthcare assistants. The trained nurse sees herself as ascertaining needs, planning their fulfilment, teaching, superintending, and assuring quality of care.

Many highly skilled practical tasks are still performed by trained nurses. Most of us have seen them at work, caring for someone who has had a heart operation or has sustained injuries requiring intensive care on a life-support system. We all recognize the special skills required of nurses in such settings.

Those of us attending hospital find that the word 'patient', with its connotation of suffering, is tending to give place to 'client'. We are likely to be greeted by a nurse who gives us her name and tells us that she will be the one in charge of us, to whom we should refer any problems. She will, with her team, plan our nursing care, work with our doctor, give us advice on health, and arrange necessary care after our discharge. Many of us are also likely to meet the practice nurse, a colleague of our general practitioner. She may run clinics of her own for immunization, diagnostic tests, child care, and minor dressings.

Nursing is influenced by social changes, medical advances, political decisions, as well as by the views of individual nurses about their respective roles. It seems likely that the next 50 years will see increased professionalism, with emphasis on planning, management, and healthcare teaching. It would perhaps be unwise, however, to preclude the possibility that the electronic technician and engineer may take over some high-tech tasks, just as surgeons envisage the employment of robotics in some routine parts of operations. Perhaps then the nurse will once again be increasingly concerned with personal care, like her medieval predecessor. WHec

**NURSING IN NORTH AMERICA** Nurses may take one of several types of educational preparation to practice as a registered nurse. There are also several kinds of advanced education available to registered nurses. The preparation required for licensed nurses and nursing assistants is also reviewed here.

### Educational preparation

In the USA and Canada, there are three different routes to becoming a registered nurse. The prerequisites for entry into these routes are a high school education, good marks, and specified required course work, usually in the sciences.

The traditional route, now becoming rare, was the 2–3 year hospital training school program. This was developed from the Florence NIGHTINGALE (p 548) model and was the primary method of achieving nursing education until the 1970s. Students are taught by faculty members employed by the hospital, and learn their skills in that hospital. The training programs prepare general duty nurses able to staff the hospital in all aspects.

The second route, which became popular in the 1970s, is the two-year community college program. Community colleges have a planned curriculum, including introductory courses in anatomy and physiology, sociology, and psychology. Colleges usually contract with nearby hospitals for student clinical experience. Faculty members are present during the clinical experience to answer questions, observe performance, and provide guidance. Some colleges also contract for preceptors in the clinical setting to assist in the teaching of students. A preceptor is an employee of the hospital or agency in which the student is placed for clinical experience.

## PUBLIC HEALTH NURSE

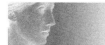

Lilian D **WALD**
(1867–1940). American public health nurse. Wald trained as a nurse and then enrolled in the Women's Medical College. During her medical student days she was asked to organize a home nursing service for immigrants on the Lower East Side of New York, and she found this so absorbing that she left medical school to make public health nursing her life work. She conceived the idea of a 'Nurses Settlement,' which she proceeded to establish in 1995. By 1913 she had assembled 91 nurses who made 200 000 home visits to the poor that year. The movement spread across the USA.

They provide the clinical supervision otherwise provided by the faculty person.

The third route, preferred today, is the baccalaureate program. Nursing is considered an applied science, and graduates receive the degree of Bachelor of Science. These programs take four years to complete, and include clinical and theoretical components. University programs, like colleges, contract with local hospitals and agencies to provide clinical experience for nursing students. Nursing subject topics include all of those available to a college student: maternal–child nursing, pediatrics, adult acute and chronic care, and psychiatric nursing. They also include community health, nursing research, and nursing theory. The emphasis in university programs is on health promotion, disease prevention, and research-based practice.

Baccalaureate education is being set as the minimum standard for the practice of nursing in both the USA and Canada. Hospital and college training programs are being phased out or are evolving into a route of entry into the baccalaureate program. The goal has been for all newly registered nurses to have this qualification as of 2000–1. Currently practicing nurses with college or hospital certificates will be allowed to continue to practice. However, there may be career implications to holding the lesser qualification. Programs are available in universities to allow previously registered nurses with less than baccalaureate preparation to upgrade their education. Students in these programs are referred to as post-basic (Canada), or registered nurse completion (USA) students.

In North America, the designation, registered nurse (RN) is reserved for those with the registration to practice general nursing in a particular state or province. Registration requires successful completion of an accredited course of studies, and satisfactory performance in the registration examination. Annual fees are paid for registration. Evidence of continuing education and/or practice hours is required to maintain registration.

Basic registration does not cover advanced practice or clinical specialization. These expanded roles, such as midwifery or nurse practitioner, require further education, clinical experience, and examination.

### Nursing assistants

To assist the registered nurse, a variety of positions were created. The roles and responsibilities of these assistants vary according to clinical setting. The licensed vocational nurse, licensed practical nurse, or registered nursing assistant have all received about one year of coursework and clinical practice. They are employed in hospitals, nursing homes, and home care agencies to give general nursing care. In some states and

provinces they are allowed to give medical treatment, dispense medications, and accept charge duties, often under minimal supervision. They are licensed by examination after completion of an approved course of studies.

In Canada, the role of the licensed practical nurse has recently been expanded, with course work now mimicking in length and content that offered previously to registered nurses in the college setting. In the USA, Veteran's Administration psychiatric hospitals nursing assistants were offered specialization programs that would allow graduates to assist the registered nurse in inpatient psychiatric care.

Nurses' aides are another category of nursing assistant. They are not licensed and education requirement varies widely, from two weeks to nine months. Aides are trained by the employing institution or through a community college for direct patient care and maintenance of the patient's environment. Responsibilities of the aide vary, from transporting patients to complete patient care. In many nursing homes, all patient care is given by aides under supervision of the licensed vocational or practical nurse.

### Clinical specialization

Graduates of generic nursing programs are considered to be generalists, able to work in almost any patient care setting. In both Canada and the USA, clinical specialization is available to any registered nurse. Specialization is achieved through experience, advanced education, or a combination of both. Two examples of specialization are the clinical specialist and the nurse practitioner.

*Clinical specialist* In North America, clinical specialization is most frequently seen as part of a graduate education in nursing. Advanced supervised practice over time may also lead to qualification. Both routes require an examination and subsequent registration. Clinical specialties are available in almost any aspect of nursing practice, including midwifery, intensive care nursing, cardiology, and community health nursing. In Canada, a further specialization is outpost nursing. Outpost nurses, usually resident in the far north, provide all healthcare services. Physician backup is often only by telephone or sometimes also by interactive television or the INTERNET. Emergency patients are flown south to the nearest medical center after initial treatment. There are advanced training programs for such nurses.

Canada also offers a psychiatric nursing specialty at the undergraduate level. These nurses are registered as general duty nurses but are designated as registered psychiatric nurses.

*Nurse practitioners* Nurse practitioners, common in the USA and becoming more so in Canada, are primary healthcare specialists. Programs for nurse practitioners are reserved for post-basic or graduate students, and vary in length from one to two years. The emphasis is on physical assessment, diagnosis, and provision of primary healthcare. Nurse practitioners are capable of examining and treating most patients, referring those with complex health problems to the physician. Nurse practitioners are found in outpost nursing stations, rural areas, and in group practice clinics, where they work with doctors and have their own caseload.

Entry into a master's program in nursing requires a bachelor's degree in nursing, or its equivalent. Master's degrees are available in clinical specialization, to research, administration, or education.

Programs in the USA are somewhat different from those in Canada. Those in the USA have a heavier class load, and most classes are required. Clinical practice is also a component. Students may not be required to complete a thesis, and may or may not have a final comprehensive examination. In Canada, more of the focus is on research. A research project or master's thesis is usually required. The core course load is lighter, and more course options may be chosen. Clinical specialization also requires clinical practice. Length of master's preparation in both countries varies among courses and foci, but is usually between one and two years.

Entry into a doctoral program in the USA and Canada is based upon successful completion of a master's degree, preferably in nursing. Again, courses differ in requirements, with the USA programs more focused on course work, and the Canadian more research-based. Required coursework in Canada is determined in consultation with the faculty supervisor. Required coursework in the USA is based on that completed at the master's level. Different degrees may be awarded, depending on the university attended. Some award a Ph.D. in nursing, others award the DNSc or DNS (Doctor of Nursing Science), or DSN (Doctor of Science in Nursing).

### Accreditation of schools

Nursing schools receive three regular examinations. All schools of nursing in the USA must receive national evaluation every seven years. New schools of nursing or new programs must be evaluated at or before the third year of the program. In addition, state boards of nursing regularly review schools in their state to determine if they are following the requirements for registration. These reviews are more frequent than the national reviews. Finally, universities and colleges regularly review programs and curricula, including nursing.

All three reviews require assessment of the goals and objectives of the school, course outlines, and student evaluations. Students, faculty, and administration are also interviewed.

In Canada, the process is the same, but national accreditation is voluntary. In both countries, lack of accreditation may mean that graduates cannot be accepted into advanced education and/or certain job placements.                    DBro

*See also* EDUCATION; WOMEN IN MEDICINE

**NUTRITION** In his earliest days man was a hunter-gatherer; he collected what he could from his surroundings and moved on when necessary. However, he did not necessarily have a poor diet; indeed, there are isolated communities in the world today that live largely on what is available around them such as fish, birds and their eggs, shell fish, small mammals, wild grain, seeds, nuts, berries, fruits, tubers, leaves — which can constitute a good diet with the variety that we now believe to be necessary — so long as the supplies are adequate.

Our ancestors began to settle down some 10 000–12 000 years ago and started farming; they tilled the soil and herded animals, selecting the 'better' crops and animals to improve yields, 'shelf life', pest resistance, etc. That process has continued over the millennia, natural and human selection giving way recently to the new science of genetic modification.

The beginning of urbanization around 1000 BC with the growth of large cities required food supplies from outside the community and called for developments in transport and food preservation. The marked increase in population and the number and size of cities during the 18th century demanded a vast expansion of agriculture and food technology, even before there was an adequate knowledge of food science on which to base the technology.

### A good diet

The ancients found dietary cures by experience and trial and error: HIPPOCRATES (p 382) wrote 'let your food be your medicine, and your only medicine be your food'. Vitamin A was discovered early in the 20th century but 1800 years earlier GALEN (p 324) had recommended the consumption of goat liver — a rich source of vitamin A — for night blindness. Galen also recommended 'swift exercise', such as running, for reducing obesity — a lesson to be learnt or relearnt by sedentary workers today.

Experimental work in the 19th and 20th centuries saw the development of the new science of nutrition. Today we define nutrition as an integrated science based on chemistry and physics, physiology, biochemistry, and micro-

**MALNUTRITION RESEARCHERS**

Christiaan **EIJKMAN** (1858–1930). Dutch physician. After training in bacteriology Eijkman was sent to the Dutch East Indies to investigate beriberi which was so widespread that an epidemic due to an infection was suspected. He noted a beriberi-like syndrome in fowls which was cured when the diet was changed from polished to unpolished rice (1888), and showed that there was some factor in rice polishings which protected against beriberi in man. He shared the NOBEL PRIZE with Gowland HOPKINS (p 855) in 1929 for his work on accessory food factors (vitamins).

*(continued overleaf)*

(continued)

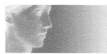

John **BOYD ORR** 1st Baron Boyd Orr of Brechin Mearns (1880–1971). British physiologist and nutritionist. He became director-general of the Food and Agriculture Organization of the United Nations (1946–47). He made notable contributions to the study of malnutrition and specific dietary deficiencies. He wrote many books on the science of nutrition and economic policy including *The national food supply and its influence on public health* (1934) and *Food—the foundation of world unity* (1948). He was awarded the Nobel Peace Prize for advocating a world food policy based on human needs rather than trade interests.

biology, as well as social sciences (although we are still trying to find out why people eat what they do).

The layman asks 'what is the perfect diet?', to which the answer is that, while there are vast numbers of good diets, there is no such thing as the perfect diet. Around the world people live healthily (so long as enough is available) on diets based largely on cassava and meat, or wheat and meat (still the basis of many western diets), or maize and fish, or rice (there are still diets today consisting of 50–75% rice) — all supplemented to extremely varied extents with fruits and vegetables.

People ate protein foods long before their role in the nitrogen metabolism of the body was elucidated during the 19th and first half of the 20th centuries, while vitamins (which must have always been consumed since they are essential to life) were discovered and their functions elucidated as recently as the first half of the 20th century (vitamin B6 was shown to be essential to man only in the 1950s).

We now know that we need 13 vitamins, around 25 mineral salts, 20 amino acids (which we consume as proteins), certain fatty acids, and enough energy from carbohydrates and fats to maintain and repair our tissues and to fulfill our daily needs for physical work. There is firm evidence for this statement since astronauts and hospital patients thrive on specific mixtures of these purified ingredients.

In early settlements, people mostly ate foods that they grew and prepared themselves and after harvest they had to preserve enough to see them through the seasons but they often suffered shortages — famines were frequent and food storage was inadequate.

### Recommended daily allowances

We know what nutrients we need but not how much of each. Attempts are made at intervals by various authorities as new knowledge or better opinions come to light to quantify the amounts of nutrients that 'should' be consumed — variously titled recommended daily or dietary allowances or intakes, dietary reference values, reference nutrient intakes, and population reference intakes. Some of these differ in their intentions, for example, a high target at which to aim, an average for the population as a whole, a high target to include the needs of all, or statistically nearly all the population, a minimum below which the average intake should not fall, and a minimum level below which an individual's intake should not fall. The problem is to set guidelines to cover the needs of everybody, with an estimated varying safety margin that differs between individuals over a 20–30% range.

Moreover, the data are inadequate so that decisions often have to be based on opinion.

The basis of recommended intakes is the avoidance of clinical or biochemical signs of deficiency. However, in recent years this criterion has been challenged on the grounds that improvements in health, including protection against some disorders, might call for higher levels. For example, some nutrients such as vitamins C, E, carotene, and selenium — antioxidants — protect the tissues from degenerative diseases resulting from oxidation by free radicals, and the amounts needed may be greater than those needed to prevent signs of deficiency diseases.

At the same time there has been considerable development of what are termed 'functional foods', those defined as foods or ingredients that confer benefits to health beyond the established function of vitamins and minerals (see Table). Apart from increased levels of established nutrients there are, for example, certain types of live microbial cultures, as are present in some yogurts, that are claimed to benefit the intestinal flora and so benefit the host (probiotics), and non-digestible polysaccharides that stimulate the growth of beneficial bacteria (prebiotics) and achieve the same results. There appears to be potential benefit from some of the non-nutrient chemicals that we consume in our diet — of which there are many hundreds or even thousands. Although functional foods are on sale in some countries, many of the claims are in urgent need of verification.

Another development is genetic nutrition, referring to nutrients, or possibly non-nutrients, that should be encouraged or shunned according to the genetic make-up of the individual. This last involves genetic disorders that may be triggered by specified dietary factors such as heart disease, diabetes, and some cancers.

### Deficiency diseases

At present the populations of most developing regions of the world suffer from chronic and acute shortages of foods manifested by specific deficiencies and general undernutrition. Even in the industrialized world there are problems caused by a shortage of certain vitamins and minerals, including iron, iodine, possibly zinc and vitamin D, although these are nothing like the scale and extent of the problems encountered in developing regions.

*Vitamin A deficiency* World-wide between a quarter and half a million preschool children in developing countries go blind each year from severe vitamin A deficiency and 190 million people are reported to be at risk. This is despite the fact that all green leaves (including grass) and colored fruits contain carotene, which is converted into vitamin A (retinol) in the body — so the remedy is all around us. However, in many regions this source of the vitamin is ignored or not realized or, ironically, regarded as food fit only for children. The problem has been tackled for over half a century by the following methods but obviously with limited success.

- Provision of massive doses of vitamin A orally or by injection at intervals throughout childhood—when the sufferers can be identified.
- Promotion of the consumption of specified fruits and vegetables and encouragement of their production.
- Enrichment of staple foods with the vitamin. This has achieved some success with foods differing as widely as sugar, salt, and monosodium glutamate, depending on local eating habits

These campaigns are ongoing and clearly still necessary.

*Iron deficiency anemia* Anemias are due to a shortage of hemoglobin in the blood; there are many types but by far the commonest is caused by iron deficiency. This may be due to low intakes of iron or high losses of blood (from causes such as bleeding due to intestinal parasites).

Shortage of hemoglobin may range from slight to extremely severe and the standard classification is a hemoglobin concentration below 85% of the average for the location population. On that basis, 10–15% of women of child-bearing age even in developed countries are classed as anemic. (This

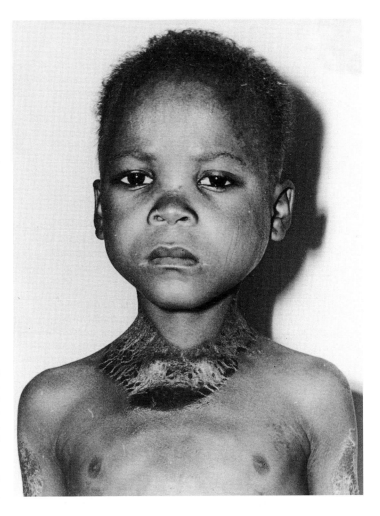

A patient suffering from pellagra, a deficiency of vitamin B which is rare in Western countries but still occurs in parts of Africa. (From Mann, J. and Truswell, S. (1998). *Essentials of human nutrition*, OUP.)

The uses of minerals in body functions

| Function | Minerals |
| --- | --- |
| Structural | calcium<br>magnesium<br>phosphate<br>fluoride |
| Nerve action | sodium<br>potassium |
| Enzymes | cobalt<br>copper<br>iron<br>molybdenum<br>selenium<br>zinc |
| Hormones or regulation | calcium<br>chromium<br>iodine<br>magnesium<br>manganese<br>sodium |
| Unknown function but essential | nickel<br>silicon<br>tin<br>vanadium |

is distinct from the apparent anemia that occurs late in pregnancy due to dilution through an increase in blood plasma volume.) In Britain one in twelve children between the ages of one and four years fall into this category.

The problem is that the amount of iron absorbed from the diet may range between 5% and 25% of the dietary iron intake, depending on its chemical form and other factors in the diet that depress or enhance absorption.

*Iodine deficiency* The metabolic rate of the body tissues is controlled by hormones of the thyroid gland, which depend on the iodine in the diet. If there is some, but insufficient, iodine (present as iodides and iodates) in the diet the gland enlarges (goiter) in an attempt to capture as much iodine as possible; in severe shortage iodine deficiency may lead to cretinism.

Almost one billion people live in regions deficient in iodine, and 200 million people are affected world-wide. The problem is common in inland areas over limestone, where there is little iodine in the soil water and so in the foods grown there. It is also found in lowland areas where the soil is water-logged and acid so that the iodine is not available to the plants. There are identified goitrogens in some foods but these are not directly a cause of goiter but may be a precipitating factor when iodine intakes are low. Since it is the local soil that is 'to blame', people consuming reasonable amounts of imported food from other regions of the world can obtain enough iodine even if their local soil is deficient. Indeed, in Britain goiter was common in Derbyshire, called Derbyshire neck, and Oxfordshire, but has now disappeared.

A solution to this problem, first employed in Switzerland in 1900, is to enrich chocolate with iodate but now iodized salt is the more usual vehicle, and in some countries, bread.

### Developing regions

There are several reasons for the widespread malnutrition in developing regions. Apart from acute shortages caused by climatic disasters and wars, there are chronic shortages due to poverty, inadequate and inefficient preservation and methods of food processing, and ignorance. So far as the science is concerned we could feed even the extrapolated growing population of the world but the science of nutrition has not been applied successfully where it is most needed.

*Food processing* Food processing, mass production, large-scale preservation, and the production of convenience foods are a feature of modern industrialized nations. Little of this is new but is rather the application of current knowledge of food science to traditional methods. For example, the ancient Egyptians dried fish and poultry (2000 BC); the Indians preserved butter by clarifying ghee (1500 BC); while refrigeration, often mentioned as a Roman practice, dates back to 1000 BC in China. Although the preparation of sugar from beet dates from the 19th century, sugar was extracted from the cane in 300 BC in India; Britain made its contribution to food technology with Cheshire cheese 2000 years ago. Ready-made noodles date back 2000 years in China, and milk was preserved by fermentation into yogurt about 1300 years ago.

Preservation with salt and with vinegar, by drying and chilling and fermenting, dates back hundreds, even thousands of years. Today we have a greater understanding of the processes involved in becoming stale and spoilage of food and the ability to preserve and so store foods more efficiently. Modern developments include the preparation of a vast number of so-called new products (mostly modifications of established products) as well as the ability to copy on a factory scale foods that 'mother used to make', and also to transport foods in bulk across the world. The industrialized world has foods of every kind throughout the year, fresh as well as processed.

Such an enormous variety — a large supermarket is said to carry some 20 000 lines — allows us to select the mixed diet that will include all the nutrients listed above — but also allows us to make a poor selection which is not always suitable.

At the same time, the relative cost of food has fallen in industrialized countries, from an average of about two-thirds of disposable income 100 years ago to about one-sixth in some communities, so we can mostly afford to pay others to prepare our dishes.

Anything the housewife can make — traditional, home-made, attractive, tasty — can be mass produced (and bought if you can afford it). The vast differences between the rich and the poor countries (where the cost of food is often the greater part of the family's income) are dramatically illustrated by the food supply.

*Public health research* So far as the industrialized countries are concerned, with increasing information on the relation between diet and health, it may become possible not only to advise the population and individuals about their diet accurately but to change agriculture in 'the right direction', to modify crops and their ingredients, and to process foods in the 'right' direction. So far as the developing regions of the world are concerned, we know the solution but the political and economic barriers appear to be insurmountable.

AEB

*See also* DIET AND DISEASE; FATNESS AND THINNESS; HEMATOLOGY; TROPICAL MEDICINE; VITAMINS

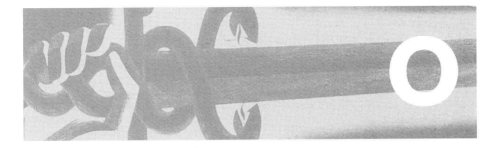

**OATHS AND CODES OF CONDUCT** A promise to adhere to the precepts and principles of the calling would have been part of the process of inducting apprentice priest-physicians in preliterate cultures; probably this soon evolved into a ceremony that included taking a formal oath. Such oaths have ancient provenance, dating back at least to Assyria (17th–13th century BCE) and in India to eight centuries BCE. The Hippocratic Oath that has come down to our time from the 4th or 5th century BCE would have had these beginnings. This is the best known of all medical oaths.

Innumerable modifications and adaptations of the Hippocratic oath exist. Devout Jews, Christians, and Moslems removed the invocation of pagan gods and substituted their own. A Jewish *Prayer for physicians*, equivalent to an oath, is attributed to MAIMONIDES (p 59), though its provenance has been questioned and there must have been precursors, probably for many centuries. Many Christian variations invoke Almighty God, the Islamic Oath of the Doctor begins, 'I swear by God the Great to regard God in carrying out my profession…'

Other changes reflect realities about the evolution of medical practice, removing obsolete allusions to cutting for the stone, or giving a woman a pessary. Modern wording responds to new views of gender equity, speaking of a duty to impart the rules of the profession to daughters as well as sons. Secular humanists and multiculturalists have composed an oath of professional commitment that removes references to deities of any kind.

It has long been customary for students in some medical schools throughout the English-speaking world to stand and recite the local variation of the Hippocratic oath in a formal ceremony, either soon after beginning their studies or around their graduation. The circumstances under which this happens are usually suitably solemn to have a lasting impact and impress on the new entrants to the profession that they have a sacred trust. In that sense, the ceremony is not merely a rite of passage or a bonding ritual, but a genuine act of commitment to honor the maxim to do no harm, to earn the trust and respect of patients and society at large by acting and behaving with due decorum in all things medical, to preserve the privacy and protect the confidentiality of the doctor–patient relationship, and to abide by all the commonly accepted principles and practice of medical ethics.

The Hippocratic oath and its derivatives spell out the duties and obligations of doctors to their patients, to their calling, to humanity at large. The growth of medical science in the 20th century and many other forces at work in this turbulent century made it necessary to create new precepts and rules to govern what may and may not be done in the course of medical research involving humans, and in the age of information technology, to protect privacy and preserve confidentiality.

The Nazi medical atrocities, in which humans were used as experimental animals, were exposed at the Nuremberg trials, and led to development of the NUREMBERG CODE (1949). This upheld

## HIPPOCRATIC OATH

I swear by Apollo the physician, by Asclepius, Hygeia, and Panacea, and I take to witness all the gods, all the goddesses, to keep according to my ability and my judgement the following Oath:

To consider dear to me as my parents him who taught me this art: to live in common with him and if necessary to share my goods with him: to look upon his children as my own brothers, to teach them this art if they so desire without fee or written promise: to impart to my sons and the sons of the master who taught me and the disciples who have enrolled themselves and have agreed to the rules of the profession, but to these alone, the precepts and the instruction. I will prescribe regimen for the good of my patients according to my ability and my judgement and never do harm to anyone. To please no one will I prescribe a deadly drug, nor give advice which may cause his death. Nor will I give a woman a pessary to procure abortion. But I will preserve the purity of my life and my art. I will not cut for stone, even for patients in whom the disease is manifest: I will leave this operation to be performed by practitioners (specialists in this art). In every house where I come I will enter only for the good of my patients, keeping myself far from all intentional ill-doing and all seduction, and especially from the pleasures of love with women or with men be they free or slaves. All that may come to my knowledge in the exercise of my profession or outside of my profession or in daily commerce with men, which ought not to be spread abroad, I will keep secret and will never reveal. If I keep this oath faithfully, may I enjoy my life and practice my art, respected by all men and in all times: but if I swerve from it or violate it, may the reverse be my lot.

the fundamental principle of respect for autonomy and human dignity. The World Medical Association, in its Declaration of Geneva (1948) and many subsequent revisions, all modeled loosely on the Hippocratic oath, begins by saying 'The health of my patient shall be my first consideration'. The World Medical Association's declaration, however, like the Nuremberg Code, deals mainly with the conditions for conducting research on humans.

The duty to protect privacy and preserve confidentiality of personal information that is explicit in the Hippocratic oath has concerned actuaries, compilers of official statistics, and epidemiologists. National and international organizations representing these professional groups have composed codes of conduct and guidelines for ethical handling of personal data files in many walks of life including medical practice. The rules are explicit, but so much personal information has to be transferred and shared among so many professional and technical support staff, that old concepts of the sacrosanct doctor–patient relationship cannot be upheld. The challenges here have continued to grow, and adequate responses to them are among the problems awaiting solution in this new millennium. It remains to be seen whether any code of conduct can cope successfully with the task of keeping medical secrets in this age of microchip and magnetic tape information storage and electronic transfer. JML

*See also* BIOETHICS; HELSINKI – DECLARATION OF; HOLOCAUST; INFORMED CONSENT

**OBESITY** See FATNESS AND THINNESS

**OBITUARIES** Short notices published soon after a person's death, are the single most important source of information on the lives and achievements of medical practitioners. Although often bland in tone and content, they function as a salve for grief, information for historians, and often moral exemplar.

Three major influences shaped late-18th and 19th century medical obituaries. Firstly, during the 16th and 17th centuries, epitaphs, elegies, and funeral sermons expressed the pious and prepared sentiment of the 'good death'. Secondly, was the mixture of Christian and Stoic ideals — the moral worth of humble beginnings, charity, piety, intellectual attainments, and fortitude — exemplified in Samuel Johnson's *Life of Sydenham* (1742). In this work, Johnson wrote that when the English physician Thomas SYDENHAM (p 721) suffered from GOUT and kidney stones, he 'never betray'd any indecent Impatience, or unmanly Dejection, under his Torments', but supported himself by the 'Reflections of Philosophy, and the Consolations of Religion'. Thirdly, was the

influence of the French *éloge*; publicly delivered eulogies, using models derived from the Greek tradition of panegyric. However, as a 1789 medical biography put it, most doctors ended up a 'humdrum Country Doctor… his merits not diffused beyond a country chronicle, and his fame confined to a country churchyard'.

From the 1780s, publications such as *The Gentleman's Magazine* and the *London Medical Journal* ran obituaries of prominent physicians, and by the 1830s, most medical journals had significant obituary sections. Sentimentality surrounding death, already in evidence in the 18th century, became more pronounced in the 19th century. Description of young and pious deaths and collections of dying words became bestsellers. Thus, the Hull physician William Gordon, who died in 1849, had his wife read to him from 'a small volume containing the dying testimonies of eminent medical men'. A colleague of Gordon's observed his last gasps, and wrote that this 'glorious spectacle lasted for about a quarter of an hour, increasing in interest to the last'.

In the late Victorian and Edwardian periods, sentimentalism gradually receded, and funerary customs became less elaborate. The Cremation Society was established in 1885, and Evangelical theology placed less emphasis on the threat of hell and the afterlife. By the 1850s, alongside the development of railways and national newspapers, obituaries became more ubiquitous. In Anthony Trollope's novel *Doctor Thorne* (1858), it was averred that a man 'is nobody unless his biography is kept so far posted up that it may be ready for the national breakfast table on the morning of his demise'.

Medical obituaries were used to measure worrying intraprofessional mortality rates. In 1861, the *London and Provincial Medical Directory* informed its subscribers that the average age at death for those doctors recorded in its obituary section was 56. A 1905 guidebook for young American doctors recorded the same average age of death from a survey of its obituaries. Some 19th and early 20th century medical obituaries were separately printed and privately circulated to family and colleagues shortly after a funeral, bound in black leather. A listing of professional and moral virtues usually included modesty, charity, a scrupulous regard for medical etiquette, piety, perseverance, wide learning, good manners and dress, prudence, self-denial, lack of ostentation, and intuitive diagnostic skills. Religion is usually invoked, especially in times of illness and approaching death, when the situation is stoically accepted with grave dignity.

Many 19th-century medical obituaries recount saintly subjects, and can be quoted *ad nauseam*. For instance, of Louis PASTEUR (p 620):

It is recorded of him that he died holding the Crucifix in one hand, and in the other his wife's hand. Here was a life, within the limits of humanity, well-nigh perfect.

and of the military surgeon Edmund Alexander Parkes:

his life was thus in all respects a pure and beautiful life, his death was that of a self-denying hero… .

In Émile Zola's *Doctor Pascal* (1893), the eponymous protagonist dies 'like a hero', and his wife, Clotilde, is grief-stricken by the 'narrative of that stoic death'.

The Edinburgh physician William Williamson died a death in 1865 with as much glory attached to it as that of a soldier.

Dr Williamson, indeed, died as he lived — at the post of duty. His death was worthy of his life. He gave himself to the service of the public, and he sacrificed his life in its service.

A young London houseman, John Baddeley, who died of typhus in 1868 at the age of 28, was similarly praised by his obituarist for displaying the 'heroic self-devotion of a soldier marching calmly on his path of duty through an unseen but not unknown death-storm'. Baddeley's obituarist further observed.

the calm manner in which, during the first few days of his illness, he assisted in the diagnosis of his disease by taking his own temperature, as well as by the quiet resignation with which he received the information that he undoubtedly laboured under typhus.

Throughout the 20th century, medical obituaries continued to be written and read widely within the medical profession. A mark of the interest in obituaries can be seen by the reaction, in 1982, and again in 1995, to editorials in the *British Medical Journal* which advocated self-written obituaries. The 1982 editorial ended with the words: 'We will welcome contributions from doctors retiring or from any who feel themselves weakening'. However, a Taunton general practitioner noted that he could 'think of no more dismal task during retirement or in an episode of "weakening" than composing one's own obituary notice'. A Norfolk doctor said in 1983 that 'when I go I hope to do so quietly, unrecorded'. Yet in a 1995 *British Medical Journal*, an editorial reported back from a questionnaire that most respondents wanted obituaries kept, although shorter, with space kept for 'ordinary' health professionals, and more on the person's failings.

Throughout the history of medical obituaries some features have remained constant. On the principle 'speak no ill of the dead', excessive praise remains commonplace, as do condolences and clichéd language. Yet for many, obituaries are compulsive reading and the section of newspapers and journals that we turn to first. The medical profession has generally shared this fascination with post-mortem remembrance.

In March 1923, Arthur Keith, anatomist at the Hunterian Museum, London, wrote to the prominent gynecologist AHG Doran, revealingly describing how he had just completed obituaries of a colleague for the *Lancet* and *British Medical Journal*:

a little labour of love — just wrote the kind of thing you would write on me or I on you…one cannot tell whose turn it may be next: it may be me, it may be you: in any case I think you should give the facts of your life to someone — if I'm alive when you go I should like to see justice done to your memory.

Most doctors and many health professionals will write, or be the subject of, an obituary. New Zealand doctors I interviewed in 1996 revealed that many found the experience of writing obituaries of colleagues to be a cathartic and emotional experience. Many must have wished, or still wish, for a friendly offer to write a 'little labor of love' in the form of a sympathetic obituary. MHut

**OBSTETRICS AND GYNECOLOGY** Despite its double name, obstetrics and gynecology is a single specialty and most of its practitioners are both obstetricians and gynecologists. Obstetrics deals with pregnancy and childbirth, the word probably deriving from the Latin *obstare*, to 'stand before': the MIDWIFE (*obstetrix*) 'stood before' the woman to receive the baby. Gynecology (from the Greek *gyne*, 'woman') deals mainly with reproductive disorders of non-pregnant women, but also includes problems in early pregnancy.

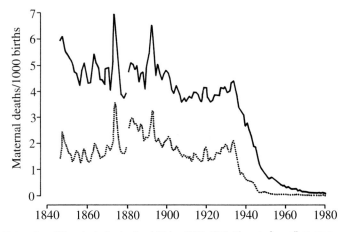

Maternal mortality rates in England and Wales, 1874–1984. The rate from all causes is shown by the bold line, and the death rate from puerperal sepsis by the dotted line. In spite of social and medical advances, both rates hardly changed between 1847 and 1937. (Redrawn from *Report on confidential enquiries into maternal deaths in England and Wales 1982–84*, p. 141, HMSO, London.)

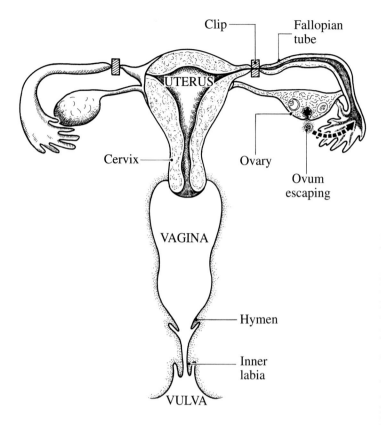

Clip — Fallopian tube

UTERUS

Cervix — Ovary

Ovum escaping

VAGINA

Hymen

Inner labia

VULVA

Diagram of the female genital tract. In the operation of sterilization, the Fallopian tubes are blocked (e.g. by clips, as shown) to prevent the sperm from fertilizing the egg (ovum).

**OBSTETRICS** In early times women in labor were attended by relatives or uneducated MIDWIVES. Some Greek and Roman physicians taught midwifery, but doctors, being men, were excluded from attending childbirth until the 16th century. The first book on midwifery was printed in 1513 in Germany. Ambroise PARÉ (p 320), a French military surgeon, founded a school for midwives in Paris. In 1572 a French Huguenot family, the CHAMBERLENS (p 493–4), fled to England with the forerunners of modern obstetric forceps, which were their family secret.

*Accoucheurs* (male midwives) became fashionable in France in the 17th century. A surgeon attended a mistress of Louis XIV in 1663 and an accoucheur, Mauriccau, published a treatise on midwifery in 1668.

In England in the 18th century the secret of the obstetric forceps became public, although their use remained controversial. The first British school of midwifery was founded in 1725 in London, and the first chair of midwifery in Edinburgh in 1726. Queen Charlotte's Hospital, Britain's first maternity hospital, was founded in 1739. In that year William Smellie, a Scottish doctor, set up a school of midwifery in London, and in 1752 he published his *Treatise on the theory*

*and practice of midwifery.* Smellie, 'the master of British midwifery', was a man of humanity and common sense but was violently opposed by some local midwives. One of his pupils, William HUNTER (p 88), a fellow-Scot and older brother of the famous surgeon John (p 398), became very popular and by the latter part of the 18th century *accoucheurs* were fashionable in England.

In the 19th century labor was still dangerous. Among the poor, rickets caused pelvic deformities. In maternity hospitals many women died of puerperal fever, whose contagious nature was recognized by Alexander Gordon of Aberdeen in 1795 and Oliver Wendell Holmes in the USA in 1843. In 1861 SEMMELWEISS (p 479) in Vienna reduced deaths from puerperal fever by reducing cross-infection with methods such as hand-washing.

Midwifery became a compulsory subject for medical students in 1833 in Scotland and 1866 in England. In 1847 James Young SIMPSON (p 43), professor of midwifery in Edinburgh, used chloroform to relieve labor pain. He met strong opposition from doctors and clergy until Queen Victoria requested it at the birth of her seventh child.

Obstetrics was limited to childbirth itself until the 20th century, when antenatal care was introduced. In 1901 R. W. Ballantyne set aside a bed for antenatal patients in Edinburgh Royal Infirmary. Antenatal clinics were opened in Boston, Sydney, and Edinburgh in 1911, 1912, and 1915, respectively. Obstetrics remained a branch of surgery until 1929, when the Royal College of Obstetricians and Gynecologists was founded.

The history of obstetrics is closely linked with that of midwifery. Midwives were mostly illiterate 'Sairey GAMPS' (p 495) until the 19th century, when several European countries introduced regulations for their training and control. Attempts to do the same in Britain failed, but in 1872 the Obstetrical Society of London began issuing certificates of competence to midwives. The Midwives Institute was set up in 1881. At last, in 1902, the Midwives Act made state registration compulsory and set up a Central Midwives Board to regulate midwifery. The Midwives Institute became the College of Midwives in 1941, the prefix 'Royal' being added in 1947.

**Maternal mortality** Throughout history, childbirth has been dangerous for women, but after 1930 there was a remarkable improvement in Britain. The maternal mortality rate — the number of women dying per 100 000 deliveries — in Britain until 1935 was around 500, but nowadays it is only 8. The mortality rate remains high in many developing countries, and in parts of Africa it is still around 500. The reasons for the fall in Britain are numerous. The health of the population has improved but the fall is probably due more to specific measures. For example, infection may now be treated with antibiotics, and bleeding by BLOOD TRANSFUSION. Legalization of ABORTION in 1967 eliminated criminal abortion as a cause of maternal death.

Since 1952 in Britain a national Confidential Enquiry into Maternal Deaths has examined each death and issued regular reports with recommendations for improvements. Hemorrhage and infection are now relatively rare causes: in recent years the commonest causes have been venous thrombosis and raised blood pressure. Death due to ANESTHESIA is now extremely rare.

*Perinatal mortality* Childbirth is 100 times more dangerous for the baby than the mother. The perinatal mortality rate is the number of stillbirths and deaths in the first week of life per 1000 deliveries. In 1935 in England and Wales it was 70, and in 1990 it was 8.3. The three main causes of perinatal mortality — low birth weight, lack of oxygen *in utero*, and congenital abnormalities — are discussed below.

*Obstetric techniques* Obstetric forceps were first used on living babies by the Chamberlens. They were modified during the 18th and 19th centuries but the forceps in use today are similar to those designed by Simpson 150 years ago. Most forceps require the baby's head to be facing towards the mother's back, but in 1916 Kjelland, a Norwegian obstetrician, designed forceps for use when the baby's head is facing to the side or to the front.

The vacuum extractor (or ventouse), invented by Malmström of Sweden in the 1950s, has a suction cup which is applied to the baby's head. After recent improvements, studies have shown that it causes less trauma to the mother than forceps delivery, although the baby may suffer mild ill-effects from bruising of the scalp.

CESAREAN SECTION got its name from the Lex Caesarea, a law dating from the 7th century BC that if a pregnant woman died, the baby should be removed and buried separately. The procedure was not done with any regularity until the 1880s, at which time 'classical' cesarean section involved a lengthwise incision in the uterus. This does not heal well and may rupture in subsequent labor. In 1906 the modern 'lower segment' operation was introduced, in which the incision is in the fibrous lower part of the uterus.

## Current practice
*Antenatal care* The emphasis in modern obstetrics is on preventing problems. The purposes of antenatal care are to treat symptoms during pregnancy, to screen for maternal and fetal complications, and to help prepare a couple for childbirth and childrearing.

At a prepregnancy clinic, checks are made on a woman's health, obstetric history, and immune status (for example, to rubella). Women with a history of genetic disease may receive counseling and, if necessary, diagnostic tests. Those with pre-existing disease such as DIABETES may need to alter their treatment.

The pattern of antenatal clinic visits varies among countries but in Britain a woman usually attends first around the 12th week of pregnancy, monthly until the 28th week, fortnightly until the 36th week, and weekly thereafter. The midwife, general practitioner, and hospital clinic share the care, depending on local arrangements and individual risk factors. The trend nowadays, for low-risk women, is towards fewer visits and less hospital care.

Investigations at booking (the first visit) include tests for anemia, syphilis, rubella, and blood grouping. If a woman's blood group is Rhesus negative and her baby is Rhesus positive, she may develop antibodies against the baby's red blood cells, leading to fetal anemia, which may be lethal. Such Rhesus isoimmunization has been almost eliminated by a national prevention program: Rhesus-negative women are injected with a small amount of antibody to destroy fetal cells in the mother's blood before they stimulate an immune reaction.

*Prenatal diagnosis* Around 2% of babies have major congenital abnormalities, such as Down's syndrome or spina bifida. The risk of some of these can be reduced. Women planning a pregnancy are now advised to take supplements of folic acid to prevent spina bifida, but for the remainder all we can do is make the diagnosis as early as possible, when the woman can be offered the option of terminating the pregnancy.

In chromosomal abnormalities, the baby's cells contain abnormal genetic material owing to failure of the chromosomes to distribute themselves correctly at conception. Most cause miscarriage but a few are compatible with life, such as Down's syndrome, in which there is an extra chromosome 21. Chromosome abnormalities may be diagnosed in various ways. Pre-implantation diagnosis can be performed after *in vitro* fertilization: in the laboratory one cell is removed from an early embryo; the chromosomes are examined and if they are normal the embryo may be placed in the womb. Chorion villus sampling may be done from the eighth week of pregnancy: a sample of placental tissue is removed via a needle inserted through either the vagina or the abdominal wall. Chromosomes from these rapidly dividing cells can be examined directly by microscopy. Amniocentesis involves removing some amniotic fluid via a needle through the abdominal wall.

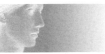
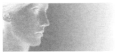

Cells shed from the fetus may be cultured and examined, which takes longer than direct examination after chorion villus sampling. Amniocentesis, formerly restricted to the 15th week of pregnancy or later, can now be done as early as the 10th week.

Anatomical abnormalities may occur in fetuses with normal or abnormal chromosomes. The most common types are abnormalities of the nervous system (such as spina bifida) or the heart: others include cleft palate or club foot. They are present from the early weeks or embryonic life but become detectable only when the structures are large enough to be seen on ultrasound scans.

*Obstetric ultrasound* During the Second World War, echoes from high-frequency sound waves were used to detect submarines. In the 1950s in Glasgow, Professor Ian Donald modified the technique to make measurements on the fetus in the amniotic fluid. In the early days a single beam of ultrasound produced blips on an oscilloscope screen, but today's machines give detailed moving images, allowing diagnosis of anatomical abnormalities and accurate assessment of fetal growth and of the position of the placenta. Ultrasound has transformed obstetrics and is now widely used in gynecology and other specialties.

*Complications of pregnancy* At each antenatal visit the size of the uterus is assessed. A large uterus may mean multiple pregnancy, excess amniotic fluid, or a large baby, and a small uterus may mean the baby is failing to grow. This may be checked by ultrasound. Checks are also made on the woman's blood pressure and urine for signs of pre-eclampsia — a condition in which the blood pressure rises and protein appears in the urine and which, untreated, may progress to eclampsia (convulsions). In the later weeks checks are made for breech presentation, which occurs at the end of 4% of pregnancies.

*Care in labor* About 600 000 babies are born in Britain every year, most in hospital. The move towards total hospital deliveries accelerated in the 1960s as doctors and women perceived hospital as safer for the baby. There is now concern that home delivery should remain as an option for women who want it, although hospitals are becoming less institutional to strike a better balance between safety and a relaxed environment.

*Normal labor* Labor has three stages, the first lasting from the onset until the uterine cervix is fully open. During the second stage (which ends at delivery of the baby), the woman feels the urge to push. The third stage is from delivery of the baby to delivery of the placenta. In Britain women in labor are cared for mainly by mid-wives, who as independent practitioners are not required to seek medical help unless they feel this is necessary.

*Pain relief in labor* There is much variation in the amount of pain experienced during labor and much debate about the best form of pain relief. Methods include psychoprophylaxis, and pain-killing drugs such as pethidine, inhaled gases, and epidural analgesia. General anesthesia is nowadays rarely used for instrumental delivery and many cesarean sections are carried out using epidural block. General and epidural anesthesia are administered by specially trained anesthetists.

For epidural analgesia a fine catheter is inserted between the vertebrae and a painkilling drug is infiltrated around the roots of the nerves leading from the uterus. This may give complete freedom from pain but may interfere with the second stage of labor by abolishing the urge to push, and therefore this increases the chance of an instrumental delivery.

*Fetal monitoring* The simplest way to monitor the baby's condition during labor is by the midwife listening to its heartbeat through a stethoscope. Electronic monitoring of the fetal heart rate became widespread in the 1970s. During labor uterine contractions may reduce blood flow to the placenta, interfering with the baby's oxygen supply and altering its heart rate, but abnormalities may have no sinister cause and an electronic monitor (cardiotocograph) can cause unnecessary concern. Cardiotocograph abnormalities can be checked by taking a sample of fetal blood for measurement of oxygen levels but this facility is not available in all hospitals.

Active management of labor also became widespread in the 1970s and 1980s. Often a woman's first labor is slow because the uterus does not contract strongly, although subsequent labors are usually much more efficient. 'Active management' of a first labor involves early diagnosis of slow progress and the use of oxytocin, a natural hormone, to strengthen the contractions. It reduces the need for instrumental delivery or cesarean section, but oxytocin has to be given by intravenous drip and some women see active management as excessive medical intervention.

*Complications of labor* Some complications such as malpresentation (for example, breech presentation) may be anticipated in the antenatal clinic, but some are unpredictable. For example, rarely the umbilical cord may drop into the vagina when the waters break, or more commonly heavy bleeding may occur immediately after delivery (postpartum hemorrhage). The most common indications for intervention nowadays are fetal distress or failure to progress.

Fetal distress means the baby shows signs of lack of oxygen, such as a slow heartbeat or the passage of meconium (bowel contents). These signs may occur, however, when the baby's oxygen levels are normal. Failure to progress in labor means the cervix fails to dilate beyond a certain point, owing either to poor contractions or to the baby being too big for vaginal delivery. 'Slow progress', however, may be a subjective diagnosis. Thus both these indications may be arbitrary.

If delivery is necessary in the first stage of labor, cesarean section is required. In the second stage vaginal delivery may be assisted by forceps or vacuum extraction, but cesarean section may be preferred to a potentially difficult instrumental delivery. Rates of cesarean section have risen steadily in many developed countries. In Britain in the 1950s, 5% of babies were born by cesarean section but by 1990–91 the rate had risen to 13%. In the USA the rate has risen to 25%. The rise has been blamed on overenthusiastic obstetricians, but recent research shows that women are unwilling to accept even a low risk to their baby, and many prefer cesarean section when a mild complication is detected.

*The puerperium* This refers to the time from delivery until the woman's genital tract returns to normal, usually around 6 weeks later. In the early days after delivery emotional lability is usual but true puerperal psychosis is uncommon. Infection of the womb, the cause of the once-dreaded puerperal fever, is now infrequent and can be treated with antibiotics. In Britain fewer than half of women breast-feed, although hospitals are now having some success in increasing this figure.

### Future trends
There is a stark contrast between the obstetric needs of countries such as Britain and those of developing countries, where the maternal mortality rate is high and many women suffer complications such as vesicovaginal fistula (bladder damage during labor). The WORLD HEALTH ORGANIZATION estimates that world-wide half a million women die every year as a result of pregnancy, one a minute. Reducing this total will not be easy. This will mean not only improving maternity services but also raising the status of women in some cultures, and providing easy access to cheap CONTRACEPTION.

In Britain, by contrast, the trend is towards reducing medical intervention without compromising safety. Research studies to distinguish useful from unnecessary intervention involve large numbers of women and complex statistical analysis, and several studies may have to be combined to obtain clear answers. Obstetric and midwifery practice is increasingly being guided by such research. At the same time, women have high expectations and any adverse outcome of pregnancy may lead to litigation. Huge awards have been made to 'brain-damaged' babies, but it is now recognized that only a small proportion of cases of cerebral palsy are due to obstetric causes.

**GYNECOLOGY** developed during the 19th century as a specialized branch of surgery. Around 1800 the vaginal speculum was first used to inspect the walls of the vagina. Dilatation of the cervix was carried out in 1832 in Edinburgh. In the 1840s James Marion Sims of Alabama developed an operation for vesicovaginal fistula. Sims was one of the founders of the Women's Hospital in New York, the world's first hospital devoted to gynecology. By 1888 an operation had been devised for the repair of uterine prolapse, a condition in which the womb protrudes through the vagina because of weakness of its supporting ligaments.

Abdominal gynecological surgery developed at the same time. In 1809 Ephraim McDowell of Kentucky carried out the first successful operation for removal of a large ovarian cyst. The mortality of such operations remained high, however, until late in the 19th century. Lawson Tait of Birmingham, England, carried out hysterectomy for uterine fibroids in 1874 and the first successful operation for ectopic pregnancy in 1883. By the end of the century surgical gynecology was established and early in the 20th century large operations were being performed, such as radical hysterectomy for cancer of the cervix, pioneered by Wertheim of Vienna. Medical gynecology developed after the discovery of the sex hormones in the 1920s, leading to innovations such as the contraceptive pill in the 1950s.

### Current practice
Gynecology now encompasses surgical operations, hormonal and other medical treatments, and broader issues — family planning, health screening, and treatment at the menopause — which demand understanding the aspirations of women in modern society.

*The menstrual cycle* The human menstrual cycle has considerable potential for going wrong, and even when normal may cause women discomfort and inconvenience. At puberty the hypothalamus (an area at the base of the brain) produces a hormone to activate the pituitary, a gland under the brain which stimulates the ovaries to secrete estrogen, a female sex hormone which thickens the endometrium (the lining of the womb). The average age at menarche (the first menses) is now

13, having been higher earlier last century. Regular ovulation begins about 15 and the ovaries fail at an average age of 51.

*Menstrual disorders* Menstrual bleeding may be too heavy (menorrhagia), absent (amenorrhea), infrequent (oligomenorrhea), or too frequent (polymenorrhea). The amount of blood lost at menstruation is normally less than 80 ml. In clinical practice the menstrual flow is not measured objectively, the gynecologist being guided by the history given by the woman.

*Medical gynecology* Most of the hormones controlling the cycle may be given pharmacologically. In cases of amenorrhea or oligomenorrhea ovulation may be induced by stimulating the ovaries. The most common menstrual disorder, menorrhagia, may be treated by suppressing the ovaries with the contraceptive pill. Endometriosis, a painful condition in which the endometrium grows outside the uterus, may be treated by suppressing the ovaries or pituitary.

*Menopause* The 'menopause' is the last menstrual period, and the 'climacteric' is the phase when the periods become irregular before stopping altogether. Menstruation ceases because the ovaries run out of eggs. Withdrawal of estrogen causes hot flushes and in the longer term increases the risk of osteoporosis (loss of bone) and heart disease. These risks may be reduced by giving estrogen as hormone replacement therapy. If this treatment were widely adopted, it could substantially alter disease patterns in older women by reducing osteoporosis and heart disease.

*Surgical gynecology* The range of gynecological operations is wide, although some, such as ventrosuspension (an operation to change the position of the uterus), are now performed much less frequently than in the past.

Hysterectomy is the commonest major operation carried out in Britain and the USA, apart from cesarean section. In Britain 66 000 hysterectomies are performed every year and in the USA 25% of women reach the menopause through hysterectomy. The most common indication is menstrual disorder, although fibroids (benign tumors of uterine muscle) are often also present.

Pelvic floor repair includes various operations performed for prolapse of the uterus or vaginal walls. Part of the vagina is removed, the muscles are tightened, and hysterectomy may be performed at the same time.

Dilatation and curettage are less frequently performed now than formerly because of better medical treatment for menstrual disorders. The cervix is stretched with graduated dilators, and a curette, a small spoon-shaped instrument, is used to remove tissue from the uterine cavity.

*Minimal access surgery* Nowadays an increasing amount of gynecological surgery is being carried out by 'minimal access' techniques.

*Laparoscopic surgery* A laparoscope is a kind of telescope which is inserted into the abdomen, usually near the umbilicus. Laparoscopy was popularized in Britain by Patrick Steptoe in the 1960s. Until recently it was mainly used for inspection of the pelvic organs and for sterilization, which involves blocking the Fallopian tubes by electrocoagulation, elastic rings, or metal clips. Recently, larger operations, including hysterectomy, have been carried out either via the laparoscope or with its help. It is still too early to say to what extent such surgery will replace conventional techniques.

*Hysteroscopic surgery* Although hysterectomy is commonly performed for menorrhagia, removal of the entire uterus is really unnecessary because only the endometrium bleeds. A hysteroscope is an instrument for looking inside the uterus through the cervix, and it may be used, along with a laser or electrocautery, to remove the endometrium, including the deepest layer, to prevent regrowth. Transcervical resection of the endometrium takes as long as a hysterectomy but, because no abdominal incision is involved, the woman can return home much sooner after operation.

*Gynecological emergencies* The most frequent reasons for emergency gynecological admission are abdominal pain or vaginal bleeding. In a woman of reproductive age pregnancy testing is usually done. Tests for human chorionic gonadotrophin, a hormone produced only by pregnancy tissue, are now so sensitive that they can detect a pregnancy before a woman misses a period.

About a fifth of all pregnancies end in clinically recognizable miscarriage, and unless bleeding stops quickly, curettage is usually carried out. Ultrasound scanning can differentiate miscarriage from ectopic pregnancy.

After conception, the fertilized egg takes 3–5 days to pass down the Fallopian tube into the uterus. One in 400 pregnancies implants in the tube — an ectopic pregnancy. The tube is too delicate to sustain the pregnancy; as it stretches, pain occurs, and tubal rupture may lead to fatal bleeding. Formerly the treatment was to remove the tube by open operation and often this is still necessary. It may be possible, however, to remove the tube by laparoscopic surgery or to remove the pregnancy and leave the tube intact, albeit with an increased risk of another ectopic pregnancy.

In the non-pregnant woman, pelvic pain is often attributed to pelvic inflammatory disease, but this is probably over-diagnosed. Ovarian cysts may cause sudden pain through rupture, twisting, or bleeding. Causes of abnormal bleeding are hormonal imbalance, heavy menstruation, or, less commonly, disease such as uterine or cervical cancer.

## Subspecialties

*Reproductive medicine* This subspecialty includes treatment of infertility, disorders of ovarian function, and the menopause.

*Infertility* About one in six couples has difficulty in achieving pregnancy. Investigation involves semen analysis and tests of ovulation and the Fallopian tubes. Little can be done to improve a poor sperm count. Ovulation may be induced with drugs, although careful monitoring is necessary to prevent multiple ovulation. Blocked tubes can be treated surgically, but the Fallopian tubes are small and delicate and if damage is severe the chances of conception are low.

In the 1980s Patrick Steptoe, working in Oldham, and Robert Edwards of Cambridge University developed *in vitro* fertilization. This involves removing an egg (or eggs) from the ovary, fertilization with sperm in the laboratory, and replacement of the fertilized egg in the uterus. The technique was difficult to develop because the egg can be fertilized only at exactly the right moment after the preovulatory surge of hormones. Even in nature, couples trying for pregnancy have no more than a one-in-three chance of conceiving in a single cycle, and it is unlikely that *in vitro* fertilization will achieve better than this. Several attempts may be needed, but *in vitro* fertilization is expensive and highly stressful for the couple.

*Gynecological oncology* Oncology is the study of cancer. Gynecological oncology is concerned with prevention, early detection, and treatment of cancer of the reproductive organs. (In Britain breast cancer is dealt with by general surgeons, not gynecologists.)

Cancer of the cervix is usually caused by the human papilloma virus, transmitted by sexual intercourse. Most cases occur after a premalignant phase lasting about 10 years, which can be detected by scraping cells form the cervix and examining them under a microscope. This is the basis of cervical screening. Formerly, cervical smears were taken when a woman happened to consult a doctor, but nowadays, with systematic screening, women between the ages of 20 and 65 have smears every 3–5 years.

If a smear is abnormal, the cervix is examined at a hospital clinic through a colposcope, a low-power binocular microscope which allows biopsies to be taken from abnormal areas. Without this it would be necessary to take a cone biopsy, which removes the entire circumference of the cervix in order to be sure of including any abnormal area. If a colposcopic biopsy is abnormal, a larger area is removed by laser or diathermy.

Cervical cancer is treated by radiotherapy, although for early disease radical surgery is an alternative.

Cancer of the endometrium (or body of the uterus) may be due to prolonged stimulation by natural estrogen, from ovarian cysts or ovarian dysfunction. Hormone replacement therapy with unopposed estrogen is also a risk factor, but nowadays if a woman has a uterus her hormone replacement therapy will include progestogen, a hormone similar to progesterone, which is produced after ovulation. Cancer of the endometrium usually reveals itself early by bleeding. Treatment is by hysterectomy, often combined with radiotherapy.

Cancer of the ovary usually does not become apparent until an advanced stage, when it presents as abdominal swelling. Treatment is by surgery and chemotherapy. Attempts at early detection involve blood tests for biochemical markers released by the cancer, and ultrasound scanning of women with raised levels. So far such screening is still experimental.

Rarer gynecological cancers include choriocarcinoma, a tumor of pregnancy tissue, which is lethal if untreated but responds well to chemotherapy. Vulval cancer usually affects older women, and treatment is wide excision of the vulval skin. Vaginal cancer is extremely rare, but cases have been reported in women whose mothers were treated for threatened miscarriage with diethylstilbestrol, an artificial estrogen.

*Urogynecology* Urinary incontinence is a common problem in women, as the muscles of the pelvic floor can be weakened by childbirth or lack of hormones after the menopause. Urodynamic investigation (measurement of bladder pressure) can distinguish different types of incontinence. Urge incontinence (oversensitivity of the bladder) is treated by drugs and bladder retraining. Stress incontinence (weakness of bladder supports) is usually treated by an operation to strengthen the bladder neck.

*Fertility control* In view of the world's problems with overpopulation, fertility control is a most important part of modern gynecology.

Contraception is best provided by general practitioners, family planning doctors, or, indeed, over the counter, but gynecologists have a role in training — particularly in the insertion of intrauterine contraceptive devices. The Royal College of Obstetricians and Gynaecologist has a Faculty of Family Planning founded in 1993.

Sterilization is popular in Britain. Every year about 90 000 female sterilizations are performed and a similar number of vasectomies. About half the couples over 40 have opted for sterilization. Female sterilization is carried out by laparoscopy under general anesthesia, often as a day-case procedure. Long-term after-effects are rare and the failure rate is less than 0.5%.

Termination of pregnancy is a more accurate term than 'abortion', which, strictly speaking, means miscarriage. In Britain the Abortion Act of 1967 allows abortion if two doctors agree that continuing with the pregnancy would be harmful to the health of the woman or her existing children. In Britain about one in three women will have an abortion at some time in her life, usually before the age of 25: about 170 000 abortions are carried out every year and the abortion rate is 13/1000 women aged 15–45. In the USA the rate is 24/1000, and in Russia, 124/1000.

*Sexual medicine* In spite of today's open attitude to sex, many couples still have difficulties. Common problems in gynecological practice include vaginismus (involuntary tightening of the vaginal muscles making penetration difficult or impossible) and lack of libido. A history of sexual or physical abuse in childhood may present in later life as sexual difficulty or pelvic pain, and such patients are best referred to a psychiatrist. For simple vaginismus, teaching a woman to use vaginal dilators may be effective.

### Future trends
The demand for surgical treatment of menstrual disorders seems likely to continue, although minimal access surgery will partly replace hysterectomy. There will be a continuing demand for assisted conception, but male infertility remains a challenge. The most urgent need is to provide realistic sex education for young people to help them avoid unwanted pregnancy and sexually transmitted disease, but this requires action from society at large. JOD

*See also* ABORTION; CESAREAN SECTION; CONTRACEPTION; ENDOCRINOLOGY; MINIMALLY INVASIVE SURGERY; SCREENING; SEXUALITY AND MEDICINE; SPECIALIZATION

### OCCUPATIONAL HEALTH — HISTORY
Occupation has always exerted a profound influence on the pattern of life and death. HIPPOCRATES (p 382) in *Airs, waters, and places*, wrote about the effects of the environment on health and the quality of life, but not specifically on the occupational environment. However, in 370 BC he described severe colic in a worker who extracted metals, and thus may have been the first to recognize lead as the cause of this symptom.

Cinnabar, the red sulfide of mercury, had been mined in Almaden, Spain, since Phoenician times. The Romans used it as a durable pigment, together with red lead and other metallic compounds, to decorate buildings. In the 1st century AD, Pliny described mercury poisoning as a disease of slaves, for the mines of Almaden, contaminated with mercury vapor, were too unhealthy for Roman citizens to work in. He also mentioned that workers handling lead oxides (used as pigments) would tie up their faces in loose bags to avoid inhaling the poisonous dust.

The Middle Ages saw the development of metalliferous mining in central Europe. Agricola published *De re metallica* in 1556, a work translated into English by Hoover, a past president of the USA, and his wife. In this book Agricola gave a detailed description of the mining, smelting, and refining of gold and silver, describing the methods used for ventilation, and illustrating primitive methods of personal protection in a series of wood-cuts. He also described mining accidents and major disasters in mines, later to become all too familiar, as well as the harmful effects of dry dust inhalation on the lungs. A little later, PARACELSUS (p 617), a Swiss physician, wrote on the occupational diseases of mineworkers, smelter-workers, and metallurgists, giving a detailed description of mercurialism.

However, Bernardino RAMAZZINI (p 583) is generally acknowledged as the father of occupational medicine. Ramazzini practiced as professor of medicine in the University of Modena, and later in PADUA (p 447). His *De morbis artificum diatriba*, published in 1700, added one important question, 'What is your occupation?', to Hippocratic history-taking. In his treatise he described 54 different occupations associated with particular diseases, and included a description of

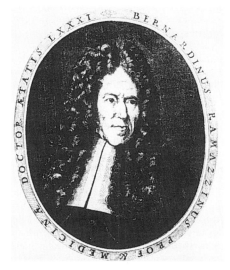

Bernardino Ramazzini, the father of occupational medicine. (Reproduced with permission from Hunter, D. (1978). *Diseases of occupations*, 6th edn, Edward Arnold, London.)

the ill-effects on surgeons of rubbing into the skin mercurial ointments in the treatment of SYPHILIS; of the diseases of the mirror-makers of Venice from mercury inhalation; and a chapter on the diseases of learned men.

The insanitary and polluted condition of the new towns, and the working conditions in the mines and factories that followed the Industrial Revolution, were eloquently described by Charles Dickens. At that time, epidemics of CHOLERA, TUBERCULOSIS, and TYPHUS, known as factory fever, were common. The pioneer of industrial medicine in Britain was Charles Turner Thackrah, who published in 1831 *The effects of the principal arts, trades and professions and of civic states and habits of living, on health and longevity, with suggestions for removal of many of the agents which produce disease and shorten the duration of life.* Thackrah was a contemporary of Addison, Bright, and the poet JOHN KEATS (p 659) at Guy's Hospital, and later was the founder of the Leeds School of Medicine. He wrote on the dust diseases of the lungs of miners and of the grinders of metals using sandstone wheels, the knife-grinders of Sheffield almost all dying before the age of 40. In his observations on the association of silica dust inhalation with tuberculosis, causing rapidly lethal silico-tuberculosis, Thackrah antedated the current concern in developing countries, where occupational exposures interact with endemic disease and malnutrition to give rise to more severe disease.

Reform of the squalid conditions in the working environment was initiated, not by knowledge of industrial disease, but by public awareness of the outrageous exploitation of child labor in mines, factories, and mills. In Britain, the humanitarian efforts of Robert Owen, Lord Shaftesbury, and others led to the first effective Factory Act of 1833. This set the minimum age of employment at 9 years, prohibited night work below 18 years, and restricted work to 12 hours a day. The Act established a Factory Inspectorate, and the Factory Act of 1844 led to the appointment of certifying surgeons.

The scandal of the climbing boys who swept the chimneys, immortalized in English literature (such as Charles Kingsley's *The water babies*), was finally brought to an end in 1875 when Lord Shaftesbury introduced a bill requiring chimney sweeps to hold a work license. One hundred years previously, Percivall Pott, through pertinent epidemiological observations, linked scrotal cancer to ingrained soot in the skin, and provided the first time evidence of an environmental cause for cancer. His work was followed by that of Sir Henry Butlin, who in 1892 showed that pitch, tar, and mineral oil also caused skin cancer, opening the road to work on experimental carcinogenesis.

At the turn of the 20th century industrial disease, in particular lead poisoning, was claiming many lives every year. In Britain Thomas Legge, appointed first medical inspector of factories in 1898, introduced the notification system for certain industrial diseases, enabling attention to be drawn to the work site for control measures to be instituted. As a result, lead poisoning, responsible for nearly 4000 notified cases with over 100 deaths annually in the early 1900s, steadily declined in frequency despite greatly increasing use of lead.

X-RAYS were discovered in 1895 and radium was isolated in 1898. At the time, physicists working with newly discovered ionizing radiation knew nothing of its biological effects. The first case of skin cancer from X-irradiation was reported in 1902. By 1922 over 100 radiologists were estimated to have died from their occupational exposures. Pierre CURIE (p 556) experienced radium dermatitis and both Marie CURIE (p 556) and her daughter died of leukemia. In a New Jersey factory between 1916 and 1923, girls pointed their brushes, dipped in radioactive paint, between their lips, in the production of luminous dials, resulting in death from aplastic anemia and bone sarcoma some years later. More recently, radiation sickness and deaths have occurred after exposure in nuclear energy establishments. An increased risk of leukemia has been observed in the children of parents working in the nuclear industry, but the evidence suggests that this is related to other environmental exposures.

While asbestos has been processed since ancient times, its increasing usage in modern technology since the late 19th century gave rise to heavy dust inhalation. This led to the progressive recognition of asbestosis, its association with bronchial carcinoma, and, in 1960, its causal relationship with malignant mesothelioma (cancer of the lining of lungs or abdominal cavity). As mesothelioma may develop 40 or more years after initial exposure to asbestos, the death rate from this condition, currently rising, is expected to rise further for some time.

Technological development makes it likely that new occupational diseases will continue to appear. To prevent or to minimize their consequences requires effective monitoring systems for new chemicals and processes, together with constant vigilance by clinicians, hygienists, and epidemiologists.                                   GK

**OCCUPATIONAL HEALTH** is concerned with the effects of work on health, and on the ability to work. It is essentially a discipline in preventive medicine. The evolution of the concept of occupational health, initially from observations on

**FOUNDING FATHERS**

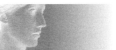

Bernardino **RAMAZZINI** (1633–1714). Italian physician. Ramazzini was appointed professor of theoretical medicine in Modena in 1682; he moved to the chair of practical medicine in Padua in 1700. Ramazzini was the first physician to be interested in occupational disease. In *De morbis artificum diatriba* (1700), he described some 40 industrial diseases. He was also a pioneer of epidemiology.

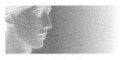

Sir James Phillips **KAY-SHUTTLEWORTH** (1804–77). British physician and pioneer of public health. Kay-Shuttleworth practiced in Manchester, where, as medical officer to the Ancoats and Ardwick Dispensary, he witnessed the horrors of the cholera epidemic of 1832. As a result he published *The moral and physical condition of the working classes employed in the cotton manufacture in Manchester* (1832). In 1835 he was appointed assistant Poor Law commissioner to implement the 1834 Poor Law Act. He inspired and administered relief during the cotton famine of 1861.

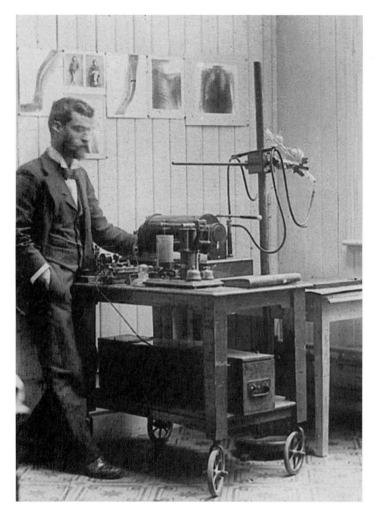

A pioneering X-ray physicist, working with unprotected equipment. (Reproduced with permission from Hunter, D. (1978). *Diseases of occupations*, 6th edn, Edward Arnold, London.)

may be confronted with exposures hazardous to reproductive health.

In developing countries the workforce is mostly employed in agriculture and other types of primary production. Heavy physical work often combined with heat stress, occupational accidents, pesticide poisoning, and exposure to organic dusts and to biological agents are the principal causes of occupational ill health. In the least developed countries such occupational factors are aggravated by poor hygiene and sanitation, poor nutrition, and poverty. Transnational corporations have opened many kinds of factories, such as oil refineries and textile mills, in industrializing regions of Brazil, Mexico, Thailand, Indonesia, etc. Often there are few or no occupational health or safety laws. The workforce predominantly comprises girls and women, is very low paid, and injured or sick workers are often dismissed without compensation.

In both industrialized and developing countries accidents in the workplace from unshielded machinery, unsafe structure, and dangerous tools are common, as are traffic accidents related to work. An estimated ten million occupational accidents with 25 000 fatalities occur annually in Europe alone. These can be largely controled with appropriate accident prevention programs. Noise-induced hearing loss is currently one of the most prevalent occupational diseases in both industrialized and developing countries. Extremes of temperature giving rise to hyper- or hypothermia, vibration, and exposure to ionizing and non-ionizing radiation are other physical factors affecting the health of workers.

Some 2000 chemicals are widely used in industry, increasingly so in developing countries. Metal poisoning is not uncommon, in particular following exposure to lead, mercury, cadmium, and arsenic compounds. The organic compounds posing the greatest occupational health hazards are aromatic, aliphatic, and halogenated hydrocarbons and the organophosphates, carbamates, organochlorine, and bipyridylium compounds used as pesticides. Pesticides are used the world over, yet despite precautionary measures, poisoning not infrequently occurs in agricultural communities. Several chemical compounds have been identified as occupational carcinogens. Among these are beryllium, cadmium, chromium, and nickel, and benzene, naphthylamine, benzidine, and 4-amino diphenyl; this last may cause cancer of the bladder.

Diverse biological agents including bacteria, viruses, parasites, fungi, molds, and organic dusts are encountered in an occupational environment. Viral hepatitis, and TUBERCULOSIS are encountered — in particular among healthcare workers; tuberculosis is a re-emerging hazard.

industrial disease, can be traced from antiquity. The pattern of occupational disease differs between industrialized and developing countries. In industrialized countries the traditional occupational diseases caused by physical, chemical, and biological agents and by heavy physical work are now less common than in the past, and tend to be restricted to small and high risk groups. Work-related musculoskeletal disorders (repetitive strain injury) have been increasing appreciably in workers required to perform more repetitive tasks at a faster pace. Such disorders remain an increasingly common problem in occupational health, as may stress-related symptoms, problems related to a progressively aging workforce and to increasing psychological stress in the work environment. Equal job opportunities are not generally available for women, who often have a double work burden of job and family care. Women may have to use machinery and work tools designed for male workers and

Exposure to certain plant and animal dusts in the work environment has given rise to allergic dermatoses and ASTHMA, among the most prevalent of occupational diseases in developing countries. Specific hazards include dusts from flour, grains, and wood products. Cotton workers and others handling hemp or flax may develop byssinosis, similar to asthma. The group of diseases known as farmer's lung, maltworker's lung, and bird fancier's lung are caused by an allergic inflammatory reaction to the fungal spores present in moldy hay or barley.

Hazardous exposures resulting from industrial activity are not, however, restricted to the workplace. Gaseous and particulate emissions from industrial plants give rise to deposition in the general environment, and industrial waste disposal may lead to leaching into waterways and to widespread pollution. As an example, gold recovery in the Amazon basin from numerous small-scale plants has given rise to mercury leaching into waterways, conversion to alkyl mercury, and uptake by fish later eaten by villagers at far away sites. Cadmium pollution of waterways irrigating agricultural land in Toyama, Japan, has caused renal dysfunction and itai-itai disease, a form of osteomalacia (softening of bones), in a population eating locally-grown rice with a high cadmium content. It has been estimated from a cross-sectional population-based study that about 10% of the general population of Belgium have an internal dose of cadmium, resulting from industrial emissions, sufficient to cause slight dysfunction of the kidney.

Identification of a health hazard in a defined group of workers with a specific, significant exposure has led to the subsequent identification of such a health hazard in the general population exposed to a lower less clearly defined exposure to the same agent.

Although occupational medicine is concerned with the diagnosis and management of occupational disease, its primary objective is the prevention of occupational disease. For prevention, occupational medicine has much in common, as a discipline, with environmental medicine, in particular using epidemiological enquiry for the purpose of identifying health risks related to exposure and life-style. There has been a move towards an integration of occupational and environmental medicine in several industrialized countries. The American and Australian colleges have adopted Occupational and Environmental Medicine in the title of their faculties. However, a move in this direction has been slower in Britain.

Environmental medicine involves the application of medical science to the study, interpretation, and provision of medical advice in the interaction

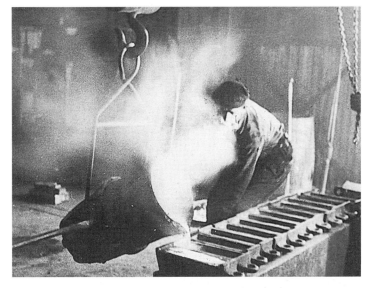

Hazardous exposure in the pouring of molten metal. (Reproduced with permission from Hunter, D. (1978). *Diseases of occupations*, 6th edn, Edward Arnold, London.)

between external physical, chemical, and biological factors and human health. Under this definition, health risks arising from smoking, diet, and other life-style factors such as poverty embrace a wider range of medical and non-medical specialties than occupational medicine alone. Occupational health is knowledgeable in risk assessment and health and safety management, whose skills are readily transferable to environmental hazards.

### Functions of an occupational health service

An effective occupational health service is mainly preventive, and essential services may be summarized as follows:

- *Job placement:* A pre-employment health questionnaire, medical examination, and in certain cases regular monitoring is necessary for determining job suitability. Jobs considered safe for a man may be hazardous for a pregnant woman and for other vulnerable groups such as the very young, the elderly, or the disabled.

- *Safety training:* An occupational health service has a responsibility to keep employees informed about workplace hazards. Workers should understand the need to comply with irksome restrictions such as wearing protective clothing, face masks, showering and changing after work, and avoiding eating and smoking at the worksite.

- *Control of recognized hazards:* A complex system of environmental and biological monitoring has been developed for the control of known hazards at work. The concentrations of toxic substances are monitored in the working environment and in certain instances by personal exposure monitoring. Safe exposure levels have been defined in terms of occupational exposure limits.

With knowledge of exposure response relationships, limits can be set in terms of an eight-hour time-weighted average or short-term exposure limits. Where an exposure–response relationship has been determined, a 'no observed adverse effect level', or where this is not possible, a 'lowest observed adverse effect level', may be set. In addition to medical examination, biological monitoring entails the examination of a blood or urine sample for an indication of absorbed dose and evidence of an effect, which result may require modification of work practice or suspension from further exposure. Thus, with regard to lead exposure, a worker is required to submit to regular blood sampling, with suspension where the blood lead level concentration exceeds 60 $\mu$g/dl in a man and 25 $\mu$g/dl in a woman.

- *Identification of unrecognized hazards:* An occupational health service should play a major part in the detection of new health hazards related to exposure or work practice. Clinical observation and epidemiological study may disclose a causal relationship between patterns of sickness absence or death in groups of workers and their occupational exposure. Such knowledge may then be applied to studies in the general environment involving more diffuse exposure patterns.

- *Treatment:* Effective on-site treatment of work injuries and poisoning where these have not been prevented can prevent complications and aid recovery. An occupational treatment service offers opportunities for specialized counseling and health education.

- *General health education and surveillance:* By advising employees on such topics as smoking, alcohol or drug abuse, exercise and diet, an occupational health service can improve worker health and efficiency and reduce illness and absenteeism. Occupational health services also provide general medical care for workers and their families in developing countries with inadequate community health services.

## Britain and the European Union

It has been estimated in a labor force survey that in 1990 some 750 000 people in England and Wales attributed illness directly to their work, related mainly to musculoskeletal, dermatological, pulmonary, psychological, or hearing loss effects. The resulting injury incidence rate for reportable injuries was about 2630 per 10 000 employed persons.

In Britain a broadly based enabling act, the Health and Safety at Work Act of 1974, aimed at covering all persons at work. This act set up the Health and Safety Commission, the operational arm, the health and safety executive being responsible for enforcing statutory provisions. The Employment Medical Advisory Service forms the medical arm of the executive, responsible for advising on health matters related to employment. In 1988 the Control of Substances Hazardous to Health regulations introduced a requirement for employers and the self-employed to assess the risks arising from exposure to substances hazardous to health. Employers are required by statute to report cases of occupational disease under the Reporting of Injuries, Diseases, and Dangerous Occurrences Regulations 1995, updated from April 1996. However, these data tend to be under-reported. The most commonly reported diseases in 1994–5 were hand–arm vibration syndrome and occupational asthma.

## Role of international agencies

A joint International Labour Organization–World Health Organizational Committee defined occupational health as: the promotion and maintenance of the highest degree of physical, mental, and social well-being of workers in all occupations; the prevention among workers of departures from health caused by their working conditions; the protection of workers in their employment from risks resulting from factors adverse to health; the placing and maintenance of the worker in an occupational environment adapted to his or her physiological equipment, and, to summarize, the adaptation of work to the worker and of each worker to the job.

This definition advances the concept of occupational health beyond the prevention of occupational diseases and introduces the promotion of positive health and the concept of fitting the job to the worker. Since its inception the WHO has played an important part in occupational health. Emphasis has been placed on 'work-related diseases' rather than purely occupational diseases, to include psychosocial hazards, reproductive hazards, and the application of ergonomics to health promotion. WHO produces a series of monographs on environmental health criteria through its International Programme on Chemical Safety and a series on the evaluation of carcinogenic risk of chemicals and processes through the International Agency for Research on Cancer.

The International Labour Organization, also based in Geneva, is best known through its occupational safety and health series of publications, and in particular, through the international classification of radiographs of the pneumoconioses, whose standard films have been widely used in epidemiological studies.

The interaction between industrial activity and the environment, between occupational health and environmental health, can be well illustrated by reference to the International Register of Potentially Toxic Chemicals of the United Nations Environment Program. A list of environmentally hazardous chemicals and processes of global significance, distributed to world governments, includes lead, mercury, cadmium, carbon dioxide, oxides of nitrogen, sulfur dioxide and its derivatives, and what has been termed the injudicious use of pesticides, which still gives rise to poisoning on a large scale in many parts of the world.

The WORLD HEALTH ORGANIZATION proposed a global strategy on occupational health for all. The objective of this strategy was that by the year 2000 the countries where trends in occupational health and safety were already positive, should demonstrate a further improvement of occupational health and safety indicators, showing a reduction of the difference between the level of health and safety of low-risk and high-risk occupations. In countries where the present trends were negative, positive development is expected and legal and other action, including the development of necessary resources and infrastructure, should be taken to make such positive trends possible. Ten priority objectives have been proposed by the strategy, which include strengthening of international and national policies for health at work and development of occupational health standards based on scientific risk assessment. For each of these objectives, both international and national actions have been specified.

Finally, to revert to one specific occupational disorder, adverse health effects related to work with display screen equipment may be considered an example of a new and increasing industrial disease related to modern technology. But then, as RAMAZZINI (p 583) observed in the early 18th century, 'where clerks incessantly drive the pen over paper, intense fatigue of the arm develops because of continuous strain upon the muscles and tendons, which eventually may lead to failure of power in the hand'. GK

**OLD MOORE'S ALMANAC** was the best known of the early English almanacs published by the Stationer's Company. Francis Moore was a physician, astrologer, and schoolmaster who published the almanac, containing weather predictions, in order to promote the sale of his pills. The first number was completed in July 1700 and contained predictions for 1701. The front cover of the edition for 1791, in the possession of W. Foulsham & Co. Ltd, carries a twopenny duty stamp and reads:

Vox Stellarum: or, a Loyal Almanack for the Year of Human Redemption M.DCC.XCI. Being the Third after Bissextile or Leap-Year. In which are contained All things fitting for such a Work: as. a Table of Terms and their Returns: The Full, Changes, and Quarters of the Moon: The Rising, Southing, and Setting of the Seven Stars, and other Fixed Stars of Note: the Moon's Age, and a Tide Table fitted to the same: The Rising and Setting of the Sun: the Rising, Southing and Setting of the Moon:

Mutual Aspects. Monthly Observations: and many other Things. useful and profitable.

There are several present versions, containing many predictions besides the weather. One edition, widely available in newsagents and cornershops, is priced at 25 pence: that of 1791 cost 'ten pence, stitched'. Its current print-run is almost 1 million copies.

**ONCOLOGY** — the study and treatment of cancer and other malignant diseases — emerged only as a coherent medical subspecialty as recently as the mid-20th century and is now one of medicine's most rapidly evolving disciplines.

### The nature of cancer

Cancer is the disordered and uncontrolled growth of cells within a specific organ or tissue type. Most cancers, though not all, begin in a single primary site such as breast, lung, or brain and, if left untreated, grow steadily, often by invading surrounding areas (that is, growing by direct extension), as well as producing secondary tumors — often termed 'metastases' — at more scattered, distant sites. These secondary cancers are the central and most feared feature of malignant disorders, particularly since conventional treatment is often unable to eliminate them entirely. They continue to pose a continuing threat to the patient's health, over many years, even after apparently successful treatment of the primary tumor. In addition to removal of the primary cancer, great effort must be directed wherever possible towards protecting patients from the possible development of life-threatening secondary deposits of tumor. In principle, this requires the use of whole-body (systemic) treatments such as chemotherapy or hormone therapy, though only a small proportion of cancers can be readily treated in this way with currently available drugs.

Although most cancers originate at a single site, this is not always the case. For example, in leukemia, essentially a malignant transformation of blood (more accurately, elements of the bone marrow which are the site of manufacture of many of the specific blood cells), the whole of this organ is apparently transformed, presumably by the single initiating process which triggered the malignant change. Little is known of the causes of human leukemia, though in animals — for example, the domestic cat — a virus is known to be responsible. Malignant blood disorders such as leukemia have a totally different pattern of behavior from most 'solid' malignancies, though even in the latter, multiple primary tumors occasionally occur in the same organ, including, for example, the previously rare Kaposi sarcoma of skin, now so prevalent in young men with AIDS, and a further rare skin condition, Gorlin's syndrome, characterized by multiple skin tumors of a very common type (basal cell carcinoma), which would far more typically occur as a single tumor.

An obvious carcinogen may result in the development of more than one primary cancer. Perhaps the most tragic example occurs in patients who smoke heavily, develop an early but curable cancer of the larynx — often cured by radiotherapy without any loss of voice or other serious side effect — but then continue to smoke and develop lung cancer a few years later, a disease with a worse outlook and a far higher fatality rate.

Cancers not only develop at a single site, but also result from malignant change within a single clone of cells. The most convincing hypothesis is that a single susceptible cell develops an irresistible pressure towards malignant change, presumably initiated by genetic, environmental, or other influences (or in most cases, of course, a combination of these) and is transformed into a malignant growth by continued cell division, producing progeny with the same characteristics and lack of cellular control. It is likely that a carcinogenic 'initiator' (the underlying event which first destabilizes the cell) is followed by exposure to one or more 'promoter' agents, which then produce further changes, initially transient, which eventually cause the cancer to develop.

## Malignant change

Several steps are required before a normal cell becomes irreversibly malignant, and cell growth and division are profoundly influenced by critical genes. Conceptually the latter fall into two groups: oncogenes, which drive the cell towards malignancy, and suppressor genes, which may mutate and result in a loss of normal regulatory or restraining function. It is often suggested that cellular oncogenes, when activated by carcinogens, initiate the events which lead to malignant transformation, and possibly certain viruses have incorporated these cellular genes into their own genetic templates, making them potential primers of malignant change occurring in mammalian or even human tissues at a much later stage. Oncogenes may be very simply activated, becoming multiplied or amplified within the chromosome, to provide additional copies, and rapidly accelerating the malignant development within the cell.

Good examples of the essential clonality of human cancer are not hard to find. In multiple myeloma, a bone-marrow cancer with some features similar to leukemia, the abnormal malignant cells are derived from characteristically large bone marrow plasma cells. Normally these produce two types of protein marker, designated kappa and lambda, whereas in myeloma it is clear that either the kappa or lambda protein chain is produced by the malignant cells, but never both. Observations such as these point strongly towards the 'monoclonal' theory of cancer, quite unlike less dangerous types of cellular growth, for example, in

A 1930s poster from the American Society for the Control of Cancer. (Reproduced courtesy of the National Cancer Institute, Bethesda, MD.)

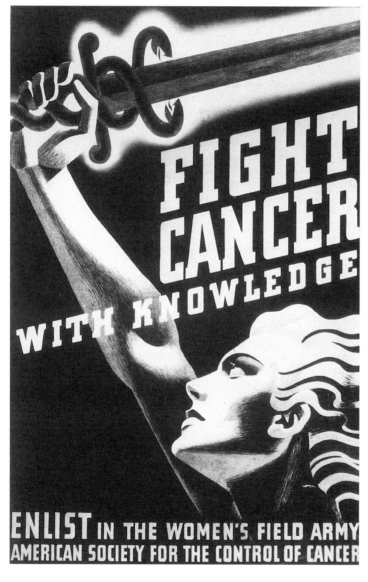

response to injury in which cell regeneration is extremely important but well controlled and regulated ('polyclonal' growth).

Despite the unchecked growth typical of cancer at the cellular level, most types of malignant or 'neoplastic' growth display some predictability in their evolution and pattern of spread. In general, there are three main patterns of behavior, and each type of malignancy tends to behave in a characteristic way, though some are more predictable than others. The major types of cancer dissemination are by local extension, by lymphatic and lymph node involvement, and finally by the blood-borne (or hematogenous) route.

## Cell markers

Cancers are truly detectable only when they have reached a substantial size in cellular terms: billions of malignant cells will by then be present within the primary mass. Early phases of cell doubling after the mutational changes described above are generally undetectable. The only exception to this is in tumors which elaborate a cell marker, generally a protein or other substance which is specific to the tumor and manufactured by it, secreted into the bloodstream, and detectable by sensitive laboratory tests. A good example is that of testicular tumors, many of which elaborate two well-recognized marker substances — alpha fetoprotein and beta human chorionic gonadotrophin — each of which can be assayed in the blood. Either (or both) of these may be detectable at abnormally high concentrations after apparently successful treatment of the primary tumor (generally by surgical removal), at a time when there is no other evidence of the continued presence or reappearance of the tumor. In these fortunate circumstances, treatment of the recurrence can start immediately before the cancer has otherwise declared itself, while the tumor burden is modest, and without waiting for other evidence of failure of the initial therapeutic approach.

Testicular tumors of this kind are an ideal clinical example, since the marker itself can be measured both reliably and at repeated intervals by a simple blood test. In addition, highly effective chemotherapy is available for relapse, regardless of where in the body that relapse might be. But for other tumors, all too common at present, there is no satisfactory answer to the problem of recurrent disease, since they either fail to produce a recognizable marker, or if they do (for example, primary liver cancer), no curative treatment currently exists.

Some apparently normal people (not yet patients, but destined to become them) have a high susceptibility to certain types of cancer. Little is known of the cellular regulating mechanisms which prevent patients who have a strong genetic predisposition from developing their cancer(s) much earlier in life. Think, for example, of the extraordinary phenomenon of colorectal (large bowel) cancer, a common condition with over 28 000 new cases a year in Britain, which can generally be cured by surgery if the tumor is detected early enough, without evidence of spread. The gene causing the disease (situated on the second main chromosome out of the twenty-three human pairs), has now been located and is known to be carried by one in every 200 people in the western population. Viewed from a different perspective, the gene is therefore present in up to 250 000 people in Britain alone, making this the most common inherited malignancy by far. Soon, this should allow large-scale testing of high-risk families (those in which several family members are known to have been affected), with the prospect of careful regular SCREENING for those who might be carrying the gene, and possibly early preventive surgery in selected cases. With straightforward means of direct examination of the whole large bowel using fiberoptic equipment, this should now prove technically possible. The difficulty will be in assessing the relative costs and benefits of such an enormous task.

## Discovery of X-rays

As with many other medical disciplines, the history of treatments for cancer is partly a reflection of emerging contemporary technology. In this case the most notable are the remarkable discoveries clustered at the end of the 19th century — of X-RAYS (by Wilhelm Conrad ROENTGEN (p 873)) in 1895, and of natural radioactivity by Marie and Pierre CURIE (p 556) in 1898. It is difficult to conceive of any observations more critical to the development of modern medicine, in both the investigational and therapeutic settings, than these remarkable and sustained efforts. Elsewhere in this volume a more detailed account is provided of Roentgen's recognition of *Eine neuer Art von Strahlen* — a new kind of ray — which he termed X-rays since their nature was entirely unknown and at the time inexplicable.

Within a few weeks of Roentgen's discovery, the French scientist Henri BECQUEREL (p 700) recognized that a recently discovered element, uranium, seemed also to have properties in some ways similar to those of X-rays. As with Roentgen, his scientific curiosity was aided by good fortune; in the case of Becquerel, the key observation was that a uranium compound, placed over a photographic plate (itself protected by a thin layer of aluminium) was unexpectedly able to fog the plate even in the presence of the aluminum filter, suggesting that uranium was also able — like Roentgen's cathode ray tube — to emit rays which

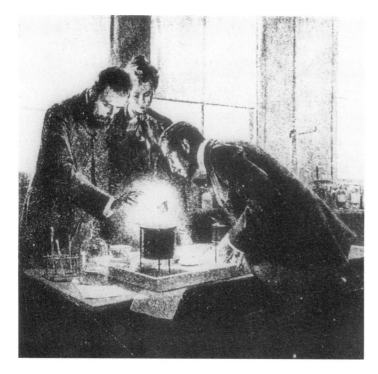

Pierre and Marie Curie experimenting with radium. (Reproduced courtesy of the National Library of Medicine, Bethesda, MD.)

tions of X-ray treatment methods led within a decade to the recognition of the major types of approach still used today: external or 'local' irradiation of the primary cancer; interstitial or 'internal' irradiation, often used, for instance, with gynecological cancers sufficiently accessible for radioactive tubes or wires to be placed within the diseased area itself; and total body irradiation, now increasingly used in conjunction with bone marrow transplant procedures for cure of leukemia, lymphoma (malignant tumor), and other blood disorders.

**Modern uses** Now, a hundred years after the discovery and initial clinical use of natural radioactivity and artificial X-rays, radiotherapy has become the most important type of non-surgical treatment for patients with malignant disease. Roughly half of all cancer patients now receive radiotherapy at some point during their illness, a figure which has risen over the past 20 years because of its rapid and widespread introduction as an important component of treatment in many diseases traditionally treated by surgical resection. The rapid replacement of mastectomy for most patients with breast cancer, in favor of local excision (with breast preservation) followed by immediate radiotherapy, is just one example of this trend in a disease whose incidence continues to rise. Other common examples include carcinomas of the bladder, prostate, and various head and neck sites, most notably the larynx. Even in colorectal carcinoma, where surgical resection remains critically important for cure, the use of pre- or postoperative radiotherapy for high-risk cases is now known significantly to improve the local control rate.

In recent years there has also been a renewed interest in internal methods of radiation treatment, often termed 'brachytherapy' from its initial Greek root (*brachy-* = close; *tele-* = from afar). Although these techniques were used within the first few years of the initial discovery of radium, improvements in choice of radionuclide, systems of delivery, three-dimensional treatment planning, and staff/patient protection have more recently permitted a much wider range of tumors to be treated with greater safety. In cancers of the head and neck, breast, cervix, and esophagus, brachytherapy is now used as a means of achieving high local doses of radiation, which can be combined with external beam irradiation as well.

One cancer particularly amenable to 'internal' radiation is thyroid cancer, a malignancy encountered most typically in young women. Since the thyroid gland is the only organ in the body which will take up and concentrate iodine — and therefore its radioactive counterpart, the radioactive iodine radionuclide $I^{131}$ — treatment of thyroid

could pass unimpeded through solid material. Somewhat surprisingly he laid the work aside, allowing his colleague Marie Curie free rein with the uranium rays — which she chose as the topic for her doctoral thesis.

Marie (originally Marie Sklodowska), together with her husband Pierre, discovered a further far more radioactive element, radium, in 1898; it took months of laborious effort to separate a few milligrams of this material from a witches' brew containing one ton of pitchblende ore, fifty tons of water, and a further five tons of additional chemicals. This Herculean effort produced a few meager milligrams of radium, the final distillate immediately presented as a gift to Professor Becquerel, but so minute in quantity that it fitted easily into his breast pocket, there producing the first known example of a severe radiation skin burn.

### Early radiotherapy

Even before this, however, X-rays such as those discovered by Roentgen had been used, in a remarkably imaginative leap, for cancer treatment as little as three weeks after the public announcement of Roentgen's discovery (in January 1896). The first patient with advanced cancer of the breast was treated in a series of extensive exposures, each lasting one hour, resulting in a surprising degree of healing — to the point where the patient died not from her primary tumor or its 'local' effects, but from distant metastases. Further ingenious applica-

cancer may be effective even if the cancer has spread through the body, as thyroid cancer cells still retain the potential for uptake and concentration of radioactive iodine, and will therefore often 'self-destruct' — a true 'magic bullet' indeed. Routine postoperative use of adjuvant I[131] therapy ('adjuvant' meaning treatment immediately after the initial surgical operation) has resulted in exceptionally high cure rates for patients with most types of thyroid cancer.

Local irradiation, often with curative intent, of a variety of primary cancers such as bladder, prostate, cervix, and larynx now represents a substantial portion of any radiotherapist's workload but equally important is the palliative use of radiotherapy for secondary cancers. Sadly, many patients develop distant or metastatic disease requiring immediate treatment, and for most, radiotherapy is the most effective treatment available. It is particularly valuable for secondary bone deposits, but may also be useful for brain, skin, and internal metastases, shrinking the secondary tumors and restoring function. For bone metastases in the spine, prompt treatment with palliative radiotherapy can prevent spinal cord compression and subsequent paralysis.

As little as ten years ago many medical oncologists (specialists in cancer chemotherapy) were predicting that with improvements in cytotoxic agents and biological therapy for cancer, the great days of radiotherapy were over. The systemic nature of most cancers was felt to imply that local therapy, however effective, would always remain inadequate and therefore become less important. Curiously, the reverse seems to have happened and we now recognize that, even though cancer is best viewed as a generalized rather than a local disorder, cure can never be achieved without a determined effort at control of the primary cancer.

## Chemotherapy

The development of drugs for effective cancer treatment has been a long sought-after medical goal. It was not until the empirical, accidental, discovery of the toxic effects of nitrogen mustard (compounds with a molecular structure similar to mustard gas) after the bombing of Brindisi harbour during the Second World War, when large volumes of mustard gas ($CH_2Cl.CH_2$) were released from an Allied armament ship, that effective anti-cancer drugs were developed. Interestingly, even as early as the immediate aftermath of the First World War, cases of bone marrow suppression after exposure to sulfur mustard agents had been reported, though the potential for cancer treatment remained unrecognized until 1943, when a patient with Hodgkin's disease (one of the lymphomas or lymphatic malignancies), treated with nitrogen mustard, showed dramatic shrinkage of the lymphomatous tissue, and the modern era of chemotherapy for cancer had finally begun.

Since then, many thousands of compounds have been screened for anti-cancer effects, and an increasing number of useful cytotoxic agents have been developed. Nearly all of the currently used drugs were initially discovered through empirical screening programs, and semi-synthetic analogs, often more active or less toxic to normal tissues, have also been developed. Although there have been real advances in our understanding of the mechanisms of action of chemotherapy, the development of an ideal drug — one that would be cytotoxic only to cancer cells, but totally safe and without effect on normal host tissues — remains elusive. No satisfactory system exists for the accurate determination of individual responsiveness, of the type which has proved so valuable in antibiotic sensitivity testing, routinely offering an opportunity for correctly choosing between a variety of potentially suitable drugs.

***Method of action*** Most anti-cancer drugs act by directly or indirectly affecting actively dividing cells, generally at the site of the cell nucleus. For instance, nitrogen mustard itself, and its less toxic though equally effective derivatives, seem to work by producing intra-strand cross-links and thereby preventing normal DNA replication and division within the tumor cell. Other anti-cancer drugs may act by a quite different mechanism, for example, the plant-extract vincristine (obtained from the periwinkle *Catharanthus roseus*), which acts as a mitotic spindle poison, directly preventing or paralyzing tumor cell division as it finally attempts cleavage into two malignant daughter cells. Taxol, a widely used anti-cancer agent also obtained naturally (from the bark of the Pacific yew tree *Taxus brevifolia*), appears to act by yet a different route, interfering with intracellular micro-tubule formation within the cancer cell, and interrupting cell division at yet another phase in the cell cycle. A full list of anti-cancer drugs, their classification, mode of action, and current usage, would require a separate large textbook — and one that would be out of date at the point of publication.

In many ways, the development of cancer chemotherapy is the most exciting oncological advance of all over the past 50 years. Before the mid-1950s, patients with leukemia, lymphoma, or disseminated testicular cancer, invariably died of it. We now regularly expect to cure many of these patients, together with an ever-increasing proportion of childhood cancers as well. Even in more common conditions in which cure is still not possible, the advent of partially effective chemotherapy has meant an improvement in survival, often with lengthy periods of remission. This large group of common cancers includes ovarian cancer, myeloma, and some types of lung and breast cancer. Most exciting of all, perhaps, is the demonstration that in tumors such as breast cancer, which are only moderately responsive to chemotherapy, its early use as 'adjuvant' therapy given directly after surgery, improves the overall outlook with an unequivocal extension in overall survival documented over at least the initial 15 years from diagnosis, even though the adjuvant chemotherapy would have been completed many years before, and generally given for a total of only six months. Other tumors such as colorectal and head and neck cancers are currently the subject of trials of adjuvant chemotherapy and also appear to show benefit (with improved chances of survival) when the chemotherapy is given at this early stage rather than much later in the evolution of the cancer, at the point of tumor recurrence. It seems clear that tumors of relatively marginal chemosensitivity respond most readily after surgical removal of the primary tumor, when the tumor burden is at its minimum.

Despite these improvements, the word 'chemotherapy' continues to strike dread in the hearts of many patients, since it is too widely assumed that the word is synonymous with intolerable treatment-related toxicity. In truth, chemotherapy side-effects are much misunderstood: in the first place, only a small proportion of these agents cause really severe nausea and vomiting, and, secondly, powerful anti-nausea agents are now available, which combat specific trigger sites of nausea and vomiting within the brain, considerably reducing the ill effects. Hair loss is a feature only of a proportion, though not all, anti-cancer drugs, and is invariably reversible when treatment is complete — indeed, hair regrowth after cancer chemotherapy is one of the few absolute guarantees that the oncologist can give. The third major group of side-effects, bone marrow suppression ('myelosuppression'), occurs with most types of cancer chemotherapy, but generally not to the point of serious danger. Advances in supportive drug therapy have helped greatly and it is usually not too difficult to tide the patient over a temporary period of bone marrow failure. Anemia can be relieved by blood transfusion if required; a lowering of the white cell count, with danger of infection, can be 'covered' — or rendered far less hazardous by highly effective antibiotics and if necessary, new biological growth factors which raise the white count significantly; and a bleeding tendency from loss of the platelet cells in the blood is usually dealt with, if required, by platelet transfusions.

Together, these methods of dealing with the various types of chemotherapy-related side-effects have permitted an increase in dosage over recent years, allowing us to test the hypothesis that dose intensification should prove increasingly lethal to the tumor without putting the patient at unreasonable danger. This and other considerations have increasingly led to the use of drug combinations, rather than single agent chemotherapy, in order not only to increase dose intensity but to capitalize on the opportunity of attacking the malignant cell via more than a single biochemical mechanism, with greater probability of lethality to the malignant clone of cells. Countless research studies have confirmed that on the whole this theory holds true and provides a significantly greater chance of cure.

*Hormonal influences* Almost as important as the radiation discoveries during the closing years of the 19th century was the observation in 1896 by Beatson that inoperable breast cancer sometimes regressed after surgical removal of the ovaries (oophorectomy). This was the first clue that cancer could be responsive to hormonal influences; some years later Huggins demonstrated that metastatic prostatic cancer in men often regressed with orchidectomy (removal of the testicles) or after treatment with estrogens. We now know that many cancer cells carry receptor proteins for steroid hormones and that an interaction between the hormone and its receptor will modify DNA activity, profoundly affecting cell growth and replication.

The use of hormones in cancer patients is chiefly limited to those with prostate, breast, or uterine cancer but in all these tumors, the remarkable feature — at least in a proportion of patients — is the relative durability of response, even in those with disseminated disease, providing excellent quality of life in a substantial number. In breast cancer, for example, patients who have estrogen receptors within the malignant cell often respond for months or even years to tamoxifen, a widely used and well-tolerated oral agent, increasingly used as adjuvant therapy. It is also being used in trials in both Europe and the USA in an attempt to reduce the risk of breast cancer development in normal healthy women — an exciting advance in a cancer which is now the most common of all in western women.

## Surgery

Initially pre-eminent as a cancer treatment, surgery remains enormously important, though its role in some types of cancer has radically altered, and diminished, over the past 25 years. As with radiotherapy, its main function is to establish local control; the surgeon has a unique contribution to cancer management, being potentially able to completely remove or debulk the primary site 'at a stroke'. If cancer were invariably a local single-site disease, without the problem of distant metastatic spread, cancer surgery would continue to reign supreme, as in the early part of this century, when heroic operations were frequently undertaken since no other approach was possible. It remains the most effective form of treatment for certain types of cancer, notably non-small cell lung cancer, many skin cancers (above all, melanoma), most forms of soft tissue tumor (sarcoma), and gastrointestinal cancers. Generally, these are tumors in which no other method has yet proved to be superior to, or even the equal of, surgery, though in many cases — bone and soft tissue sarcomas are good examples — operations are now very much less radical than they used to be. Indeed, this general point holds true for much of cancer surgery today.

Radical surgery has given way to conservative procedures in which tissue preservation is a key objective. The success of this approach requires routine use of pre- or postoperative radio- and/or chemotherapy. In many tumors, including limb sarcomas and head and neck cancers, for example, the use of early, postoperative radiotherapy has dramatically reduced the scope and extent of the surgical operation required. To give just one example, cancers of the larynx are now generally treated by radical radiotherapy (with or without chemotherapy) in an attempt to retain surgery as a secondary or 'salvage' approach. The intention, of course, is to retain the larynx, and thereby the patient's normal speech function.

*Laser surgery* Laser surgery is frequently used. This is not surgery in the usual sense, since a focused light beam has been substituted for the surgeon's traditional scalpel. Lasers may now be employed to remove areas of malignant or premalignant tissue, for example, in accessible cancers such as the tongue and cervix. Exciting advances have also been made with laser treatment of lung and esophageal (gullet) cancers, since conventional surgical treatment may be hazardous or impossible, and the laser can burn through areas completely blocked or obstructed by the cancer growth. Local radiotherapy can then be given to a patient in a far better condition, with greatly improved nutrition and with at least the possibility of more long-term control. Internal (or 'interstitial') laser therapy can also be used, for example, to deal with secondary liver deposits from colorectal cancer.                    JST

*See also* CELL AND CELL BIOLOGY; HEMATOLOGY; MOLECULAR BIOLOGY; NUCLEAR MEDICINE; PHARMACOLOGY, CLINICAL PHARMACOLOGY, AND THERAPEUTICS; SMOKING AND HEALTH; SPECIALIZATION

**OPERA** was long thought of as the least profound of the arts. As such, any relation with medicine would be superficial, shown, say, by those doctors who stand by helplessly and merely pronounce characters dead (*La Traviata*) or diagnose a case of madness beyond their treatment (*Lady Macbeth*). Doctors are even figures of fun: 'Dr' Dulcamara, an itinerant quack (*L'elisir d'amore*), sells the hero a love potion, which, though successful, is in reality a bottle of red wine. And lovesick heroines tend to go mad, usually to be miraculously restored without medical help when misunderstandings had been resolved.

### Serious themes

Nevertheless, opera has always had its more serious side. Published correspondence between composer and librettist — Verdi and Boito, or Strauss and Hofmannsthal, for example — shows how much trouble both took to attain depth. Opera has sometimes had a political slant; Verdi had a role in the Risorgiomento (the cries of Viva Verdi at performances of his operas also meant Viva Vittore Emmanuele, Rei d'Italia, and the chorus of the exiled Israelites in *Nabucco* had a resonance for an Italy partly occupied by the Austrians; and, as Bernard Shaw argued, there are good grounds for regarding Wagner's *Der Ring des Nibelungen* as a tract against capitalism). Not surprisingly opera has also addressed serious themes in medicine. Given that this art form was at its zenith in the 19th century, we should examine this era first for the evidence. Two prominent medical fears of the time were TUBERCULOSIS and SYPHILIS. Tuberculosis figures prominently in causing the deaths of the heroines, Violetta and Mimi, in *La Traviata* and *La Bohéme*. Linda and Michael Hutcheon have discussed in *Opera, desire, disease, and death*, how the disease is handled significantly differently in both. At the time of the first (1844), nobody knew the cause of consumption — as it was widely called — but it was ascribed to temperament, a riotous life, and, crucially, to heredity. By the second (1897), KOCH (p 455) had found the infecting organism, *Mycobacterium tuberculosis*, and it was known to be associated with poverty, overcrowding, and malnutrition, but particularly to be contagious, the infection being spread by droplets in coughing. As a result, at one point in *La Bohéme* the hero takes care to distance himself physically from the heroine.

Superficially, Wagner's *Parsifal* deals only with the redemption of a religious community by a 'pure fool'. Parsifal overcomes an evil magician using the latter's spear to heal the abbot's wound and enable the community to resume its normal worship. However, in an era when fear of syphilis was rampant (and the same year that Ibsen's *Ghosts* appeared), audiences were hardly

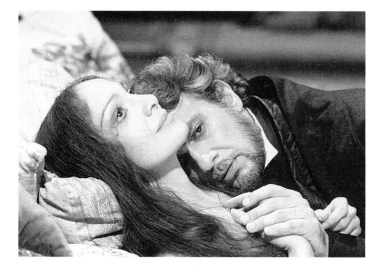

Teresa Stratas and Placido Domingo in the 1983 Universal production of *La Traviata*. (Reproduced courtesy of the Kobal Collection.)

likely to misinterpret the nature of the abbot's symptoms and signs. His wound (which Wagner originally sited in the genitals, but then altered to the side) refuses to heal and he has excruciating night pains (a characteristic of tabes, a form of late syphilis). And Wagner emphasizes this association by surrounding the magician with flower maidens (who, as their titles suggest, are prostitutes).

Syphilis also features in two 20th century operas, Alban Berg's *Lulu* and Stravinsky's *The rake's progress* (where the hero Tom Rakewell ends up demented in Bedlam). And, curiously, another 19th century preoccupation, CHOLERA, also had to wait until the 20th century before it was dealt with in opera. From the 1830s until the end of the century epidemics of cholera were another theme for general anxiety, with its various linkages to the East (its original source), divine retribution for immorality, and association with contaminated food and water. Again, it was Robert Koch who in 1882 showed that the illness was due to a microorganism, a vibrio, and spread by food and water contaminated by sewage.

All these associations are featured in Thomas Mann's novella *Death in Venice*, on which Benjamin Britten based his last opera. The protagonist, Aschenbach, a famous writer, falls in love with a handsome Polish youth, also on holiday in the Lido, but can never speak to him and dies during a cholera outbreak. Such a theme found a resonance in Britten, himself a withdrawn homosexual, and the darkness of the music (written while he was suffering from heart disease, which killed him two years later) draws the strands together in a masterly fashion.

At least four 20th century operas other than *The rake's progress* have medical associations. Alban Berg's *Wozzeck* is, like the ballet, based on George Büchner's play of the same name. In it, the sadistic doctor pays Wozzeck to be a guinea pig in experiments on a diet rich in beans. (Just as this is an anticipation of the discovery of vitamins, so more trivially is what happens to the gods in Wagner's *Ring*: in *Das Rheingold*: deprived of Freia's golden apples, they rapidly, but reversibly, lose their youth.) And in Berg's second opera, *Lulu* (whose first husband is a professor of medicine), the heroine develops both cholera (from which she recovers) and syphilis. In Richard Rodney Bennet's *The mines of sulfur* the dénouement occurs when the heroine, a member of a group of strolling players, discloses that she has the PLAGUE. Janáček's *The Mackropoulos affair* has a heroine who has lived 387 years as a result of being a guinea pig. Her father, physician to Rudolf II at Prague, was ordered by his royal master to devise an elixir of life — but then had to try it out on his daughter to show that it was not lethal.

Given that a few operas have managed to mirror the medical preoccupations of their time, surprisingly none has yet tackled one of today's: HIV/AIDS. There is little doubt, however, that an article in a future edition of this Companion will report that one has been written.      SPL

*See also* DANCE; MUSIC

**OPHTHALMOLOGY** Vision is the most important of the traditional five senses, and eyesight is responsible for almost half of the total sensory input from the external world to the internal world of the conscious human being. As a result, loss of vision or the prospect of loss of vision can cause great anxiety and can greatly exacerbate mental stress or mental illness. As early as 1550 BC, the Egyptians had outlined in the EBERS PAPYRUS a list of recognized eye diseases and in 327 BC, Alexander during his campaign along the Indus River, commented on the knowledge of eye disease among Indian physicians. The Chinese were also aware of ocular disease and had described cataracts even before the Indian physicians. HIPPOCRATES (p 382) described the anatomy of the eyeball and the optic nerve, and for some 2000 years his teachings held sway. In 1847 Charles Babbage, the Englishman who invented the computer, suggested that it would be possible to view the back of the eye through the pupil, using a perforated mirror. This was elaborated on by von HELMHOLTZ (p 372) in 1851, triggering a massive increase in the knowledge of ocular disease. In the last 30 years, advances in electrophysiological techniques, and the use of intravenous dye markers and advanced imaging techniques, have further increased our understanding of both normal and abnormal ocular conditions.

## Anatomy and physiology

The eye converts the images of the external world into electrical signals. The electrical impulses from the eye are transmitted up the optic nerve to a junction with the optic nerve from the other eye, where at least half of the nerve fibers cross to relay to the opposite side of the brain. This crossing is called the optic chiasma. The nerves then travel as a bundle of fibers called the optic tract, until they come to a relay station (called the lateral geniculate ganglion), where a rearrangement of the fibers takes place. The messages are then transmitted through another fan-shaped bundle of nerve fibers (called the optic radiation) to the occipital (back) lobe of the brain, where more processing is carried out by the visual cortex. At this level, vision consists of very crude images of light and dark, and for vision to occur as we know it, the messages have to be passed on to several other areas in the brain. These include an area in the temporal (side) lobe of the brain, where visual memory is situated, and the parietal (front side) lobe of the brain, where vision is related to other forms of sensory input and where our ability to recognize symbols needed for reading and writing are situated. There are also connections to the anterior part of the brain, the frontal lobe, where conscious imagery is processed further.

The eyeball consists of three separate concentric layers, modified in the front to form the transparent cornea, which allows the passage of light. The outermost layer, the sclera, is a tough, fibrous, protective envelope consisting of protein, collagen, and referred to in lay terms as 'the white of the eye'. The innermost layer, the retina, is designed to be light sensitive and can convert these light signals to electrical coded signals for transmission to the higher visual centers. The intervening layer, the choroid, is rich in blood vessels. In its interior part it forms the ciliary body and part of the iris. The bulk of the space in the eyeball is occupied by a transparent gel, the vitreous humor, while in the front part of the eyeball there is a cavity between the cornea and the lens called the anterior chamber, filled with clear circulating fluid, the aqueous humor.

## Refractive errors

About one-third of the population do not see clearly because of refractive errors, resulting either from differences in the size of the eyeball in relation to the focusing power of the eye, or from changes in the curvature of the cornea or lens. Under normal circumstances the cornea and the lens focus the object of regard clearly on the macular area (small yellow spot on the retina). If this does not happen, a blurred image results. There are three main types of refractive error — hypermetropia, myopia, and astigmatism.

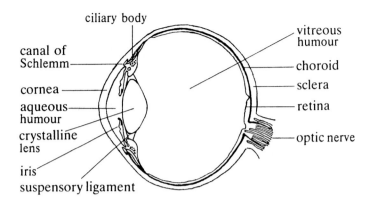

Vertical section through the eyeball.

In hypermetropia (long sight) the eyeball is smaller than normal, in myopia (short sight) it is larger than normal. In both conditions the image of an external object is not focused properly on the macular area and blurring of vision results. These refractive errors can be corrected by spectacle lenses or contact lenses, which refocus the image on to the macular area. More recently it has become possible to change the curvature of the cornea and hence its focusing power using advanced laser surgery. At present myopia seems to be more amenable to this treatment rather than long sight, but the results are not as predictable as those using spectacles or contact lenses.

Astigmatism occurs when one meridian of corneal curvature is different from the other, again leading to blurring of an external image on the macular area. This refractive condition can be corrected by spectacle lenses and less frequently by contact lenses or corneal surgery. Long sight is associated with acute narrow-angle glaucoma (high pressure in the eye) and myopia with retinal detachment, macular hemorrhage, and chronic open-angle glaucoma.

## Visual failure

In the developed world this occurs more commonly in the elderly and in many cases is age-related. In the developing world visual failure occurs in the younger age groups, often related to infection and malnourishment. The three main causes of visual failure in the elderly in the developed world are cataracts, age-related macular degeneration, and chronic open-angle glaucoma.

*Cataracts* The lens in the eye, about the size of a pea, is totally transparent and made up of proteins. As age progresses, the proteins break down and opacities begin to develop in the lens, sometimes in the center (the nucleus) and sometimes in the lens material surrounding the nucleus (the

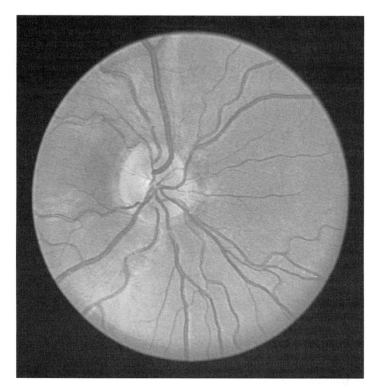

Normal fundus. View of fundus to show normal optic nerve and retinal blood vessels. The macular area is on the extreme right of the picture. (Reproduced courtesy of Ayerst International Inc, NY.)

Macular degeneration is age-related and develops insidiously, often making itself manifest by distortion of central vision which progresses to a blank spot in the center of vision. The patient is unable to read, but yet can see around and about and can navigate fairly easily. In one type of macular degeneration, small new blood vessels grow, and occasionally this is amenable to treatment using a laser, but the vast majority of cases are untreatable. In myopia, macular degeneration results from macular hemorrhage more frequently than in the non-myopic population.

***Chronic open-angle glaucoma*** In some individuals the drainage of aqueous humor becomes defective and the intraocular pressure slowly rises to somewhere in the region of 30–40 mm of mercury, compared with the normal intraocular pressure range of 15–22 mm of mercury. This pressure, if continued for several years, causes the blood vessels supplying the optic nerve, as the optic nerve enters the eyeball, to be squeezed and the optic nerve suffers as a result. This optic nerve damage manifests itself as deficiencies in the field of vision which relate to nerve fiber damage. Over the age of 40, 1% of the population develop open-angle glaucoma in the fullness of time, and the incidence rises with age. The treatment may be medical or surgical. Medical treatment consists of drops which improve the efficacy of the drainage mechanism in the eye, and surgery takes the form of an artificial drainage system created by a carefully sculpted gap in the sclera called a fistula, which is covered by conjunctiva. There is a move to earlier surgical intervention by ophthalmic surgeons rather than very long-term medical treatment.

### Acute visual failure

Usually affects one eye, but may occur in both as a result of head injury or obstructions in the blood supply to the visual cortex in the occipital lobe of the brain. There are three main causes of uniocular acute visual failure: acute narrow-angle glaucoma, in which there is a marked increase of intraocular pressure over a short period of time; as a result of a sudden shutdown of circulation within the eye; or acute inflammation of the optic nerve.

***Acute narrow-angle glaucoma*** Acute narrow-angle glaucoma occurs in small eyes (hypermetropic) and is the result of an abnormality in the basic architecture of the drainage mechanism, whereby this mechanism shuts off suddenly and the intraocular pressure rises to about 50–60 mm of mercury. This causes acute pain and a diminution of vision — the cornea becoming cloudy as a result of water being forced into it and making it less dehydrated. The treatment is medical in the

cortex). As the opacities increase, the ability of light to pass through the lens decreases and slow visual failure occurs. Present techniques of cataract surgery involve removing the lens through a small incision in the cornea, but leaving the posterior capsule of the lens — the envelope which surrounds the lens matter — intact. A plastic lens is inserted into the space to compensate for the lens that has been removed. The power of the lens to be inserted has to be accurately determined usually with ultrasound. If it is not possible technically to insert an intraocular lens, the loss of the natural lens can be compensated for by a contact lens or by spectacle lenses, these last being somewhat unsatisfactory because of magnification of the image and problems of distortion. Occasionally the posterior capsule of the implanted lens thickens again and a hole has to be made in the capsule to allow good vision to return; this may be carried out using a laser on an outpatient basis. Cataracts may also occur as a result of injury to the eye and may occur at birth as a result of maternal infections in pregnancy, for example, rubella (German measles), or as a hereditary trait in certain families.

***Age-related macular degeneration*** The macula depends solely on diffusion from the choroid (layer outside the retina) for its nutrient supply and if this diffusion is impaired, degeneration can result, with consequent impaired central vision.

first instance to reduce the formation of aqueous humor and to try to improve the outflow so that the pressure becomes normal, at which time the pain decreases and vision improves. However, the condition is likely to recur if surgical intervention is not undertaken; modern techniques use a laser to make a small hole in the peripheral iris, allowing free drainage of aqueous humor from behind the iris to in front.

*Retinal vascular occlusions* Obstructions in the blood supply to the retina cause sudden visual failure. The most common is a central retinal vein occlusion, which may be related to high blood pressure, arteriosclerosis, raised intraocular pressure (which makes the circulation sluggish), or any condition which thickens the blood, such as an increase in protein or blood cells. When a central vein is occluded there is appreciable congestion of the blood vessels as they leave the eye and loss of vision, usually permanent, ensues. Much less common is obstruction of the central retinal artery, which causes sudden visual loss as a result of it being occluded as it enters the eye, more commonly as a result of emboli — small particles of blood clot or degenerate arterial wall which are carried into the small blood vessels resulting in blockages.

*Inflammation of the optic nerve* The most common inflammation of the optic nerve, resulting in visual failure, is optic neuritis, usually due to multiple sclerosis. In this condition, inflammation of the optic nerve results in the loss of special sheaths around the nerve fibers that allow them to conduct impulses at a rapid rate. The condition is usually unilateral, the patient is young, and complains of loss of central vision with occasional slight pain in the eye on movement because the coverings of the optic nerve are inflamed and stretched. Vision recovers usually in 6–8 weeks in most cases, but inflammation may recur over several years.

## Retinal detachment

Retinal detachment is more frequent in short-sighted people. Retinal detachment is the result of a hole occurring in the peripheral retina, allowing fluid from the vitreous to escape and strip the retina off the underlying deeper layers like wallpaper off a wall. The hole, which can be caused by trauma or degeneration, is usually related to a strand of vitreous pulling on the peripheral retina and tearing it. The patient is aware of an area of poor vision which slowly gets larger, and if the hole is not sealed, total visual loss may occur. Treatment aims at sealing the hole to stop further leakage of fluid underneath the retina. This may use extreme cold (cryotherapy) laser treatment or other surgical procedures that push the retina on

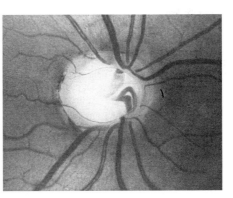

Open-angle glaucoma. View of the cupped optic disc, indicating vascular damage to the optic nerve as it enters the eye.

to the underlying deeper layers using an injection of gas into the vitreous, or silicone sponges applied to the outside of the eye to indent it and, as it were, to bring the wall to meet the wallpaper. Over the past decade the results of retinal detachment surgery have improved considerably.

## Retinopathy of prematurity

Survival rates for premature babies have increased greatly over the last 40 years, so that now 65% of babies with a birth weight of under 1000 grams and 90% of babies with a birth weight between 1000 grams and 1500 grams survive. Babies with these birth weights often require oxygen and a side-effect of this treatment can be retinopathy of prematurity, in which developing retinal blood vessels constrict and new abnormal blood vessels grow from the retina into the vitreous. This condition of abnormal vessels in the premature baby's eye, if not screened for and if necessary treated by an ophthalmologist, may lead to visual impairment in a few cases. Virtually all low birth weight babies are now screened for this condition, and the incidence of visual impairment is low.

## Squint (strabismus)

In the human, both eyes look ahead and the field of vision of one eye coincides to a marked degree with that of the other and overlaps by some 85%. This allows stereoscopic vision to take place and is usually the rule in hunting animals that need precise perception of depth to catch their prey. The ability to move the eyes together depends on complex centers in the mid-brain relaying messages from the eyes to the muscles that move the eyes. If this process is disrupted in any way, the eyes do not move together and a squint will result, so that the eyes are not directed at the same point. A squint may be due to a paralysis of one or more of the six muscles responsible for moving the eye (causes include injury, raised intracranial pressure, or thyroid eye disease); a poor retinal image in one or both eyes, so that the images cannot be superimposed properly because of, for example, refractive error cataract; or a disturbed relationship between accommodation, that is, the ability to focus and the ability of our eyes to converge, such as happens when reading (concomitant strabismus).

This last type of squint is more usual in children. In an eye which squints, the brain is faced with a double image and in children under the age of 7 the brain can blot out the image from the squinting eye. If the squint is not detected, the vision in the squinting eye becomes poorer and poorer until it is amblyopic (blind) — a lazy eye. After the age of 7 the prospects of restoring vision to an amblyopic eye are poor. Treatment aims at making the child use the lazy eye by patching the good eye under close supervision until the vision is as good as it was before the squint. If a squint is still present at that stage, surgery may be necessary.

### Systemic diseases

Many systemic diseases have effects on the eyes; DIABETES is one of the most common.

*Diabetes* Both types of diabetes — namely, insulin-dependent and non-insulin-dependent — may affect the eye. Cataracts are more common in both types than in the general population. Small retinal blood vessels are susceptible to damage in long-standing disease. There are two forms of retinopathy: non-proliferative,

which is far more common, and proliferative. In non-proliferative retinopathy, the small blood vessels leak and cause fluid and fat to accumulate in the retina, disturbing vision; in proliferative retinopathy, because small blood vessels become occluded and low oxygen levels result, the growth of new blood vessels is stimulated. These blood vessels are much less robust than normal and can cause bleeding and thus a great deal of internal damage both to the retina and to the eye as a whole. As a consequence, patients with diabetes are now regularly screened for ocular complications, and if diabetic retinopathy is diagnosed, many such patients receive laser treatment on an outpatient basis. Treatment aims at obliterating the new blood vessels and at destroying areas of the retina where oxygen levels are low; this is successful provided the condition is diagnosed early enough. There is increasing evidence that good control of diabetes can postpone the onset and lessen the severity of diabetic retinopathy.

### World-wide problems of visual failure

Total blindness is rare in the developed world, but much more common in the developing world. An estimated 100 million people in the developing world are suffering from blindness. In the developed world, the bulk of visual loss is borne by the elderly because of degenerative diseases, whereas in the developing world many young people suffer blindness related to untreated infections, vitamin deficiencies, and lack of ophthalmic medical and surgical care. Cataracts are widespread and surgery is often not available, so many millions of cataract sufferers do not have vision restored because of lack of resources. Trachoma, a chlamydial infection (a virus-like bacterium), infects 500 million people in the world, 2 million of whom are classified as blind. This disease, spread by flies, is accentuated by poverty. In undernourished populations, VITAMIN A deficiency is widespread, leading to opacification of the cornea as a result of drying of the eyes. A small vitamin supplement in the daily diet obviates this visual failure and if instituted world-wide, would prevent blindness in 250 000 children annually. River-blindness (onchocerciasis) is a parasitic infection, spread by flies, which occurs in central tropical Africa and in central America. The parasite causes inflammation in the eyes and their blood vessels. LEPROSY, which is curable, accounts for about 500 000 cases of blindness in the world each year. It is a chronic bacterial infection, leading to invasion of nerves by the bacteria. This leads to problems in closing the eyes, so that the cornea becomes dry and opaque, while in other cases inflammation in the eye leads to blindness.

ALCrom

Diabetic retinopathy. View of retina showing diabetic exudates and hemorrhages.

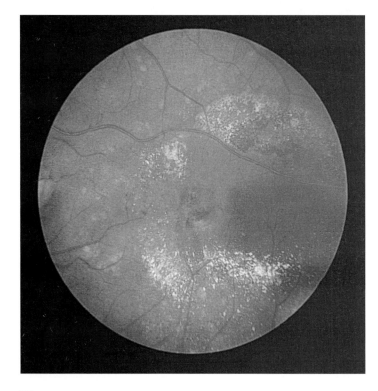

## ORTHOPEDIC SURGERY (ORTHOPEDICS)

deals with affections of the motor apparatus, mainly the bones, joints, muscles, tendons, and ligaments. Before the 19th century it dealt mainly with deformities and congenital anomalies of the skeleton, but nowadays it encompasses fractures, arthritis, osteoporosis, and its scope is constantly widening.

The first appearance of the word 'orthopedic' is attributed to Nicholas André, in a book (1741), of which Whitman in 1896 wrote: 'André is sometimes called the father of the speciality, and there appears to be a very general misapprehension as to the object and scope of his book…[which] was what might be called a nursery guide…intended only for parents and nurse'. The term at first applied to conditions affecting children (hence the Greek root *ped*), and only in this century has it become applicable to conditions in adults as well.

Institutions with 'orthopedic' in their title were founded early in the 19th century — such as the orthopedic infirmary in London (1838), the London Orthopaedic Institute (1840), the Boston Orthopedic Institution (1838) — but the physicians manning those institutions did not specialize — they were general surgeons, or even those who today are called general practitioners. As a surgical specialty, the beginning of orthopedics had to await on the availability of techniques that allowed operations to be carried out safely and painlessly, that is, asepsis and anesthesia. These followed LISTER'S (p 473) development of antiseptic surgery in 1867, but even so, orthopedic surgery as practiced until the turn of the century included only the simplest of procedures — amputations, excisions, tenotomies (division of tendons), and draining of abscesses. There was greater emphasis on non-surgical therapy (bracing, splinting, manipulation, and traction), as applied to the deformities such as club foot, scoliosis (lateral curvature of the spine), and later to other orthopedic conditions such as fractures. The use of X-RAYS, after ROENTGEN'S (p 873) discovery of 1895, strongly influenced the application of orthopedic treatment, both surgical and non-surgical. However, general availability of radiology for orthopedics did not occur until after World War I.

Organizations of societies of orthopedic surgeons, in the developed countries, began at about the turn of the century (American Orthopedic Association 1887, British Orthopaedic Association 1898). Along with other medical specialties, these reflect the changes in practice as well as in relationships between government and medical services to the people and have differed considerably in the different countries. They are now often integral in the planning and implementation of training programs, monitoring of training, certification of specialty status, and even delineation of what constitutes good practice. As circumstances change in different countries — for example, the development of the National Health Service in Britain, or the advent of managed care and health maintenance organizations in the United States of America — changes occurred inevitably in the character of orthopedic practice.

Another change, most evident in the United States of America but now extending to all the developed countries, is what might be called 'ultra-specialization'. There are now groups of pediatric orthopedic surgeons (with their own societies and periodicals), hand surgeons, spine surgeons, etc. Most numerous among the ultra-specialists are the sports medicine men, who serve not only as orthopedists treating athletes with sports injuries, but also as counselors on training for fitness-minded individuals and for teams ranging from the professionals to elementary school students.

The treatment of fractures of the upper end of the femur provides an illustration of the changes in the practice of orthopedic surgery. At the end of the 19th century, the diagnosis would be made by a history of injury and the physical findings of a rotational deformity and marked limitation of hip motion (by pain). X-rays might be taken (rarely, and only in the few centers where facilities existed). The patient would then be hospitalized and the leg splinted or placed in traction. Several splints were popular, as were traction devices. Only a handful of surgeons in the world might attempt open reduction of the fracture fragments, and each might try to apply a nail (of various compositions — ordinary steel, or aluminum, or a bone peg usually derived from beef) to immobilize the fracture fragments. They would justify this procedure on the likelihood that the patient had little chance of recovering an ability to walk, would be bedridden for months, and finally die.

Only when X-rays became readily available was it recognized that fractures could differ one from the next from the anatomical (mechanical) standpoint, leading to differences in what would be needed, particularly for fixation of the fracture fragments. A two-fragment fracture through the middle of the neck of the femur might require the use of one, two, or three nails or pins (or bone pegs). A three-fragment fracture, or a comminuted fracture, would necessitate the use of a more complex device, perhaps including a plate fixed to several inches of the femoral shaft.

X-rays also showed at least one element in the fracture that might so increase the risk of failure of fixation treatment as to make any surgical procedure ill advised. It was well known, at the end of the 19th century from post-mortem studies, that a

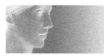
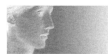
fracture of the femoral neck close to the hip joint often resulted in death (necrosis) of the proximal bony fragment. This fact, during more recent times, has led to a major change in the rationale of treatment for such cases.

By the end of World War I there was a distinct change in how fractures of the upper end of the femur were treated. Many army surgeons were experienced in diagnosing and treating fractures, and schools were formed to train military surgeons in handling injuries. Also, among the military related researches, the discovery of formulas for stainless steel proved important in devising devices for implantation. These special steels were much less irritating than were the earlier substances, and ways were found for fixation of femoral fractures, using hardware devised for any mechanical situation which might arise, with little fear that tissue intolerance to the implanted fixation device would constitute a contraindication to surgical treatment.

## X-ray screening

Another technological development was an X-ray fluorescent screening device, with which the surgeon, during the operation, could see what he was doing, instead of having to take repeated intraoperational radiographs. Radiographs were not only extremely inconvenient in a surgical theater, with the need for asepsis, repositioning of the patient and of the film cassettes, but also the added minutes of operating time for developing the radiographs.

Likewise, there was an appreciable increase in doctors experienced in caring for injured patients after World War II. Upon returning to civilian life many became orthopedic surgeons. The war also stimulated much research and was responsible for further developments in metallurgy. The implanted metallic devices thereafter included two new alloys, one based on titanium and the other on cobalt, both of which would show improved tolerance by tissues.

A noteworthy discovery was made in 1962 by Sir John CHARNLEY (p 601), who found that he could replace a damaged hip joint with a polyethylene socket on which a stainless steel ball articulated. To fix the two components firmly in the pelvis and femur, he used a polymer, methyl methacrylate, which acted as a grout, polymerized *in situ*. There had been numerous attempts previously at 'total replacement arthroplasty' (with metal components), or even hemiarthroplasty (replacing just the femoral head or just its articulating surface), but at best those attempts yielded limited success. Charnley's discovery could be applied to fractures of the upper end of the femur, particularly in the elderly, and also when the fractures had characteristics adverse to healing

(callus formation) by the traditional treatment (reduction, fixation, and immobilization). Total hip replacement (for acute fractures or their sequels and other affections of the joint) has now become so common an operation that it often is listed as the most frequent in many hospitals, even outnumbering appendectomies. Its success has led orthopedic surgeons to attempt similar replacement arthroplasty for other joints — knees, fingers, shoulders, and so on.

Charnley's success also encouraged a multitude of research efforts, such as improvements in the design of the implant, and alterations in its surface (making it porous, so that the methyl methacrylate, which occasionally deteriorated or fractured, would not be needed). The surgeon about to perform a total replacement of the hip now has numerous options — many designs of femoral implants made of different metals (a special stainless steel, or a cobalt chromium alloy, or titanium, or even ceramic). He may decide to fix the two articulating components with methyl methacrylate to allow the patient to be up and about after a minimal stay in the hospital — a week or two. Eliminating the methyl methacrylate by making the metal surface porous brings with it the disadvantage of limited loading while the callus grows into the pores — a matter of months with the patient using crutches.

## Computerized tomography

Two other important developments should be mentioned: one is computerized tomography, in which the doctor uses X-rays, aided by a device to obtain images of thin slices of tissue; those images are then computerized to yield a three-dimensional representation. The other, magnetic resonance imaging, is the use of high energy magnets to activate specific ions in the tissues. The release of the applied energy then can portray the physical properties of the tissues. Each of these techniques now is indispensable in diagnosis (of fractures of all sorts, and of other orthopedic conditions), planning, and treatment.

Advances in other specialties have also had important influences on orthopedic practice. In the operating theater, the anesthesiologists now have an array of machines with which they monitor continually many of the patient's physical signs (blood pressure, electrocardiograph, body temperature) and also chemical data (serum carbon dioxide, pH, blood hemoglobin, etc.) so that they can detect, quickly and early, most complicating abnormalities indicative of trouble and can institute counter-measures. Besides the avoidance of serious intraoperative mishaps such as anemia or shock through blood loss, these anesthesia-related advances have allowed operations to be prolonged, often for hours, so that the traditional premium on speed no longer applies. Operations requiring hours-long manipulations (for example, microsurgery, massive reconstructions) can now be carried out routinely.

Another new influence is the collaborative handling of conditions which were formerly managed by general physicians practicing solo. An example is cancer, in which patients are usually under the care of general physicians or oncologists. If such cancers spread to the bones by metastasis, orthopedic surgeons may relieve pain or restore the patient's mobility by resorting to surgical measures. Orthopedic surgeons are likewise frequently asked to help manage patients with back pain, a major diagnostic and therapeutic concern with important industrial and economic implications. The range of lesions that affect the back includes arthritis, gout, and other conditions, but it also includes prolapsed intervertebral disc, spinal stenosis, and even ordinary, common ligamentous sprains; the symptom that all of these may have in common is backache. That symptom also characterizes many non-orthopedic lesions involving one organ or another, or, perhaps, in psychosomatic cases, no organ at all. Given the very high prevalence, the many possible etiological lesions, the inordinate number of diagnostic tests that may be required, and the different types of treatment to go with each distinctive lesion, the cause of many backaches cannot be diagnosed, and in such patients the treatment prescribed by the orthopedic surgeon along standard principles, based on anatomical and biomechanical considerations, may be ineffective.

Painful feet, while not the major socioeconomic problem that backache represents (that is, not a frequent cause for loss of work days, or compensation because of work-related injury), nevertheless have many causes and often are the symptom that drives the patient to the orthopedic surgeon. The conditions requiring treatment include the common (and minor) lesions such as bunions, hammertoes, ingrown toenails, and the life-threatening — for example, gangrene of the toes in an elderly (arteriosclerotic) or diabetic individual.

Fractures, however, constitute probably the largest fraction of many orthopedists' practice. The mounting numbers of individuals injured in vehicular accidents (as well as sports, such as skiing or football) have brought in train a massive refinement in the characterization of fractures. Hence a detailed treatise on all fractures, written in 1950, might be a 500-page book, but today would require five such volumes.

The scope of orthopedic surgery ranges from simple procedures to complex ones. 'Simple' pro-cedures need not be technologically simple, even if they are conceptually simple. For instance, an amputation of part of a leg injured in an accident, and deemed to be beyond repair, might, as an emergency, be treated as in centuries past, by tying off major blood vessels and removing all tissues beyond the ligatures. An orthopedic surgeon today would consider how best to salvage the involved tissues (bone, muscle, and skin) so as to maximize the function of the residual part of the leg. If the injury is at a level which demands the use of a prosthesis for walking, the surgeon must consider how the patient's weight is to be borne, that is, how best to tailor the skin and soft tissue covering to avoid pressure sores where the prosthesis will rub or press. Thus, the emergency measures serve best as a prelude to medical measures aimed at restoring maximal function in the shortest time possible. Often those two variables — functional restoration and economy of time needed — are somewhat at odds. Hence a surgeon might choose to do the amputation at a level to aim for quick healing of the stump, and fitting of a prosthesis within a week or two. In contrast, the salvage of a longer fraction of the leg (perhaps retraining the knee joint) might mean months of treatment and repeated procedures, but ultimately a vastly superior limb. One even might envisage the insertion of an artificial knee joint.

A complex procedure most often is a 'customized' regimen aimed at restoring maximum function to the arm or the leg or to the spine. The regimen usually includes only one operation, which in itself may be complex (for example, implantation of a large bone graft to replace a massive tumor of bone, or a delicate reconstruction of tendons, nerves, and blood vessels, each being sutured microsurgically).

Finally, some developments affect not only the surgical process, but also other aspects of orthopedic practice — antibiotics to cure or prevent infections; steroids to combat immunological mishaps; chemical approaches to alleviate disturbances in mineral or enzymatic metabolism (osteoporosis or Gaucher's disease, for example); and the several hematological advances (control of postoperative or genetic abnormalities in clotting).

Where complexity exists, the regimen usually is a team effort and also involves physical therapists, occupational therapists, and occasionally others, such as, prosthetists. The widening application of orthopedic treatment also has necessitated collaborative approaches to patients whose disease would not involve the orthopedic surgeon primarily, such as those with deformities caused by rheumatoid arthritis, under the primary care of rheumatologists (or internists, or general practitioners). Another example might be the hematol-

(continued)

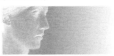

John **CHARNLEY** (1911–82). English surgeon. He worked in the orthopedic department at Manchester Royal Infirmary for some years before going to Wrightington Hospital to develop the Centre for Hip Surgery. Although best known for his pioneering contributions to operations for replacement of the hip joint, Charnley had already contributed notably to orthopedic surgery in his work on compression arthrodesis, and with his book on *The closed treatment of common fractures* (1950). For his work on hip replacement, he supplemented his surgical skill by meticulous studies on engineering, on materials science, and on the control of infection during surgical operation. He received a knighthood.

ogists caring for hemophiliac patients, whose recurring hemorrhages into joints often destroy them. Hence, the role of urban centers in treatment is increasing, given that teams of specialists can administer programs impossible for solo practitioners in rural settings.                    JCoh

*See also* ARTHROSCOPY; IMAGING; RHEUMATOLOGY; SPECIALIZATION; SPORTS TRAUMA

William **OSLER** (1849–1919). Canadian physician. Born in Ontario, the son of a clergyman who had emigrated from Falmouth, Cornwall, Osler began his medical training at Toronto, moving to Montreal, where he graduated at MCGILL (p 139) in 1872. After touring the European medical centers for two years he returned to Canada as professor of the Institutes of Medicine in McGill University, becoming physician to the Montreal General Hospital in 1878. His reputation grew so rapidly that after six years he was invited to take the chair of medicine in the University of Pennsylvania and five years later to become the foundation professor and physician at the JOHNS HOPKINS University Hospital (p 840) at Baltimore.

During his 15 years in this post he influenced medical teaching throughout the USA, combining the bed-side methods of the English school with the laboratory associations of the German. Here to he wrote his work *The principles and practices of medicine* (1892), which is now in its 20th edition and has been the model for all later TEXTBOOKS.

In 1904, he moved to the more peaceful atmosphere of the Regius chair of medicine at Oxford, where his antiquarian and literary tastes had leisure in which to develop. His success was no less than it had been in the USA. He expanded the preclinical departments at Oxford and helped to overcome the university's traditional suspicions of 'the sciences'. He was largely responsible for founding the Association of Physicians of Great Britain and Ireland and the *Quarterly Journal of Medicine*. He received a knighthood.

At the time of his death the *Lancet* obituary described him as 'the greatest personality in the medical world'. His influence upon the teaching and practice of medicine in the USA and elsewhere is incalculable, but he was also an outstanding clinical observer. He was among the first to study the platelets (1874), to describe hereditary hemorrhagic telangiectasia (Osler-Rendu-Weber disease, 1901), polycythemia vera (Vaquez-Osler's disease, 1903), and infective endocarditis (Osler's nodes, 1909). His biography was written by Harvey CUSHING (p 537).

**OSTEOARTHRITIS** See RHEUMATOLOGY

**OSTEOPATHY** — from the Greek *osteo* (bone) and *pathos* (disease) — is the system of medicine concerned with the diagnosis and manipulative treatment of structural problems within the musculoskeletal system. Its premises are that the structure and function of the human body are reciprocally and mutually interdependent; that any mechanical restriction may directly affect the organs and systems related to that area; and that when the mechanical structure of the body is normalized or improved, function will also improve. Osteopathy originated in the United States in the last quarter of the 19th century as a result of the work of Dr Andrew Taylor Still, who founded the first College of Osteopathy in Kirksville, Missouri, in 1892. Many USA colleges of osteopathy now offer a 4-year curriculum resembling a conventional medical course but emphasizing massage and physical treatment rather than pharmacology and therapeutics.

Osteopaths in Britain are now statutorily registered and undergo a 3–4 year full-time training program at registered colleges of higher education. Osteopaths in the USA possess an equivalent qualification to medically registered doctors. Though practicing conventional medicine, they do emphasize the 'laying on of hands' in diagnosis and treatment.                    GL

*See also* COMPLEMENTARY AND ALTERNATIVE MEDICINE

**OSTEOPOROSIS** See RHEUMATOLOGY

**OTORHINOLARYNGOLOGY** See ENT

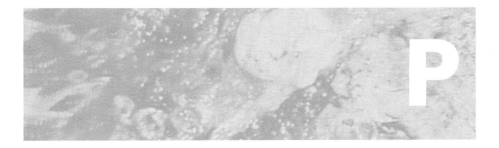

**PADUA, UNIVERSITY OF** See ITALY

Sir James **PAGET** (1814–99). British surgeon. Born in Great Yarmouth, the eighth of 17 children, Paget was apprenticed to a local surgeon, Charles Costerton, at age 16 and in 1834 he enrolled at St Bartholomew's Hospital, London. He was admitted as a member of the Royal College of surgeons in 1836, but, unable to afford the fees for surgical pupillage, he never served as a house surgeon. Instead, he supported himself by teaching, writing, and editing. In 1837 he was appointed curator of St Bartholomew's Hospital's pathological museum, and lecturer in anatomy and physiology in 1843. The same year he also became one of the original fellows of the Royal College of Surgeons, and warden of the residential college for students at St Bartholomew's. Despite having been neither a surgical pupil nor house surgeon, Paget was elected assistant surgeon in 1846, and in 1861 he became full surgeon. He retired from St Bartholomew's in 1871 after a serious illness, but nevertheless was elected president of the Royal College of Surgeons in 1875, and vice-chancellor of the University of London in 1883. Since 1858 he had been surgeon-extraordinary to the Queen and the Prince of Wales, and received a knighthood.

**PAIN** is an unpleasant sensory and emotional experience associated with actual or potential tissue damage or may be described in terms of tissue damage. Pain is the prerogative of humans because they perceive pain, whereas animals respond to a noxious stimulus (nociception). This basic difference was reinforced by PAVLOV (p 729) in the early part of the 20th century, when he gave dogs electric shocks before he fed them. Initially this produced a painful response, withdrawal, and vocalization, but with time the painful response was replaced by a joyful response — salivation. Thus he proved that in dogs the response to a noxious stimulus could be changed from nociception to pleasure. This difference between pain and nociception has important connotations when research in animals is extrapolated to man. Pain and nociception are not the same: they are related but not necessarily directly.

The basis of research into pain had been the relationship between the stimulus and the response, not the perception of pain. However, in only one of the three different types of pain — operative, acute, and chronic — is this relationship direct. The patient's response to surgery, a noxious stimulus, is followed by a response in an almost graded fashion. As most, if not all, surgery is performed under general ANESTHESIA (therefore the patient's response to the noxious stimulus is assessed by the anesthetist who infers that the patient is or is not feeling pain), this situation is also nociception. During surgery there is progressive damage and the pain provides some protection.

The second type of pain is acute. A good example is the pain associated with a broken limb, made worse by movement but not necessarily relieved by rest. Movement-associated pain is protective in that the fracture may heal more quickly and effectively if the limb is rested. In this instance, the stimulus is related to the response. However, another pain is associated with the fracture: a dull aching pain which is not associated with any external stimulus but must be related to the trauma itself. It is difficult to see a protective function for this pain, apart from reminding the patient of the injury. Postoperative pain is similar.

Chronic pain is the third type in which there is no relation between the stimulus and the response. For example, there is no correlation between the pain of arthritis and the degree of arthritis found on radiographs. Chronic pain provides no protective function for humans. Acute pain provides some advantages, whereas chronic pain seems to provide only disadvantages and may be a random error in the system.

There are numerous variations of each of these themes, and there are also theories that encompass elements of both. The Gate theory of pain is a pattern theory which has stood the test of time. This states that the perception of pain could be modified at the first junction — the spinal cord; modification of the pain was a result of all the information available from within and outside the patient. It was the first theory that included chronic pain as part of its basis. Interestingly it

## THEORIES OF PAIN

There are two theories of pain perception:

- specific theory: pain is a specific sensation with specific receptors (nociceptors), that is transmitted along specific neural pathways to specific areas of the brain.
- pattern theory: pain is perceived as a result of all the information available to the brain at that time. Thus most if not all receptors can transmit pain and there are no specific neural pain pathways within the central nervous system.

was proposed by a psychologist and an anatomist/physiologist, thus highlighting the importance of the two elements of pain — physical and emotional. This theory has been shown to be correct in that both pain and nociception can be modified at the first junction of the spinal cord (Fig. 1).

### Acute pain

The most common acute pain is that after surgery (postoperative pain). Most acute pain resolves with time as part of natural healing. There is no evidence that treating the pain has any effect on its duration. Thus the treatment of acute pain is of the symptom while the body's 'healing' process resolves the underlying cause — the surgery. Usually there are two different types of postoperative pain: the dull ache present all the time and pain related to movement. With the dull ache there is no obvious relation between the stimulus and the response; it is presumably related to the local trauma of the operation, whereas with the second type there is an obvious stimulus. A wealth of evidence supports the importance of early mobilization after surgery and so there is a need for pain control to enable this. Dull aching pain lasts longer than movement pain. There is a third type of pain, which uncommonly follows any trauma, that is, neurogenic pain. It is related to nerve damage, and may not be relieved by conventional analgesia; hence this pain may persist and become chronic.

Roughly one third of patients do not require postoperative analgesia irrespective of the operation. The explanation for this observation is

unknown; at one end of the spectrum patients may have no pain and at the other do not wish to have any treatment for it. The latter expect to have pain postoperatively and prefer it to the possible complications of therapy. Most patients are in the middle of this spectrum, with varying combinations of these attitudes.

*Movement pain* Physical methods, such as acupuncture and electrical stimulation, are not very effective for treating this type of pain. However, in a small group of patients these techniques are effective. The usual method of dealing with pain is pharmacological, the most common drugs used being the opiates (narcotics). Morphine, the standard for such drugs, is usually given as an injections, either intermittent or continuous. Intermittent intramuscular injection is the most common technique in hospitals, but there has been a tendency towards continuous infusions of morphine or similar drugs usually given intravenously and, most commonly, via patient controlled analgesia machines. These circumvent most of the disadvantages of intermittent injections and give individual patients control over their pain and pain relief. Most patients do not give themselves complete relief: they titrate themselves to an acceptable level of pain which is different for each patient.

Patient-controlled analgesia aims to maintain a steady blood concentration of the opiate to provide background analgesia and then when the patient is about to move, or when the pain increases, the patient administers a boost of the drug to prevent or control the pain. It is generally very effective, but because there are so many variables (including the patient, the operation, the pain, and the drug used), it is not totally effective in all patients. Patients controlling their analgesia are more satisfied with their pain relief than those using conventional, as required, dosing of the same opiates. Most large hospitals commonly have a pain control team to supervise the use of patient-controlled analgesia machines, comprising at least a doctor and a nurse. The doctor's role is to control the prescription of the drug and to liaise with other medical staff, while the nurse ensures that patients and machines are being monitored effectively and liaises with the nurses on the wards.

It is possible to use injections of local anesthetics around the appropriate nerves to provide analgesia for movement pain or a catheter may be placed near the nerve to provide continuous blockade. This provides good pain relief but has the disadvantage of numbness and weakness in the distribution of that nerve. In theory it is possible to block any nerve to provide pain relief but it is unusual for the pain after surgery to be limited

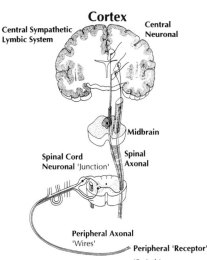

Fig. 1 The areas where the physical components of pain may be interrupted, which may be at the receptors (switch), axonal (wires), or neuronal (junctions). The emotional components of a patient's pain may be modified in the brain but the precise area or areas remain to be defined.

**Cortex**

Central Sympathetic Lymbic System

Central Neuronal

Midbrain

Spinal Cord Neuronal 'Junction'

Spinal Axonal

Peripheral Axonal 'Wires'

Peripheral 'Receptor'

'Switch'

to the distribution of one nerve. Hence the most common technique used for postoperative pain is epidural catheterization. Most of the nerves pass from the spinal cord via the epidural space to supply various parts of the body and so local anesthetics can be placed in the space to block them. Epidural catheterization is most commonly used in childbirth. Two significant improvements in this technique are the use of epidural opiates in conjunction with the local anesthetic and the use of constant infusions of local anesthetic and opiates, sometimes with patient-controlled analgesia machines.

### Therapy

The two components of pain, physical and emotional, are always present, but both do not always need treatment. Pure physical pain probably does not exist (Fig. 2) because there is always an emotional component. Similarly, pure psychogenic pain probably does not exist because there is always a physical component (albeit very small).

There are four basic mood dimensions — *arousal* (how alert or drowsy the patient is), *anxiety* (how relaxed or tense the patient is), *depression* (how happy or unhappy the patient is), and *aggression* (how angry or comfortable the patient feels towards others). All these mood factors have an unpleasant component which is therefore painful and so will need treatment.

The physical component always requires treatment because patients believe that there is a physical basis for their pain and they are correct. However, the physical component may not be the major element. The art of treatment is to identify which is the more important element and then to design treatment to deal mainly with it while also treating the other components. There are four strategies for dealing with the physical component of a patient's pain: physical, for example, electrical stimulation; pharmacological; injections; and surgery. There are three strategies for dealing with the emotional component of pain: reassurance, pharmacological, and professional counseling.

All therapies have potential side-effects and therefore all decisions on therapy should be based on a risk–benefit ratio.

### Operative pain

Most patients commonly require general or local anesthesia to prevent operative pain. However, simple operations have been performed using electrical stimulation, acupuncture, or a strong magnetic field. Electrical stimulation, acupuncture, and magnetic fields are somehow related to physical therapy; general anesthesia is based on the use of drugs; and local anesthesia requires

injections. There are no operations which provide analgesia for surgery. Some patients can use self-hypnosis to control their pain during surgery and in susceptible patients operations may be performed under HYPNOSIS.

General anesthesia is believed to have its effects on the neuronal synapse (junctions), whereas local anesthesia has its effect on the axons. Under general anesthesia the patient's physiological responses to the stimulus are assessed. The anesthetist infers from these responses that the patient is or is not feeling pain and takes action. The mechanisms underlying general anesthesia have not been defined. It is at least one stage deeper than SLEEP and we do not yet fully understand sleep. Most probably general anesthetics have their effect throughout the central nervous system, probably via a non-specific (global) effect on synaptic transmission. Electrical stimulation presumably has its effect via the axons, and the magnetic field via the central nervous system (being analogous to general anesthetics). Acupuncture possibly has its analgesic effect via a similar mechanism to that underlying hypnosis. It is not understood how self-hypnosis and hypnosis provide analgesia but it is probably at a cortical level (Fig. 1).

The emotional component of operative pain is awareness (arousal).

Movement-related pain generally resolves within the first 48 hours of surgery and so the patient is left with the aching type pain, which also resolves with time.

*Aching pain* This pain is generally relieved by orally administered drugs. The two main groups used are opiates and non-steroidal anti-inflammatory drugs. The physical therapies such as acupuncture and transcutaneous electrical nerve stimulation may also be effective.

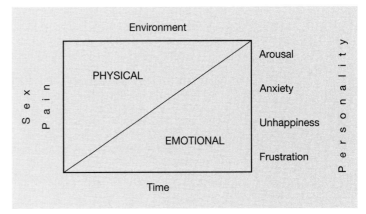

**Fig. 2** The two components of pain, physical and emotional (the patient's response to the pain), as well as the other factors which affect the patient's perception of pain.

*Neurogenic pain* This pain may be relieved by transcutaneous electrical stimulation and acupuncture. It may respond to unconventional analgesics, such as antidepressants, and anticonvulsants. It does resolve with time, but the sooner the patient is given a clear explanation of the cause of the pain and provided with effective therapy, the sooner it will resolve.

There are surgical procedures for specific acute pains, for example, the removal of a lumbar disc pressing on a nerve root and causing pain in the leg.

The unpleasant emotional component of acute pain is the patient's anxiety and unhappiness about its connotations, and they should be informed of the possible causes and their meaning. Patients may need pharmacological treatment or counseling to help them cope with the information, although generally they respond to reassurance.

## Chronic pain

Chronic pain is pain which has persisted for at least a month despite all conventional treatment and investigation. Chronic pain may be acute pain which persists despite appropriate treatment. The pain may persist because the patient is intolerant of the correct treatment or does not wish to partake in it. The treatment prescribed for patients with chronic pain is symptomatic, as carried out at pain clinics — groups of health professionals who specialize in treating patients with chronic pain symptomatically.

## Treatment

Transcutaneous electrical nerve stimulation provides adequate analgesia in a third of the patients in whom it is used. Acupuncture is effective for chronic pain. All injections, be they acupuncture, PLACEBO, or active drugs can produce long-term pain relief. Unfortunately, it is not possible to predict in whom these techniques will provide analgesia. It is worthwhile trying the conventional analgesics, but some patients are insensitive or intolerant to these. The unconventional analgesics, antidepressants and anticonvulsants, are commonly effective in chronic pain. Anticonvulsants have been used effectively to treat trigeminal neuralgia for 30 years because conventional analgesics were ineffective. Many other types of pain respond to these drugs, either individually or in combination.

Axonal blockade involves the injection of local anesthetics to abolish the pain, albeit briefly, in those patients who are made numb. If patients do not achieve analgesia while they are numb, the pain cannot be coming from where the patient is feeling it. Thus axonal blockade is diagnostic, and occasionally it is also therapeutic in that the pain does not return when the effect of the local anesthetic wears off. In those patients who do not have pain relief while numb it is possible to stop their pain with the injection of drugs, such as morphine, around the spinal cord — neuronal blockade. Catheters may be implanted around the spinal cord to provide a continuous infusion for long-term pain relief. The present technology may not be good enough to recommend its routine use in non-malignant pain. Nevertheless, these systems will improve. The most complete form of neural blockade is general anesthesia, but this is inappropriate for patients with chronic pain. Operative procedures for the relief of chronic pain are time limited because the nervous system is designed to overcome interference such as destructive procedures. Therefore these procedures should be reserved for patients with limited longevity. Unfortunately even in these patients the success rate of surgery for chronic pain is not 100%, at best, 80–90%.

A clear explanation of the emotional component of chronic pain may be enough to enable some patients to cope with this aspect. It is normal to be chronically anxious, unhappy, and frustrated by the pain (Fig. 2). The decision in an individual patient whether the emotional components need specific treatment should be discussed with that patient. Drug therapy for this revolves around the use of antidepressants, which should help the anxiety and the unhappiness. There are no drugs for frustration, the only treatment being professional counseling, which is also an option for the anxiety and unhappiness. The object of this is to enable the patient to cope with the pain and the problems it creates. It is not designed to relieve the pain *per se*.

## The future

Operative pain can be relieved in all patients. Adequate pain relief can be provided for most patients with acute pain, remembering that patients with acute pain do not wish to be totally pain free. Effective short-term pain relief is achievable for most patients with chronic pain; long-term relief awaits technological advances. With increasing knowledge the medical profession will improve its ability to treat patients with pain more effectively.                    CJG

**PAKISTAN** is a country of 130 million people situated in the north-western part of the Indian subcontinent. Although it emerged as a political entity in 1947, this region has been a cradle of some of the most vibrant and progressive of civilizations in the past. The ruins at Mohenjodaro (*c.* 3000 BC) show extraordinary skills of town planning, public health engineering, and waste disposal. The streets are paved with bricks, with covered drains on the sides. Manholes have been provided for cleaning. The houses have bathrooms with wells and latrines. There are clay pipes to carry wastewater. Such elaborate arrangements reveal the concern of the Indus Valley people about water supply, hygiene, and sewage disposal. Ironically, many people in Larkana, the modern town near the ruins, do not have the facilities that the residents of Mohenjodaro enjoyed 5000 years ago.

The Aryans started colonizing this area in the second millennium BC. It was here that their civilization first developed. Panini, who formulated grammar for Sanskrit, was born here and so according to one tradition was Kautliya, the author of Arth Shaster. By the 6th century BC, Taxila had developed into a great center of learning, attracting students from far and wide. One such student, Jivaka Kumarabhytia, came all the way from Magdh, in Eastern India, to learn from the famous medical teacher Atreya. His training lasted seven years, and included the science of removal of disease from the skull through surgery. Another Atreya disciple, Charaka, was author of a famous medical text, and his sermon to physicians who complete their training remains valid even today.

The Ayurvedic system of medicine developed in various centers in the subcontinent has survived to this day. It is based on the concept of balance of HUMORS maintaining health; although it is no longer commonly practiced in Pakistan, such ideas of humors, hot and cold effects of food, and vital points in the body are firmly rooted in popular perception and indigenous medicine.

Emperor Ashoka (269–232 BC) undertook to provide health services not only for the people but also for animals. His edict carved on a rock has been discovered in Shahbaz Garhi. This concept of state responsibility for healthcare has survived over the centuries, and attempts to levy user charges in the government-run institutions generate more resentment than funds.

The ancient Gandhara, the present-day northwestern Pakistan, was a meeting place of the East and the West. It has been claimed, perhaps with some justification, that Hellenic medicine borrowed from the advanced system of medicine developed there. This belief is based on similarities between the two systems and the probability that the development of medicine in the subcontinent antedated that in Greece. It is, however, difficult to judge who borrowed from whom, and perhaps safer to conclude that all benefited from those exchanges.

There were other occasions when medical skills and knowledge were transferred abroad. After the Arab conquest of Sindh in the 8th century, many local scholars went to Baghdad to join others who were engaged in collecting, processing, and disseminating medical and other knowledge. They commanded considerable respect at the Abbasid court and in medical circles, translating many of the medical treatises such as Sushruta and Charaka's samhitas into Arabic. Maneka was an expert toxicologist and the author of a book on poisons called *Kitab ul Samoom* or book of poisons. Dhashtak worked as a physician at the famous Jandi Shapur hospital. Salah bin Bahla Hindi was appointed royal physician to Caliph Haroonul Rashid and was considered very close to him. The Unani system developed as a result of interaction among subcontinental Greek, Persian, and Arabic medicine, being introduced into the subcontinent with the Muslim conquest in the 11th century. Its name refers to its Hellenic roots.

Muslim rule saw well-organized medical services provided for the population. The hospitals had different specialists including eye specialists; many of the prominent physicians had been trained abroad and were attracted by better opportunities in the Muslim Empire. They were well rewarded and many rose to occupy high government offices. In later periods, many European physicians also enjoyed this patronage. William Hamilton, at the court from 1711–1714, successfully treated King Farukh Siyar. He was offered an elephant, a horse, two diamond rings, five thousand rupees, a jewelled aigrette, a set of gold buttons, and models of all his instruments in gold. He also obtained important trade concessions for the East India Company.

Medical knowledge made steady progress, with attempts to incorporate local drugs and remedies into the Unani system. Many books were written drawing upon the information available from local literature. One by Bhawa bin Khawas Khan, completed in 1512–13, reviewed the ancient medical literature of the subcontinent and employed local terminology to make it more useful. One chapter was devoted to military surgery.

Many kings such as the Tughlaqs were themselves interested in medicine. Emperor Akbar (1542–1605 AD) ordered experiments to be conducted on tobacco to see if it was of any use. His court physician recommended that the smoke should be made to pass through water to dissipate its toxic effects. His son Emperor Jehangir was also a keen observer, recording in his diary the relationship of plague with rats and rabies with animal bites.

### British rule

The British ruled the subcontinent from about the middle of the 19th century. They can be credited with introducing the modern medical system, with its network of hospitals and teaching institutions. A medical school was started in Lahore in 1860, and admitted 49 students in the first class, with the first to pass the subassistant surgeon examination being in 1865. The first woman student was admitted in 1883. The school was renamed the King Edward Medical College in 1912 and has had an important role in training generations of students, as well as providing the teachers who were to start other medical institutions in the country.

Not surprisingly, the initial and major concern of the British was to keep their troops in good fighting order in the hostile and disease-prone environment of the subcontinent. They were provided with better facilities than the civilian population, trained nurses being first posted to the military hospital at Rawalpindi in 1883. The first ever use of Roentgen rays in the field was in the Tirah campaign in 1898. Even now this region is very remote and inaccessible, and the troubles which the medical officer had in transporting his delicate equipment can be imagined.

In the initial years soldiers lived under terrible conditions. Florence NIGHTINGALE (p 548), who herself never visited the region, started a relentless campaign to improve their lot. A commission set up in 1859 to study the problems issued a comprehensive 2000-page report, and the death rate declined substantially after the implementation of its recommendations. The value of good sanitation and hygiene could not have been better demonstrated. The lessons learnt in the army were applied by the Indian Medical Service doctors to civilian problems. Established in 1896, this élite service played a vital part in setting up the medical services in the country.

When the British left in 1947, British India was divided into India and Pakistan, with great upheavals at the time of independence. The results were profound for the practice of medicine in Pakistan; in particular, medical resources, which were inadequate to begin with, were appreciably depleted because of the emigration of non-Muslim doctors and medical staff to India. The challenge to rebuild the medical infrastructure was great. A lack of material and human resources together with rising expectations of the people compounded the problem. It was further complicated by friction with India, with Pakistan having to fight three wars over the disputed region of Kashmir and over its former eastern half. The limited available resources had to be diverted towards defence, and as a consequence improvements in social welfare and health projects suffered.

In 1947 Pakistan had only two barely functioning medical colleges. To increase the supply of doctors, four new medical colleges were established in various parts of the country. Many of these doctors went to Britain, North America, and the Middle East. In an effort to increase the training of doctors even further, six new medical colleges were started in 1974, and the number of student vacancies was increased in the existing medical colleges. This led to a great fall in educational standards, at least initially, while a serious effort was made to provide for the absorption of the newly qualified graduates. The third phase in the provision of doctors and allied staff began when non-governmental organizations arrived. The Aga Khan university was established in 1985, and two more medical schools in Karachi and five more colleges in the rest of the country followed. Unlike public institutions that are heavily subsidized, such private colleges charge very heavy tuition fees, but their academic standards vary.

Significantly, two of the medical colleges are exclusively devoted to women students, and women now constitute a substantial proportion of students in other medical colleges as well. This not only reflects the concern for the lot of women, but is also due to the conservative nature and orthodox religious views of the people. Pakistan is still a male-dominated society, where in general women lead secluded lives and have less access to health facilities.

A further problem some decades ago was that the facilities for postgraduate training were even more limited. Although the universities granted diplomas after one year's training, most doctors preferred to go abroad, especially to Britain, for specialization, as there was also a great shortage of teachers in the newly established medical colleges. An important initiative was taken by setting up the Basic Sciences Institute at the Jinnah Postgraduate Medical Center in Karachi in 1955. Established with the collaboration of University of Indiana, USA, this institute helped to train many medical teachers, and in 1962 the College of Physicians and Surgeons of Pakistan was entrusted with the task of organizing and supervising postgraduate education.

Health policy has evolved mainly through the five-year planning process, with the main emphasis being on increasing the number of medical colleges, doctors, and hospital beds. The costly curative side was thus emphasized, while the primary and preventive services remained neglected. In the 1970s and '80s greater attention was paid to the basic rural health services, where the vast majority of people live, though doctors remained reluctant to work in these areas because of the lack of amenities.

Pakistan today is a country with a rich potential but poor in material resources. Its per capita income is only about 420 $ US. The bulk of the population subsists on agriculture, living in rural

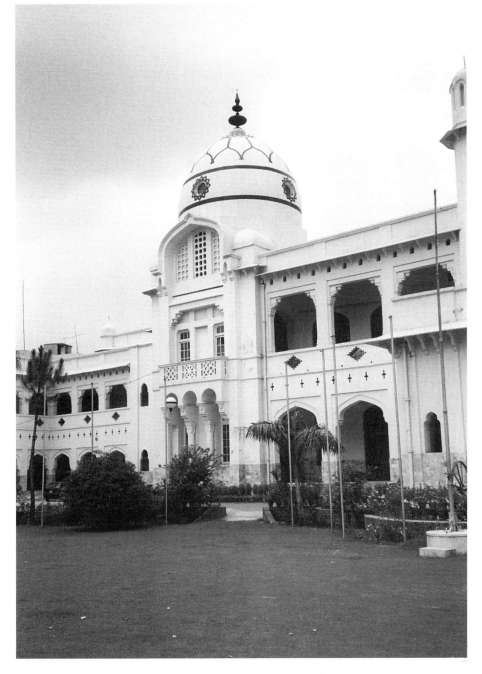

The King Edward Medical College, Lahore.

areas where the facilities are few: electricity is not available to 56%, safe drinking water to 49%, and proper sanitation to 84%. There is a highly inequitable system of land ownership; despite attempts at land reforms, most farmers remain tenants working for feudal and absentee landlords. The unemployment and poor living conditions in the rural areas have resulted in large-scale migra-

tion to the cities, further straining the already inadequate health and sanitation facilities

High fertility, high infant and maternal mortality, malnourishment in women and children, high incidence of infectious and communicable diseases, and low life expectancy characterize the health scene in Pakistan. The population has increased rapidly, having more than quadrupled in 50 years since independence, with children and the young comprising a large proportion. Nevertheless, with the implementation of the extended program of immunization and the use of oral rehydration salt therapy, childhood survival should increase, and hence the age structure of the population may change in future. The disease pattern due to increasing longevity is already changing, with heart disease, DIABETES, and cancer emerging as major problems. Although CHOLERA, PLAGUE, and other epidemics no longer occur, the classic conditions of MALARIA, TUBERCULOSIS, respiratory infections, intestinal infections, and hepatitis continue to cause concern. AIDS mercifully has not emerged as a problem so far. There is one doctor for 1880 persons, one nurse for 5810, and one hospital for 1538.

## Medical manpower and education

Medical education is controlled by three agencies. The government provides funds for public institutions and controls recruitment and employment of staff. The universities are responsible for conducting examinations and granting degrees. The Pakistan Medical and Dental Council is a statutory body which is responsible for licensing, and setting and enforcing standards.

There are currently 18 medical colleges and three medical universities, with several further private medical colleges being established. The number of doctors is more than can be absorbed in the public and private sector, though conversely nurses and paramedical staff are in short supply.

## Health delivery system

Pakistan is a federation comprising four provinces: Punjab, Sindh, Baluchistan, and NorthWest Frontier Province. According to the constitution, health and education come under the purview of the provinces. The federal government is responsible only for formulating national policies, coordination, laying down medical standards, and running a few postgraduate institutions and some special programs.

There is a basic health unit for every 10 000– 15 000 population, staffed by one physician and seven paramedics and providing both preventive and curative services. It is supported by secondary and tertiary facilities at the district and provincial level; the hospitals attached to the medical colleges offer specialized services. Treatment at the government hospitals is free, but it has become increasingly difficult to provide for it, given that health insurance does not exist for the general population. The private sector accounts for about 60% of expenditure on health. Urban based, it mostly provides curative services through outpatient clinics and a few hospitals, and is unable to affect the adverse health picture given that it cannot change the underlying poor environment, unsafe water supply, and parasitic and infectious diseases.

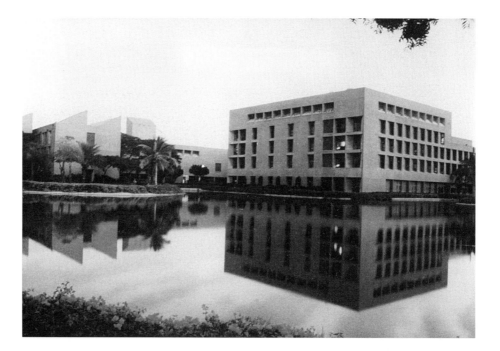

The Aga Khan University, Karachi.

A large segment of the population uses traditional or alternative systems of medicine because of their accessibility and low cost. About 36 000 registered tabibs practice Unani medicine, using herbal medicines.

Pakistan has come a long way since its independence over 50 years ago. The health delivery system, however, is still in a poor shape. Over 5000 years, the practice of medicine in Pakistan has seen many highs and lows. It is hoped that the progress since independence represents a trend towards emerging from the present low.    MA

**PALEOPATHOLOGY** is the study of disease in ancient human and animal remains. A less restricted view is to consider it as that part of medical history which deals specifically with the history of disease, and to use all the relevant information — documentary, pictorial, or pathological.

For many years, ancient human remains were treated as curiosities. Serious study did not begin until towards the end of the 19th century and the beginning of the 20th. After this time the subject became established as an academic discipline. Interest in paleopathology was stimulated by two factors: the push westwards in the USA which brought army surgeons into contact with Indian burial mounds; and the excavations in Nubia, which took place in advance of the raising of the Aswan Dam in 1909. Many hundreds of mummies and skeletons were examined in work associated with Grafton Elliot Smith and Frederick Wood Jones. In the early years, the greatest contribution was made by Sir Marc Armand Ruffer, who also worked in Egypt. Ruffer is often credited with having coined the term 'paleopathology' but he was anticipated by R. W. Schufeldt, writing in the *Popular Science Monthly*, an American magazine, in 1893.

In the 1930s and 1940s, paleopathology languished, but was revived in the 1950s in Europe and North America. In the past 20 years, the discipline has become much more rigorous, and epidemiological techniques are used, with more concentration on diseases in populations than on skeletons with interesting pathology, as was formerly the case.

Several problems beset paleopathologists. The most obvious is that they can deal mostly with only those diseases that affect the skeleton; this is a very small number of those in the International Classification of Disease (ICD) and includes few which cause death. Work with mummified remains offers at least the possibility of being able to examine soft tissues. The number of mummies available for study is small. To try to overcome this deficiency, an ambitious, multi-centered study of the prevalence of schistosomiasis has been set up and a reference tissue bank of mummified tissue is being established in Manchester.

The nature of the material available for study means that most paleopathologists must concentrate on the diseases which affect the skeleton, such as joint diseases, and osteoarthritis in particular. Osteoarthritis is abundant in any group of skeletons and some features of the disease have remained unchanged over thousands of years. It is closely age-related, rather more common in women than in men, and does not affect all joints equally. There are some interesting differences, however. Thus, osteoarthritis of the hip was more common than of the knee in the pre-medieval period, whereas the converse is true thereafter and probably osteoarthritis of the medial tibio-femoral joint is a very recent phenomenon. Likewise, in the early period, it was much more likely to affect only a single joint (or a single group of joints of the hand), whereas after about 1500, multifocal disease of the hand is much more common. In examining joints, paleopathologists enjoy one advantage over their clinical colleagues in being to examine all the joints of the body, and for this reason the distribution of affected joints may show some differences from what might be expected from clinic-based studies.

Erosive diseases of the joints are found in skeletons, but are uncommon and their diagnosis is problematical. Rheumatoid arthritis has been reported, but the number of recognizable cases conforming to modern clinical criteria is small. Claims for a high prevalence among some North American indigenous populations have not been accepted by all authorities and only a few cases have been reported in Britain. Some authentic cases have been reported in France in skeletons dating from the Roman period, which suggests that the disease is not 'modern', as has often been proposed.

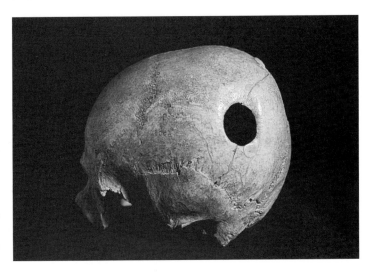

Trepanned skull, Bronze Age, from the Grotta della Scoglietto, Toscana, Italy. (Reproduced courtesy of John Robb, University of Southampton.)

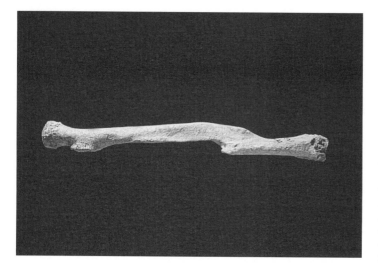

Healed fracture (radius) Bronze Age, from the Grotta della Scoglietto, Toscana, Italy. (Reproduced courtesy of John Robb, University of Southampton.)

Both deliberate and accidental injury to the skeleton is commonly encountered. Much can be learned about the practice of bone-setting in earlier populations by the state of healing of fractured bones and their alignment, and by whether they have become secondarily infected. From the good results that appear to have been achieved, evidently many former populations had access to individuals with considerable skill in reducing and setting broken limbs, and presumably few of these would have had any formal medical or surgical training. Injuries received in fights, brawls, and battles are relatively common in some periods, and judicial injury in the form of beheadings and hangings may also be observed. Evidence for surgery and for anatomy are found with increasing frequency after the 18th century. Several skeletons from those who were subject to a post-mortem examination have been found in London, for example, as have skeletons with evidence of amputation. These skeletons provide interesting information about the techniques which were used by early surgeons and anatomists. The practice of trephining, or trepanning — cutting or chipping a disc-shaped hole in the vault of the skull — dates back to neolithic times if not earlier, and may have mystic or religious significance (release of evil spirits). Many trephined skulls show evidence of healing.

### Difficulties in diagnosis

Another difficulty with which paleopathologists have to contend concerns diagnosis. There is little to help them other than the morphology of the changes in the bone, supplemented in some cases by radiography. This greatly limits the ability to reach a diagnosis in the first place and makes it difficult to compare prevalence rates in contemporary populations in whom diagnosis can be substantiated. Comparing the frequency of osteoarthritis in a skeletal population with that from either a hospital or a general practice population is extremely problematical since the groups are similar in almost no respects. Moreover, ancient remains are unlikely to be representative of community-wide prevalence. Nor is the comparison with data obtained from radiological surveys reliable since it has been shown that the paleopathologist can detect many more lesions than are visible on X-RAYS.

Not much can be gained by comparing data with those of earlier workers. Wood Jones's account of the pathology in Nubian material stated that rheumatoid arthritis was the most common disease. He was actually referring to osteoarthritis, not what is now known as rheumatoid arthritis. Older writers used many synonyms for the same condition and some of these are no longer understood; this and inadequate descriptions of the lesions and poor (or no) illustrations frequently make it impossible to recognize the diseases referred to. Since there are few or no agreed diagnostic criteria to apply to bony lesions, it is far from certain that modern paleopathologists are referring to the same entity when they attach a diagnostic label to it. This makes comparisons between studies if not impossible, then certainly imprecise. Studies of the prevalence of disease in the past are similarly hindered by diagnostic fluidity and by problems associated with finding the correct denominators to use when calculating the prevalence of a disease in a group of human remains. Some attempts have been made to introduce operational definitions into paleopathology; this is true for osteoarthritis and work is proceeding to introduce some for the more common and important infectious diseases such as SYPHILIS and TUBERCULOSIS. The suggested operational definitions for osteoarthritis have met with much criticism and we are a long way from agreeing how to diagnose even this, the most common condition met with in ancient skeletons.

Despite the inherent difficulties in the subject, paleopathologists have made important contributions to understanding disease in the past and have made significant contributions to the knowledge of pathological processes in bone. Perhaps the most notable example is the work of Møller-Christensen, who described the bone changes in LEPROSY based on his study of skeletons from a leprosy hospital in Denmark.

### Survival of bone

The most interesting development in paleopathology in recent years has been the realization that the organic matrix of buried bone survives much better than had been thought. This has resulted in the extraction of various proteins, albumin, IgG, hemoglobin, osteocalcin, and myeloma protein from bone. It has also been possible to extract and amplify mitochondrial and genomic DNA using the polymerase chain reaction. The extraction of genomic DNA has applications for sexing skeletons where this is not possible by anthropological means and is particularly helpful in sexing fetal or juvenile skeletons, which are otherwise difficult — if not impossible — to sex. Several workers have been able to extract bacterial DNA from bone, including DNA from *Mycobacterium tuberculosis* and *M. leprae.* For the first time there is the opportunity to provide absolute confirmation of these infections in bone. Rather gratifyingly, the positive results have tended to confirm the diagnoses made on morphological grounds alone. The technique can be used only to *confirm* a diagnosis; a negative result does not rule it out since the DNA may not have survived in sufficient quantity or may be too degraded to be extracted.

The ability to extract bacterial DNA provides a potential means whereby several interesting questions about disease in the past can be answered. For example, it is very likely that brucellosis was common at some periods but it is extremely difficult to differentiate the changes caused by brucellosis from those of tuberculosis; extraction of DNA from doubtful lesions should enable this differentiation to be made and as it is possible to distinguish between the human and bovine forms of tuberculosis using the polymerase chain reaction, we will be able to determine which of the two forms was the more common at different periods and to say when the human form superseded the bovine, if indeed the two were not always contemporaneous. There is no reason to suppose that the polymerase chain reaction will not be able to detect DNA from other organisms or that proteins which are biomarkers of disease or antigens will not be extracted from bone. The future paleopathologist may rely as much on laboratory methods as on morphology when determining which diseases affected our ancestors.

Dental disease — caries, and missing teeth, malocclusion, and periodontal disease — have been extensively studied. Some ancient populations were relatively free of caries, others were quite severely affected. Some inferences about ancient diets can be made on the basis of this evidence (sometimes reinforced by cerements such as offerings of food in grave sites).

Slowly, paleopathologists are assembling the record of ancient ills to which mankind is heir.

HAW

*See also* MUMMIES; RHEUMATOLOGY

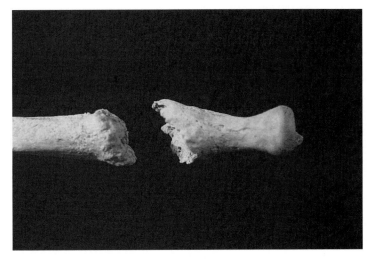

**PALLIATIVE CARE** Attitudes to death and dying have changed over the centuries. An abrupt change occurred in the 20th century (perhaps after the bloodbath of the First World War) when death became a forbidden subject, a new taboo. The tendency not to tell a dying person the truth, the likelihood of an impersonal death in hospital or nursing home, and the inability of society to allow any display of emotion in public (other than in the media) have made dying and BEREAVEMENT intensely lonely experiences. The old acceptance of destiny has gone, and a new sense of outrage that modern advances cannot finally halt the inevitable creates a negative climate among dying people and their families. The challenges of their care are thus more demanding as well as more rewarding if they are truly faced and people are to find any meaning in the situation.

Such care was considered an essential part of the family doctor's commitment, yet it has rarely had the attention in medical education that it warrants. The needs of the dying in hospital may be crowded out of attention of those responding to the urgent demands of acute care. A great deal has been learned, and much published, during the past four decades, but the attitudes and skills of the hospice and palliative care movement are only slowly spreading. Recently, chairs in palliative medicine have been established and the situation is improving.

### On making decisions

Doctors are committed to giving appropriate care to their patients, not to every treatment that may be technically possible. The prolongation of life should not in itself constitute the exclusive aim of medical practice, which must be concerned equally with the relief of suffering. These two

Healed fracture with pseudoarthrosis (ulna); late Roman period, from Isthmia, Greece. (Reproduced courtesy of John Robb, University of Southampton.)

aims must be balanced as the doctor and the whole multidisciplinary team aim to act in a patient's best interests. Many interventions in themselves serve only to increase suffering without a balance of benefit. Such decisions are not easy, especially where a patient is no longer competent to discuss and make an informed choice as to which treatments he wishes. If he is already unconscious, a document previously drawn up, preferably with a designated proxy, may help the clinician in making a judgement in this situation.

The doctor may not embark on any conduct with the primary intention of causing a patient's death, and if a terminally ill patient expresses a desire to commit SUICIDE a doctor may not in law facilitate the suicide. Nor can he respond to suggestions from a family to end life, although he does not have to continue futile treatment. In a few states in the USA physician-assisted suicide is becoming legally possible, while the situation in the Netherlands from November 2000 is that if certain guidelines are adhered to it is legally allowable. There is evidence, however, that these guidelines are not always observed but there is the possibility of an alternative in the developing work in palliative care now available in that country.

Skilled control of the physical, social, and emotional problems of far-advanced and terminal disease does not necessarily have to wait until all other treatment ceases, but may indeed make it more effective. When the clinician is involved with active treatment such as chemotherapy, with the control of pain and other symptoms, and with support to both patient and family, it will be easier to recognize diminishing returns in the former and to discontinue it without any member of the family or of the caring team feeling that now no treatment is being given. To accept a situation where treatment is directed to the relief of symptoms and the alleviation of general distress will no longer mean an implicit 'there is nothing more that we can do' but an explicit 'everything possible is being done'. This should in no way be termed 'passive euthanasia'. and nothing would undermine such good practice more than any form of legalized direct and intended killing. A 'right to die' could all too easily become a 'duty to die' and discourage the development of this important branch of medicine.

## The evolution of hospice and palliative care

Hospices 'for the dying' were founded in France in 1842 and, with no connection, in Ireland in 1879. Mme Jeanne Garnier and the Irish Sisters of Charity both took the early Christian word which, from the 4th century onwards, had meant hospitality for the sick and destitute, and for pilgrims and travelers. They had no particular connection with dying. Several homes with different titles — Catholic, Jewish, and Protestant — were founded on both sides of the Atlantic during some 20 years at the turn of the 20th century. Caring for only a fraction of those in need, they had a very limited impact upon general medicine, which by the 1950s was becoming increasingly able to lengthen the time between the diagnosis of malignancy and the patient's death. The modern hospice movement grew out of the need to address better long-term control of pain and other symptoms, together with concern for the patient as a person and for his family at such a time.

Unusually effective pain control with the regular giving of oral opioids was observed by the author in St Luke's Hospital (founded in 1893 as a home for the dying poor) from 1948 onwards; it was introduced and developed from 1958 in St Joseph's Hospice (founded 1905). The decade between was spent in medical training, but also saw the introduction of many of the drugs that were to be used in the increasingly effective control of symptoms. To the basic principle of giving analgesic drugs regularly to prevent pain occurring, rather than to allow a patient to suffer before receiving relief, could be added an ever-more detailed analysis of often complex problems with increasingly effective

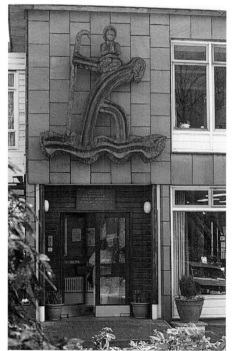

Entrance to St Christopher's Hospice, London. (Reproduced courtesy of St Christopher's Hospice.)

specific adjuvant treatments. With such an approach, patients were able to remain alert and often surprisingly active, and to be free to address all the other pressures of a mortal illness. Opportunity was given for a deepening of family communication and relationships, and to attend to unfinished business of all kinds. Possibilities of more ready access to the truth of the situation opened up as confidence in relief to the end developed. This, in turn, gave greater control to the patient and more choice as to where he spent his last days.

When St Christopher's Hospice opened in 1967 as the first modern hospice dedicated to research and education as well as to care, it set out to lay the scientific foundations for practice in this subject that could be interpreted in the home as well as in other settings, and could become a part of medical, nursing, and other teaching. In 1969 it pioneered both a hospice home-care team, complementary to the local primary care teams in the community, and drug studies in pain control. Systematic bereavement support began in 1971, and a study center opened in 1973 to accommodate the increasing number of visitors, from both Britain and elsewhere. Many of these set out to interpret the basic hospice principles in their different cultures and settings. A Hospice Information Service grew from these demands and today is in contact with a widespread network among more than 80 countries, supplies information packs (contributed by members) about many different developments in the subject, newsletters, and regularly-updated British and overseas directories.

Professionals from North America came on sabbaticals to St Christopher's in the early 1970s, and in 1974, established a home-care team with no back-up beds in New Haven and a similar consulting hospital team in New York. The following year the Palliative Care Unit and Service was established in Montreal. These three different patterns have developed world-wide, while in Britain both independent and NHS units and home care and hospital teams have proliferated. Government support has gradually increased, but nearly all capital and well over half of funding comes from public support. Hospices are major fund raisers in the voluntary sector.

Various professional associations and national and international organizations now set guidelines and standards. In Britain the title 'The National Council for Hospice and Specialist Palliative Care Services' illustrates the different names that have been chosen. It is becoming the accepted single voice for a movement that is now a recognized medical specialty with recognized principles.

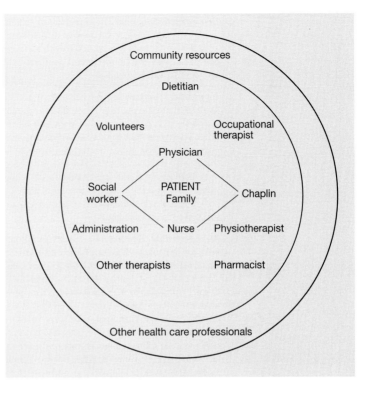

Diagram showing possible composition of an interdisciplinary palliative care team. (From Doyle, D. et al. (ed.) (1994). *The Oxford textbook of palliative medicine*, OUP.)

## Principles of palliative care

*Maximizing potential* Until death, patients should be enabled to live at their own maximum potential, performing to the limit of their physical activity and mental capacity, with control and independence wherever possible. They should be recognized as unique persons and helped to live as part of their family and in other relationships with some awareness from those around of their hopes and their expectations and of what has deepest meaning for them.

*Place of choice* Patients should end their lives in the place most appropriate for them and their families, and where possible have choices in the matter. If the patient is given some insight into the serious nature of their disease, this will help them to make realistic decisions.

*The patient and family as the unit of care* When a person is dying, his family finds themselves in a crisis situation, with the joys and regrets of the past, the demands of the present, and the fears of the future all brought into stark focus. If this time is to be fully used, there needs to be some degree of shared awareness of the true situation. In general, sharing is more creative than deception.

*Bereavement follow-up* The family has to recover. A bereavement follow-up service will identify and support those in special need, working in co-operation with the family doctor and any local services that can be involved.

*Competent symptom control* The patient and his family will not use the time left to them to the full unless there is good control of pain and all the other symptoms that may arise. All doctors and nurses should be aware of the development of these skills, and special units have a responsibility to initiate research and disseminate such knowledge. Once good symptom control is achieved it is then easier to become aware of the mental and social aspects of suffering.

*An experienced clinical team* A multidisciplinary medical approach is as important in the later stages of the management of disease as in the earlier phases. A group of consultants in a hospice unit or team may act merely as a resource while the patient remains in the care of his family doctor or of the clinicians who were involved with his initial treatment. A team may, however, take over the management completely, particularly if there is some special need, such as intractable physical distress or complex family problems.

*Supportive team nursing* The particular character of the nursing of dying patients includes the time given to do things at the patient's pace, to listen to the fears that are often revealed first to the helper in an intimate situation, to offer tenderness, understanding, and humor alongside practical deftness, and to greet and include the family both as cared for and as carers.

*An interprofessional team* Teams are particularly needed by those who are grappling with emotional as well as with practical demands. Psychiatrists, social workers, and chaplains have frequently been involved as support. Volunteers may have an important role, but must receive sensitive selection, training, and support.

*Home care* Families in the developing world, and still many in the developed countries, will care for their dying members but often need the skilled support of an experienced team. This is an important component of the now world-wide spread of the movement, complementary to any medical practice that may exist.

*Teaching in all aspects of terminal care* Teaching in this aspect is much in demand by students and graduates of all the disciplines concerned, as it has only a meager place — if any — in general curricula. Although much of the future development must be more closely integrated with general teaching centers, the academic units are likely to maintain their role of stimulating interest, organizing courses, and initiating research.

*Support for staff* All members of staff will at times become drained by the work, and need both formal and informal support.

Efficiency is comforting, and competence in administrative detail gives security to patients, families, and staff. It eases the liaison with outside contacts that is so essential for the small specialized team, and supports those who are managing such work among other pressures.

*The search for meaning* The work will at times cause pain and bewilderment to all members of the staff. Those who commit themselves to remaining near the suffering of dependence and parting find they are impelled to develop a basic philosophy, part individual and part corporate. This grows out of the work undertaken together, as members find that they each have to search, often painfully, for some meaning in the most adverse circumstances, and gain enough freedom from their own anxieties to listen to another's questions of distress.

This search for meaning can create a climate in which patients and families can reach out in trust towards what they see as true and find acceptance of what is happening to them. CS

*See also* EUTHANASIA, PAIN

**PAMPHLETEERING** During the centuries after the invention of printing, pamphleteering became a popular means of disseminating information and opinions, a pamphlet being a privately printed short booklet either unbound or bound loosely in paper covers. The views thus promulgated were mostly religious or political, usually controversial, but some of medical interest. Among the latter were, for example, Thomas PERCIVAL's (p 629) exposition of medical etiquette (*Medical ethics*, 1847), John SNOW's (p 48) account of the true mechanism of cholera transmission (*On the mode of communication of cholera*, 1849), and the contemporaneous pamphlet 'concocted on sanitary subjects' by which Sir Edwin Chadwick was said to have established himself in a position of absolute power on the General Board of Health. The importance of pamphleteering declined towards the end of the 19th century with the growth of newspapers, magazines, and journals.

*See also* BOOKS AND LIBRARIES; JOURNALS.

Maurice Henry **PAPPWORTH** (1910–94). British physician and ethicist. Pappworth held junior posts in Liverpool and served in the Royal

---

**VICTORIAN PAMPHLETEER**

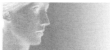

Samuel **SMILES** (1812–1904). British physician and writer. Smiles studied at Edinburgh, and served his apprenticeship and later practiced in Haddington. In 1838 he became editor of the radical *Leeds Times* and from 1854–66 was secretary to the South-Eastern Railway. Thereafter he was occupied in writing, chiefly biographies and tracts. His best known publication was *Self-help* (1859), which sold 250 000 copies in 25 years.

Army Medical Corps during the Second World War before going into private practice and private teaching. The anxiety of many of his pupils about the human experimentation going on in teaching hospitals in Britain at the time led him to document published examples of seemingly unethical practices, particularly where procedures carried no benefit to the patient and no INFORMED CONSENT had been obtained. In 1967 he expanded an earlier article into a book *Human guinea pigs*, in which he documented experiments on residents of institutions, prisons, and hospitals; named the experimenters responsible; and criticized ethical standards. The book caused outrage amongst the medical establishment of the time, but Pappworth had nothing to lose over his brave stance, and he was supported by similar work published from Harvard by the professor of anesthesiology there, Henry K. BEECHER (p 94). The resultant public furore led to professional reports and the belated establishment of a code of medical ethics and the setting up all over the world of research ethics committees to vet applications for therapeutic research involving humans. In many countries the procedure was extended to animal research as well.

Theophrastus Philippus Acreolus Bombastus von Hohenheim **PARACELSUS** (1493–1541). Swiss physician. Paracelsus, always known by this assumed name, was taught by his father, a cultivated physician. He later attended several universities and may have received the MD Ferrara, although this is not known for certain. He began practice in Strasbourg but in 1527 was appointed town physician and professor of medicine in Basle. He so outraged his colleagues by burning the works of GALEN (p 324) and AVICENNA (p 60) and by admitting BARBER-SURGEONS to his lectures, which were delivered in the vernacular, that he was forced to flee in 1528. Thereafter he wandered through Central Europe as an itinerant practitioner vigorously propounding his iconoclastic doctrine. He died, it is said, in a drunken brawl in Salzburg at the age of 48.

Paracelsus has been called the 'Luther of medicine'. Coarse-fibered but violently articulate, he defied the authority of Galen and Avicenna, condemning all medical teaching not based on experience. In so doing he opened the door to the renaissance of medical thought. An able doctor and a competent chemist, he introduced laudanum, sulfur, lead, and mercury into western therapeutics and popularized tinctures and salts. He associated cretinism with endemic goiter and distinguished mental defect from acquired mental illness.

**PARASITOLOGY** is the scientific discipline dealing with the association of two organisms that may result in disease in one of the species. The word 'parasite' is derived from Greek; it means 'situated beside'. Parasite was used in ancient Greece to describe people who ate beside or at tables of others. In spite of this 'social' background of the word, scientists started to use it in a specific way: parasites are defined as organisms residing on or within another living organism. Parasites may, therefore, be organisms that are either animals or plants, including a diversity of species such as bacteria, yeasts, fungi, algae, viruses, protozoa, helminths, and arthropods. From a biological point of view, parasitology may be defined as that branch of ecology in which one organism constitutes the living environment of another. This broad definition of parasites is not, however, the one that is in common use. From the medical point of view, parasitism is a specialized, dependent mode of life. Furthermore, parasitism represents a subgroup of symbiosis; there are thousands of species that use the symbiotic way of life and only some of these may cause disease in man, animals, or plants. Further restriction of the domain of parasitology occurred between the 17th and 19th centuries. Parasitology became the science dealing with zooparasites — that is, organisms that belong to the animal kingdom. In contrast, organisms such as bacteria, viruses, and fungi that have been classified as of plant origin are dealt with in the discipline of MICROBIOLOGY.

## History

The history of parasitology does not give a clear idea of the development of the discipline. Anthony van LEEUWENHOEK (p 489) has been credited with seeing the first protozoan using a simple microscope. Between 1674 and 1716 he described many free-living protozoa and also the first parasitic protozoan, *Eimera stiedai*. The description of the first human parasitic protozoon was made in 1681 by van Leeuwenhoek; he found *Giardia lamblia* in his own diarrheic stools. The major discoveries of parasitic protozoa were, however, delayed for over a century. During the 19th century the trypanosomes, amebae, and malaria parasites were described. WORMS or flukes, on the other hand, comprised almost all known parasites until the 1870s. In retrospect, evidence for several worm infections have been found in ancient Egyptian MUMMIES (1210–1000 BC). The famous EBERS PAPYRUS of 1550 BC indicates that in Ancient Egypt at least four worm infections were recognized, including *Ascaris lumbricoides*, *Taenia saginata*, *Dracunculus medinesis* (guinea worm), and *Schistosoma haematobium* (biliharzia). Reference is made to hematuria as a manifestation of disease in Ancient Egypt. The papyrus also includes information on arthropods such as fleas, flies, and lice. More recently, evidence was obtained from examining tissue sections of ancient Egyptian mummies that *Trichinella spiralis* existed as an infection during that period. Worms also were mentioned by Assyrian, Babylonian, and Greek physicians. The two most prominent historical discoveries of worms occurred in 1379 (*Fasciola hepatica*) and in 1558 (*Cysticercus cellulosae*), but it was not until the 18th and first half of the 19th century that many species of worms and arthropods were identified and classified. The latter part of the 19th century and early 20th century witnessed consolidation of the discoveries of many human parasites in general, identification of their life cycle, and recognition of their related disease syndromes.

Parasitology as a science is now undergoing a fundamental change because of the major biomedical revolutions that led to important discoveries in molecular biology and biochemistry. These tools are now being applied to the study of human parasites; the day may be close when we shall see molecular biology paving the way for the development of antiparasitic vaccines and new methods of controlling these infections.

Zooparasites are widely spread in the animal kingdom; parasitic members have been described in every major phylum. Among the protozoa, several species of amebae, flagellates, and ciliates and all of the sporozoa are parasitic. Metazoa include species that are common parasites of marine invertebrates. Parasitic representatives of the helminths, flat- and round-worms, are numerous. In addition arthropods are represented by many parasitic species or they may be involved in disease transmission as vectors.

The three major groups of organisms now recognized as falling within the scope of parasitology are protozoa, helminths, and arthropods. They vary greatly in many biological characteristics. Protozoa are unicellular organisms that are microscopic in size and that share with other micro-organisms such as bacteria and viruses the capability of dividing and multiplying within their mammalian host. In contrast, worms are *multicellular*; all adults can be seen by the naked eye and may reach huge dimensions — for example, some tapeworms may reach 10 m in length. Furthermore, worms generally cannot multiply within the mammalian host, re-exposure must occur. The third group of zooparasites, the arthropods, represent a heterogeneous collection of vectors of disease or they themselves may parasitize mammalian hosts causing varying degrees of discomfort or disease. Recently the term microparasites has been introduced to include viruses, bacteria, and protozoa. They are small in size, have high rates of direct reproduction within the host, and result typically in a short duration of infection. Macroparasites, on the other hand, include worms and arthropods, are larger, have much longer generation time as multiplication in the host usually does not occur, and produce infections that tend to be prolonged.

### Origin of parasites

Parasites originated from their free-living ancestors; they evolved along with their hosts. Consequently certain groups of parasites are limited to specific groups of hosts. This evolutionary relationship between parasites and their hosts may give valuable information about the relationship between different groups of hosts. For example, the moderately evolved monogenetic trematodes parasitize only fish, while the highly evolved digenetic trematodes are found not only in fish but more commonly in higher vertebrates. Furthermore, the more advanced digenetic trematodes tend to occur in the highest host groups.

Parasites may need more than one group of hosts. A definitive host is the one that harbors the adult stage of a parasite while the larval forms are located in an intermediate host. Some parasites may have more than one intermediate host. A vector is an arthropod, mollusc, or other agent which transmits the parasite from one vertebrate host to another. If parasite development occurs within the vector it is called biological to differentiate it from mechanical vectors, where parasites are simply passively transmitted.

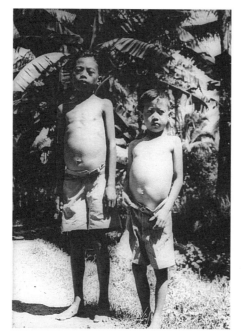

Schistosomiasis: two young sufferers of this debilitating waterborne parasitic disease. (Reproduced courtesy of the WHO/ National Library of Medicine, Bethesda, MD.)

## Host–parasite relationship

Entry of a specific parasite into a specific host is called infection. The outcome of such a process determines the survival of the parasite and occurrence of untoward effects, such as disease. Parasites invade their hosts through skin or mucous membranes, or by ingestion, or they may be transmitted through the placenta from the mother during birth, or by blood transfusion. On entry into the host, parasites may die or be killed, or may go through the host unchanged; in both cases no major pathological consequences of infection can be detected in the host. Alternatively, parasites may survive within the host or may proceed to develop and multiply. In both circumstances disease may occur. It is, therefore, important to differentiate between infection and disease due to zooparasites. The etiology of disease due to parasite invasion of mammalian hosts is almost always multifactorial: both parasite and host contribute to a delicate balance that may either arrest infection or lead to pathological sequels. Parasites result in disease because of their specific physiological or nutritional needs; disease may also occur because of mechanical destruction of host tissues. The host in turn attempts to reject the foreign invader using a multiplicity of immunological and non-immunological mechanism. A by-product of some of these host responses is a chain of immunopathological reactions that ultimately results in illness.

The host–parasite relationship is a dynamic process; the host uses several natural (innate) and acquired protective mechanisms. The complex structure of zooparasites in contrast to bacteria and viruses poses a significant challenge to host immune responses. Furthermore, not all of these responses are protective. In fact, protective immunity is the exception rather than the rule after a specific parasitic infection. Successful

Table 1  Major parasitic infections of man

| | Species | Disease | Estimated prevalence (millions) | Major endemic areas |
|---|---|---|---|---|
| Protozoa | *Plasmodium falciparum* <br> *P. vivax* <br> *P. ovale* <br> *P. malariae* | Malaria | 800 | Latin America, Africa, Asia |
| | *Entamoeba histolytica* | Amebiasis | Ubiquitous | World-wide |
| | *Trypanosoma gambiense* <br> *T. rhodesiense* | African sleeping sickness | 20–40 | Tropical Africa |
| | *T. cruzi* | Trypanosomiasis Chagas's disease | 40 | South America, Central and South America |
| | *Leishmania donovani* <br> *L. tropica* | Kala-azar Cutaneous leishmaniasis | 10–20 | Latin America, Africa, Asia |
| | *L. mexicana* <br> *L. braziliensis* | Mucocutaneous leishmaniasis | | |
| | *Toxoplasma gondii* | Toxoplasmosis | Ubiquitous | World-wide |
| Helminth | *Ascaris lumbricoides* | Ascariasis | 1000 | World-wide |
| | *Necator americanus* <br> *Ancylostoma duodenale* | Hookworm disease | 750 | World-wide |
| | *Schistosoma haematobrium* <br> *S. mansoni* <br> *S. intercalasum* <br> *S. mekongi* | Schistosomiasis (bilharziasis) | 200–300 | South America, Caribbean, Africa, Asia |
| | *Wucheria bancrofti* <br> *Brugi malayi* | Lymphatic filariasis | 200–300 | South America, Africa, Asia |
| | *Onchocerca volvulus* | River blindness (onchocerciasis) | 50 | Central America, West Africa |
| | *Taenia solium* <br> *T. saginata* | Teniasis | ? | World-wide |

survival of parasites has dictated that several mechanisms of evasion of host protective mechanisms have been developed to ensure their propagation. Parasites evade their host's immune responses either by simple mechanisms such as intracellular location or by more elaborate processes involving changing their antigenic structure or altering the host responses in a way that favors their survival.

Zooparasites constitute a major group of infectious diseases of humans and animals. Their prevalence and intensity have not been drastically changed in most of the developing world. The major parasitic protozoan and helminthic infections of humans and their estimated prevalence and the main endemic areas are summarized in Table 1. The burden of illness from these infections is staggering and the available methods of control are limited. Table 2 summarizes major arthropods that are medically significant because they act as vectors for parasitic or other infections.

The prevalence, intensity, and clinical significance of parasitic infections vary in different parts of the world. They are generally more prevalent in warm climates, in less developed areas, and in the socially deprived sections of any given society. Environmental and economic factors are prominent among those responsible for endemicity of parasitic infections in many parts of the world. Attempts to control the major parasitic infections have yet to demonstrate the effectiveness of any given strategy. In the 1940s and 1950s vector control and chemotherapy were thought to be the effective measures against the spread of malaria. Short-term successes were achieved but soon drug resistance developed in the mosquito vectors and in the parasite. Newer tools, whether chemotherapeutic or immunological, are therefore urgently needed to bring containment of these major health problems. Furthermore, their close relationship to socio-economic development and the role of cultural factors must be taken into consideration in formulating control strategies.                    AAFM

*See also* ANTIBIOTICS AND ANTI-INFECTIVE DRUGS; MALARIA

**PARKINSON'S DISEASE** See NEUROLOGY

Louis **PASTEUR** (1822–95). French chemist and microbiologist. Born at Dôle, in eastern France, Pasteur was educated at Besançon, and the École Normale in Paris, where he studied chemistry. For two years, he was professor of physics at the Lycée at Dijon, before moving to the University of Strasbourg as professor of chemistry and in 1854 being appointed dean and professor of chemistry in the faculty of sciences at Lille. In 1857 Pasteur returned to Paris as director of scientific studies

**Table 2** Major arthropod vectors of human parasitic diseases

| Class | Genus | Etiological agent |
|---|---|---|
| Crustacea | *Diaptomus* | *Diphyllobothrium latum* |
| | *Cyclops* | *Dracunculus medinensis* |
| Insects | *Anopheles* | *Plasmodia* |
| | *Triatoma* | *Trypanosoma cruzi* |
| | *Rhodnius* | |
| | *Culex* | *Wucheria bancrofti* |
| | *Phlebotomus* | *Leishmania* |
| | *Simulium* | *Onchocerca volvulus* |
| | *Glossina* | *Trypanosoma* |

at the École Normale and from 1867 was professor of chemistry at the Sorbonne.

Pasteur first gained recognition for his crystallographic research in 1848, in a paper on racemic acid, but he is best known for his biological investigations. Whilst at Lille, his interests were focused on the process of fermentation and the causes of diseases of wine and beer, and as a result of his experimentation he was able to declare that fermentation was the result of micro-organisms. He carried out a series of experiments to disprove the doctrine of spontaneous generation, demonstrating that the micro-organisms were derived from micro-organisms in ordinary air and that they could be destroyed by heat — 'pasteurization'. He applied this process to vinegar, wine, and, some years later, to beer. In 1865, Pasteur was commissioned by the government to investigate a silkworm disease which was ruining the French silk industry. After three years he had found the parasitic and bacterial causes of the disease and recommended action to save the industry. This research in addition to the results of his fermentation and spontaneous generation experiments led him to develop the germ theory of disease. In 1880 he turned his attention to the animal diseases of chicken cholera and anthrax; for both he isolated the bacillus and produced an effective inoculation. He then focused his investigations on rabies and in 1885 successfully inoculated a patient with the virus. In 1888 the PASTEUR INSTITUTE was established in Paris to continue his research into rabies and other microbiological diseases; he headed this until his death in 1895.

**PASTEUR INSTITUTE, THE,** in Paris was founded in the lifetime of Louis PASTEUR, and he was its first director. In 1885 he administered rabies vaccine to a person for the first time. In 1886 the results were so good that he advocated that an institute should be founded against rabies. Money poured in and the Institute began in 1888.

Pasteur attracted many top-class scientists and set up five departments: for microbe research in general; for microbe research applied to hygiene; for microbial morphology; for microbe technology; and for rabies. Among the first five researchers were Roux and METCHNIKOFF (p 412). Other now world-famous names from the Institute are Yersin, Bordet, Nicolle, d'Hérelle, CALMETTE (this page), Guérin, LAVERAN (p 480), Bovet, Jacob, Lwoff, and Monod, eight of whom won NOBEL PRIZES in physiology or medicine.

Now the Institute is a private state-approved foundation, which helps generate total intellectual freedom. There are eight departments: bacteriology and mycology; ecology; virology; immunology; molecular biochemistry and genetics; molecular biology; experimental physiopathology; and a clinical department. The hospital facilities were started in 1900 and it is private and non-profit-making. The Institute was instrumental in assisting the Institut du Radium to apply Marie CURIE's (p 556) discoveries to medicine. There is an intensive teaching program for students from many parts of the world. The influence of the Institute spreads far beyond its walls, not only through its students, but because there are Pasteur Institutes in Lille and Lyon, and also throughout the world, which, although independent, have associations with the Paris one.

*See also* FOUNDATIONS; RESEARCH INSTITUTES

**PATHOLOGY** is the study of disease processes and how they affect the cells, tissues, and organs of living things. Diseased cells, tissues, and organs are studied for many reasons, but the principal motive is to discover in what ways they have become abnormal and whether they could be returned to normal, and/or whether the abnormality could have been prevented.

Pathology is a wide concept, and its range is different in different contexts and in different parts of the world. In many countries 'pathology' is used to mean solely histopathology (microscopic investigation of diseased tissue). In Britain, it has become divided into five medical topics: chemical pathology (clinical chemistry), HEMATOLOGY, IMMUNOLOGY, medical MICROBIOLOGY, and histopathology. Sometimes pathology is qualified as anatomical pathology or tissue pathology, particularly in the USA. In central Europe, for administrative reasons, pathology developed separately from medical microbiology, medical immunology, and clinical chemistry, and covers macroscopic and microscopic examination of tissue as in biopsies and autopsy practice (anatomical pathology). Anatomical pathology in medicine is practiced almost exclusively by medically qualified pathologists.

## Morbid anatomy and histopathology

Used in the sense of anatomical pathology, pathology encompasses the study and dissection of diseased organs and tissues at the level of the naked eye (macroscopic). This type of study has fascinated scholars from CELSUS (p 806) in ancient times, through Michelangelo and MORGAGNI (this page), who was the first to correlate symptoms in life with anatomical changes, to the present. It has long been referred to as 'morbid anatomy', that is, anatomy that has become deranged, distorted, or disturbed over time. Today most morbid anatomy departments have changed their names because 'morbid' is regarded as a distressing word, too much associated with death and dissection.

Morbid anatomy is particularly the province of the post-mortem room. The post-mortem examination (synonyms: AUTOPSY, first used 1678; post-mortem (1850); necropsy (1856)) establishes which disease processes were present at the time of death. Together with microscopic examination of selected tissues and organs and any other information or evidence that may be collected, the 'cause of death' may be deduced.

Since post-mortem examinations began to be performed routinely in some countries, particularly Germany and Austria, at the beginning of the 19th century — correlation of the pathological findings with the clinical signs, symptoms, and test results has contributed a great deal to medical knowledge of individual diseases. Deaths from unnatural causes, including homicide, poisoning, road accidents, come into the realm of forensic pathology (part of forensic science) that employs specially trained pathologists.

Histopathology, the term that is often used to replace morbid anatomy but actually complements it, is the study of diseased cells, tissues, and organs microscopically. Its normal counterpart is histology, which has the same relationship to histopathology as anatomy to morbid anatomy.

Although fresh and even living cells and tissues can be observed microscopically, they are virtually translucent and devoid of detail. It is usually more convenient to 'fix' them in a preservative such as 10% formaldehyde solution, cut them into thin slices or sections (usually 5–10 $\mu$m thick for light microscopy or less than 0.1 $\mu$m for electron microscopy), stain them to pick out the components of interest, and mount them on glass slides with a glass coverslip to maximize their optical properties. For electron microscopy the sections are mounted on copper grids. From VIRCHOW's (p 853) time (c. 1858) until recently staining was largely empirical, but first histochemical and enzyme histochemical techniques and then monoclonal antibodies capable of labeling special antigens (immunohistochemistry) became available

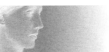

(*continued overleaf*)

(continued)

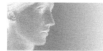

Matthew **BAILLIE**
(1761–1823). British
physician and morbid
anatomist. Baillie married the
sister of John (p 398) and
William (p 88) HUNTER and
worked at the Great
Windmill Street School,
which he inherited on the
death of William Hunter. He
was the greatest of the early
British morbid anatomists
and published the first work
on the subject *The morbid
anatomy of some of the most
important parts of the human
body* (1793).

(continued opposite)

for identifying cellular and tissue components. In the 1980s the development of molecular biology produced the technique of *in-situ* hybridization to identify specific lengths of DNA and RNA. Research in pathology is also applying computerized image analysis, advanced statistical and epidemiological methods, quantification of staining, analysis of shape, size, and distribution of tissue structures, and automatic or interactive cytometric instruments applying visible or ultraviolet light. Pathology workstations designed for making such measurements easier and automatic measuring and screening instruments have been developed.

## Exogenous (including iatrogenic) disorders

Pathological effects are frequently the result of injurious influences from outside the body. Physical agents include heat, cold, accidental, deliberate, or occupational injuries from blunt or sharp objects, and various forms of radiation, such as sunlight and ionizing radiation. Chemical agents include all forms of chemical substances, including poisons and substances that are abused, such as alcohol and the constituents of glue, or inhaled or ingested at work, such as asbestos fibers or coal dust. Microorganisms, including bacteria, viruses, protozoa, and fungi, and the toxins they produce are important exogenous causes of disease. Finally, an important and easily forgotten part of, sometimes unavoidable, exogenous damage is that caused to patients by treatments such as surgery, radiotherapy, prescription of the wrong dosage of drugs and medicines, or side-effects or adverse reactions to the correct dosage — this form of disease is termed iatrogenic. Iatrogenic disease may therefore be of physical, chemical, or microbiological origin.

## Congenital disease

Congenital disease includes inherited disease, determined by the genome inherited from the parents, such as hemophilia; developmental abnormalities and syndromes, such as congenital heart disease; and sundry abnormalities acquired before birth, such as heart failure due to rhesus incompatibility, or during birth, such as brain damage due to lack of oxygen. Developmental abnormalities are often multiple.

## Inflammatory conditions

Inflammation is the reactions of tissues and organs to various agents, including infecting organisms such as bacteria, viruses, protozoa, and fungi, and injuries such as wounds or fractures. It may be acute, as in abscesses or pneumonia, or chronic and scar forming, as in tuberculosis or chronic ulceration. Some of the body's reactions to injury are mediated by immune processes designed as defense mechanisms; however, these may themselves become disturbed and cause inflammation, especially if the immune process wrongly comes to regard body components themselves as inimical. Rheumatoid arthritis is believed to be an example of such an 'autoimmune' disease.

## Circulatory disorders

Diseases of the circulation include bleeding (hemorrhage), which may result from injury or have a hereditary origin as in hemophilia, and inappropriate clotting (thrombosis). A thrombus (blood clot) may obstruct the blood supply to an organ, as when it occurs in one of the coronary arteries that supply the heart muscle, with severe or fatal consequences. Alternatively a thrombus, particularly in a leg vein, may break off into the blood stream and circulate until it is caught in a branching or narrowing blood vessel and, again, the blood supply is blocked; circulating material is called an embolus, which may consist of thrombus or other substances. Pulmonary embolism (a blood clot blocking the main artery to the lungs) is a feared and potentially fatal complication after surgical operations and injuries. After much study by clinicians and pathologists, deep leg-vein thrombosis and consequent pulmonary embolism have been greatly reduced by using rhythmically inflated boots during surgery, and making patients move their legs and walk much earlier than used to be the practice.

## Metabolic conditions

Abnormal metabolism or handling of nutrients and chemical substances by the body, such as DIABETES or GOUT, generally have a genetic basis but may be initiated by additional factors, such as viral infections. Some, such as phenylketonuria, should be screened for in early life. Others, such as uremia, are the result of damage to specific organs, in this case the kidneys, but can affect a wide range of organs and tissues.

## Degenerative conditions

Degenerative pathology is the result of wear and tear, and therefore occurs in older people. For example, the cartilage that covers bone ends in joints is prone to wear out, especially in people

## CATEGORIES OF PATHOLOGICAL CHANGE

All anatomical pathology is included within seven disease categories: (1) exogenous, (2) congenital, (3) inflammatory, (4) circulatory, (5) metabolic, (6) degenerative, and (7) neoplastic. These categories are not mutually exclusive; for example, the pathology of cirrhosis of the liver includes aspects of all seven categories. Nevertheless, to be able to categorize a disease pathologically greatly enhances one's ability to think constructively about it and to devise ways of studying diagnosing, treating, or preventing it.

who have had injury to their joints or through being overweight. This can lead to osteoarthritis, which is not the same as rheumatoid arthritis, an inflammatory autoimmune disease of the joints. The tissue changes associated with aging are usually considered degenerative. These changes may contribute to the emergence of disease conditions. Better understanding of changes associated with aging may expand the number of diseases that can be considered degenerative.

## Neoplasia

The mechanisms that control cell division are complicated and are still being worked out (see also ONCOLOGY). It is obvious that very fine control is needed to build a human being from a fertilized egg, and that many things may go wrong. Similarly, after development is complete, cells in the various organs and tissues are constantly dividing to replace worn out and dying cells, particularly in the blood, skin, and intestinal tract. Cells that are lost through injury or disease are replaced by cell division, which then stops. Sometimes cell division occurs inappropriately, so that too many cells are produced; this is called hyperplasia. Sometimes the cell division gets completely out of hand and does not stop; this is called neoplasia (new growth). The usual lay term for a neoplasm is a tumor, although 'tumor' is also used less precisely to mean a swelling of any sort. If the neoplastic cells infiltrate the surrounding tissues and/or are carried to other parts of the body through the lymphatic, venous, or arterial vessels and continue dividing there (a metastasis, metastases), this is malignant neoplasia or cancer. If they merely divide locally without spreading into neighboring tissues or further afield, this is benign neoplasia. Benign tumors may have deleterious and even fatal effects, but technically they are not cancers. It is believed that neoplasia arises as a result of a change, or series of changes, in the genome of a single cell, the progeny of which then behave in a neoplastic way, that is generally irreversible. Neoplasms, including malignant tumors, can be produced experimentally in animals and in cell culture by physical means, ionizing radiation, chemicals, dietary substances, drugs, and viruses, thus tending to confirm with varying degrees of conviction that similar associations in man are causal. Changes that influence the process of cell death (apostasis) or multiplication of cells (as revealed by mitosis, division of chromosomes) are important in the progression of cancer. Damage of mitotic mechanisms, leading to aneuploidy, may explain the fast accumulation of changes in cancer cells.

A vast amount of clinical, experimental, and epidemiological research is devoted to the study of cancer, to find ways of preventing, curing, and

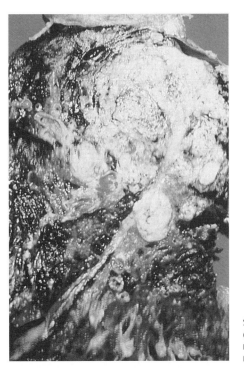

Section of cancerous lung. (Reproduced courtesy of the National Cancer Institute, Bethesda, MD.)

alleviating or palliating the suffering it causes. For the individual patient and for this research effort it is imperative that cells and tissues are examined microscopically to ensure that it really is cancer that is being dealt with and not another form of tissue pathology. This form of diagnosis, together with the identification of other features indicating how one may expect the tumor to behave, requires the skill and experience of the surgical pathologist. Cells and tissue taken for diagnosis are called a biopsy. The development of surgical pathology has taken place especially at university pathology departments, and consultation centers such as the Armed Forces Institutes of Pathology in Washington DC.

## Etiology and pathogenesis

Research in pathology and pathologists are particularly called upon to explain the causation of diseases. Etiology investigates the causes and origins of diseases. Pathogenesis is the term used to describe the progression or development of pathological changes once something has gone wrong with the normal structure or function of the cells. It is, therefore, one thing to try to elucidate the cause of a disease, but quite another to study its progression or natural history, and how the latter may be altered by different factors, including treatment. The useful terms etiology and pathogenesis should not, therefore, be used loosely or interchangeably.

*(continued)*

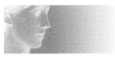

Sir William Boog **LEISHMAN** (1865–1926). British bacteriologist and army medical officer. Leishman joined the Army Medical Service in 1887 and served under Sir Almroth Wright at Netley, succeeding him as professor of pathology in 1900. He was adviser in pathology to the army in the First World War and in 1918 became director of pathology at the War Office, being promoted director-general of the Army Medical Service in 1923. Leishman devised the familiar modification of Romanowsky's stain (Leishman's stain); he described the causal organism of kala-azar (*Leishmania donovani*); and he elucidated the life cycle of the cause of endemic relapsing fever (*Borellia duttoni*).

TEXTBOOK AUTHOR

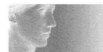

William George
**MACCALLUM**
(1874–1944). American
pathologist. Although born in
Canada, MacCallum spent his
entire professional career in
the department of pathology
at JOHNS HOPKINS (p 840),
succeeding W. H. Welch as
professor. MacCallum made
several important
observations, including:
showing endothelial lining of
lymphatic vessels, the relation
between parathyroid glands
and blood calcium
concentration, and careful
studies of the cardiac lesions
resulting from rheumatic
fever. He wrote a textbook of
pathology that was widely
used for many years.

### Relative frequency of pathological categories

Epidemiological studies on the frequency of various types of diseases are important for the planning of health services. Frequencies of diseases in different groups in different societies change with the health associated habits, including diet. In developed countries, heart disease (cardiac infarct) and cancer are today the most common causes of death followed by strokes, respiratory disease, and violence (traffic accidents, suicides etc.). Other disease conditions are responsible for the remaining 25% of deaths. In developing countries infective diseases, famine-associated diarrhea, and malnutrition still dramatically influence the cause-of-death statistics.

### Specialization

Until the 1930s many physicians and surgeons not only carried out post-mortems but also many of the simple pathological tests that were then available. General or all-purpose pathologists had, however, been gradually emerging during the early 20th century, alongside pathologists specializing in microbiology and anatomical pathology, particularly in the universities, medical schools, and teaching hospitals. Since 1948 the activities of the anatomical pathologists have traditionally included casework with living and dead patients, usually together with teaching and research, in collaboration with virtually every other medical specialist and general practitioner, since anatomical pathology underlies all their work.

With the enormous expansion of pathological knowledge in this period, however, anatomical pathologists have begun to form subspecialties, that is, after a general postgraduate anatomical pathology training, to concentrate on one specific part of anatomical pathology. Forensic pathology was the first subspecialty. Cytopathology is emerging as a separate subspecialty and merits further consideration below. Perinatal and pediatric pathology have become an acceptable subspecialty. Otherwise, apart from neuropathology, which is concerned with the central nervous system, peripheral nerves, and voluntary muscles, only enthusiasts have been able to establish a career in the pathology of a single organ or system, usually in specialist hospitals. After postgraduate general training further expertise may be gained through concentrating on narrower aspects of pathology. In this fast advancing subject today's pathologists must be prepared to retrain in understanding and studying emerging issues throughout their postgraduate life.

### Cytopathology

In histopathology the diagnosis calls for the study of both the cells and the extracellular structures in the tissues and their relationships to each other.

Cytopathology, on the other hand, is a branch of histopathology that deals with cells obtained in such a way that their normal histological or histopathological relationships are lost. Cytopathological preparations obtained by scraping the cells off the surface of the uterine cervix (neck of the womb) with a spatula — cervical smears — are the best known. PAPANICOLAOU (p 740) popularized this technique in 1928, and the stain named after him is still widely used. But cells may be obtained if necessary from almost any surface by scraping, brushing, or irrigating, from inside organs and tissues by sucking with a syringe and needle (fine-needle aspiration cytology), and from urine or body fluids, such as cerebrospinal fluid (lumbar puncture), followed by centrifugation. However obtained, the cells are stained on slides, covered with a coverslip, and studied microscopically.

Cytopathology is used particularly for the initial diagnosis of cancer. The recognition of cells, sometimes just a few cells, among many non-malignant cells as being malignant is, however, subjective and not easy. Before a patient undergoes irreversible surgery or potentially harmful radiotherapy or chemotherapy, most clinicians confirm the diagnosis by taking a piece of tissue (biopsy) for histopathological examination as well.

*Cervical screening* In the initial stages of cancer of the cervix the premalignant or malignant cells are confined to a small area of the surface. At this stage the cancer can be completely eliminated and therefore cured. The authorities in British Columbia were the first to try to perform cervical cytology on all the women in their population at regular intervals and to see if the incidence and mortality of cancer of the cervix fell. By 1964 the incidence had fallen. However, the work is labor intensive and a proportion of false positive and false negative results is inevitable in spite of quality control and quality assurance procedures. Another drawback is that many women, often those most at risk, are not reached by the screening programs.

*Breast screening* Deaths from cancer of the female breast are increasing in the developed countries. Many of these cancers can be recognized in X-RAY pictures (mammography) before they can be felt, and, after confirmation of the diagnosis by fine-needle aspiration cytology and/or biopsy, excised. In Sweden the mortality has been lowered through the breast cancer screening programs.

### Conclusion

The medical specialty of anatomical pathology complements anatomy and/or histology and, encompassing morbid anatomy and histopathology (including ctyopathology), underlies the whole practice of medicine. In most countries training and practice are regulated by the government, local medical unions, or scientific societies. In Britain the regulatory body is the Royal College of Pathologists. Pathologists are to be found in every general hospital, teaching hospital, and medical school world-wide. In addition to their day-to-day casework, pathologists are usually enthusiastic teachers of undergraduates and postgraduates, and also do an immense amount of research work, usually in collaboration with clinical colleagues. There are several prominent journals devoted to pathology, some of them general, others focused on narrower aspects of pathology. As the subject started to develop in the 19th century and to be particularly associated with post-mortem work, it has acquired an old-fashioned aura, which, in the era of molecular biology, is not justified.

The old tasks of pathology (tissue diagnosis, prognosis, elucidation of etiology, and pathogenesis) are even more important and powerful today than they used to be. The best and most modern methods of light and electron microscopy, immunohistochemistry, molecular biology (molecular pathology), computerized image analysis, advanced statistical analysis, quantification of staining analysis of shape, size, and distribution of tissue structures, and automatic or interactive cytometric instruments applying visible or ultraviolet light, usually in association with microscopy, are all used. Through such methods the science of pathology — in addition to improving the general understanding of disease conditions — is able to have an immediate influence on decisions on treatment and on treatment research for various types of diseases, including cancer. WFW, YC

*See also* CELL AND CELL BIOLOGY; CLINICO-PATHOLOGICAL CONFERENCE; ONCOLOGY; SCREENING

**PATIENTS' ASSOCIATIONS** Groups set up by people with a common medical problem are described by health professionals as 'patients' associations', though the organizations themselves usually prefer terms such as self-help or mutual aid groups. These organizations have a variety of interests, ranging from providing information, support, and practical help for the victims of a disease and their relatives to fund-raising for research. Some associations act as pressure groups to try to change public attitudes to a disease or the social restrictions and legal regulations affecting the lives of families with the disorder. A few self-help groups are critical of the medical establishment and some are positively hostile (the People's Medical Society in the United States claimed in 1983 that 'the enemy is the doctor'). Most, however, work closely with health professionals.

The earliest organizations to help the victims of disease were religious orders, but the victims themselves had a passive role. Secular organizations began to participate in the care of the sick in the 18th century with the growth of trades unions and friendly societies, which were self-help bodies in that they were managed by the same people as were being helped. The main role of these societies was to provide a system of health insurance to give financial help during the sickness of members and their families. In Britain, the friendly societies and a range of local and national bodies such as the Hospital Saturday Fund continued to act as health insurers for the poor until the introduction of the National Health Service in 1948, when most were wound up. A few survived as medical insurance bodies, but in the early years of the Health Service private medical care formed only a small fraction of the total. In the past 20 years it has grown substantially, so that the private sector now carries out around one quarter of all elective surgery. Since the 1970s the financing of this private medical care has come mostly from non-profit associations, such as the British United Provident Association and the Private Patients Plan. These schemes lack several of the essential features of self-help groups, however, and the subscribers take little part in their management.

Self-help groups can trace their origins to a few pioneers in the middle of the 20th century. They began mostly with a single person affected by a disorder or experience who had the energy and enthusiasm to set up a support and information group. Examples in Britain include Cruse (an association providing support for the bereaved) and the Mastectomy Association (which gives practical and emotional help to women who have had a breast removed for cancer).

Although ALCOHOLICS ANONYMOUS (p 626) was one of the prototypes, it chose a narrow range of activities when compared with many other groups. These may include support and befriending; providing information (including setting up lectures and workshops), maintaining a stock of leaflets, books, and videos, publishing literature and newsletters; campaigning; and fund-raising.

The characteristic features of a self-help association are that its members should share a common experience in the health field that causes them continuing difficulties; its members should own and run the group; the people who attend its meetings should benefit from its activities; the group should have some formal structure and organization; and, though members may make contributions to the running costs or may raise funds for research, they should not be asked to pay fees.

# ALCOHOLICS ANONYMOUS

World-wide, one of the earliest and certainly the best known self-help groups is Alcoholics Anonymous, founded in the United States in 1935. Local branches can be found in nearly 100 countries. Membership is open to anyone with a drinking problem who wants help. No fee is charged, the costs of the local groups being met by voluntary contributions from their members. Meetings are of two types. At open meetings, which can be attended by anyone including the families of alcoholics, speakers describe their lives as alcoholics and the help they have received from Alcoholics Anonymous. At closed meetings new members are encouraged to describe their drinking problems, and other members then give practical advice based on their own experiences.

This association limits its activities to providing practical help to alcoholics. It does not maintain membership records, engage in or sponsor research, provide professional psychiatric treatment, or provide vocational counseling. In response to requests from the families of alcoholics it has set up support groups called Al Anon for the relatives of problem drinkers and more recently a further type of support group called Alateen for the adolescent children of problem drinkers.

The numbers of groups grew rapidly in the last third of the 20th century to cover most of the common causes of physical illness and disability and mental illness and many of the more rare disorders, too. In part, this rapid expansion in numbers was inspired by theoretical reappraisals of the role of medicine put forward by medical philosophers and SKEPTICS such as Thomas McKeown, René DUBOS (p 247), and Ivan Illich. They argued that the contribution made by medicine to health had been overrated and that patients should take far more responsibility for their own health. Many of the early self-help groups questioned medical definitions of health and disease, and criticized the stigma attached to conditions such as alcoholism and obesity. They called for a holistic approach to health and wanted patients to be given rights to take part in making decisions about their management.

## Formation of subgroups

As more groups were established it became apparent that no single association could hope to satisfy all the needs of patients and their carers. The experience of Alcoholics Anonymous, which led to its setting up subgroups for the families of alcoholics, is evidence of one problem encountered by many self-help support groups: it often proves difficult for the same organization to provide emotional support for people with a chronic disease and for their carers. Finding others with the same problem as oneself seems to provide comfort: it is often easier to talk about the practical and social problems associated with many diseases in a setting where others have had the same experiences. But organizations which have as their prime objective the support of people with a disease can only rarely also provide support for their families, who need to be able to discuss their problems and offer sympathy to each other in a setting which excludes the victims of the disease. Recognizing this, groups such as Headway have as their primary aim support for the families of patients recovering from head injuries, which may have had profound psychological effects.

Several thousand self-help groups are now listed in directories and databases available on the internet (http://www.cmhc.com/selfhelp/). Most of them provide a simple practical service: they supply information and advice about a disease (or group of diseases such as arthritis) and its management. They usually also act as a source of detailed advice about the benefits and services provided by statutory and other agencies. Someone recently diagnosed as having a long-term illness such as DIABETES or ASTHMA will find that joining the British Diabetic Association or the Asthma Society will give them access to an explanation of their illness and practical advice about living with it. Often this information will be available in several versions, some simple and some more complex.

Joining a group will also help a newly diagnosed patient make contact with other people with the disease. For common diseases there are often local branches, and for diseases such as diabetes which are more frequent in some ethnic groups there are often organizations for Asians, Afro-Caribbeans, for example. Members of self-help groups commonly find that they eventually know more about the practical management of their condition than do many general practitioners, or even hospital specialists. One of the skills learned from self-help groups is how to make best use of a doctor who has little interest in a disease he or she regards as rare and of specialist concern.

Second only to the groups for people with a chronic disease are organizations for people who want practical help in dealing with a problem. The pattern of Alcoholics Anonymous has been followed by people addicted to tranquilizers and to gambling. People who have repeatedly tried and failed to lose weight may join slimming groups, some with a strong commercial bias, with others being closer to conventional self-help groups. They all share the aim of encouraging participants to take more responsibility for their own condition, rejecting the old-style assumption that it was the doctor's role to oversee the management of an addiction or other problem.

Groups for both patients and carers may also provide practical direct services, such as transport pools, babysitting, and details of holiday destinations which welcome people with disabling or disfiguring disorders. Some organize trips abroad for special treatments, such as visits to the Dead Sea for people with psoriasis. They may also

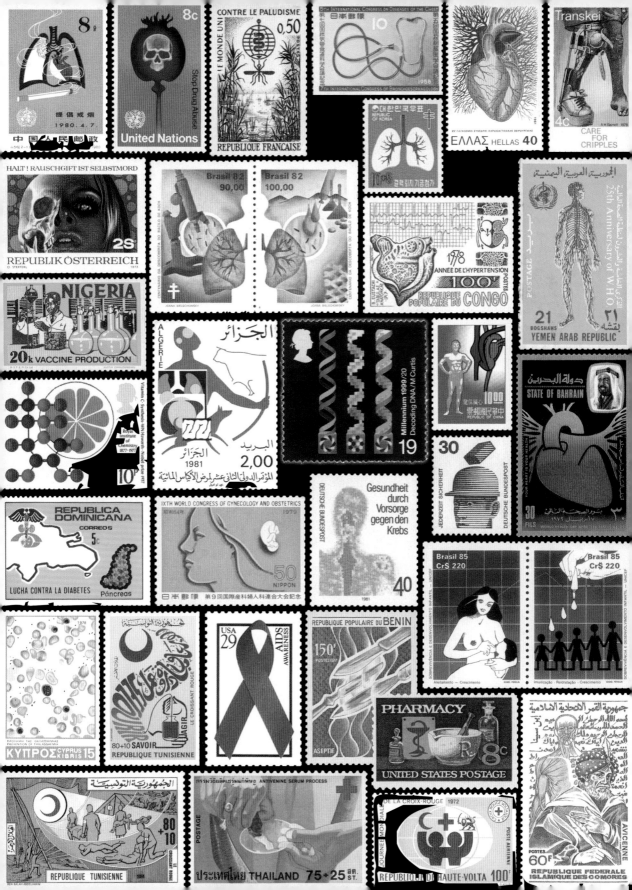

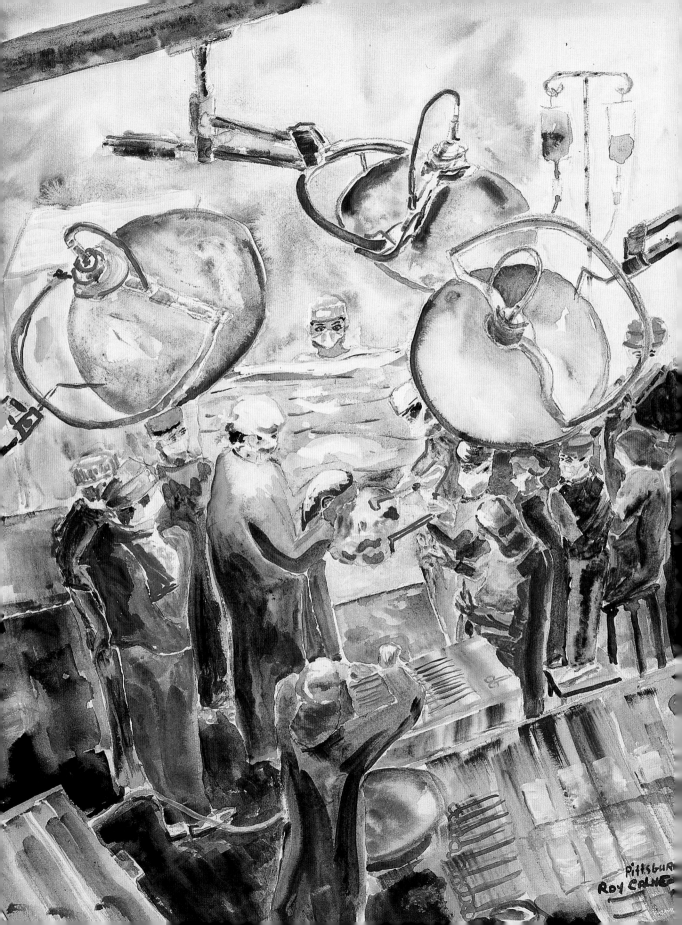

Pittsburg
Roy Calne

organize social activities for people with the disease, carers, or both.

Some organizations have as their main objective fund-raising for research into the disease: the Imperial Cancer Research Fund and the Cancer Research Campaign employ large numbers of scientists in their laboratories and provide university research departments with grants for specific projects.

Finally, many self-help groups act as pressure groups campaigning to change public attitudes to a disorder or group of disorders and to improve the benefits and services provided by statutory authorities. Organizations concerned with chronic mental illness such as schizophrenia, and with HIV infection and AIDS, have achieved much in combating ignorance and prejudice against people with the diseases. Action for Victims of Medical Accidents (founded in 1982) has campaigned for information to be made more easily available to patients who have been damaged by a medical or surgical error during their treatment.

In Britain two national organizations, the Patients' Association and the College of Health, claim to speak for patients and may often be heard commenting on the broadcast media about new initiatives in health care or advances in understanding disease. They provide the public with information services and practical help in dealing with the bureaucracy of the National Health Service, and they maintain comprehensive listings of the autonomous self-help groups for individual disorders. It is these small groups, often still managed by a single dedicated individual with a small band of helpers, that have given so much support to patients and their families in the past two or three decades.                    ASmi

## PATIENTS, NOTABLE (ILLNESSES OF THE FAMOUS)

A tiny number of individuals have a claim to historical immortality solely because of their medical conditions. The name of James Phipps would be entirely forgotten but for the fact that he was the first individual to be vaccinated against smallpox by Edward JENNER (p 452). Alexis St Martin, a French-Canadian fur trapper, is remembered because a gunshot wound created a gastric fistula that exposed the workings of his stomach and enabled the American doctor, William Beaumont, to make pioneering observations upon the physiology of digestion.

But if sicknesses have won very few people celebrity, the ailments of the illustrious have been of perennial interest; eminent physicians have written at length about their distinguished patients (Lord Moran on Winston Churchill being a prime instance), and medical historians, amateur and professional, have published widely on the maladies of the mighty. The reasons for this are many. All the trivia of eminent people attract attention. As we know very well in these days of media voyeurism about AIDS, the private lives of prominent people become appropriated into the public domain. Along similar lines, it was noted two centuries ago that the sicknesses of the eminent create fashions in complaints. 'Various distempers in certain ages and countries have had the fashion on their side, and have been thought reputable and desirable', observed the notable clinician, William HEBERDEN (p 628):

> some maladies have been esteemed honourable, because they have accidentally attacked the great, or because they usually belong to the wealthy, who live in plenty and ease … when Louis XIV happened to have a fistula, the French surgeons of that time complained of their being incessantly teased by people, who pretended, whatever their complaints were, that they proceeded from a fistula: and if there had been in France a mineral water reputed capable of giving it them, they would perhaps have flocked thither as eagerly as Englishmen resort to Bath in order to get the gout.

The medical histories of the great also attract attention because they are exceptionally well-documented, affording rare shafts of light into the generally poorly recorded practice of medicine in former centuries. We know, for instance, that only after the death of Queen Victoria did her physician, Sir James Reid, discover that she had a ventral hernia and a prolapsed uterus — clear proof that he had never once given her a full physical examination. This instance may well indicate just how recently physical examinations have become a normal aspect of medical practice — although, equally, it might point to an eccentricity of the queen and the power of the throne to command physicians.

Or take James Boswell. Because he kept such copious diaries we know that Dr Johnson's biographer was a habitual sufferer from venereal infections. Boswell was 'clapped' on no fewer than 19 occasions. What forms of treatment did he undergo? For his youthful bouts of 'Signor Gonorrhea', Boswell religiously went to regular surgeons, such as Andrew Douglas in Pall Mall. Douglas initially treated him with purges, put him on a light diet, and ordered bed rest; many years, many claps, later, having changed his strategies, Douglas was to try injecting fluids into the urethra.

When he was infected in Italy, Boswell went to the very best surgeon — James Murray, personal physician to the Old Pretender — and secured an audience with no less eminent a man than MORGAGNI (p 621), the father of pathological anatomy. On later occasions, Boswell waited upon regular surgeons, such as Peter Adie in Edinburgh and Daniel Johnstone in Ayr. By 1767, Boswell, still

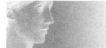

William **HERBERDEN** the younger (1767–1845). British physician, son of William Heberden the elder. In 1793 Heberden became physician to St George's Hospital and two years later physician-extraordinary to the Queen and in 1805 to the King, being later promoted to physician-in-ordinary. He was a sound physician, but after the death of his wife in 1812 he retired from all except his Royal appointments to educate his nine children. He took a particular interest in rheumatic diseases.

only 25, had his seventh attack, and paid a visit to the Edinburgh surgeon, Duncan Forbes. On a later occasion he consulted the great Percivall Pott, perhaps the most illustrious surgeon in Britain. On the point of marriage, he consulted a whole gaggle of doctors to ensure he was infection-free.

But Boswell also, just to make sure, travelled to London to purchase some bottles of Kennedy's Lisbon Diet Drink, a popular nostrum vended by Gilbert Kennedy, graduate of both of Rheims and Oxford. The Diet Drink consisted of sarsaparilla, sassafras, liquorice, and guaiac wood, and cost half a guinea a bottle; Boswell was instructed to drink two bottles a day.

When his regular doctors, such as Sir John Pringle, tried to dissuade him from taking it, Boswell mounted a defence of Kennedy's mixture. 'It is amazing', he recorded in his journal, 'to see a man of Sir John's character so impregnated with partiality as to refuse its just credit to a medicine which has undoubtedly done wonders'. Boswell noted that Pringle had been equally 'prejudiced' against Keyser's pills, another remedy for venereal disease that he had mooted taking. Boswell wanted to believe that self-interest underlay the doctors' distrust of such proprietary cures. As early as 20 January 1763, when being treated by Douglas, he had reflected his doubts. Douglas was his 'friend'; yet he behaved not as a friend, but in the 'opposite character' of a surgeon, 'Douglas as a surgeon will be as ready to keep me long under his hands, and as desirous to lay hold of my money, as any man.'

Matrimony did not put a conclusion to the clap, and subsequent attacks saw Boswell often consulting Pringle and Douglas, who, despite being orthodox, by now had his own personal injection fluid ('a secret known to only a few'). But by this stage — maybe less sanguine about the doctors, or simply feeling that intimate familiarity had made him an expert — Boswell also took to self-medication, something probably connected with reading in 1786 John HUNTER's (p 398) *Treatise on the venereal disease.* Boswell modified his views in course of time. As with whores, so with cures, Boswell tried them all. Here, Boswell's eminence, his contacts, and the fact that he was a compulsive recorder of his own experiences, enable us to piece together a scene of the medical jigsaw all too often lost.

### Effect of gout

Studying the ailments of the great is also fascinating because it provokes speculations as to how far the diseases of the great have changed the course of history. The Ottoman leader, Bajazet, was deterred by an attack of gout from marching into central Europe; upon this, Edward Gibbon (himself a sufferer) observed in his *Decline and fall of the Roman Empire* that 'an acrimonious humour falling on a single fibre of one man may prevent or suspend the misery of nations'. In 1920, King Alexander of Greece died from the bite of his pet monkey. His death triggered a series of events that led Churchill, obviously recalling Gibbon, to comment that 'a quarter of a million persons died of this monkey bite'. Others would, of course, counter that it is not the accidents of the individual but grand impersonal forces that are the true agents of historical change. Had Lenin not died prematurely in 1924, following three strokes, Stalinist totalitarianism would not have been averted; rather, it would now be known as 'Leninist'.

Not least, the diseases of the famous entice attention because they provoke questions as to how far the personalities and careers of notable people were affected by such ailments and infirmities. It has been suggested, for instance, that on his later voyages James Cook (who successfully ensured adequate vitamin C for his sailors) was suffering from serious dietary deficiencies: WORMS may have deprived him of niacin and thiamin. To these have been attributed an increased tetchiness and failure of judgement that may have precipitated the series of blunders that led to his death at the hands of the Hawaiians in 1779.

Even with extremely conspicuous and often well-documented individuals, it is often hard to formulate a retrospective diagnosis upon their illnesses and cause of death, to say nothing of the possible effect of ailments upon their lives and minds. Despite the spilling of a vast amount of ink, there is absolutely no agreement as to the cause of Mozart's death; kidney disease and heart disease are widely suggested, but some still believe that he was poisoned, perhaps by the rival composer, Salieri. Both Friedrich Nietzsche and Robert Schumann died insane, but autopsies did not clearly establish the causes of their conditions. Although it is widely assumed, there is no convincing proof that Nietzsche's growing paralysis was the long-term aftermath of a syphilitic infection picked up from prostitutes (although Nietzsche himself seems to have given currency to this view).

In many cases, confusion seems to proliferate rather than to become resolved. Undoubtedly Charles DARWIN (p 214) suffered, in the last 50 years of his life, from seriously debilitating conditions, including headache, vomiting, dyspepsia, nausea, lassitude, palpitations, and other nervous afflictions. Some historians and biographers believe his condition was organic, perhaps the consequence of Chagas's disease, contracted from a bite from an insect, *Triatoma infestans*, suffered while on the pampas in South America, or perhaps the result of self-dosing with proprietary medicines containing arsenic. Other psychobiographers suggest that Darwin's malady was essentially psychogenic. Some have argued that the morbidly oversensitive Darwin never successfully mourned the early death of his mother. Others believe that the strain of developing the scandalous theory of evolution by natural selection precipitated nervous collapse. Still others suggest that Darwin's invalidism, whatever its cause, was an instance of 'creative malady', a disorder not too serious to preclude work but sufficient to protect the naturalist from official appointments and other interruptions and calls on his time. Indeed, no small number of eminent people have probably been the beneficiaries of such therapeutic 'creative maladies' — Florence NIGHTINGALE (p 548), for instance, who took to her bed soon after her return from the Crimea, and exercised power during the rest of her extremely long life as an invalid whose malady was never satisfactorily diagnosed.

Certain disorders have long been seen as top people's diseases. At least since the Renaissance, gout (as William HEBERDEN (p 628) noted) was viewed as a mark of good living and fine pedigree (it was regarded as a hereditary disorder). 'Gout is the distemper of a gentleman', insisted Lord Chesterfield, 'whereas the rheumatism is the distemper of a hackney coachman'. The great English clinician, Thomas SYDENHAM (p 721), himself a sufferer, noted of gout, 'what is a consolation to me, and may be so to other *gouty* persons of small fortunes and slender abilities, is that kings, great princes, generals, admirals, philosophers and several other great men have thus lived and died'. In *Bleak house*, Dickens' old county baronet, Sir Leicester Dedlock, reflects that 'all the Dedlocks in the direct male line through a course of time during and beyond which the memory of man goeth not to the contrary, have had the gout'. Gout was widely seen as one of the 'diseases of civilization' — others included hypochondria, nervous disorders, and neurasthenia — that supposedly occurred disproportionately in wealthy rather than poor nations, in the upper rather than the lower classes, and especially amongst gentlemen and ladies of talent, sensibility, and imagination.

Associations between eminence and sickness were particularly stimulated by the theory of the 'mad genius'. Originating in Plato's concept of 'divine furor' and the Aristotelian notion of black bile (one of the HUMORS), the notion became popular in the Renaissance that geniuses were typically afflicted with melancholy. It required a malady of the soul to fire the imagination to that pitch of intensity and unworldliness required to produce great art or poetry, or indeed to be a distinguished religious prophet. In his *Lives of the artists*, Vasari noted the oddities of many of the distinguished painters of the Renaissance. Much

was later made of the idiosyncrasies of Sir Isaac NEWTON (p 544) as a typical absent-minded scientist. The 'mad poet' appeared in Georgian England with William Collins, Kit Smart, William Cowper, and William Blake, rather as the 'mad king' appeared with George III in Britian and Christian VII in Denmark. Many early 19th century Romantics positively celebrated the idea that it was the artist's fate to soar spiritually only at the cost of physical decomposition and a premature death. TUBERCULOSIS and SYPHILIS became the fashionable disorders of Romantic and Bohemian intellectuals and artists (Keats, Chopin, Schubert, Baudelaire, Flaubert, the Brothers Goncourt, Alphonse Daudet, and so on).

Two new twists were added to these concepts around the turn of the 20th century. On the one hand, 'degenerationist' psychiatrists, notably followers of Cesare Lombroso, began to suspect the sanity of almost anyone eminent in the arts. And, at the same time, FREUD's (p 321) investigations of the workings of the unconscious claimed to confirm that there was something neurotic about the urge to produce great art, and furthermore cast suspicion upon the very urge to greatness, leadership, and power. Freud's study of LEONARDO (p 40) implied that his artistic creativity arose from sexual confusion, which had its roots in immature homosexual tendencies; and his investigation of Woodrow Wilson seemed to attribute the American President's need to exercise power to unresolved personal and sexual tensions with his father. The one-time colleague of Freud, Alfred ADLER (p 675), focused his attentions upon the psychopathology of power, and Wilhelm Reich analyzed fascism as a form of megalomania. Over the past 50 years, there has been a plethora of studies purporting to explain the public careers of politicians, statesmen, generals, artists, and media stars in terms of their supposed unhappy childhoods, sexual inadequacies, neurotic disorders, or physical defects. Eminent people, nevertheless, remain willing to expose themselves in the psychiatrist's chair, perhaps revealing that the chief disorder of famous people is exhibitionism.    RPor

*See also* DEGENERATION; 'ROYAL MADNESS' AND PORPHYRIA

**PEDIATRICS** See CHILD HEALTH

**PENNSYLVANIA, THE MEDICAL COLLEGE OF** See USA

Thomas **PERCIVAL** (1740–1804). British health reformer and ethicist. Educated at Edinburgh and then a prominent member of the Manchester Industrial and Philosophical Society, he holds an important place in the history of epidemiology for his analysis of the Bills of Mortality from 1772–6, and for his code of medical ethics. The latter was initially circulated privately as a book on jurisprudence in 1794 and as a result of solicited comments from colleagues then published in an expanded form with a change in title to *Medical ethics* in 1803. Percival had been asked by the Manchester Royal Infirmary to help with an internal dispute and became particularly concerned with the divisions that had arisen among the different branches of the profession — the physicians, surgeons, and apothecaries with their different backgrounds of training (university, hospital, and apprenticeship respectively). But he did not merely concern himself with intraprofessional relationships: he also laid down a code for conduct towards patients, whether rich or poor, and his ideas were rapidly taken up by the USA, Australia, and Canada — in fact, the ethical code introduced by the newly formed American Medical Association in 1847 used several passages taken directly from his book.

**PHARMACEUTICAL INDUSTRY** The pharmaceutical industry manufactures substances used for medical treatment — especially medicines, but also vaccines, artificial foods, disinfectants, and other ancillary materials. Its products are sold to governments for health services and through wholesale distributors to pharmacies and other shops. In developed countries, medicines are subject to extensive controls. Many can be obtained only on prescription by doctors, while the sale of others is restricted to registered pharmacies. These restrictions have a major influence on the trading practices of the industry.

Until about 1600, medicines were supplied by local collectors and tradesmen. Then explorers brought new materials from the New World and the Orient, some of them with medicinal reputations. Many exotic remedies became available, and businesses were set up to trade in them. Some prospered and others did not. All relied on raw materials produced at home or imported by traders and on public demand, focused through physicians, apothecaries, and direct requests for self-medication.

The science of chemistry advanced rapidly in the 19th century, and was applied to the isolation of pure, potent drugs from, mostly, botanical sources. Commercial advantages were seen in supplying alkaloids and other purified products,

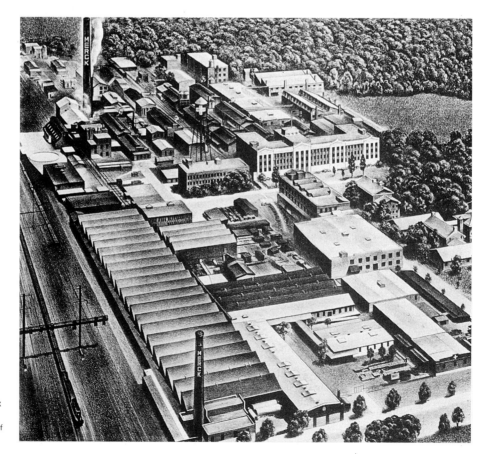

The Merck industrial complex in New Jersey. (Lithograph by Louis Lozowick/National Library of Medicine, Bethesda, MD.)

and individual firms set up laboratories to undertake such work.

At the same time, the Industrial Revolution created large businesses, which began to take advantage of scientific progress in heavy chemicals, and gradually in more refined products — including dyestuffs, which began to be made synthetically. Many substances never previously known now existed, and some were discovered, by accident or deliberate trial, to be medicinally useful. So a market was developed for purely synthetic drugs as well as chemically purified 'natural' products. An industry was born with mixed parentage, partly from purely chemical firms and partly from the more innovative of the traditional medicine suppliers.

### German lead

The first major pharmaceutical firms developed in Germany, largely as a consequence of a German lead in applying the results of research in chemistry. H. E. Merck of Darmstadt, inheritor of a pharmaceutical family business founded in 1668, worked with and was inspired by the famous chemist Justus von Liebig to set up a small laboratory in his own business. He adopted the newly discovered methods of purifying morphine and other alkaloids and produced them on a commercial scale. The business flourished, and in 1900 established a branch in New York, which was separated from the parent firm when America entered the First World War in 1917. Many years later it merged with another company to form a leading pharmaceutical company, Merck Sharp and Dohme in New Jersey. Other German firms, including Hoechst and Bayer, both later absorbed into I. G. Farben, started as chemical businesses and developed pharmaceutical divisions later.

In Switzerland both J. R. Geigy (1758) and E. Sandoz (1886) were manufacturers of aniline dyes, and turned to making drugs only because of wartime needs, Sandoz in 1919 and Geigy in 1940. Ciba was formed by a merger of smaller firms in 1884, and Hoffmann La Roche (1896) was concerned with pharmaceuticals from its beginning.

In Britain the old established London drug firm of Allen and Hanbury (1715) remained well known after most of its contemporaries disappeared, but was ultimately absorbed by Glaxo Laboratories. Jesse Boot, of Nottingham, expanded his mother's 'Household Stores' to deal with patent medicines. He formed a limited company in 1883, manufacturing for and supplying the public from his own shops. A new business was established in London in 1880 by two young American pharmacists, Silas Burroughs and Henry WELLCOME (p 316), notable for setting up research laboratories in chemistry, physiology, and later tropical medicine. A branch was established in New York and became a second

headquarters of what ultimately became a worldwide group of companies, deeply engaged in research as well as production.

In 1907, 'drugs, medicines, and medicinal preparations' accounted for about one fifth of the selling value of the British chemical industry. By 1924, the output of the industry had more than doubled and with a larger proportion medicinal. During this period Glaxo Laboratories evolved from the New Zealand business of Joseph Nathan & Co., and initially specialized in milk products for infants ('Glaxo builds bonny babies'). It was innovative in preparing vitamin D and supplying it as a dietary supplement. The research activities expanded, and ultimately Glaxo acquired Burroughs Wellcome and became Glaxo Wellcome. The major British chemical firm Imperial Chemical Industries did not become involved with drugs until the Second World War, when pharmaceuticals were developed from the dyestuffs division. Among other activities, an important program was developed for inventing antimalarial drugs. ICI Pharmaceutical flourished, and ultimately became the separate company Zeneca.

In North America, as in Europe, the pharmaceutical industry grew partly from firms which supplied simple medicines and then embarked on larger scale manufacture (for example, Smith Kline in Philadelphia, 1830; Eli Lilley in Indianapolis, 1876) or from businesses primarily interested in chemical manufacture (such as Charles Pfizer in Brooklyn in 1849 to manufacture fine chemicals; E. R. Squibb, also in Brooklyn, 1858, to manufacture ether, which was suddenly in demand when general anesthesia became widespread). In 2000 two new giants were created by the merger of Glaxo Wellcome with Smithkline Beecham and Pfizer with Warner-Lambert.

Wherever medicines are prepared, the quality of the product is very important. Remedies made from natural sources vary greatly according to the season in which they are collected and the care with which they are handled and stored. Distinguishing good from weak, decayed, or substituted material is a job for an expert. Remedies of known chemical composition are easier to define precisely but not necessarily easier to purify and free from unwanted, sometimes damaging, ingredients. To produce high quality medicines is expensive, and commercial pressures for corner cutting and short-term gains can have serious consequences.

The most reputable firms set up laboratories simply to control the quality of their products. Such laboratories were also useful to assess the stability of products, and to find ways of improving their appearance and ease of administration. Development was gradually separated from quality control. Less reputable firms produced remedies more cheaply, and showed more interest in their profits than their products. Their activities, particularly in the United States, brought discredit on the industry and had much to do with the introduction of legislative controls on the goods supplied.

In the last quarter of the 19th century the practice of medicine was deeply altered by discoveries leading to the 'germ theory of disease' and associated new ideas about how diseases might be prevented or cured. The first therapeutic material to result from these theories and discoveries was diphtheria antitoxin. As soon as it was shown to save lives, the demand for it grew. Facilities for its production in hospitals or academic laboratories on such a scale simply did not exist. Especially in the United States, the public health departments of certain large cities undertook a manufacturing process (which required a large stable of horses to be inoculated and bled for the serum which contained antitoxin, or did not if the horses were not responsive enough), but the difficulties of such extensive innovation within the confines of a social service were overwhelming. American firms (H. K. Mulford in Philadelphia and Parke Davis in Detroit) embarked on antitoxin production, and in Britain Henry Wellcome used the physiological research laboratory as a base for its development and production.

Use of live animals and manipulating their immune responses presented unfamiliar problems to a predominantly chemical industry, and promptly involved severe conflicts with some public opinions, and with naturally cautious government. The need, particularly for effective treatment for diphtheria, prevailed, and its production paved the way to other biological activities within the industry. When insulin was isolated from dog pancreas by BANTING (p 236) and BEST (p 236) in Toronto in 1923, the alert research director of Eli Lilley recognized that production of insulin was soon going to be needed urgently. He acted vigorously so that his firm was in a pre-eminent position to obtain adequate supplies of bovine pancreas and to manufacture the new medicine, vital for the survival of diabetics.

The pattern of following academic developments and undertaking the development and production of new remedies at the right time remains an important aspect of the industry. But increasingly the industry developed its own more basic research laboratories. A great future lay in finding out if any of the chemical substances, newly synthesized in a firm's laboratories, might become useful medicines. Direct testing on man or woman of substances with unknown properties was unacceptably hazardous. Experiments, often known as screens, involving animals or parts of animals, became an essential, extensive, and expensive part of the research activity. Such methods had already

been used by the great immunologist and pharmacologist Paul EHRLICH (p 260). They resulted in 1910 in the discovery of the first potent drug active against SYPHILIS, named salvarsan, and have led to many later discoveries.

Much ingenuity, combined with a detailed knowledge of pharmacology, has been spent on designing compounds for a particular purpose, such as curing pneumonia or malaria, preventing heart failure, or achieving any other desirable result. An early success produced safe local anesthetics, which replaced cocaine, then the most effective agent but liable to cause sudden death. After years of discouragement, new antibacterial agents were found, especially (at the time) the outstandingly important sulfonamides. Of these, 'M & B 693' (sulfapyridine) was perhaps the most famous, partly because it was used to treat Winston Churchill's pneumonia in 1943. During the 1950s very many new drugs were identified by synthesizing and screening and were introduced into medical practice. But the problems of adequate assessment of safety of the remedies introduced were not clearly appreciated.

### Drug tragedies

Tragedies, sometimes related to technical errors in production of particular drugs, occurred from time to time, but the hazards of unforeseen toxicity to patients were underestimated both inside and outside the industry. The new drug THALIDOMIDE, introduced in the late 1950s as a safe hypnotic, was discovered, too late, to cause severe damage to the fetus when taken at a certain stage of pregnancy. No regular system existed for notifying and recording centrally the occurrence of fetal abnormalities, so many isolated cases occurred before the epidemic was identified and the cause investigated. The large number of cases and the tragedy for each individual caused deep and widespread concern, exacerbated by attempts of the original manufacturer to conceal information about early cases.

It became increasingly clear that animal tests, though essential, did not provide complete assurance of safety, and that surveillance for some years at least of all new drugs brought into clinical use was as essential as the precautions necessary when they were introduced. For a decade, both industry and government became more concerned with the safety of medicines than with any further advances in discovery of new drugs, and obsession with safety testing delayed the introduction of numerous remedies, some of life-saving value.

Throughout the 20th century, the overall picture of the industry was one of growth and amalgamation. Any new medicine, especially one for a familiar disorder, is likely to have a world-wide market. The profits from even a single new medicine may be very large indeed, enough to have a major influence on a firm's prospects. Profits depend greatly on patent rights, and on the skill and luck of competitors in their own research. Some are absorbed in recouping unrewarding research expenditure and in financing future research, which has become increasingly expensive, but without which a firm may fail to maintain a substantial part of its business. All these factors have driven the industry to make international agreements or mergers, creating a few very large companies and many smaller ones, which confine themselves to uninnovative manufacturing.

The basic problem remains, how can the industry judge its own products? Purity is quite distinct from efficacy — does the medicine actually do any good? — and safety — does it do any harm, even when it is used correctly? A pharmaceutical manufacturer is well equipped to guarantee the purity of its product, but needs medical collaboration to justify claims of safety and therapeutic virtue. The market for pharmaceuticals depends entirely on their use for therapeutic purposes, and success in the business requires such claims to be made. So pharmaceutical firms developed clinical research divisions, often very large, staffed by physicians specially trained both in clinical pharmacology and in the difficult problems of evaluating the efficacy and the safety of remedies.

The science of evaluating medicines has developed greatly. Methods for detecting adverse effects are much improved, but are still far from perfect. Assessment of the effectiveness of medicines is often problematical and commercial opportunism in promoting medicines is consequently difficult to restrain. The tension between therapeutic judgement and commercial efficiency has been moderated but has not disappeared, and the industry still has to balance with the utmost care procedures which are commercially acceptable with those which are ethically tolerable.                      MWea

*See also* ANTIBIOTICS AND ANTI-INFECTIVE DRUGS; DIABETES MELLITUS

## PHARMACOLOGY, CLINICAL PHARMACOLOGY, AND THERAPEUTICS Pharmacology is
the scientific study of the effects of chemical substances on living systems. The chemicals which pharmacologists investigate include normal constituents of the body, compounds extracted from other animals or plants, as well as substances synthesized by chemists. Clinical pharmacology is the study of the effects of drugs in man, especially those which might lead to therapeutic benefits or adverse effects. Therapeutics is the branch of medicine concerned with the treatment of disease. Rational therapeutics uses chemicals to counteract, or reverse, the effects of those pathological processes which cause disease and is based

on the disciplines of pharmacology, clinical pharmacology, and toxicology.

When a chemical is to be used as a drug the Pharmacopoeial Commission assigns a trivial name, which is chosen for its relative simplicity, its resemblance to the scientific name, and its chemical origins. These names such as paracetamol for the chemical *N*-acetyl *para*-aminophenol and aspirin for the chemical acetylsalicylic acid, are known as 'generic' names or 'non-proprietary' names. The pharmaceutical company which sells the drug frequently does so under a 'proprietary' or 'brand' name, which is a registered trademark and the property of the company. As such, a drug will have only one 'generic' name but may have several different 'brand' names.

### Historical development
For thousands of years, rational therapeutics was based on either logic or empiricism. Where physicians claimed knowledge of the cause of a particular disease, and where they believed (usually on theoretical grounds) that a substance could reverse the disease process, they applied the remedy — logically — as a treatment. Alternatively, where (by chance) a remedy was observed — empirically — to exert a favorable outcome in patients with a particular condition, other patients with the same disease were given the treatment in anticipation of a similarly favorable outcome.

In general, neither of these approaches produced medicines of much clinical value. Until the 19th century, beliefs about the causes and nature of disease were at best simplistic, and often theological or metaphysical rather than biological, so that the 'logical' approach to therapeutics was usually flawed. The 'empirical' method also suffered from serious defects because the natural history of many conditions was so poorly understood that spontaneous remissions were frequently mistaken for therapeutic success. It is hardly surprising, therefore, that many of the remedies used by Egyptian, Greek, Roman, and Arab physicians were at best useless and at worst harmful. Even the great advances in medical sciences after the Renaissance failed to be paralleled by substantial progress in pharmacology and therapeutics. Nevertheless, some pharmacologically active substances were known to ancient civilizations even though they were used indiscriminately. They included copper salts as an emetic, castor oil as a purgative, and opium as an analgesic and hypnotic.

Modern therapeutics dates largely from the work of the Birmingham physician William WITHERING (this page). He learned of the virtues of the foxglove (*Digitalis purpurea*), in treating heart failure, from an old Shropshire lady. Rather than use this 'empirical' treatment indiscrim-

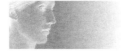
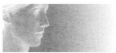

*(continued)*

**Oswald SCHMIEDEBERG**
(1838–1921). German pharmacologist. One of the earliest and greatest of German pharmacologists, he had many distinguished pupils including J. J. Abel and A. R. Cushny. He showed the vagus to contain accelerator fibers (1871); extracted muscarine from *Amanita muscaria* (1869); carried out important studies on digitalis (1883); and deduced the formula of nucleic acid (1896).

inately he embarked on a series of clinical studies with the drug — a crude preparation of digitalis glycosides — which culminated in the publication of his pharmacological classic *Account of the foxglove* in 1776. Digitalis (either as digoxin or digitoxin) is still widely used today: but its therapeutic propeties, and adverse effects, were carefully documented by Withering over 200 years ago.

The advances in pharmacology since Withering's time are in stark contrast to the slender progress made during the preceding 3000 years. Four influences have made this possible. First, the development of chemistry in the 19th century, and of biotechnology in the latter part of the 20th century, have allowed the preparation of a range of new compounds in pure form. Secondly, the increased understanding of human biology has provided pharmacologists with a framework for studying the effects of chemicals on living systems. Thirdly, knowledge of the origins and basis of disease has encouraged pharmacologists and physicians to seek ways of reversing pathological processes by chemical means. Finally, the techniques of experimental therapeutics have permitted the rigorous evaluation of new medicines prior to their introduction as routine forms of treatment.

### Basis of drug action

The two fundamental mechanisms by which drugs produce pharmacological effects are either by binding to specific cellular targets including receptors, ion channels, and enzymes, or by their physico-chemical/physical effects.

*Cellular targets* Many drugs, as well as those chemicals which are mediators of physiological processes within the body including neurotransmitters and hormones, produce their effects by interacting with specific and discrete cellular components known as receptors. These large proteins are located either within the membrane or the nucleus of the cell. Upon binding to a receptor, a compound which initiates a train of events resulting in a characteristic response such as muscle contraction or glandular secretion is known as an agonist.

By contrast, an antagonist binds to a receptor but in doing so does not stimulate the tissue. Drugs which act as agonists mimic the action of endogenous substances and examples include the anti-ASTHMA drug, salbutamol and the analgesics codeine and morphine. Antagonists produce their effects by displacing naturally occurring agonists and thus prevent the action of the latter. Examples of drug receptor antagonists include the anti-ulcer drug ranitidine, which antagonizes the endogenous transmitter substance histamine, and the anticancer agent, tamoxifen, which antagonizes endogenous estrogens.

One of the most important observations in modern pharmacology is that receptors which are specific for a particular endogenous chemical mediator may also be tissue specific or functionally specific. Subpopulations of almost all endogenous transmitter substance receptors have now been identified either by the use of specific agonists and antagonists and more recently with the use of molecular biological techniques. Such knowledge enables the development of ever more functionally specific drugs.

The transport of ions across cell membranes is mediated by two kinds of ion channels, ligand-operated and voltage-operated. Whereas the former represent a type of receptor to which an agonist binds to initiate an opening of the channel, the voltage-operated ion channels open in response to a change in electrical potential. Some drugs produce their effects by facilitating the action of the endogenous agonist at the ligand operated ion channel. For example, the anxiolytic/ sedative compound diazepam enables the neurotransmitter gamma aminobutyric acid (GABA) to open the chloride ion channel associated with GABA receptors. In contrast, local anesthetic agents block voltage-operated sodium ion channels in nerve cell membranes to prevent the conduction of nervous impulses from the site of administration of the local anesthetic to the central nervous system.

The formation and breakdown of most body components are catalysed by proteins known as enzymes. Many important therapeutic agents are enzyme inhibitors and thus prevent their normal action. Inhibition of the formation of biologically active substances within the body provides the basis for the action of aspirin and the other 'non-steroidal anti-inflammatory drugs (NSAIDs)'. Such drugs inhibit the enzyme cyclo-oxygenase, which is involved in the formation of a family of chemicals known as eicosanoids. Since these chemical mediators participate in the processes of inflammation, pain, and fever, inhibition of their synthesis by non-steroidal anti-inflammary drugs reduces these symptoms.

*Physico-chemical/physical effects* Some drugs exert their effects as a consequence of their physicochemical properties. For example, alkali mixtures containing sodium bicarbonate or aluminum hydroxide will chemically neutralize excess acid in the stomach and in so doing relieve the pain of gastric ulceration. Many commonly used therapeutic agents produce their effect by their physical action alone. Thus substances such as ispaghula husk and lactulose, which passively alter the volume and consistency of feces, are used to treat constipation.

## Drug handling

The intensity and duration of effect of many drugs depend upon their handling within the body, which in turn is regulated by the processes of absorption, distribution, excretion, and metabolism.

*Absorption* Most drugs are given by mouth and must pass through the stomach before undergoing absorption in the upper small intestine. Intestinal absorption of most drugs occurs by simple diffusion across the mucosal lining of the gut. From the gut, drugs are transported in the hepatic portal vein to the liver and then into the systemic circulation.

*Distribution* Once in the bloodstream, drugs are distributed, to a greater or lesser extent, to various tissues and organs. The degree to which drugs penetrate individual organs and cells is governed by many factors including the chemical properties of the drug, the structural characteristics of the tissue, and its blood supply. Penetration of drugs into the brain is restricted by 'tight junctions' between cells lining the cerebral blood vessels, and only those compounds which are sufficiently soluble in the lipid membrane of this so-called 'blood–brain barrier' are capable of producing pharmacological effects in the central nervous system.

*Elimination* Once drugs are circulating, various physiological processes act to eliminate them from the body. Most are eliminated either by renal excretion or by metabolism.

*Renal excretion* Some drugs are excreted in unchanged form from the kidneys, but the rate of renal elimination varies for different drugs. However, provided that renal function is normal, the rate of renal excretion of a particular drug shows little variation between individuals.

In the presence of renal disease, renal drug excretion rates fall, half-lives become longer and, as a consequence, higher blood levels and more intense pharmacological effects (including adverse reactions) may occur. Thus if toxicity is to be avoided in patients with reduced renal function, it is necessary to reduce the dosages of drugs undergoing renal excretion. The immature kidney of the newborn infant, and the normal decline in renal function which occurs with advancing years also renders the very young and the elderly susceptible to drug toxicity.

*Metabolism* Most drugs used in clinical practice are lipid-soluble and must undergo metabolism in the liver to water-soluble degradation products (metabolites) before they can be excreted in the urine. Often these metabolites are pharmacologically inactive and drug metabolism is therefore regarded as a detoxication mechanism. There are exceptions, however, and some drugs (prodrugs) require metabolism to be pharmacologically active, others are converted to metabolites which show greater pharmacological (and sometimes toxicological) activity than the parent compound.

Although a wide variety of drug metabolic pathways exist, metabolism has been divided broadly into two phases, I and II. The former consists of 'functionalization' reactions, in which a functional group is introduced into or unmasked in the drug molecule. This chemical group then provides a 'handle' for the phase II 'conjugation' reaction. Conjugates are almost always pharmacologically inactive and sufficiently water-soluble to be excreted by the kidney.

There are appreciable interindividual variations in the rates at which people metabolize drugs via specific pathways of biotransformation. Among healthy individuals these are largely due to both genetic and environmental factors, but are also influenced by gender and age. It may be difficult to predict how liver or other major organ disease may affect the ability of a person to metabolize a particular drug, especially when that person is ill. Where the margin between therapeutic failure (due to a relative underdosage) and toxicity (due to a relative overdosage) is large, such differences may be important only for a few individuals lying at the extremes of metabolism. Where the margin of safety is small, special steps must be taken to ensure therapeutic efficacy or safety.

## Scientific basis of therapeutics

It is now almost universally accepted that before a drug is brought into routine use its efficacy, safety, and the balance between the two (sometimes called the 'risk-to-benefit ratio') need to be formally demonstrated.

*Efficacy* The efficacy of new drugs is, nowadays, almost invariably established with a technique known as the RANDOMIZED CONTROLLED TRIAL. This method for assessing a drug's efficacy aims to eliminate bias and involves the random allocation of patients with a particular disorder, and who are reasonably alike in their relevant characteristics, to two (or more) groups. One (the 'test') group receives the study drug, and other groups receive either an inert 'placebo', an established 'active comparator', or both. The outcomes of the patients in each group are then compared statistically.

*Safety* Unwanted and unintended effects of medicines, occurring under normal conditions of use, are known as adverse drug reactions or (incorrectly) side-effects. All medicines have the potential to cause ADVERSE DRUG REACTIONS, at least in some people, and they belong to one of two types:

*Type A reactions* are the exaggerated, but otherwise predictable, pharmacological actions of a drug. Examples include low blood pressure in patients taking antihypertensive medication, or a hangover after a hypnotic. They occur either because of an increased sensitivity of the particular organ where the drug acts, or because the patient 'handles' the drug in an unusual manner. People who metabolize, or excrete, a drug more slowly than normal will be at particular risk. Many, if not most, patients with Type A adverse reactions can be managed by an appropriate reduction in the dose of the drug.

*Type B reactions* are bizarre responses that are totally unrelated to a drug's normal pharmacological profile. Examples include rashes with antibiotics or liver damage with anti-tuberculous drugs. They are often unpredictable, and few can be reproduced in experimental animals. Many Type B reactions have an immunological or genetic basis, with potentially serious outcomes, and their occurrence is usually an indication to stop taking the drug. Fortunately Type B reactions are generally uncommon.

The principal difficulty posed by adverse drug reactions, both in individuals and in the community at large, is their prediction and detection. Almost all mimic some naturally occurring disease and attribution therefore requires considerable expertise. Type A reactions are most easily recognized because they manifest themselves as an exaggeration of the normal pharmacological profile of the drug. Indeed, many can be prevented if the patient possesses features that are likely to predispose to their development. The elderly, for example, are particularly vulnerable to certain Type A reactions and these may usually be avoided by prescribing lower doses than those given to younger people. Type B reactions pose a greater difficulty. Liver damage due to a drug, for example, is often difficult to distinguish from other causes of liver damage (such as viral hepatitis) and, in the absence of any specific tests, the diagnosis may be made only by excluding other causes.

A causal relationship is made more likely if the suspected adverse drug reaction (such as liver damage) resolves on withdrawing the drug but in this instance it has to be remembered that most forms of viral hepatitis also resolve spontaneously. A positive 're-challenge' (a return of the reaction when the drug is re-instituted) is often regarded as the ultimate diagnostic test, but such a step is rarely in the best interests of the patient and is seldom undertaken.

Common (usually Type A) reactions may be recognized during randomized controlled trials. Investigators record all adverse medical events (including suspected adverse drug reactions, in both control and test groups: an increase in the frequency of particular symptoms or laboratory tests among patients treated with the test drug strongly suggests an adverse reaction). Rarer reactions are more difficult to identify, and practical limitations on the numbers of patients who can be enrolled into randomized controlled trials mean that adverse reactions occurring in 1 in 1000 or less will be detected only by other means. Indeed, less common adverse reactions can generally be detected only during widespread use, and the study of the safety of marketed medicines is now referred to as 'pharmacovigilance'. Three main pharmacovigilance methods are available:

*Spontaneous reporting schemes* Most developed countries have systems whereby doctors (and other health professionals) are asked to report suspected adverse drug reactions they encounter during routine clinical practice. In Britain it is known as the 'yellow card' system (because of the color of the reporting card). The scheme has proved invaluable in identifying possible adverse reactions to particular drugs but, because of under-reporting, and its inherent biases, it often has to be complemented by other approaches.

*Case-control studies* In this method the frequency of use of a particular drug, among patients with a suspected adverse drug reaction (the 'cases'), is compared with the frequency of use in a group of patients without it (the 'controls'). The method is especially suitable for studying rarer, but important, adverse drug reactions such as blood clots in women taking oral contraceptives or hormone replacement therapy.

*Cohort studies* This approach involves studying the fate of patients taking a particular drug, with those who have not, during routine clinical practice. As with case-control studies, however, considerable care needs to be taken to eliminate potential sources of bias.

**Risk versus benefit** It is self-evident that patients should, on average, be better off taking a particular drug than not. It is obvious, therefore, that a drug should be used only to treat a particular condition if it has been shown to be effective. Furthermore, these benefits should have been shown to outweigh the risks of treatment. In the management of otherwise lethal conditions randomized controlled trials may show whether there is favorable balance. In many situations, though, the balance is more difficult to strike and the severity of the disease will inevitably influence the degree of risk that patients can be expected to accept. Thus, for drugs merely providing symptomatic relief for self-limiting conditions (such as the common cold, or a sprained ankle), the degree of acceptable risk will be very small.

## Development of new drugs

Once potential new therapeutic agents have been developed in the laboratory, they undergo further extensive (and expensive) development.

*Preclinical studies* Before new drugs are given to humans they are subjected to detailed toxicological study in experimental animals. The purpose is to eliminate those agents that are likely to pose particular hazards if given to volunteers or patients. They may be expected to identify most Type A adverse drug reactions but they are of little value in predicting Type B reactions.

*Clinical studies* Clinical studies with new drugs involve three phases:

*Phase 1* Single doses of the new drug are given to patients or, more usually, healthy volunteers. The primary purposes are to confirm whether the pharmacological effects seen in animals also occur in man and, if so, at what dose. In the first human experiments very small doses are given to start with. The dose is then gradually increased until the estimated therapeutic level has been reached.

*Phase 2* A preliminary examination of a drug's efficacy is made to define the optimum dose. Such studies generally take the form of randomized, placebo-controlled trials comparing efficacy (and safety) at various dose levels. They usually involve 200 to 500 patients.

*Phase 3* Investigation of the new drug's performance in a larger population often in comparison with existing treatments. Studies are conducted as randomized controlled trials with continuing emphasis on both efficacy and safety. The results of such studies are critical in evaluating the new drug's risk-to-benefit ratio.

If the national drug regulatory authority (such as the Medicines Control Agency in Britain, or the FOOD AND DRUGS ADMINISTRATION in the USA) is satisfied that the drug is of satisfactory quality, is effective in the conditions for which it is to be promoted, and relatively safe, the manufacturer will be granted permission to place it on the market. Even then the assessment of a new drug's safety can only be provisional and a period of intense *postmarketing surveillance* begins. The methods adopted will invariably include careful scrutiny of 'yellow card' reports of suspected adverse drug reactions by both the manufacturer and the national regulatory authority, and may involve the use of other methods if these are warranted. A small proportion (around 3%) of new drugs are withdrawn for safety reasons within a year or two of marketing.

## Conclusions

Therapeutics has been revolutionized by the new drugs introduced over the past fifty years. The explosion in biological knowledge and understanding promises that the next fifty years will see no less a revolution.　　　　　MDR

*See also* ADVERSE DRUG REACTIONS; MISADVENTURES

**PHARMACY** is concerned with the preparation and dispensing of medicines. The word comes from the Greek *pharmakeus* meaning druggist. Today, its scope extends from the scientific expertise of isolating and identifying drugs, and knowing their actions and uses, to the social and behavioral skills involved in advising patients when and how to take them. The science and practice of pharmacy are now international, although enormous differences still remain in the numbers, training, and roles of pharmacists.

## Origins

Pharmacy is among the oldest of professions, and the earliest prescriptions, written by the Sumerians, date back to at least 2700 BC. The practitioners of healing at this time combined the roles of priest, pharmacist, and physician. Chinese pharmacy traces its origins to the emperor Shen Nung, in about 2000 BC, who investigated the medicinal value of several hundred herbs. The most important Egyptian pharmaceutical record is the EBERS PAPYRUS, of about 1500 BC, a collection of around 800 prescriptions. In Greece, Theophrastus, the father of botany, observed and wrote about the medicinal properties of herbs in about 300 BC.

The transition of pharmacy into a science received a major boost with the work of Dioscorides in the 1st century AD. He described how to collect, store, and use drugs, and his texts were considered basic science up to the 16th century. But the greatest influence on pharmacy was GALEN (p 324) (130–200 AD), who practiced and taught both pharmacy and medicine in Rome. His principles for preparing and compounding medicines remained dominant in the western world for 1500 years, and he gave his name to pharmaceuticals prepared by mechanical means (galenicals). Between the 5th and 12th centuries, western knowledge of both pharmacy and medicine was preserved in monasteries. Manuscripts from many countries were translated or copied, and the monks gathered herbs in the fields, or grew them in their own gardens.

The professions of apothecary and physician were differentiated by the Arabs, who established the first privately owned drug stores in Baghdad in the 8th century. They built on knowledge acquired from Greece and Rome, developing a

### PHARMACIST-EDITOR

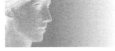

William **MARTINDALE** (1840–1902). London pharmacist. Martindale was president of the Pharmaceutical Society of Great Britain in 1899–1900, and compiled and edited the first edition of the *Extra pharmacopoeia*, published in 1883. Martindale's name has been perpetuated by its attachment to successive editions of this work, which has continued to provide a much valued reference source of information about the properties, actions, and uses of drugs and medicines. Martindale himself had been responsible for producing ten editions by his death, after which his medically qualified son William Harrison Martindale continued the family association until 1933. Subsequent editions have been produced by the Pharmaceutical Society of Great Britain. William Martindale was a practicing pharmacist, who became lecturer in pharmacy at University College Hospital, London, and who was the first pharmacist appointed to that institution (in 1868) to possess a statutory qualification in the subject. He later left to set up his own pharmacy in nearby New Cavendish Street.

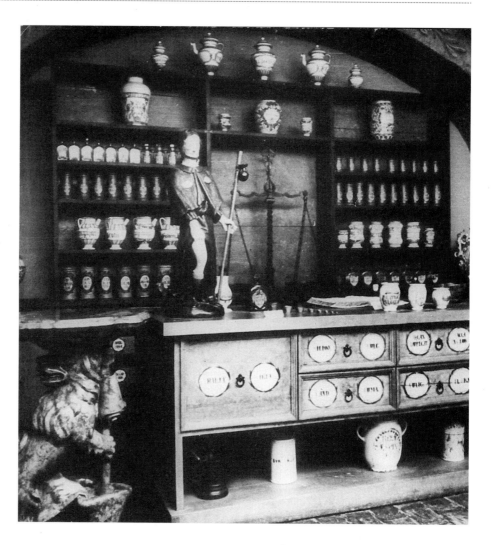

An 18th century pharmacy from Köszeg, Hungary, as displayed at the Semmelweis Museum of Medical History in Budapest. (Reproduced courtesy of the WHO/National Library of Medicine, Bethesda, MD.)

wide range of novel preparations, including medicinal syrups and alcoholic extracts. These new ideas became assimilated into the practice of pharmacy across western Europe following the Muslim advance across Africa, Spain, and southern France. One of the great contributors to the science of medicine and pharmacy during this period was the Persian Ibn Sina, known by the western world as AVICENNA (p 60). He wrote in Arabic, and his teachings were treated as authoritative in the West well into the 17th century. They remain dominant influences in some eastern countries to this day.

## Organization

In European countries exposed to Arab influence, pharmacy shops began to appear around the 11th century. Pharmacy first became legally separated from medicine about 1240 AD in Sicily and south-

ern Italy. Frederick II of Hohenstaufe, Emperor of Germany and King of Sicily, provided a link between the east and west. At his palace in Palermo he presented the first European edict separating pharmacists from physicians, and he laid down regulations for their professional practice.

In most European countries, the apothecary or pharmacist developed from pepperers and spicers. In France the *apothicaire* of the 14th to 18th centuries prepared medicines and administered clysters (enemas). As a result largely of the efforts of caricaturists, the word became associated with ridiculous, and in the 17th century the word *pharmacien* made its appearance. This became official with the establishment of the Collége de Pharmacie in 1777, which ushered in modern French pharmacy. During the 17th and 18th centuries many people in Europe passed the examinations for both pharmacy and medicine, and practiced both. In some countries, regional developments took place. In Italy, for example, Austrian regulations for the Lombardy district in 1778 provided the stimulus for changes in pharmacy practice in the north. But uniform arrangements were established across Italy only after the setting up of the new Italian Kingdom in 1870.

In Germany, pharmacists in Nuremberg formed themselves into a society as early as 1632. A regional organization for north Germany was formed in 1820, and for southern Germany in 1848. After the federation of German states these two societies amalgamated to form a national German pharmacists' society, the Deutscher Apothekerverein, in 1872. A few years later, in 1890, the Deutsche Pharmazeutische Gesellschaft was established to promote pharmaceutical science and research. In England, Wales, and Ireland, however, unlike other European countries, a profession based entirely on the art of pharmacy, with the objective of improving the professional and social standing of its members, did not exist before the 19th century; in Scotland, it did not exist before the 18th century.

In 1841 a large group of chemists and druggists in Britain joined with those apothecaries still practicing pharmacy to form the Pharmaceutical Society of Great Britain, with a view to improving standards of education and practice. The modern history of pharmacy in Britain may be traced from this time. Early American pharmacy was heavily influenced by immigrants from Europe. An Irish apothecary, Christopher Marshall, established the first such shop in Philadelphia in 1729. The American Pharmaceutical Association, open to 'all pharmaceutists and druggists of good character', was established in 1852.

## International pharmaceutical organizations

A long-standing dream of many pharmacists around the world had been the establishment of an international pharmacopeia, or book of standard medical ingredients and preparations. German pharmacists took the initiative to convene an international congress of pharmacy to exchange information and plan such a volume, but also to tackle the problems created by quackery and self-medication. This first congress took place in Brunswick, Germany, in 1865. International congresses continued to be held every few years in different countries. The International Pharmaceutical Federation (or Fédération Internationale Pharmaceutique), founded in 1911, has as its objective the development of pharmacy at an international level, both professionally and scientifically, and the extension of the role of the pharmacist in healthcare.

Although for most of its history pharmacy has focused on the drug rather than the patient, in recent decades professional organizations have promoted the benefits of having pharmacists, and of supporting the services they provide to patients. Internationally they have worked with the WORLD HEALTH ORGANIZATION in laying down minimum levels of pharmaceutical services, and in defining the education and training of pharmacists. Today, many pharmaceutical organizations exist to support and promote the role of the pharmacist, and to assist colleagues elsewhere. The Commonwealth Pharmaceutical Association, for example, based in London, organizes an annual pharmaid scheme. In this, superseded editions of the *British National Formulary* (produced twice a year) are collected from pharmacists and doctors in Britain for onward distribution to health professionals in Commonwealth developing countries. There are also regional pharmaceutical organizations for the Americas (the Pan-American Congress of Pharmacy and Biochemistry) and Asia (the Federation of Asian Pharmaceutical Associations).

## Support staff and education

Pharmacists in all countries have employed assistants since the earliest times. But the training received by these assistants, and what they are allowed to do once they are qualified, vary greatly. Some receive no training and simply work as pharmacy assistants. Others receive varying degrees of training and may qualify as pharmacy technicians or dispensers: in this case they may dispense prescription medicines, but only under the supervision of a pharmacist.

In some countries there is a level of qualification of pharmacy technician, that is not as great as that of the pharmacist. In Sweden, for example, many people train as prescriptionists; they are educated in schools of pharmacy, but not to the level of pharmacist, and they cannot carry out the full range of pharmacist duties; they may, however, become pharmacy managers. Similarly, in Holland there are two groups, the druggists and the pharmacists, with druggists being allowed only to sell and supply medicines available without prescription.

The idea of two levels of qualification in pharmacy is not new. In France, legislation in 1803 provided for six higher-level schools of pharmacy for the education of pharmacists of the first class, who were authorized to practice pharmacy throughout the country; pharmacists of the second class were allowed to practice only in the district where they had passed their examination. Having pharmacists at two different levels of qualification is not without problems, however, and the second-class category of pharmacists was abolished in 1909. In Britain, there were two routes to qualification as a pharmacist until 1953.

In most countries, the education of pharmacists underwent a great transformation during the 20th century, from an apprenticeship system to one based on graduate entry. This represented both a shift away from practical skills to knowledge, and a step in the professionalization of pharmacy. In western countries the pharmacist was traditionally trained by means of apprenticeship until around the 1960s, and the apprentice usually provided the pharmacist with a cheap source of labor.

In Britain, the first degree course in pharmacy was recognized by the University of London in 1925. Degree courses were offered by other schools of pharmacy in later years. The option of taking an apprenticeship followed by a period at college ended in 1967. From that year, entrants to the profession had to attend a three-year degree course, followed by one year of pre-registration training, which could be undertaken in any branch of pharmacy. Since 1997, all new entrants to the profession have been required to take a four-year degree course at a British school of pharmacy, followed by one year of pre-registration training.

In the USA a confusing range of qualifications in pharmacy were available for many years, although by the 1930s most colleges of pharmacy awarded either a Bachelor of Science (BS) or a Bachelor of Science in Pharmacy (BS in Pharm.). A six-year professional doctorate qualification in pharmacy (the Pharm.D) was first offered by the University of Southern California in 1950. Today in the United States many schools of pharmacy offer only this qualification, and it seems set to become the norm in many countries in future.

Pharmaceutical education in Commonwealth countries has generally followed that in Britain, but standards have varied across the different countries, from university degrees equivalent to British ones, to diplomas little more advanced than those of pharmacy technicians in other countries. The Commonwealth Pharmaceutical Association works with member countries in raising the standards in the poorer countries. Britain has agreements with Australia and New Zealand for the mutual recognition of pharmaceutical qualifications. A Directive of the EUROPEAN UNION for the mutual recognition of pharmaceutical qualifications throughout the community has been in force for some years, although movement of pharmacists within the community has so far been limited.

Around the world, most pharmacists work in shops. There are considerable variations in community pharmacy both among continents and within the various European countries. In Scandinavia, Austria, and the countries of eastern Europe, for example, pharmacies tend to be restricted to purely professional activities, dealing only in medicines, and medical, surgical, and related health products. In others, including Britain, a wide range of commodities tends to be sold, including toiletries and cosmetics, photographic, baby products, and health foods. In some countries, community pharmacy has become dominated by large pharmaceutical chains, which have often become general stores. However, dispensing medicines is generally kept separate, and remains a professional activity. Today, in most western countries, up to three quarters of the turnover of many privately owned pharmacies comes from dispensing prescriptions written by doctors.

## Europe and USA

Since the end of communism, formerly nationalized pharmacies in eastern European countries have been increasingly privatized. However, in a reverse tend, Swedish pharmacies were nationalized into a single company from 1 January 1971. The National Corporation of Swedish Pharmacies, two thirds of which is owned by the Swedish government, has responsibility for maintaining the supply and distribution of medicines around the country. Nationalization has enabled the planned distribution of pharmacies, and ensured uniformity in practice, usage, and image.

In the USA, the term drug store is used to denote a shop owned and run by someone other than a pharmacist. Such stores sell proprietary medicines which need not be sold from pharmacies, medical and surgical sundries, health foods, and related items. Similar arrangements exist in most European countries, including *drogeries* in France, *drogerias* in Germany, *drogherias* in Italy, and *drogerias* in Spain. The number and size of registered pharmacies vary from country to country. In Britain there are about 12 000 registered pharmacies, each of which must be under the personal control of a pharmacist.

Although most pharmacists are employed in the community, a wide range of other employment opportunities exist. The second largest group are employed in hospitals. Pharmacies are to be found in all types of hospital, from large teaching, to local general, to specialist hospitals, such as those for children and the mentally ill. The largest departments in the USA may employ several hundred staff, many of whom have specialist roles, such as providing drug information; preparing formularies, purchasing, and computers; manufacturing sterile solutions for parenteral nutrition; and making up solutions for cancer chemotherapy.

One of the most important developments in hospital pharmacy practice was the development of ward or clinical pharmacy in the 1970s, originating in North America but rapidly implemented in many European countries and Australasia. This represented a shift in the location of practice from the pharmacy to the ward, as pharmacists increasingly gave advice on the prescribing and administration of drugs at ward level. Most hospital pharmacists now act as clinical pharmacists, often for a particular specialty such as cardiology or intensive care.

The 1990s has seen diversification in the range of career opportunities for pharmacists. In Britain, increasing numbers of pharmacists work directly for health authorities, monitoring prescribing and dispensing, and advising on measures to increase the effective and economic use of medicines. Others are employed directly by groups of medical practitioners to develop formularies, and advise on the better use of medicines. Similar trends are apparent in other European countries and in North America.

Many hundreds of pharmacists are employed by the PHARMACEUTICAL INDUSTRY, in the research and development of new drugs, and in the marketing and promotion of existing ones. Some are employed on drug regulation, and in the provision of information by medical departments. Smaller numbers of pharmacists are employed in academic institutions in research and teaching, and others work for the armed forces and in the prison service.

### Challenges

Throughout the world, many of the challenges faced in the 21st century by pharmacy are already apparent. There are both significant threats and great opportunities. The supply function of the pharmacist will be transformed by the development of original pack dispensing, where the pharmacist will supply packs as received from manufacturers. The range of drugs available will increase, and they will become more targeted, safe, and effective. The number of drugs which pharmacists will be able to supply without prescription will grow, and the public will demand more information and advice about their use. Nurses and other health professionals will achieve rights to prescribe medicines previously obtainable only on the prescription of a doctor.

Both community and hospital pharmacy will increasingly focus on pharmaceutical care, a concept originally developed in the USA. Pharmaceutical care — 'the responsible provision of pharmacotherapy for the purpose of achieving definite outcomes that improve a patient's quality of life' — has three basic components: assessing a person's drug related needs; developing a plan for meeting those needs; and following up to see if those needs have been met. This has recently been endorsed by the International Pharmaceutical Federation, representing pharmacists throughout the world.

Whatever the uncertainties of the future, the need for highly-trained pharmacists, able to assist doctors with prescribing decisions, able to offer advice on a wide range of ailments, and able to supply a wide range of effective remedies to the public, world wide, will be as great in the future as it has been in the past.                SA

**PHRENOLOGY** Interest in phrenology has existed since the concept was advanced in Paris in the 1790s by the Viennese physician Franz Joseph GALL (this page). Although the word was not coined until 1815, by then Gall's 'physiognomical system' or 'craniology' was already the subject of dozens of books, pamphlets, and articles in journals and newspaper. The century-long debate over its anatomical, physiological, and craniological propositions was under way, and so was the philosophical, theological, and social controversy over its materialist and fatalistic implications. In one way or another, phrenology would impinge on virtually every aspect of 19th century life and thought, capturing the interest of everyone from Thomas WAKLEY (p 453) to A. R. Wallace, from Metternich to Marx.

What Gall proposed, so controversially, was both a theory of brain and a science of character. His contentions were fivefold:

- the brain was the organ of the mind
- the brain was not a homogeneous unity, but an aggregate of mental organs with specific functions
- these cerebral organs were topographically localized
- the relative size of any one of the mental organs could be taken as an index to that organ's power of manifestation
- since the skull ossifies over the brain during infant development, external craniological topography could be used to diagnose the internal state of the mental faculties.

Individually and collectively these were startling propositions. By addressing the basis of mind and brain and, hence, thought itself, Gall contributed fundamentally to the Enlightenment debate over man's place in nature and society. At the same time, by providing a practical means to character analysis, he generated a new kind of astrology-cum-popular psychology.

The main audiences for phrenology varied over time. During the first phase of its history, up to the 1820s, those involved were mostly men of science, medicine, philosophy, and 'letters', along with sections of fashionable society seeking instruction and amusement. From the

**PHILOSOPHER'S STONE**

A putative object or mineral substance capable of effecting the transmutation of base metals into gold. It was the ultimate goal of alchemy and the quest for it chief among the preoccupations of alchemists ('philosophers'). Some felt that the stone, when found, would also prove to have the power to cure all diseases and to prolong life indefinitely.

**FOUNDER FIGURE**

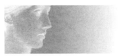

Franz Joseph **GALL** (1758–1828). Austrian physician, who, with J. C. Spurzheim, devised the pseudoscience of cranioscopy, later called phrenology. They claimed that the brain consisted of 27 (later increased to 37) organs responsible for traits of character and revealed by palpable protuberances on the surface of the skull.

mid-1820s to mid-1830s its center of gravity shifted to a generation of middle-class ideologues and social activists, most of whom were drawn from the legal and medical professions. Influential in disseminating phrenology among the medical profession in particular was John Elliotson, the redoubtable professor of medicine at University College, London. In 1823 Elliotson founded the London Phrenological Society, over which he presided for two decades. In the early 1840s, like many other phrenologists, Elliotson ventured into MESMERISM, founding in 1844 the journal *The Zoist* for its investigation and propagation.

To these persons — well informed on the subject by the itinerating disciple of Gall, J. G. Spurzheim, and, in turn, by Spurzheim's disciple, the Scottish lawyer George Combe (the Huxley of Victorian phrenology) — phrenology became a practical and ideological resource in the reform of the social order. The knowledge provided a would-be scientific justification for emergent and idealized social relations with women, savages, and the politically recalcitrant working class. More practically, it was applied to the reform of education and to the treatment of the insane and the criminal, as well as to the hiring of servants. As a means to all of these ends, phrenological societies were established and an extensive popular literature disseminated. The most famous phrenological text, George Combe's *Constitution of man* (1828), ran through dozens of editions, was widely translated, and is said to have existed in homes where the only other books were *The Bible* and *The pilgrim's progress*.

Although the phrenological movement ebbed towards the middle of the 19th century, a two-pronged revival and transformation of sorts took place in the 1860s. The American 'phrenological Fowlers' largely took over its popular cultivation, spawning a new generation of practical head-reading 'professors,' many of whom lasted well into the 20th century. At the same time, the declining scientific fortunes of Gall's ideas underwent a surprising reversal. In the work of Jean-Baptiste Bouinaud and Pierre-Paul Broca in France, G. T. Fritsch and E. Hitzig in Germany, and John Hughlings Jackson and David Ferrier in Britain, clinical support emerged for the theory of cerebral localization. Although only a small proportion of the many publications resulting from these men's research can be reckoned 'phrenological', it nevertheless encouraged and gave new legitimacy to head-reading anthropometric studies of 'primitive' peoples and schoolchildren — projects which also lasted into the 20th century.

The science of phrenology is no more, but its fascination persists. Its imagery is pervasive in the world of advertising; porcelain phrenological busts remain sought after; and historians of science, medicine, and society continue to debate its impact.                    RC00

*See also* CULTS AND QUACKERY

**PHYSIOLOGY — HISTORY** This is the study of how the body works and nowadays includes or is closely related to other scientific specialties, including biochemistry, neuroscience, pharmacology, and molecular biology. At the end of the 19th century and throughout the first half of the 20th, physiology was *the* dominant medical science: in addition to functional studies of the body, it embraced histological and pathological work, bacteriology, chemical analysis of living tissues, and often plant physiology. The creation and naming of the NOBEL PRIZE in physiology or medicine in 1901 indicates its central importance to medicine. Although the word *physiologia* was first used by Jean Fernel, physician to Henri II of France, it was not until the middle of the 19th century that the subject, and the word, emerged as an independent experimental science. Until then, studies of function were included as anatomy, the 'Institutes of Medicine', or materia medica. As plant physiology has increasingly been recognized as a botanical specialization, 'physiology' has become synonymous with 'animal physiology'. From the late 19th century the discipline matured, developed, and diversified, and contributed to the further subdivision of modern biomedical sciences.

### Before the 19th century

In the Ancient World it was recognized that many living creatures were warm, whilst the dead were cold, and the preservation of this living heat, and its destruction by disease and death, were issues of concern and discussion for medical philosophers and practitioners. The Hippocratic Corpus (written before *c.* 350 BCE) emphasized the significance of four bodily HUMORS, each with different physical characteristics. GALEN (p 324) provided an account that endured for over a thousand years, teaching that the liver absorbed nutriment and transformed it into blood, which was then transported to the heart, passed through invisible pores in the septum from the right to the left side, and mixed with *pneuma*, or life spirit, drawn in by the act of breathing. The vitalized blood then ebbed and flowed in the major arteries and veins. Throughout the early Middle Ages these views were preserved in Arab lands, and, recovered by the western world in the late medieval period, they were incorporated into Christian traditions of creation, and became accepted, unquestioned, dogma. Challenges to these concepts did not occur until the Renaissance.

By then, the working of the body in health and disease was recognized as the theoretical basis of practical medicine. Advances, both conceptual and technical, in other aspects of science, such as chemistry, mechanics, thermo-dynamics, optics, and ARCHITECTURE, led to the realization that new knowledge could have practical significance. William HARVEY (p 363), physician to King Charles I of England, challenged the Galenical view, and suggested that blood circulated constantly around the living body. He established that blood was ejected from the right ventricle into the pulmonary circulation, and on being returned to the left side of the heart was pumped around the body, returning to the heart through a system of veins. Harvey's work stimulated others to experiment: the English clergyman Stephen Hales measured the blood pressure, an assessment that is now a routine diagnostic tool, and observed that the arterial pressure of a living horse was much greater than the venous pressure.

There was also increasing recognition that the *measurement* of biological values might be relevant in understanding physiological processes. SANTORIO (p 743) examined fluctuations in normal human functions by inventing an instrument to count the pulse rate, and a THERMO-METER to measure the body's temperature. With a specially constructed chair balance, he also charted his own body weight, food intake, and excreted output, and revealed the regular loss through 'insensible perspiration' of a small amount of body weight, the theoretical basis of all modern metabolic investigations.

At the beginning of the 18th century, influenced by the ideas and values of the Enlightenment, Hermann BOERHAAVE (p 121), from LEIDEN University (p 257), suggested that functional systems within the body operated both independently and together to form a coherent whole. He was strongly influenced by René Descartes, who likened the body to a clockwork mechanism that functioned according to mechanical laws and principles. Boerhaave postulated that the body was a series of vessels, through which vital body fluids ebbed and flowed, and their movement, obstruction, or stagnation accounted for health or disease. His teachings influenced generations of medical practitioners and theorists, including Albrecht von Haller, who proposed that the solid parts of the body were composed of fibers. Connective fibers formed the vasculature, membranes, and supportive tissues of the major organs; nerve fibers and muscle fibers were endowed with vital properties, of sensibility or responsiveness to painful stimuli (nerve fibers), or irritability, the property of contractility in response to stimulation (muscle fibers). Haller's theories ascribed physiological sensitivities to the

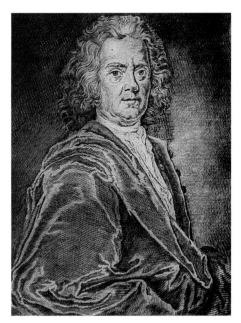

Hermann Boerhaave (1665–1738).

fibers to account for their responses to stimulation, and the concepts of irritability and sensibility achieved widespread acceptance, although they remained qualitative.

Towards the end of the 18th century experimental approaches became more routine, including those of the French naturalist René RÉAUMUR (p 433), who trained a pet kite to swallow and regurgitate small fenestrated tubes filled with food, and examination of these indicated that the stomach digested meat more fully than starchy foods. Lazzaro SPALLANZANI (p 743), extending Réaumur's observations by swallowing and regurgitating linen pouches himself, emphasized that gastric function was only one component of digestion. Luigi Galvani, from an observation that a frog muscle contracted when a metal pin in its spinal cord was stimulated, postulated the existence of animal electricity and that the muscle was a reservoir of electricity that caused contraction. A lengthy and acrimonious debate developed with Allessandro Volta, who maintained that electricity had to be applied to a muscle to make it contract. The debates continued long after Galvani's death and were not resolved until Emil Dubois-Reymond integrated Galvani's concept into a theory of the electrical nature of the nervous impulse.

### The 19th century

Medical practitioners became increasingly aware that disease processes involved dynamic pathological changes which affected how physiological

## PIONEER PHYSIOLOGISTS

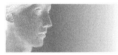

Carl Friedrich Wilhelm **LUDWIG** (1816–95). German physiologist. Ludwig was successively professor at Marburg (1846), Zurich (1849), the Josephinum in Vienna (1855), and Leipzig (1865). One of the creators of modern physiology and a teacher of immense influence, he sought to explain all vital processes in physicochemical terms. His own researches were concerned with the circulation and secretion. A man of great ingenuity, he invented the kymograph (1849), the mercurial blood pump (1859), the stream gauge (1867), and devised a method of maintaining the circulation in isolated organs (1865).

*(continued on p 646)*

questions were recognized, and addressed. Within European medicine, attention began to shift away from the medical schools of universities such as those of Leiden and Edinburgh, to newer establishments which emphasized more practical approaches and the application of physiological knowledge. These were often associated with key figures, such as Claude BERNARD (p 102) in Paris and Carl LUDWIG (p 643) in Germany, and students began to travel to learn new attitudes and methods for the promotion of physiology.

Physiology's growth and differentiation into an independent experimental and professional science may be clearly identified from this period onwards: new institutions were established; full-time research and teaching positions were created; and specialist journals and societies started. Other factors became associated with, and in turn influenced, this diversification, most notably the deliberate and systematic manipulation of natural processes. These were facilitated by the increasing acceptability of using of animals in experiments, an approach considerably accelerated towards the end of the century by the routine use of reliable anesthetics. Microscopes became more powerful and accurate, and also increasingly available, and the use of complex equipment became accepted not only for the pursuit of scientific activities, but also later for use in diagnosis.

The most consistent and successful attempts to provide facilities for the new scientific physiology were taken in France and in Germany, represented here by Claude Bernard and Carl Ludwig. In France, hospital medicine in Paris fostered a revolution in medical practice, which encouraged practitioners to formulate and test explanations of disease processes. From this medical tradition arose several of France's most distinguished physiologists, including Bichat, François Magendie, and his pupil Claude Bernard. In the German states, there was ready recognition that this new experimental approach required an infrastructure of support, and Breslau, Heidelberg, Leipzig, and Munich all developed laboratories and institutes for the support and promotion of physiology. In France, however, the absence of such well-equipped institutes and laboratories hampered the development of physiology for some time.

For much of his career, Claude Bernard worked in a cramped basement in the Collége de France, from which his visitors returned to their own countries to reproduce his methods, set up their own laboratories, and teach the next generation. He is important in the history of physiology for two main reasons: firstly, as an experimentalist in his own right; and secondly, as a teacher of new ideas and techniques. He developed new methods

and techniques in animal surgery, which attracted his laboratory students from across Europe and America, and from his work came much physiological knowledge: the digestive function of pancreatic juice in fat metabolism; the biosynthetic capabilities of the liver in carbohydrate breakdown; and the differentiation of sensory and motor properties of mixed nerves. Bernard's experimental and philosophical approach to physiology and medicine was guided by the principle of coherence — organs and tissues functioned in an integrated manner, and organic functions followed a determined pattern to maintain an environmental constancy that he termed the *milieu intérieur*, later developed into the theory of homeostasis by the American physiologist Walter Cannon. Bernard's advocacy of investigative physiology as the intellectual and practical basis of medical education and practice was equally significant. In his *Introduction to the study of experimental medicine* (1865) he emphasized that disease states such as diabetes were malfunctions of fundamental mechanisms, and that detailed knowledge of physiology should be recognized, supported, and incorporated into routine medical teaching.

In Germany, Johannes Müller devised a theory of specific nerve energies, which stipulated that stimulation of any given sense organ gave rise to its own peculiar sensation and no other. In 1843 his pupil, Emil Dubois-Reymond showed that a flow of electric current was involved not only in muscle contraction, as suggested by Galvani, but also in nerve conduction, and he proposed that the transmission of excitation between a nerve and muscle was due to this flow. The versatile Hermann von HELMHOLTZ (p 372) established a law of the conservation of energy — that energy was neither created nor destroyed. He measured the speed of conduction in a nerve fiber; recognized that a delay occurred at the neuromuscular junction; and proposed a mechanism of color vision involving retinal cones that were differentially sensitive to red, green, and violet (blue). Equally versatile was Ernst von Brücke, who also studied sense organ physiology, intestinal mobility, salivary secretion, and fat metabolism.

Carl Ludwig occupies a similar niche in the hierarchy of physiological deities to that of Claude Bernard, although his own research career is often overshadowed by his role as mentor to the next generation of physiologists. But it was Ludwig's skills and talents in experimental methods that drew students: work on the blood and the innervation of blood vessels; studies of renal and respiratory physiology, including the proposal of a filtration–reabsorption mechanism for kidney function. His scientific belief was determinedly anti-vitalist, demanding that physiological phenomena be explained by reference to the laws of physics and chemistry. Ludwig's views spread from his laboratory during the final decades of the 19th century to most countries of continental Europe, across the English Channel to Britain and beyond to North America, and his intellectual 'family' includes practically every notable physiologist practicing at the turn of the century.

In Britain, the early promotion of physiology, stimulated by the work of Bernard and Ludwig, depended on the enthusiastic endeavors of a few highly committed men. William Sharpey, professor of anatomy and general physiology at University College, London, advocated new methods, approaches, and ways of thinking about functional organization, emphasized by his use of histology. His pupils included Michael Foster, who, in 1870, became the first praelector in physiology at Trinity College, Cambridge, and 13 years later the first professor of physiology in Cambridge. When Foster departed for Cambridge, another Sharpey student Edward Schäfer developed the teaching of histology at University College London, while John Burdon Sanderson, organized courses in 'practical physiology', which included chemical, mechanical, and functional experiments. Ten years later Sanderson became the first professor of physiology in Oxford and Schäfer became professor at University College, later to move to Edinburgh. Thus the three most influential positions in British physiology were filled by Sharpey's protegés.

Physiology, at the end of the 19th century, was organized into three main topics: histology; chemical physiology (concerned with the chemical analysis of body fluids and constituents); and practical physiology — which most closely resembles what is thought of as physiology today; the experimental manipulation of organs and tissues, the investigation of their innervation and vascularization, and studies of integration, coordination, and regulation within the body as a whole. These approaches, especially for research, required the use of living animals, and in Britain this brought physiology and its practitioners to the attention of a wider public. A Royal Commission in 1875, on the use of experimental animals, recommended legislation, the 1876 Cruelty to Animals Act, which required people and places involved in such work to be registered with the Home Office. Experimental procedures, except in special cases, had to be conducted entirely under terminal anesthesia; and official reports of experiments had to be provided every year.

By the end of the 19th century physiology was accepted as an important component of medical teaching. Physiologists were poised to promote,

develop, and shape the discipline in unprecedented ways as they attempted to understand the functional integration and control of living systems at several different levels of analysis — from that of the whole animal, via a physiological system, a specific organ, or tissue, down to the cell, subcellular component, or molecule.    TT

*See also* ANIMAL RIGHTS/ANTI-VIVISECTION MOVEMENTS; CLINICAL CHEMISTRY

**PHYSIOLOGY** Twentieth-century physiology included detailed examinations, at several levels, of the functioning of particular organs or systems both in the laboratory and in the intact animal investigations into the intrinsic and extrinsic control mechanisms of those systems by neural or blood-borne factors; broader studies, of the interaction and integration between different systems; and analyses of multi-organ, whole-body, integration and regulation. Some specific examples of notable advances will be briefly reviewed.

### The gastrointestinal system

Experiments on animals, assisted by advances in surgical techniques and chemical anesthesia, revealed new levels of complexity in every system examined, and gastrointestinal physiology demonstrates many of these features. The Russian physiologist, Ivan PAVLOV (p 729), did much to elucidate functional mechanisms of different parts of the upper part of the digestive system, and the integrative controls of the system, especially the role of the vagus nerve. Pavlov was particularly expert in devising surgical approaches such as pouches and fistulae for studying the function of the stomach and pancreas, although his interests in the control mechanisms of the system eventually diverted almost completely into physiological psychology. Human studies were occasionally undertaken by physicians, the first being that by the American William Beaumont, whose patient Alexis St Martin had suffered a shotgun accident that rendered direct access to his stomach possible, allowing Beaumont to make fundamental observations about gastric motility and the flow of gastric juice in different conditions.

The American physiologist Walter Cannon devised a technique, now in routine diagnostic use, of examining the internal workings of the body without recourse to surgery. He used newly discovered X-RAYS to follow the passage of radio-opaque food pellets along the digestive system, and he analyzed the mechanical properties of every region of the tract. His resulting 'J'-pictures, of the shape of the stomach and pylorus during gastric emptying, were originally traced onto lavatory paper held over the Roentgen screen, and are still the classic illustrations in many textbooks.

(continued)

Schack August Steenberg **KROGH** (1874–1949). Danish physiologist. Krogh was appointed professor of zoological physiology in Copenhagen in 1908. His researches included the chemical regulation of respiration, the pH of blood, the oxygen consumption of tissues, and the chemical changes in muscle. He is best known, however, for his studies on the physiology of the capillaries, for which he was awarded the NOBEL PRIZE in 1920.

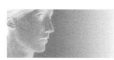

Sir Hans Adolf **KREBS** (1900–82). Anglo-German biochemist. After working in Freiburg Krebs came to Britain in 1933 as a refugee and became a research student at Cambridge. In 1935 he was made lecturer in biochemistry at Sheffield and in 1945 professor; he moved to the chair in Oxford in 1954, where he was director of the Medical Research Council unit for research in cell metabolism. His two most important discoveries were the cyclic formation of urea (1932) and the citric acid cycle (Krebs cycle, 1937), the chief source of metabolic energy. He was awarded the NOBEL PRIZE for physiology with F. A. Lopman in 1952.

(continued opposite)

Cannon's interest in integrative physiology led him to examine the effects of different foods on how fast the stomach empties and then into an examination of emotional influences on gut function; from this came an extensive study of the control mechanisms of the autonomic nervous system (that part not under conscious control). His work on the interaction and control of different regulatory components resulted in his most famous book *The wisdom of the body*, an exposition of his theory of homeostasis, a direct but more advanced descendant of Claude Bernard's proposal of the constancy of the *milieu intérieur*.

## Cardiovascular physiology

W. H. Gaskell studied frog and tortoise hearts, and showed that motor impulses from nerve endings in the large veins influenced heart rhythm but not the cardiac movements, which were due to muscle contraction. To perform similar studies in the more rapidly beating mammalian heart, attempts were made to isolate it from control by the nervous system, first achieved by Michael Foster's student Henry Newell Martin in 1884. His approach lasted well into the 20th century, until superseded by Starling's heart–lung preparation. Ernest Starling deduced his eponymous 'Law of the heart', which related the contractile energy of a cardiac muscle fiber to its resting length. Later refinements included the development of more advanced perfusion pumps; the discovery and introduction of anti-clotting agents; and general improvements in perfusion and irrigation media. These all contributed to the creation of the apparatus for first successful heart bypass surgery in the early 1950s. In the same period, a technique devised by Adolf Fick for calculating the output of the heart was used successfully for human diagnosis.

The heart's specialized conduction system was thoroughly investigated by F. W. Stannius, who demonstrated vagal inhibition and the intrinsic pacemaker (how the heartbeat is regulated). In 1893 Wilhelm His discovered the auriculo-ventricular bundle of special conducting tissue that bears his name, often coupled with that of A. F. Stanley Kent, who discovered the bundle independently in the same year. Willem Einthoven, following the British physiologist Augustus Waller, provided the classic description of the electrocardiograph using a capillary electrometer, and developed a string galvanometer that could accurately portray the electrical changes in the human heart. This instrument permitted laboratory and clinical examinations of the heart, such as investigations of the damage to the bundle of His that dissociated auricular and ventricular beats, and was important in the creation of modern electrodiagnostic techniques.

## The respiratory system

John Scott HALDANE (p 510) combined interests in public health and respiratory physiology, and his early experiments were on mine gases and physiological function in miners. Like many physiologists, he also studied high-altitude responses. Claude Bernard's pupil Paul Bert discovered from studies of balloonists that the respiratory gases dissolved in blood exerted their effects not in proportion to their concentrations, but to their partial pressures, and the Italian, Angelo Mosso, determined that respiratory distress at high altitudes among mountaineers was accused by a lack of carbon dioxide. Haldane calculated that oxygen tension in the blood was higher than in pulmonary air, and, erroneously, that the lungs secreted oxygen, which led to a protracted dispute with the Danish physiologist August KROGH (this page), who believed that the exchange of gases in the lungs could be explained by diffusion.

As in many emerging physiological specialties, respiratory work needed new, increasingly sensitive, and more portable, analytical equipment. Many eponymous pieces resulted, for example, the 'Haldane' gas analysis apparatus measured oxygen and carbon dioxide, and was a cornerstone of respiratory physiology until superseded by the 'Scholander' apparatus, which combined the same level of sensitivity but required a smaller volume gas sample; the 'Van Slyke' for the manometric analysis of dissolved gases; and the 'Douglas' bag for collecting gas samples.

Respiratory research extended beyond investigations of gas exchange in the lungs. The airways themselves were examined by K. E. R. Hering and J. Breuer, who delineated two important nervous reflexes, mediated through the vagus nerve (which supplies both the heart and the lungs). They showed that inflation of the lungs delayed the next intake of breath, but that a maintained deflation increased the rate and depth of inspiration. Different approaches to respiratory function were also developed among members of what became identified as the biochemical community, and include insights into the cellular mechanisms of respiration and intermediate metabolism, by Otto Warburg, Otto Meyerhof, and Hans KREBS (this page), among others, all of which contributed greatly to functional understanding of living organisms.

## The nervous system

The British physiologist, Charles SHERRINGTON (p 647) exemplifies the transition of physiology from a medical interest at the end of the 19th century to a well-defined, scientific specialty by the middle of the 20th century. Sherrington qualified in medicine in 1885 after studying with Michael Foster in Cambridge, and became the first specialist lecturer in physiology at St Thomas's Hospital, London. In 1895 he moved to the chair of physiology in Liverpool and in 1913 to Oxford. During the First World War he combined academic work with shifts in a munitions factory, studied fatigue, and devised an influential laboratory course. It is for his careful analysis of the function of the nervous system that he is best remembered, work that began in the late 1880s and occupied his entire career. The discrete *anatomical* unit of the nervous system was defined by Santiago Cajal as the neuron and Sherrington defined the *functional* unit of the nervous system as the reflex arc. Many complex activities such as walking or breathing may be reduced analytically to a series of reflex arcs. He established the basis of modern physiological understanding of the nervous system and deduced that inhibitory mechanisms operated in the nervous system. All of these led to, and were subsumed in, two major concepts, 'the final common pathway', and the 'integrative action' of the nervous system. The former referred to the convergence of reflex arcs originating from several sensory inputs onto one efferent neuron (carrying impulses away from the central nervous system), whose motor nerve forms a final pathway to the effector muscle.

In 1932 Sherrington shared the NOBEL PRIZE with E. D. (later Lord) Adrian, who had also been trained in the physiological laboratory at Cambridge. After the First World War, Adrian worked on the nervous impulse, a critical factor in his success being his development of new techniques to record nervous activity, and he constructed a system to amplify the neural signal, using the thermionic valve amplifier, then in use in telegraphy and radio work. Simultaneously, the Americans H. S. Gasser and J. Erlanger incorporated valve amplification and also introduced the cathode ray tube, thus heralding the electronic age in the physiological laboratory. Adrian's sensitive recording apparatus allowed him to record electrical impulses coming from muscles, cutaneous nerves, and autonomic nerves, and he refined the technique to record them from a single nerve fiber. This work confirmed that there was only one kind of nervous impulse, and that sensory and motor information was produced by variation in its frequency. He also studied the electrical activity of the human brain using electro-encephalography, a technique now used in the diagnosis and study of human neurological disease.

David Hubel and Torsten Wiesel directly continued Adrian's sensory research by analyzing the successive stages in the process of vision.

The autonomic division of the nervous system was expertly examined by two Cambridge physiologists, J. N. Langley, and W. H. Gaskell. Langley dissected the anatomical pathways of the two major component parts of the autonomic (a word he introduced) system, and delineated much of its function. He was influential in developing one of the most powerful concepts in 20th century biomedical sciences, the 'receptor' theory, used to account for cell–cell and cell–drug interactions in living tissues.

A student both of Gaskell and Langley in Cambridge in the 1890s was Sir Henry DALE (p 212), who discovered that the mechanism by which nerves communicate across the gaps where they link (synapses) was due to the release of specific chemicals. He showed that autonomic ganglia, the end organs of the parasympathetic nervous system, and the neuro-muscular junction could all be stimulated by acetylcholine, which he also identified as a natural constituent of the animal body. Later, G. Burnstock suggested that ATP (adenosine tri-phosphate, a compound known to be involved in metabolic pathways), might act as a neurotransmitter, and then expanded his ideas into a theory of co-transmission, that nerve terminals release a complex cocktail of two or more active chemicals. Henry Dale realized that as pharmaceutical and therapeutic dependence on natural substances increased during the 20th century, new analytical techniques and concords would be necessary to provide a coherent framework in which medical research and practice could progress, and he promoted national and international agreements on biological standards, as important a contribution to 20th century medical science as his experimental work.

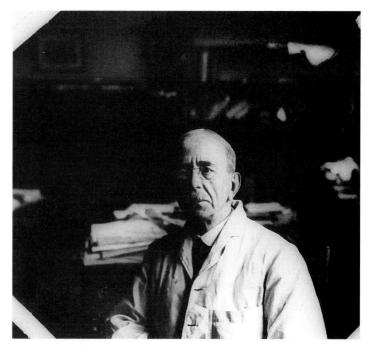

Sir Charles Sherrington (1857–1952).

*(continued)*

Sir Charles Scott **SHERRINGTON** (1857–1952). British neurophysiologist. In 1932, jointly with Lord Adrian, he was awarded the NOBEL PRIZE in physiology for this work on the nervous system. His researches over a period of 50 years explained reflex action and laid the foundation of our present knowledge of neurophysiology. They were embodied in his book *The integrative action of the nervous system* (1906). He received a knighthood.

*(continued overleaf)*

(continued)

William **RUTHERFORD**
(1839–99). British
physiologist. Rutherford was a
Scotsman, known for his
theory of hearing, as well as
other physiological researches.
The resonance theory of
HELMHOLTZ (p 372) noted
the varying fiber lengths of
the cochlear membrane, so
that notes of varying pitch
were assumed to cause
vibration of selected fibers.
This accounted for only some
of the observed phenomena.
Rutherford proposed a
telephone theory in which the
whole membrane was
thought to vibrate in response
to sound, as in the diaphragm
of a telephone microphone,
which then generates
electrical impulses in bursts. It
seems likely that hearing is
dependent both on peripheral
and central analysis in the ear
and brain to interpret sounds.
Rutherford qualified in
medicine in Edinburgh,
studied in Berlin with Dubois-
Reymond and in several other
continental cities. In 1869 he
was appointed professor of
physiology at King's College,
London, and he returned to
Edinburgh as professor in
1874.

## The endocrine system

At the beginning of the 20th century Ernest Starling and William Bayliss, of University College, London, showed that the inner lining of the upper part of the intestine, stimulated by the presence of food, released a chemical factor (which they called secretin) that induced enzyme secretion from the pancreas. They developed a generalized theory for this type of secretory process, and coined the word 'hormone' to describe such substances. They were not the first to observe the effects of such internal secretions, since an earlier account from the same laboratory (of Schäfer and Oliver in 1894) had reported that extracts of the medulla of the adrenal gland could raise the blood pressure. This substance, later called adrenaline, became the centerpiece of a debate, as commercial interests represented by Parke, Davis and Co. became involved in physiological progress. Claims to have patented adrenaline and to have exclusive commercial rights to it, exacerbated worsening relationships between pharmaceutical manufacturers and scientists in America. Such tensions were still evident in 1921, when two Canadians, F. BANTING (p 236) and C. H. BEST (p 236), made perhaps the most famous endocrinological discovery, of pancreatic insulin as the treatment for diabetes.

The classic approach to endocrine research was established quite early: the removal of the suspected source of an internal secretion; the charting of the consequent signs and symptoms of resultant disease; and their reversal by the injection of a crude extract prepared from the removed gland. The French physiologist and neurologist Charles BROWN-SÉQUARD (p 708) followed a similar protocol in his controversial organotherapy, in which testicular extracts from animals were injected into men, including himself, with a claimed 'rejuvenating' effect. During the first four decades of the 20th century testosterone and several ovarian hormones were isolated and recognition that hormone levels altered significantly during pregnancy led to the development of a reliable pregnancy test by S. Aschheim and B. Zondek in 1928. By 1936 the plethora of work on endocrine mechanisms allowed the biochemist A. Doisy to propose four firm scientific criteria for the identification of a hormone: confirmation that a gland produced the secretion; the availability of precise methods to detect the secretion; the production of an extract from which a purified hormone could be obtained; and, finally, the chemical isolation, chemical identification, and synthesis of the hormone.

Observations that disease or damage to the pituitary gland might result in glandular malfunction encouraged investigations into higher control mechanisms. Work by Aschheim and Zondek revealed the presence, in the anterior pituitary, of gonadotrophins, hormones that stimulated further glandular hormone release, and yet a further stage in the control hierarchy was recognized by G. W. Harris, who determined that the hypothalamus released 'factors' which either stimulated or inhibited pituitary function. This work led to the discovery of many integrated control mechanisms, such as the hypothalamic-pituitary-gonadal axis. Understanding these stages in the control of sexual function has had widespread significance in the development of medical and social attitudes towards questions of fertility, infertility, contraception, and abortion.

Bayliss and Starling's recognition of hormones as chemical messengers implied the existence of a target, a hormone receptor site. In the 1970s and 1980s membrane preparations were used to study these sites, and revealed that most water-soluble polypeptide hormones bind to specific sites on the surface of the cell membrane, in line with what had become the traditional view of cell–drug interactions. However, steroid hormones, soluble in lipid, could penetrate the membrane to act as specialized sites inside the cell, on either cytosol or nuclear receptors, and by interacting with DNA, evoke messenger RNA, and consequently protein synthesis.

## Membrane physiology

The availability of increasingly complex physical and chemical techniques stimulated investigations into membrane structure in the latter part of the 19th century. A specialized boundary mechanism, the cell membrane, that contained protein and lipid had been proposed, and in 1935, J. Danielli and H. Davson published their theory of a permeable membrane, whose dynamics and transport mechanisms have provided one of the most fruitful aspects of modern physiological research.

Physiologists knew from studies of injured nerve and muscle fibers that an electrical potential difference existed across their membranes, and in 1902, Helmholtz's pupil, Julius Bernstein, having found that the interior of these fibers was rich in potassium but contained little sodium or chloride, suggested that it was this ionic imbalance that resulted in a voltage across the membrane. The discovery in 1933 of the giant axon of the squid by the British zoologist J. Z. Young provided large fibers, up to 1 mm in diameter, which were used by A. L. Hodgkin, A. F. Huxley, and B. Katz to derive a mathematical hypothesis of the nerve action potential, which depended upon the external concentration of sodium ions.

As in many topics, technical advances were critical: membrane physiology was greatly facilitated by the availability of radioactive isotopes as tracers, just before the Second World War; and the development of the flame photometer in the early

1950s eased the tedious analysis of measuring sodium and potassium ions. In 1951 the Dane, Hans Ussing, proposed that there was a cyclical carrier mechanism of permeability, linking active sodium and potassium transport across the membrane and during the following decade active transport of sodium ions was demonstrated across many membrane preparations. Further experiments led to the concept of the sodium pump, which maintained the ionic imbalance across the membrane.

At the beginning of the 21st century, several shifts and developments in physiology may be discerned. Its close relationship to medical practice, prominent at the end of the last century, is no longer so apparent, although therapeutic utility is often proclaimed as a justification for experimental research. Interest has progressively moved: from the whole animal to the integrated system; from the organ to the cell; from the cellular component to the ion. Associated with these movements has been the breakdown of 'traditional' departmental barriers and the growth of new disciplines such as biophysics, neurosciences, etc. However, the physiological approach as the study of the function of living matter has retained its identity, even if the boundaries of the subject itself are becoming increasingly indistinct. TT

*See also* ANTI-VIVISECTION; BIOETHICS, DIABETES MELLITUS; ENDOCRINOLOGY; INFORMED CONSENT;

**PLACEBO** The earliest known medical definition of 'placebo' (from the Latin word meaning 'I shall please') is found in George Motherby's *New medical dictionary* (1785): 'a commonplace method of medicine', a definition that does not suggest the modern meaning of the word. However, in Robert Hooper's *Medical dictionary* (1811) it is defined as 'any medicine adapted more to please than benefit the patient'. This suggests that a change in meaning took place around the start of the 19th century. Since then the concept has broadened further.

There are two types of placebos: those that contain pharmacologically inactive ingredients, and those whose contents have pharmacological activity. Although the former are always knowingly used as placebos by physicians, the latter may be given either in the knowledge that their pharmacological action is not appropriate or in the mistaken belief that it is. Here are some examples of the uses of a placebo.

### Clinical trials

The most common use of the inactive placebo is as a dummy for the active treatment in clinical trials. Some patients receive the active treatment, some the dummy. This reduces the element of subjective bias: if the patient and doctor do not know whether or not the active treatment is being used, the outcome will not be influenced by expectations of efficacy.

Occasionally an inactive placebo is given to a patient who is incessantly complaining of some symptom and who is thought to be exaggerating. Pain is the symptom usually involved. If the pain responds to the placebo it is often assumed that the patient was making an unnecessary fuss. However, it is wrong to assume that because the patient's pain was relieved by, say, an intramuscular injection of saline, the symptom did not exist or was not severe. About one-third of people are placebo reactors and will report symptomatic relief of real pain after the administration of an inactive compound. So, on occasion, and despite real pain appropriate to real pathology, relief can be obtained from a placebo. Placebos should not be used in this way.

The issue of a prescription is a common way of ending a patient's visit to the doctor, who, lacking an effective treatment, will sometime prescribe an active compound whose pharmacological action is irrelevant. The doctor may be well aware of this, for example, giving the patient a vitamin formulation, with the information that it is 'a tonic'. On other occasions a doctor may find it difficult to

---

## PINK DISEASE

Pink disease (acrodynia, erythredema), named because of the skin colour of the sufferers, was once a serious disease of infants and young children. It appeared in the western world about the turn of the 20th century, particularly in English-speaking countries. Babies turned bright pink and became ill, intolerant to light, lost their appetites, and became utterly miserable, often rejecting even their mothers. Some lost fingers and toes from gangrene and, on average, 7% of sufferers died.

The disease baffled the medical profession for 50 years. There were many theories about its origins, most of them following the latest fashion. The most popular was that it was due to a virus, then that it was nutritional, perhaps a form of pellagra. It was observed to occur near water courses, it was a 'peculiar neurosis of the vegetative nervous system in young children', and some blamed long winters. Little rigorous thought was given to the causes, explanations were casual, and the only writer to consider mercury poisoning immediately rejected it. No one asked why, in German-speaking countries, the patients were usually over 4 years old whereas among English-speakers they were between 10 months and 2 years.

The cause was almost certainly poisoning from mercury in teething powders (and worming powders in some countries), which mothers bought over the counter. Paradoxically this was at the very time when the British Medical Association was examining patent medicines and campaigning against them, yet no one made the connection. Even when faced with strong evidence, powerful pediatricians refused to believe it or even to test the evidence. Eventually questions were asked in Parliament and the manufacturers, sensing what was likely to happen, voluntarily withdrew mercury from their teething powders. The disease then virtually disappeared, apart from a few isolated cases, which were mostly traced to mercury — perhaps in a broken thermometer or from an old stock of teething powders on a chemist's shelf. AD

*See also* ADVERSE DRUG REACTIONS; MISADVENTURES

## THE NOCEBO EFFECT

Just as an inactive or inappropriate treatment may be beneficial if administered with positive expectations, so it may be harmful if administered with negative expectations. The concept of the placebo has therefore led in turn to the obverse concept of the nocebo (from the Latin word meaning 'I shall do harm'). In the nocebo effect the expectation of a harmful effect leads to the undesired outcome. The classic example is the harmful, sometimes fatal, effect of a hex in voodoo. The nocebo effect is seen in patients who are given negative expectations before surgery — they require more painkillers postoperatively than those who have been sympathetically prepared.

accept that there is no effective treatment and may feel constrained to try something. There are many examples of pseudotherapy, based on apparently good ideas that do not survive scientific examination, such as the use of 'cerebral vasodilators' in the treatment of dementias. Similarly, some patients cannot believe that there is no medicine to cure their disease, and sometimes no amount of talk will persuade them otherwise. Often, in exasperation, the doctor will prescribe something that, however tenuously, could be interpreted as being rational treatment, such as the misguided use of diuretics in the treatment of obesity.

### Factors affecting the response

The doctor's attitude when prescribing a placebo is important for its success: a placebo that is prescribed with enthusiasm and some show of belief in its efficacy is more likely to be effective. A good rapport between doctor and patient also helps.

The placebo response can be affected by the way in which the drug is presented. For example, in one study the pain-relieving effect of red placebo was as good as that of white aspirin; in another study, green was good for anxiety, yellow for depression. The larger the tablet the better, and a capsule is better still.

The way in which placebos produce symptomatic relief is not known. Undoubtedly the expectation of an effect may increase the likelihood that the effect will occur, and patients' expectations and doctors' expectations can reinforce one another. However, the physical basis of this is not known, although it has been suggested that endorphins and enkephalins might be involved.

Just as a placebo can relieve real symptoms so it can cause real adverse effects. Even if a patient expects benefit, incidental unwanted events may be attributed to an otherwise inactive placebo and labelled as adverse effects. For example, in one survey of placebo studies, common symptoms were dry mouth (9%), nausea (10%), fatigue (18%), difficulty in concentrating (15%), and headache (25%). Competitive, aggressive patients are more likely to suffer placebo adverse effects.

There may be other unwanted outcomes of inappropriate prescribing. If a doctor uses placebos unthinkingly, he may ignore the patient's real problem, and that may lead to delayed diagnosis of a treatable condition. Delay in diagnosis, and hence in instituting proper treatment, will particularly be prolonged if the patient initially responds to the placebo.

One outcome of the placebo effect is that if an ineffective remedy is touted as being effective, it will be apparently effective until proved otherwise. This is the origin of Armand TROUSSEAU'S (p 29) observation that one should use a new remedy while it has the power to work. It is also the basis of the success of many popular remedies that are marketed over the counter without formal proof of efficacy.　　　　JKA

**PLAGUE** is a severe bacterial infection due to the organism *Yersinia pestis* (formerly known as *Pasteurella pestis*). It is endemic in parts of South-East Asia and Africa, and occurs sporadically elsewhere. Primarily a disease of wild rodents, transmission to man usually occurs through the bite of a rat flea, causing the variety known as bubonic plague, in which regional inflammation of the lymph nodes (bubo) is prominent. When the condition becomes septicemic and pneumonic, person-to-person transmission occurs by droplet infection. Untreated, the mortality rate is high; but it responds well to early antibiotic therapy.

*See also* BLACK DEATH

**PLASTIC AND MAXILLOFACIAL SURGERY — HISTORY** Plastic surgery is a medical specialty with ancient roots. The Egyptian papyri describe physicians who specialized in the treatment of fractures of the facial bones, war injuries, and accidents. Their methods of repair have been studied by students of medicine.

Plastic surgery is sometimes defined as 'that branch of medicine which seeks to correct congenital or acquired deformities in order to improve function, appearance, or both'. It deals with defects of the body surface and the underlying bones and muscles. Although it is, in large measure, concerned with deformities involving the face, the head, and the neck region, it also includes the treatment of deformities of the hands and feet, the breast, body contours, and the external genitalia. Deformities inhibit function by making an individual feel that his or her physical image is inadequate. The word plastic basically means 'form', and it is the form of the human face and body that primarily concerns the plastic surgeon.

Aristotle, in his treatise *On the parts of animals*, stated, 'Art indeed consists in the conception of the result to be produced before its realization in the material'. That ability is a quality much needed by the plastic surgeon. It is a quality that should distinguish the artist from the technician. In 1798, Desavit first used the term 'plastique' in a medical paper and, in 1838, Zeis published the first *Handbuch der plastischen Chirurgie*. Plastic surgery was entirely reconstructive until the 20th century. In recent decades, the reliability and safety of this branch of surgery have advanced to such a degree that elective cosmetic (esthetic) surgery is now highly reliable and extremely popular. Such surgery always carries some risk and should not be undertaken unless that patient's sense of deformity is producing significant emotional problems. These problems may lead to inhibitions that significantly affect the patient's behavior and personal relationships — inhibitions that are often eliminated by appropriate surgery.

During the 8th century AD, Arabian scholars, with the rise of Islam, provided Arabic translations of the work of the famed Indian practitioner, Sushruta. Thus, Europeans and, in particular, Italians, including the Branca family of Sicily and Gaspare Tagliacozzi of Bologna, became familiar with ancient methods of plastic surgery that had been developed on the subcontinent of India.

In 1597, Gaspare Tagliacozzi published his treatise entitled *De curtorum chirurgia per insitionem.* This marvellous work established him as the first modern plastic surgeon. He described the use of flaps of skin and fat taken from the upper arm to reconstruct the nose. He employed a technique of moving these flaps of skin in stages to make the operations more successful. Tagliacozzi, like William HARVEY (p 363), another great medical pioneer, was ridiculed and persecuted for his 'heresies'. Following his death, there was a decline in science and medicine throughout all of Europe, including the practice of plastic surgery. This lasted throughout the 17th and 18th centuries. During these dark times, surgeons reported the mythical use of reparative tissue taken from a slave or person other than the patient and used for grafting.

In the 13th century, it was common practice in India to punish convicted criminals by amputation or mutilation of body parts. A frequent punishment for adultery was amputation of the nose. As in modern times, adultery was not limited to the poorer classes and, as a result, demand emerged for physicians with skill in the surgical replacement of the human nose. The cost of surgery was no problem for the prince or maharajah who had lost his nose. This 'demand' produced specialists in what we now call 'plastic surgery'.

Hindu religious law prohibited those belonging to the higher levels of the caste system from touching human blood. It was left to the lowly tile makers (belonging to the seventh caste) to develop the necessary surgical skills for rebuilding the nose. Over a period of many generations, these surgical skills were developed and passed down from father to son, unbeknown to the western world of medicine.

### Indian procedure

In 1794, two British physicians, traveling in India, were invited to witness one of these nasal reconstructions, performed in the Indian foothills of Mahvatta. They were astonished when they saw this operation. The patient was held on the ground by four strong men as the surgeon quickly cut free most of the skin from his forehead, leaving it attached only by a small bridge at the medial eyebrow region. The skin was then turned, folded, and roughly shaped into the form of a nose before fastening it to the scarred skin in the central face. Stitches and thorns were used to fasten the new nose into position and the patient's forehead was then dressed and allowed to heal over a period of weeks. The pedicle of skin remaining between the eyes was divided 25 days later. When this dramatic operation was reported subsequently by those English physicians in the *Gentleman's Magazine* in London (1794), it was met with disbelief and ridicule. Only after some years was the validity of the report established. To this day, we know this technique of transferring forehead skin to reconstruct the nose as the 'Indian method of rhinoplasty'.

Dr Joseph Carpue, a noted English surgeon, intrigued by this report from India, devoted the next 20 years of his life to confirming the details and methods that were used. Finally, he attempted the operation himself in September in 1814. His patient had been an officer in the Egyptian army who had been treated for syphilis by the use of mercury. This medication had caused the loss of his nose.

In an operation lasting exactly 37 minutes, Dr Carpue cut and elevated skin from the forehead and sewed it into new incisions that he made into that part of the patient's face which surrounded the

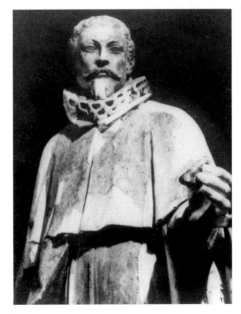

Sculpture at the University of Bologna showing Gaspare Tagliacozzi as he holds the model of a human nose and contemplates the problem of its reconstruction. He is known today as the father of modern plastic surgery.

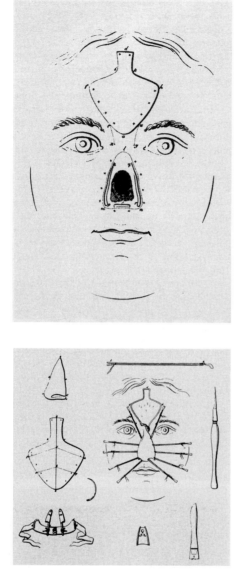

Illustration from Von Graefe's book, *Rhinoplastic* (1918), showing his diagram on the forehead to outline the shape of the skin needed to rebuild the nose.

The forehead flap has been transferred into the nasal defect. Small fish-tailed wooden sticks are used to allow daily tightening and loosening of the stitches. The lower left-hand corner pictures a splint to maintain the nostril air-passages during the healing period. This is a modification of the ancient Indian method of rhinoplasty described in Sushruta.

In France, Dupuytren (1832) developed new methods for treating burns and for relieving severe contractures of the hands. At the same time, von Langenbeck was making major contributions to the closure of congenital clefts of the palate in children.

On 8 December 1869, Reverdin gave the first demonstration of free skin grafting in the human. Ollier, in 1872, and THIERSCH (p 653), in 1874, published extensions on this technique to show that larger grafts and grafts containing dermis (the deepest layer of the skin), as well as epidermis, could also be used. In 1876 in England, Wolfe first described the use of the full-thickness skin graft for the treatment of eyelid deformities.

### Early plastic surgery in the USA and Britain

In the USA, specialization in plastic surgery appears to have developed as a result of the stimulation by William Stewart HALSTED (p 746) at the JOHNS HOPKINS University School of Medicine (p 840). He encouraged one of his younger associates, Dr John Staige Davis, to limit his practice to plastic surgery. Dr Davis published, in 1919, the first textbook in English on plastic surgery, entitled *Plastic surgery — its principles and practice.*

When the First World War broke out in 1914, Dr Davis and Dr Morestin of France were the only two recognized specialists in plastic surgery among the allied forces. Trench warfare in France produced a staggering number of maxillofacial wounds, and most military surgeons did not know how to deal with these problems. Morestin, a native of Martinique, conducted an active plastic surgery program at the military hospital of Val-de-Grâce in Paris. He died, prematurely, in the great influenza epidemic in 1917, but not before he had interested a British physician Sir Harold Gillies, in plastic surgery. Gillies subsequently established a military plastic surgery centre at the Queen Mary Hospital in Sidcup, Kent. At this hospital, many young plastic surgeons, such as Kilner and McIndoe, Ferris Smith from the USA, Waldron and Risdon from Canada, and Pickerill from Australia, learned many of the operative methods and skills of reconstructing patients who had received severe war injuries.

During the First World War, Varstad Kazanjian, a dental surgeon from the Harvard Dental School, was working at Etaples near Boulogne. He applied his knowledge of prosthetic DENTISTRY to the early treatment of gunshot wounds of the jaws, and perfected new methods of splinting jaw fractures that were associated with massive loss of bone. He developed principles that are still in use many years later. When the USA entered the First World War in 1917, Surgeon-General GORGAS (p 824) organized a section on oral and plastic surgery for the US military forces. Vilray P. Blair,

defect caused by the missing nose. When the dressing was removed three days later, the patient exclaimed, 'My God, there is a nose'. This operation and a second one performed by Carpue in 1815 marked the introduction of major reconstructive plastic surgery into western medicine.

During the 19th century, several other European surgeons made great contributions to the specialty of plastic surgery. These included von Graefe and his publication of *Rhinoplastik* in 1818 in Germany. His younger contemporary, Dieffenbach (1845), ingeniously extended the principles of nasal reconstruction to other types of defects, especially those involving the face and lips.

of St. Louis, headed that section and chose Robert H. Ivy as his assistant. Five years earlier (1913), Blair had published a classic book entitled *Surgery and diseases of the mouth and jaws*.

In the 1920s and 1930s, John Staige Davis and Vilray Papin Blair, in the USA, and Harold Delf Gillies in England, were the best-known leaders in the developing specialty of plastic surgery. Each made important and original contributions to the application of plastic surgical principles to correct the deformities of civilian life. In 1920 Gillies helped to pioneer the development of the tube pedicle flap, while in 1929 Blair and his associate, Barrett Brown, developed the technique of cutting and using large, thin sheets (split thickness) of skin to resurface the open wounds of patients with major burns. In 1939, Earl Padgett and an engineer, George Hood, developed the first mechanical dermatome that could be used for taking large sheets of split-thickness skin grafts. The invention of the dermatome made it possible for surgeons with only modest surgical skill in plastic surgery to harvest skin grafts for covering large skin defects. During the Second World War, this device saved many lives and limbs.

Cosmetic, or esthetic, plastic surgery began to develop during the period between the World Wars. A German surgeon in Berlin, by the name of Joseph, was developing the modern method of corrective rhinoplasty, permitting the operation to be carried out by means of incisions hidden within the nose. Two surgeons from the USA, Aufricht and Safian, observed and further developed his methods.

In 1937, Vilray Blair and 12 other senior American plastic surgeons established The American Board of Plastic Surgery. At the end of the Second World War there were still only 200 American surgeons who could meet the qualifications for certification by that board.

By 1951, only two plastic surgeons had been appointed as full-time heads of plastic surgery divisions in American medical schools (Robert McCormack at the University of Rochester in New York and Milton Edgerton at the Johns Hopkins University in Baltimore, Maryland). Academic plastic surgery was still in its infancy. During the ensuing 40 years, 6000 additional American and Canadian plastic surgeons have received plastic surgery board qualified training, and over 100 American medical schools now have appointed full-time specialists in plastic surgery. Several universities have given plastic surgery full departmental status. Hospitals in Canada, England, Scotland, Ireland, France, Italy, and Japan have also established postgraduate training programs for plastic surgeons.

One of the largest medical centers during the Second World War was The Valley Forge General Hospital at Phoenixville, Pennsylvania. The chief of its plastic surgery section, Dr Barrett Brown, and his associate, Dr Bradford Cannon, trained many young general surgeons in reconstructive surgery. When those medical officers returned to civilian life, they applied these wartime surgical techniques to civilian problems, such as cancer of the head and neck, industrial and automobile injuries, esthetic and body contour surgery, and even to correction of deformities caused by metabolic and vascular diseases such as arthritis and stroke. It is noteworthy that Dr Joseph E. Murray, one of the plastic surgeons trained at Valley Forge during the Second World War, was later awarded the 1900 NOBEL PRIZE in medicine for his continuing contributions to organ transplantation — the first plastic surgeon so honored.

During the years just before the Second World War Drs Sterling Bunnell, Alan Kanavel, and Summer L. Koch had pioneered advances in surgery of the hand in the USA. Enormous progress was made during that war in rebuilding the injured hand. For the first time, hand surgery became a major part of the work of plastic surgeons throughout the world. In the 1950s, William Littler inspired many young plastic surgeons to become serious students of surgery of the hand. In the 1960s, Paul Brand, working in Vellore, India, first demonstrated that the hand and facial deformities of LEPROSY could be greatly relieved by techniques of plastic surgery. This gave millions of leprosy victims new hope.

After the Second World War many new medical centers sprang up in Europe to recognize the specialty of plastic surgery. Burian established a department at Charles University in Prague in 1948. In Vienna, Eiselsberg, Pichler, and Esser developed facilities in the specialty. In Germany, Schuchardt established a plastic clinic in Hamburg to treat soldiers who had been injured on the Russian front. Wassmund, in Berlin, continued the plastic surgery methods originally started by Axhausen.

Several French surgeons had been trained in plastic centers, either in Britain or in the USA immediately following the Second World War. They then established a new French school of plastic surgery under the leadership of Morel-Fatio and Claude Dufourmental. At about this same time, in South America, plastic surgery was being developed and demonstrated by Hector Marino and Malbec. This world-wide activity led to the founding of the first International Association of Plastic Surgeons in 1960. The new and burgeoning specialty of plastic surgery in Japan soon developed too, as a result of the leadership of Sechii Ohmori.     MTE

*See also* SPECIALIZATION; TRAUMA; WAR

## SKIN GRAFTER

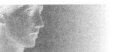

Karl **THIERSCH** (1822–95). German surgeon. Thiersch became professor of surgery in Erlangen in 1854, moving to the chair in Leipzig in 1867. He served as a surgeon in the Schleswig-Holstein war of 1864 and as consulting surgeon to 12 Corps in the war of 1870. Thiersch was a strong supporter of Listerian doctrine and reawakened interest in the subject by his method of skin grafting (Thiersch graft), introduced in 1874. He wrote on cancer (1865) and he also described phosphorus necrosis of the jaw ('phossy jaw') in 1867.

PLASTIC SURGERY continues to expand its boundaries and explore new frontiers of medical science. The 1960s saw the advent of craniofacial surgery by Tessier in France and by Edgerton and Converse in the USA. The 1970s ushered in the use of muscle flaps, which became widespread in the 1980s and is typified by the transverse rectus abdominis myocutaneous flap for reconstruction of the breast. A natural extension of this work was to combine the technique of microsurgery to flaps, thereby revolutionizing the reconstructive surgery for oncology and trauma. The 1990s saw a focus on healing at the cellular level and tissue engineering. The latter was pioneered by Green with the development of cultured skin and later cartilage. Esthetic surgery has also seen dramatic changes in techniques, equipment, and popularity. The result is that plastic surgeons can now dramatically improve the outcome and lives of many more people, in both reconstructive and esthetic surgery.

To master this broad specialty requires extensive diversified training. The American Board of Plastic Surgery requires a long period of training in general surgery and a further two to three years of plastic surgery residency. There are over 100 training programs in the USA and many more in Britain, Europe, and Asia. Facilities providing plastic surgery have multiplied and training programs have likewise spread to all parts of the world.

A further impetus to the spread of operative and teaching facilities has been the international humanitarian efforts of many plastic surgeons. Organizations such as Interplast, Operation Smile, and Physicians For Peace go well beyond the scope of medical relief efforts. These groups and dozens of others have allowed the interchange of ideas and furthered training while caring for hundreds of thousands of patients around the world.

### Wound and burn care

Problem wounds from arterial insufficiency, venous stasis, DIABETES, radiation therapy, and pressure ulceration affect millions of people and consume vast resources annually. Increasingly, these wounds are being treated by plastic surgeons. Basic scientific research and clinical studies have led to a better understanding of the wounding and reparative processes. Specific agents to influence these processes, such as cytokines and growth factors, have begun to be used in an effort to facilitate healing. Hyperbaric oxygen therapy has been used for these conditions and its exact role is being refined.

Improvements in critical care, antibiotics, and the creation of specialized units for treating burn patients have improved survival. In the 1960s, patients with 50% body surface area burns had a 50% chance of survival; today that survival rate is seen in patients with a 75% burn. Early debridement of burn eschar (removing the sloughs) with skin grafting has shortened hospitalization and improved recovery rates. In patients with massive burns, the technique of cultured epidermal autografts has allowed the sites to be covered. This involves growing sheets of cells called keratinocytes in artificial culture from a 2 cm² biopsy specimen of the patient's skin. More durable results are now achieved by coupling this with cadaveric dermal grafts, and new synthetic dermal substitutes are in various stages of development.

### Craniomaxillofacial surgery

This specialty arose in World War I, where the means of mass destruction produced devastating deformities of the head and jaws. At that time plastic surgeons could still not effectively address these injuries or those of congenital origin. The years after World War II saw a renewed interest led by Gillies, who performed the first reconstructions of this area but thought them too dangerous and abandoned the procedure. Nevertheless, Tessier built upon this experience and launched the revolution seen in craniofacial surgery.

These principles removed the last barriers to reconstruction of the skull and facial bones for trauma and congenital conditions. Further advances allowed the anatomical restoration and stable fixation of the craniofacial skeleton. Metallic plating systems with screws as small as 1.0 mm have made this possible. Recent concerns about the use of these devices in growing skulls and the possibility of their movement within the skull has spurred the development of newer materials. These include fixation plates and screws that are bioabsorbable over a year. Tissue adhesives are in use in parts of the world for soft tissue closure and are being investigated for bony stabilization.

'Distraction osteogenesis' is now changing the way that many craniofacial conditions are treated. This is based upon the principle of gradual separation of bone that allows the intervening gap to be bridged by new bone, and eliminates the need for new grafting. Distraction over some weeks also lessens the skin's tendency to counteract the advancement by taking advantage of its ability to be gradually stretched (for example, tissue expansion in pregnancy). The technique is currently being used to correct deformities of the jaws and facial bones with excellent results. Further technical advances will allow distraction to be applied to deformities of the skull and other tissues.

### Flaps

Modern plastic surgery is characterized by the ability to use all types of tissues (skin, connective tissue (fascia), muscle, bone, and nerve) in a reliable manner to provide the needs of reconstruction. Using flaps taken from all over the body the plastic surgeon can now transfer large amounts of tissue in a single stage, and effectively manage even the largest and most complex defects. Flaps of muscle or skin and muscle (myocutaneous) have been particularly helpful in dealing with ischemic, contaminated, or deep wounds, where dead space may inhibit healing. Other types of flaps include cutaneous, fasciocutaneous, osteocutaneous, and specialized flaps that may include tendon, nerve, bone, cartilage, or bowel, the choice being dictated by the defect to be reconstructed. The ability to transfer flaps as 'free' tissue using microsurgical techniques has further expanded the importance and use of flaps in all surgical specialties.

## Microsurgery

Alexis Carrel in the early 1900s pioneered the techniques of vascular and microsurgery that are still in use today. The 1960s saw many investigations into experimental replantation of limbs and microsurgical tissue transfers. In 1962 successful replantation of severed arms was reported and in 1968 that of digits. Nakayama described the first free-tissue transfer in 1964 with microsurgical transfer of intestine to the esophagus. Since then, advances have been made in both the operative microscopes and the microsurgical materials. Transfer of tissue by microsurgical means may greatly simplify treatment and obviate the need for the previously used cross-leg flap or amputation. In cancer and trauma reconstruction, for example, free tissue transfer has allowed plastic surgeons to replace 'like with like'. Examples of this include reconstruction of the mandible with fibular or iliac bone free flaps while providing oral lining with an attached skin paddle. The application of free flaps has also been extended to genital reconstruction and gender reassignment, with the forearm skin transferred for reconstruction of the phallus and creation of a neourethra. The free transfer of tissue may be reliably performed with an expected success rate of 95% or better.

## Breast reconstruction

Perhaps no part of the human anatomy has such psychological and social importance as the female breast. In the United States, for example, legislatures have gone so far as to pass laws requiring insurance companies to pay for breast reconstruction and surgeons to discuss the options for reconstruction with the patient. The ability to recreate an esthetically pleasing breast that imitates the natural one has been an important improvement. Successful reconstruction using the technique of tissue expansion followed by insertion of a silicone or saline filled implant is possible and remains effective. However, autologous tissue reconstruction has become increasingly popular, using the woman's own muscle. This is especially useful at present because of the media misrepresentation of dangers associated with silicone gel filled mammary prostheses and the public's natural concerns. Moreover, muscle flaps tolerate radiotherapy for cancer better than the breast reconstructed with artificial material.

## Tissue expansion

First used in the 1950s and refined by Radovan in the 1970s, tissue expansion is a technique that takes advantage of the skin's inherent elasticity. An expandable silicone balloon is placed under the subcutaneous tissues, which is then intermittently inflated with saline injected through a port buried beneath the skin. The result is a gradual stretching of the overlying tissues, which may then be used to correct areas of deficiency. Tissue expansion is most commonly used in breast reconstruction after mastectomy. It is also widely used by plastic surgeons to reconstruct the scalp in alopecia or smallness of the ears and when it is desirable to increase the area or quality of skin coverage.

## Esthetic surgery

The primary goal of esthetic surgery is to improve the patient's appearance and self-image leading to enormous psychological and vocational gain. The public has come to appreciate this, as the demand for esthetic (cosmetic) surgery has continued to increase exponentially. Many of the advances were initially developed for reconstruction, including subperiosteal dissection, endoscopic surgery, and the use of grafts, implants, and lasers. Esthetic procedures are performed in an office, an office-based operating room, a free-standing surgery center, or a hospital. Many surgeons operate in specialized centers, which are more economical than the traditional hospital setting, commonly with local anesthesia and intravenous sedation, which also minimizes the expense and allows many procedures to be performed on an outpatient basis.

Breast augmentation was a common procedure in the USA until the Federal Drug Administration placed a moratorium on silicone implants in 1992 because of health concerns in a few patients. Several large studies in the USA and Europe have refuted these claims and demonstrated their safety. With their fears allayed, women have been undergoing augmentation in greater numbers than ever. Saline implants are the type most commonly used in the USA, although silicone implants are still available.

Alteration of the body shape by removal of fat, skin, or both has become the most popular plastic surgical procedure. Until the 1970s, the technique consisted of removing large amounts of fatty tissue through long, but concealed, incisions. Later, surgeons began to use suction in combination with sharp curettes to remove fat through smaller incisions, and the technique has undergone several modifications to improve it. The most recent advance has been the addition of ultrasonic energy to disrupt the fat cells, creating an emulsion that can be evacuated by applying a vacuum. This technique is reported to lessen bleeding and bruising, and also provides an easier removal of fat, and a more thorough removal of fibrous fatty deposits as found in the upper abdomen, back, and enlarged breasts in men.

### Endoscopic and laser surgery

Like general surgeons, plastic surgeons have also started to operate through small incisions using endoscopes (small tubes passed into body structures). Carpal tunnel release was one of the first applications, but the technique has now been extended to endoscopic brow-lift, face-lift, and breast augmentation. Using specialized instruments and viewing the surgical field on a video monitor, the plastic surgeon can now perform many standard procedures through much shorter incisions that are located in favorable locations. Examples of this include the endoscopic placement of breast implants through small incisions hidden in either the armpit or the umbilicus. Raising the forehead and brows may also be accomplished with a few small incisions in the scalp hair.

Lasers produce powerful beams of synchronized energy that can be visible or invisible. Many types of lasers with medical applications exist and each has a particular wavelength that defines its interaction with human tissues. Hence differing tissues can be selectively 'targeted' by choosing an appropriate wavelength. Current lasers in plastic surgical use are directed at smoothing wrinkles, tightening skin, and removing vascular birthmarks, spider veins, and unwanted hair. Some surgeons also use lasers to cut skin or tissues precisely in operations on the eyelids and hair transplantation.

Laser resurfacing of the face removes crowsfeet and wrinkles from around the mouth, chin, and cheeks. This is accompanied by a generalized tightening of the facial skin that stimulates to a lesser degree the effects of a standard facelift. In many practices laser resurfacing has replaced the techniques of chemical peeling and dermabrasion for treatment of wrinkles and acne scarring. The technique avoids the postoperative hypopigmentation that characterizes peels and dermabrasion.

Port-wine stains and other disfiguring birthmarks were initially treated by argon lasers, with results that were tempered by the accompanying scarring. The tunable dye laser was specifically designed to treat these lesions by selecting, or tuning, the wavelength produced by the laser so that it would be absorbed by blood cells. This process, known as 'selective photothermolysis', is responsible for the laser energy being preferentially transferred to the abnormal blood vessels rather than surrounding tissues. The heat generated within the vessel causes it to coagulate, which results in a clearing of the birthmark. Newer solid state lasers have improved these results and are cheaper.

### Implants and augmentation materials

Plastic surgeons have a long history of transplanting tissues for reconstructive purposes, and they generally prefer tissues taken from the patient's own body. In some cases, however, artificial material may be used. Examples of this include augmentation of the facial skeleton with material such as silicone, hydroxyapatite, polypropylene, and polytetrafluorethylene. Such implants are used to alter the contour of the cheek bones, chin, and jaw lines and are available in many shapes and sizes.

### Modern practice

Although the public and media tend to think of the esthetic aspect of plastic surgery, most surgeons are actively involved in reconstruction as well. Today the distinction between the two is less clear than before. The patient with a facial palsy after cancer resection may have a muscle transfer to restore closure of the eyelids, but the same muscle may be used to reanimate the face. One might ask, is the restoration of that most human of elements, the smile, a matter of reconstruction or cosmesis? Techniques initially developed for one purpose are often later applied in the other. Patients may begin treatment for reconstructive surgery and later have concerns about their appearance. In the end, the surgeon realizes that the distinction is unimportant; that despite technological advancements, little has changed since the days of Tagliacozzi, as the plastic surgeon strives to restore *both* form and function. MTE, TJG

*See also* MINIMALLY INVASIVE SURGERY; SPECIALIZATION

**PNEUMA** was a supposed all-pervading vital principle central to a Greco-Roman theory of medicine widely accepted during the 1st centuries BC and AD. Pneuma was carried around the body in the nerves and underwent changes in particular organs; at death it left to rejoin a universal stockpile. The doctrine was promulgated by Erasistratus and others.

**POETRY** In Shelley's *Hymn of Apollo*, which takes its myth from Ovid, the god says:

> I am the eye with which the Universe
>     Beholds itself and knows itself divine;
> All harmony of instrument or verse,
>     All prophecy, all medicine are mine.

The notion of a common basis for such contrasted activities as medicine and poetry is paradoxical, but for the ancient Greeks and Romans both poetry and medicine were the fruit of inspiration from APOLLO (p 359). Today we use the word 'inspiration' meaning the mental processes that evoke and make for excellence, not only in works of art but also in scientific discovery and medical diagnosis; so the claims of Apollo in Shelley's *Hymn* still make good sense.

Some years ago I was asked to compile an anthology of poems by doctor–poets. I defined 'poets' as those who had published poems of acclaimed value, and 'doctors' as those who (a) were medically qualified, whether or not they had practiced medicine, or (b) had practiced, whether or not they had a medical qualification, or (c) had made a significant contribution to medical science. My anthology, which I called *Apollo*, soon had its available space filled with works by 67 doctor–poets. Most of the chosen poems were written in English, but there were also poems in ancient Greek, Hebrew, Italian, French, Spanish, German, Swedish, Russian, Czech, and Japanese, for which translations in English were provided.

The earliest poems in *Apollo* are three epigrams from *The Greek anthology* by Nicias of Miletus (fl. 250 BC). In his 11th Idyll, Theocritus addresses Nicias as 'both physician and favorite of the Muses'. There were other doctor–poets, and there is a large body of Latin verse on medical subjects from Roman times to the Renaissance; verse must have seemed the natural medium for doctrines inspired by Apollo, but the purpose of the metrical treatises was didactic, so they are not represented in *Apollo*.

After Nicias, *Apollo* takes a long leap forward to the Gospel of St Luke, 'the beloved physician'. Luke might have been surprised to find himself called a poet, but passages such as the familiar verses on the birth of Christ gain rather than lose their freshness through frequent recall — a hallmark of true poetry. Another long leap carries *Apollo* to the school of Hebrew poetry that flourished in Spain during the 11th century. The most famous of these poets, Judah Halevi (1075–1141), was for a time physician to King Alfonso VI in Toledo. His poems are mystical and sensuous,

with some surprising thoughts, as when he praises God who causes both the strengths and the weaknesses of his medicaments.

After these brief visits to antiquity and to the Middle Ages, *Apollo* makes its definitive landfall in the Renaissance. Medicine was then an art steeped in literary culture, and it was no anomaly for RABELAIS (p 700) (1490–1553), a medical graduate of Montpellier, to become one of the giants of French literature. *Gargantua et Pantagruel*, a prose work, contains some elegant passages of verse, such as the introductory lines inviting the reader to laugh with the author, '*Pour ce que rire est le propre de l'homme*'.

Thomas Lodge (1558–1625: DM Oxford) was a general practitioner of letters — pamphleteer, novelist, poet, dramatist. His romance, *Rosalynde*, which gave Shakespeare the story of *As you like it*, contains some pleasing lyrics. Thomas Campion (1567–1620) was poet, composer, art theorist, physician, and Latinist, a true Renaissance man. T. S. Eliot praised him as 'after Shakespeare, the most accomplished master of the rhymed lyric of his time'. The delicacy and wit of such lute songs as 'When to her lute Corina sings' and 'It fell on a summer's day' are among the miniature glories of English poetry and music. Campion took an MD degree at Caen in Normandy and practiced in London.

Medical knowledge in Campion's time was very limited. The situation changed with the rapid growth of science and the divergence of scientific and artistic spheres that came later, but there continued to be an unexpectedly large number of doctor–poets. This should not seem surprising, for the human experience gained in medical practice will nourish a literary imagination, and the sensibilities of an artist are not out of place in one who practices the art of medicine. Anton CHEKHOV's (p 84) double life as doctor and dramatist illustrates the point well; he told a friend that he would probably not have been a writer if he had not practiced medicine. An even more obvious factor which drives poets to lead double lives is economic: few poets can live on their earnings from poetry.

The major preoccupation of poets in the Elizabethan age was amorous; both Lodge and Campion excelled as writers of love poems. In the 17th century, however, religion came to be the central theme of poetry. *Religio medici*, the prose masterpiece of Sir Thomas Browne (1605–82), contains some memorable poetry — the colloquy with God, which ends:

> O come that hour when I shall never
> Sleep again but wake for ever.

A similar preoccupation drew from Henry Vaughan (1622–95) such visionary poems as

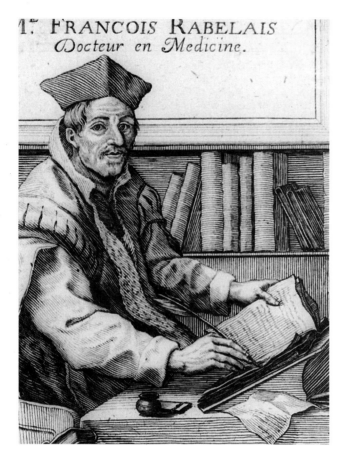

Francois Rabelais (1490–1553), doctor of medicine. (Reproduced courtesy of the National Library of Medicine, Bethesda, MD).

'They are all gone into the world of light' and *The retreat*, which anticipates the doctrine Wordsworth expressed in his Ode, *Intimations of immortality*. Vaughan's 'Metaphysical' paradoxes are sometimes disturbing, as when, in his poem *Affliction*, he sees illness as a sort of medicine to cure man of his behavioral disorders. Vaughan also published love poems and a translation of a German treatise on the medical ideas of PARACELSUS (p 617). He practiced medicine, but it is not known where he took his medical degree. Two German contemporaries of Vaughan were Paul Fleming (1609–40: MD Leipzig) and Johannes Scheffler (1624–77: MD Padua). Fleming has been called the only good poet in Germany during the Thirty Years' War, and Scheffler (known as Angelus Silesius) wrote a famous collection of mystical epigrams. For a time he was court physician to the Austrian Emperor.

A very different contemporary of Vaughan was Abraham Cowley (1618–67: DM Oxford). He was one of Milton's three favorite English poets (the others were Spenser and Shakespeare). Dr Johnson regarded him as the peer of Milton and 'undoubtedly the best of the Metaphysicals'. He wrote in various forms — Pindaric Odes, love poems, an epic on King David — and translations of Anacreon. There is some eloquent verse in Cowley's substantial output, but also much bombast and bathos, so it is not surprising that his poetic reputation, unlike Vaughan's, faded in the century after his death. He did not practice medicine, but his scientific writings were influential in the genesis of the Royal Society.

The leading Italian poet of the 17th century was Francesco Redi (1626–98), physician to the Medici grand dukes in Florence and also a biologist, whose experiments helped to demolish the prevailing belief that worms appear by spontaneous generation in rotting meat. In contrast with the God-intoxicated poetry of Vaughan, Redi's poetry was wine-intoxicated. His long dithyrambic poem, *Bacco in Toscano*, describes, in unsteady but melodious verse, a voyage in search of the 'King of all wine'.

The late 17th and early 18th centuries in Britain were the 'Augustan' age, when heroic couplets and classical decorum were in fashion and epics were in demand. Sir Richard Blackmore (1650–1729), physician to King William III, published four long epics, one of which (*Prince Arthur*) became very popular. Dr Johnson devoted a chapter in *Lives of the English poets* to Blackmore, but found his epics dull. Sir Samuel Garth (1661–1719) drew upon his medical experience in a mock heroic poem, *The dispensary*, which anticipates Pope's *Rape of the lock* in some respects. His portrait of a physician is unflattering:

> The sage, in velvet chair, here lolls at ease
> To promise future health for present fees.
> Then, as from tripod, solemn shams reveals,
> And what the stars know nothing of, foretells.

John Arbuthnot (1667–1735), physician and friend of Pope, speculates on his own nature with an anatomist's particularity and perplexity:

> The pipes through which the circling juices stray
> Are not that thinking I.

Another poet–physician was John Armstrong (1709–79), whose long blank verse poem, *The art of preserving health*, had some success. Two doctor–poets whose literary reputation is still fresh are Oliver Goldsmith (1728–74) and Mark Akenside (1721–70). Goldsmith's famous poem, *The deserted village*, is written in heroic couplets but gives glimpses of a post-'Augustan' sensibility as it laments the passing of an age of supposed innocence:

> Ill fares the land to hastening ills a prey
> When wealth accumulates and men decay.

**Plate 11** Cardiac catheterization. (Reproduced courtesy of Science Photo Library.)

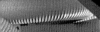

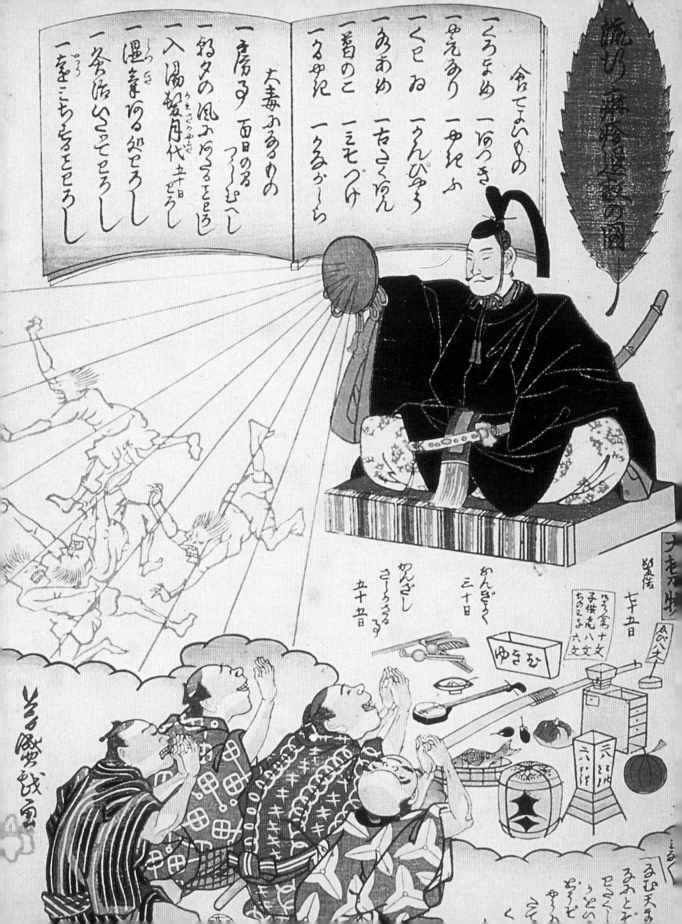

His wry, whimsical humor is shown in some other poems. Akenside, a physician at St Thomas's Hospital in London, was a more eminent doctor than Goldsmith, but, though his writings are less highly regarded than Goldsmith's, his long poem *The pleasures of imagination* was very popular. Like Goldsmith, Akenside seems to be pointing the way towards the coming Romantic era, anticipating Wordsworth's nature mysticism. The novelist Tobias Smollett (1721–71) wrote some poems which pre-echo those of his compatriot, Sir Walter Scott; Smollett, a Glasgow graduate, practiced for a time in London.

Erasmus DARWIN (p 214) (1731–1802), grandfather of the great biologist, was a polymath who poured his thoughts, discoveries, and fancies on botany, chemistry, medicine, steam power, infusion of digitalis leaves, the Portland vase, and much else into a huge poem, *The botanic garden.* He practiced medicine in Lichfield and presided over that great institution, the Lunar Society of Birmingham, whose members met on the night of the full moon to discuss their latest scientific thoughts and discoveries. From the prosy and sometimes unintentionally funny profusion of *The botanic garden* true poetry sometimes erupts, as in the invocation to spring, starting:

> Ethereal cohorts, Essences of Air!
> Make the green children of the Spring your care!

Edward JENNER (p 452) (1749–1823), the pioneer of smallpox vaccination, wrote some attractive light-hearted verses which are well crafted and might easily be taken for unfamiliar minor poems of Wordsworth.

The two greatest poets of Germany have a place in *Apollo*: Goethe (1749–1832) studied anatomy and discovered the intermaxillary bone of the human skull; Schiller (1759–1805) qualified in medicine at a military academy and was, for a time, surgeon to a brigade of grenadiers. By including these German masters *Apollo* gained the inclusion of two great English poets as translators, — Shelley, who made an English verse translation of the Prologue to Goethe's *Faust*, and Coleridge, whose *Visit of the gods* is a metrically apt version of Schiller's *Dithyrambe*. A fine German poet of the next generation was Justinus Kerner (1786–1862), an associate of Mörike, Uhland, and the other poets of the Swabian school; he was an eminent physician who also published medical textbooks. Meanwhile in Britain, George Crabbe (1754–1832) was a successful, unqualified, medical practitioner and a prolific poet who used heroic couplets to project, in *The borough*, an almost 21st century image of Aldeburgh and its people. His comments on medical colleagues are shrewd:

> Helpers of men they're call'd, and we confess
> Theirs the deep study, theirs the lucky guess.

Charlatans and quacks he trounced:

> Some, too, admitted to this honour'd name
> Have, without learning, found a way to fame…
> There are among them those who cannot read,
> And yet they'll buy a patent, and succeed.

John KEATS (this page) (1795–1821) was a Licentiate of the Society of APOTHECARIES, but he did not practice. Suffering from TUBERCULOSIS, in his short life he wrote and published much poetry, including the great odes, *The eve of St Agnes* and the unfinished *Hyperion*. Medical insights may be noticed in *La belle dame sans merci*, and in those oft-quoted lines from the *Ode to a nightingale*, lamenting human suffering in a world

> Where palsy shakes a few, sad, last grey hairs,
> Where youth grows pale, and spectre-thin, and dies.

Thomas Lovell Beddoes (1803–49) wrote and re-wrote his verse drama, *Death's jest book*, under the influence of reading Elizabethan and Jacobean drama. Some of his lyrical poems have a haunting beauty — for example, *Dream pedlary*, which starts

> If there were dreams to sell
> What would you buy?
>
> Some cost a passing bell;
> Some a light sigh.

After taking his MD in Göttingen, Beddoes emigrated to Germany and stayed there. He was morbidly fascinated by death and poisoned himself with curare.

Oliver Wendell Holmes (1809–94), professor of PHYSIOLOGY at Harvard, wrote witty and ingenious poems, like the story of the 'wonderful one-hoss shay,' which was built so logically that it could not break down but wore out, all parts turning simultaneously to rubble and leaving the stunned passenger sitting on terra firma. Holmes was one of the cultured 19th-century doctors who could turn their hand to elegant verse when this seemed appropriate: others were Sir Charles SHERRINGTON (p 647) (1861–1952) and Sir Ronald ROSS (1857–1932) (p 481) (both NOBEL laureates) and the eminent neurologist Sir Henry HEAD (p 745) (1861–1940). Robert Bridges (1844–1930), a physician at St Bartholomew's Hospital, retired in his 40s to devote more time to writing, and became Poet Laureate in 1913. He was one of the most gifted poets of his time; he rarely wrote on medical subjects, but there are a few moving poems (for example, *On a dead child*) about medical experiences.

Very different from Bridges was the American avant-garde poet, William Carlos Williams (1883–1963), who distanced himself from the British poetry scene in verses called *The testament of perpetual change*, which consists of the grandiose opening lines of Bridges' *Testament of beauty* alter-

### DOCTOR-POETS

John **KEATS** (1795–1821). British physician and poet. Keats, the son of the head ostler at the Swan and Hoop public house, Moorgate Pavement, London, was apprenticed to a surgeon at Edmonton in 1810 and later studied at Guy's and St Thomas's Hospitals. He ceased to practice in 1817, died in Rome in 1821 of pulmonary tuberculosis, as had his mother and his brother. His chief works were *Poems* (1817); 'Endymion' (1818); 'Ode to a nightingale' (1819); and 'Hyperion' (1820).

*(continued overleaf)*

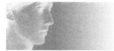

**John MCCRAE**

(1872–1918). Canadian physician and poet. McCrae became a member of the department of pathology at McGill University. During the First World War he served in France and in 1916, at a field dressing station, he wrote the poem *In Flanders fields*, He died of pneumonia in Boulogne in 1918, and his verses were published posthumously.

nating line by line with snippets of colloquial chatter. He practiced medicine and wrote some moving poems on medical themes. The Mexican poet Enrique Gonzalez Martinez (1871–1952) was a physician and an ambassador; under his influence Spanish poets reacted against the Romantic tradition. In Germany Hans Carossa (1878–1956), a physician, and Gottfried Benn (1886–1956), a surgeon, were leading poets, as were Oliver St John Gogarty (1878–1957), an ear, nose, and throat surgeon in Ireland, and Mokichi Saito (1882–1953), a psychiatrist, in Japan; and many others at that time led such double lives, among them Havelock ELLIS (p 747) (1859–1940), Sir Arthur Conan DOYLE (p 233) (1859–1930), and Rancis Brett Young (1884–1954) who wrote *The island*, a long poem on British history. John MCCRAE (this page) (1872–1918), a Canadian pathologist, was famous for one poem, *In Flanders fields*. The eminent neurologist, Russell Brain (1895–1966) published a small book containing *Hiroshima*, a poem which starts with an image that is both apocalyptic and scientific:

> Now the trumpet of the atomic gale
> Blasts through the interstices of flesh

Though a master of words, Brain was an exceptionally silent man, as I well remember from my time as his house physician. Another neurologist–poet, John Penman (1913–92), was a classical scholar before he studied medicine. A French doctor, Paul Noël (1904–79), published a book of love poems, for which he was awarded the Prix Verlaine by L'Academie Française in 1951.

Among the poets in *Apollo* who were alive then several are well known, including Miroslav Holub (1923–98), the Czech immunologist whose poems in translation are familiar to many readers in Britain, Dannie Abse (b. 1926), formerly President of the Poetry Society, whose poems, some of them medical, often have a disturbing intensity, and John Stone (b. 1936), an American cardiac physician who has published several collections, in one of which appears this miniature triumph:

> Death
>
> I have seen come on
> slowly as rust
> sand
>
> or suddenly as when
> someone leaving
> a room
>
> finds the doorknob
> come loose in his hand

The poems of Alex Comfort (1920–99) seem to have sprung from the same soil that nourished his career as a medical biologist.

For many doctors poetry has been something more than a hobby; this applies, for example, to

Kenyon Alexander (b. 1921), Gael Turnbull (b. 1928), and J. R. Heron (b. 1932); also to the Gambian surgeon, Lenrie Peters (b. 1932), to a Swedish woman doctor, Eva Ström (b. 1947), and to a Russian, Alexander Rosembaum (b. 1951), who is a popular singer of his own song-poems.

A few years after *Apollo* appeared, Yann Lovelock published a scholarly essay entitled *Furor Apollonis: an occupational disease*. My comment in *Apollo* that writing poetry must be an occupational hazard of doctors had prompted Lovelock to scan the relevant literature in Latin, Spanish, Portuguese, French, Italian, Romanian, Modern Greek, Arabic, Dutch, Swedish, German, and English; and he found 85 doctor–poets who are not represented in *Apollo*. Some are eminent poets, including the Dutch psychiatrist R. van der Hoofdaker, whose pen name is Rutger Kopland (b. 1934), and Tomas Tranströmer (b. 1931), a leading Swedish poet who is also a psychiatrist. There must be many other doctor–poets of whom neither Lovelock nor I were aware; one who came to my notice recently was Emil Aarestrup (1800–56), a well-known Danish poet and general practitioner.

In both lists, Lovelock's and mine, Germany and England are well represented, and it seems that some factor, perhaps the importance of the Romantic tradition, accounts for the prevalence of the doctor–poet syndrome in these countries. There are very few women among the doctor–poets, perhaps because many women who practice medicine already lead double lives, as mothers and doctors. The high incidence of psychiatrist–poets should not seem surprising, because doctors who have made a special study of the mind and its disorders are likely to be interested and even involved in that tantalizing disorder, the compulsive urge to write poems. Poetry, like MUSIC, may also interest doctors because of its potential therapeutic value. The doctors who would seem least at risk of developing the 'syndrome' are specialists in laboratory medicine, but there have been some notable writers in that category, among them the Egyptian bacteriologist, Abu Shadi (1892–1955), Miroslav Holub, and, most recently, an American pathologist, Lenny Emmanuel (b. 1932).

As a microbiologist who has for much of his life endured (and enjoyed) the doctor–poet syndrome, I have been struck by the similarities between the conceiving of thoughts for scientific research and the conceiving of thoughts which lead to the composition of poems. Another link between these activities is expertise with LANGUAGE, by which both scientific ideas and poetic images are formulated. Although the purposes of science and art are quite distinct, the emotions that drive people to do these things (the 'role of Apollo') are much the same, whether the outcome is a scientific experiment or a sonnet sequence.                                          EL

*See also* AUTHORS; LITERATURE; TRUANTS – DOCTORS IN OTHER WALKS OF LIFE

---

[Edward Lowbury himself is also a distinguished poet, whose collections include *Time for sale* (1961), *Daylight astronomy* (1968) *The night watchman* (1974), *Collected poems* (1993), and *Mystic bridge* (1997).]

**POISONING** The word poison is derived from the same source as potion, being something taken by mouth. It is defined as a substance that damages the body no matter how it may gain access.

Colorful as many of these stories may seem, they mostly lack scientific validation, for sudden death, presumably as common then as now, was often suspected to be the result of poisoning. Moreover, the application of chemical analysis to identify poisons in organs and tissues post-mortem did not become feasible until the beginning of the 19th century. Quantitative factors must also be taken into account: PARACELSUS (p 617), a Swiss physician, first enunciated the principle that 'It is only the right dose that differentiates a poison from a medicine'. Arsenic, for example, is often found in the body, but in such small quantities as to have no toxic significance. All too frequently this factor is disregarded, to make more impressive those warnings issued by the media, politicians, and pressure groups about the dangers of pollutants in the environment, in our drinking water, and in our food.

**Toxicology** is the study of poisons and poisoning in the broadest sense. First of all, it is essential to know if a substance is toxic at all and to what extent. In earlier and more inhuman days, prisoners and slaves might be sacrificed as test subjects; now the information comes from experiments on laboratory animals, chiefly mice, rats, guinea pigs, and rabbits, sometimes dogs and occasionally anthropoid apes, in the face of vigorous protests from members of the animal welfare groups.

But it is imperative to generate reliable data for designing policies to safeguard human health and to formulate effective measures for treating anyone who may get poisoned.

**Poisoning in practice**
Any knowledge of willful poisoning must depend very largely on the resources available and the efforts mobilized to bring the perpetrators to account. Over a large part of the world, uncertainty prevails. Nevertheless, one should always be on the alert for these transgressions, since deliberate poisoning may be motivated politically, as an act of vengeance, or in the furtherance of some other crime.

Despite all the precautions ostensibly taken to prevent it, poisoning continues to occur globally in some form or another. Extensive areas still exist in which venomous creatures roam at large to inflict their bites. Mushroom poisoning remains common, ironically, among amateur enthusiasts collecting wild fungi for cooking. In addition, mycotoxins, formed on damp grain and other foodstuffs, take their toll, notably in Asia, and the aflatoxins on ground-nuts are carcinogenic. More perplexing are those unforeseen epidemics that may suddenly erupt, frequently from human carelessness or neglect. Thus, rice purveyed in Taiwan and Japan for human consumption was subsequently found to be contaminated with commercial polychlorinated chemicals, but not before some thousands of victims had fallen ill or died. In Spain the 'toxic oil syndrome', which came to notice in 1981, was associated with the consumption of a low-priced 'olive oil' that was in fact rape seed oil, mysteriously containing some toxic ingredients, that were never identified. This claimed thousands of casualties before the offending material was withdrawn from the market. Dramatic, too, was 'Minimata disease' on the coast of Japan. Factory effluent found its way into the waters, contaminating them with salts of mercury, but as these were in the inorganic form they were rated as having low toxicity to humans. What was not foreseen was that the marine microorganisms in this bay could convert this mercury into the organic form. This, in turn, concentrated in the marine food chain through plankton to crustacea and ultimately in people living in the area. In consequence they were stricken with organo-mercury poisoning, a severely crippling disease affecting the developing fetus as well as others, which for some time eluded diagnosis.

The natural presence of inorganic fluoride in the groundwater on which the local population depends for drinking is essentially environmental. When the concentration is modest, it can be beneficial in mitigating dental decay. But when the levels are higher these lead to discoloration, with 'mottling', of the teeth, while higher levels still, as in East Africa and parts of India, may cause excessive and disabling calcification of skeletal bones.

In the Andes, the subterranean strata are endowed with ores of arsenic, but are also the only source of drinking water for the people living above. Among these people chronic arsenical poisoning is endemic; manifested by the involvement of many body organs, notably the nerves and the skin, which is prone to develop cancerous changes. For these unfortunate people there is no escape, unless an adequate, alternative supply of potable water can be provided or they themselves can be uprooted to other surroundings.

## POISONING IN HISTORY

Poisoning was once a widespread hazard, notably among the poor, who in need of food were obliged to gather wild plants and fruits without knowing if they were safe, and who were also prey to all the venomous creatures then at large. For the more privileged members of the community, deliberate poisoning served as a means for eliminating adversaries and enemies, even for disposing of inconvenient relatives. History is replete with such accounts of poisoning, not least by the Borgias, in 14th-century Italy, when it was the custom to 'carry pure death in an ear-ring, a casket, a fan-mount, and a Filigree basket'. It should be remembered, too, that Socrates suffered judicial homicide by drinking the hemlock cup.

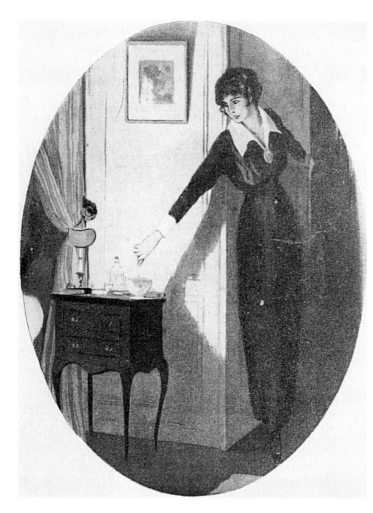

A melodramatic representation of poisoning, from Octava Feuillet's *La morte* (c. 1910). (Reproduced courtesy of the Mary Evans Picture Library.)

Another risk of mass poisoning arises at many industrial locations, where a sudden explosion may disperse toxic material over the neighborhood. Once this happens the emergency services are often at a loss to know what, if anything, they should do; chaos reigns, fears are magnified, and over-reaction ensues. It is incumbent upon the authorities and the factory management to have exigency plans prepared in advance.

In the more developed countries chronic poisoning assumes a peculiar form, in the persistence of habits which are inimical to health, for example, tobacco SMOKING and over-indulgence in ALCOHOL, as outright SUICIDE with a massive overdose of a poison. The majority, on the other hand, are simply making a gesture, or seeking no more than an escape, albeit temporarily, from a situation which they fear will otherwise overwhelm them. Commonly, for this purpose they choose medicaments in tablet or capsule form, prescribed either for themselves or for other members of the family and which seem readily to hand in most homes.

Those which are thought to act upon the brain are most popular: hypnotics, analgesics, tranquilizers, or antidepressants. An estimated 100 000 episodes of this poisoning occur each year in Britain alone, and form over 10% of all acute, medical, hospital admissions. Elsewhere the pattern is much the same, for example, in Scandinavia, Central Europe, and the USA, although alcohol features more prominently in Finland and hard drugs such as cocaine or heroin in the United States. Among the white population of South Africa the picture is more or less the same, but among the blacks, kerosene and traditional medicines are more popular.

Customarily, on presenting at hospital, most overdose patients are admitted, if only as a precaution, for all but about 1% of them enjoy rapid and complete physical recovery but, as 'parasuicides', they require ongoing psychiatric and social support.

**Medical management**

No time must be wasted on delving deeply into the precise diagnosis. The priority is to maintain the vital systems — the respiration, heart, and circulation. This regimen is continued until the patient is judged to be out of danger. In serious cases the resources of an intensive care unit may be demanded. According to the patient's condition and the response, measures to clear the toxin from the gut before it is absorbed may avail, as by induced vomiting, gastric aspiration and lavage (the 'stomach pump'), purgatives, or introducing adsorbents, such as activated charcoal, by mouth. In addition, elimination may be promoted by augmenting the output of urine (forced diuresis), by hemodialysis (the artificial kidney), or by hemoperfusion, when the blood flow is diverted externally to percolate through a column of adsorbent material before being returned to the circulation.

Contrary to popular belief, specific antidotes are seldom appropriate, although sometimes they may be salutary — e.g. oxygen for carbon monoxide exposure, cobalt edetate for cyanide, acetylcysteine for paracetamol overdose, naloxone for opiates, and a few others. Meanwhile, the nonspecific supportive measures must be maintained. When antidotes are indicated they should be administered without delay. These are among the few occasions when chemical analyses of the blood and/or urine may be needed.

**Information**

Doctors may not be familiar with the recognition, appraisal, and specialist management of patients thought to have been poisoned. Less still are they familiar with the composition and toxicity of the wide range of potentially toxic substances — medicines, household products, cosmetics, or industrial and agricultural chemicals. For this reason poisons information or control centers have often been set up, either governmentally or as local initiatives, which will answer questions about poisons by telephone.

Coordination of these activities takes place nationally, as through the American Clearing House for Poisons Control Centers, and internationally, as through the European Association of Poisons Centers and Clinical Toxicologists. Meetings, congresses, and publications provide for the exchange and dissemination of case reports, together with research findings upon the subject generally.

On a global scale, the International Programme on Chemical Safety, a tripartite operation between the WORLD HEALTH ORGANIZATION, the International Labour Organization, and the United Nations Environmental Program, provides for separate countries to formulate their own policies on an informed basis.

### Statutory control

For both personal and communal safety it is the rule, in most developed countries, for statutory control to be imposed over the storage, sale, supply, and labeling of hazardous substances — namely, poisons. Within Europe, the pattern is set by directives issued by the Commission in Brussels and, within the UK, effect is given to these by, primarily, the Environmental Protection Act, 1990, with guidance offered by an independent advisory committee on hazardous substances, serviced by the Department of the Environment. Also relevant is the Health and Safety at Work Act, 1974, concerned with poisoning that may arise from working practices. More specifically, rigid controls are applied under the Misuse of Drugs Act, 1974, to drugs of addiction, such as morphine, heroin, and cannabis. Internationally, coordination of these measures is also advanced by the International Programme on Chemical Safety.

Perhaps surprisingly, the statistics indicate that the death toll from poisoning is generally below that from other diseases, although the incidence varies quite widely between one country and another according to the extent to which such deaths are investigated and determined.      RG

*See also* ADVERSE DRUG REACTIONS; MISADVENTURES; PHARMACOLOGY, CLINICAL PHARMACOLOGY AND THERAPEUTICS

**POOR LAW** See BRITAIN, WORKHOUSES

**PORPHYRIA** See 'ROYAL MADNESS' AND PORPHYRIA

**POST-TRAUMATIC STRESS DISORDER** is a chronic disabling psychological condition which develops as a reaction to a life-threatening or other horrifying event. Described originally after exposure to extreme violence and death in war, it may be seen in civilian life, after personal assault, or torture; rape and sexual abuse; involvement in a disaster or act of terrorism; industrial accident; road, rail, or air accident; a bad experience in childbearing; and other situations in which an individual's bodily integrity is seriously threatened. It can also be brought on in someone, not in personal danger, who witnesses the death or injury of a loved one. (The proximity of time, place, and relationship between the onlooker and victim is a matter of legal debate.)

The symptom of this disorder may include intrusive recollections of the scene, such as flashbacks, nightmares, and disturbing dreams; raised anxiety, irritability, poor concentration, poor sleeping, exaggerated startle response; avoidance of reminders of the stressful event, blunting of the warmth of relationship with family and friends, loss of interest in and expectation of the future. The symptoms are likely to appear between one and six months after the event, they can last indefinitely if not treated, and can make it difficult for the sufferer to hold down a job. There may also be varying degrees depression, anxiety, panic attacks, and heavy smoking and drinking.

Treatment is a task for the specialist with particular psychological skills and not for the well-meaning counselor or doctor. Such treatment will begin after the initial distress is past, probably after about two or three weeks, but for practical reasons it regrettably often starts much later. No one treatment has been shown to be superior to the others. There is psychodynamic therapy (talking and exploring in depth), group therapy, and family therapy (important when children are affected, directly or indirectly).

Children and adolescents may react to psychological trauma just as adults do, but with less ability to articulate their distress. They can react by regressing and functioning poorly at school. Their needs must be anticipated after accidents and deaths in the family circle.

Rescuers too may suffer from prolonged contact with the death and suffering after a disaster, and being a 'professional' (for example, police, armed forces, fire brigade) does not confer immunity. Their likely needs must be anticipated.

Well-motivated people who are able to confront the traumatic experiences in their treatment, are likely to do well in terms of diminution of their symptoms and improvement in social functioning.

This condition was formally described after the Vietnam war, but the clinical features have long been recognized in wars under different names, such as shell shock, combat neurosis, battle fatigue, and lack of moral fiber. Unusually for a medical condition, it is tightly defined in the Diagnostic and Statistical Manual of Mental Disorders, 4th

**POLIOMYELITIS** is an acute virus infection, also known as infantile paralysis, spread from person to person by the fecal–oral route. In many people infection produces no symptoms at all, and in others a minor illness, but in some it destroys many nerve cells in the spinal cord and base of the brain, producing paralysis that may threaten life and lead to subsequent crippling disability. An ancient disease, polio was represented in Egyptian art 3000 years ago, but was described at the end of the 18th century. One of the first cases to be recognized was Sir Walter Scott, whose lameness in adult life has been ascribed to the disease. Devastating epidemics occurred from the end of the 19th century; 50 000 people a year were affected in the USA and President Franklin D. Roosevelt was crippled by an attack in 1921.

The life-threatening paralysis in the disease was one of the factors leading to the development of CRITICAL CARE, which aimed at supporting life while the patient recovered from the paralysis, which not only affected movement but also breathing. Early in the 20th century Simon FLEXNER (p 257) produced the illness in monkeys injected with nasal secretions from patients, and the virus had been grown in the laboratory by 1949. Effective vaccines followed from 1955, at first given by injection (introduced by Jonas SALK (this page)) and later on a sugar lump by mouth (introduced by Albert SABIN (this page)). With intensive immunization campaigns the virus was declared eradicated from the Western hemisphere in 1994 — so that the CHARITY The March of Dimes (started originally in 1935 to combat the disease) was able to switch its target to research into birth defects.

Currently pockets of disease remain in 10 countries in Africa and Asia, with India accounting for over half the childhood cases. Building on its success with the world-wide elimination of SMALLPOX, the WORLD HEALTH ORGANIZATION has started an intensive campaign to eliminate polio from these countries in the early 2000s. However, because the virus can survive only in human hosts, success entails eliminating the virus from entire populations by immunizing everyone. The campaign's efforts are hampered by civil war in several countries, particularly Angola, Sudan, Sierra Leone, and the Congo. Hence, until the combatants agree to a brief cease-fire to enable universal immunization to take place, polio is likely to persist and form a threat to the nonimmunized in the rest of the world. (In the West there are still occasional outbreaks in small groups that refuse to allow their children to be immunized on religious grounds as occurred, for example, in 1993 in the Netherlands.) SPL

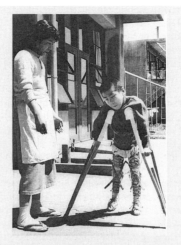

A young Japanese boy with polio is struggling to walk with the aid of crutches and a leg brace. (Photo courtesy of Dominique Darbois/WHO.)

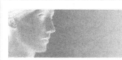

Cecil Kent **DRINKER** (1887–1956). American physiologist. Drinker's professional career was mainly spent in the physiology laboratory at the Harvard School of Public Health, where he carried out extensive studies of pulmonary function with emphasis on lymphatic circulation in the lungs. Later, with his brother Philip, he developed the Drinker respirator, or 'iron lung', which was used in management of patients with poliomyelitis who had respiratory paralysis. He also made studies of oxygen toxicity and of decompression sickness in divers and submarine personnel.

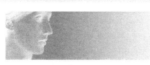

Albert Bruce **SABIN** (1906–93). Russian-American pediatrician and microbiologist. Sabin was born in Bialystock (now in Poland). He migrated to the United States in 1921, graduated from high school the following year, and then from New York University medical school. After service in the US Army, he returned to Cincinatti, concentrating his attention on live attenuated vaccines for oral use. He developed an oral polio vaccine in the mid 1950s, and, although early experience with this was disastrous, with paralytic poliomyelitis in some healthy volunteers, he persevered. After successful field tests in 1958–60, the Sabin oral polio vaccine came into widespread use in the USA and many developing countries, soon superseding the Salk vaccine.

Jonas **SALK** (1914–95). Salk's parents were uneducated Russian-Jewish immigrants to the USA. He was the first member of his family to go to college, where he intended to study law, but was attracted instead to medicine. As a medical student at New York University he was invited to spend a year doing microbiological research on influenza. After graduating he continued to work on influenza and developed a method of reducing the capacity of the influenza virus to cause infection in humans. This became the basis for his later work on poliomyelitis. In 1947 Salk moved to the University of Pittsburgh Medical School, where he concentrated on developing a vaccine against polio. After eight years the research yielded the first vaccine, which was successfully tested in human trials in 1955. Salk refused to patent his discovery so his vaccine became freely available world-wide. The Salk vaccine used killed poliovirus and was superseded in the USA and other countries a few years later by the live oral poliovirus vaccine subsequently developed by Albert SABIN (this page), despite evidence that the live virus actually caused polio in some persons. In countries where the Salk vaccine has remained in general use, poliomyelitis has been eradicated, Jonas Salk received many awards, (not including the NOBEL PRIZE) and used the money from these awards to endow the Jonas Salk Institute for Biological Studies. He remained an active research worker as well as a prominent thinker and passionate advocate for peace and international harmony until the end of his life. In his later years he became active in world-wide social and public health issues such as the problem of the growing imbalance between expanding populations and shrinking resources. These interests are eloquently described in his monograph, *World population and human values: a new reality* (1981) and in subsequent writings and speeches.

Edition (DSM IV) of the American Psychiatric Association, and in the International Classification of Disease, 10th Edition (ICD–10). This is partly because acceptance of the condition is relatively new, and partly because of its medicolegal importance in personal injury claims.　　　GB

*See also* BATTLE NEUROSIS; DISASTERS

**POVERTY AND HEALTH** Absolute poverty refers to a standard of minimum requirement, and relative poverty refers to falling behind most others in a given community. Poverty is usually held to include social dimensions — for example, the inability to participate fully in the social life of a community or country. Impoverished people experience powerlessness, their bargaining power reduced by work insecurity, lack of resources, and lack of income. They are often vulnerable to external risks, including natural disasters.

The many reasons for the relationship between poverty and disease include educational disadvantage; lack of healthcare; inadequate nutrition, clean water, and shelter; cultural beliefs about the causation of disease; and the deleterious effects of war and conflict on the infrastructure of society. Although income is important in determining health, economic growth does not invariably lead to improvements in health. The disparities in income between and within many countries have grown in recent decades, and despite overall economic growth on a global scale the number of people in absolute poverty is increasing. At the start of the 21st century about 1.3 billion people live in absolute poverty having incomes of under US$1 a day. Since 1980, 100 countries have suffered economic stagnation or decline, resulting in reduced incomes for 1.6 billion people. In 1960 the richest 20% of the world population had incomes 30 times greater than the poorest 20% of the world's population. By 1995 the difference had increased to around 82-fold. The 1998 UN World Development Report stated that the world's richest 225 people combined possessed more wealth than the income of the poorest 47% of the world's people.

Many of the mechanisms linking economic growth and human development at the national level are missing at the international level. Within countries, income tax and expenditure policies on education, social security, and health help to redistribute wealth, enhance the well-being of deprived sectors of the population, and ultimately benefit the whole of society. Such mechanisms do not operate at an international level. Continuing international debt is an important factor inhibiting the development of some of the poorest countries. In the early 1980s structural readjustment programs were proposed by the World Bank and the International Monetary Fund to overcome the severe economic and financial crisis affecting

## POST-TRAUMATIC STRESS DISORDER
### BEHAVIORAL AND PHARMACOLOGICAL TREATMENTS

- **Desensitization**. The aim is to help people confront their experiences, especially those which trigger flashbacks and lead to nightmares, and to bring them out in the open, and then to integrate them into their ordinary awareness and so deprive them of their power to cause distress.

  The affected person may make a detailed tape recording of the traumatic experience, which can then be played back over and over again, which similarly brings the experience out into the open.

- **Cognitive therapy**. The patient is taught how to change the dysfunctional ways of thinking that have been maintaining the disabling symptoms, and so to come to view the symptoms in a new way.

  The philosophy of this approach is that the individual has established faulty assumptions (cognitions) which perpetuate the disability, and that changing these assumptions will lead to improvement.

- **Drug treatment**. Antidepressants are often used with good effect,

preferably in conjunction with some other therapy. Potential habit-forming drugs should be avoided as the treatment may be long-term.

- **Eye movement desensitization and reprocessing**. This is a new approach, becoming widely accepted, in which the patient concentrates on a traumatic image, while the therapist rapidly moves a finger across their visual fields. Statements about the distress being experienced are replaced with more positive statements.

- **Early care**. Common kindness leads us to give comfort to those in distress, and to give them a chance to talk, perhaps repetitively, about their experiences. Mild sedative drugs may also be given.

  More intense early intervention, 'psychological debriefing', in which people are helped to process their experiences, has not been shown to lessen the likelihood of later post-traumatic stress disorder, but the evidence is still unclear.

many developing countries. In these countries there was frequently a dramatic impact of reduced public spending on health. The excesses of early structural readjustment programs have been acknowledged, particularly by the World Bank; and its recent president, James Wolfensohn, has stated that the bank's prime objective is now to reduce poverty. Nevertheless, it has not yet proved possible to cancel the debts of the highly indebted poorest countries. Accordingly, between 1990 and 1993, Africa transferred 13.4 billion dollars each year to its creditors, four times more than the spending by those governments on health services. Sub-Saharan Africa contains 34 of the 41 countries defined by the World Bank as heavily indebted. The 1999 Cologne G8 summit meeting resulted in an additional $70 billion dollars reduction in the total debts of the poorest countries, on top of $30 billion debt relief cancelled under pre-existing arrangements. This occurred after extensive campaigning made clear the depth of public concern. However, many indebted countries will not see their annual payments reduced and the economic conditions imposed on the countries in return for debt relief have yet to be clarified. Much remains to be done to alleviate the burdens on poor countries.

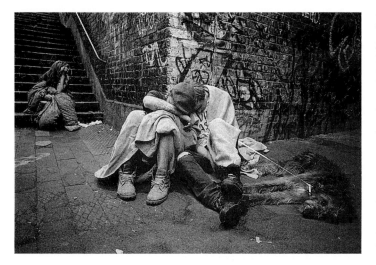

Three homeless people with a dog. (Reproduced courtesy of Tony Stone Images.)

To try to counteract the decrease in public spending on health by generating other funds for such services, many countries introduced cost sharing through mechanisms such as user fees. Many studies have analyzed the impact of these fees and have concluded that in general they tend to reinforce existing inequalities in access to health services, unless exemption policies are introduced to protect the poor.

### Poverty and health in industrialized countries

Between 1990 and 1993 average income fell by 20% or more in several industrialized countries, particularly in eastern Europe and the former Soviet Union. This was accompanied by declining life expectancy and an increasing gap in life expectancy between western and eastern Europe. Between 1970 and 1995 the gap in life expectancy between the best performing countries in western Europe and the poorest performing countries of eastern Europe increased from about three to 15 years for men and from four to ten years for women. In Russia, in 1995, the life expectancy for men dropped to 59, below retirement age. Why such gaps are widening over such a short period is still open to debate. Increases in alcohol consumption and in violence were contributory factors, in addition to dramatic falls in income for many people.

In the United States and Britain income distribution became more unequal in the 1980s and the early 1990s. According to the United Nations Development Program income distribution in these two countries is now among the most unequal of industrialized countries in the world. In Britain, for example, the proportion of people with an income below half the national average

rose from under 10% in 1982 to over 20% in 1993. The class difference in mortality between rich and poor has increased, because death rates have fallen faster in the rich than in the poor. The proportion of children living below the official poverty line trebled over a ten-year period. The 1980 Black Report on inequalities in health concluded that if the death rates of occupational class I (professional workers and members of their families) had been experienced by classes IV and V (partly skilled and unskilled manual workers and their families), 75 000 deaths of people aged under 75, including nearly 10 000 children, would have been avoided annually. The report had a negative reception from the then Secretary of State for Health, and the government at the time attempted to minimize its impact because it was unprepared to consider the additional expenditure recommended.

Income and social class differentials in health in industrialized nations are accompanied by gradients in death rates for several causes. For infants up to 1 year, British experience shows definite disparities in deaths from accidents and respiratory disease. Between the ages of 1 and 14 the differences between social classes narrow but are still in evidence, accidents showing the sharpest social class gradient in mortality. Among adults the social class difference is particularly large in those in their 20s and 30s, and gradients are steep for accidents, poisoning, and violence, particularly in men. Gradients in mortality are also seen in diseases of the respiratory system and circulatory, digestive, and genitourinary systems.

A major study of over 17 000 civil servants in Whitehall showed that men in the lowest employment grade had three times the mortality of those in the highest grade from coronary heart disease and from other causes. Conventional risk factors such as smoking, obesity, physical inactivity, blood pressure, and blood cholesterol concentrations explain only part of the observed difference in mortality. Subsequently, it was suggested that lack of control over work environment might explain some of the difference between the higher and lower grades in coronary disease death rates.

### Early environment

The early environment may also influence later expression of disease. Studies by Barker and colleagues have suggested that factors operating *in utero* and early life may increase cardiovascular risk. For example, among men born 70 years previously, those with lower birth weights and weights at 1 year had higher death rates from coronary heart disease. Since low birth weight is commoner among women from lower social classes, this may explain how deprivation has an impact on health in the long term. Other studies have also shown that disadvantage in childhood may contribute to the higher risk of death in later life.

Investigations of illness or general health and poverty have also been undertaken. In Britain the General Household Survey, conducted by the Office of National Statistics, asked people about both chronic and acute sickness. A social class gradient is most pronounced for long-standing illnesses that limit activity, particularly in those aged 45–64. Self-reported disease and psychosocial ill health (including inability to sleep, concentrate, etc.) are also more likely among individuals from the lower social classes.

Unemployment has also been associated with poor health in several studies. For example, after adjusting for social class, Moser and colleagues (1987) found an excess mortality of 20–30% among the unemployed, which did not seem to result only from health-related selection for unemployment. Raised standardized mortality ratios were noted for suicide, lung cancer, and ischemic heart disease. The death rate of wives of unemployed men was also higher than that of other married women. Studies of the health effects of unemployment in Calne, Wiltshire, by Beale and Nethercott showed an overall increase in ill health which did not seem to be explained by lower symptom tolerance. They suggested that unemployment led to chronic ill health and increases in consultations for cardiovascular disorders and other chronic complaints, which may have been in part psychosomatic.

Four types of explanation for health inequalities were mentioned in the Black Report: artefactual, selection, cultural or behavioral, and materialist. An artefactual relationship might occur, for instance, if social class were recorded differently on death certificates and at the census. Also, if the size of lower class groups were to decrease, these might contain a greater proportion of individuals at high risk of premature death. If unhealthy people moved down the social scale this might explain the association between poor health and economic status. Though behavioral components of the social gradient are important for health — clearly, cigarette smoking is partly responsible — it seems unlikely that lifestyle is the whole explanation of the differences, because the gradient in mortality is higher for many causes, including diseases not thought to be related to life-style.

The Black Report described as materialist those explanations for socio-economic differences in health which involve differences in exposure to hazards with which poor individuals are more likely to come into contact. These might include occupational exposures, physical and chemical hazards, poor quality housing, and exposure to environmental factors operating *in utero* or early

life. Behavioral and materialist explanations are probably both relevant to understanding the socioeconomic differences in health. Differential access to healthcare probably explains only a little of the socio-economic gradient in health, although the proportion is likely to vary by country.

Four main approaches to reducing health inequalities related to poverty have been proposed: improving the physical environment; addressing social and economic factors; reducing barriers to adopting healthy life-styles; and improving access to appropriate and effective health and social services. There may not always be a clear distinction between interventions that address poverty itself or health inequalities related to poverty. For example, a government program that provides subsidized or free food has the effect of income redistribution to address poverty directly, and also by improving nutrition may improve health. Improvements in the physical environment that may be relevant include improving housing stock — for example, by improving insulation of housing occupied by the elderly, who in countries with cold winters suffer raised mortality in the winter months.

## Public policies

Public policies to improve the social environment and reduce income inequalities may be highly effective. A randomized trial in Gary, Indiana, suggested that increasing the income of poor expectant mothers on welfare resulted in an increase in the birth weight of their babies. Education, particularly schooling for mothers, has had a dramatic impact on health. In Peru mothers with seven or more years of schooling have a nearly 75% reduction in child mortality compared with mothers with no schooling. Studies in several countries have shown that mothers with secondary or higher education are much more likely to treat childhood diarrhea appropriately with oral rehydration therapy. Families are also likely to be smaller when women are more highly educated. In several countries, including Bangladesh and Zimbabwe, credit schemes have enabled the poor to improve their economic condition. One of the best known is the Grameen Bank, in Bangladesh, which since 1983 has been giving credit to the landless and to poor women. The repayment rate is extremely high (around 98%), and villages which have adopted the scheme have benefited from a lower poverty rate, higher employment, and higher asset levels compared with villages which have not participated. However, credit schemes may be insufficient to guarantee an escape from grinding poverty. Ill health may be important in increasing personal and family indebtedness. Thus credit schemes need to be accompanied by effective, affordable healthcare, and in Bangladesh such a low cost health insurance scheme is being developed by a non-governmental organization.

The combination of poverty and illiteracy has a particularly devastating impact on the health of women and their children. In many poor developing countries, the struggle for survival is so fierce that education is a very low priority, especially for girls. They are married off, at or very soon after puberty and begin having babies. In some African countries many men migrate to the cities in search of work, returning all too often infected with HIV. But the illiterate village girls and women, lacking even vestiges of education and lacking power or influence, must cope with all: frequent pregnancies, often difficult childbirth, ailing, poorly nourished children, no money, no resources, no healthcare, no hope ultimately of a better life.

Rather than seeing the poor as passive recipients of aid, many non-governmental organizations and community groups have a participatory approach, which involves the poor themselves in developing local policies and activities for improvement.

### Intervention

Large-scale multidisciplinary interventions involving a range of agencies and programs may be cost-effective. For example, the special supplemental food program for women, infants, and children was initiated in 1972 in the USA and combined giving healthy food, nutrition, education, and health services to low-income women and their children. Analysis of the outcomes suggested substantial reductions in low and very low birth weight babies, and the project paid for itself through savings in medical care. Project Head Start, also in the USA, provided pre-school children and their families with education, health and social services; short-term and long-term benefits were shown in health development and social outcomes.

Costa Rica, Sri Lanka, and Kerala in India have considerably improved health by political, social, and economic interventions affecting society as a whole, but in many cases actively involving communities in the process. Additionally, they have provided access to government-funded health services giving basic healthcare. Around the world about 800 million people are likely to be without adequate health services, and even in a rich nation such as USA the number of uninsured people is increasing.

Primary care interventions — including measures to reduce childhood malnutrition, improve immunization against childhood diseases, provide chemotherapy against TUBERCULOSIS, provide condoms and education to combat AIDS, and interventions to reduce smoking (including consumer taxes on tobacco) — are all cost-effective.

Over 50 years ago the United Nations published its Declaration on Human Rights, which mentions access to food, shelter, and clean water as well as to basic health care. If we are to be successful in reaching its goal, substantial changes in political will and public policy will be necessary.                                    APH

**PRIMARY MEDICAL CARE** See GENERAL PRACTICE

**PRIONS** See CREUTZFELT-JAKOB DISEASE; INFECTIOUS DISEASES; MICROBIOLOGY

**PRISON MEDICINE** Winston Churchill said that a society could be measured by the way it treats its prisoners. On any one day between 30 and 50 million people around the world are in prison. These prisoners present a huge challenge to health authorities because they tend to have high rate of health problems, particularly SUBSTANCE ABUSE, mental disorders, SUICIDE, and communicable diseases. In addition, providing a high quality health service in prison is difficult because conditions are often exceedingly poor; resources are scarce; the needs of security often conflict with the needs of health; attracting high-quality staff may be difficult; and separation from the health service for the ordinary community may mean that the prison health service sinks to a lower standard. Prisons are also places where abuses of human rights are common.

Prisoners in all countries tend to be male, young, of low social class, poorly educated, and commonly from marginal groups. Many move backwards and forwards regularly from prison to unemployment, homelessness, or life in mental hospitals. Prisoners have been categorized as 'bad, sad, and mad,' and in most prisons in most countries the sad and the mad outnumber the frankly bad.

HIV infection, hepatitis, and tuberculosis are all found in prison populations. HIV infection and hepatitis occur because intravenous drug abusers make up a high proportion of prisoners. Injection of drugs is common in prisons, and some prisoners begin injecting while in prison. Needles may be shared, and authorities in many countries are reluctant to run needle exchange schemes or make sterilizing equipment available. HIV infection and hepatitis are also spread by sexual contact in prisons.

Infections among prisoners may be important for the public health. Historically prisons were an important source of TYPHUS, and today prisons encourage the spread of HIV infection. Currently, prisons in the former Soviet states are major sources of drug-resistant tuberculosis.

Abuse of alcohol and illegal drugs is common among prisoners because addiction often leads people to crime to support their habit: intoxication may lead to crime; substance abuse itself may be a crime; and drugs are freely available within many prisons. Treating substance abuse in prison is difficult — as no drugs (even alcohol) are supposed to be available and abstinence within the highly abnormal environment of prison may not lead to abstinence on release.

Many prisoners have mental health problems. Poor mental health, particularly what psychiatrists call personality disorders, may lead to crime, but in many societies prison also serves as a sump for people with chronic mental disorders who have nowhere else to go. Furthermore, the appalling and frightening circumstances of most prisons aggravate and create mental health problems.

Suicide among prisoners is several times higher than in the community, and prison health services have made many attempts to reduce the suicide rate. One strategy is to identify and observe closely prisoners at risk of suicide, but this strategy has not proved particularly successful because those at risk are not easy to identify and even if identified and observed a determined prisoner can still kill himself. An alternative strategy has been to try to humanize prisons, making it less likely that prisoners will be driven to suicide.

Although most prisoners are adult men, adolescents and women may also be imprisoned. Most authorities try hard to keep young people out of institutions, recognizing that many become 'schools for criminals' with three-quarters or more of the young people reoffending after release. Women in prison are likely to be treated on a medical rather than punitive model — but often with little success. The same high rates of mental disorder, substance abuse, and HIV infection are seen among women, and there are additional problems of genitourinary infection (many are prostitutes) and of what to do with prisoners who are pregnant or have young children.

Doctors working in prisons face formidable clinical and ethical problems. Accurate diagnosis may be difficult as some prisoners deliberately exaggerate their symptoms in order to obtain drugs or be moved away from the cells to the prison hospital; yet early symptoms of serious disease may be missed if the doctor leans too far towards dismissing the prisoner's complaints. Treating chronic disease that requires taking medicine regularly may also present logistic problems in terms of having the medicines delivered to the patients.

Most prisoners see doctors as members of the prison system and are unbelieving of doctors' assertions that their first priority is to their patients. Problems arise, for instance, when doctors have to declare prisoners fit for punishment or when they are asked to force feed prisoners on hunger strike. There are also severe problems with confidentiality, and research in prisons may be very difficult because of doubts over the validity of informed consent.

In many countries, far from trying to improve the poor health of prisoners, authorities deliberately TORTURE them. Doctors find themselves under pressure to either declare patients fit for torture or to become involved in torture. If they attempt to resist they may find themselves tortured. Sadly, more doctors around the world seem to be participating in inflicting torture than in managing the severe and prolonged health problems of patients who have been tortured.     RS

*See also* AIDS; BIOETHICS

**PROFESSIONAL REGULATION** Students in a health profession will find, after many years of study and passing numerous examinations, that they may not yet start practicing. Most countries require registration with a licensing body, usually insisting on a year of supervized training. Although the detailed structure and function of these bodies varies considerably, most have the following remit:

- setting educational standards and accreditation of educational institutions
- registration of successful candidates
- setting standards of practice and of professional conduct
- exercise of disciplinary powers in the event of complaints
- intervention if a professional's health is impaired to the extent of being a risk to patients.

Some licensing bodies also try to ensure that health professionals maintain their skills throughout their careers.

### Nature of licensing bodies
Licensing bodies commonly take one of the following forms. The self-regulatory model is usually a council or board set up by the national or state government. It comprises members of the profession, some nominated or elected by the profession and some chosen by the responsible minister, often representatives of the public. The scope of the board's activities is limited by the government and professionals can appeal through the courts against board decisions. This model is found in Britain and countries once colonized by English-speaking nations.

The European (or government-regulated) model is usually part of a government health

**PENAL REFORMER**

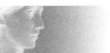

John **HOWARD** (1726–90). British sanitary and penal reformer. Howard's father left him well endowed and in 1773, after travels abroad, he became high sheriff of Bedfordshire. Part of his duties involved visiting the local prison, where he was appalled by the conditions of detention. He visited many other countries and their prisons and found that all were insanitary, overcrowded, and disease-ridden. He correlated the incidence of gaol fever (TYPHUS) with the density of the prison population. He advocated sanitary reforms, the regular whitewashing of walls, the making of smooth floors so that they could be washed, the isolation of the sick from the healthy, and the baking of clothes in ovens. Bills were passed through Parliament as a result of his findings and lobbying. He started the whole range of prison reforms and his work had an effect on the design, cleanliness, and sanitation of hospitals for lepers and other sick poor in Europe. He died in 1790 of what was called camp fever, which may ironically have been typhus.

department or ministry, managed in accordance with national law. Appeals against disciplinary decisions are heard by administrative appeals bodies, and the final say may lie with the minister. This model is found in most European countries and their former colonies.

In 1983 Ralf Dahrendorf, a German graduate who became Director of the London School of Economics, suggested that the differences between the 'European' and 'English' models lay in their differing understanding of the 'contract' between individual professionals and society at large. Professionals in Britain have a direct obligation to serve the public and are expected to regulate their behavior accordingly, by themselves. In Europe, the contract is between the professionals and the state, and the public expects the state to exercise control over them.

## Evolution of licensing bodies

The self-regulatory style had its origins in the British colonies. There was probably a greater need to differentiate qualified doctors from unqualified 'quacks' when communication between the universities and the colonies was by sail, than in Britain itself, where qualifications could be checked within days. Medical licensing had a false start in New York in 1760, when legislation established a licensing examination, but died out as local medical qualifications became *de facto* licenses to practice.

It reappeared in modern guise in Tasmania and New South Wales. The former made history in 1837 by passing *An Act to provide for the attendance of medical 'witnesses at inquests'*, and establishing a Court of Examiners which could grant letters testimonial.

The British House of Commons, meanwhile, struggled with many medical reform Bills between 1840 and 1858, when an Act was finally passed establishing the General Council of Medical Education and Registration (after 1951 the General Medical Council). New Zealand followed suit in 1867.

Medical boards returned to the United States with an Act in Texas in 1873, and all states had medical boards by 1912. Despite almost 100 years of continued attempts at national uniformity, today the United States has 70 medical licensing bodies and has yet to achieve interstate uniformity. Australia and Canada, also federations have been more successful. In 1992 all Australian states and territories agreed to recognize doctors registered in each jurisdiction. The Medical Council of Canada conducts an examination, granting a licentiate which is licensing requirement in most provinces.

The development of licensing boards for other health professions has generally followed those established for doctors.

## Functions of modern licensing bodies

The reasons for establishing the self-regulatory model have varied. Whereas the Australian colonial administrations wanted to know who was qualified to give evidence at coroners' inquests, those in the United States wanted to know who was qualified to treat the sick. In Britain, professional overcrowding, jealousies between the branches of the profession, and rivalry between the universities and colleges had much to do with the calls for reform. Today, many bodies worldwide see the protection of the public as their prime concern.

The reputations of medical boards have not been unsullied. At times, frank professional jealousy has resulted in qualified persons not being registered. Shortly after World War II, for example, only eight foreign doctors were allowed to register each year in New South Wales.

*Registration* The registration of persons of good character who, after completing a course of medical studies, have satisfied the examiners at a local university, is obviously the first function of a licensing body. Registration might be limited to the duration of an internship, might be full or unconditional once the internship has been satisfactorily completed, or might be subject to some conditions following a finding of unsatisfactory professional conduct or professional misconduct.

Since 1996, New Zealand has taken an innovative approach. Practitioners progress through three stages from 'probationary' — subject to supervision; through 'general' — subject to oversight by a vocational (specialist) practitioner and not able to practice independently — to 'vocational'. A substandard vocationally registered practitioner may be relegated to general registration.

A second registration function relates to foreign graduates. The self-regulatory bodies are generally required to assess applicants' proficiency in English and their medical competence by formal examinations. Passing the US Medical Licensing examination, the Medical Council of Canada examination, or the Australian Medical Council examination will permit a foreign graduate to seek registration in any of the jurisdictions of those federations.

The European model usually requires a foreign doctor to be a citizen of the country to be eligible for unconditional registration, proved ability to use the language (with the exception of graduates from fellow-European Union countries), and satisfactory performance in an examination set by the national health authority.

Both models usually have provisions for temporary recognition of foreign graduates undertaking further studies or participating in research or exchange programs. Some countries depend heavily on foreign doctors for staffing their hospitals. Both Britain and the USA recognize large numbers of Indian and Egyptian graduates, and the USA employs many South American graduates, while some Australian states, in turn, depend heavily on British graduates.

***Discipline*** The second traditional remit of licensing bodies relates to complaints made about registered practitioners. Those in the European countries are handled according to standard principles and practice of administrative law, often without a right of appeal to the courts. The self-regulatory model allows for considerable variation among jurisdictions. Some bodies, such as the British General Medical Council, receive complaints, conduct investigations, and then hold enquiries, the more serious in public. In other jurisdictions, such as in New South Wales, the medical board merely administers the Medical Practice Act. Complaints are received and investigated by an independent healthcare complaints commission, responsible to the state parliament. Hearings of serious charges are conducted, in public, by a judge of the district court, with two doctors and a lay person comprising the medical tribunal. Appeals lie with the supreme court of New South Wales. Lesser charges, generally over professional or technical standards, are heard in private by a committee of two doctors and a lay person. The medical board, itself, does not enquire into disciplinary matters or pass judgement.

The practices of medical boards across the English-speaking countries vary considerably, but usually lie somewhere within the spectrum between the British General Medical Council model and that of the New South Wales Medical Board. Some jurisdictions have an independent health *ombudsman* or commissioner, who, by receiving and investigating complaints about health professionals, relieves aggrieved patients of the burden of carrying forward their complaint at their own expense.

***Impaired practitioners*** A third aspect, actively undertaken by some of the medical boards in the United States, has been to prevent danger to the public by doctors who are themselves unwell. 'Impaired doctor programs' are becoming widespread through the English-speaking jurisdictions. The problems commonly dealt with are habituation to drugs or alcohol and psychiatric illness, which result in the gradual deterioration of a doctor's capacity to practice safely. Every effort is made to encourage the doctors to acknowledge their problem and to undertake therapy and rehabilitation, usually under close supervision and with regular monitoring of urine or blood specimens. In some cases, the doctor might leave practice for some months while undergoing rehabilitation. The European model also provides for possible action to protect the public. Licensing bodies registering other health professionals have also started taking a similar interest in such problems.

***Assessment of performance*** The newest aspect of medical board activity, perhaps most advanced in Ontario, Canada, is supervision of clinical performance. Until recently, most licensing bodies saw their authority as ceasing with the issuing of a license to practice, unless complaints were made about that doctor. It now appears that such doctors often share certain attributes, being older and practicing in isolation. Hence, the College of Physicians and Surgeons in Ontario has started performance assessment, initially choosing doctors at random, but also looking at older and isolated practitioners and at representative samples of doctors in different specialties.

The United Kingdom Medical Act has been amended to allow the General Medical Council to assess a doctor's performance, where there is a reasonable suspicion that this is below standard. Similar powers were given to the New Zealand Medical Council in 1995, whether or not a doctor is the subject of a complaint. Self-regulatory boards in other countries are now looking at the possibility of having their Acts amended.

To function effectively, any licensing body needs money. Whereas the European model is funded by government, the self-regulatory body usually relies on annual fees paid by registrants. As a result, the larger bodies, which are better resourced, are better able to carry out their functions and able to experiment.

### The future of licensing bodies

Recently, the public expectation of the role of registering bodies has become more demanding. Trust in the professions has been eroded and governments are increasingly expected to exercise more control over professions which sometimes seem unable to discipline themselves, to handle complaints fairly, or to deal equitably with all their members. Such public disquiet, often magnified by the media, has been reflected in government responses in a number of geographic areas. Thus of 13 members of the Rhode Island Medical Board, six are public members, while in Michigan public members are in the majority on disciplinary tribunals, casting into doubt the notion that the profession there is self-regulating.

***Discrimination*** Allegations of racial discrimination, or discrimination against foreign graduates, are increasingly forcing licensing bodies to review their processes for the recognition of foreign graduates. Most jurisdictions recognize people as medical graduates if they have completed a full course of study at a medical school recognized by the WORLD HEALTH ORGANIZATION. Other than graduates of European Union countries being automatically entitled to registration in other European Union countries, foreign graduates face language and examination hurdles. Not infrequently, their inability to master the language, to pass the examinations, or to become familiar with the medical culture leads to claims of discrimination.

The spread of consumerism has fueled allegations that the domestic medical establishment is using such procedures to protect its own commercial turf. Racism is also alleged to account for disproportionate numbers of disciplinary findings against foreign graduates, and even against local graduates of foreign ethnicity. With less serious complaints often handled in private in the self-regulatory model, the way is open for allegations of bias. While discrimination-based complaints have not generally succeeded in the courts, their defense has become a significant financial drain on the licensing bodies.

*Competition policy* National competition policy is challenging licensing bodies in many countries, obliging them to prove that the restrictions of trade in their medical practice act in the public interest. With a steadily growing overlap between different health professionals, many non-medical professionals are challenging the doctors' claims to exclusivity. A few examples are nurse anesthetists in the USA, podiatrists in Britain, pharmacists in Australia, and nurse practitioners in Canada, and, for dentistry, dental technicians in Australia.

Some jurisdictions have adopted an innovative approach. In the Netherlands, the health professionals' licensing authority (the 'BIG' Register) was established in 1993. Eight health professions are recognized: doctors, dentists, pharmacists, clinical psychologists, psychotherapists, physiotherapists, midwives, and nurses. Although the practice of medicine is open to all, certain procedures are restricted to certain categories of professionals. The restricted procedures are: surgery, obstetrics, catheterization, endoscopy, punctures and injections, general anesthetics, the use of radioactive substances and radiation, cardioversion, defibrillation, electroconvulsive therapy, lithotripsy, and artificial insemination. A reserved procedure may be carried out by an authorized professional or by another health professional working directly on their instruction. 'The rule of thumb is: those not proficient to perform a procedure are not legally authorized to do so.' Performance by an unauthorized person is a criminal offence.

Ontario's 1994 *Regulated Health Professions Act* established a registering and disciplining college for each of the recognized professions. Like the Dutch law, it sets out specific procedures which may not be carried out by any person unless registered.

The state of Massachusetts in the USA has responded to public criticism of lack of access to information about individual medical practitioners by legislating for the Medical Board to publish an internet website which details doctors' qualifications, training, appointments, awards and publications, participation in health insurance plans, and information about malpractice claims and disciplinary actions.

*Impact of healthcare funding arrangements* The way in which healthcare is funded in different countries is influencing the traditional roles of licensing bodies. Bodies responsible for funding are deciding on the allocation of funds for healthcare which may conflict with the priorities of those who deliver that care. When things go wrong, the patient or relatives look first to the immediately involved health professional as the person about whom to complain. However, increasingly clearly, in an era of deliberate cost-cutting and implicit rationing, the fault may lie within management and administration. Disciplinary bodies are increasingly finding that the causes of misadventure are systemic problems rather than the fault of any one individual. However, the remit of the licensing body does not generally extend beyond the registered professionals themselves.

In some countries with a fee-for-service payment system, competition law permits non-medical persons to own corporations which sell medical services through the employment of health professionals. These corporations determine policy, aimed primarily at ensuring profits. They are not constrained by the profession's traditional views on ethical behavior, on advertising, commercialization, or self-promotion. These corporations, like the health funding entities, are beyond the remit of the licensing bodies.

In those countries where health insurance is not conducted by government agencies, insurers are limiting the services they will pay for. Contracts may exclude certain conditions, disabilities, or diseases; the range of services covered by the policies may be limited; and the range of health professionals may be restricted. Under such 'managed care', the insurers are effectively displacing the licensing bodies in determining the scope of an individual's professional work.

*Risk minimization by professional indemnity organizations* In some jurisdictions, the law requires health professionals to carry indemnity insurance, as a prerequisite for licensure. The organization offering indemnity cover can then assume some of the roles of the licensing authority. By refusing a health professional indemnity cover related to certain procedures, that professional's scope of practice can be effectively limited. Such decisions are based on the financial risk which that individual poses to the organization, rather than on a concern for public safety. Doctors working in high-risk disciplines might find insurance prohibitively expensive or unavailable. Although this might improve standards by stopping some less than adequate doctors from harming the public, it might also prevent significant medical and surgical advances in high-risk disciplines, such as heart–lung transplantation, and may lead to a diminution of doctors willing to work in high-risk areas, such as in obstetrics in rural Australia.

In many countries, patients and their lawyers regard professional indemnity cover as a form of insurance if things go wrong, whether or not the outcome was caused by the intervention or the carers were negligent. This chasm, between public expectation and the reality of professional indemnity cover, translates into political demand for 'no fault' insurance.

By contrast, the Massachusetts Board's listing of the medical negligence record of each doctor runs the risk, despite the board's extensive disclaimer, of patients making adverse selections on the basis of isolated cases, where the fact of negligence was established on a point of law or procedure in an adversarial legal system.

Dahrendorf saw the extent of the public's trust in the professions as being crucial to the maintenance of self-regulation in the 'English' model. This trust is strained when a profession appears not to be keeping its house in order, or when it seems to be abusing its privileged status to preserve financial self-interest. To the extent that the public loses confidence in the ability of a profession to self-regulate, it will turn to the state to exercise control. The challenge for the self-regulatory licensing bodies, at the beginning of the new century, is to find ways to demonstrate to the public that they deserve their confidence. In this way, they might avoid coming under the direct state controls which characterize the European model.                    PCA

**PROHIBITION** Discussion of changes in policies dealing with illicit drugs, alcohol, or smoking is often prefaced with the statement that prohibition does not work; it is ruled out as an untenable policy option. This belief rests largely on historical analogy — the effects of the prohibition of alcohol which operated in the United States from 1919–1933, and the prohibition of medical prescription of opiates, which was US policy from the 1920s until the 1960s.

So far as US alcohol prohibition is concerned, this indeed was the view in historical writing until the 1960s. Temperance was seen as an old-fashioned moral movement which had failed; prohibition led to more drinking, more crime, flouting of the law, and ultimately repeal of the legislation. But recent historiography has taken a more sympathetic view of prohibition and its proponents. Temperance was part of the broad reform movement in early 20th-century America known as Progressivism; the prominent role of the Women's Christian Temperance Union revealed feminist influence and a reforming outlook on social problems.

The impact of prohibition was also different from the conventional view. An initial period of effectiveness in 1919–22 was followed by widespread violation in 1925–7. But effectiveness varied according to the local situation, and the automatic connection with the growth of criminal activity cannot be fully substantiated. There was widespread corruption and gang warfare in American cities before 1910. 'Alcohol and Al Capone' were nevertheless connected: criminal elements did organize and exploit the liquor business. However, the central criminal-directed activity was gambling, not liquor. Prohibition was, contrary to received opinion, effective, and this may be measured through figures for direct and measurable effects of alcohol consumption — arrests for drunkenness, hospital admissions for alcoholism, and death rates for cirrhosis of the liver all declined.

Consumption figures also provide a measure of effectiveness. Recent calculations reinforce much earlier estimates that liquor consumption dropped to about a third of pre-prohibition levels in the early 1920s, but then rose by the late 1920s to around two thirds. The belief that more people were drinking is probably not valid. But a shift in patterns of drinking occurred. Working-class drinking declined, and prohibition led to the end of the old-time saloon and its culture. But drinking also became 'smart', part of a new culture of conspicuous consumption among the sons and daughters of middle-class people, a revolution in manners fed by the rise of the media and mass advertising in the 1920s. Prohibition also affected the distribution of consumption among different types of liquor. Beer consumption, bulky and less easily concealed, declined, while wine sales boomed. But the greatest impact was on spirit consumption, which strengthened its hold and was particularly associated with party or speak-easy drinking rather than with more sociable drinking at meal times, patterns

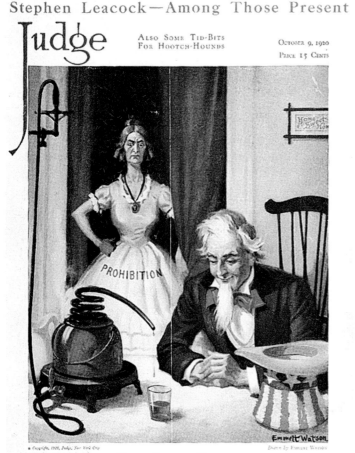

Stephen Leacock — Among Those Present

**Judge**

ALSO SOME TID-BITS
FOR HOOTCH-HOUNDS

OCTOBER 9, 1920

PRICE 15 CENTS

HAPPY THOUGH MARRIED

'Prohibition' and 'Uncle Sam' from a cartoon by Emmett Watson which appeared in *Judge* in 1920. (Reproduced courtesy of the Mary Evans Picture Library.)

local states and legislators did not cooperate in the concept of 'concurrent enforcement'. Compromise might have brought about a different solution; some historians have argued that legalization of beer and light wines might have pacified the wet forces.

### End of prohibition

But the end of prohibition was not a signal for a rise in consumption and for more drinking than ever. The repeal movement promoted moderate use and wanted restraining liquor laws. Some states retained prohibition in the 1930s, or had local options. Many established state dispensary systems. Alcohol consumption remained below pre-World War I figures. The repeal of prohibition was certainly not a triumph for drink.

The other major historical example of prohibition also dates from the USA in the same period — the prohibition of medical prescription of opiates to addicts. Here again older and more recent revisionist historiographical views have to be considered. The 'standard' view is that, beginning in 1909 with the enactment of the Smoking Opium Exclusion Act, a series of laws was passed which made access to opiates increasingly difficult. The key legislation was the Harrison Act of 1914, which required physicians, pharmacists, and others who dealt in narcotics to register with the US Treasury, pay a nominal tax, and keep records of the opiates they dispensed. The issue of 'maintenance' prescription to addicts was tested in the courts and judged illegitimate. Doctors suspected of maintaining addicts were prosecuted and most of the municipal clinics established to supply and treat addicts closed by the early 1920s. Addicts turned, so it is argued, to the black market as supplies dried up, and were forced into crime to raise the money they needed. More recent historical work has, as has the work on alcohol prohibition, emphasized that the connection between these legal changes and the growth of criminal activity was more complex. Changes in the patterns of opiate use were occurring before 1914 and the association with lower-class criminal activity predated the 1914 Act. The anti-maintenance policy accelerated rather than started the trend towards criminalization.

The older view of narcotic prohibition was of political use in the USA in the 1960s and '70s and served as the rationale for the introduction of methadone and other forms of medical maintenance which found favor during that period. In general, the argument that prohibition failed, that it increased crime and usage of alcohol and drugs, has had continuing political utility. A more balanced assessment would point to the successes as well as the failures of alcohol prohibition and would emphasize that broader cultural and econ-

which were established in southern European countries.

Why, then, was prohibition repealed? It was not simply, as in the older interpretation, because it failed. The changing economic context had more to do with repeal. The Great Depression of 1929 shifted public concern to questions of tax revenues and employment, and prohibition became a convenient scapegoat. The focus in the prohibition movement on a national constitutional amendment was also a strategic error. Earlier political aims, before 1910, had involved a range of different strategies — including partial prohibition and local option. In the 1890s, sections of the temperance movement had considered plans for government control and ownership. Realization of the national legislative goal was both a success but also a potential weakness in that this was an 'all or nothing' venture. It proved difficult, also, to maintain a truly national system of prohibition in a country with a federal political structure, and

omic changes lay behind some of the effects ascribed to it — and to narcotic prohibition. It is also clear that other forms of strict alcohol control — for example, in Australia and Britain during the First World War — achieved much the same in terms of the reduction of per capita consumption and cirrhosis mortality. Some commentators have linked the two historical models, arguing that the change from prohibition to regulation in the 1930s and after offers a model for future change in a similar direction for drug control policy. The political utility of prohibition continues. VB

See also ALCOHOL; PATIENTS' ASSOCIATIONS; SUBSTANCE ABUSE

**PROSTATE CANCER** See ONCOLOGY; SCREENING; UROLOGY

**PSYCHIATRY — HISTORY** The treatment of mental illness has not always been the province of doctors. For long periods of recorded history, mental disorders have been thought of, not as illness, but as the result of divine or demonic possession. It is true that Greco-Roman medical writings contain some references to mental illness and that these illnesses were generally regarded by the writers as having bodily causes and requiring medical treatment. However, in the ancient world generally and throughout the Middle Ages, mental illness was more often ascribed to possession by supernatural forces. As such it was not generally thought to be the concern of doctors. Instead, many mentally ill people were either given religious help or persecuted as witches.

### New beginnings

In the 16th and 17th centuries a more scientific approach to mental disorders began to develop. Several doctors wrote about the less severe mental disorders that physicians encountered among their patients. For example, Timothy Bright published a *Treatise on melancholy* in 1586, Thomas Willis referred to melancholia and hysteria in his lectures in 1663, and Thomas SYDENHAM (p 721) wrote about hysteria and hypochodriasis. However, most doctors had little to do with the care of patients with severe mental illness, and there were hardly any hospital provisions for such treatment. Indeed, until the beginning of the 18th century the only hospital in England devoted solely to the care of the insane was the BETHLEM HOSPITAL (p 103). At this time, most psychotic patients were not treated in hospital, but lived as best they could in the community, often as beggars or vagabonds. Others were in prison.

In the first half of the 18th century, small signs of progress began to appear. In England three other hospitals began to provide for the mentally ill. These were Bethel Hospital (1724) in Norwich, and Guy's Hospital (1728) and the French Protestant Hospital (1737) in London. In Ireland, a mental hospital was founded in Dublin with money left for this purpose in the will of Jonathan Swift, who died in 1745.

In 1751 St Luke's Hospital was opened in London. The physician to this new hospital was William Battie, a distinguished medical man who served as president of the Royal College of Physicians from 1764 to 1765. He instituted courses of clinical instruction in psychiatry at St Luke's and later published them. His book was the first significant English medical text devoted solely to psychiatric disorders. In the introduction, Battie explained that one purpose of the founders of St Luke's was to 'introduce more gentlemen of the faculty to the study and practice of one of the most important of branches of physick'. In his writings, Battie warned against the excessive use of many of the treatments of the day, such as emetics, purges, and blood-letting. He stressed that even severe mental illness often recovers spontaneously if the patient received good nursing.

Battie's book was followed by others which reflected a growing interest among doctors in the problems of mental illness. Meanwhile the interest of the general public in psychiatry was increased by the news of the illness of George III, whose first mental illness occurred in 1788–9. At the same time, a few psychiatric hospitals were founded by public subscription. Many of these were associated with a general hospital — foreshadowing arrangements that are thought desirable today. In addition, small private ASYLUMS for the mentally ill (called 'mad-houses') flourished in many parts of the country. Some of these were supervised by doctors, others by laymen. Although a number were the subject of scandals, many provided efficient and humane care.

### Hospital reform

It was not only in Britain that many mentally ill people were treated in poor conditions. In France conditions in the mental hospitals of Paris were equally unsatisfactory. In 1793 Philippe PINEL (p 77) set out to reform the Bicêtre, a hospital in which many patients were restrained in chains. Pinel released them from their chains and instituted a more liberal form of care. He made the important observation that the abnormal behavior of mentally ill patients can be caused as much by unsuitable treatment as by illness.

In Britain, the pioneer of similar reforms was a layman QUAKER philanthropist, William Tuke. In 1796 he established a new kind of institution in York, calling it The Retreat. Here, restraint was seldom used, neither were any of the harsh physi-

**FOUR FOUNDING FIGURES**

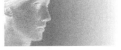

Eugen **BLEULER** (1857–1939). Swiss psychiatrist. Bleuler became professor of psychiatry in Zürich and is best known for his studies of schizophrenia. He was responsible for suggesting this term instead of dementia praecox, which it had hitherto been called.

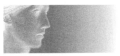

Alfred **ADLER** (1870–1937). Austrian psychiatrist. He was a close associate of FREUD (p 321) and president of the Vienna Psychoanalytical Society. In 1911 he seceded and formed his own movement of 'individual psychology'. He developed the notion of the 'inferiority complex' and held that the driving force was not sex, as Freud believed, but the need for superiority and power.

*(continued overleaf)*

(continued)

Carl Gustav **JUNG** (1875–1961). Swiss psychiatrist. Jung could be said to have a religious background, with a grandfather, a father, and eight uncles all pastors of the Basle Reformed Church. He read widely, studied medicine, and later turned away from formal religion, partly by way of spiritualism. Following correspondence with FREUD (p 321), a relationship began, which lasted for seven years, before dissolving in acrimony. In 1914, Jung severed his connection with psychoanalysis and formed his own school of analytical psychology. This placed less emphasis on sexual drives starting in infancy, and more on a theory of symbolic archetypes and the collective unconscious. Whatever may have been going on inside his head, Jung's outer life was stable and calm, and he lived to a good age with his wife and five children, becoming known as the 'Sage of Zürich'.

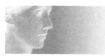

Anna **FREUD** (1895–1982). Austrian psychiatrist. Anna Freud was born in Vienna, the youngest daughter of Sigmund Freud. She extended her father's work in psychoanalysis to children and adolescents and therefore contributed to education and the development of psychiatry in these age groups. When Austria was annexed by Nazi Germany she fled with her father to London, and cared for him until he died. She wrote several books, notably *Normality and pathology in childhood* (1968).

cal treatments of the day. Instead, patients were nursed in quiet, friendly surroundings in which they stayed until their illness abated. This 'moral' (i.e. psychological) treatment was intended to foster self-control, so reducing the need for external restraint.

Despite this example, conditions in many hospitals continued to be very unsatisfactory. Those in the Bethlem Hospital eventually provoked a public inquiry in 1807. The subsequent report was followed in 1808 by legislation for England and Wales. This allowed each county to provide, at public expense, an asylum for the mentally ill.

Although the County Asylum Act of 1808 encouraged the building of asylums, progress was slow. For this reason, a further Act was passed in 1845, requiring counties to take action. In the new county asylums that resulted, patients were at first managed with 'moral' treatment. As time passed, more and more were admitted because the public was becoming less willing to tolerate the mentally ill in the community, or to pay for their maintenance in Poor-Law institutions. The resulting overcrowding led to less satisfactory care and to an increasing use of restraint in inadequately staffed wards. It therefore became necessary to restate the liberal ideas of the earlier pioneers. Between 1835 and 1837 Charlesworth and Hill, working at Lincoln asylum, showed once again that mental hospitals could be conducted without the use of restraint. Similar principles were subsequently expounded by John Conolly in an important book *The treatment of the insane without mechanical restraints*, published in 1856.

In the early 19th century the academic study of psychiatric disorders developed most strongly in France and Germany. In France, Pinel published his *Traité de la manie* in 1801. This influential text was followed in 1838 by another important book written by Pinel's pupil Esquirol. Pinel's book was notable for the quality of the descriptions of disease and for the use of simple statistics of the frequency of various forms of mental illness. However, it was in Germany that psychiatry first became firmly established as a subject for university study. In 1811, J. C. A. Heinroth was appointed to the first chair of 'mental therapy' in Leipzig, a post renamed the chair of psychiatry in 1828. In 1865 William Griesinger was appointed first professor of psychiatry and neurology in Berlin and developed a university department for the study of mental disorders. Other chairs were established in Göttingen (1866), Heidelberg (1871), Leipzig (1882), and Bonn (also 1882); and in Zürich (1869) and Vienna (1877).

With these academic developments, the study of psychiatric disorders began to flourish in German-speaking countries. Several themes were important. First, study of the natural course of

psychiatric disorder, notably by Kahlbaum and KRAEPELIN (p 355). It was mainly on the basis of these outcome studies that Kraepelin developed a comprehensive classification of mental illness which is the basis of schemes now in use throughout the world.

The second theme was concerned with the relationship of psychiatric disorder to brain pathology. Enquiries of this kind were encouraged by the progress then being made in identifying pathological lesions in NEUROLOGICAL disorders. Among similar studies applied to mental disorders, the work of and Wernicke was particularly influential. The discovery of general paralysis of the insane encouraged this line of research. However, the scientific methods of the day were not adequate, and further progress was limited.

The third theme was also concerned with the causes of mental disorder. It developed from the work of a Frenchman, Morel, who in 1809 proposed ideas which came to be known as the 'theory of degeneration'. This postulated first that mental illness is inherited, and secondly that it tends to appear in an increasingly severe form as it is transmitted to successive generations. These ideas flourished for a time. They had the unfortunate effect of encouraging a pessimistic approach to treatment, and supported those who wished to remove the mentally ill from society. Partly as a reaction, the last part of the 19th century saw an increasing interest in the psychological causes of mental disorder.

### The rise of psychoanalysis

The most important step in developing ideas about psychological factors in mental illness was taken by a neurologist. Sigmund FREUD (p 321) began his professional career as a research worker, changing to the clinical practice of neurology in his late twenties. In his new work, he often saw patients whose symptoms could not be explained by organic disease. Some had HYSTERIA, and were particularly difficult to treat. Freud therefore visited the clinic of the distinguished French neurologist CHARCOT (p 400) to learn about his use of HYPNOTISM in hysteria. When he returned to practice in Vienna, Freud began to use hypnosis with similar patients. However, he was not a natural hypnotist and experimented with an alternative technique of his own. In this, no attempt was made to induce a hypnotic trance; instead, patients simply spoke aloud the thoughts that came into their minds (free association). From this simple beginning, Freud gradually developed the elaborate techniques of PSYCHOANALYSIS.

These broad aspects of Freud's theories have had a great influence on the arts and literature, as well as on the ways in which ordinary people think about the mind. In psychiatry they were important in directing attention to the role of psychological factors in mental disorder. In addition, his practical discoveries about the technique of psychoanalysis laid the foundation of modern psychotherapy. These were important contributions. However, the details of Freud's theory were less satisfactory. Despite frequent revisions, the theory has not provided a satisfactory explanation for most mental disorders. Furthermore, it was not constructed as a set of scientific hypotheses which could be tested, so that it has not fitted easily with the scientific ideas on which medicine is generally based.

Freud's own contributions were outstanding in their breadth and ingenuity, but several of his colleagues and successors also did important work. Among these, JUNG (p 676) made the most significant independent contribution. Jung had read some of Freud's papers and decided to apply the ideas to the study of schizophrenia. Before long the two men were collaborating closely, but in 1914 Jung left the psychoanalytical movement as he disagreed strongly with some of Freud's most important ideas, notably his emphasis on sexual motivation. Jung's 'analytic psychology' has not equaled psychoanalysis in its influence on psychiatry and psychology, partly because his writings were often less clear and compelling than those of Freud. Another distinguished Swiss psychiatrist, Eugen BLEULER (p 675), resigned from the International Psychoanalytic Association in 1930. He made important contributions to the understanding of the symptomatology of schizophrenic patients. His departure from psychoanalytical circles removed from Freud an important early opportunity to establish psychoanalysis in the universities. It was not until the 1930s, and in America rather than Europe, that this came about.

In France, Pierre Janet developed another psychological theory of the neuroses. In this theory, mental functions are arranged in a hierarchy, part of which is outside conscious awareness. Neuroses develop when the normal integration of these mental processes breaks down. This breakdown is caused by stressful events but it occurs more readily in people who have a constitutional lack of 'mental energy'. Unlike Freud, Janet did not emphasize sexual causes either of the predisposition to neurosis or among the precipitants. Janet's theories were influential around the turn of the century but they were overtaken by those of Freud and are little known today.

## Psychiatry between the wars

Inevitably the First World War interrupted the development of psychiatry. The return of peace marked the beginning of a period of increasing interest in prevention and treatment of mental disorders. In Britain a most important event was the opening of the Maudsley Hospital. Henry MAUDSLEY (p 484) had worked as a psychiatrist at the Manchester Lunatic Asylum (Cheadle Royal) before becoming professor of medical jurisprudence at University College, London. He wrote three important textbooks and was most influential in his day, but his lasting achievement was an imaginative plan for a new kind of psychiatric hospital concerned with early treatment, teaching, and research. Maudsley gave a substantial endowment which helped establish the hospital which now bears his name and the associated academic developments.

In the post-war years, gradual progress was made in opening outpatient clinics for treatment with psychotherapy of the less severe mental disorders. Some such — child guidance clinics — were devoted to the care of children. As well as seeking to relieve their immediate problems, it was hoped that treatment in childhood would prevent mental illness in adult life. Unfortunately, these hopes proved over-optimistic.

In the 1930s three new forms of physical treatment were developed. In 1933 insulin coma therapy was introduced by Sakel as a treatment for schizophrenia. Insulin was used to produce a fall in the blood sugar concentration sufficient to produce a temporary impairment of consciousness. Repeated treatment with insulin seemed to benefit some schizophrenic patients but subsequent research showed that the effects were non-specific and probably related to extra nursing care. Insulin coma therapy was abandoned soon after these findings were published in 1962.

In 1935 Egas MONIZ (p 538) performed the first leukotomy, a neurosurgical operation on the white matter of the frontal lobes of brain. The operation led to a striking reduction of aggressive behavior, anxiety, depression, and obsessional symptoms. However, the procedure was followed in some cases by undesirable changes in personality and in others by epilepsy. These adverse effects brought the original procedure into disrepute, but more limited operations were developed with greatly improved results. However, these surgical improvements were overtaken by the discovery of drugs which produced similar benefits and the new operations were not widely used. These procedures have fallen out of use, except in a few specialist centers, where they are offered to a tiny minority of patient whose long-standing and incapacitating symptoms have not responded to any other treatment.

In 1938, Cerletti and Bini introduced a treatment that is still in use in a modified form. It was known at the time that when patients had both a serious mental disorder and epilepsy, they often improved dramatically immediately after a seizure. Cerletti and Bini found that induced convulsions had the same beneficial effect. At first a drug, cardiazol, was used to produce the convulsion; later electrical stimulation was used so that the method became known as electroconvulsive therapy. With improvements in anesthesia it was possible to obtain the therapeutic effect with the patient lightly anesthetized and the motor seizure controlled by muscle relaxant drugs. Although the procedure was made more acceptable in this way, it was a controversial treatment since it appeared to be a blunderbuss approach lacking a scientific rationale. More recently, controlled trials have shown that electroconvulsive therapy has a specific therapeutic effect in severe depression, and biochemical investigations have shown the likely basis of this effect. Because its effect is more rapid than that of medication, it is still used in urgent cases of severe depressive disorder, though for other purposes it has been replaced by drug treatments.

The 1930s was also a decade in which psychoanalysis developed in important ways. Several influential analysts migrated from Europe to the United States to escape Nazi persecution. Franz Alexander, Erich Fromm, and Karen HORNEY (p 686) helped to establish psychoanalysis as a dominant influence in American psychiatry. They also modified Freud's theories by placing more emphasis on contemporary social influences and less on sexual instincts and events in early childhood. Psychoanalysis in both its original and this modified form was to dominate American psychiatry for the next 40 years, until advances in neuroscience led to new approaches to treatment.

Britain also received many psychoanalysts fleeing from Nazi persecution and they, too, found opportunities to re-establish their work. Nevertheless, psychoanalysis never assumed the dominant place in British psychiatry that it attained in North America. That a more eclectic view prevailed in Britain was, no doubt, partly a reflection of national temperament, but it also reflected the influence of two outstanding teachers. These were D. K. (later Sir David) Henderson of Edinburgh and A. J. (later Sir Aubrey) Lewis of the Maudsley Hospital in London. Both had trained in America with Adolph Meyer, a Swiss psychiatrist who was professor of psychiatry at JOHNS HOPKINS Medical School (p 840). Meyer was an influential teacher who championed an approach to psychiatry which stressed the interplay of psychological, social, and physical causes of mental disorder and discouraged an excessive preoccupation with any one set of theories. These ideas, known as psychobiology, became the mainstay of British psychiatry through the teaching of Henderson and Lewis.

## Psychiatry after the Second World War

The post-war period was marked by two important therapeutic advances. The first, which originated in experiences gained from the practice of psychiatry in the armed forces, was the use of social rehabilitation using small and large groups. These methods were increasingly used to treat the schizophrenic patients resident in overcrowded mental hospitals. Reforms were introduced which in many ways repeated those of the early 19th century. Locked doors were opened, restrictions removed, and patients encouraged to take more personal responsibility. These liberalizing steps were aided in 1952 by the second therapeutic advance: the discovery in France of the beneficial effects of chlorpromazine. This drug suppresses many of the most troublesome symptoms of schizophrenia, including the overactive and aggressive behavior which had been the main reason for restrictions imposed on schizophrenic patients in earlier years. As a result of these two advances, the number of inpatients in psychiatric hospitals in England and Wales, which had been rising progressively, began to fall. Similar changes took place in other countries as these new methods were introduced.

The discovery of chlorpromazine was soon followed by the development of other valuable drugs. In the early 1950s, isoniazid was being used to treat tuberculosis. Related compounds were tested and one of these — iproniazid — was found to produce euphoria in some patients, although it was less effective as an antitubercular agent (see CHEST MEDICINE). Subsequently iproniazid and similar compounds were used to treat depression. In 1957 Kuhn found that another drug, imipramine, also had antidepressant properties. Since that time, imipramine and related drugs have transformed the treatment of depressive illness, which can now often be treated in its early stages by family doctors. Soon after this, it was discovered that lithium carbonate can prevent relapses of manic-depressive disorders. This was another important milestone.

Another feature of the post-war period was the development of community services designed to enable mentally ill patients to live outside hospital. Such people need help with work and accommodation as well as continuing psychiatric treatment. To provide this help, rehabilitation units, hostels, and sheltered workshops were developed (see PSYCHIATRY).

In Britain, a most important feature of post-war medicine was the development of a comprehensive system of good general practice. This was becoming well-established by the time that safer and more effective drugs enabled general practitioners to undertake the treatment of many people with less serious mental disorders, including many who in other countries would be treated by specialists. At the same time, the new policies of treating patients in the community involved family doctors increasingly in the care of people with chronic mental illness and with the mentally handicapped. Indeed, a survey showed that general practitioners refer to specialists only about 1 in 20 of the patients who consult them with problems which have an important psychiatric component.

The successful discharge in the 1950s of patients who had lived for many years in large mental hospitals, led to ambitious plans to close these institutions. Care was to be mainly in the community with short periods of treatment in small units attached to general hospitals. These changes brought benefits to many patients but the level of community provisions was inadequate for the needs of others. There were two main reasons for the failure of community care to deal adequately with the needs of the most ill patients. First, the costs of care were underestimated, so that there were too few staff and inadequate provision of hostels, day centers, and sheltered workplaces. Second, patients who had been in hospital for only a few weeks under the new system were not all as willing to accept care as had been patients who had spent many years in hospital under the old system. This minority of discharged patients required frequent and intensive attention, which reduced the already inadequate levels of staffing available to others. The failures of the system for this minority of seriously ill patients became evident in the increasing number of homeless mentally ill people in the streets of large cities, and in occasional but highly publicized cases of extreme violence by a tiny minority of the patients living in the community. In the last decade it has been recognized that some patients require long-term secure accommodation in special units, but little progress has been made in providing for their needs.

## The mentally retarded

Until the second half of the 19th century few provisions were made for the mentally retarded. By the end of the century many of these people were confined in large hospitals in which they were segregated from society, partly with the intention of preventing them from having children. Many such hospitals were understaffed, and provided insufficient variety and stimulation for their patients. While hospital provisions were often inadequate, arrangements for care in the community were generally lacking and many of the mentally retarded remained in hospital for much of their lives.

These conditions persisted until well after the Second World War, when attention was given to the possibility of discharging mentally handicapped people as well. Gradually, hostels, special schools, and sheltered work were provided. These plans have been more successful than those for the closure of the mental hospitals, and most mentally retarded people now live outside hospital either with their family or in sheltered accommodation. In many countries the main responsibility for care has passed from the medical profession to the social services, since most mentally retarded people need social support rather than medical treatment. Nevertheless, specialist psychiatric care is still needed for the minority of mentally retarded people who develop mental disorder or who have periods of disturbed behavior. Many of those with the most severe mental retardation also have physical handicaps which require care from specialist medical services.

## Developments in psychiatry and the law

The law is concerned with mentally ill and mentally handicapped people in two ways. First, there are provisions concerned with mentally ill offenders whose illness appears to have reduced their responsibility for illegal actions. Those which most often come to public notice are concerned with the killing of another person by someone who is, or is claimed to be, mentally disordered. Second, the law defines circumstances in which mentally disordered or mentally handicapped people can be admitted to hospital and kept there against their own wish. In general, this is permissible by law when a person is suicidal or dangerous to others as a result of mental illness (or, in certain circumstances, severe personality disorder or mental handicap). This legislation has two aims: it prevents the improper admission to a psychiatric hospital of a person who does not need to go there; and it ensures that people who do not realize that they are ill receive the treatment they require. It has always been difficult to balance these considerations. In the 19th century public concern was aroused by reports of cases in which people had been admitted to mental hospitals against their will and without adequate reasons. This led to the requirement that all admissions to a mental hospital must be 'certified' by a magistrate. This requirement continued until 1930, by which time it had become clear that it was preventing the admission to hospital of other people whose illness was in an early stage and who were likely to benefit if they could enter hospital in a more informal way. The Mental Treatment Act of 1930 allowed the admission of voluntary patients, though retaining the requirement that a magistrate should be involved in the admission to a psychiatric hospital of those unwilling to enter.

In 1959, a new Mental Health Act was introduced in England and Wales. A magistrate was no longer involved in compulsory admission; instead, the procedure was usually completed by the nearest relative (or a social worker) and two doctors. By this time, more effective methods of early treatment had reduced substantially the need for compulsory admission. Thus in the 1980s, only a few patients were admitted in this way to a psychiatric ward, most being voluntary admissions carried out with no more formality than entry to a medical or surgical ward. In 1983 a further Mental Health Act came into force requiring, for example, a statutory second opinion prior to the administration of certain forms of treatment in patients incapable of giving informed consent.          MGG

*See also* ASYLUMS; HOSPITALS; 'ROYAL MADNESS' AND PORPHYRIA

**PSYCHIATRY** is the branch of medicine concerned with mental disorders. In this article, psychiatry is considered from five points of view: the principal psychiatric disorders; the work and training of psychiatrists; the treatments they use; the organization of psychiatric services; and psychiatric research.

### Mental disorders

Mental disorders are divided into three groups: mental retardation, personality disorder, and mental illness. The groups are not mutually exclusive; for example, personality disorder and mental illness may occur together.

*Mental retardation* Mental retardation (also called learning disabilities or mental handicap) is present from the earliest years. It is characterized by abnormally low intelligence and retarded development of other aspects of psychological functioning evident at or soon after birth. People with mental retardation often have physical handicaps as well as, for example, problems in walking or controlling the bladder. They also have problems in coping with the demands of everyday life — in milder cases with shopping and traveling, in severe cases even with personal hygiene. In the most severe cases the person may be unable to speak or to control the bladder or bowels. However, most people with mental retardation can live reasonably normal lives provided that they or their families receive some help.

*Personality disorders* Personality disorders become apparent from the teenage years. The person is of normal intelligence but his or her behavior is persistently unusual in some way. Many kinds of personality disorder have been described and two examples will be given. People with antisocial personality disorder (sometimes called psychopathic or sociopathic) are self-centered and heartless, and do not make loving relationships. They are impulsive and do not strive consistently for goals in life. Such people do not feel guilt, and may be callously indifferent to the effects of their actions on others. They make poor parents and may neglect or abuse their children. Another example of a personality disorder is the paranoid type. These people are unduly suspicious and sensitive. They are constantly on the lookout for attempts by others to deceive or play tricks on them. They appear secretive, devious, and jealous, and have little capacity for enjoyment.

*Mental illnesses* Mental illnesses are disturbances of behavior appearing after a period of normal development. They may be divided into two groups, psychoses and neuroses, according to two distinguishing features. Firstly, psychoses are generally more severe (they correspond, more or less, to the layman's idea of madness), while neuroses are less severe (corresponding to the layman's idea of nervous problems). Secondly, in psychosis the person is generally unaware of the extent of his or her illness (he 'loses insight'), while in neurosis he or she retains this awareness. Each of these two broad classes of mental illness is divided into several further categories, of which some examples will be given.

There are three principal types of psychosis. The first type is called *organic* (this term refers to the presence of a structural abnormality in some organ of the body — in this case in the brain). Organic psychosis is caused by physical disease either affecting the brain directly (for example a brain tumor) or indirectly (for example, toxic substances in the blood resulting from kidney failure). When an organic psychosis develops quickly the patient is muddled and uncertain of his whereabouts (he is 'delirious'). When an organic psychosis develops slowly there is a gradual decline in all intellectual functions (dementia), often evident first as poor memory.

In the other types of psychosis, no physical disease can be discovered, so that they are called functional psychoses (the term functional is a term used in medicine to indicate the absence of organic pathology). There are two types of functional psychosis: affective disorders, which are primarily disorders of mood (affect is a technical term for mood), and schizophrenia. Recently it has become apparent that the distinction between organic and functional psychosis is not absolute. Thus brain imaging and modern techniques of neuropathology have revealed subtle structural changes in the brain in schizophrenia.

Schizophrenia is a serious mental illness affecting thinking, perception, mood, and initiative. When the illness is acute, the common symptoms include auditory hallucinations (hearing voices) and delusions (false ideas) which are often to do with imagined persecution. In its chronic stage, these symptoms are still present but are often overshadowed by chronic apathy, loss of drive, and social withdrawal.

Affective disorders are of two kinds, mania and depressive disorder. Some patients experience only the one or the other; some alternate between the two. These alternating disorders are called manic-depressive psychoses. A depressive disorder consists of much more than feelings of sadness. The mood is of profound pessimism often accompanied by thoughts of suicide and severe but inappropriate self-blame, sleep is disturbed (the patient often wakes very early and cannot go to sleep again), appetite is impaired, and activity is reduced. The picture of mania is the opposite. The mood is usually elated but sometimes irritable, and the person is overactive and inappropriately confident. Some manic patients enter into unsound business schemes, go on spending sprees, or commit other rash and mistaken acts.

Neuroses are subdivided into anxiety disorders, obsessional disorders, and dissociative disorder. Anxiety disorders are dominated by anxious feelings and worrying thoughts, together with the bodily accompaniments of anxiety such as racing heart, dry mouth, and sweating. These sensations are familiar to everyone; the patient with an anxiety disorder experiences more severe and persisting distress in circumstances in which there is no objective reason to be afraid. Obsessional disorders are characterized by repeated intrusive and distressing thoughts, for example, blasphemous thoughts and preoccupations with spreading disease by contamination. Such ideas are often accompanied by actions which produce temporary relief from distress: for example, a person with thoughts about contamination may wash his or her hands repeatedly.

In dissociative disorder (also known as conversion disorder, or HYSTERIA), symptoms characteristic of physical illness occur without any physical cause. For example, patients may be unable to move an arm however hard they try, even though the nerves, muscles, and other structures involved are healthy. Dissociative disorder arises from emotional conflict in the unconscious part of the mind, so that patients are unaware of the emotional causes of their symptoms.

Psychiatrists treat some conditions which do not fall within this scheme of classification. The first is dependence on ALCOHOL or drugs. The second is the disordered pattern of eating found in anorexia nervosa and bulimia nervosa. In anorexia nervosa the patient, often a teenage girl, engages in relentless attempts to lose weight through extreme dieting, exercise, and other means. In bulimia nervosa there are episodes of gluttonous eating followed by self-induced vomiting to avoid weight gain. Psychiatrists also give help to people who, although not mentally ill, are passing through a period of intense personal difficulties which have caused emotional distress. Such conditions are referred to as adjustment disorders.

Children suffer mental disorders. In pre-school children these usually involve difficulties with sleeping, eating, and control of aggressive feelings. In older children, most psychiatric disorders fall into two groups. Emotional disorders are characterized mainly by anxiety, unhappiness, and excessive worries. Conduct disorders are characterized by stealing, truancy, and aggressive behavior.

Mental disorders of these kinds have been found in all countries. Neuroses are more frequent than psychoses, and adjustment disorders are more common still. It has been estimated that about one-sixth of patients attending general practitioners in Britain have some kind of mental disorder, either on its own or accompanying physical illness.

The view has been expressed that mental disorders do not really exist: they are medical labels attached to unusual behavior that society cannot tolerate. Three sets of observations indicate that mental disorders are real entities. The first observation will have been made by readers who have met a person suffering from schizophrenia: the severity of the disorder and its sudden appearance in someone who has up to that time lived a socially conforming life are exceedingly difficult to reconcile with the idea that mental illness is merely a label attached to unconforming people. The second observation is that identical forms of mental illness occur at the present time in places with widely different social structures (for example, rural areas of China and large cities in the USA). The third observation is that the forms of mental illness recorded in the medical writings of previous centuries closely resemble those seen today. There are also observations of a more technical kind, such as the finding of structural changes in the brain of some patients with schizophrenia, which indicate that mental disorders are more than behaviors that society finds inconvenient. Nevertheless, it is true that people can be called mentally ill when they are not. This can happen when a doctor does not examine his patient adequately, or fails to use generally agreed criteria for diagnosis.

Thus there have been reports of the detention in hospital in some countries of political dissidents who are mentally healthy.

### The work of psychiatrists

Psychiatry is a major medical specialty which is divided into subspecialties of general adult psychiatry, child and adolescent psychiatry, psychotherapy, forensic psychiatry, and mental retardation.

Psychiatrists providing general psychiatric services for adult patients work with nurses, occupational therapists, psychologists, and social workers, who together make up a 'mental health team'. In the care of the elderly, the team often includes physiotherapists as well; and in the care of children, teachers. Although most patients are now treated outside hospital, the most severely ill patients still require periods of inpatient care, either in a psychiatric ward of a psychiatric hospital or in a general hospital. Psychiatrists are in charge of these inpatient care units but much of their time is spent in treating patients in the community, consulting with general practitioners and with staff looking after patients in hostels or day centers.

Child psychiatrists work mostly with outpatients since few children need to be treated in hospital. They advise parents, schoolteachers, and the staff of children's homes about the care of children with emotional problems, and work alongside pediatricians in helping handicapped children and those with serious physical illness.

Forensic psychiatrists treat mentally disordered offenders. They see people who are remanded for psychiatric reports by the courts, advise the courts about matters such as the effects of mental disorder on responsibility for illegal actions, and provide treatment especially for the small number of mentally ill or mentally retarded patients who may be dangerous.

Psychiatrists who treat people with mental retardation are concerned mainly with the treatment of mental disorder and behavior problems (these occur more frequently in people with mental retardation than in other people). They help to plan services for these people and for their families, although the provision of many of these services is the responsibility of the educational and social services and of family doctors.

### Education and training

All psychiatrists are qualified in medicine and most have undertaken a further period of general medical work before specializing in psychiatry. In Britain, the training of a specialist in psychiatry lasts for at least six years. During the first three years, the trainee passes through an organized series of posts, chosen to provide wide experience in treating all kinds of psychiatrist disorder. At the same time the trainee undertakes a course of academic study leading to an examination. In Britain the final three years of training is more specialized, with increasingly greater clinical responsibility and a requirement for some training in research. Similar arrangements exist in other countries, although the details of length of training and timing of professional examinations are not all the same.

At the end of training, most psychiatrists in Britain enter a consultant post in the National Health Service. In many other countries the fully trained psychiatrist enters private practice, often combining this with a part-time hospital appointment. Consultant psychiatrists keep their knowledge up to date by regular attendance at postgraduate meetings and by reading professional journals.

Some laymen confuse the training of psychiatrists and clinical psychologists. Clinical psychologists are not medically qualified; they begin their training with a three-year degree course in psychology instead of the five-year medical course, with its subsequent preregistration year. They then undertake a course in clinical psychology, usually for 2–3 years, instead of the 5–6 years' training of psychiatrists. Many also obtain a research degree before entering clinical practice.

### Psychiatric treatments

Psychiatric treatments can be divided into three groups: physical, psychological, and social. Sometimes a patient requires only one of these methods; for example, psychotherapy to help with difficulties in personal relationships. In other cases, a combination is needed: for example, drugs to relieve severe depressive symptoms and psychotherapy directed to emotional problems that might lead to further depression. It is a common misconception that there is an inherent conflict between the prescription of drugs and the use of psychotherapy or social measures. On the contrary, a combination is not only compatible in principle but also often necessary in practice.

*Physical treatment* This term used to describe the prescription of drugs, the use of electroconvulsive therapy, and the (now very rare) use of neurosurgical operations. In practice nowadays, most physical treatment is with drugs.

Drugs that alter psychiatric symptoms are of four kinds: anxiolytic, which reduce anxiety; antidepressant, which modify depressive disorders; antipsychotic, which relieve symptoms of psychosis; and mood regulators, which prevent relapse in manic-depressive disorders. Each of the main groups of drugs contains many different compounds, most of which differ more in their side-effects than in their therapeutic effects.

Psychotropic drugs provide an effective and safe way of controlling many of the symptoms of illness. Antidepressant drugs have transformed the treatment of depressive disorders. Patients who, in the past, would have remained depressed for months or even years, now usually improve within a few weeks with antidepressant drug treatment. Antipsychotic drugs have also brought about substantial changes in the well-being of schizophrenic patients. Although these drugs do not cure the condition, they calm the patient and reduce the most troublesome symptoms, so that patients can return to life outside hospital, while continuing to take the drugs. However, more than other kinds of psychotropic drugs, antipsychotic drugs have unpleasant side-effects so that some patients are unwilling to take them, and relapse.

Electroconvulsive therapy is mainly used in treating the most severe forms of depressive disorder. Antidepressant drugs have replaced it for most purposes, being generally as effective. However, their beneficial effects do not appear as quickly as those of electroconvulsive therapy, which is the best treatment for the most severe and urgent cases. In addition, some patients who fail to respond to antidepressant drugs improve with electroconvulsive therapy.

**Psychological treatment** Psychological treatment includes counseling, cognitive-behavior therapy, and dynamic psychotherapy. All three treatments can be given to a single patient or to a group of patients with similar problems, but the following account will deal only with individual treatment.

*Counseling* This is the simplest form of psychological treatment and the one used most often. The essential steps are to relieve distress by allowing patients to talk about their feelings; to help them clarify their ideas and plans, correcting misunderstandings (for example, unduly pessimistic views of the outcome of illness), and encouraging self-help. When patients feel overwhelmed by many problems, a 'problem-solving' approach is valuable. In this the problems are defined, possible solutions are considered one by one, a plan of action is worked out with the patient, the plan is acted on, and the results are reviewed. This systematic approach is valuable not only in reducing current feelings of distress and hopelessness but also in preparing the patient to deal better with future problems. Counseling can be given by all doctors or by paramedical staff; it lasts usually for six sessions or less.

*Cognitive-behavior therapy* deals with ways of thinking or behaving that exacerbate or prolong a disorder. The behavioral procedures are simpler to carry out, for example, assisting patients to return repeatedly to situations that provoke anxiety and which they have been avoiding. The cognitive methods include ways of changing irrational fears and beliefs. For example, if the patient is convinced that physical sensations are evidence of serious physical illness, the therapist examines the evidence on which the patient supports his beliefs, helps the patient to see that the ideas are irrational and that there is a more rational way of thinking. Cognitive-behavioral treatment is carried out by psychiatrists, clinical psychologists, and psychiatric nurse specialists.

*Dynamic psychotherapy* helps patients understand the origins in earlier life of their present problems, and the unconscious elements of these problems. This aim is achieved by encouraging patients to talk about their problems, and encouraging them to identify occasions in the past when they experienced similar feelings. Hypotheses are made about the ways in which past experiences (for example, rejection by a parent) explain present problems (for example difficulty in establishing close relationships); hypotheses of this kind are called interpretations.

Dynamic psychotherapy is carried out mainly by psychiatrists and clinical psychologists. For most patients, treatment is weekly for 6–9 months (so-called brief dynamic psychotherapy). A few patients need more intensive and prolonged treatment lasting for 18 months or more. When dynamic psychotherapy is intensive and lengthy and closely modeled on the methods developed by FREUD (p 321), it is called psychoanalysis.

**Social treatment** The term social treatment is used in two ways. First, it refers to methods in which the influences of a social group are used to bring about beneficial changes in patients. The second is to describe attempts to arrange a suitable environment for the patient, for example, by finding suitable work and living conditions. Social treatment in either of these senses is to be distinguished from social work, which is the name for the various activities carried out by social workers. The latter are concerned with people with social difficulties (especially children and old people); they organize and supervise community resources such as hostels and old people's homes; they arrange the provision of services such as meals-on-wheels for the old; and they provide counseling for people who need this.

A special form of social treatment is called a therapeutic community. This term is used to describe a group of patients (usually about 20) who share a common problem, such as difficulty in relationships or drug dependence. These people live together, take part in communal activities, and engage in group discussions. The focus of the discussions is the patients' problems in their relationships with one another, for example, inappropriate aggression or unwillingness to take responsibility. Because the patients are resident, it is possible to arouse strong emotional responses in group therapy that might be hazardous in people returning home from outpatient treatment. It is the hope that changes brought about in these problems within the therapeutic community will generalize to everyday life when the patient is discharged.

### Psychiatric services

In every branch of medicine, the provision of services depends on social conditions as well as clinical considerations. This is particularly true of psychiatry, because the scale and type of provision required for mentally ill people are determined in part by the willingness of a society to tolerate unusual behavior and to care for its handicapped members. The number of hospital places needed for people with chronic mental disorder depends crucially on these social factors.

*The organization of services* Patients with chronic psychiatric disorder treated outside hospital require accommodation, occupation, supervision, and treatment. Accommodation may be with the family, or in a hostel or shared house (a 'group home'). Occupation may be in ordinary employment but often sheltered work is needed; patients who cannot undertake even sheltered work require occupational therapy. These activities may be provided in a center in the community or at a hospital. Supervision and treatment are provided by general practitioners and psychiatrists, community nurses, and social workers, working in clinics in the community, or in day hospitals. Clinical psychologists and occupational therapists are other members of the 'community team', which aims to provide in the community most of the treatments available in hospital, and to support and counsel the families of patients living at home. When these provisions work well, treatment in hospital is needed for only the most ill patients who require intensive nursing or a degree of security for their own safety or that of other people.

### Psychiatric research

In Britain there are academic departments of psychiatry in every medical school. In this short article, it is possible only to consider the subject very briefly from three viewpoints; subject matter, advances in knowledge, and educational activities.

Psychiatric research is concerned with the description, causes, and treatment of psychiatric disorders, and with their distribution in the community. Effective enquiries into these issues involve the use of the research methods of epidemiology, genetics, pharmacology, biochemistry, brain imaging, experimental psychology, and sociology. Psychiatric research contributes to the solution of some of the problems in these other topics of knowledge; for example, to questions about the ways that drugs act on the healthy brain; and psychiatric research groups often include members of one of these other disciplines.

EPIDEMIOLOGY is the study of the distribution of disease in the populations. Differences in this distribution can point to the causes of psychiatric disorder; for example, attempted suicide is more frequent among people living in areas with overcrowding and poor social amenities, suggesting that social factors may play a causal part.

Genetic studies begin with inquiries into the frequency of a disease in people with different degrees of kinship to patients with the disease in question. For example, finding that schizophrenia is more common among identical twins of schizophrenics than among non-identical twins of schizophrenics points to a hereditary cause because identical twins have identical genes whereas non-identical twins do not. When a genetic cause is likely, molecular genetics may be used to try to identify the relevant genes. Molecular genetic studies of schizophrenia and affective disorder are being carried out in many countries and, although the causative genes have not yet been identified, it is likely that substantial progress will be made before long.

Genes act through biochemical mechanisms and for psychiatric disorders these mechanisms are in the brain. The brain is inaccessible to direct study because it is encased in the skull and indirect methods have to be used, with consequent uncertainty. Recently new methods of brain imaging have been developed which, although indirect, have provided a much more detailed and certain picture of the abnormalities of brain function in mental disorder. These methods are referred to collectively as brain IMAGING. They use short-lived radio-isotopes or nuclear magnetic resonance to measure the activity of specific parts of the brain and to study biochemical processes within it. These methods provide insights into the functioning of the healthy brain as well as the abnormalities in various kinds of mental illness.

Even when the genetic and biochemical basis of mental disorders becomes known, it will be necessary to explain how these changes are translated into the abnormalities of emotion, thinking, and behavior that characterize mental disorders. To achieve this, psychological and social investigations are needed and these studies can progress before all the details of the genetic and biochemical changes become known. Methods of experimental psychology have been used to identify the precise abnormalities of thinking that occur in affective and anxiety disorders and to find ways of changing them. Also psychological studies can identify specific abnormalities of function that are known to be organized in particular areas of the brain. Such investigations can guide and supplement studies using brain imaging.

Much psychiatric research is concerned with developing better treatment. As in other branches of medicine, it is not necessary to wait for a complete understanding of the causes of a disorder before an effective treatment can be devised. Indeed, finding an effective treatment often leads to a better understanding of the condition treated. Basic pharmacological research into the mechanisms of drug action have led to the discovery of more specific drugs with fewer side-effects. Clinical trials have established which drugs are effective for particular groups of patients, for how long treatment needs to be continued, and whether a sequence or combination of treatments is more effective than one alone. There are now many studies to guide the clinician in the best treatment for the various psychiatric disorders.

### Some recent advances in knowledge

Because psychiatric research is advancing rapidly it is impossible to review here even a small proportion of the recent findings. Instead, four examples will be given with the caveat that even these may be overtaken by discoveries made after the time of writing.

Modern imaging techniques have shown structural changes in the brains of schizophrenic patients. The nature of the changes suggests strongly that they result from faulty development of the brain around the time of birth. The idea that the predisposition to schizophrenia is established early in life is supported by the finding that people who develop the disorder as adults are more likely than others to have shown minor abnormalities of behavior in childhood. These findings show the need for further studies of genetic and environmental factors that might account for this abnormal brain development and they suggest possibilities for prevention.

Important progress has been made in finding the causes of ALZHEIMER'S DISEASE, the most frequent cause of dementia in the elderly. Genes have been identified which predispose to the disease and biochemical studies have shown which chemical messengers become insufficient as the disease develops. These studies have led to the production of drugs to augment the function of these depleted messenger molecules and clinical trials are being carried out to determine their value in arresting or delaying the progress of the condition.

New forms of psychological treatment have been developed to treat severe anxiety disorders without the need for the prolonged use of medication. These treatments have a sound scientific basis in experimental studies of the patterns of thinking and behavior present in states of abnormal anxiety and they have been shown to be effective in clinical trials. In this way psychological treatments are acquiring the same scientific status that drug treatments have had for many years.

Much progress has been made in the treatment of depressive disorders. New drugs have been developed that avoid the unpleasant side-effects of the earlier compounds and are much safer if taken in overdose — an important consideration since many depressed people have suicidal impulses. Also clinical trials have shown that combinations of antidepressant drugs can improve the condition of patients whose disorder has not responded to a single drug. Depressive disorders sometimes recur after successful treatment and other research has shown how recurrence can be prevented with medication and psychological treatment.

### Conclusion

It is important to end by emphasizing the close links that exist between psychiatry and the rest of medicine. These are most apparent — and most important — in the area of professional standards, education, and training. They are also evident in the use of common methods of research. (for example, biochemical methods). Finally, methods of treatment are moving closer as psychiatrists develop new and effective drugs, and physicians pay increasing attention to psychological and social aspects of care, which are a central concern of psychiatrists.                    MGG

**PSYCHOANALYSIS** was the name originally given by Sigmund FREUD (p 321) to his method for treating neurotic disorders. Quite early in its history, psychoanalysis became a general theory of human nature rather than merely a method of treatment. It soon became the established idiom for discussing childhood development, human motivation, and personal relationships. During the first half of the 20th century, psychoanalysis sought to throw light upon sociology, anthropology, art, literature, religion, and the occult. For some, it became a secular faith; a way of making sense out of life and giving it meaning.

Psychoanalysis was born in the 1890s in Vienna. In April 1886, Freud, who had been a poorly rewarded research worker in the Physiological Institute of Ernst Brücke, reluctantly embarked upon medical practice in order to make enough money to get married. During the previous winter, he had studied with CHARCOT (p 400) in

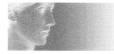

Karen **HORNEY**
(1885–1952) disciple of
Freud, soon departed from
orthodox psychoanalysis and
founded her own school of
psychoanalysis in New York
City in which she emphasized
the sociocultural factors
operative in neurosis and
especially their importance in
the psychology of women.
She founded and edited the
*American Journal of
Psychoanalysis* (1941).

Sigmund Freud, the Austrian
neurologist and founder of
psychoanalysis at his desk in
1938. (Reproduced courtesy of
the Mary Evans Picture Library.)

Paris. Charcot was particularly interested in HYPNOTISM, which he used as a method of distinguishing 'hysterical', neurotic paralyses and similar symptoms from those caused by organic disease of the nervous system. Freud learned from him that hypnosis could be used to abolish such symptoms, and could also implant suggestions of positive health. From his colleague and erstwhile friend, Josef Breuer, Freud also learned that hypnosis could be used to make the patient recall the exact moment at which a particular hysterical symptom appeared. If the patient could re-experience the emotion accompanying this, the symptom often disappeared. In the first psychoanalytic publication, *Studies on hysteria* (1893), Breuer and Freud jointly announced 'Hysterics suffer mainly from reminiscences' (Standard Edition, II. 6, 7).

Because these reminiscences were usually painful or shameful, they were not easily accessible to conscious recall. Freud was led to postulate a mental mechanism which tended to banish unpleasant memories from consciousness, which he named *repression*. But he also discovered that it was generally not necessary to hypnotize the patient in order to recover traumatic memories. By 1896, Freud abandoned hypnosis as unreliable. Instead of urging his patients to recover memories, he encouraged them to relax on a couch and reveal whatever thoughts and fantasies spontaneously occurred to them. This technique became known as 'free association' and had momentous consequences, for it compelled the patient to take the initiative, and thus reduced the patient's need to rely on the doctor's authority. Psychoanalysis and all its derivatives have in common that they

are techniques of helping patients to understand and help themselves rather than obeying doctors' orders or carrying out instructions. In spite of this, Freud discovered that his patients tended to put him in the position of a father-figure, an idealized lover, or even a savior. Freud's discovery of what he called 'transference' has affected every subsequent type of analytical psychotherapy.

### Role of sex

As his psychoanalytic thinking progressed, Freud concluded that many of the traumatic incidents which apparently caused hysterical symptoms were comparatively trivial, and concluded that such incidents had really provoked memories of earlier, more deeply buried experiences which had taken place in infancy. On the basis of 18 cases of hysteria, Freud asserted that 'Whatever case and whatever symptom we take as our point of departure, *in the end we infallibly come to the field of sexual experience.*' (Standard Edition, III, 199). This was Freud's last attempt to provide figures supporting his conclusions. He later abandoned the idea that premature sexual experience was the prime cause of neurosis, but continued to believe that what was wrong with neurotics was their failure to develop a normal sex life. Freud remained convinced that sexual satisfaction was the key to happiness.

In November 1899, Freud published *The interpretation of dreams.* Freud's original view was that most DREAMS were disguised, hallucinatory fulfilments of repressed infantile sexual wishes. This theory cannot now be sustained; but this important book established dreams as phenomena deserving serious study, and encouraged painters, sculptors, and writers to value the irrational and make use of their inner worlds of dream and day-dream in their creation. Psychoanalytic ideas have had a major, permanent effect on 20th-century art and literature. Psychoanalysis has entered the language we use, and it would be difficult to discard from our writing and speaking such words as 'repression', 'sublimation', 'ego', 'id', 'superego', 'unconscious', 'projection', and 'defence mechanisms' — to take but a few examples.

Psychoanalysts have written several bad biographies in which the subject's behavior and peculiarities are traced back to hypothetical infantile experience for which there is often no evidence. But, because psychoanalysis rightly emphasized sex as a prime mover of human conduct, it has become impossible for any conscientious biographer to omit consideration of his subject's sexuality.

Psychoanalysis became popular partly because it was in line with the new biology. DARWIN (p 214), by showing that man was not a special

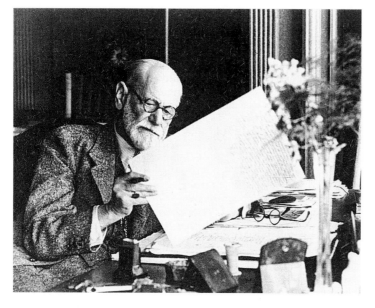

creation, but simply the most highly evolved primate, paved the way for a psychology based on our kinship with other animals. Psychoanalysis supported this by claiming that man was primarily driven by instinct. People were more governed by emotion and irrationality than they commonly realized; and even man's loftiest achievements in the arts and philosophy were regarded as sublimations of primitive drives. Psychoanalysis reduced the mental to the physical, and therefore appealed to those who liked to think of themselves as hard-headed realists.

Although psychoanalysis has probably increased tolerance of those who are sexually unconventional, it has made us suspicious of what used to be considered virtues. Celibacy is interpreted as fleeing from sex; altruism as a wish to patronize; self-sacrifice as masochism; religious faith as an infantile longing for paternal protection. Psychoanalysis taught that people are governed by drives of which they may be entirely unconscious.

Even if every theory which Freud originally advanced could be proved wrong, there is no going back. Psychoanalysis has been disappointing as a method of treatment of neurosis; but it has had an inescapable and powerful influence upon the way people think about themselves, which we now take so much for granted that we may not even be aware of it. ASto

**PUBLIC HEALTH** Public health is a set of scientific disciplines, practical skills, and beliefs (values), all of which are directed to the maintenance and improvement of the health of all the people through collective or social action. Typically, though not in all nations, public health services function nationally, regionally, and locally with coordination, collaboration, and interaction among them. Public health work is conducted by teams of physicians, nurses, dentists, epidemiologists, social workers, behavioral scientists, health inspectors, sanitary engineers, statisticians, administrators, and supporting clerical and secretarial staff. Efficient and effective public health practice probably demands more harmonious teamwork than any other aspect of the health and medical services in society. The teams vary greatly in size, complexity, levels of skill, financial support, and political (that is, government) commitment to the perceived importance of public health.

National leaders from Disraeli and Bismarck to Franklin D. Roosevelt and John F. Kennedy have eloquently recorded their recognition that public health is of paramount importance — indeed, is at the foundation of national security: protecting the health of a nation's people is as important as protection against invasion by a foreign adversary. Yet public health services command only a tiny fraction of the total national expenditure on all medical and health services — typically, less than 5% of the health budget from all public and private sources. In the world's poorest nations, where the public health problems are most oppressive, the proportion is seldom as much as 1 or 2% of all health expenditure. Many of the poorest nations spend far more of their slender resources on armaments, sometimes used against their own people, than on public health services.

Internationally, the WORLD HEALTH ORGANIZATION plays a crucial part in protecting the health of all the people of the world. Its functions include provision of leadership as well as specialized training for public health workers in all the disciplines and professions required in public health practice.

An illustration of the leadership role of the World Health Organization is a series of worldwide discussions in 1997, conducted primarily by e-mail and fax, and involving 145 prominent leaders of public health in 67 nations from all regions of the world. The discussions aimed at defining essential public health functions. What is the minimum absolutely necessary to protect the health of the population? The list has expanded from the six basic requirements that were identified in the USA in the middle of the 20th century, described in an adjoining article. Not all are the exclusive domain of the health sector; indeed, some belong wholly or in part in other sectors of society.

Essential public health functions are a set of fundamental, indispensable activities carried out to protect the population's health and treat diseases of public health importance. They are so important that countries at all levels of development must ensure they are performed to minimum acceptable standards.

Nine categories of essential public health functions were defined by the international panel in 1997. Each has several component parts. They are:

- Monitoring: morbidity and mortality; determinants of health (such as smoking); effectiveness of public health programs; effectiveness of public health functions; and population needs and risks.

- Protecting the environment: producing, protecting and ensuring access to safe water; control of food safety and quality; provision of adequate drainage, sewerage, and solid waste disposal services; control of hazardous substances and wastes; provision of adequate vector control measures; ensuring protection of water and soil resources; ensuring environmental health aspects are part of development policies, plans, programs, and projects; prevention and control of atmospheric pollution; ensuring adequate preventive and promotive environmental services; ensuring adequate inspection, monitoring, and control of environmental hazards; and control of ionizing radiation.

- Health promotion: community involvement in health; provision of information and education for health and life skill enhancement in school, home, work, and community; and maintaining links with politicians, other sectors, and the community in support of health promotion and public health advocacy.

- Prevention, surveillance, and control of communicable diseases: immunization; disease outbreak control; disease surveillance; and prevention of injury.

- Public health legislation and regulation: review, formulation, and enactment of health legislation, regulations, and administrative procedures; ensuring adequate legislation to protect environmental health; health inspection and licensing; and enforcement of health legislation, regulations, and administrative procedures.

- Occupational health: setting occupational health and safety regulations; ensuring safety in workplaces; and medical and health services for workers.

- Specific public health services: school health services; emergency disaster services; and public health laboratory services.

- Public health management: ensuring health policy, planning, and management; use of scientific evidence in formulation and implementation of health policies; public health and health systems research; and international collaboration and cooperation in health.

- Care of vulnerable and high-risk populations: maternal health care and family planning; infant and child care; displaced persons, refugees, and aboriginal people.

Clearly some of these essential public health functions have higher priority than others. In a well-run state, nation, or community, all should be available. When they are not, or when they have previously existed and have fallen into disrepair (as has happened in the former Soviet Union), epidemic diseases such as DIPHTHERIA and POLIOMYELITIS soon return, endangering not only the local people but all people everywhere. Moreover, the fact that many of these essential functions require participation of other sectors of society helps to reinforce the notion that public health not only calls for teamwork and collaboration; it is everybody's business. JML

**PUBLIC HEALTH — EUROPE** In Europe, the concept of public health is confused. In some countries the term is used to distinguish services provided by government, that is, the public purse, from those provided privately such as expenditure by the individual or insurance-based. A modified form of the definition proposed by WHO aids this discussion: 'Public health is the science and art of preventing disease, prolonging life and promoting health through the organized efforts of society.'

The achievements of improvement in the health of populations in Europe have been very great. In spite of many obstacles and vested interests, including governments and industry, the 19th and early 20th century were the 'golden years' for health improvement in all countries. The scourges were infectious disease and poverty leading to malnutrition associated with exploitative working conditions. The solutions included a safe water supply, improved housing, and better conditions of work with more pay and fewer hazards. These gains were made possible through the leadership of such individuals as Johann Peter Frank and VIRCHOW (p 853) in Germany and Central/Northern Europe, Bertillon in France, and Chadwick and John Simon in Britain.

With their co-workers and successors, they were able to achieve these results by careful assessment of the size and causes of the public health problems, possible effective means of controlling the hazards and promoting the introduction of changes which would eliminate the problems. The books by SNOW (p 48) on cholera in London, RAMAZZINI (p 583) on industrial health, and more recently Evans on typhoid in Hamburg all give good examples of how public health problems were identified and tackled.

Most of the easily amenable changes have now been made and public health measures offering such dramatic improvements are no longer feasible. Our present problems are due to chronic diseases, for example, cancer or coronary heart disease; behavioral problems, such as smoking cigarettes, drinking too much alcohol, and taking too little exercise, or demographic reality, for example, aging of the population. Of course, the problems of infectious disease, and, above all, poverty still exist.

Public health in Europe has been impeded by three major factors:

- Advances in curative medicine and technology have overshadowed the contributions that public health can, does, and should make.

- The advent of microbiology has obscured the need to consider the causes of disease from a multi-factorial perspective — for example, we tend to forget the effect of poverty on the incidence and severity of tuberculosis.

- The main determinants of disease continue to be associated with social factors, such as unemployment and deprivation; risk-taking behaviors, such as cigarette smoking and overconsumption of alcohol; environmental factors, such as housing or the lack of fluoride in drinking water; genetic predisposition; and the availability and quality of clinical services.

The role of public health in finding a way through the jungle of determinants of disease is complex. Many of the determinants are inextricably linked to political, professional, and economic realities. Their identification and correction may well antagonize one interest group or another. But, whereas in the past, correction of a problem, such as cleaning of the water supply, would lead to an immediate, dramatic improvement in health, this is only rarely the case now, since most diseases have a long time course and thus the effect of correction takes many years — as may the development of harm, for example, BSE and its human manifestation, new variant CJD.

For public health to function it must be involved in appropriate studies — whether epidemiological, sociological, psychological, or statistical — which enable hypotheses to be tested and solutions formulated and implemented for the control of ill health and the promotion of better health. Public health needs the means and freedom to identify and disseminate knowledge of the factors that lead to ill health or promotion of better health. It requires an independent voice and must use it if it is to influence public health policies. Many of the factors that influence health are under the control of local or central non-health departments, such as education, agriculture, and environment. Thus it is essential that public health considerations are taken into account in the policies of these departments or agencies, and that public health practitioners participate and guide the deliberations of these non-health bodies.

Thus, the major functions of public health are:

- surveillance of the health of the population centrally and locally
- encouraging policies which promote and maintain health
- ensuring that the means are available to evaluate existing services.

There is an important distinction between public health activities directed to populations and public (non-private) health activities that are directed at individuals. The latter are clinical functions. In Britain and most European countries, particularly those with an organized general practitioner service, public health assures, but does not provide, clinical, personal services to general or specific groups such as infants,

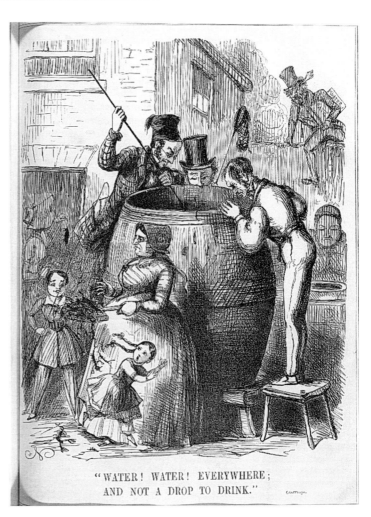

"WATER! WATER! EVERYWHERE; AND NOT A DROP TO DRINK."

mothers, refugees, children, aborigines, etc. This has removed many of the past sources of friction between clinical and public health medical practitioners. It also ensures that services to 'at risk' groups are not stigmatized and are delivered by specifically trained medical practitioners having a clear role in the delivery of preventive care and health promotion messages.

A recent publication, reviewing the development of public health in Britain in the last 100 years, has examined how the present structure meets the needs of the present and future. It concluded that there are deficiencies in the way that public health functions and that structural, organizational, and attitudinal changes are required for it to fulfil its role.

Public health medicine is reasonably well defined in Britain. There is an educational and training structure and a system of accreditation and specialist recognition. Public health specialists work at all levels of the NHS and in the central

'Water, water, everywhere; and not a drop to drink': *Punch's* comment on the impurity of drinking water in London in 1849. (Reproduced courtesy of the Mary Evans Picture Library.)

health ministry. However, only at central, governmental level does public health impinge on policy in education, environment, welfare, and so on. There is no formal link between public health and decisions, for example, on housing, education, transport, at a local level. Furthermore, although many other disciplines, such as nurses or health educators, work in public health services they have no recognized qualifications for this, nor is their contribution sufficiently recognized. There is separation in the function of environmental health officers (sanitary engineers) and public health medical officers in the investigation and control of outbreaks of disease (particularly infections), with no clear legal responsibilities or accountability. Several outbreaks of disease, such as food poisoning from *E. coli* 157, have shown the need for greater co-operation and clear lines of accountability. Current public health practitioners also have difficulties in the freedom they require to be

forthright in the identification and dissemination of health hazards because of the terms and conditions of employment as members of health authorities. Thus, even in the country which in Europe is considered to be the most advanced in training and performance of the public health function, there are problems and difficulties.

The problems are as great at European Commission (EC) level. Although the European Treaties of Maastricht and Amsterdam state that the Community has a role in the prevention of disease, health information, and education, and that 'health protection shall form a consistent part of the community's other policies', its major activities and programs are limited to AIDS, drugs, and cancer. The EC has recently announced that it will develop appropriate information systems and networks, particularly for surveillance of infectious disease. However, the Public Health Directorate (DGV) at this time lacks an adequate core of pro-

## PUBLIC HEALTH IN SOME EUROPEAN COUNTRIES

**Belgium** Public health started in the mid 19th century with the establishment of inspectors of hygiene. There has been little evolution since then. There is little formal organization, most responsibilities being exercised by the Ministry of Health and regional councils.

**Denmark** There is a long tradition of state-employed local medical officers of health, who in each county have a responsibility to advise on environmental health, social medicine, and the health of the local population. There is no formal accreditation or specialist training program.

**France** Public health is practiced at various levels in the French healthcare system. The Ministry of Health, with regional and departmental administration (through the prefect), has responsibility for planning and regulating hospitals and independent practitioners. The social security funds have a separate regional and departmental structure, linked to the regional and departmental general councils.

Prevention is divided between these two systems. Infectious disease is the responsibility of the ministry, whereas child health is that of social security. Information and surveillance systems are being developed, particularly for infectious disease, and formal, structural methods of training, specialist recognition, and so on are being developed.

**Germany** Public health services are controlled by local state governments and are financed from local taxes. Every administrative district

has a health office, in which there is a medical officer and a variety of other workers, such as sanitary engineers and nurses. These officers perform traditional tasks in the control of environmental hazards, communicable disease, and food hygiene as well as certain clinical functions, as in mental health.

**Greece** Although public health was established in 1918 to combat malaria and dengue, and provide traditional environmental health services (water and sewage) as well as clinical services in rural areas, it has gradually declined. Current reforms in the Greek health system encourage the establishment of regional public health units, with practitioners trained to perform modern public health tasks.

**Ireland** The Irish system of training for public health is similar to that of Britain, with public health being located at all levels within the health system.

**Italy** Provincial National Health Service hygiene departments are responsible for monitoring environmental health, including ensuring that services keep within environmental health laws, while laboratories undertake necessary analyses and are responsible for communicable disease control. Each region has an 'epidemiological observatory' to determine health needs and assist in planning.

**Netherlands** Public health is mainly decentralized with central inspectorates for food and environmental priorities. Many of the organized preventive services, for

example, immunizations and screening, are carried out at municipal level, as is environmental health. Many of the functions are carried out by non-medical staff. There is no recognized public health medical specialty, the nearest approach being general healthcare, a subspecialty of social medicine. Its practitioners cover a wide spectrum ranging, from hospital directors and policy advisors in central government, to specialists in preventive care at municipal level.

**Portugal** Public health doctors played a leading part in the reforms of the health service in 1970. The new specialty has responsibility for communicable disease control; environmental health; health promotion and prevention; and health services planning and policies.

**Spain** With the decentralization of services, public health has largely been recognized as a function at municipal levels. There are, however, wide variations. Specialists are usually attached to administrative bodies or hospital preventive medicine departments. Most of their roles are concerned with infectious disease control and occupational medicine.

This description of the place and organization of public health in some of the European countries shows how deficient this subject is and how varied the interpretation of the needs. Not all countries have been described, but the organization and functions in the remaining European Union countries — such as Finland, Sweden, and Austria — are similar to those included.

fessionals trained in public health to perform the required co-ordinating function to influence the policies of the European Union to consider public health other than implicitly. This is best exemplified by the European Union, on the one hand, subsidizing tobacco production through the system of agricultural subsidy, and, on the other, introducing a ban on cigarette advertising.                                   WHOl

**PUBLIC HEALTH — USA** The first formal efforts to protect the health of the public in the new nation of 13 states were initiated in response to the YELLOW FEVER epidemics of 1793–1806. The major port cities enacted various quarantine and/or isolation regulations for travelers to prevent the introduction of epidemic diseases into their jurisdictions. Public health, however, remained largely a local concern for almost a century. The first federal effort to support the health of the public was the enactment by the first congress of the United States of a law establishing the Marine Hospital Service for merchant seamen. This service gradually evolved into the US Public Health Service, which is now the backbone of federal public health efforts in the United States.

With growing industrialization and the consequent urban poverty, crowding, and poor sanitation during the early 19th century, TUBERCULOSIS and other respiratory diseases, and enteric diseases became the major health problems. These have now been largely, but by no means totally, controlled — first through sanitary measures and later by advances in MICROBIOLOGY and engineering which resulted in the development of vaccines and techniques for reducing air pollution and safely processing sewage. The 20th century, however, spawned the 'chronic disease epidemic', especially cardiovascular disease and cancer. Now the cardiovascular diseases have been reduced to a small fraction of their peak death rates, and even cancer as a whole is yielding. Control of infections and reduced cardiovascular mortality have resulted in a dramatic extension of the average life span from under 50 years a century ago to over 75 years. People now need to think about improving the quality of the life that has been extended.

Since the US constitution does not explicitly assign health responsibility to the federal government, the matter is officially left to the states. Taking advantage, however, of authority over interstate and foreign trade, as well as their greater tax powers, the federal administration has taken increasing leadership in protecting the health of the public. They have provided funds and skills to the states for specific activities aimed at health improvement, and have supported health research.

Meanwhile, the states have established administrative structures for sanitary regulations and other protective health functions. In 1869, Massachusetts became the first state to form a state board of health to guide its public health activities after the landmark 1850 report of the Massachusetts Sanitary Commission headed by Lemuel SHATTUCK (p 692). That report recommended surveys of local health conditions and supervision of water supplies and sewage disposal, as well as the establishment of a state board of health. Other states followed Massachusetts's lead in creating such boards, with varying powers, until that became the pattern across the nation.

Although the states possess the primary public health authority in the United States, they exercise it largely through local health departments that the cities and counties have formed in their jurisdictions. The heavily populated areas are generally served by substantial well-organized local entities, but less formal organizations prevail in the rural regions, where the states usually provide more direct services.

Thus all three tiers of government in the United States — federal, state, and local — have assumed public health roles that have become stabilized over the years. As new health problems arise, for example, HIV infection, they tackle those cooperatively.

### Voluntary efforts

In addition to governmental efforts for public health in the United States, an extensive voluntary effort has developed. In 1872, Stephen Smith called together a group of professional colleagues in New York City and announced the formation of the American Public Health Association, now the most important non-governmental organization supporting public health in the USA. Other medical, academic, and voluntary organizations, such as the American Cancer Society, American Heart Association, and American Lung Association, have been formed to mount campaigns to deal with specific health problems. Generally, these societies seek to persuade the public to fund research and model programs, and to lobby for governmental support at the federal state, and local level for their particular disease or health issues. They are funded by voluntary contributions.

As the communicable diseases came under increasing control during the early part of the 20th century, attention slowly turned to other health problems. For example, the US Children's Bureau, which was formed in 1912, developed strong public support, resulting in the passage of the Sheppard-Towner Act of 1921. The Act provided funds for state programs in maternal and child health that met federal standards, thus setting the federal–state pattern of cooperation in

## SURVEY AUTHOR

Lemuel **SHATTUCK**
(1793–1859). Shattuck was the principal author of the *Report of the Sanitary Commission of Massachusetts, 1850*. The subjects included the formation of State Boards of Health; periodic census enumerations; uniform nomenclature for recording diseases; periodic local surveys and analyses of causes of sickness in various localities among persons of different occupations; control of the sale and use of unwholesome, spurious, and adulterated articles intended for food, drink, or medicine; vaccination against smallpox; promotion of health in infancy and childhood so that a good foundation will be laid for a vigorous adulthood; protection of health of school children; measures to reduce the evils arising from the use of intoxicating drinks; town planning, control of over-crowded tenements, new housing for the poor; institutions to educate and qualify females for nursing; training of physicians to be preventive advisers and the establishment of sanitary professorships in all colleges and medical schools; the importance of mobilizing support among the public for health measures; the extension of health awareness into every home. The report was neglected for nearly two decades; however, many of its detailed recommendations have since been absorbed into the public health movements in the USA.

public health programs. Money appropriated by Congress flows to the states under national supervision and the states in turn allocate them to local jurisdictions for specified purposes.

At the end of World War II public health had matured sufficiently for the American Public Health Association to specify the six basic functions of a health department: vital statistics, communicable disease control, environmental sanitation, laboratory services, maternal and child health services, and health education of the public. State public health directors were heavily committed to guiding local departments in carrying out these functions and, where rural areas did not maintain their own departments, supplying direct state services as needed.

Although medical associations generally supported five of these functions, they organized resistance to maternal and child health on the grounds that it constituted governmental interference with the heretofore exclusive medical profession domination of individual patient service. That tension between medicine and public health concerning services to individuals, originating early in the 20th century, has continued and still creates difficulties. The health needs of pregnant women and their children, however, especially among the poor, were put forward so effectively that the programs gained strong support and overcame the resistance from medical circles.

Recognizing the importance of medical care for pregnant women and their offspring, and assuring it through governmental aid, has led to providing comparable medical services for almost all people, including the poor, who in the USA have often not received such services. Public health officials have sometimes taken responsibility for administering these indigent medical care programs, but generally they have rebuffed that responsibility, insisting that provision of medical service is 'not public health' and that it jeopardizes medical profession support for other health department programs. Hence, medical services for the poor have typically been handed over to welfare departments that provide income and other support for the poverty-stricken. In recent times public heath and welfare departments have often been combined, for example, at the federal level in the US Department of Health and Human Services, and in several states.

Around the mid-20th century, just as the six basic functions were becoming widely accepted as the public health paradigm, the health picture changed. The 'chronic disease epidemic' hit with full force. Cardiovascular disease and cancer, which in 1900 had accounted for only 18% of all deaths, were now causing 55% of deaths. Meanwhile, pneumonia and influenza, and tuberculosis, which had occupied the first and second

places on the mortality list in 1900, had dropped to sixth and seventh, from causing 23% of all deaths to only 7%.

The federal government responded to the new situation by building the National Institutes of Health, beginning with the National Cancer Institute, in 1937. The states, however, approached the chronic disease epidemic gingerly. Their health officers took this position because of their commitment to the six basic functions and because of strong influence by organized medicine bodies. Physicians opposed public health chronic disease control programs because they worried about possible encroachment on their private practice domain. Massachusetts, once again, led the way in governmental efforts; as early as 1928 the legislature established a cancer control program, specifying in the legislation, 'with or without the cooperation of the medical profession'. In 1946, the states across the nation with funds appropriated for the purpose by the US Congress, began cancer control activities such as statistical services, epidemiological studies, public education, and screening. During the past few decades, state and local chronic disease control endeavors have expanded slowly, often with legislatively established specific aims, such as tobacco control.

### Other agencies

State and local authorities have recently tended to place responsibility for what many regard as public health problems in agencies other than health departments; for example, air pollution in separate boards, substance abuse in police departments and prisons, and domestic violence in welfare and police departments. These problems exemplify the complexity of current health challenges and the necessity of coordinated multi-agency responses. The general weakness of public health agencies to address the current health concerns effectively led the Institute of Medicine, National Academy of Sciences, in its 1988 report on the future of public health, to assert 'that this nation has lost sight of its public health goals and has allowed the system of public health activities to fall into disarray. Public health is what we, as a society, do collectively to assure conditions in which people can be healthy. This requires that continuing and emerging threats to the health of the public be successfully countered'.

The public's view of public health's effectiveness is suggested by a 1996 poll of California residents, in which at least three-fourths placed priority on ensuring safe drinking water and foods free from contamination, and protecting against exposure to toxic chemicals and other hazardous materials, as well as against the spread of communicable diseases. Only one-third or fewer, however, thought that delivery of these services was 'very effective'. That same poll showed that over three-fourths of adults favored tax increases on tobacco products and alcohol beverages to fund 'community health promotion and disease and injury prevention programs and environmental health services'.

Federal support of public health in the United States at present is administered through many different agencies, but the two lead agencies are the United States Department of Health and Human Services, which provides grants to states for public health initiatives and sets public health goals, and the United States Public Health Services. The latter, which evolved from the Marine Hospital Service founded in the first decade of the nation, includes the National Institutes of Health, which is responsible for selecting and funding research projects and is the main provider of funds for research in the United States, if not the world. It also includes the Centers for Disease Control and Prevention, which respond to requests from states for assistance in disease control, support public health research projects, provide laboratory testing services, conduct surveillance for diseases of public health importance, provide short-term training programs, and recommend national health goals. The centers also include the National Institute of Occupational Safety and Health, which sets regulations for the protection of workers, the Food and Drug Administration, which regulates food safety, and other agencies concerned with the health of the public.

## National objectives

One tactic to re-direct and re-invigorate public health in the United States was adopted by the Department of Health and Human Services in 1980 — namely, setting national health objectives for 1990. These took the form of 15 quantifiable objectives, such as reducing infant mortality to 9 deaths/1000 from a baseline in 1978 of 13.8, and reducing motor vehicle fatalities to 18 per 100 000 from a baseline of 24. For 1990, 2000, and 2010 the department has carried out a similar exercise and also mid-course reviews of progress toward the objectives. The set of objectives has expanded over the years, with the draft 2010 objectives specifying 26 objectives, including several not listed in the 1990 version, such as access to quality health services (preventive, primary, emergency, long-term, and rehabilitative), more efficient public health infrastructure, improved health communication, and reduced mortality from selected diseases such as cancer and diabetes.

Schools and communities are increasingly generating health report cards, in which they present data concerning health conditions in their areas, including comparison with national or other data. There is increasing conviction that public health should define and meet objectives regarding current health problems, delineate quantitative objectives and measures, and report progress.

In the United States, in contrast to other countries, schools of public health have constituted an important element in this reformulation of the discipline from the decades-old six basic functions. In 1916 the Rockefeller FOUNDATION pioneered these institutional ventures by founding a school of hygiene and public health at JOHNS HOPKINS UNIVERSITY (p 840), and in 1922 supporting the Harvard School of Public Health, which had emerged from a joint Harvard–Massachusetts Institute of Technology program for health officers established in 1913. By 1936, ten schools had appeared in larger universities, both private and public.

For many years after the Second World War, schools of public health were subsidized with funds from the federal government, which stimulated the growth of many new schools. By the mid-1980s, however, direct support for schools of public health had ceased, and schools had to rely on other sources of funding, including tuition, research grant overhead, and state and private support.

By 1998 the number of schools of public health had grown to 28, 18 of them in state universities and 10 in private universities, with a half dozen additional states in the process of establishing schools. Thus public health schools now constitute the most rapidly growing segment of professional health education in the United States. In general, they not only provide training in public health work for medical and other personnel, but also conduct research on many problems. The schools are usually linked to their state and local public health agencies. Typically, they emphasize epidemiology, biostatistics, environmental health, population-oriented medical services, and behavioral sciences. Many also include nutrition, laboratory sciences, and other aspects of public health.

## Privatization

During the past few years public health, along with other public services in the United States, has been under pressure to 'privatize'. This has taken the form of relinquishing public control of services to private enterprise or contracting for private operation of services using public funds. Recently, managed care organizations have become very popular. These recruit participants to their plans, which provide care through specific physicians and medical providers. Typically, access to specialized care is regulated by a physician/gatekeeper and a panel, which approves all special care beyond the routine. Premiums for the plan are usually paid by employers or public agencies. The rapid growth of these organizations has appreciably affected both the practice of medical care and public health.

The emergence of these new for-profit organizations has created considerable turmoil in both medicine and public health, since profit, not health, becomes the most important aim. Although seen by many leaders as a strategy for containing rapidly escalating healthcare costs in the United States, and for providing care for traditionally underserved populations, many managed care organizations are now refusing to accept these underserved populations, such as the elderly, at the reimbursement rates currently provided by federal, state, and local governments. Public health leaders and political leaders must now come to some understanding with these for-profit health providers or set up an alternative system for ensuring that the poor, the elderly, the uninsured, and other under-served populations have access to quality healthcare.

Public health in the United States now faces resurgent old problems, such as the re-emergence of drug-resistant tuberculosis and other agents as major health problems, the emergence of new public health problems, such as HIV/AIDS; the continuing epidemic of chronic diseases; the problem of improving the quality of extended life for the elderly and their families; the problems of continuing urbanization, such as violence; and the problems that population growth create; as well as the unforeseen problems that technical advancement will present to workers, and possibly to the public through changes in the environment. Finally, it will be important for public health leaders in the United States to join with public health professionals from both the developed and developing world as new communications techniques continue to 'shrink' the world and increase interactions and interdependence of peoples throughout the world. It will be interesting to see how a capitalist-oriented confederation of states can meet these challenges.     LBres, RD

*See also* FOOD AND DRUG ADMINISTRATION; MANAGED CARE; USA

**PULMONOLOGY** See CHEST MEDICINE

Half of what you are taught as
medical students will in ten years
have been shown to be wrong,
and the trouble is, none of your

# Q

**QUACKS** See CULTS AND QUACKERY

**QUAKERS AND MEDICINE** Since the foundations of the Society of Friends, which followed the
teachings of George Fox from the middle of the
17th century, Quakers have always been interested
in philanthropic ventures and the welfare of
mankind. Believing that there is a spark of divinity, an inner light, in every human being, they
have been concerned throughout their history
with the unfortunate — the poor, those living in
conditions of confinement, the inhabitants of
hospitals, mental asylums, or prisons. Many
Quakers were also strong opponents of slavery in
the years that led up to its abolition. Not unnaturally, medicine with its concern for the sick and
afflicted provided particular opportunities for
Quakers as doctors as well for non-medical
Friends with their commitment to philanthropy.

There were, from the earliest years of the
Society of Friends, Quakers who practiced medicine. George Fox himself had a reputation as a
healer. Charles Lloyd and his brother Thomas,
both doctors, came from the landed gentry, but
most Quakers during those early years were artisans, workmen, or shopkeepers and they lacked
the necessary education for entering medicine.
Nor had they the financial security to undertake
philanthropic endeavor. Furthermore, the early
Friends not only suffered persecution and often
imprisonment for their beliefs, but they were also
debarred from the English universities and therefore from the professions.

By the 18th century, however, Quakers were
becoming increasingly prosperous. In seeking to
establish themselves in contemporary society,
younger sons of yeomen farmers and minor gentry who were Friends took advantage of the newly
established school of medicine in Edinburgh,
founded in 1726, to study medicine. There, unlike
Oxford or Cambridge, there was no religious bar
to entry. The Quaker physician John FOTHERGILL
(this page), graduate of Edinburgh in 1736, became
one of London's most sought-after physicians and
he was rich enough to support many philanthropic causes. A French eulogist wrote at his

death that he had given 200 000 guineas for
helping the poor, no doubt something of an exaggeration. He opposed slavery and strongly
supported emancipation. Robert Willan, from
Quaker stock, founded the specialty of dermatology. Fothergill's Quaker protegé, John Coakley
LETTSOM (p 242), like Fothergill barred from the
Fellowship of the Royal College of Physicians
because he had been educated at neither Oxford
nor Cambridge, founded the Medical Society of
London in 1773, providing dissenters with an alternative forum for discussing medical matters.
Deeply concerned with the vicissitudes of the poor
in the expanding and overcrowded parishes to the
east of London, he also founded the first DISPEN-
SARY for the London poor at Aldersgate in 1770,
where dissenters often chose to work. The dispensaries took the brunt of medical treatment for the
poor in those days, their doctors visiting patients
and their families in their own homes, often contracting fevers which might be fatal. Inheriting
property in the West Indies after his father's death,
Lettsom at once freed all his slaves.

During the 19th and 20th centuries many
Quakers chose medicine as their career, since
there were no longer any social barriers for the
members of a society which had become synonymous with philanthropic endeavor. Thomas
Young, according to HELMHOLTZ (p 372) the most
erudite physician of his generation; Thomas
Hodgkin, the pathologist who described the
disease that bears his name; and Sir Jonathan
Hutchinson were all Quakers. Joseph LISTER
(p 473), pioneer of modern antiseptic surgery, was
born a Quaker, son of Joseph Jackson Lister, who
invented the achromatic lens that made modern
microscopy possible. More recently, Sir George
Newman, one of the greatest public health
reformers and first chief medical officer to the
Ministry of Health when it was founded in 1919,
also found time to edit the *Friends Quarterly
Examiner* for 40 years.

At the same time, the Society of Friends
became increasingly involved in evangelism and
in foreign missions. The first Quaker MISSIONARY
was William Wilson and his successors played a

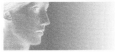

John **FOTHERGILL**
(1712–80). British physician.
Fothergill was a Quaker who
practiced in London with
great success and developed
a botanical garden at Upton,
Essex, 'second only to Kew'.
He described 'putrid sore
throat', which was either
diphtheria or malignant scar-
latina in 1748, and trigeminal
neuralgia (tic douloureux) in
1773. Fothergill co-operated
with Benjamin Franklin in
attempts to reconcile the
American colonies and Great
Britain. He wrote a pamphlet
advocating repeal of the
Stamp Act (1765).

particularly important part in bringing medical care to remote areas of China.

In view of the pacifist testimony of Friends, they did not bear arms, and this led to the formation during the First World War of the Friends Ambulance Unit. There were few Quaker doctors in the Unit's early days but many Friends, later to be distinguished in other disciplines, served in the unit, which became widely respected for the courage of its members and for their contribution to the care of civilian populations afflicted by war.

### Medical dynasties

Another feature of Quaker involvement in medicine was that whole dynasties were involved in one way or another with medical care. Perhaps the most famous of these was the Fox family. Joseph Fox, surgeon of Falmouth, was the ancestor of some 21 doctors and three pharmacists in seven succeeding generations of this remarkable family. They included R. Hingston Fox, author of an important biography of Dr John Fothergill. In our own times, (Sir) Theodore Fox belonged to the sixth generation. One of the most celebrated medical editors of modern times, he was widely respected for his independence, wisdom, and unfailing courtesy. He served in the Friends Ambulance Unit during the First World War, before studying medicine at Cambridge. He worked on the editorial staff of the *Lancet* from 1939, the last twenty years as editor.

One of the most important contributions of Friends to medicine was their involvement in the care of the insane, particularly with pioneering the moral treatment of the afflicted, which rejected traditional methods of management such as restraint. In the 1790s, several Friends who were members of York Meeting, dissatisfied with the care of the mentally ill at the York Asylum, were moved to consider founding a new establishment. This led to the opening on 11 May 1796 of the Retreat at York. Founded by William Tuke, a tea merchant who was a descendant of William Tuke — one of the original followers of George Fox, who had suffered imprisonment for his beliefs — the Retreat has never been closed since.

Not surprisingly, in view of its foundation as a Quaker Colony, Quakers played an important part, both as doctors and as members of colonial society, in the development of medicine in Pennsylvania. Quakers such as the Pembertons were closely involved in the founding in 1751 of the Pennsylvania Hospital, whose first board of managers included four Quakers, as well as the American scientist, philosopher, and sage, Benjamin Franklin. American Friends, like their English cousins, were also deeply concerned with the care of the insane. In the beginning, treatment at the Pennsylvania Hospital was not entirely in accord with the principles of humanity later developed in York, orders for shackles and chains appearing in the board minutes. In 1799, however, a Quaker minister from Philadelphia, Thomas Scattergood, visited the Retreat in York. He and later his son went on to play an important part in establishing the Friends Asylum for the Insane in Philadelphia in 1817. This was the forerunner of other institutions for the mentally ill throughout the one-time American colonies. Quakers have continued to be part both of medical and philanthropic endeavor. In our own time, Dr Jonathan Rhoads, professor of surgery at the University of Pennsylvania, has been President not only of the College of Physicians of Philadelphia but also of the American College of Surgeons and the American Philosophical Society, America's oldest learned society.

Quakers of today feel that members of their Society have made an important contribution, both as healers and as responsible citizens of the world. As Russell Elkington, another distinguished medical editor, has put it: 'We who are Quaker physicians and healers have a great responsibility to carry forward this precious heritege … to apply it to the building of the Kingdom of God'.                              CCB

*See also* RELIGION, PHILOSOPHY, AND MEDICINE; RELIGIOUS SECTS

**QUARANTINE** Quarantine is defined as restriction of the activities of well persons or animals who have been exposed to a communicable disease. The aim is to prevent transmission of the disease from potentially infected to healthy persons during the incubation period.

The word derives from the Italian, *quaranta dei* (forty days) and reminds us that the custom of segregating putatively infected persons and the ships on which they were traveling originated in the maritime empire of Venice in the 14th century. This length of time probably relates to the biblical story of the forty days Jesus spent in the wilderness, not to knowledge of the mode of transmission of infection — although the rise of the practice suggests that there was some understanding of the concept of contagion even if not empirical knowledge of infective periods and incubation times of the plagues that were raging in Europe in those days. Few infectious diseases have an incubation time or infective period greater than 40 days. An exception is rabies, which may not declare itself for many months. That is why non-immunized animals that may have been exposed to rabies are quarantined for many months when they arrive in countries where rabies does not exist.

Animal and plant quarantine procedures are often more important than human quarantine

There are two varieties of quarantine:

● Absolute or complete quarantine, with limitation of freedom for a period equal to the longest usual incubation period of the disease.

● Modified quarantine, with selective or partial limitation of movement, based on known differences in susceptibility. Examples of this are exclusion of children from school and confining military personnel to their base. Modified quarantine includes personal surveillance, medical supervision and segregation of the individual or group, or establishment of a *cordon sanitaire*, that is, a boundary zone between uninfected and infected (or exposed) persons.

now that many of the most dangerous contagious diseases can be kept under observation without such draconian restrictions as formerly required; but the economic importance of agriculture and animal husbandry in many countries makes it essential to spare no effort to exclude diseases that might wipe out valuable cattle herds or destroy a harvest. A very important human disease with an incubation time that can and probably usually does exceed 40 days is HIV infection, but for reasons that have more to do with human rights than epidemiological insights, there is no quarantine for persons exposed to HIV infection.

Quarantine as a way to control the spread of contagious diseases is an extreme form of isolation, which has several less severe variations. Bedside isolation, in which patients suffering from an infectious disease are 'barrier nursed' to break the chain of transmission, is the mildest variation. More dangerous varieties of contagious disease such as pulmonary tuberculosis with excretion of tubercle bacilli, diphtheria, or cholera, are preferably isolated in a special hospital or closed ward. Until recently, patients with such diseases as typhoid, paralytic poliomyelitis, and meningococcal meningitis, were strictly isolated and every effort was made to preserve a *cordon sanitaire* around them; and their contacts were quarantined under public health laws in some jurisdictions, even though epidemiologically this made little or no sense as a means of preventing transmission of infection. Powerful antibiotics and better understanding have made quarantine unnecessary for these and many other diseases: infected patients are often treated nowadays in a general hospital rather than in one dedicated to infectious diseases. The practice of *universal precautions* is a modified form of quarantine, in which patients with a contagious disease (such as HIV/AIDS) are barrier-nursed and otherwise cared for (for example, by extreme care in avoiding contact with the patient's blood or other body fluids) so as to minimize the risk of HIV transmission.

## Compulsory segregation

Quarantine goes further than isolation because it includes the compulsory segregation of contacts of infectious cases, that is, people who are themselves healthy but because they are or may be carriers of infection, having been in contact with a contagious case, there is a risk that they could be incubating the infection, or even if they are not, that they may transmit the disease to others.

Quarantine may involve infringing the liberty of outwardly healthy people, and this has both legal and ethical implications. Any restriction on freedom to move of apparently healthy people must be justified, and it is sanctioned by public

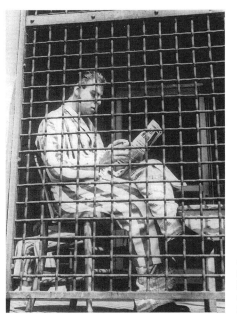

A man reading a newspaper at the Ellis Island Quarantine Detention Center. (Reproduced courtesy of the National Library of Medicine, Bethesda, MD.)

health laws and regulations in many nations. In the early 20th century most industrial nations had lengthy lists of contagious diseases to which quarantine laws applied. By the 1960s most of these diseases could be controlled without such severe restrictions, and in 1969 the WORLD HEALTH ORGANIZATION issued International Sanitary Regulations for just six designated quarantinable diseases: CHOLERA, PLAGUE, YELLOW FEVER, louse-borne relapsing fever, louse-borne TYPHUS, and SMALLPOX. Smallpox was proclaimed eradicated by WHO in 1980, and most of the other diseases on the list (except cholera in some parts of the world and occasionally yellow fever in others) are now rarely encountered or respond well to medical treatment, or both. The quarantine stations that were formerly a feature of large seaports around the world have been abandoned, dismantled, or turned into holiday resorts.

Quarantine law and regulations still apply in many countries and regions within countries, however, to protect animals and plants from exotic diseases of economic importance.

Public health officials who invoke quarantine laws or regulations must justify this action ethically, on the grounds that it is in the interests of the greater good of the community. In the past, this 'police power' of public health officials was accepted by most people as a necessary measure to control the spread of contagious disease. Community values changed in the late 20th century; now there is emotional and political resistance to restricting freedom in the interests of safeguarding the public's health. It is regarded as ethically unacceptable to quarantine promiscuous persons who are HIV-positive, even though it might be in the best interests of the general public to do so. In some places, public health officials have invoked the 'police power' of their quarantine regulations and, sometimes with the assistance of local police forces, they have incarcerated incorrigibly promiscuous persons infected with HIV/AIDS. AIDS activists and civil rights advocates oppose this, and a debate that played out in relation to detention of polio contacts in the early 20th century is being reprised. JML

*See also* INFECTIOUS DISEASES

### QUOTATIONS

Life is short, the art long, opportunity fleeting, experience treacherous, judgement difficult,
Hippocrates, *c.* 460–357 BC, *Aphorisms* I, 1

Physicians wishing to make a point, to emphasize the truth of their statement, or to call the ancients in support of their theory, may quote

HIPPOCRATES (p 382), Sir William OSLER (p 602), Oliver Wendell Holmes or some other illustrious physician from the past. It may be that all lecturers are fond of pressing their point with a pithy quote from others, but there is a very long tradition of this in medicine, perhaps because of the breadth of their involvement in the complexities of the human condition, and the need to capture the essence of these interactions and events.

Every first year medical school class is greeted by a sobering quotation, although the speaker usually doesn't know its origin:

Half of what you are taught as medical students will in ten years have been shown to be wrong, and the trouble is, none of your teachers knows which half.
C. Sydney Burwell (1893–1967) *British Medical Journal* **2**, 113, 1956

Many a lecture, learned talk, research presentation, journal article, or clinical presentation carries at least one quotation from an authority in the recent or distant past. Never mind that it is often inaccurate, and perhaps attributed to someone else — the point is made and strengthened by the voice of an authority. If Osler didn't say it, well, he certainly could have.

The medical lecturer is not confined to quoting physicians, and just as often finds support for his point of view from the Bible, Shakespeare, Jefferson, or Shaw. Through their words Charles Dickens, John F. Kennedy, Oscar Wilde, Samuel Johnson, and the great philosophers are regular attenders at medical meetings and rounds. Great LITERATURE provides a lively source of quotations, as writers tell us more of the human condition, of relationships, emotions, suffering, hope, birth, death, the travails and the frailty of life than any medical TEXTBOOK or JOURNAL. Quotations can open our minds to an idea or concept, hammer home a point, make one pause and think, provide an aura of erudition, or just give us pleasure.

Medical journal articles are not only replete with abundant references, but often quote passages that capture the author's meaning especially well. It seems more secure to have the voices from the past make our point than to make it ourselves, even though we would never accept the general state of medical knowledge of that era. It is as if those voices might have had less knowledge but had greater wisdom.

Like John Bartlett, the 19th-century bookseller of Cambridge, Massachusetts, some physicians keep their own personal collections of favorite quotations. Henry Southgate, who published an early collection of quotations, called them *The flowers of intellect* and his book a *Bouquet of thought*. The collection of a physician's personal favorite quota-

## SOME FAVORITE MEDICAL QUOTATIONS

Physician, heal thyself.
Bible: *Luke* 4:23

Physicians, like beer, are best when they are old.
Thomas Fuller (1608–61), *The holy state and the profane state*

Cur'd yesterday of my disease,
I died last night of my physician.
Matthew Prior (1664–1721)
*The remedy is worse than the disease*

The best doctors in the world are Doctor Diet, Doctor Quiet, and Doctor Merryman.
Jonathan Swift (1667–1745)

The art of medicine consists of amusing the patient while Nature cures the disease.
Voltaire (1694–1778)

Physicians think they do a lot for a patient when they give his disease a name.
Immanuel Kant (1724–1804)

The only sure foundations of medicine are, an intimate knowledge of the human body, and observation on the effects of medicinal substances on that.
Thomas Jefferson (1743–1826)

The medical student is likely to be one son of the family too weak to labour on the farm, too indolent to do any exer-

cise, too stupid for the bar, and too immoral for the pulpit.
Daniel Coit Gilman (1831–1908)

PHYSICIAN: n. One upon whom we set our hopes when ill and our dogs when well.
Ambrose Bierce (1842–*c.*1914)

Medical education is not completed at the medical school: it is only begun.
William H. Welch (1850–1934)

The fact that your patient gets well does not prove that your diagnosis was correct.
Samuel J. Meltzer (1851–1921)

The secret of the care of the patient is in caring for the patient.
Francis Weld Peabody (1881–1927)

A physician is judged by the three A's: Ability, Availability, and Affability.
Paul Reznikoff (b.1896)

Fifty years ago the successful doctor was said to need three things; a top hat to give him Authority, a paunch to give him Dignity, and piles to give him an Anxious Expression.
Anonymous:
*The Lancet*, 1951, 1, 169.

tions starts early, first as a medical student, capturing the essence of the teacher's lesson and pithy *bon mots* in marginalia or in small notebooks. Later the young physician sets aside a notebook (these days a floppy disc) specifically for that use, and such 'commonplace books' were indeed common centuries ago, long before Bartlett published in 1855 for the general public 'quotations familiar or worthy of being familiar'. Some personal collections were published and became valuable sources for broader collections. William Bennett Bean mined the papers of the eminent 19th-century London physician Peter Mere Latham for aphoristic observations on a wide range of clinical topics. Aphorisms of Bela Schick, the eminent New York pediatrician, were collected and published by I. J. Wolf. Many of Eugene Stead's pithy observations on medical care, the university, medical edu-

cation, and other topics made up the entire content of *Just say for me*. Over a century after Bartlett, Maurice Strauss and his medical colleagues followed Bartlett's example and selected for publication familiar quotations relevant to medicine, ones that would be recognizable to most, if not all, physicians.

Authority is important in medicine, and reflects our history, our constant advancement and evolution of knowledge, and our respect for those who came before us. Quotation of our forebears is also an act of filial respect, an acknowledgement of our heritage, and a picture of the continuity of the profession. These quotations help us recognize whence knowledge and tradition came, and how we came to where we are today. It can be the history of medicine writ small.                                   TJM, EJH

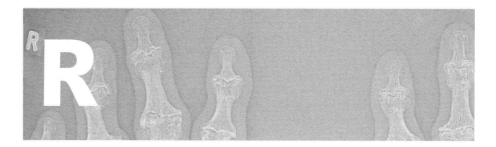

# R

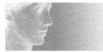

Antoine Henri
**BECQUEREL** (1852–1908).
French physicist. He was
appointed professor of physics
at the Polytechnique in 1895
and demonstrated the
radioactivity of uranium salts
(1896). He suggested the
possibility of radiotherapy
after sustaining an accidental
burn from carrying radium in
his pocket. In 1903 he shared
the NOBEL PRIZE for physics
with Marie and Pierre CURIE
(p 320).

François **RABELAIS** (*c*.1494–1553). One of
the greatest French writers of the 16th century
and undoubtedly the funniest. Born near
Chinion, he took orders at a Franciscan abbey
(1521), studied Greek (then forbidden by the
Sorbonne) and translated Herodotus, but joined
the Benedictines, apparently on the pretext that
his Greek books had been confiscated. Later he
became secretary to a bishop; graduated bachelor
of medicine at Montpellier (1530); and was lectured on Greek texts of HIPPOCRATES (p 382) and
GALEN (p 324) (1531); and was doctor at Hôtel
Dieu hospital in Lyons (1532–5), where he edited
medical texts and wrote *Gargantua* and
*Pantagruel*. His medical reputation growing, he
left Lyon as physician to the cardinal Du Bellay,
whom he accompanied to Rome. In 1537 he
became a licentiate and then doctor of medicine
at the University of MONTPELLIER (p 319). His
works being proscribed by the Sorbonne, he spent
time abroad but seems to have died of natural
causes in Paris around 1553.

His books, purporting to be the biographies of
two giants, are some of the funniest satires ever
written, referred to this day as Rabelaisian, In the
first book the giant Gargantua is born by entering
the hollow vein and climbing through the diaphragm to a point above the shoulders where this
vein divides in two, taking the left fork and
coming out by the left ear, immediately crying
'Give me a drink! a drink! a drink!' When later
sent to Paris, he picked up the bells of Notre
Dame to hang around his horse's neck on the
way to continue his education. When his son
Pantagruel was about to be born and the midwives were waiting to receive the child, there first
came out of his mother sixty-eight mule drivers,
each one leading by the halter a mule loaded with
salt, nine dromedaries loaded with hams and
beef-tongues, seven camels loaded with eels, and,
finally twenty-four cartloads of leeks, garlic,
onions, and shallots, all of which greatly frightened the midwives. Later Pantagruel thought of
becoming a doctor, but decided that the work was
too wearying and that physicians smelt of suppositories like old devils. Later, medical advice is

given by Dr Rondibilis, who describes the various
causes of loss of sexual desire as: (1) the intemperate use of alcohol, which causes a certain
cooling of the blood, letting down of nerves, stiffness of the senses, and a certain misfire in physical
movements; (2) certain drugs, such as the pond
lily, American willow, mandragora, hemlock, and
hippopotamus skin; (3) assiduous labor, which
causes a great dissolution of bodily substances
and diversion of the blood; and (4) ardent study,
which causes an incredible dissolution of animal
spirits so that none are left to be sent pulsing
down to those places reserved for the propagation
of humankind.                                    GD

**RADIATION, IONIZING** Ionizing radiation is
part of the electromagnetic spectrum; it includes
X-RAYS (p 319), gamma rays, and ionized particles
(electrons, protons, neutrons, and alpha and
other atomic particles). In contrast to other forms
of electromagnetic radiation such as infrared and
visible light, ionizing radiation imparts enough
energy to living tissue into which it is absorbed to
cause ionization and excitation of atoms and
molecules. This is the underlying cause of the biological effects of ionizing radiation. These effects
have been studied in great detail, leading to development of principles and procedures to protect
against radiation injury; generalization from these
principles has led to means of coping with other
kinds of environmental health hazards.

There are three main natural sources of ionizing
radiation: cosmic rays that come from outer space;
terrestrial radiation from radioactive elements in
the earth's crust (radium, uranium, radon, etc.,
including their radioactive breakdown products
such as radon 'daughters'); and radiation, such as
potassium-40 and carbon-14, that emanates from
radioactive isotopes of elements that commonly
are incorporated in living tissues. These three
natural sources expose every one of us to about
one milliSievert (mSv) of radiation each year.
Artificial sources of exposure include diagnostic
X-rays, radioactive trace elements in building
materials, radiation-emitting components of TV
sets, computer screens, smoke detectors, and other

domestic appliances and equipment, radioactive fallout from nuclear tests, and leakage from nuclear power plants.

## Evidence of harmful effects

Soon after ROENTGEN'S (p 873) discovery of X-rays, the occurrence of skin ulcers and cancer after exposure to X-rays and radium persuaded physicians and the general public that, although X-rays could be very beneficial, these and related forms of ionizing radiation also were dangerous. Descriptive epidemiological studies after the atomic bombs were dropped on Hiroshima and Nagasaki confirmed that there is a dose–response relationship, and raised doubts about a threshold below which exposure to ionizing radiation is harmless.

As ionizing radiation penetrates living tissue random collisions with atoms and molecules in its path cause the formation of ions and reactive radicals, which in turn break chemical bonds and cause other molecular changes that produce biological injury. The distribution of ionizing events along the path of impinging radiation depends on the energy, mass, and charge of the radiation as well as the density of the absorbing tissue. X-rays and gamma rays produce ions sparsely and tend to penetrate deeply, whereas charged particles produce ions densely and penetrate poorly. For example, alpha particles generally cannot even penetrate the skin. The production of injury is correlated with the density of energy deposition in the affected cells, so protons and alpha particles are generally higher in relative biological effectiveness than X-rays and gamma rays.

The anatomical distribution of the dose delivered by an internally deposited radionuclide depends on its uptake, tissue distribution, retention, and metabolism, which tends to be specific to a particular radionuclide. For example, radioactive iodine is taken up and retained by the thyroid gland in such a predictable manner that this radionuclide is used clinically to assess thyroid function.

At the cellular level radiation takes several forms — inhibition of cell division, chromosomal damage, gene mutation, neoplastic transformation, and various other changes. A large enough dose of ionizing radiation kills any kind of living cell. Radiation can alter any molecule within a cell, but the deoxyribonucleic acid (DNA) molecule is the most critical target, because damage, even to a single gene, may profoundly affect the cell. Many changes in DNA are reparable but the type of damage caused by a densely ionizing radiation is less reparable than that from a sparsely ionizing radiation.

Radiation may cause the breakage and rearrangement of chromosomes and may interfere with the normal segregation of chromosomes

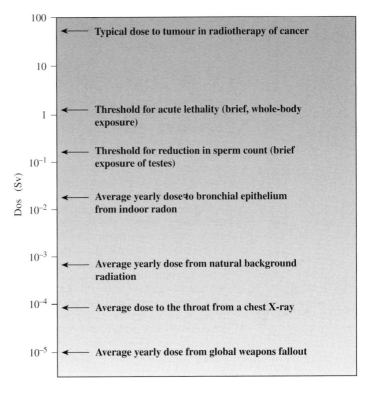

Levels of exposure to ionizing radiation (in sieverts; Sv) from different sources, in relation to the thresholds for various forms of acute radiation injury.

to daughter cells at the time of cell division, thereby giving rise to changes in chromosome number and structure. The frequency of such chromosome aberrations increases as a linear non-threshold function of the radiation dose, approximating 0.1 cell Sv in human blood lymphocytes irradiated in culture. However, only a small proportion of all chromosome aberrations is attributable to natural background radiation, other causes include certain viruses, chemicals, and drugs.

Mutagenic effects of ionizing radiation have been extensively studied in many organisms since MÜLLER'S (p 338) pioneer work on fruit flies in 1927. In mouse spermatogonia and oocytes the frequency of mutations is increased about 100% per Sv, depending on the conditions of irradiation. Heritable effects of radiation on human germ cells remain to be shown. The numbers exposed to radiation from the atomic bombs in Japan in 1945 were too small and the average dose (0.5 Sv) to parents also was too small, to demonstrate a significant effect. The available evidence suggests that the dose required to double the frequency of mutations in humans probably exceeds 1.0 Sv. We infer from this that only a small percentage (0.1–0.2%) of all genetically related diseases in the general population can be attributed to natural background radiation. The percentage that could be attributed to manmade sources has been a subject of debate, but there is no evidence to suggest it is a cause for concern.

### Effects on cell survival

The susceptibility of cells to irradiation increases with their rate of proliferation, a relationship that accounts for the radiosensitivity of cancer cells as a class. In most tissues, 1–2 Sv suffices to reduce the number of dividing cells by half. In tissues characterized by relatively rapid cell proliferation, such as bone marrow, gonads, lymphoid system, skin, lining of the gastrointestinal tract, and lens of the eye, inhibition of cell division may be detected immediately after intensive irradiation, to be followed months or years later by fibrosis and other degenerative changes. Because cells depleted by irradiation may be replaced in time by the compensatory proliferation of uninjured cells, a given dose generally causes less damage to tissue if it is accumulated over a period of days or weeks than if it is received in a single brief exposure. For the same reason, a given dose generally causes greater injury if delivered to a whole organ or the whole body than if delivered only to a small part of the organ or of the body.

Intensive irradiation of the bone marrow or of the gastrointestinal tract may kill enough cells in these tissues to cause radiation sickness, known as acute radiation syndrome. Nausea, vomiting, and loss of appetite typically occur within a few hours after intensive irradiation, and are followed by a symptom-free period until the main phase of the illness. In the intestinal form, associated with a dose exceeding 10 Sv, this begins 2–3 days after irradiation and is characterized by severe diarrhea, prostration, and death. A radiation dose that exceeds 1–2 Sv causes radiation sickness that affects the blood-forming organs (bone marrow), typically 2–3 weeks after exposure, with reduced white cell counts, and platelet damage that causes bleeding and bruising. If exposure is sufficiently severe death, occurs after about 4–6 weeks from bleeding or infection. A third form of the acute radiation syndrome affects the brain; this occurs after a rapid exposure of the brain to a dose in excess of 50 Sv. There is almost immediate severe vomiting, nausea, and loss of appetite, followed by drowsiness, loss of balance, confusion, convulsions, loss of consciousness, and death.

### Effects on embryo

The cells and tissues of the developing embryo and fetus are highly radiosensitive. For this reason even dental and chest X-rays should be avoided altogether or kept to the absolute minimum in early pregnancy, preferably before pregnancy begins if it is planned and expected to occur. Long-term epidemiological studies of the offspring of women who had minimal exposure to X-rays (for example, a single chest radiograph)

during early pregnancy have shown that they have elevated rates of anomalous development in adolescence and early adult life as well as a small but significant increase in the incidence of cancer and leukemia in early childhood. These studies suggest that if there is a threshold dose it must be very small.

### Ionizing radiation and cancer

The early 20th century pioneers of X-rays and radium treatment had very high incidences and death rates from cancer. So did patients who were treated with radiation for a variety of conditions, including ringworm, ankylosing spondylitis (a severe form of arthritis of the spine), and the 'condition' that was called status thymolymphaticus. This was particularly tragic because healthy adolescent children irradiated to 'cure' this mythical disease almost all died later of leukemia or other kinds of cancer. Malignant neoplastic diseases typically do not occur until some years after exposure to ionizing radiation, the latent period varying inversely with dose. High exposure doses increase the risk of leukemia, with a latent period of five years; medium doses are associated with increased risk of soft tissue sarcoma and lymphoma after a longer latency; smaller exposure doses increase the risk of cancer in other cancer-prone organs and tissues such as the female breast, with a latent period of 20 years or more; but these approximations conceal irregularities in the target organ, the observed dose–response relationships and the latency periods. The evidence from numerous observational studies over many years suggests that there is probably no threshold dose below which exposure to ionizing radiation is entirely without risk — but of course it is impossible to avoid exposure to natural background radiation, and up to 3% of all cancers are thought to be attributable to this. Medical sources of exposure to ionizing radiation now are so well shielded that those at occupational risk, for example, the staff in hospital X-ray departments, have cancer incidence rates no higher than the general population. Modern X-ray machines, and precautions taken to avoid unnecessary exposure to ionizing radiation, have reduced the risk to a minimum.            ACU, JML

*See also* CHERNOBYL; EPIDEMIOLOGY; IMAGING

**RADIOTHERAPY** See ONCOLOGY

**RANDOMIZED CONTROLLED TRIAL** The ascendancy of the randomized controlled trial became the hallmark of progress in clinical investigation during the second half of the 20th century. The randomized controlled trial is considered the necessary evidence that a medical intervention works, that is prevents or ameliorates the natural course of a disease. All types of medical interventions may be subject to a randomized trial: vaccines, sera, dietary supplements, surgical, radiological, or drug treatment. In practice, most randomized controlled trials concern drugs or vaccines. The principle is thought so important that investigations in which a randomized trial is applied usually carry the words 'randomized controlled trial' in the title of the scientific publication. The justification is genuine uncertainty about the best way to prevent or treat a condition (a state of mind known as equipoise). It is unethical to carry out such a trial in the absence of uncertainty.

## Comparisons

The principle that the randomized trial aims to achieve is an old one: the comparison of 'like with like', in Latin 'ceteris paribus', a time-honored principle of causal reasoning. The idea is that one can attribute an effect to a certain intervention if and when all other influences are ruled out. This principle was one of John Stuart Mill's 1862 canons of causality. It took some time, however, before the principle was applied to study the effect of medical interventions. The principle was somewhat earlier applied in laboratory experiments in which the investigator sought to 'control' all other factors that might influence the outcome. The problem with medical investigations on patients is that it is usually impossible to control 'all other factors' that influence the course of the disease (also called 'prognostic factors'), or determine the success of a treatment. As a means to achieve the same end, physicians who wanted to study the merit of one treatment against another have tried to achieve 'comparability': they have tried to form two (or more) groups with a comparable prognosis. If the overall prognosis of the groups was the same at the onset of the study, any difference in true outcome at the end of the study will be due to the only difference that exists between the groups: the administration of different treatments.

The earliest clinical trial (a comparison of diets) is reported in the *Old Testament* in the first chapter of the book of Daniel. Perhaps James LIND (p 853) was thinking of this story when he gave six pairs of sailors each a different diet and compared the effects of each on the scurvy, reporting the results in *A treatise of the scurvy* (1753). More systematic attempts to achieve comparability were developed by Pierre Charles Alexandre LOUIS (p 780), who founded the movement called *Médecine d'observation* in Paris in the 1830s. However, at that time, judgement about the comparability of the patients relied on the judgement of the physician. For example, in the treatment of TUBERCULOSIS, patients who were judged to have had an equal prognosis were com-

pared. In the first half of the 20th century, attempts were initiated to make the principle of comparability more objective: the judgement of the physician was deemed fallible and not reproducible or insightful to outsiders. For example, it was proposed that in addition to ranking patients with tuberculosis according to the severity of their disease, and then taking them pairwise to different treatments, a 'random' element of flipping a coin would be added: to decide which of the two patients with similar disease severity — as judged by the physician — would receive the treatment. Such 'flipping of the coin' would be an objective guarantee against the fallibility and irreproducibility of the judgement of the treating physician: any remaining incomparability would become equally distributed in both groups. Instead of flipping coins, other devices were also used, such as dividing patients according to odd or even dates of birthdays, days of admission, or the statistical table of random numbers.

## Breakthrough

The breakthrough came from another discipline of investigation in which the problems of unknown variability were at least as great as in medicine: agriculture. In the 1920s Sir Ronald Fisher introduced and promoted research designs in which plots of land were 'randomly' allocated to different treatments, for example with fertilizers. The principle was adopted as alternation in medicine. Firstly, in trials of gold treatment of tuberculosis and the serum treatment of lobar pneumonia in the 1930s, and then in the Medical Research Council streptomycin trial on the treatment of tuberculosis of 1948, which still stands as a milestone of the first successful published trial with individual randomization in modern medicine. Randomizing tuberculosis patients was acceptable because there was a shortage of the drug: patients were either put on active treatment with the new drug, or received standard care. Since then, however, randomization has become the pivotal principle to prove that an innovative treatment improves the outcome of patients: it is required that the drug is compared with placebo (inert or inactive substance) to assess objectively whether it has any effect. Strong movements were started to promote this form of more objective scientific medicine, mainly in the USA and Britain, advocated by among others Sir Austin Bradford HILL (p 381), who had helped design the early MRC trials and the streptomycin trial. As government agencies started to require evidence from randomized trials in order to approve new drugs on the market, not relying on randomized trials was soon seen as a backward form of medical reasoning.

In the end, this meant that 'chance' was invoked to achieve scientific comparability. The next question became: how good is chance to achieve comparability? In principle, it is perfect for infinitely large groups, or for endless repetitions of trials. The principle of randomization assures that the average trial has comparable groups. What about a single moderately large trial? From early on, randomized trials were plagued by problems of inference. The most interesting example was the University Group Diabetes Program: it was a randomized trial in which several treatment modalities of diabetes (diet alone, insulin, oral hypoglycemic agents) were compared. The group of patients taking oral hypoglycemic agents was ended prematurely and published in 1970 because of an increased death rate through myocardial infarction. Given the nature of the randomized trial ('all other things being equal'), the conclusion seemed inescapable that this must be due to these drugs. A heated controversy followed, that took over 20 years to resolve. Basic in the controversy was that at the start of treatment, the patients that had been randomly allocated to the oral hypoglycemic agents had 'by chance' a less favorable cardiovascular profile. Much was made of that finding. It led to a re-analysis of the trial in which patients were regrouped according to their baseline profile (by statistical stratification procedures), which did not alter the findings to any considerable degree. The major lesson was that in interpreting the results of a randomized trial it is imperative to verify whether 'chance' has indeed resulted in prognostically comparable groups. So, final judgement about comparability falls back on the physician who reads the report.

An even more difficult notion is whether the results of the randomized trial denote 'causality', that is, causal mechanisms whereby the drug works. A word of caution against overly causal interpretation came from another British epidemiologist, Archie COCHRANE (p 79), who was a champion of promoting the randomized trial. In his book *Effectiveness and efficiency* he proclaimed that 'All effective treatment should be free', and that effectiveness of treatments was proved only by randomized trials. A movement called the 'Cochrane Collaboration' that promotes 'EVIDENCE-BASED MEDICINE' carries his name. He recounted how he tried out a randomized treatment when he was a prisoner of war, to see whether he could abate signs and symptoms of 'hunger edema' in his fellow prisoners for whom he was the medical officer. His idea was that hunger edema was caused by lack of vitamins, a form of 'wet beri-beri'; he randomly gave a two spoonfuls of yeast daily to his fellow prisoners of war who suffered from edema. The symptoms resolved in the treated group and he concluded that this experiment proved that hunger edema was caused by lack of vitamin. Only much later

did he realize that protein deficiency was the real cause, and that the spoonfuls of yeast might have given just enough extra protein to abate the worst symptoms of hunger edema.

The randomized trial has evolved into a major instrument in medical scientific reasoning. In addition to the randomization principle, the trials are often carried out 'double blind'. 'Double blind' means that neither the treating physician, nor the patients, know whether they receive the active drug or the inactive placebo. This extra caution is introduced to rule out any subjectivity in assessing the effect. In summary, the randomized controlled double-blind trial is the most objective form of clinical investigation on patients, and therefore rightly receives a proper independent place in the medical scientific armamentarium. We should never forget the philosopher Hume's dictum, however, that causality cannot be directly inferred from observations, but that it resides in the interpretation. Any result of a randomized trial has to be incorporated into existing medical reasoning; otherwise, it has no basis to exist. Finally, all randomized trials are experiments on humans, and ethical standards must be maintained, with INFORMED CONSENT from all the participants.                    JPV

**RECORDS** Medical records could be taken to include any information relating to the practice of medicine, but the term is usually understood to refer to the case records of individual patients made and used by those responsible for their clinical care; as such they have a long and interesting history.

The earliest case records of individual patients are those that have survived from the Hippocratic school of medicine in Cos, and date from the 4th century BC. Like all subsequent case records they describe the onset and course of illness in an individual patient, the observations and actions of the doctor, and information supplied by the patient. A vivid sense of occasion enlivens these ancient case histories. 'Philiscus lived by the wall. He took to his bed with acute fever on the first day, with sweating; night uncomfortable'. We are immediately interested in what happens to Philiscus. These case histories demonstrate the rational approach to the diagnosis and treatment of disease which characterized GREEK MEDICINE. For the first time disease is seen as due not to magical influences, but to natural events that could be understood by appropriate observation. These qualities made the case histories of the Hippocratic corpus an ideal model for clinicians for the next two thousand years. Throughout this time the principal purpose for recording and preserving case histories was an educational one. They were intended to advance the understanding of disease and its treatment, and to assist doctors in their clinical practice.

In the 19th century the humoral theory of disease that had dominated medical thought since Hippocratic times was gradually replaced by our current concepts based on pathological anatomy and physiology and on the application of new knowledge from the basic medical sciences. Clinical practice underwent profound changes as a result of this new understanding. Physical examination became a necessary basis for diagnosis. Evidence from both the patients' history and the physical examination had to be recorded in a systematic way and analyzed together with the results of many special investigations to achieve a diagnosis. Follow-up notes were required to document and manage the continuing care of patients. The medical record then became an important instrument in the actual process of medical care.

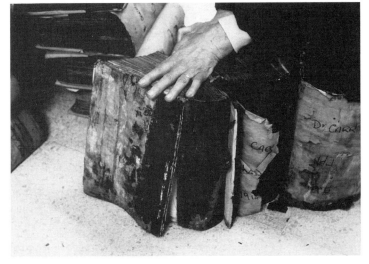

## Storage and communication

The increasing technical complexity of medicine, and the wide range of different professionals involved in the care of an individual patient during the 20th century, made the medical record indispensible, not only for collecting and storing information, but also as a means of communication. The doctor has become dependent on the patient's medical records for the effective management of the consultation and is likely to become disabled without it. Unfortunately as the need for the record has grown its quality has deteriorated. The volume and complexity of information needing to be recorded have overwhelmed the capacity of the traditional medical record.

In the 1960s a number of proposals were made for improving the medical record. Perhaps the most influential of these was the 'Problem orientated medical record' suggested by Lawrence Weed. In his writing he advanced the concept of the 'defined database'. This was the range of information needed to accomplish a particular medical task. The database, Weed suggested, should be clearly defined, collected, and recorded so that it was permanently available, and would not need to be continually reconstructed, as happened in the traditional hospital record. Weed also suggested an 'active problem list'. This would occupy a prominent place in the record and would list all problems needing attention. He pointed out that doctors most often deal with problems rather than diagnoses, and that problems on the list should be expressed at the doctor's 'honest level of understanding'. This was a timely plea for intellectual honesty in the use of diagnostic labels. He stressed that many problems of great importance to patients cannot be expressed in traditional diagnostic terms, but

nevertheless needed to find a place on the problem list if they were not to be forgotten. He suggested that problems might appropriately be described in physical, psychological, or social terms, and also that problems might be the doctor's problem rather than the patient's; an unexplained abnormal finding for instance. All follow-up notes were to be written in relation to a specific problem on the problem list so that, 'the logic pathway of the doctor's problem solving' would be made evident. In this way the medical record would facilitate assessment of the quality of the doctor's work and form the basis for continuing education.

Although the problem orientated medical record was not widely adopted in its pure form, the ideas it proposed have stimulated many efforts to improve and extend the function of the record, both in hospital and in general practice.

## Role of computers

A reorganization of the structure of the record has become particularly important at a time when clinical medicine is moving towards the replacement of manual records by COMPUTERS. Such a move requires that the information is presented for storage in an appropriate form. At the present time most medical institutions use both manual and computerized record systems. One reason for the persistent use of manual records is that the computer cannot provide the same flexibility as the traditional hand written record. Some clinicians await the future with misgiving fearing that the computer will impair the personal quality of the traditional medical consultation. Others feel that only with their help can the huge amount of information now carried by the medical record be organized and made available to the doctor when it is needed.

Unfortunately, too often old hospital records are decayed and rotting, and therefore useless for research. (Reproduced courtesy of the Wellcome Trust.)

Undoubtedly, the computer has become an intrusive new element in the medical consultation. This can have some significant disadvantages. It can impair other important aspects of the doctor–patient encounter. Eye contact and the sense of personal attention that comes with it are made much more difficult, and with it the doctor's ability to recognize when the direction or style of the consultation needs to change. Computers do not encourage the asking of facilitating questions, or sensitive reflection, or the attentive toleration of silence.

Computerized medical records are here to stay and they offer huge benefits to medical practice, but their use in the intimate world of the consultation needs critical evaluation.

Whatever form the record takes, it will maintain its function as a unique record of the medical history of the individual patient. As such its role is becoming more important. Access to the record is now not confined to those caring for the patient. It is also sought by many other individuals or institutions; the courts, employers, and insurance companies, for example. Important ethical issues are involved in allowing access to personal medical records. What is or is not recorded may profoundly affect the lives of individuals. In the past the record has been considered the property of the doctor, who has controlled access to it. Patients were not expected to read their notes, or know what had been written about them. Today patients not only have the right to see what is recorded in their medical record but are often encouraged to comment on and agree its content.

With the advent of computers, protecting the confidentiality of the record has become of great concern. It is now possible to link information extracted from very large numbers of individual records. The research implications of such technologies are exciting. Schemes for mutual access to records kept in hospitals and general practice exist and can include other medical services, raising the possibility of better communication of vital medical information at critical moments. But such linkages increase the difficulties of protecting the confidentiality of the record.

Improving access to important information is also the reason for providing patients with their own personal health record to be carried by them and available in case of need.

In all these recent developments the patient is becoming a much more active partner in the construction, maintenance, and use of the personal medical record. Thus the function of the record in the process of medical care is extending and will continue to do so as new technologies are developed. What is also evident is that many important ethical issues will have to be confronted, and new methods developed to protect the individual from harm.

Not only attending personal doctors but nurses, receptionists, accountants or business managers, technicians in laboratories and X-ray departments, and all others who encounter patients or their body parts or specimens, keep records; and all records contain useful information that can be extracted and statistically analyzed. The information in medical records falls into several well-defined categories: clinical, demographic, sociological, economic, and behavioral.

Medical AUDITS are based on analysis of medical records. These can reveal a great deal about the quality of medical care.

Finally, medical case records are themselves an important primary source of the medical historian. I have drawn attention to the Hippocratic case histories, but those of any age provide similar intimate insights into the day to day practice of medicine and into the thoughts and behavior of doctors and patients, and the society in which they lived. We have a responsibility, I think, to preserve at least a selection of today's medical records for the historian of the future. To do so will need more positive planning than has been our habit in the past                    IT

*See also* DIAGNOSIS; HIPPOCRATES

**RED CROSS, RED CRESCENT** On the evening of 24 June 1859 Jean-Henri DUNANT (this page), a young Swiss, found himself by chance in the Lombardy village of Castiglione, during the Italian Campaign to free Italy from Austrian occupation. Throughout the day some 300 000 soldiers, with accompanying horses and artillery, had been engaged nearby in battle. Fought in a confined space surrounded by hills, the main thrust had been in and around the village and heights of Solferino which was to give the battle its name. When the fighting ceased abruptly in the late afternoon some 40 000 men were dead, wounded, or missing.

Although the medical services of the victorious French were well organized by the standards of the day, the scale of the casualties was beyond their ability to cope. The addition of enemy wounded abandoned by fleeing comrades completely overwhelmed them. To speed their retreat, the Austrians had commandeered most of the carts in the district, thus adding to the difficulties. Those wounded who could neither walk nor crawl had to depend on the few ambulance wagons the French had in the field. Hundreds did not survive the wait.

Castiglione became a huge casualty clearing station with the wounded packed tightly wherever there was space for a man to lie. Of those lying in the streets or gardens, many were without shelter from the burning sun. There was a shortage of food, medical supplies, water — everything.

Above all, there was a shortage of people to look after the casualties.

Aghast at the conditions, Dunant was tireless in tending the wounded and persuading others to help. At first the villagers were reluctant, afraid of reprisals should the occupying power regain control and find they had helped the enemy. 'Tutti fratelli,' Dunant repeated again and again, explaining that we are all brothers and that, once wounded, a man became a victim deserving of help regardless of the side he had been on.

Afterwards Dunant could not forget the suffering he had witnessed and to exorcize his ghosts wrote a book called *A memory of Solferino*. In it he pleaded for neutral status for the wounded, those tending them, and whatever was used to transport and house them. Mindful, too, that the resources of military medical services are seldom unlimited, he also suggested that each country should train volunteers in peacetime to supplement the medical services of armies in time of war. The book captured the imagination of the rich and influential of mid 19th century Europe. On 26 October 1863 a small committee, of which he was secretary, hosted an international congress in Geneva at which Dunant's proposals were accepted. Before the year was out the first National Relief (to become Red Cross or Red Crescent) Societies had been formed. Recognizing that more than pious hopes would be required to make sure that the neutral status of the wounded would be respected at all times, the committee persuaded the Swiss government to convene a Diplomatic Conference in Geneva the following year. It was attended by representatives of many European countries, among them Great Britain. Two weeks later, on 22 August 1864, an international treaty, the Geneva Convention for the Amelioration of the Condition of the Wounded of Armies in the Field, was signed.

In the course of its deliberations it had become apparent to the conference that something would be needed to differentiate members of the medical services — and their volunteer helpers — from combatant troops, keeping them safe from attack: an immunity they had not enjoyed hitherto. A similar immunity was required for hospitals, permanent and temporary, and ambulance wagons. The emblem chosen, and incorporated into the 1864 Convention, was a red cross on a white field — the Swiss flag in reverse. Although it had no religious significance and was not intended to have any, a crescent was substituted in certain Muslim countries, where the red cross was seen as a symbol of Christianity. With a third emblem, no longer in use, the crescent was legalized and officially adopted in 1929 at a diplomatic conference. At the same time, the signatory governments stipulated that no further emblems would

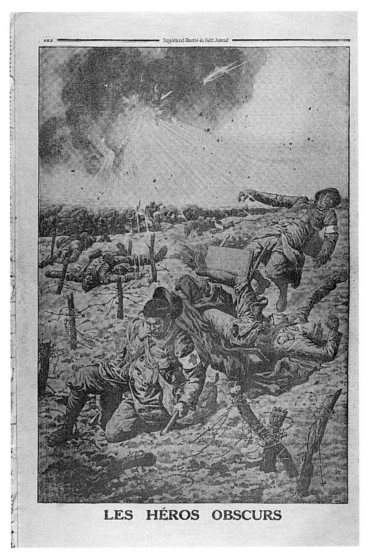

LES HÉROS OBSCURS

be considered as a visible sign of protection accorded by the Geneva Conventions.

In 1919, the International Red Cross extended its activities to include help for the victims of natural disasters. A League of Red Cross Societies was set up to coordinate this work and to help new societies to develop.

By its 120th anniversary, in 1983, the Red Cross movement had over 200 million members: practically every independent state in the world was a signatory to the Geneva Conventions — which by that time numbered four — and most signatory countries had a national Red Cross or Red Crescent Society.

Although national societies are autonomous they are bound by the principles and statutes of the Red Cross, which oblige them to support

Red Cross stretcher-bearers under fire at the front in World War I, as portrayed in *Le Petit Journal*. (Reproduced courtesy of the Mary Evans Picture Library.)

each other, and by the Red Cross objectives for war and peace which are common to all societies. Individual societies engage in peacetime programs appropriate to their national needs. Primary medical care has an important role in developing countries, for instance. Disaster preparedness programs have a vital part in countries which lie in natural disaster belts. In some countries the blood donor service is one of the principal activities, while in others welfare services predominate.

In 1901, Henry Dunant was joint recipient of the first Nobel Peace Prize. Subsequently, it was awarded to the International Red Cross in 1917, 1944, and 1963.                                    HiK

*See also* WAR

**REGULATION OF THE HEALTH PROFES- SIONS** See PROFESSIONAL REGULATION

**REJECTION, GRAFT** See TRANSPLANTATION

**REJUVENATION** For almost all of recorded history, human beings seem to have searched for ways to prolong their lives and augment the vitality of the aged — effects which, for the want of a better word, can be described as rejuvenation. The EDWIN SMITH PAPYRUS (dating from *c.* 1600 BC and probably a copy of a work from 3000 BC) contains an ancient Egyptian recipe for transforming an old man into a youth; the Greek philosopher Empedocles claimed to know of drugs that could reverse aging; and Gilgamesh, the hero of the 650 BC epic whose sources go back to 3000 BC, sought a thorny plant growing at the bottom of the sea that was supposed to confer immortality.

Later, Roger Bacon, the celebrated Doctor Mirabilis, recommended pearls, coral, the bone from a stag's heart, and, most important, the breath of a young virgin to renew the waning vitality of an aging man. The alchemists were convinced that the philosopher's stone, apart from transforming base metals into gold, would make an old man young and cure all illnesses. The discovery of Florida in the early 16th century was an unexpected byproduct of Juan Ponce de León's search for the fabled Fountain of Youth, whose waters would bestow youth and long life. Finally, the first reports of successful blood transfusion in animals in 1650 emphasized that it rejuvenated them. Not all techniques of rejuvenation depended on the exotic: scoffing at alchemy, the German physician Christoph Wilhelm Hufeland asserted that the prolongation of life depended on conserving the body's vital powers by moderation in all things, especially diet.

From the 19th century onwards, quests for youthfulness and longevity became increasingly

'scientific'. Many techniques were proposed for the retention or restoration of youthful vitality, often linked with the endocrine system. This part of the story begins with Charles-Edouard BROWN- SÉQUARD (this page), the peripatetic French- American physiologist, who at the age of 72, announced that he had regained strength and energy by injecting himself with extracts of the testicles of dogs and rabbits. Although Brown- Séquard's work is always mentioned in any history of ideas of rejuvenation, its contemporary impact was greater in triggering a craze for treating innumerable ailments (not simply senility) with extracts from all kinds of organs, ranging from the sex glands to the brain (organotherapy) and, simultaneously, inducing a new interest among physiologists in investigating the functions of the ductless glands.

Later Brown-Séquard's experiments were resurrected as pioneering contributions to rejuvenation, most notably by the Viennese physiologist Eugen Steinach and French-Russian surgeon Serge Avramovitch Voronoff in their efforts to establish a scientific genealogy for their own hugely (albeit transiently) popular procedures for rejuvenation. Steinach evolved a simple operation, almost identical to a standard vasectomy, which, he argued, destroyed the sperm-producing cells of the testes and freed space for the hormone-secreting interstitial cells to proliferate. This proliferation led to increased hormone secretion, which, by augmenting blood flow to all regions of the body, energized the aging person.

Countless men across the world had the Steinach operation, including the poet W. B. Yeats, who claimed to have regained his sexual as well as poetic prowess after it, and Sigmund FREUD (p 321), who resorted to it in the hope of halting the progress of his oral cancer but did not think it had done him any good. Voronoff's equally popular operation involved grafting testicular tissue from primates into senile men — hence the evocative phrase by which it became known: the 'monkey-gland' operation. Although Steinach attempted to rejuvenate women by low-dose irradiation of the ovaries, most modern techniques of rejuvenation have been designed for men.

One well-known modern technique for rejuvenation, however, has been exceptional in avoiding surgery as well as male bias. The Russian biologist Elie METCHNIKOFF (p 412) (Il'ia Il'ich Mechnikov) was convinced that senility was ultimately caused by the disharmonious physiological effects of certain bacteria harbored by the human large intestine, which could be destroyed by the consumption of large quantities of sour milk preparations. With those potent sources of disharmony removed, human beings, Metchnikoff promised, could live for many more years and do so in good

**SELF-REJUVENATION**

Charles Edouard **BROWN- SÉQUARD** (1817–94). Mauritian physician. Trained in Paris, he roamed the world, practicing in Philadelphia, New York, Virginia, London, Boston, and Paris. A single-minded research worker, he described the results of hemisection of the spinal cord (Brown-Séquard syndrome, 1849), elucidated the function of the adrenal glands, and attempted his own rejuvenation with 'testicular fluid' from animals.

health. Yet another innovative procedure was pioneered by the Swiss physician Paul Niehans in the 1950s. Niehans, an elusive figure whose work has been explored only by sensationalistic journalists, claimed to rejuvenate the elderly by injecting cells taken from fetuses of sheep or calves, infant bulls, or pigs. This 'cellular therapy,' according to its originator, was not merely rejuvenative in a general sense but was useful in almost any non-infectious malady, with some effect even on cancer.

Today, quests for rejuvenation are again turning toward ENDOCRINOLOGY or so, at least, one suspects from press reports hailing the miraculous powers of dehydroepiandrosterone, melatonin, and growth hormone. Simultaneously, increasingly complex forms of PLASTIC SURGERY offer an array of procedures to remove the outward signs of aging. The dietetic methods proposed by Hufeland have not died out either, as evinced by growing concerns with nutrition, exercise, and the avoidance of habits such as smoking.

To leave aside dietary measures and surgery, there is no unequivocal evidence that any medical method of rejuvenation actually works — except, of course, by suggestion. Nevertheless, the medical historian has much to learn from the subject: each theory of rejuvenation is rooted in specific ideas about the physiological cause of aging; the social utility (or lack of it) of the elderly; the regulation and the biological potential of the human body; and the capacity of 'science' to determine the extent, form, and quality of human existence. In strictly medical terms, rejuvenation might be no more than a dream but when properly interpreted, the dream, to paraphrase FREUD (p 321), can open a royal road to the social and cultural history of medical beliefs and practices.                              CSEN

## RELIGION, PHILOSOPHY, AND MEDICINE

Religion has been and is a factor in healing for various reasons and in a variety of ways. At a primitive level it is the substitute for an empirically grounded theory of causation in malfunction or disease. Illness is brought about by powers external to man or the world; by the gods, the stars, spirits of evil or of the dead. It is the function of religion to manipulate or to neutralize these powers — the task of priests, diviners, astrologers, soothsayers, exorcists, witch-doctors. Not all gods are indifferent or malign; some are beneficent, the healer gods: Gula, Kurak, Thoth, IMHOTEP (p 412), ASCLEPIUS (p 710), Hygieia. Religion could invoke these and prepare the patient in mind and body to receive divine aid. Healing would come from some adjustment between the patient and his environment, diverting hostile forces, invoking the benign; strengthening the patient against the one, making him

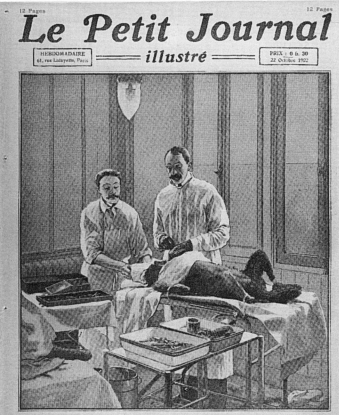

L'Homme qui rend la Jeunesse

Cette photographie unique a été prise dans un laboratoire dépendant du Collège de France. Elle montre le docteur Voronoff et son assistant expérimentant sur un chien âgé la méthode de rajeunissement qui fit la célébrité du savant praticien.

Voronoff tries out his rejuvenation method on an old dog at the Collège de France. (From *Le Petit Journal*, 1922. Reproduced courtesy of the Mary Evans Picture Library.)

receptive of the other. Some physicians went along with this: it was convenient for heavenly agents at the shrines to incur the odium of painful manipulations. Some were skeptical. Others saw plain quackery and resented it, as inimical to the search for knowledge of cause and outcome.

### Hebrew ethical monotheism

Such in general was the picture — overlooking significant variations — of religion and medicine in Egypt and Mesopotamia, among the Hittites, Assyrians, and Babylonians, and of ancient Greece. The ethical monotheism of the Hebrews gave men a new creed, a new theory of causation, and new ethics. None of these emerged fully grown; the revelation or perception grew over time. In its fullness, as found in the Psalms and the major prophets, the Lord alone was God, the Creator of heaven and earth. He therefore was supremely responsible for all that is, all that occurs, in the world, whether by permission or by the direct hand. But since His nature was right-

## GOD OF MEDICINE

**ASCLEPIUS**. Greek god of medicine. Asclepius is first mentioned in the *Iliad* as a king of Thessaly and a healer. Later in the *Eoeae of Hesiod* he was a mythical hero, the son of APOLLO (p 359) and the nymph Coronis, who was taught the art of healing by the centaur Chiron and struck down by a thunder-bolt from Zeus, fearing he might make all men immortal. The worship of Asclepius was introduced in Athens and spread throughout Greece; temples and shrines were erected, often near springs, the most famous being that at Epidaurus (Epidhavros) dating to around the end of the 6th century BC. These temples offered instruction in medicine and treatment for the sick, and were the forerunners of hospitals and medical schools. Asclepius is frequently depicted in sculpture holding a staff entwined with a serpent, the symbol still in use for medicine today.

eousness and steadfast love, all events, all His acts, had moral significance. The nation's sufferings were occasioned by the nation's sins; and so personal suffering was occasioned also by personal sin. Job contested this doctrine, protesting his innocence the more as his comforters loaded him with guilt. But the doctrine persisted. Despite theological change, it persists in popular emotion to this day. 'Why should it happen to me? What have I done to deserve this?' Repentance would bring forgiveness and restoration both to divine favor and to health. The doctrine was promulgated regularly by bishops in the later Middle Ages, calling for repentance and works of devotion in face of natural calamities — pestilence, foul harvest, weather, war. The language of their mandates was translated into the English of the *Book of common prayer* in the exhortation to be read (but now never read) to the sick man upon his bed.

The doctrine, behind its limitations and distortions, had three merits. Firstly, it assumed that the natural universe was ordered, not capricious, and could therefore be studied; science in such a world was possible. Secondly, it assumed the priority of good, of health and well-being; evil and suffering were departures from the primary good and were not absolute; suffering could indeed effect redemption from evil. Thirdly, it is in part compatible with the understanding of psychosomatic disorder and of the therapies which go beyond physical treatment: some maladies — not all — are the product of guilt, as some guilt is the product of religious indoctrination; and release from guilt can contribute to the cure. Jesus lived and worked with this faith. Like Job, he denied the universal and inevitable connection between calamity and sin (*Luke* 13: 1–5; *John* 9: 2–3); but he associated some of his healings with forgiveness of sin; and in some he employed methods used by healers of his day — touch, anointing, exorcism. His earliest apostles did the same.

### The compound of Hebrew theology, Greek philosophy, and Hippocratic medicine in Christian tradition

In the New Testament we have the Gospel according to St Luke, 'the beloved physician' (*Colossians* 4: 14), St Paul's companion on his journeys, which he narrated in the *Acts of the Apostles*. Christianity, therefore, launched into the Hellenistic world by St Paul (who himself, in the first two chapters of *Romans*, validated for Christian theology the Gentile conscience and Gentile reasoning), was well equipped to take Hippocratic medicine into its system. This it did, accepting the empirical and philosophical base, excising the appeal to pagan divinities, and strengthening the ethical impulse with motives

derived from its own faith. The Church became one carrier of Greek medicine into the modern world. It was a conservative carrier, more of a mind to care than to cure, and dissuading from rather than promoting radical advance in the science or the art. These had to wait for the new men of the Renaissance — for the curiosity and matchless eye and hand of LEONARDO da Vinci (p 40) in dissection, the challenge of VESALIUS (p 846) to GALEN (p 324), the wild essays of PARACELSUS (p 617) into chemotherapy.

### Present-day Christian practice

In Christianity today the elements in its tradition remain with varying emphases in different Churches. Orthodox medicine is commonly accepted, though RELIGIOUS SECTS, like Jehovah's Witnesses and Christian Scientists, reject parts of it. Prayer for the sick, and for doctors, nurses, and hospitals, and thanksgiving after recovery, are universal. Unction, the anointing of the sick, raised to the status of a sacrament in the late medieval Church, is administered routinely in the Roman Catholic Church and selectively in the Anglican and Episcopalian. For some centuries it became Extreme Unction administered as part of the last rites in immediate preparation for death. Now it is regarded as a sacramental ministry to the soul in sickness, contributing either to recovery, or to a creative patience in chronic disease, or to preparation for death. Confession of sin, and absolution, would normally accompany it.

*Roman Catholic Church* The Roman Catholic Church associates healing cults with particular shrines. These were many in the Middle Ages, originating in the veneration of the outstanding sanctity of a local man or woman. The tomb of Edmund Lacy, for instance, the 15th-century bishop of Exeter, was the center of a therapeutic cult until it was desecrated at the Reformation. In his lifetime Lacy had compiled a liturgical office of St Raphael, the angel of healing in the Book of Tobit, and promoted his cult, with papal approval. Modern shrines are associated with visions, as of the Blessed Virgin Mary, vouchsafed these. Of the most notable in western Europe is LOURDES (p 478), visited by pilgrims in thousands, some sick, some to pray for the sick; cures and remissions are reported. These cults are controlled liturgically and by canon law, and tests for 'miracles' are increasingly stringent. A more cautious theology, recognizing that in the New Testament the healings performed by Jesus and the Apostles were written of as 'signs' of the coming of God's kingdom, does not look for them as direct divine interventions in the same way now.

The laying on of hands has, in some congregations, passed from the private ministration of the priest or minister into the open as a congregational event, accompanied by corporate expressions in sound and action called 'charismatic', and evocative of what adherents believe to be the practice of early Christian congregations. Exorcism, reduced to a harmless ritual in Catholic wisdom, erupts occasionally in other churches in its more intense forms, sometimes with terrifying and even fatal results. After notorious outbreaks in the recent past, Anglican bishops, halting between a wavering conviction as to the objective validity of the process and pressure on prudential ground, to forbid it, contented themselves with the pious language of 'regulation'.

The corporate activity of the Church, however, engaging lay strength, initiative, and enthusiasm, issues in the founding and support of Christian communities and institutions in which orthodox medicine can find its place in the care of the whole person, his spiritual as well as his physical and mental reality. When the municipal hospitals of the Roman Empire decayed, the Church was ready to replace them: hospitals for the sick, for lepers, and for the aged poor were founded and sustained throughout the Middle Ages, and were supplemented by lay or liberal philanthropy in the centuries before a state health service was conceived to be a national responsibility. Hospitals and medical care were, with education, the spearhead of missions overseas; in the confident expansion of the 19th century they were the main carriers of western medicine abroad. The same impulse sent Albert SCHWEITZER (p 504) to French Equatorial Africa, Mother Teresa to Calcutta, and (Dame) Cicely Saunders to establish the hospice movement — the one to care for destitute children, the other to enhance effective PALLIATIVE and general medical CARE for the terminally ill, and a positive concept of the value of dying.

**Contribution** Orthodox Christianity claims no prerogative in healing or in medical care. It contributes to the care of the sick in offering communities in which orthodox medicine can be practiced at the highest level locally attainable. It contributes to the forming of character and motive in doctors and nurses — a factor felt so strongly by some as to impel them into specific Christian associations such as the Christian Medical Fellowship, guilds of Catholic doctors, or the Guild of St Barnabas for nurses. It contributes to the philosophy and ethics of medicine from its own theology. These insights and emphases were summarized by a recent Archbishop of York, Lord Habgood: belief in God as Creator and in man as his creature on the one hand sets limits to man's assumption to himself of godlike powers and on the other gives man a stewardship in the natural order, in which his responsibility advances with his power. Belief in the incarnation of the Son of God, and a doctrine of salvation, give man new dignity, imprinting on him the capacity to bear the image of God; while the doctrine of original sin warns him of a bias towards evil and frustration in all human activities, when even good can be exploited for evil. The Christian is both committed to and skeptical of all effort for human betterment.

## Rabbinic Judaism

Jewish medical ethics stand in a tradition of centuries in which rabbinic guidance is given on the interpretation of the Jewish law with regard to birth, death, and, above all, the preservation of life by permissible medical treatment. The Rabbis, like the Christians, took Hippocratic and Galenic medicine into their system, but maintained a strict independence of judgement. The method is the application to particular cases of the Law, as contained in the Pentateuch and interpreted by the Targums (the early Aramaic translations and paraphrases), the Talmud (the binding precepts of the elders, with commentaries), and the Responsa of other Rabbis. The moral tradition is developed, as new demands and cases require, but always under the control of principles. The strongest of these is the overriding duty to save life, derived from the theological belief that every human life is infinitely precious to God. The work of a recent Chief Rabbi of the British Commonwealth, Sir (now

---

### PRAISE FOR THE PHYSICIAN

The regular practice of medicine, orthodox with the orthodoxies of each age, continued within this pattern of belief. In *Ecclesiasticus*, one of the books of the Old Testament written in Greek and not in Hebrew (and therefore relegated by some Churches of the Reformation to the Apocrypha), the son of Sirach wrote the celebrated paean of praise for the physician, with the theological overtones clear:

> Honor a physician with the honor due unto him for the uses which ye may have of him: for the Lord hath created him.
> For of the Most High cometh healing, and he shall receive honor of the king.
> The skill of the physician shall lift up his head: and in the sight of great men he shall be in admiration.
> The Lord hath created medicines out of the earth; and he that is wise will not abhor them.
> Was not the water made sweet with wood, that the virtue thereof might be known?
> And he hath given men skill, that he might be honored in his marvellous works.

> With such doth he heal [men], and taketh away their pains.
> Of such doth the apothecary make a confection; and of his works there is no end; and from him thee is peace over all the earth,
> My son, in thy sickness be not negligent: but pray unto the Lord, and he will make thee whole.
> Leave off from sin, and order thy hands aright, and cleanse thy heart from all wickedness.
> Give a sweet savor, and a memorial of fine flour; and make a fat offering, as not being.
> Then give place to the physician, for the Lord hath created him: let him not go from thee, for thou hast need of him.
> There is a time when in their hands is good success.
> For they shall also pray unto the Lord, that he would prosper that which they give for ease and remedy to prolong life.
> He that sinneth before his Maker, let him fall into the hand of the physician.

(*Ecclesiasticus* 38: 1–15)

Lord) Immanuel Jakobovits, demonstrates the method and its application to some contemporary questions concerning the beginning and ending of life, the control of pain, euthanasia, abortion, sterilization, and contraception.

### Islam

Islam, the third great religion of the West, first received its medicine from Greece, having the Hippocratic and Galenic texts, especially the Oath and commentaries on it, translated into Arabic. There was close rapport also with Jewish practitioners; and a major work of practical medical ethics, *Adab at-tabib*, was written by a Jewish author in the 10th century AD. This tradition was then overlaid — as it has been again locally in recent years — by an interposed Koranic or 'prophetic' orthodoxy, varying in intensity from place to place. This would permit, for instance, medical participation in the castration of eunuchs and in penal mutilation. Where western medicine has penetrated, however, western attitudes, both strict and lax, tend to accompany.

### Hinduism

The basic texts of *Ayurveda*, Hindu medical lore, date from before AD 700. They describe ethics of mutual obligation between physician and patient, though the physician was not obliged to treat the incurable, the king's enemies, or certain disqualified classes of people. The ethics were highly protective of the physician; but he was liable to fine if guilty of incompetence, negligence, or malice. The taint of impurity or of unpropitiated sin infected his fee: he could not use it for charitable purposes. In the tradition, only when used to save the mother's life was abortion without sin. Experiments on animals or men were unknown. Ayurvedic and Unani medicine and homeopathy are still taught and widely practiced; they coexist with western practice, and only practitioners qualified in the latter may operate under the Medical Termination of Pregnancy Act 1971. Indian doctors today are deeply involved in campaigns for sterilization promoted by central and state governments; even in the short-lived imposition of compulsory abortion and sterilization for parents of more than an allowed number of children in the state of Maharashtra in 1976.

### Buddhism

The Buddhist Path of Life enjoins the purification of the mind and compassion for all creatures. The Buddha is believed to have been a healer. Hospitals were set up as early as the 3rd century BC. By the curing or relieving of their physical ills men are freed to cultivate their minds. But the mind itself, calm and trusting, is also an instru-

ment of healing and of health. Strict adherents to the tradition of reverence for life find abortion and contraception unacceptable.

### Chinese medical ethics

The organization of medical care in the People's Republic of CHINA and the therapeutics of ACUPUNCTURE and the Chinese *materia medica*, are considered elsewhere. Official policy in both the Nationalist and the Communist revolutions was to deliver medicine from its traditional attachments: first to the cult of the ancestors; then, since the last five centuries BC, to the conflict of demons; then to the Confucian doctrine of correspondence, the balancing of influences internal and external as the way to health; and lastly to the Tao, which ambiguously both disdained medicine and cultivated it in the utmost prolongation of life. In practice, the aim is to combine the best of western medicine with the best of traditional practice, taking acupuncture, for instance, into the arts of anesthesia. Convulsive changes of political and social ideology in recent years make the recognition of a characteristic medical ethic difficult. Whereas at one period all western philosophy of medical science and practice was denounced as bourgeois, now western philosophy of medical science and technology are under invitation to expand. The stern battle with population growth has entailed the sacrifice of some human liberties, including the free choice of family size.

### Shinto

Shinto in Japan is like Buddhism in that it offers more the ethics of a community life than of a professional practice, and in that it extends the mercy of God to all creatures, animal as well as man. It has hygienic value, in its enjoining cleanliness of body and soul, to be attained by bathing and by rituals of the cult. A conscious search for a pure Japanese medicine (Wano-igaku) and its attendant ethics began at the beginning of the 19th century with the rejection of prevailing medical knowledge, partly Chinese, partly European. Atsutane Hirata (1776–1843), in his book *Shizu-no-iwaya* (1811), required a high standard of ethical conduct from so solemn an undertaking as the practice of medicine. Today western practice and concepts of medicine are fully integrated in Japanese medical practice, and Japanese students of medical law and ethics are fully conversant with developments in Europe and the USA. The concept of brain death is not widely accepted in Japanese culture, and the insensitivity of an impetuous transplant surgeon to deeply held beliefs about the beating heart and the recently dead still inhibits organ donation over two decades later.

## Conclusion

From time immemorial the practice of medicine has been bound up with religion and philosophy. Does 'time' include the present with the past? Is the statement still true? In one sense it is no longer true. Medicine has freed itself from the cultic prescriptions of religion; and most of the religions which claimed to possess therapeutic powers have died with the nations that practiced them. In another sense the present is continuous with the past. The religions which still claim men's intellectual, moral, and spiritual allegiance, notably Christianity and Judaism in the West, Hinduism and Buddhism in the East, show a capacity, while cleaving to their fundamental theology and derived principles of behavior, to accommodate new knowledge and formulate a new ethic for conditions and possibilities unknown before. For this reason, more than surviving, they flourish: commitment to medical science and practice is compatible with the practice of religion; indeed, the one may be deepened by the other. Contemporary Islam is divided. Part continues to accommodate western medicine as once it took in the Hippocratic. Part imposes a new Islamic orthodoxy hostile to that liberality which the West regards as humane. Islam is old enough to change yet again.                GRD

*See also* BIOETHICS; JUDAISM; MISSIONARIES; QUAKERS

## RELIGIOUS SECTS

**RELIGIOUS SECTS** Sects have evolved out of all of the world's major religions, having different beliefs and practices from the mainstream believers. Sometimes these departures from orthodoxy have implications for health or medical care. The following examples of religious sects illustrate this.

### Christian Science

Christian Science was founded by Mary Baker EDDY (this page) in 1875. Its basic premise is that physical and spiritual well-being are inseparable. Therefore the most dedicated believers in Christian Science assert that one can cure physical illness, even dangerous life-threatening illness, by the power of prayer. Fortunately, few believers in Christian Science take their beliefs so far as to prefer prayer to surgery for such conditions as acute appendicitis, though there are occasional tragedies when someone does. Because many diseases have a large emotional component, the spiritual well-being that is an integral part of true belief in Christian Science may have a desirable therapeutic effect.

### The Church of Jesus Christ of the Latter Day Saints (Mormons)

The Church of Jesus Christ of the Latter Day Saints was established by Joseph Smith at Palmyra, New York, in 1830 after he received revelations detailed in *The book of Mormon* and later works. Members of this church are known as Mormons. Their unorthodox beliefs, regarded as heresies by Christians, led to persecution of many early converts, and they migrated west to Utah, where they settled in what has since become Salt Lake City. Mormons, now numbering several million, actively promote conversion to their beliefs. Missionaries pursue this task all over the world in their schools and clinics.

Several features of Mormon beliefs are relevant to health. The Mormons abstain from alcohol, tobacco, coffee, tea, and generally they are encouraged to adhere to a vegetarian diet. This combination of abstemiousness and dietary practices might account for the low incidence of certain cancers and coronary heart disease among Mormons. It is an article of faith among Mormons that salvation of their ancestors can be achieved by their retroactive baptism. Mormons, therefore, are much preoccupied with genealogy, and maintain at their world headquarters in Salt Lake City a rich resource of genealogical information, not only about the members of their own sect but also about the population at large. They have assembled a unique store of ancient records, such as parish registers from medieval Europe and comparable (sometimes even more ancient) family records from China, Japan, and Korea. These records are useful in genetic studies of diseases such as certain kinds of cancer. Soon after establishment of this sect it became notorious for polygamous marriages, but this practice is now rare.

### Seventh Day Adventists

As the name denotes, this sect celebrates Saturday rather than Sunday as its holy day. Based on Calvinist ideas dating from the 17th century, it was founded in the 1840s by William Miller after failure of his prediction that the world would end in 1845 (or in 1846). Adventists believe devoutly in the Second Coming of Jesus Christ as the savior of the world. They eschew meat, alcohol, tobacco, coffee, and tea, and drugs other than those strictly necessary for medical diseases. Their strict adherence to a vegetarian diet and their abstention from alcohol, tobacco, tea, and coffee are associated with a lower incidence of coronary heart disease and several common varieties of cancer compared with others living in the same communities and pursuing similar occupations. Recruits to the sect are actively sought among young adults who are entering tertiary education, so this sect tends to be weighted towards members with above-average educational levels. Another of their characteristics is 'health consciousness' — they are well informed about determinants of good health, and take seriously the admonitions of spe-

**DISCOVERER OF CHRISTIAN SCIENCE**

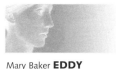

Mary Baker **EDDY** (1821–1910). Mary Eddy was the discoverer and founder of Christian Science. In childhood she suffered much invalidism, but was able to marry and have one child. That marriage was dissolved, as was a subsequent one, but in 1877 she married Asa G. Eddy, by whose name she has since been known. From 1866 until about 1875 while partially incapacitated by 'an incurable spinal illness', she studied the New Testament extensively; this led her to formulate the principle of Christian Science, the basic tenet of which is that the only realities are God, Mind, and Matter, and that most of the ills of mankind can be either mitigated or cured by recourse to the philosophy of Christian Science. Her first book, *Science and health*, was published in 1875. It was revised several times and the later versions were called *Science and health with key to the scriptures*. She held many public meetings, attracting followers to her gospel, and eventually established the Christian Science Church. The 'Mother Church' in Boston was completed in 1906. In 1908 the great national US newspaper, the *Christian Science Monitor*, began publication in Boston. Many churches and public reading rooms have since been established, not only in the USA but also in other parts of the world.

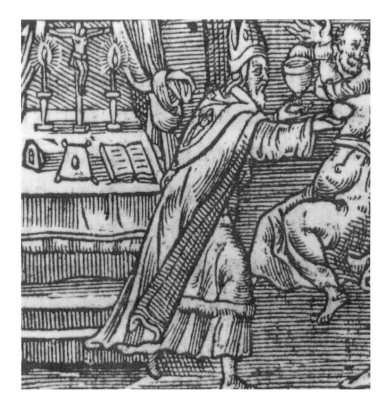

A priest healing a possessed women. (Reproduced courtesy of the National Library of Medicine, Bethesda MD.)

**ROCKEFELLER WORKER**

Rufus **COLE** (1876–1966). American physician. At the New York Rockefeller Institute he implemented his ideas for a clinical research center in which a few diseases were studied intensively in scientific laboratories located close to the patient care area. This is regarded as the forerunner of a modern clinical research center. Cole collaborated in work which led to development of antisera effective in treating the more common pneumococcal infections.

cialists in preventive medicine to partake of SCREENING procedures aimed at early detection of departures from good health. They run many hospitals and clinics in their missions in developing countries and have a highly regarded medical school at Loma Linda, California.

### Jehovah's Witnesses (The Watchtower Bible and Tract Society)

This fundamentalist sect was founded about 1879. Its practices, based on an interpretation of certain passages in the Bible, include prohibition of blood transfusions even when essential to save life. Therefore when a dependent child of a Jehovah's Witness requires a blood transfusion, legal steps are sometimes taken to make the child a ward of the court so that treatment can be given. Since the HIV/AIDS epidemic, interest in blood substitutes has increased, and some of the work of adherents of this sect on blood substitutes for transfusion has been applied with benefit to a wider population.

### Scientology

Scientology is a system of beliefs supposedly based on the study of knowledge, founded by L.R. Hubbard in 1951; the founder's own definition is 'an applied religious philosophy dealing with the study of knowledge, which, through the application of its technology can bring about conditions of life'.

### The Hutterites and Old Order Amish

The Hutterites and Old Order Amish are among the Anabaptist communities which settled in North America to escape persecution in Europe. They adhere to simple, rural ways of life, and resist modern innovations such as cars and television. They often perceive themselves as closed communities in which individuality can be subservient to the wishes of the collectivity. This perception has implications for informed consent procedures: in Hutterite and Old Order Amish communities informed consent for medical interventions or participation in research may have to be obtained from the collectivity as a whole rather than from individuals or responsible relatives. These communities also incline towards consanguinous marriages, so certain genetic disorders are sometimes expressed among them. JML

*See also* GENEALOGY; INFORMED CONSENT

**RESEARCH INSTITUTES** Independent medical research institutes emerged in several countries in the late 19th and early 20th century. The first such body, founded in 1888, was the PASTEUR INSTITUTE (p 620) in Paris, which became the model and inspiration for similar ventures across Europe and North America and very soon across the world. The impetus behind most of these institutes was to develop bacteriological research and to diffuse its practical benefits. The Pasteur Institute sought to institutionalize the achievements of Louis PASTEUR (p 620) and initially acted as an antirabies serum dispensary as well as a research institute. The Koch Institute for Infectious Diseases in Berlin was created to allow the further development of KOCH's (p 455) ideas and techniques, opening with the announcement of a purported remedy for TUBERCULOSIS. Both were created apart from existing universities and medical schools and linked medical innovation to national, if not imperial, social, and economic progress. The Pasteur Institute was the product of a populist newspaper campaign and voluntary fund-raising, while the Koch Institute was formed and funded by the state. All the other institutes followed one or other of these patterns, though it soon became common for private institutes to rely upon large donations from wealthy benefactors, as was the case with the Lister (London) and Rockefeller Institutes.

The thinking behind this burst of institution building was that if such recent achievements in medical science as the germ theory of disease, antisera, antitoxins, and vaccines had been achieved by the *ad hoc* activities of individuals, what more might come from organized, well-supported, and perhaps mission-oriented team work. A second assumption was that the future understanding and control of disease would emerge from the work of laboratory-based, biomedical scientists rather than clinicians or public health doctors. In other words, one could invest in and expect results from research, and the place to invest in was the laboratory.

The Rockefeller Institute was the first to adopt the term 'medical research' in its title. The idea for such an agency came from a board of scientific directors called together by John D. ROCKE-FELLER (p 316) to advise on the creation of a permanent arrangement for his philanthropy in medicine. For a short time Rockefeller money was distributed to individuals, though the scale of the resources available soon led to the introduction of research boards and institution building. The Rockefeller Institute opened its laboratories in 1904, moved to permanent quarters in 1906, and produced its first notable innovation — the spinal injection of cerebrospinal meningitis serum — in 1907. A permanent endowment of $2.6 million followed, which allowed an associated hospital for clinical research to be opened in 1910.

The Rockefeller Institute was deliberately established without a link to a university or medical school. The aim was to avoid the competing pressures of teaching and administration, while also freeing researchers from having to undertake private clinical practice. The provision of full-time posts in medical schools had been an issue in the United States, as medical schools broke with the tradition of employing local practitioners on a part-time basis to teach preclinical subjects. American medical schools were mostly recently formed and did not have the stability that their European counterparts enjoyed through state support, endowments, and affiliation with universities. Most American schools were private colleges that relied almost exclusively on student fees for income and in the late 19th century they were finding it increasingly difficult to keep up with the expertise and equipment demanded by laboratory medicine. The first full-time post was that of Henry P. Bowditch at Harvard, but the real break came in 1893, when JOHNS HOPKINS (p 840) created the first full-time departments to teach the preclinical sciences. This new cadre of medical scientists, with both time and facilities, became a focus for the development of research in subjects such as physiology, experimental pathology, bacteriology, and immunology.

As a dedicated research agency, the Rockefeller Institute differed from medical institutes in Europe as well as from earlier public health laboratories in the United States. The European model was for institutes to service PUBLIC HEALTH measures, for example, the production of antisera, vaccines, and regulatory functions with research supporting and developing these activities. The Pasteur Institute quickly produced a spectacular innovation in diphtheria antitoxin, becoming involved in its production and standardization. The Koch Institute, besides tuberculin, also worked on the development of diphtheria and tetanus antitoxin. Paul EHRLICH (p 260), whose work was integral to these successes, left the Koch Institute to establish rival institutes with similar missions, first to head the State Institute for the Investigation and Control of Sera and then to the Institute for Experimental Therapy at Frankfurt in 1899. In its early years the Lister Institute could not claim similar successes from research programs, though its teaching of preventive medicine and production of vaccines and sera was highly valued. In 1904, a second medical research institute was founded in London, when the Imperial Cancer Research Fund charity opened laboratories with the specific aim of identifying the cause of cancer and hopefully a solution to this growing problem.

In the late 1900s the fate of medical research institutes was caught up in the wider reform of medical education as, with the carrot of Rockefeller money and the stick of the criticisms of Abraham FLEXNER (p 258) and others, attempts were made to place the training of doctors on a more rigorous scientific basis. The strategy, as part of the wider philanthropic gospel of applied science, was to create high-powered institutions that would train doctors and give them the necessary weapons to become effective in the fight to improve the health and hence the wealth of nations. However, it was acknowledged that a medical school could not simply relay knowledge; it also had to be engaged in its creation and development. Hence, medical education and research became increasingly linked with universities, a trend exemplified by such new foundations as the Otho S. A. Sprague Memorial Institute, which went to the University of Chicago (1911), and the George Williams Hooper Foundation for Medical Research at the University of California, San Francisco (1913).

The Rockefeller model of independent medical research found few emulators. The founders of other institutes felt it essential to link applied research to a university, medical training, or a hospital. A new type of research institute emergent in the United States were those established by clinicians, usually to support research into a particular treatment or disease, for example, Edward L. TRUDEAU'S (p 831) Saranac Laboratory for the Study of Tuberculosis based on the Adirondack Cottage Sanatorium. A more entrepreneurial and important venture was the MAYO CLINIC (p 841), founded in Rochester, Minnesota, by William J. and Charles H. MAYO (p 841). With finance accumulated from their highly successful and lucrative practice, the brothers created the Mayo Foundation for Medical Education and Research (p 841) at the University of Minnesota in 1915.

In Europe in the early part of the 20th century, there was far less private and philanthropic support for medical research, universities and medical schools were less entrepreneurial, and the state played a far more important part. In Britain, state support and policies were developed through the Medical Research Committee (later Council) established in 1913. With responsibility for medical research in the country as a whole, the Medical Research Council had to wrestle with two issues that would loom ever larger as time went on: the balance between funding research work at a central research establishment (intramural) as against funding work at institutions across the country (extramural); and whether to fund the long-term work of individuals and groups (grants) or to support only mission-oriented projects with specific outcomes (contracts). In 1914 the Medical Research Committee decided to create a central institute independent of both medical schools and universities. The First World War delayed matters and not until 1920 did the National Institute for Medical Research open in its own buildings. Initially, there were departments of bacteriology, applied physiology, biochemistry and pharmacology, and medical

statistics, all of which pursued lines of research largely chosen by their staff.

The Council's extramural support was influenced by the ideas of its secretary, William Morley Fletcher, who saw its primary role as supporting fundamental research, with clinical research largely secondary. The council in general, and Fletcher in particular, tried to direct the whole of medical research in Britain and worked closely with philanthropists and the Rockefeller Foundation. However, there was friction with other bodies — such as the Royal Colleges; interest groups such as the cancer charities; and even the Ministry of Health, all of which had other ideas about the aims and organization of medical research.

### Industrial research

Another important development was the growth of industrial research laboratories devoted to medical research, especially in what became the PHARMACEUTICAL INDUSTRY. The most notable in Britain was the Burroughs Wellcome and Company Research Laboratory, whose first head, Sir Henry DALE (p 212), following work on insulin, moved directly to head of the National Institute of Medical Research in 1928. Also between the wars, important work was performed

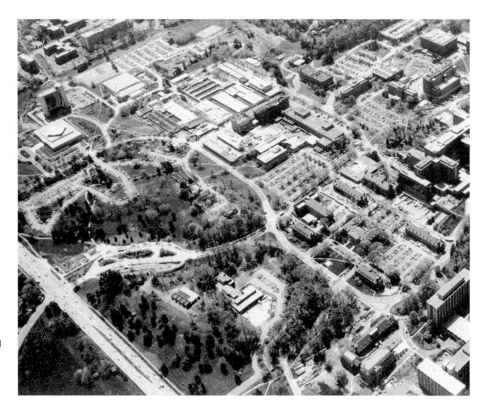

An aerial view of the National Institutes of Health, USA. (Reproduced courtesy of the National Library of Medicine, Bethesda, MD.)

in Britain by the May and Baker Company, which with Lionel Whitby (based at the Middlesex Hospital) developed the new sulfonamide drug — sulfapyridine or M&B 693. Similar developments were evident elsewhere, especially in Germany and the United States. The Bayer Company had supported a research group in experimental pathology which explored antibacterial drugs. After many false dawns in the early 1930s, the group, headed by Gerhard DOMAGK (p 50), identified a substance that killed streptococci in mice, which was the basis for the development of the sulfonamide range of drugs. The links between drug companies and medical research institutes grew at every level, including work in academic departments funded by companies, as with Merck's support of Waksman's research on antibiotics in the 1940s.

The Koch Institute remained at the center of German medical research in the early decades of this century, a role which continued during the Nazi period. Its only rival of note was the Kaiser Wilhelm Society for the Promotion of Sciences, intended as a German version of the Rockefeller Foundation and established with donations from industrialists. However, this concentrated on promoting the 'pure' sciences and sought to preserve the unity of the sciences by avoiding the support of specialized institutes. Its role in the development of medical research institutes was small until after the Second World War. In France the Pasteur Institute system also continued to hold center stage. However, the system lost its dynamism in the 1910s and 1920s and took many years to re-establish itself as a world center of medical research, which began again after 1945. Indeed, in the inter-war period the work of the central institute was often outshone by that of colonial institutes, most notably Charles Nicolle's NOBEL PRIZE winning work on TYPHUS undertaken in Tunis.

An enduring problem for medical research institutes was the linking of research to clinical practice. The Pasteur Institute had opened a hospital for clinical investigation in 1900 and the Rockefeller a similar facility in 1910. In 1914 the Medical Research Committee anticipated that the National Institute for Medical Research would have a hospital for clinical research. However, for reasons of cost, likely public resistance to an 'experimental hospital', and fears of a divorce from higher teaching the hospital was not developed. Instead, a department of clinical research and experimental medicine was supported at University College Hospital, London, and the Medical Research Council followed the policy of promoting the establishment of academic units in teaching hospitals across the country to provide both research and higher postgraduate teaching.

However, in the 1930s this policy was challenged by leading clinicians notably, (Sir) Thomas LEWIS (p 188) and Lord Moynihan, who called for the creation and long-term support of clinical researchers. Several important issues concerning medical research were at stake. Firstly, there were differing weights to be placed on the basic sciences ancillary to medicine and laboratory work, as against studies of disease and treatment in clinical settings. Second, how far was it appropriate to associate research and education? Third, who was qualified to undertake medical and especially clinical research — doctors or scientists; and should careers and full-time posts in clinical research be fostered? Ultimately, these issues were settled, though not resolved, by the expansion of support for medical research after 1945, when it became possible to support many of the diverse interests that had previously competed for scarcer resources.

### Government involvement

Central government also moved into medical research in the United States in the 1930s, when the Roosevelt administration transformed the hygiene laboratory of the Public Health Service into the National Institute of Health. In 1937 the National Cancer Institute was added to the Washington medical research scene, such that by 1940 the National Institute of Health budget was $700 000, though still barely a seventh of the $4.7 million given by foundations. But this was soon to change. The success of the investment in science and technology during the Second World War ushered in what has been called the era of 'big science' — large-scale state support of research and development across the scientific spectrum, summed up in Vandevaar Bush's phrase, 'Science: the endless frontier'. In the United States most of the new federal money went to the physical sciences and was linked to defence aims. However, medicine benefited, too, being able to boast its own research successes of the war — penicillin and antimalarial drugs, BLOOD TRANSFUSION, and innovations in subjects such as TRAUMA and PLASTIC SURGERY. By 1946 the National Institute of Health budget had increased to $3 million and in 1948 it was $26 million, having had the National Heart Institute added to its portfolio. It also became plural, the National *Institutes* of Health. Its home, Bethesda in Maryland, became, if not quite a 'science city', then certainly a large medical research suburb, which in the late 1960s employed 13 000 full-time researchers and took about 20% of the total National Institutes of Health budget of over $1 billion.

In the post-war period the National Institutes of Health, through its award of grants and contracts, took on an important role in the development of the biomedical sciences and the support of medical schools. By the end of the 1960s, a third of all medical school income came from external research grants and much of this from the National Institutes of Health. The growth of state funding was matched by that from philanthropy and industry, though in the late 1980s the National Institutes of Health accounted for a third of all health research and development spending. The 1940s and 1950s saw a proliferation of privately endowed, medical research institutes, which relied on mixed sources of funding — endowments, federal grants, research contracts for private, voluntary, and public bodies. The role of in-house research by pharmaceutical and other industrial corporations grew in importance, as did their support of research in institutes and universities.

One of the most famous new medical institutes in the post-war period was the Salk Institute for Biological Studies in California, which opened in 1960. Like many of the earlier institutes this was based on the work of a distinguished researcher — Jonas SALK (p 664) and his polio vaccine — and once again sought to provide the opportunity for the pursuit of fundamental research without the distractions of routine university or clinical work. However, it was modern in the sense of being a diverse, multi-department institute, without a single goal or particular disease problem in view. While this was happening on the west coast, on the east coast the Rockefeller Institute was moving the other way, seeking to integrate its research into postgraduate training, a position formalized in 1977 when it became the Rockefeller University.

### New funding pattern

The aims of the Salk Institute can be seen as a reaction to the new pattern of post-war funding of medical research. One change had been the relative loss of autonomy, which had previously allowed institute staff to decide or governors to allocate. There was never a golden age of complete autonomy. Institutes always had their own internal policies and financial controls, but often, and within the limits of their overall mission, staff had been able to set their agenda and to follow this with some flexibility. However, since 1945 support increasingly came from external agencies as contracts usually with a fixed time and on a fixed budget. The quantum rise in the scale of funding brought calls for greater accountability. Several aspects of this new situation caused and continue to cause concern. First, whether long-range and long-term research is neglected. Second, the growing bureaucratization of research as medical scientists spend ever more of

their time writing research grant applications, refereeing the applications of others, and serving on research policy and grant committees. Third, the link between laboratory and clinic as the typical medical researcher at the new millennium held a Ph.D. rather than a MD. The original aim of medical research institutes had been to free medical researchers from the pressures of teaching and clinical practice, though, as discussed already, neither of these proved wholly possible or desirable and it subsequently proved possible to associate research with postgraduate training and clinical research in productive ways.

The post-war growth in medical research coincided with a switch in emphasis from attempts to understand and combat infectious diseases to the problems of chronic, degenerative diseases. For many years after 1945 researchers maintained that to deal with these problems the basic biological processes of chronic diseases needed to be first understood, and that research in the biomedical sciences was the key to unlocking these secrets. However, political, public, and medical faith in this model of medical research is still apparent in the level of private and public support for medical research institutes.

### Cost-benefit concerns

Nevertheless, the unease, evident from the cost–benefit concerns of the mid-1960s, and which became more challenging in the 1970s and 1980s, cannot be ignored. First, it was asked whether reductionist research was the best means of improving the quality of life and longevity, as the supporters of life-style changes, especially diet and exercise, pointed to the importance of non-medical factors in the prevention of disease. Second, ethical issues came more and more to the fore at every level, from vivisection and animal rights through to asking about the personal and public costs of the search for perfect physical health and the postponement of death. The community health center might make a greater contribution to well-being than the medical research institute. Third, and relatedly, there was the claim that advanced, industrialized medical science offered little that was applicable or transferable to the health needs of most of humankind in third world countries. Finally, and as a consequence of one of the recent and more promising subjects of biomedical research — genetic engineering — people questioned the ecological and moral dangers of altering genetic material, while some went so far as to ask what right biomedical scientists have to 'play God'. Clearly, the work of medical research institutes in the late 20th century — for economic, social, and moral reasons — was more public than when they were founded a century earlier. But the underlying issues are little changed: basic versus mission-oriented research; freedom and accountability; competing pressures of research with teaching, clinical practice, and administration; linking research with clinical medicine; ambivalent public perceptions of medical science; and strong interests in alternative means of improving health.                    MWOR

*See also* BIOETHICS; EDUCATION; FLEXNER REPORT; FOUNDATIONS

**RESEARCH MISCONDUCT** On 26 March 1974 Dr William Summerlin, an immunologist at the Sloan-Kettering Institute, New York, used a black felt-tip pen to darken a transplanted skin patch in two white mice. His hope was to show that he had overcome the normal difficulties of rejection of a foreign tissue transplant by its recipient. Nevertheless, when the deception was discovered he confessed to the distinguished head of the institute, Dr Robert Good, that he had faked his results. A subsequent inquiry censured not only Summerlin but also Good for not providing sound experimental planning and guidance.

At the time, Summerlin's behavior was perceived as an aberration — so much so that he was sent on a year's sick leave with full salary. But the episode began an era of realization that some deception had always been a feature of medical (and general scientific) research, that it was occurring regularly throughout the world, and that, whatever the difficulties, the scientific community had a duty to try to prevent it and to deal with suspected cases fairly.

Of the reported cases, there seem to have been two principal backgrounds to the misconduct (which is also termed fraud, dishonesty, or deception). One was greed — to obtain money paid by a pharmaceutical company, say, for each patient entered into a multicenter trial of a new drug by inventing data for non-existent patients. The other was to obtain prestige, promotion, and tenure by publishing a large number of papers. Such research workers tend to be found in prestigious highly active departments working on 'hot' topics, such as molecular biology, cancer, and cardiology. Others in the department, including the bosses, were caught up in the misconduct by accepting 'gift' or 'honorary' authorship (putting their names on papers for which they could take no responsibility).

Of three other factors in research misconduct, possibly the 'Messianic complex' is the most important. This is an inner conviction of the righteousness of one's view on a theory to such an extent that no experimental proof is necessary. It probably explains the misconduct of William McBride, an Australian obstetrician who had been among the first to recognize the harmful effects of

thalidomide on the unborn child. Convinced thereafter that other drugs given to pregnant women could also produce deformities in their babies, he falsified data to show that this happened when Debendox (an effective antiemetic) was given to pregnant rabbits. Two other causes of misconduct are frank mental illness and crookedness (in the words of a Nobel Laureate, Sir Peter MEDAWAR (p 819), a small proportion of humankind is crooked and there is no reason why researchers should be any different).

Research misconduct can take various forms — from the most serious (invention of data) to the regrettably common practice of gift authorship. Among the first are piracy (stealing ideas without attribution) and plagiarism (possibly overall the most common type, because the least detected): copying ideas, data, or text without acknowledgement. Other practices include a failure of declaration of conflict of interest (not mentioning that when asked for advice on an article or research grant application as a referee that you hold stock or are a paid adviser to a rival company, for example). Another is to pursue an initial research protocol, which has subsequently been allowed by a research ethics committee only on condition that certain modifications were introduced.

### Initial reactions

At first the scientific community reacted to any disclosure of scientific misconduct with disbelief and shock. Even worse, given that cases usually came to light through whistleblowers, was the treatment of the latter, who almost invariably came off far worse than the alleged or actual miscreant. (Whistleblowing has been the principal means through which these cases have come to light. Audit of records, particularly as required in the PHARMACEUTICAL INDUSTRY, is another mechanism.) Nevertheless, after reports in the scientific press showed that misconduct was a reality, official bodies reacted with a series of reports, recommending measures for prevention and for dealing with a possible case. These have come from various countries — the USA, Australia, Britain, and the Nordic countries, in particular — and generally follow three principles. Firstly, the onus rests on the university or hospital department concerned to investigate the allegations. Secondly, the process should be carried out in stages (usually three: receipt of complaint; investigation to see whether these are warranted; and formal inquiry), so that proceedings may be stopped if they disclose no need for any further action. Thirdly, natural justice ('due process') should prevail, including speed, strict confidentiality, and respect for the rights of both the whistleblower and the accused. If a finding of serious misconduct is made, then several bodies need to be informed: the medical or other

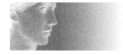

**EARLY PLAGIARIST**

Everard **HOME** (1756–1832). British surgeon. As John Hunter's brother-in-law and executor, he destroyed all Hunter's notebooks and manuscripts in 1823 having used their contents in preparing papers he claimed as his own.

licensing body; the employers; grant-giving bodies; and editors of JOURNALS, who should arrange for articles to be retracted from the literature if they are based on proved fraud. If, however, the integrity of the accused is vindicated by the inquiry then he or she should be offered the opportunity of public vindication.

Perhaps even more important, however, is the prevention of the early stages of research misconduct, by the elimination of sloppy science. Many organizations have now drawn up guidelines for standards in research, covering such aspects as data recording and storage, authorship, and citation of previous work (the document by the Harvard Medical School is exemplary). And many countries now also have national committees on research misconduct. These act as a resource, advising and protecting whistleblowers, holding regular courses on good research practice, and publishing annual or more frequent reports.

One of the difficulties has always been that nobody has any idea how frequent research misconduct is: estimates vary widely from 0.001% to 20% of projects being tainted in some way. Certainly there are probably fewer than 1000 cases in the public domain, yet most people suspect that these represent only the tip of a largish iceberg. When questioned, between a quarter and a third of academics know of a case, and audit of research documents suggests that the proportion is somewhere around 0.25% of research projects. Nevertheless, compared with only a few years ago, at least today the scientific community has come to terms with dealing with what is probably a small but important blemish in its midst.     SPL

**RHEUMATOLOGY — HISTORY** Rheumatic diseases have been recognized since early times. HIPPOCRATES (p 382) referred to joint conditions in 18 of his aphorisms. The term 'rheuma' dates back to the 1st century AD, its meaning resembling the Hippocratic Catarrhos. Both terms refer to substances which flow, and are derived from the term phlegm, which was one of the four primary HUMORS. Rheumatic diseases, including chondrocalcinosis and GOUT, were found in Egyptian mummies. Intervertebral disc calcification was common in mummified specimens, and osteoarthritis has been found in archeological specimens. The first clinical description of rheumatoid arthritis is credited to Landre-Beauvais (1880). He described a series of women with a disease he considered to be a variant of gout. Examination of Flemish paintings between 1400 and 1700 show a few people with rheumatoid arthritis, demonstrated by swelling of the interphalangeal joints.

AVICENNA (p 60), a famous and skilled Arabian physician whose *Canon of medicine* was a leading medical text of the time, mentioned gouty attacks, pain in the joints, and sciatica. Alexander of Tralles first used the word gout in the 6th century — gout being derived from the Latin word *guttae*, droppings from the nose. Interestingly, this was similar to the term Balonius, a graduate of the University of Paris, first used — rheumatism — coming from '*rheuma*', Greek for watery or catarrhal discharge. In the 17th century, tumor albus (white tumor) which probably referred to tuberculosis of joints was described. Thomas SYDENHAM (p 721) was responsible for clearly separating gout from acute and chronic arthritis. He wrote a vivid account of gout, more vivid since he suffered from the disease and died from the effects of nephrolithiasis (uric acid stones in the kidney).

Haygarth described in 18th century some 10 000 patients on whom he kept careful clinical records, a disease which he referred to as acute rheumatism or rheumatic fever. Unfortunately, he lacked, by two decades, the advantage of the stethoscope and therefore did not recognize heart disease in patients who subsequently died. To quote: 'on the tenth day the swelling of the hands receded, her breath became shorter with cough and spitting of blood which soon terminated fatefully. The rheumatic inflammation seems here to have been translated from the joints to the lungs'.

Sir Archibald Garrod first used the term rheumatoid arthritis widely in the late 1850s. In the latter part of the 19th century, European rheumatologists — including Bechterev, Strumpel, and Pierre Marie — described a particular form of arthritis affecting the spine and causing stiffness. This was later known as ankylosing spondylitis, but may have been associated with other forms of arthritis.

During the 20th century, further classification of the rheumatic diseases occurred. This was made possible through careful clinical observation, for example, by Verna Wright, who categorized the sero-negative arthropathies (those with negative blood tests) and Barbara Ansell, who defined a classification for juvenile chronic arthritis. Crystal joint disease underwent a similar differentiation, with the development of assays for specific crystals other than uric acid, including calcium pyrophosphate and calcium hydroxyapatite. Immunological testing with the human leukocyte antigen (HLA) tissue typing, and radiological techniques, such as sacroiliac scanning, helped in our understanding of these diseases.

Since the discovery of rheumatoid factors by Waller in 1940 and Rose in 1948 and the observation by Hargreaves of the lupus erythematosus cell phenomenon, immunological and clinical differentiation of the lupus erythematosus subgroups have become possible. Radio-immunoassay procedures have been developed for measuring particular DNA and antinuclear antibodies, and these antibodies have been further subdivided by immuno-precipitation techniques.

Rheumatic diseases cover many pathologies from the degenerative or regenerative process occurring in bone and cartilage and seen in osteo-arthritis, to infectious forms of arthritis such as Lyme disease or viral arthritis, or the more common forms of inflammatory arthritis, such as rheumatoid arthritis and the sero-negative arthropathies. Undoubtedly there is a genetic component, certainly in determining the severity of these inflammatory forms of arthritis, if not their actual precipitation. Inflammatory forms of arthritis seem to have both an initiating and a perpetuating event. The most likely initiating event is an infection — probably a virus or viruses attacking a genetically susceptible host.

The rheumatic disorders are among the most fascinating diseases known. Though investigations are helpful, the basis of diagnosis rests, to a large extent, on careful history taking and examination.

DJ, PMB, RJRM

**RHEUMATOLOGY** is the branch of medicine dealing with the causes, pathology, diagnosis, and treatment of rheumatic disorders. In general, rheumatic disorders are those characterized by inflammation, degeneration, or metabolic derangement of the connective tissue structures of the body, especially the joints, joint capsules, tendons, bones, and muscles. There are over 150 different forms of rheumatic or musculoskeletal diseases. These conditions may be acute or chronic, and no age or racial group is spared. Some conditions, such as systemic lupus erythematosus or scleroderma, have multi-system involvement; others, such as osteoarthritis, may affect single or many joints.

The expansion of knowledge in rheumatology has paralleled that in medicine. The disciplines of IMMUNOLOGY and MOLECULAR BIOLOGY have led to a rapid increase in the understanding of rheumatological disorders. For some reason, in inflammatory arthritis, the immune system is activated and joints and surrounding structures appear to be the target. For years, infection has been a common etiological theme. Infectious agents may stimulate inflammatory and immuno-logical processes in genetically predisposed hosts. Causative infectious agents for rheumatoid arthri-tis and systemic lupus erythematosus are specula-tive, whereas spondyloarthropathies and Lyme disease have well-defined infectious triggers.

The rheumatologist deals primarily with the treatment of musculoskeletal disorders. Some dis-orders affect the muscle; some, such as osteoporo-sis, affect the bones; but most involve the joints. Though some disorders are localized to a few joints, others affect many and also the internal organs, and are associated with constitutional symptoms such as fatigue, fever, and weight loss. The pattern of such involvement aids the rheumatologist in diagnosing a disorder.

Since many rheumatic diseases are chronic and show increased prevalence in the aged, their inci-dence will increase with the rising age of the population. Musculoskeletal disorders are more prevalent, and a more frequent cause of disability, than either heart disease or cancer. Rheumatic diseases are among the most common reasons for visiting a family doctor, and the drugs prescribed for rheumatic diseases are among the most common prescription drugs.

### Rheumatic disorders and their treatments

*Osteoarthritis* This is the most common bone and joint disorder. By 60 years of age, some 80% of people have radiographic changes of osteo-arthritis in at least one joint. Osteoarthritis is more common in women than men. There is a poor correlation between radiological changes and symptoms. Osteoarthritis has multiple causes, including mechanical (trauma, obesity, developmental abnormalities, and joint laxity) and biological factors (immunologic, metabolic, and genetic). The characteristic joint abnormal-ities begin with an increasing stiffness of the cart-ilage, with subsequent micro-fracture and an increasing density and remodeling of the under-lying bone to form bony spurs (osteophytes). Osteoarthritis is generally progressive, although its clinical course is variable and unpredictable. Significant numbers of patients show very little progression over time. The primary complaint is joint pain. Patients develop bony deformities (the most obvious being hard swelling — osteophytes) over the finger joints. There is limitation in range of motion with reduced function, particularly if the hip and knee are involved. The outcome depends on the site and extent of joint involve-ment. If the primary problems involve the fingers, the effect on function is less than if there is involvement of a weight-bearing joint such as the hip or knee. Other common regions affected include the neck and lower back. Lower back and neck osteoarthritis may lead to persistent pain, and may be associated with nerve entrapment, where there is referred pain radiating down the arm and the leg.

A most important factor in preventing osteoarthritis is to maintain ideal body weight and good muscles around the joint. Exercise pro-grams are necessary to preserve joint function and may be very useful in reducing pain and stiff-ness around the hip and knee. Physical therapy —

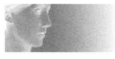

directed at improving motion, increasing strength, and reducing pain — is an important element of any treatment plan.

The medical treatment is broad. Pain control with acetaminophen is a good first step. Often this is more beneficial if taken regularly rather than only with a flare of pain. Acetaminophen is safe when taken in appropriate doses and may be quite effective. If pain or disability persists, non-steroidal anti-inflammatory drugs such as aspirin and aspirin-like drugs (for example, naproxen and ibuprofen) may be used. These drugs should be used with caution as they may cause stomach irritation or stomach ulcers. Patients who are over 65, or patients who have had problems with stomach ulcers, are particularly at risk and therefore, if possible, these drugs should be avoided. The risk may be decreased significantly by using these agents in combination with drugs that protect the stomach. Newer and safer agents are now available.

Local treatment of joints such as the knee may include injection with corticosteroids. This may help control pain and inflammation for up to several months. An alternative is injection of the joint with a hyaluronate supplement. The theory is to replace the depleted joint synovial fluid with a similar material in an attempt to decrease joint pain. Some patients find this beneficial for early and mild osteoarthritis. If pain and disability cannot be controlled by medical management, surgery for the affected joint may be an option. Replacement of knee and hip with artificial joints has become common and has excellent results of reducing pain and restoring function.

***Rheumatoid arthritis*** This is a chronic systemic inflammatory disorder of unknown cause. It affects 1–2% of the population and is 2–3 times more common in women than men. Rheumatoid arthritis usually occurs between the ages of 20 and 50, although it may affect children and the elderly. Often it occurs in genetically predisposed individuals and probably it involves some type of environmental trigger, perhaps an infection. This trigger in some way activates the immune system, which results in infiltration of the joint lining (the synovium) with inflammatory cells producing tender and swollen joints. The activated cells of the immune system produce antibodies known as rheumatoid factors which may be found in the blood of 80% of patients with rheumatoid arthritis. These may also be found in some people who do not have rheumatoid arthritis.

The joints involved may become damaged if the inflammation is not well controlled. Because of the intense joint inflammation, enzymes are released which can destroy cartilage and bone. The smooth joint surface becomes irregular with damage of cartilage and bone especially at the joint margins. These changes, called erosions, can be seen on radiographs.

Patients with rheumatoid arthritis generally experience a gradual onset of fatigue, feeling unwell (malaise), stiffness, pain, and swelling of many joints. The joints often appear enlarged, and may be warm to touch. The most common joints involved are the wrists and the small joints of the hands and feet, but any joint may be affected. The disease typically affects both sides of the body in a symmetric fashion. It may also cause anemia and weight loss. A fifth of patients develop nodular swellings on the forearms or other places, called rheumatoid nodules. Less commonly, it may be associated with internal organ inflammation, presenting with chest pain on breathing due to inflammation of the lining of the lung, or nerve involvement with pins and needles sensation in the feet.

To make the diagnosis of rheumatoid arthritis, several joints on both sides of the body, including the hands, must be painful and swollen for at least six weeks. The presence of rheumatoid factor in the blood or finding erosions on X-rays of the joints helps with the diagnosis. Similar but less common types of inflammatory arthritis must be excluded. Over time persistent joint inflammation leads to joint damage. Once damaged, the involved joints develop deformities, which appreciably impair functioning. Not all patients progress to this stage and the rate of progression is extraordinarily variable. To prevent patients from reaching this state of deformity and disability, it is important to attempt to keep the disease under control with treatment.

Treatment involves many disciplines. Many patients benefit from assessment and guidance of physical and occupational therapists. Regular exercise with the goals of maintaining maximal range of motion and joint function is important. Medical treatment usually includes multiple medications. Anti-inflammatory medications such as naproxen or ibuprofen are helpful in controlling pain and inflammation of joints. These drugs control the symptoms of the disease but probably do not modify the damage caused by the dysfunctional immune system. Many options of disease-modifying anti-rheumatic drugs may be used. Patients, when discussing treatment with their physician, should consider their quality of life, their functional requirements, and the implications of leaving the disease untreated and balance these with the potential side-effects of the treatment they choose.

Rheumatologists differ on choice or order in which to use these drugs. Many different regimens including single or combination drugs may be effective. These include antimalarial drugs,

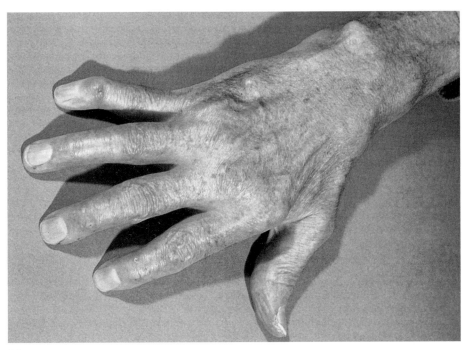

(a)

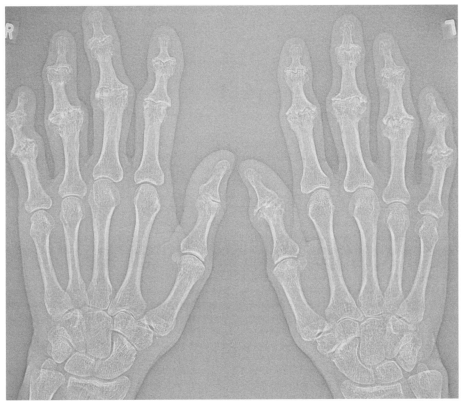

(b)

(a) Hand showing signs of
nodal osteoarthritis; (b) X-ray
of hands with nodal
osteoarthritis, showing
destruction of parts of the
small bones (erosions).

hydroxychloroquine or chloroquine, gold salts — which must be given by intramuscular injection — and immunosuppressive drugs, methotrexate, azathioprine, or leflunonmide. These medications have significant potential adverse effects. To make these drugs as safe as possible, patients are monitored closely with frequent blood samples, urine samples, and physician visits. The patient must be aware that by no means everyone is affected by the side-effects. Most patients take these drugs for years without problems. New 'biologic agents' which should control the disease are being developed. These target the dysfunctional immune system using the body's own chemical mediators (manufactured by recombinant DNA technology) to reduce the immune mediated inflammatory response. Examples include tumor necrosis factor, soluble Fc receptor, and interleukin 1 receptor antagonist. These medications are aimed at specific targets of the inflammatory process which we know are involved in rheumatoid arthritis.

Corticosteroids such as prednisone are quite effective in controlling inflammation, but their long-term side-effects (such as thinning of the bones (osteoporosis), diabetes, and cataracts demand either short courses of medication to control disease flares, or the lowest dose possible. To avoid systemic effects, steroids may also be injected into a joint to control local inflammation. Occasionally surgery may be needed to improve a patient's functional capacity; total knee and hip replacements are remarkably successful in improving functional limitations.

### Connective tissue diseases

This term describes a group of systemic inflammatory disorders in which tissue injury is caused by an immunological mechanism. The initial disease trigger, as in rheumatoid arthritis, is thought to be a viral infection in a genetically predisposed host. Diseases in this category include systemic lupus erythematosus (SLE), presenting with joint inflammation, rash, fever, thrombocytopenia — reduced blood platelets — or kidney and nervous system dysfunction; scleroderma or systemic sclerosis, presenting with skin tightening, lung inflammation, and scarring or acute renal failure, a swallowing disorder, and color change in the fingers on cold exposure (called Raynaud's phenomenon); dermatomyositis — polymyositis (inflammation and weakness of the muscles with rash); and types of vasculitis — manifested by organ damage due to inflammation of the blood vessels.

All these are multi-system diseases, a term that reflects the wide range of tissues and organs affected by the underlying immunological process. The goal in all of these conditions is to control the inflammatory state, and thus prevent organ damage. In systemic lupus and scleroderma, the joint inflammation is treated with non-steroidal anti-inflammatory drugs, and various disease-modifying anti-rheumatic drugs. Antimalarial drugs, such as hydroxychloroquine (plaquenil), may be highly effective in systemic lupus erythematosus for the control of joint inflammation and fatigue and in preventing disease flares. In more severe cases (for example, with kidney disease), dermatomyositis, and types of vasculitis such as polyarteritis nodosa, corticosteroids may be used in an attempt to control the inflammatory process. In cases unresponsive to steroids, immunosuppressive drugs, such as methotrexate, azathioprine, or cyclophosphamide are used to further suppress the damaging immunological reaction.

### Gout and pseudo-gout

Uric acid is a normal breakdown product of body tissues and food. In genetically predisposed persons, or those with kidney disease, uric acid may build up and precipitate in the body to form crystals. These crystals may trigger severe episodes of joint inflammation and produce the clinical manifestations of GOUT. In gout, the crystals are composed of uric acid, and in pseudo-gout they are composed of calcium pyrophosphate or other calcium products. The clinical manifestations of both conditions include rapid onset of pain — with features of inflammation; redness, heat, and swelling. Gout usually affects the big toe, while pseudo-gout more commonly involves the knee. Other joints may be involved, sometimes more than one at a time. The diagnosis of these conditions is dependent on obtaining a small amount of fluid from the inflamed joint, examining it under a special microscope (polarized), and identifying the characteristic crystals in that joint fluid. Treatment and prevention of these disorders involve reversing the acute inflammation with either a non-steroidal anti-inflammatory drug or colchicine. In patients with recurrent episodes of gout, drugs which lower the serum uric acid (allopurinol) or a so-called uricosuric agent, which increases the renal excretion of uric acid (probenecid) may be used.

### Other diseases

*Spondyloarthropathies* are a group of disorders which include ankylosing spondylitis, reactive arthritis, psoriatic arthritis, and the arthritis associated with inflammatory bowel disease. These diseases have some features in common; they all have the potential to affect the back and sacroiliac joints. They also share a common genetic marker (human leukocyte antigen) called HLA B27. Although this marker may be found in perfectly healthy people, it is found more frequently in patients with these diseases, especially ankylosing spondylitis. It is not certain whether this genetic marker has anything to do with the pathogenesis of these disorders. Ankylosing spondylitis involves the back more frequently than the related diseases. Inflammation causes back pain which is typically relieved by activity, often aggravated by rest, for example, at night. In severe cases the back inflammation may lead to decreased back and neck mobility.

All of these types of arthritis may also affect other joints. Usually the large, weight-bearing joints such as the knee, ankle, or hip are involved in an asymmetric fashion. Reiter's syndrome is distinguished from the others by the associated symptoms of conjunctivitis and urethritis. Very distinctive rashes may also be seen with this disorder. Psoriatic arthritis is generally associated with cutaneous psoriasis or nail changes of psoriasis. Treatment for spondyloarthropathies starts with non-steroidal anti-inflammatory drugs. Other drugs such as sulfasalazine or methotrexate may be used in more active cases.

*Fibromyalgia syndrome* This is a common syndrome characterized by diffuse aches and fatigue. Over three-quarters of cases occur in women with a peak incidence between 20 and 60. Patients most frequently complain of generalized aching or diffuse stiffness, which may vary in intensity from day to day. In association with the musculoskeletal symptoms, patients may complain of tension headaches, pins and needles sensation in hands and feet, and the sensation of swollen hands. It may cause or be caused by dysfunctional sleep. In some studies patients with fibromyalgia syndrome have lacked the normal electrical brain wave pattern during sleep. The syndrome is diagnosed from the clinical symptoms along with findings of point tenderness in specific areas on physical examination

The treatment is often challenging. Poor sleep tends to be a consistent feature, which exacerbates the symptoms of the condition. Restoring sleep to normal may be an important therapeutic strategy. Simple measures such as keeping a regular routine — rising and going to sleep at the same times every day — are a place to start. Keeping physically active on a daily basis is of utmost importance. Vigorous physical activity is often not tolerated, but less strenuous activities such as stretching, aquafitness, or walking have been beneficial. Medications to achieve a normal quality of sleep and reduce chronic pain are commonly prescribed. Amitriptyline used as an antidepressant medication may be helpful, but doses used are much smaller than those used for depression. Similar medications such as cyclobenzeprine may also be beneficial. Other treatments

with anti-inflammatory medications or steroids are not useful. This condition is chronic but is uncommon in older individuals. It is important that patients should remain as functional as possible with their normal routines, as pain may persist.

## Arthritis caused by infections

*Rheumatic fever* is an acute inflammatory condition that follows a sore throat due to streptococcal infection, usually occurring initially in childhood. Because of the introduction of antibiotics to treat streptococcal throat infections, the frequency of this disease has decreased significantly in developed countries. Nevertheless, this is still a major health problem in some areas of the world with poor access to healthcare. The infection is not in the joint itself but, rather, the body reacts to the throat infection by causing inflammation in the joints, skin, heart, and nervous system. Treatment involves penicillin to eradicate the infection as well as controlling the symptoms with aspirin or other anti-inflammatory medications. To prevent recurrences, monthly penicillin is given to those at risk for several years after the initial rheumatic fever event.

*Septic arthritis* unlike rheumatic fever occurs when there is direct infection of the joint. The bacteria usually get into the joint from an infection which starts elsewhere in the body. The most common bacteria include gonococci (in the setting of gonorrhea), staphylococci, and streptococci. Septic arthritis most commonly involves one joint, and is associated with fever and chills. The joint is markedly inflamed, with severe limitation in the range of motion. The most commonly involved joint is a hip or a knee. The diagnosis is usually made by taking fluid from the joint and looking for evidence of infection. This type of infection requires the rapid administration of intravenous antibiotics. With such medication in combination with drainage of fluid from the joint, an optimal outcome of normal function and range of motion is expected.

*Lyme disease* is another type of infection which may cause arthritis. The infectious agent is an organism called *Borrelia* which is transferred to a patient through the bite of a deer tick. Patients may present with a characteristic rash in association with fatigue, low-grade fever, aches, and pains. Many months after the initial infection, patients may develop problems with their heart, nervous system, and/or develop arthritis. Despite the fact that this is a true infectious arthritis and often involves a single joint, such as the knee, it differs from infectious arthritis in that it is not associated with a septic presentation (fever and chills) but is more a chronic inflammation. The diagnosis is usually based upon the history of a tick bite or travel to an area known for Lyme-infected ticks in combination with the clinical presentation. Unlike other forms of septic arthritis the causative organism cannot be cultured from the joint fluid. Blood tests can usually detect evidence of a prior infection with the *Borrelia* organism. Most patients with Lyme disease respond to treatment with tetracycline, penicillin, or penicillin-like antibiotics.

*Viral infections* may also cause significant joint inflammation. Hepatitis B, hepatitis C, parvovirus, and rubella are among the more common causes. Multiple joints are commonly affected. These are usually self-limiting but may in some cases persist to cause a chronic arthritis.

*Tendinitis and bursitis* The soft tissues surrounding the joint include tendons (connecting muscles to bones), bursae (sacs of fluid cushioning the space between skin and bone), and muscles. All of these structures may become inflamed if overused. Such overuse may occur in one's occupation, sports activities, or with wear and tear over time. The most common areas of tendinitis and bursitis include the shoulder (rotator cuff tendinitis or bursitis), the elbow (tennis or golfer's elbow), and the outer aspect of the thigh (trochanteric bursitis). X-rays of the affected areas are usually normal but may show small amounts of calcium at the area of inflammation. Treatment of these disorders involves avoidance of overuse and physiotherapy in combination with medications to try to control the inflammation. Anti-inflammatory medications are often used or a local corticosteroid injection into the affected area may help significantly.

## Osteoporosis

Osteoporosis is a metabolic bone disease characterized by low bone mass and structural deterioration of bone tissue, with a consequent increase in bone fragility and susceptibility to fracture. Fractures that are commonly attributed to the low bone mass affect the hip, wrist (Colles's fracture) and vertebral compression. One third of women between the ages of 60 and 70 have osteoporosis, and 70% of women after the age of 80. Common risk factors for osteoporosis are increasing age, a family history, decreased estrogen or testosterone, low activity level, cigarette smoking, alcohol, and certain drugs (for example, steroids). Osteoporosis itself is usually asymptomatic. If a fracture occurs owing to the thin and fragile bone, only then will a patient experience pain. The diagnosis may be made with a test of bone mineral density, and women or men at risk should be evaluated with this test. To help prevent osteoporosis or fractures,

several precautions can be taken. Daily intake of elemental calcium should be 1000–1500 mg. This can be taken through the diet although supplements are often necessary to take an adequate amount. Exercise, particularly weight bearing, strengthening exercises, are good for remaining active and preventing falls which can lead to fractures. Avoidance of cigarette smoking and reducing alcohol consumption are beneficial. Medications such as steroids should be used with caution in the lowest dose and shortest duration possible. In many diseases, patients require long-term treatment with steroids, in which case measures to help limit bone loss should be implemented. In women, hormone replacement therapy is generally the first line of treatment. When started within three years of the menopause, this reduces the risk of osteoporotic compression fractures by 50–60%. For some women hormone therapy is contraindicated or unacceptable and alternatives may be considered, such as the bisphosphanates (etidronate and alendronate). These help prevent further bone loss and may even increase bone mass. DJ, RJRM

*See also* INBORN ERRORS OF METABOLISM

**ROCKEFELLER FOUNDATION** See FOUNDATIONS; RESEARCH INSTITUTES

Benjamin **RUSH** (1746–1813). American physician and political figure. He studied medicine as an apprentice in Philadelphia and later obtained a medical degree at Edinburgh. Returning to Philadelphia, he was appointed professor of chemistry and then of medicine, and began to take an interest in matters of public policy, including the abolition of slavery and the temperance movement. He was a member of the Continental Congress and a signatory of the Declaration of Independence. For a year he served in the War of Independence as surgeon-general and physician-general of the Middle Department of the Continental Army, but resigned in 1788 because he considered that his superior was mismanaging medical care. In 1797 he was appointed Treasurer of the Mint, an appointment he held until his death.

A hyperactive state of the arteries (which he called hypertension) was, in Rush's view, the key to disease and he was an advocate of 'depletion,' which could be obtained with copious bleeding and purgation. He was convinced of the value of drastic purgation, particularly with calomel (which he called a safe and nearly a universal medicine), and engaged in a violent controversy with his colleagues over the use of this in patients with yellow fever (he had remained in Philadelphia during the terrible epidemic of 1793, caring for hundreds of victims). Rush was prominent in the movement to

# 'ROYAL MADNESS' AND PORPHYRIA

Between January 1765 and 1820 the English King, George III, suffered from at least four major and four minor attacks of an illness with severe constitutional and mental disturbances. The former included malaise, constipation, pins and needles in the arms and legs, tremor and difficulty in swallowing, flushing and headache; the latter insomnia, delirium, illusions, delusions, and hallucinations. Self-evidently at a time when the British king's influence on British politics was paramount, the effects of such an illness were considerable – in particular, the Regency crisis in 1788 (when Parliament almost passed a Bill appointing the Prince Regent as the ruler before the king began to recover) and the loss of the American colonies in 1776. Despite much public medical controversy at the time, the consensus was that the king was subject to recurrent episodes of madness and from 1788 he was treated by the Reverend Dr Francis WILLIS (this page), 'a mad-doctor' from Lincolnshire.

In 1967, the received wisdom was shaken when a mother and son, Ida Macalpine and Richard Hunter, both psychiatrists and medical historians, claimed that George III's condition had been due to the rare inherited disease porphyria. This inborn error of metabolism is caused by aberration of the purple pigment present in every cell of the body, and responsible for the red color in the hemoglobin of the red blood cells. Porphyria exists in two main forms, one affecting mainly the skin, the other general bodily functions and particularly with delirium and even mania. Attacks are provoked by sunlight, some drugs (particularly the sulfonamides and the anesthetics), and childbirth, and during them the urine turns a distinctive blue-purple color; prevention is by avoiding known participants.

Macalpine and Hunter based this thesis on studying a vast number of records of the king's illness. Not only did the clinical features fit the textbook descriptions, but crucially they found mention of a change in the urine colour to blue during the attacks. Given the hereditary nature of porphyria, they then examined the clinical history of other members of the British Royal family, claiming to find likely cases in Mary Queen of Scots (thought to have been 'hysterical'); James I (who had attacks of melancholy, abdominal crises, and 'bloody urine', and died suddenly); his son Henry, Prince of Wales (who had a similar illness and died suddenly, with allegations that he had been poisoned); the Duchess of Orleans (who died of a sudden episode of excruciating abdominal pain); Queen Anne (who, all her life a victim of the 'flying gout', died suddenly in a coma aged 49); George IV (often dangerously ill with mysterious attacks, which he concealed); and Princess Charlotte (who died suddenly after childbirth). There were seven other cases in descendants of Mary Queen of Scots, including Frederick the Great, with descriptions of similar clinical features in all and the documentation of the blue urine in two. Finally, in two living family members Macalpine and Hunter found the biochemical abnormalities of porphyria.

This thesis attracted a lot of publicity, both when it was published in the *British Medical Journal* (and a subsequent pamphlet) and a much fuller book. Several years later the story formed the basis of a play by Alan Bennett and a film based on it. Yet many doctors remained skeptical. For one thing, PALEOPATHOLOGY (historical diagnosis) is notoriously difficult, and before the rise of modern medicine a century ago, retrospective diagnosis is subject to great error. Again, the manifestations of porphyria described in George III, his ancestors, and his descendants were not the same as those in the classic descriptions. In any case, doctors resented possible suggestions that the diagnosis of a physical condition vindicated the monarch from the taint of madness. Hence most doctors regarded the thesis by Macalpine and Hunter as interesting but far from proved.

*(continued overleaf)*

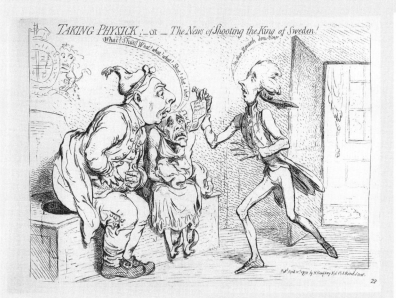

The grossly agitated King George III and Queen Caroline, seated in a latrine to receive news of the King of Sweden's assassination from William Pitt. Blue urine and agitation are both features of porphyria. (Etching by Gillray J., (1972). Reproduced courtesy of the Wellcome Institute Library, London.)

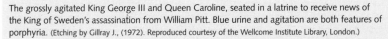

Francis **WILLIS** (1718–1807). British physician and clergyman. Willis was educated at Oxford, where he attended medical lectures but then took holy orders. He is said to have practiced first without a license. He was awarded an MB and MD from the University of Oxford, and in 1769 was appointed physician to an asylum in Lincoln, where he successfully treated several cases of mental disorder. In 1788 Willis was called to attend George III after his first attack of madness. He received considerable opposition from regular physicians, but maintained that the King would recover, which he did in 1789. Willis based his treatment on two main measures: restraint (usually with a strait waistcoat), and a mixture of vomits, purges, bleeding, and the application of leeches. Willis returned to private practice with a high-standing reputation and a large number of patients.

(continued)

Nevertheless, in the 1990s a historian and two geneticists (John Röhl, Martin Warren, and David Hunt) vindicated the thesis. Re-examining the archives and medical records of many more European royal houses, they also did DNA tests on several bones from exhumed bodies, proving the existence of porphyria in the one person whose skeleton could be identified beyond question.

They also showed that Queen Victoria's eldest daughter, Vicky, who married the future German emperor, carried the porphyria gene, passing it on to her daughter, Charlotte (who had the symptoms and passed purple urine) — who passed it to her daughter, Fedora, Princess of Reuss. In Britain, Prince William of Gloucester, killed in an air crash in 1972, was found to have been treated for porphyria;

however, it is not present in the immediate British Royal family. Hence the description of porphyria as a royal malady has finally been proved to be no exaggeration.          SPL

*See also* ASYLUMS; HOSPITALS; INBORN ERRORS OF METABOLISM; PSYCHIATRY – HISTORY

---

produce a code of ethics for doctors, and emphasized the need to take a patient's history in his own words. His fame was due not only to his public prominence, but also to the large number of students he had taught and a large literary output. For many years his *Medical inquiries and observations upon the diseases of the mind* was the only American textbook on the treatment of mental illness. He also wrote a pioneer text on geriatrics, listing the factors favoring longevity as: descent from long-lived ancestors, temperate eating and drinking, matrimony, and equivocality of temper.

**RUSSIA** The name Russia is used throughout this entry to denote what was formerly the Russian Soviet Socialist Republic, largest of the republics of the former USSR, and what is now the Russian Federation. It covers an area of 17 075 400 km² and at the beginning of 1997 had a population of 147.5 million, of which 73% were classified as urban and 27% as rural.

In Russia today the public provision of medical care has been badly affected by the weakness of central government and the country's chaotic transition to a free market economy. Compounding these factors is the negative legacy bequeathed by the communist regime. It caused lasting damage through chronic underfunding and organizational strategies which eventually, during the years of political restructuring (perestroika) came to be officially rejected as inappropriate or counter-productive.

Under the Soviet administrative command economy, a key defining feature of health service planning was the heavy emphasis on quantity rather than quality. Equally important were the ideological and bureaucratic controls, which the masters of the one-party state exercised over personnel in this as in every sector.

Soon after seizing power in 1917, the Bolsheviks made it impossible for independent professional groups to influence government policy. By the 1930s, under the role of Joseph Stalin, Soviet medicine had become a tool of the state. Although doctors occupied the key positions in the health ministry and elsewhere in the administrative hierarchy, they subordinated specialist knowledge, expertise, and ethics to the *political* demands of the day.

In the early 1930s, as one concomitant of forced industrialization, a vast increase in the number of medical graduates was ordered, and obtained, by means of crash courses with lowered standards. The number of women doctors rose rapidly; by the early post-war years they accounted for some three-quarters of the medical profession. Another development which left an indelible imprint was the heavy emphasis on providing healthcare for the rapidly growing industrial labor force at factories, mines, and other workplaces. The doctors who staffed the units were obliged to enforce labor discipline, a function which manifested itself especially in the certification of short-term illness.

At that time healthcare in rural areas normally comprised little more than the services of the local midwife and of the *feldsher*, who had sub-medical training and who, as in Tsarist days, acted as the peasants' doctor-surrogate. After World War II, access to inpatient treatment improved fairly rapidly but for many villagers the '*feldsher*-midwife point' even now remains the first stop for treatment.

Most medical research was retarded and to a degree perverted by the combination of ideology, party controls, and the literal isolation of most scientists from the intellectual life of the non-communist world. Sadly, this is no mere academic point; among the medical specialties, particular harm was done to the practice of psychiatry. For example, during the post-Stalin years, Marxist-Leninist dogma was applied to justify the abuse of diagnostic categories (mainly schzophrenia) in connection with the incarceration of peaceful dissidents in special prison hospitals.

Throughout the Soviet era the practice of medicine suffered from generally low levels of clinical competence, poor quality buildings, and shortages of modern instruments, equipment, and pharmaceutical products. These deficiencies all reflected the low priority assigned to a 'non-productive' sector of the economy. After the Second World War, the introduction of sulfonamide preparations and antibiotics probably made an important contribution to an improvement in average expectation of life at birth. However, modern drugs for the advanced treatment of illness, by then taken for granted in the West, were frequently unobtainable, because of the systemic failures of production and distribution.

After 1991, partly as a consequence of moves towards a free market economy, the health service became heavily dependent on imported products. The proportion of Russian-made medical technology in healthcare units had fallen from 70% to 10% between 1992 and 1997. Furthermore, 100 named drugs and substances had ceased to be manufactured and home production accounted for only 45% of the pharmaceutical market. Licenses were given to 7028 imported drugs, compared with only 3038 made in Russia.

The essentially quantitative approach to healthcare planning persisted until the implosion of the Soviet Union, when the nationality-based republics became independent. In Russia, specifically, the supply of doctors in 1989 was at the huge total of 697 700; this represented 47.3 doctors per 10 000 population.

The supply of doctors in relation to population was over twice the ratio for Japan and not far from twice that for France. Inevitably, these cross-national comparisons are broad brush; the figures have not been adjusted to take account of the interpretation of 'doctor' in Soviet statistics or the fact that Russian doctors had to undertake a range of administrative and other duties from which their counterparts in non-communist countries were partly or wholly exempt.

By 1989, the supply of hospital beds in Russia had reached the huge ratio of 138.7 per 10 000 persons. This level of provision, unsurprisingly, was associated with a heavy emphasis on inpatient treatment; the equivalent of almost a quarter of the population (24.9%) were admitted to hospital during 1989.

In the 'new Russia' by 1997 the Health Ministry had become convinced of the need for major restructuring, which would result in a reduction of the hospital bed to population ratio from 120 to 102 per 10 000 persons. Given that the annual average occupancy rate was only 301 days, there was an evident opportunity for savings to make; in 1996, according to a government official, some 700 billion roubles had been expended 'ineffectively'.

The planners also considered that the optimum ratio was 41 doctors as against the existing 44.9 per 10 000 persons. That average for Russia as a whole conceals great variation among the many regions of the vast land mass. Indeed, regional disparities can be shown to have increased since the communist era — excluding the data for Moscow and Leningrad/St Petersburg because of the concentration of medical research institutes there. Thus the standard deviation in respect of the doctor to population ratio was slightly higher in 1994 than in 1985, having increased from 7.21 to 7.60. The all-Russia average stood at 45.1 per 10 000 persons in both years.

A range of strategies have been planned to reduce what is now recognized as an excessive reliance on inpatient treatment. (In 1995 the equivalent of 21.2% of the population were admitted to hospital and the average duration of stay was as high as 16.8 days.) Thus the Health Ministry envisages the provision of day and short-stay units and, most importantly, a strong development of specialist and generalist care in the community.

Central to the latter strategy is a concept which can be construed as revolutionary. It entails something which communist Russia did not have — namely, a single type of doctor of first contact whom patients could consult irrespective of their age, sex, and presenting symptoms. By taking the decision to train what is officially termed 'a doctor of general practice' (family doctor), the planners implicitly admitted the inadequacies of the Soviet policy of delivering first-line care with 'specialist' care based in polyclinics and other units in the community.

In connection with training large numbers of doctors to work essentially as technicians, the Soviet regime abolished the traditional single-door entry to medicine and disaggregated the curriculum into separate, if overlapping courses. In Russia today most doctors still obtain their initial qualification in one of the following aspects: therapeutics (*terapiya*); pediatrics; dental surgery; hygiene, sanitation, and epidemiology. After obtaining their diploma (not degree), many undertake postgraduate courses hoping to rise in the pyramid of specialization which has the 20 000 or so 'ambulatory-polyclinic' units at its base and the most prestigious hospitals and research institutes at its apex.

The statistical yearbook assigns most doctors to one of fourteen basic specialties and together these account for 84% of the total. The residual category almost certainly includes medical biochemists or biophysicists and probably also interns, those in full-time administrative posts, and non-practicing doctors who have yet to reach pension age.

Many doctors identified as specialists in general medicine provide first-line care for adults in 'sectors' — microdistricts of urban communities and/or at the place of work. (Many pediatricians

## IMPORTANT FIGURES

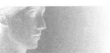

Ivan Petrovich **PAVLOV** (1849–1936). Russian physiologist. After working with Heidenhain and with Ludwig, in 1890 Pavlov became professor of pharmacology at the Military Medical Academy and director of the Experimental Medical Institute in St Petersburg. His early work was on the circulation and control of blood pressure, but he soon turned to the physiology of digestion, where his skill as an animal operator enabled him to make notable advances., For this work he was awarded the NOBEL PRIZE in 1904. The latter part of his working life was occupied by his researches on 'conditioned reflexes', the subject for which he is now particularly remembered.

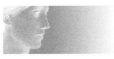

Nikolai Ivanovich **PIROGOFF** (1810–81). Russian surgeon. After training in Moscow Pirogoff studied and graduated in Germany. He was made professor of surgery in Dorpat in 1836 and in St Petersburg in 1840. Pirogoff was in charge of the medical services during the Crimean war and served at Sebastopol in 1854. One of the most important figures in Russian medicine, he was a medical educationalist and a supporter of women's role in medicine. A skilled surgeon he is known for his osteoplastic amputation of the foot (Pirogoff's amputation, 1854) and for his attempt to induce anesthesia by administering ether rectally (1847).

## FICTIONAL DOCTOR

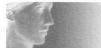

Dr **ZHIVAGO** is the eponymous young doctor and poet of the novel by Boris Pasternak (1890–1960). *Dr Zhivago*, which in the Russian original is partly in verse, recounts the experiences of Yuri Zhivago during the Russian Revolution; it contains some explicit anti-Marxist passages, particularly in the conversations between Yuri and his uncle Kolya. Publication was initially suppressed in the Soviet Union, and the first version to appear was an Italian translation. An English translation was published in 1958, the same year that Pasternak was awarded, but felt obliged to reject, the Nobel Prize for literature.

perform the same function for child populations.) Although intended to be the linchpin of the health service, these general physicians never had overall responsibility for the patients in their sector, who are free to refer themselves to other specialists such as ophthalmologists, also based in the community, possibly in the same polyclinic. Furthermore, the sector doctors hardly act as 'gatekeepers', since they simply refer many of the patients, reportedly up to half of all those who consult them.

Given that background, it is not surprising that one of the health planners' top priorities is the reform of primary medical care on the basis of general practice. To be fair, some credit for initiating the moves in this direction should be given to Yevgenii Chazov, one of the USSR's last Ministers of Health and the first to examine western health services with a view to learning from them. During his term of office, Russia's first postgraduate training scheme for general practitioners commenced in Leningrad (now St Petersburg), in January 1989.

From articles in newspapers it is evident that the notion of a generalist has wide public appeal, not least because it seems to promise the sort of personalized service which is idealized in the old Russian saying that a doctor should give the patient a part of his heart. By 1992 the Russian Health Ministry was presumably convinced that, among other advantages, the continuity of care desired by patients would also give rise to significant benefits for running the health service. In August 1992 it issued an order with the self-explanatory title: *Concerning the gradual transition to the organization of primary medical care on the principle of the doctor of general practice (family doctor).*

But that was not all. In 1993 the government enacted the law, *Concerning the fundamentals of the Russian Federation's legislation on health care,* in which article 22 confers on all families the right to choose a family doctor who provides a service based on their place of residence. At the time, such a commitment could be little more than a utopian aspiration, if only because so few personnel had the requisite training. Subsequently the Health Ministry drew up a plan to phase in this massive reform over eight years. During 1997–98 work was to take place on the appropriate 'normative-legal, material-technical, and organizational base'. Next, in 1999–2000, the emphasis was planned to shift to developing general practice at the operational level, taking account of plans which the regions have themselves drawn up for their territories. It is intended that the third and final phase should be completed during 2001–5, with a gradual transition to 'family medicine' through the length and breadth of the Russian Federation.

## Deterioration

In the meantime, a truly distressing picture of the people's health emerges from the illness and death rates. It is true that pre-revolutionary Russia had some of the worst rates in the Europe of those days, and that the same held true of the country during the last period of communist rule. All the same, the situation has deteriorated sharply during the subsequent years. Thus official figures report a large increase in new cases of diphtheria between 1990 and 1995 — from 0.8 to 23.1 per 100 000 population. The number of new cases of TUBERCULOSIS rose over the same period, from 34.2 to 57.8 per 100 000 population and in some regions this grim scourge is beginning to reach epidemic proportions. That is to be explained in part by reference to factors operating outside the control of the health service, such as the general fall in living standards, poor diet, and a substantial inflow of refugees (from Chechnya and former Soviet republics) who are infected with the tubercule bacillus.

For sexually transmitted diseases, the incidence of new cases of gonorrhea increased from 128.0 to 173.5 per 100 000, while new cases of SYPHILIS soared from 5.3 to 177.0 per 100 000 population. Death from all types of infectious and parasitic diseases increased from 12.1 to 20.7 per 100 000 population over 1990–95.

Virtually no reduction has occurred in the infant mortality rate, that litmus test for the general level of a country's socio-economic development as well as for the standards of its maternity and child health services. In 1990 the infant mortality rate stood at 17.4 per 1000 live births, peaking at 19.9 in 1993, and then fell back to 17.0 by 1996. In that year the British rates were 6.8 for boys and 5.4 for girls.

The level of maternal mortality, already very high by the standards of developed countries, actually increased somewhat over the years 1990–95, rising from 47.4 to 53.3 per 100 000 live births. As in Soviet Russia, the main form of family limitation continues to be the legal termination of pregnancy rather than contraception. In 1995 there were 73.9 legally induced abortions per 1000 women aged 15–49, with abortions exceeding births by a ratio of two to one.

Although 'the capitalist revolution' has given rise to great wealth for some, it has also much increased the numbers for whom uncertainty about their future and crushing poverty are a daily reality. Societal dysfunction has been compounded by the widespread lawlessness and inability of central government to collect tax revenues, whose absence leads to massive underfunding of public services and non-payment of salaries for months on end. Moreover, public sector personnel, including doctors, generally have salary levels below the average industrial wage. The implications for morale and work efficiency are self-evident.

## Non-natural deaths

Given the turmoil of the times, it is small wonder that a marked increased has occurred in the rate for all deaths from non-natural causes over the years 1990–95. For this category, which includes suicide, murder, accidents, poisonings, and trauma, the standardized mortality rate per 100 000 population rose from 239.6 to 394.7 for men and from 55.7 to 93.6 for women.

The foregoing offers some background for understanding the decline which has occurred in the summary social indicator; the average expectation of life at birth (based on projected mortality rates for the year in question). This measure fell by as much as five years — from 69.2 to 64.0 years — within the short period 1990–94, thereafter recovering to 65.9 years in 1996.

The average life expectancy for male babies declined from 63.8 to 59.6 years in 1996, when the figure was just under 75 in Britain. Life expectancy for baby girls fell from 74.3 to 72.7 years in 1996, when it was nearly 80 years in Britain. The very large differences between the sexes would have been less but for the lethal consequences of the traditional macho drinking culture, which entails a heavy consumption of vodka. Nor is the situation likely to get better quickly. A devastating report by the United Nations on World Aids Day (1 December) 2000 showed that Russia was the country with the fastest growth rate in HIV/AIDS in the world, given the rapid rise in drug abuse from heroin smuggled from Afghanistan.

The objective of reducing the territorial disparities in illness and death will prove all the more difficult to achieve because the federal constitution has devolved so much power to the regions (including the 'autonomous republics', which are the homelands of ethnic minorities). Another constraint is the existence of over 20 separate health services owned by various government departments (for example, the railways). Created in the Soviet period, they largely duplicate the main service and are seen by the Health Minister as a wasteful use of resources.

## Financing

Even more critical is the absence of a single system of healthcare financing which can provide sufficient revenue and under which, to quote Aneurin Bevan, 'poverty is not a disability and wealth is not advantaged'. That civilized moral imperative clearly implies that medical care should be free at time of receipt.

In Russia today, patients or their relatives are obliged to pay often considerable sums out of their own pockets when they use the publicly provided health service. According to data collected by the Health Ministry, the amount may be 'up to 50%' of the cost of treatment, when account is taken of all items, including medicines, food, hospital bedding, etc. Directly associated with these payments is the desperate shortage of public funds for the health service. At the end of the 1980s, its income from budgetary sources accounted for only 3.6% of the gross national product but by the mid-1990s the proportion had slipped back to about 2.0%.

Intended to provide a supplementary source of finance, a scheme of compulsory medical insurance is now being introduced throughout the country. Enacted in 1991, it has encountered many teething troubles and continues to be modified in detail. All the same, it was fairly strongly established by the start of 1997, covering a total of 121.9 million persons, or 77% of the employed and 69.5% of the non-employed population. Some 15 000 healthcare units fell within its scope and its payments accounted for 35–40% of the total income of the health service — in several regions up to 80%.

At a high level of generality, the emergence of this and other schemes of social insurance constitutes an important feature in the development of a post-socialist economy. In Russia, as in other former communist countries, such institutional innovation can be construed as marking a 'return to Europe' which has followed the failure of the 'Soviet experiment'.                    TMRy

*See also* HEALTHCARE SYSTEMS

# S

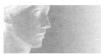
**SAINTS** Early Christians invoked medical saints in much the same way as the Greeks and Romans had invoked their gods, healing having been a specific function of the Church since the power to cure was conferred on the 12 disciples (*Luke* 9:1); and the tradition persisted until modern times. Even at the beginning of the 19th century, for example, Scottish patients with mental disturbances were treated by immersion in the waters of St Fillan's pool, St Fillan being one of the heavenly psychiatrists (another was St Dymphna, who specialized in mental subnormality). The list of saints associated with particular conditions includes: St Margaret of Antioch and St Dorothy were called on during the discomfort of labor; St Petronilla looked after fevers (as did the mythical St Febronia, descended from the Roman goddess Febris); St Roche and St Sebastian dealt with the prophylaxis and cure of plague; others were St Vitus (nervous diseases), St Lawrence (burns and scalds), St Erasmus (abdominal complaints),

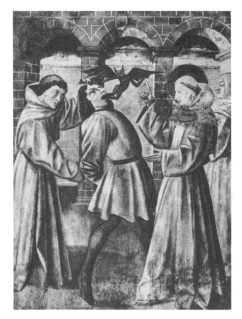

Saint Antony of Padua in a fresco by Mezzasti, 1192.
(Reproduced courtesy of the Wellcome Institute Library, London.)

St Clare (ophthalmic diseases), St Apollonia (toothache), and St Antony (scurvy). No fewer than four were assigned to chorea (involuntary jerky movements) — St Guy, St John, St Antony, and St Vitus — and two to erysipelas (skin infection commonly affecting the face) — St Francis and St Antony.

*See also* STIGMA

**SALERNO** See ITALY

**SANITARIUMS** Sanitariums (or sanitaria) were institutions for treating respiratory TUBERCULOSIS that enjoyed great popularity in the western world from the mid-19th to the mid-20th centuries. The sanitarium movement was based on the premise that tuberculosis was curable through the regimen practiced at the institutions. This included rest, exercise, nutritious food, and lots of fresh air, and from the 1920s and 1930s some surgical intervention. The location of the sanitarium was all-important in the treatment.

The first sanitarium to gain a world-wide reputation was that established by a German physician, Hermann Brehmer, in the South German Alps at Goebersdorf, Silesia, in 1859. Like many a proprietor of sanitariums after him, Brehmer himself suffered from tuberculosis. He confidently believed that fresh air and exercise, with their beneficial effect on the heart and lungs, could cure tuberculosis. Other institutions to follow Brehmer's model included that founded in 1888 by Otto Walther at Nordrach-in-Baden, located 1500 feet above sea level in the Black Forest. Sanitariums based on the 'Nordrach principles' sprang up all over Europe, North America, and the Antipodes in the late 19th and early 20th centuries, generally in places said to have a bracing climate.

Between 1892 and 1903 in Germany alone, 69 institutions were modeled on the Nordrach system. Sanitariums in the Swiss ski resort of Davos became a popular destination for wealthy tuberculosis patients from the 1880s. Davos boasted about 27 sanitariums by the 1930s. The most famous of the early American sanitariums was that founded by Dr Edward Livingston TRUDEAU (p 831) at Saranac Lake in the Adirondack Mountains. Having gone to this famous 'cure spot and hunting region for the wealthy' to treat his own tuberculosis, Trudeau subsequently opened the Adirondack Cottage Sanitarium in 1884 (renamed Trudeau Sanitarium in 1917).

## Characteristics in common

All sanitariums shared certain characteristics. They aimed at attracting early 'curable' cases of tuberculosis. Some cases were so 'early' that in all probability they were not tuberculosis at all. Hans Castorp, the main character in Thomas Mann's *The magic mountain*, set in a sanitarium at Davos, was probably not that unusual in being admitted without suffering from active tuberculosis. However, most institutions did not succeed in confining admissions to early cases, and death rates remained depressingly high.

Sanitariums also shared a belief in the value of fresh air, rest, exercise, and good food. However, private sanitariums were very different from the public or charitable sanitariums set up by philanthropists or public health authorities from the early 20th century. Sanitariums for the rich, such as those at Davos, were more like hotels than hospitals. In between indulging in lavish meals accompanied by good wines and brandy, patients rested, played games, or went for long walks. The British tuberculosis authority Sir James Kingston Fowler wrote in 1923 that walking exercises were suitable for private sanitariums, but that patients in sanitariums for the 'industrial class' 'cannot be given unlimited freedom of movement for reasons upon which it is not necessary to dwell'.

Working-class sanitariums introduced a system of 'graduated labor', by which the patients contributed to the upkeep of the institution through work, which was carefully controlled and monitored by medical attendants. These establishments were generally run on authoritarian lines, with the medical superintendent reigning supreme. A 1912 textbook on tuberculosis claimed that manual labor was now recognized as an essential part of sanitarium treatment. Attempts to introduce this new form of treatment to private sanitariums failed.

When disillusionment set in concerning the results of sanitarium treatment around 1920, the educative value of the institutional stay was emphasized: patients were to be taught how to keep their disease under control and how to avoid passing it on to others. However, this was not enough to attract patients. New inducements came in the form of surgical interventions. These were popular with medical attendants, nurses, and patients, all of whom regarded the conservative sanitarium regimen as no substitute for 'real'

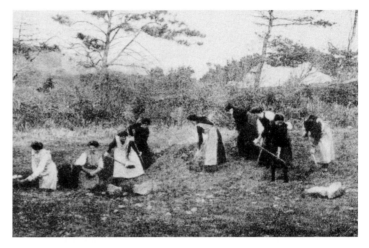

treatment. Artificial pneumothorax was a way of temporarily collapsing the lung, thereby resting and helping to heal it. Permanently collapsing the lung by rib resection (thoracoplasty) was a more invasive operation. Yet there is no evidence to suggest the superiority of surgery over the more conservative methods of treatment. The demise of the sanitariums occurred with the introduction of chemotherapy for tuberculosis from the 1950s. Prolonged stay in a specialist institution was no longer necessary, and from the 1960s most of the sanitariums either closed or were converted for other purposes.

Female patients at a sanitarium doing 'graduated labour'. (From the *British Journal of Tuberculosis*, 1910, Bodleian Library, Oxford.)

## Literary accounts

Thomas Mann's *The magic mountain*, written in 1924 but set in pre-war Europe, is the most famous novel immortalizing life in the sanitarium. The sanitarium experience was romanticized and used as a backdrop for philosophical musings. Other literary accounts adopted a much more realistic view of experiences in a sanitarium — the best known include Betty MacDonald's autobiographical account, *The plague and I* (1948), A. E. Ellis's *The rack* (1958), and Erich Maria Remarque's *Heaven has no favourites* (1961). Nearly every novel set in the first half of the 20th century with a tubercular hero included a stay in a sanitarium. Many were semi-autobiographical; sanitariums appear to have had a profound impact on those who experienced them. In both fiction and real life, sanitariums served as a setting for romance, filled as they were with young adults of both sexes in their prime of life, who remained in the institutions for a considerable length of time ranging from three months to a year or more. Yet it was romance made all the more poignant because of the ever-present threat of death. Such narratives were above all personal encounters with tuberculosis. Little of the enthusiasm of the doctors who established the sanitarium movement is echoed in these patient accounts.　　　LBry

*See also* CHEST MEDICINE

**SCANDINAVIA** Strictly speaking, the Nordic countries comprises Denmark (population, 5.2 million), with the Faroe Islands (44 000) and Greenland (56 000); Finland (5.1 million), with Åland (25 000); Iceland (267 000); Norway (4.4 million); and Sweden (8.8 million). Nevertheless, loosely they are often referred to as Scandinavia — strictly, Denmark, Norway, and Sweden) and this is the usage followed in the article.

The political structure and the strong ties existing between the Nordic countries have influenced the development of medicine in Scandinavia. Denmark and Norway formed a political union between 1380 and 1814, with Copenhagen as the political and medical center. Finland was part of Sweden from 1154 until 1809, when it became an autonomous grand duchy subordinated to Russia. Norway and Sweden were forced into a political union in 1814. Norway again became independent in 1905, Finland in 1917. Iceland was first an independent nation, then became part of Norway, following it into the Danish–Norwegian kingdom, persisting as a part of Denmark until 1944, when the country again became independent. The Faroe Islands and Greenland are politically integrated with Denmark, but have some degree of independence. Åland Islands are part of Finland, but have their own government, which has the overall responsibility for the entire public health service. Denmark, Finland, and Sweden are members of the European Union; Iceland and Norway are not.

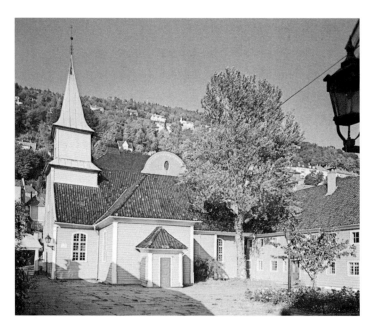

St Jørgen's Hospital, Bergen, Norway (now a medical museum).

### History of medicine

Trepanned skulls from prehistoric times have been found in Denmark, Norway, and Sweden. In 1939 a Neolithic skull was found during excavations near Kirkenes in Finmark, Norway. Similar operations were performed all over Europe, using the same and similar techniques, apparently with some knowledge of anatomy. Accordingly, an exchange of professional knowledge must have taken place in prehistoric times.

The earliest sources of information about the history of medicine in Scandinavia are based upon the Edda, a collection of old verses and sagas (850–1050), the sagas (1050–1350), and written laws (1050–1350). The most famous doctor in the saga period was Hrafn Svein-Bjornsson in Iceland, who was killed in 1213. He had traveled extensively in Europe and is known to have removed concretions from the urethra and performed venesection and cauterization.

In northern Europe, medicine grew up mainly in religious institutions such as monasteries and abbeys. Scandinavia became Christian around AD 1000 and medical institutions were therefore slow to develop. Several monasteries were built in Scandinavia during the 12th and 13th centuries. Archeological excavations at Vadstena in Sweden and Öm and Æbeltoft in Denmark have shown that care and treatment of patients were part of their activities. Although the Church opposed the practice of medicine by monks, especially surgery, several skeletons found at the Cistercian abbey at Öm indicate that surgical treatment had been given. Surgical instruments were found in both Öm and Æbeltoft in Vreta and Gudhem in Sweden, and at Varna in Norway. The oldest monastery in Norway to offer medical treatment was the Augustine abbey at Halsnoy, an island south of Bergen. It was founded in 1164 and closed at the Reformation.

LEPROSY was widespread in Scandinavia during the 13th century. Patients were excluded from social life by law, but were taken care of at St George's institutions. Denmark had 35 institutions dedicated to St Jørgen (St George). They were all closed with the Reformation. The first leprosy hospital in Bergen was established in 1266, but St Jørgen's hospital was first mentioned as a leprosarium in 1411. It remained a hospital for leprosy until the disease was eradicated from Norway, and is today a medical museum.

The order of St Antony was known for the care and treatment of diseased people, especially those suffering from ergotism (*ignis sacer*) and others crippled by disease or injury. Nonneseter abbey in Bergen and Maarkor in Denmark belonged to this order.

With the Reformation in 1536 all monasteries were closed. The first hospitals to be built in Scandinavia after the Reformation were established for academic purposes. Uppsala in Sweden had the first, Nosocomium academicum. It was built in 1717 and was followed by the Serafimerlasarettet (Seraphim Lazaret) in Stockholm in 1752. Serafimerlasarettet had eight beds but could take 15 patients, two in each of seven of the beds. In 1765 the number of beds was increased to 40.

The Royal Fredrik Hospital in Copenhagen was opened in 1757 and had 158 beds. It was not built for academic purposes but became an important center for training surgeons. The General Hospital in Copenhagen was opened in 1769 with 300 beds, mainly for the poor. Untrained washerwomen were used at first to nurse hospitalized patients. NURSING was slow to develop. The organization of deaconesses was founded in Germany in 1836 and had branches in Stockholm (1851), Copenhagen (1863), and Oslo (1868).

The University of Uppsala was founded in 1477 but had no chair in medicine until the 17th century. Therefore, Sweden did not train academically qualified physicians in the 16th century. The University of Copenhagen was founded in 1479 during the reign of Christian I. It had four faculties, one of them medicine. However, no physicians graduated before the Reformation in 1536. The university was reopened by King Christian III in 1537. It soon had a dominating position in Scandinavia, with anatomists such as Nicolaus Stenonius and Thomas Bartholin. They and several of their colleagues had been students at various universities in Europe, such as Rostock, Paris, Leiden, and Montpellier, and they integrated Copenhagen in the common European medico-cultural tradition. Oluf Rudbeck in Uppsala was equally prominent in Swedish medicine. He built the first anatomical theater in Uppsala in 1662 and he is remembered as the first to describe the lymphatic vessels.

The University of Åbo (Turku), Finland, was opened in 1640 and Lund, Sweden, in 1666. However, Lund remained for a long time mainly a theological school. As in most European countries, surgery was from the beginning performed by a heterogeneous group of academically unqualified men. In Scandinavia the surgeons organized guilds of surgery just before, or during, the 16th century — in Stockholm, 1496; Copenhagen, 1506; and Bergen, 1597. A three-year apprenticeship followed by four years abroad were required to qualify as a surgeon. Surgeons could treat cutaneous lesions, perform venesection and cupping, and remove stones from the bladder and urethra. They were not permitted to treat internal diseases. On the other hand, surgery could be performed only by those trained in the discipline.

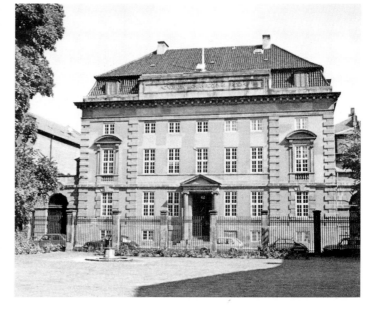

The Royal Surgical Academy, Copenhagen, Denmark.

Surgeons were not admitted to the universities. The training of surgeons was reformed during the 18th century. A separate academy of surgery, independent of the university, was opened in Copenhagen, and a director general appointed. The faculty of medicine protested vehemently. However, in 1785, the first professor at the Academy of Surgery was accepted as equal to the professor of medicine. The Academy of Surgery was closed in 1842 and all medical training transferred to the faculty of medicine. In Sweden, surgery was accepted by the medical collegium in 1797. The Karolinska Medico-surgical Institute in Stockholm was founded in 1810 and was coordinated with the faculty of medicine in 1874. The 18th century was important for medicine in Scandinavia. Maternity clinics were built in Copenhagen in 1750 and in Stockholm in 1775. The first such clinics were established to provide homes for unmarried pregnant poor women and to prevent the killing of newborn babies, which was not uncommon. The first medical acts of Denmark (and with it, Norway) were written in 1674, declaring that only those who graduated and defended a doctoral thesis at the University of Copenhagen were allowed to practice as physicians. This was changed in 1788, when physicians became civil servants and did not need a doctor's degree. The first hospital in Norway was the Rikshospitalet (National Hospital) in Oslo. It was opened in 1826 as a university hospital for the first Norwegian university, which opened in 1813.

Towards the end of the 19th and the early 20th centuries social security and medical treatment became the official health policy of the Scandinavian countries. Many earlier hospitals were private, owned by religious organizations, but the state, and then the counties, expanded the hospital system and took over the private hospitals. Contacts between the Scandinavian countries have been very close and their hospital systems have developed in parallel, leading to a similar, often identical, structure.

## Organization of health services

Some features of the health services in Scandinavia are common to all countries. Services are financed by the government or through compulsory insurance schemes. The health and social security systems are similar in terms of benefits, services, and their availability. Health services are based on a combination of municipal primary health systems, county-based hospital services in both general secondary care and psychiatry, and advanced medicine (tertiary care) associated with the regional hospitals, which are also university hospitals and research centers.

In all Scandinavian countries an amount is charged for treatment and drugs. Wages or a cash allowance are given during sickness to employees. All countries have well-developed hospital services with advanced specialist treatment. Hospitalization is free. Specialist treatment outside hospitals is also offered.

Primary healthcare is a public matter in all Scandinavian countries. In Finland, Iceland, Norway, and Sweden most treatment takes place at publicly provided health centers; in Denmark it is provided by general practitioners and specialists.

All countries have programs of prevention for mothers and infants, school healthcare, and dental care for children and young people, preventive occupational health services, and general measures of environmental protection. In recent years, the health services have undergone rationalization and new methods of treatment have come into use. These initiatives have contributed to reducing the length of hospital stays, and there has been a fall in healthcare expenditure.

*Denmark* The health service has a decentralized organization. The state is responsible for legislation and bears overall responsibility for healthcare and supervision. Responsibility is divided among several ministries. The Ministry of Health is responsible for hospital care, public healthcare, training of nurses, postgraduate medical education, and the part of the national health insurance which finances the general practitioners, dentists, etc. The Ministry of Social Affairs is responsible for nursing homes and housing for old people, the Ministry of Labor for the occupational health services, the Ministry of Education for the university education of health professionals, and the Ministry of Environment for environment hygiene.

The county authorities are responsible for hospital service, health insurance, and special nursing homes. According to the Hospital Act, all general and psychiatric hospitals are run by the counties. The hospitals in the City of Copenhagen and Fredriksberg municipalities, and the State Hospital (Rigshospitalet) are merged into the joint metropolitan hospital service. Highly specialized hospital functions are centralized to five major hospitals in the country. Hospital treatment is free of charge.

Private, non-profit hospitals have so far been run as a part of the public hospital service, according to an agreement with the counties. At the end of the 1980s, however, a private profit hospital was set up, and more were planned. A few private hospitals operate independently of the public hospital service.

National health insurance is financed by taxes. It ensures that patients who do not need hospital treatment get a number of services, either free of charge or with a reduced fee. Furthermore, the cost of many medicines is partly covered.

The municipalities are responsible for the primary and public healthcare systems, home nursing, child dental care, and child and school healthcare. Most nursing homes and other local services for the elderly are also run by the municipalities. Drugs are sold by public, controlled pharmacies. Greenland Home Rule took over the responsibility for health services from the Danish government in 1992. In 1996 a research council was set up to review health research in Greenland. Common diseases are treated at district health centers. In a few centers more or less complicated surgery is carried out. For more complicated courses of illness, patients are transferred to the central hospital in Nuuk or to hospitals in Denmark.

*Finland* The health services come under the Ministry of Social Affairs and Health, via the National Agency for Welfare and Health. The Ministry of Education is responsible for the university education of health personnel and the National Board of Education, under the Ministry of Education, for postgraduate medical education. The Ministry of Environment is responsible for environmental hygiene.

For regional administration the country is divided into 12 provinces, each with its own Department of Social Affairs and Health. These departments administer state appropriations and form an administrative intermediate authority in public healthcare, as well as approving regional plans. The specialized central hospitals are run by a federation of municipalities. Each hospital handles the most common clinical specialties. There are five university hospitals: in Helsinki, Turku, Oulu, Kuopio, and Tampere.

The municipalities are responsible for organizing health and social services and for general public health (environmental health). The municipalities have established health centers that operate either independently or in collaboration with adjoining municipalities.

The primary healthcare system is based on health centers. It includes the primary healthcare, such as maternal and child services, school and student health services, care of those engaged in active employment, healthcare of the elderly, health information, other preventive measures (such as vaccination and screening), primary medical and nursing services and medical rehabilitation, dental care, and ambulance services. Most dental care for adults is performed by private practitioners. The budgeting procedure of the healthcare section was reformed when new municipal legislation came into effect on 1 January 1997. Public health sector accountancy is now based on the same principles as in the case of the private sector. The aim of this reform was to increase knowledge about municipal spending and hospital expenditure. It also makes municipal and hospital data more comparable.

*Iceland* The Icelandic Ministry of Health and Social Security has the responsibility for health affairs. This includes all general matters, primary medical care, preventive measures, the appointment of physicians, the Directorate General of Health, the Medico–Legal Council, hospitals and sanatoria, nursing homes and homes for old people, dental treatment, sales and control of drugs, insurance, and the State Assurance Institute (Riksforsikringsanstalten).

Except for a few private institutions, the hospitals are run by the state. The two main hospitals are the State Hospital and the Municipal Hospital in Reykjavik.

In 1990 the operation of independent health centers was entirely subordinated to government administration. Since 1991 the state has taken over other health centers, as well as the municipal hospitals. Today the state is responsible for almost all health services and covers all expenses for their daily operation, while the municipalities still pay 15% of all expenditure for investment and maintenance. However, the actual administration of health services has been decentralized to a great extent to special boards in the districts. Primary healthcare is divided into eight regions, which are subdivided into 31 areas with a total of 83 health centers. Of these, nine are in Reykjavik. Dental treatment is usually given by dentists in private practice in their own clinics. The Ministry of Education is responsible for health education. Postgraduate medical education takes place mainly abroad.

*Norway* Political responsibility for the national health services in Norway rests with the Ministry of Social Affairs and Health, which bears the main responsibility for assessment and planning within the health sector. The Directorate of Health is in charge of the overall professional supervision of the health service in Norway. Each county has a state-employed county medical officer, with responsibility for supervision of health and health services in the county. The county medical officer is also an advisor to local and central health authorities.

The health system is regionalized. There are five health regions in Norway, each with its regional hospital, which is also a university hospital. All regional hospitals are owned by the respective counties, except for the State Hospital in Oslo (Rikshospitalet), which is the regional hospital for health region I, but is owned by the state in close collaboration with the county. The state also runs a few specialized hospitals. The regional hospitals are dependent upon substantial block grants from the state, which cover up to half of the running costs.

The counties are responsible for the operation of specialist and dental treatment. They are authorized to plan and run health institutions, specialist health services, medical laboratories, and ambulance services, and to provide advice and guidance to the local health services in aspects such as pediatrics, geriatrics, etc. The county authorities also have a duty to ensure that dental health services are available to all living in the county. Dental services are performed either by the counties' own employees or private dentists, who work according to an agreement with the county.

The municipalities are responsible for primary healthcare: health promotion and the prevention of disease or infirmity through environmental healthcare, family health services, school health services and health information, diagnosis and treatment of sickness, injury, and infirmity, medical rehabilitation, nursing, and care. The local health authorities may organize these services by employing their own staff or by making an agreement with professionals in private practice. The responsibility for the prevention of disease and for treatment of patients rests with the local authorities, but patients are referred for specialist treatment in hospitals or university clinics whenever needed. Pharmacies are mainly private but subject to strict public control.

*Sweden* There are three political administrative levels in Sweden: central government, county councils, and the municipalities. The state bears the political responsibility for the hospitals and health services. The National Board of Health and Welfare is the central supervisory authority for the health and hospital services. The central supervisory authorities within environmental and health protection are, in addition to the National Board of Health and Welfare, the National Environmental Protection Board, the National Board of Occupational Safety and Health, the National Food Administration, the National Institute of Radiation Protection, the Chemical Inspectorate, and the National Drug Inspectorate. The corresponding regional responsibility lies with the provincial authorities.

The health and hospital services under the 23 county councils are divided into the regional hospital service, the provincial hospital service, and the primary health service. The county councils and the independent municipalities bear the final responsibility for the health and hospital services.

There are six regional hospitals, each associated with a university. However, the universities are run by the state, whereas the university hospitals are regional. These hospitals provide advanced and specialized diagnostics and treatment, as well as general central hospital functions.

The provincial hospitals comprise both more specialized hospitals covering all the province and hospitals covering only part of the province. Medical treatment is provided within most specialties, both for inpatients and at outpatient clinics. Psychiatric treatment, which is often divided into sectors, belongs under the provincial hospital service.

Private health and sickness care exist on a limited scale. There are a few places at private nursing homes. About 15% of all medical consultations take place with private practitioners. In addition, there are physiotherapists in private practice. Half of the dentists are private practitioners.                                             JAA

*See also* HEALTHCARE SYSTEMS

**SCIENTOLOGY** See RELIGIOUS SECTS.

**SCREENING** Screening involves testing people for early signs of disease. Sometimes the purpose of screening may be to protect other people, for example, in testing the contacts of patients with INFECTIOUS DISEASES such as TUBERCULOSIS, TYPHOID, or AIDS, to prevent spreading the infection to others. More usually, in developed societies, screening is performed to identify a disease in its very early stages to prevent it from developing into its full-blown form. This article is concerned solely with this latter purpose.

In screening, unlike normal clinical practice, it is not the patient who goes to the doctor, but rather the doctor who goes to the public, recommending that they be tested for their own good. This proactive role, like that of a missionary or a salesman, puts a particular ethical responsibility on the doctor or PUBLIC HEALTH authority to be

sure that the benefits from screening exceed the prospect of harm.

The main benefit of screening is an improved prognosis for those found to have early signs of a serious disease that can be cured by early treatment. The disadvantages of screening accrue mainly to the screened people who do *not* have the disease in question, who usually outnumber the diseased people by thousands to one. Some may suffer from hazards of the test itself, for example, accidental miscarriage after amniocentesis; others may suffer anxiety caused by a false positive result and morbidity from its further investigation, such as an unnecessary biopsy. These side-effects of screening are usually minor, but because they may affect so many people the total sum of morbidity must be weighed against the benefit to a few. Moreover, screening is usually expensive because so many people have to be tested for every one helped.

Therefore before introducing screening it should be fully evaluated to measure how many people will benefit, to quantify that benefit, to measure how many people will suffer harmful side-effects, and to assess its costs.

An important factor influencing both benefit and cost is the validity of the screening test. In diagnosing a patient with an overt complaint the doctor uses information derived from several sources — the history, physical signs, and investigations, which he may order and may repeat. But in screening he has only the result of a single test and on the basis of this has to sort out those who probably have the disease, 'positives', from those who probably do not, 'negatives'. People with positive results need a diagnostic work-up to clarify whether they have the disease or are false positives. A test which gives many false positives is said to have a low *specificity*. Conversely, a test may fail to detect some people with the disease, thereby giving false negative results, and is said to have a low *sensitivity*. Many screening tests measure a continuously distributed variable, such as blood pressure or serum phenylalanine concentrations, and so the cut-off point to distinguish positives from negatives can be varied. If made less stringent, specificity will improve but sensitivity will be lower, giving more false negatives.

In seeking the earliest indicators of disease, even a full diagnostic work-up may not tell which individuals with positive results will develop overt disease, and which will not — there is a borderline group whose future is uncertain, and the size of this group is usually much larger than the group with obvious early disease. The management of people in this borderline group poses problems because it is impossible to distinguish those with progressive

# SCHISTOSOMIASIS

Schistosomiasis was probably the most widespread serious worm infestation at the end of the 20th century. Its two main variants affect over 200 million people in Africa, and South and East Asia. Infestation causes chronic ill-health, chiefly due to anemia, and a variety of specific, often serious, complications. The agent is a blood fluke, a flatworm that is 6–25 mm long. The life cycle involves stages in snails and mammals and there are two distinct intermediate stages in which the parasite swims as a free-living creature. The adult worm lives in and feeds on blood in veins around the bladder or intestine. The Egyptian (African) variety usually inhabits veins around the bladder, the Oriental variety is harbored mainly in veins around the large intestine. In the Nile delta, and in the new irrigation regions developed since the Aswan High Dam was completed, and elsewhere in Africa where livelihoods depend on irrigation of crops by people whose bare skin is exposed to contaminated water, almost everyone has schistosomiasis, also called bilharziasis in honor of Theodor Bilharz, who identified the parasite.

The eggs of bladder flukes are excreted in the urine, and those of the intestinal variety are excreted in the feces. The eggs develop into free-swimming larvae, which invade and pass the first developmental stage of their life cycle in freshwater snails. The larvae reproduce asexually in the snails to give rise to large numbers of free-swimming tiny worms called cercaria that are released in periodic bursts through the snail's skin. The cercaria swim free until they encounter bare human skin, which they penetrate (causing itching and a rash); once in the human host the cercaria develop further into adult worms that migrate to the veins around the bladder or large bowel. Adult schistosome worms may live many years, a male and female together in permanent copulation, laying millions of eggs.

Schistosomiasis is difficult to control. Attention has been aimed mainly at the snails: if these can be eliminated, the life cycle is broken. Education to prevent people defecating and urinating in the water helps, but water buffalo and other mammals may also be hosts to schistosomes, so education alone is not enough. In China, where manual labor is cheap and plentiful, successful control was achieved in many places by turning over

sods of wet mud to allow it to dry in the sun, thus killing many snails. Another strategy was to cut vertical walls in the banks of irrigation canals and ponds; the snails breed at the water's edge on sloping surfaces and cannot breed if the land-water junction is vertical. Alternative irrigation methods such as sprays rather than canals, and lining canals with cement, have worked well in other parts of the world such as Japan. Poisons that kill

snails are less effective for oriental schistosomiasis than for the African variety. Treatment of schistosomiasis is mainly directed at people from outside endemic regions, though if its costs could be covered in places where virtually everyone is infected, it might help to break the transmission cycle.

JML

*See also* WORMS

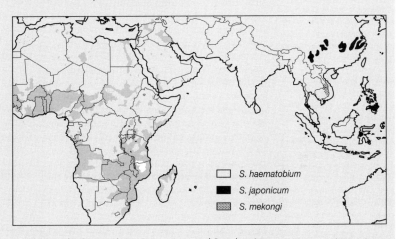

Distribution of *S. haematobium, S. japonicum,* and *S. mekongi.* (From Eddleston, J. and Pierini, S. (1999). *The Oxford handbook of tropical medicine,* OUP.)

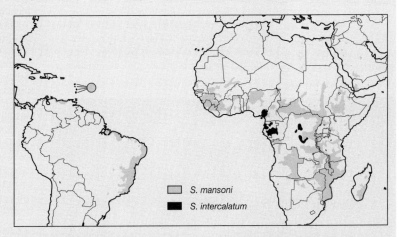

Distribution of *S. mansoni* and *S. intercalatum.* (From Eddleston, J. and Pierini, S. (1999). *The Oxford handbook of tropical medicine,* OUP.)

disease requiring treatment from those with non-progressive disease. Hence all must be treated even though some will not benefit from it, and may even be harmed by being incorrectly labeled as having the disease in question.

Developments in molecular biology offer hope that this problem may be overcome in future with much more precise identification of those people truly at risk, using DNA tests that are completely sensitive and specific.

Ultrasound scan of a normal
fetus at 16 weeks of
pregnancy.

### Prenatal screening

The long-revered system of repeated prenatal visits is itself a form of screening, although it was introduced long before the need for evaluation was recognized. Its precise role in bringing down maternal, fetal, and infant mortality cannot be ascertained because many other factors, such as improved nutrition and better housing, have been happening at the same time.

In recent years several screening tests for specific fetal abnormalities have been developed. This subject is rapidly expanding as a result of developments in imaging and in molecular genetics, enabling identification of fetuses with severe inherited diseases and other congenital abnormalities. Some of the tests, for example, ultrasound detection of intestinal non-development, enable treatment *in utero* or in the immediate neonatal period. But most are directed against conditions for which there is no effective treatment and in which the prognosis for the fetus is so poor that termination of pregnancy is offered to the prospective parents. The benefits of this policy are avoidance of a lifetime of handicap in the child, and greatly improved quality of life for the parents. This form of screening raises ethical issues for some, but is easy to evaluate in terms of the number of handicapped children avoided; it has been shown, for neural tube defects and for Down's syndrome, that it is cost-effective for society, the saving in costs of care for affected children being greater than the costs of screening. Its unwanted side-effects are serious, but fortunately very rare, being the loss of a normal fetus either because of a false positive result or as a result of physical trauma from the screening and follow-up procedures. For inherited autosomal recessive conditions, such as cystic fibrosis, it is now possible to screen both parents by a simple DNA test, and investigate the fetus only if both parents are carrying the relevant gene mutations.

### Screening in infancy and childhood

Phenylketonuria and congenital hypothyroidism, two important causes of severe mental handicap, can be prevented by screening blood samples taken from infants at 6–10 days of age. The screening tests measure serum phenylalanine, and thyroid-stimulating hormone concentrations, respectively. Infants with confirmed positive results can be successfully treated for phenylketonuria with a low phenylalanine diet, and for hypothyroidism by thyroid hormone. The screening program in Britain reaches 99% of new born infants, and most patients with each of these conditions are now of normal intelligence. The only drawback to these highly cost-effective screening program is overdiagnosis (and consequent overtreatment) of some children who would have developed normally. This is evidenced by the incidence of known cases of both these abnormalities having nearly doubled since the introduction of screening.

Infants are also routinely screened at 6 weeks for congenital dislocation of the hip, although the effectiveness of treatment (by immobilization or traction) in preventing later hip disease has never been tested. Screening tests for hearing impairment and for squint are routinely applied later in infancy, and early correction of these conditions is accepted as being beneficial, even though they too have not been formally researched. Other tests, for example, for motor development, congenital heart disease, and undescended testicle, are also widely used. In older children the emphasis of screening shifts away from congenital and inherited diseases to acquired conditions, such as dental caries and chronic ear infections. Screening schoolchildren for spinal scoliosis by visual examination is advocated by some, but there is considerable doubt about the efficacy of treatment and probably most cases are non-progressive. It is unfortunate that, given the uncertainty about much screening in children, RANDOMIZED CONTROLLED TRIALS of effectiveness have never been carried out.

### Screening adults

Screening for the major life-threatening diseases of middle age, such as cancer, heart disease, and stroke, has been extensively researched with somewhat disappointing results.

***Cancer of the uterine cervix*** Cytological examination of cells scraped from the surface of the cervix enables detection of pre-cancerous changes that are easily removed by biopsy. This is probably the most successful screening program in adults.

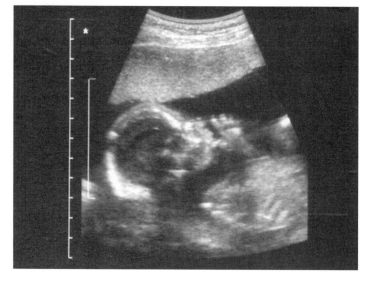

Theoretically the test should prevent about 90% of cancers and thus make a large impact. Its main constraint is that those women who are most at risk are least likely to come forward for screening. Its principal disadvantage is overdiagnosis of minor degrees of abnormality, that would never develop into invasive cancer. This problem is exacerbated by over-frequent screening and it has been shown that annual, as opposed to 3-yearly, screening identifies few new invasive cancers.

**Breast cancer** Because it is the most common cancer of women in most developed countries, there is intense interest in early detection of breast cancer. Methods of early detection include physical examination of the breasts either by a health professional or by the woman herself (breast self-examination), and X-ray mammography. The value of physical examination in detecting early aggressive cancers while they are still curable has never been proved, but several randomized controlled trials of mammography screening, repeated at 2–3 year intervals, have shown that subsequent mortality from breast cancer can be reduced by 20–40%. This benefit applies only to women who are over the age of 50 when first screened, possibly because there are many false negatives in younger women because of the greater density of premenopausal breast tissue. Most European health services recommended routine mammography screening only for women over 50, but, owing to political pressure rather than epidemiological evidence, the National Cancer Institute in the USA recommends regular mammography for all women over 40. This issue may be resolved when the results of a British randomized controlled trial of annual mammography starting at age 40 become available. Further research is also ongoing into other imaging methods (such as magnetic resonance imaging) of breast tissue in premenopausal women.

**Prostate cancer** Screening for prostate cancer is the subject of much debate and illustrates many of the dilemmas of screening. Prostate cancer is increasing in frequency and its death rate is also rising, so it has priority for better control. It can be detected in asymptomatic men by measurement of prostate-specific antigen (PSA) in serum, followed, if positive, by transrectal ultrasound-guided biopsy. There is uncertainty about the level of prostate-specific antigen to use as the cut-off point, whether this should vary with age, whether the ratio of free to protein-bound prostate-specific antigen would be better than total prostate-specific antigen, and whether changes in prostate-specific antigen level over time should indicate when to biopsy. But more crucially there is also uncertainty about the optimum treatment of early prostatic cancer,

some urologists advocating total radical prostatectomy or radical radiotherapy, others adopting a 'watchful waiting' policy with no intervention until the tumor shows signs of progression. Various case-series of symptomatic patients have reported very good survival rates for early cancers managed by these different policies but there is no guarantee that the case-mix of patients was the same in all of them.

Unfortunately, no randomized controlled trials of radical versus conservative treatments have yet been completed, although several are in progress. There seems little point in introducing screening until it is known whether active treatment by surgery or radiotherapy carries a better prognosis than passive observation. A further difficulty is that radical prostatectomy is a major operation with an operative mortality rate of at least 1%, and both surgery and radiotherapy cause intermittent incontinence in up to 20% of men, and impotence in at least 75%. Because of lack of more definitive evidence on who is likely to benefit from radical treatment, some urologists recommend this (usually total prostatectomy) for relatively young men with early tumors of high histological grade and 'watchful waiting' for older men and those with low-grade tumors.

The rationale of the wait-and-see approach is that many prostate cancers are so slow-growing that the patient will probably die of some unrelated condition before the cancer starts to spread. Moreover, autopsy studies have shown that around one third of men over the age of 65 harbor latent prostate cancer that was undiagnosed in life. If screening were to uncover this vast pool of borderline cases, many men who would not otherwise know they had cancer would be subjected to the anxiety of a cancer diagnosis and the possibility of radical treatment, and some would suffer the morbidity of its side-effects. How these undesirable consequences balance against lives saved by early treatment can be determined only by a randomized controlled trial in which mortality and morbidity in a population of men invited for screening are compared with a control population; a few such trials are now underway in North America and in Europe but it will be many years before their results become available. Meanwhile uncontrolled case-finding, using prostate-specific antigen in investigation of benign prostate hypertrophy, is likely to spread without evidence of the balance between its benefit and its cost. It has therefore been recommended that before ordering a prostate-specific antigen test, the doctor should fully inform the potential patient about the possible consequences of a positive test and the uncertainty surrounding its outcome, and to encourage him to decide for himself whether he wishes it.

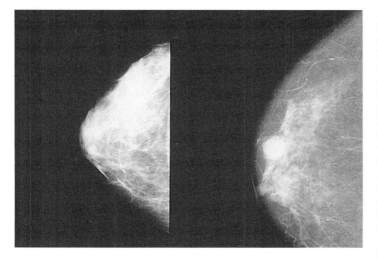

Mammogram, showing normal breast (left) and breast cancer (right). (Reproduced courtesy of National Cancer Institute, Bethesda, MD.)

*Colorectal cancer* There are two potential benefits of screening the large bowel. The first, and most obvious, is to identify and surgically remove early cancers before they have had a chance to spread and become incurable. The second is to find and remove adenomatous polyps that carry a high risk of progressing to invasive cancer, thus reducing the incidence of cancer and its mortality. Two screening tests are available, testing for occult blood in the feces, and direct observation of the bowel by endoscopy. Three trials of fecal occult blood screening have shown a modest reduction in subsequent mortality. The test requires collecting a small sample of stool and sending it to a laboratory, a procedure which many of the middle-aged and elderly people who are most at risk reject because they find it distasteful or threatening. A further constraint is that the test is not very sensitive, detecting only about half the cancers destined to present with symptoms within two years. Investigation of the 1–2% of people with positive results reveals a number with adenomatous polyps, but there is no evidence yet that their removal results in a fall in future incidence. Endoscopic screening has been shown to reduce cancer incidence in people with the rare condition of familial polyposis coli, but its value in the general population is still the subject of ongoing trials.

*Other cancers* Trials of screening for lung cancer, using chest X-rays and sputum cytology, repeated as frequently as 6-monthly, have shown that even this intensive screening cannot influence the prognosis of this aggressive form of cancer. Screening programs for other cancers, including ovary, skin melanoma, mouth, and neuroblastoma in children, are still being evaluated.

*Heart disease and stroke* Unfortunately, direct tests (electrocardiogram and carotid bruit) to detect early coronary or cerebral arterial disease lack both sensitivity and specificity. The physician therefore has to fall back on screening for earlier risk factors such as HYPERTENSION, hypercholesterolemia, obesity, and smoking. While blood pressure and serum cholesterol level are valid tests for their respective risk factors, judged by their ability to predict future coronary and cerebrovascular events they, too, lack sensitivity and specificity. Nevertheless, screening for mild to moderate hypertension does result in a modest reduction in the incidence of stroke, but not heart disease, and similarly, among people with very high cholesterol levels, early treatment has been shown to reduce heart attacks.

The main drawback to these two screening tests is that most people with positive results are not going to suffer heart attacks or strokes, but nevertheless have to undergo long-term drug treatment and endure the anxiety and side-effects accompanying it, a similar problem to that of screening for cervical cancer. Most authorities now recommend screening for hypertension in middle-age, at intervals of 3–5 years, but there is more controversy about hypercholesterolemia as a 'stand alone' screening test. A cautious approach is to include serum cholesterol in a package of risk-factor tests, but to regard as positive only those people who have at least one other risk factor.

### Conclusions

Most of the disorders for which screening can clearly be recommended are identified very early in life. The benefits can be quickly realized, they result in cost savings which offset the costs of screening, compliance (of parents) is good, and often a single screen is all that is needed. By contrast, in screening adults the benefits tend to be limited and do not appear for many years, compliance is lower, the test needs to be repeated at intervals and hence is much more costly, and over-treatment of people, who in the absence of screening would not develop overt disease, is a common problem.

Future developments in genetic testing may reduce the problems of false positives and uncertain borderline results, and also open up other diseases for possible screening, but the challenge of finding and proving effective treatments is likely to remain.                                JC

*See also* BREAST CANCER; INBORN ERRORS OF METABOLISM; RANDOMIZED CONTROLLED TRIAL

**SCURVY** results from a deficiency of vitamin C (ascorbic acid) in the diet. It is now rare except in groups at special risk, such as the isolated elderly and the mentally handicapped. The clinical manifestations of frank scurvy (as opposed to the non-specific symptoms ascribed to putative 'subclinical' states) include follicular, thickening of the skin and pinpoint bleeding into it bruising, swollen gums which bleed easily, hemorrhages around the bones (in children), hypotension, and anemia. Ascorbic acid is widely available in most foods of vegetable origin.

*See also* VITAMINS

**SCUTARI** (now Uskiidar) was the suburb of Constantinople (Istanbul) in which were situated the military hospitals serving the Crimean battle-fields, and the scene of Florence NIGHTINGALE's (p 548) first and greatest achievement. The accommodation, for over a thousand men, had not been secured until many months after the war had started and was in a parlous condition when Miss Nightingale, with 38 nurses, arrived on 4 November 1854. Of the main hospital, Lytton Strachey later wrote:

> In these surroundings, those who had long been inured to scenes of human suffering — surgeons with a world-wide knowledge of agonies, soldiers familiar with scenes of carnage, missionaries with remembrances of famine and of plague — yet found a depth of horror which they had never known before. There were moments, there were places, in the Barrack Hospital at Scutari, where the strongest hand was struck with trembling, and the boldest eye would turn away its gaze (*Eminent Victorians*, London, 1918).

The transformation brought about by Miss Nightingale during the succeeding six months represents a landmark in British history, military, medical, social, and administrative.

*See also* NURSING; WAR

**SELF-EXPERIMENTATION** has a long history among doctors and medical scientists. At one level, it is a variety of the more general phenomenon of human experimentation, but with its own special characteristics. Using oneself as the experimental subject may be a public demonstration of the importance and/or safety of the experiment; it allows the experimenter direct access to the subjective results of the experiment; it neutralizes some of the ethical ambiguity surrounding the use of a new technique, drug, or procedure; it ensures the reliability of the subject; and it may seem 'natural' even if it is uncomfortable, painful, or even dangerous. Animal experiments may establish the relative safety, effectiveness, or importance of a new discovery, but if the results are to be applied to a human situation, someone must go first. Ethical protocols governing human experimentation are recent and revolve around the issue of INFORMED CONSENT. No one is better able freely to give informed consent than the actual investigator, although recently special protocols have been devised even here.

Although certain branches of medicine, for example, surgery, do not readily lend themselves to self-experimentation, most aspects of medical knowledge and practice have been influenced by a few classic, and hundreds of routine, examples. Many of these relate to what Claude BERNARD (p 102) described as the three pillars of medical science: PHYSIOLOGY, PATHOLOGY, and PHARMACOLOGY.

## Physiology

One of the most disciplined of all self-experimenters was Sanctorius (Santorio SANTORIO) (this page). His quantifying impulse led him to devise an elaborate balance chair, where for 30 years he took frequent careful measurements of his body weight, and the weight of his food, drink, and excreta. From this he calculated the amount of fluid lost in insensible perspiration. He also routinely recorded his pulse and temperature. Sanctorius's balance chair was the forerunner of the advanced metabolic chambers which Theodore Bischoff, Carl Voit, and others constructed in 19th-century Germany, using themselves in relating controlled diets and exercise to measure oxygen consumption and the elimination of carbon dioxide, urea, and other waste products through the lungs, kidneys, and bowels.

Many of the basic principles of respiratory physiology and adaptation to high altitude were established from the 1870s by Paul Bert, both in a pressure chamber and in the Peruvian Andes. Bert's self-experiments on respiration were continued by J. S. HALDANE (p 510), who habitually used himself as his principal subject, and made important contributions to the identification of the occupational hazards of miners and sewage workers, invented the hemoglobinometer, and developed the decompression chamber to treat caisson disease in divers.

Cardiac catheterization has become a routine diagnostic procedure and has led to a variety of minimally invasive therapeutic innovations. The German surgeon, Werner FORSSMAN (p 147), who first developed the technique, was discouraged by his superiors from that line of inquiry. Instead, after animal experiments, he used himself as his first human subject, in 1929. His work led to much condemnation and little immediate interest and he abandoned it, although he later shared the NOBEL PRIZE with two other investigators who carried on his work in the early 1940s.

A classic investigation of the physiology of pain was carried out by Sir Henry HEAD (p 745) and Wilfred Trotter, who had nerves in their arms severed so that they could observe the gradual return of sensation. Trotter's colleague at University College Hospital, Sir Thomas LEWIS (p 188), established the sequence of events occurring after

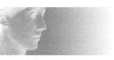
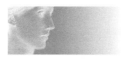
(*continued on p 745*)

local skin irritation (the 'triple response') and, with J. H. Kellgren, conducted an elaborate series of self-experiments, aimed at providing a classification of the varieties of pain and the patterns of referred pain.

Long before William Beaumont's creative use of the gastric fistula in his patient Alexis St Martin in the 1830s, Lazzaro SPALLANZANI (p 743) had investigated his own digestion, training himself to swallow bags of food tied to a string and to regurgitate food at will. A modern parallel was W. B. Castle's search for the cause of pernicious anemia. He showed through regurgitating minced beef that his own normal stomach secreted a substance ('intrinsic factor') missing in patients

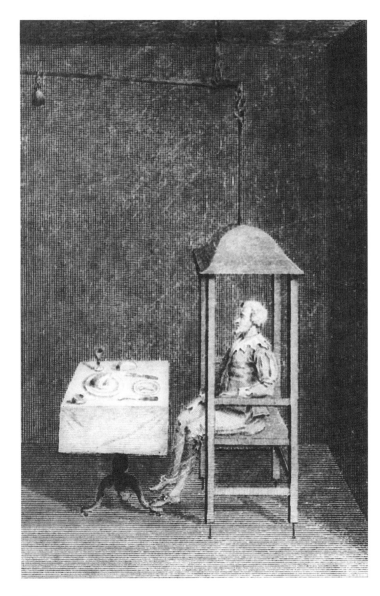

Sanctorius in his balance chair. (Reproduced courtesy of National Library of Medicine, Bethesda, MD.)

suffering from pernicious anemia. Vitamin and nutrition research have also lent themselves to self-feeding (and deprivation) experiments. Modern pioneers in this approach include Robert McCance and Elsie Widdowson, Victor Herbert and John H. Crandon. Joseph Goldberger tried to convince dubious colleagues that pellagra is a nutritional rather than an infectious disorder, by injecting himself with blood and swallowing capsules containing urine, feces, and skin from patients suffering from the condition.

## Pathology

Goldberger's experiments show how close physiological and pathological methods can be, and are one series in many aimed at elucidating the causes, mechanisms, and/or prevention of disease. A classic instance is John HUNTER's (p 398) report of a man (probably himself) whom he inoculated with some pus taken from a patient suffering from gonorrhea. When the subject subsequently developed signs of both gonorrhea and syphilis, Hunter concluded that these two are simply stages of a single venereal disease.

KOCH's (p 455) postulates specified an animal model in establishing the bacteriological causes of disease, but diseases spread through insect vectors have produced some of the most dramatic self-experiments. Several early advocates of the mosquito hypothesis of MALARIA transmission allowed themselves to be bitten by mosquitoes which had fed off malarious patients, or injected malarious blood into themselves. YELLOW FEVER was without known treatment, but the same mosquito procedure was used by an American team in Havana, with the accidental death of Jesse Lazear and the permanent incapacitation and premature death of James Carroll, two of the team. More recently, Ralph Lainson's work on LEISHMANIASIS and Claude Barlow's investigations of SCHISTOSOMIASIS involved deliberately contracting the disease.

Vaccine development has been another common source of autoexperimentation, to test whether the vaccine is safe and actually protects. Louis PASTEUR (p 620) volunteered to test rabies vaccine on himself. In the end, he did not, although Jacques Graucher, who accidentally stuck himself with a syringe containing rabies virus, and two other of Pasteur's assistants, did. Waldemar Haffkine tested his CHOLERA and PLAGUE vaccines on himself; Almroth Wright tried out his brucellosis and TYPHOID vaccines; and several workers first tested the variety of polio vaccines which were produced from the 1930s.

## Pharmacology

Observing and measuring the effects on oneself of ingested or injected drugs have long been mainstays of experimental pharmacology. During the 19th century, many anesthetic agents were first used on the experimenter: the subjective effects of nitrous oxide were described long before the substance was actually employed during surgery, and Crawford Long had experienced either socially before he used it professionally. In the 1860s, Benjamin Ward Richardson used himself in investigating a series of compounds of known chemical composition. Amyl nitrite was one of them, later taken up for the treatment of angina pectoris because Richardson reported intense flushing and other signs of dilatation of the blood vessels.

Other 19th-century self-experimentalists include Enoch Hale Jr, who injected himself with castor oil; J. E. Purkinje, who described digitalis toxicity; and P. J. Touéry, who showed that charcoal was a useful antidote against arsenic and strychnine poisoning. In the 20th century, A. Hoffmann reported the hallucinogenic effects of LSD; H. Osmond worked with amphetamine, mescaline, and other hallucinogens; and S. M. Smith and F. Prescott allowed themselves to be completely paralyzed with curare, under monitored conditions.

These examples represent merely the tip of a large iceberg. The circumstances are usually routine, but occasionally extreme. The results, too, are generally simply part of normal science. Nevertheless, self-experimentation is embedded within the fabric of research and, governed by the ethics of human experimentation, is certain to retain its importance.                                    WFB

*See also* CARDIOLOGY — HISTORY; PHARMACOLOGY, CLINICAL PHARMACOLOGY, AND THERAPEUTICS; PHYSIOLOGY; SEXUALLY TRANSMITTED DISEASES; TROPICAL MEDICINE

**SERENDIPITY** is the fortuitous discovery of things one was not looking for. The word was coined in 1754 by Horace Walpole, fourth Earl of Orford, in a letter to Horace Mann, referring to the three princes of Serendip (Sri Lanka), who displayed this knack. Serendipity has played so important a part in scientific discovery, including biomedical research, that a book (*Serendipity: accidental discoveries in science*, by Royston M. Roberts) and numerous articles have been written about it.

Pharmacology has a particularly rich history of serendipity. The discovery of penicillin by Alexander FLEMING (p 50) is the best known example. Similarly, the concept that certain chemicals can be used to cure cancer developed after soldiers exposed to mustard gas in World War II developed reduced numbers of white cells in the blood, leading to the use of the chemically related nitrogen mustard as an anti-leukemic drug. The hallucinogenic properties of LSD unfolded when

Albert Hoffmann ingested some accidentally while working to develop a drug to control hemorrhage after childbirth and migraine. Serendipity even has a major role in Arthur Hailey's novel *Strong medicine* in the discovery of an aphrodisiac. In an example of life imitating art, the ability of the new anti-impotence drug sildenafil (Viagra) was discovered accidentally during a search for a cardiovascular vasodilator.

Examples of serendipity also exist in surgery. Microvascular surgery originated when Julius H. Jacobson II had to join small blood vessels in a dog during an experiment. Realizing that this required the help of a microscope, he proceeded to use one — but also recognized its potential for surgical practice. Another example of serendipity is the surgical glove, developed by William HALSTED (p 746) to prevent his operation-room nurse (whom he subsequently married) from developing dermatitis due to the mercuric chloride used for asepsis. Halsted asked the Goodyear Rubber Company to fashion thin rubber gloves for her. That post-operative infections decreased following the use of gloves was a later but much more useful offshoot of this invention.

Entire disciplines have benefited from one single serendipitous discovery. Charles Richet's observation that dogs surviving an initial dose of extract from the tentacles of sea anemones reacted violently and died from a second much smaller dose led to the concept of anaphylaxis. The observations by Crawford Long in 1842 and Horace Wells in 1844 that inhalation of ether or nitrous oxide lead to a sensation of painlessness gave rise to the discipline of ANESTHESIA. A chance remark by a milkmaid that she could not get SMALLPOX because she had had cowpox, led Edward JENNER (p 452) to the discovery of the smallpox vaccine and the beginnings of IMMUNOLOGY. That gastric juice contains hydrochloric acid and that this rather than a mechanical process digested food was the discovery of William Beaumont, who recognized the opportunity to study the functioning of the stomach when his famous patient, Alexis St Martin, accidentally shot himself in the stomach and developed a gastric fistula (1822). X-RAYS were discovered accidentally by Wilhelm ROENTGEN (p 873) while looking for the emission of cathode rays from the Crookes tube in 1895.

The Pap smear used in the diagnosis of cancer of the womb is an application of a technique developed by George PAPANICOLAOU (p 740). Remarkably, he developed the technique while working with Charles Stockard on the influence of alcohol on the germ cells of developing embryos of guinea pigs. Likewise, Oscar Minkowski and Joseph von Mering were studying fat absorption in a dog from which the pancreas had been removed when they found that the dog

(continued)

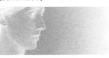

Sir Henry **HEAD** (1861–1940). British neurologist. Head was elected physician to the London Hospital in 1896, and carried out experimental studies on the return of sensation after a cutaneous nerve in his forearm had been divided and sutured. From these he described 'epicritic' and 'protopathic' sensibility. His classic work *Aphasia and kindred disorders of speech* was published in 1926.

produced more urine than normal, and that this contained sugar. Further experiments by Minkowski showed that dogs from which the pancreas had been removed always developed DIABETES MELLITUS, leading to the discovery by Frederick BANTING (p 236) and Charles BEST (p 236) of insulin in 1921.

Serendipity is important even in clinical practice. It is also significant that the NOBEL PRIZE, the ultimate accolade for scientific development, has been awarded to many, including Roentgen, Minkowski, and Fleming, for their serendipitous discoveries. So perhaps students should be taught to develop this art. Investigators should likewise keep an open mind when encountering expected and unexpected findings. Above all, it is essential to maintain an insatiable curiosity, for as Louis PASTEUR (p 620) — who himself discovered the vaccine for chicken cholera when he accidentally used an old and forgotten bacterial culture for inoculating fowl, only to find that the fowl became ill but did not die — said, 'In observation, chance favors the prepared mind'.                SAP

**SERPENT** See EMBLEMS

**SEVENTH DAY ADVENTISTS** See RELIGIOUS SECTS

**SEXUALITY AND MEDICINE** Medical disorders and their treatments often interfere with sexuality and may cause persistent sexual problems. Such problems may arise because of the direct effects of illness or treatment on the anatomical or neurophysiological components of sexual function. In some cases sexual difficulties develop because of emotional responses to illness or treatment. Commonly both types of association are relevant. Thus, a patient who suffers from a disorder which partially interferes with sexual function may react to this with anxiety or embarrassment such that the sexual problem is amplified. Illnesses sometimes precipitate sexual problems because of poor previous sexual adjustment. Thus how a couple adjusts sexually to a physical disorder in one partner will depend partly on the quality of their sexual relationship before the illness.

A further important influence on sexual adjustment to illness is the way this topic is addressed by doctors and their colleagues. For example, lack of discussion or advice about sexuality following a heart attack may result in a couple abandoning their sexual relationship because they fear, albeit usually erroneously, that sexual activity is likely to be dangerous because it might precipitate another heart attack.

### Types of sexual problems
Sexual difficulties may affect any of three aspects of sexual function: sexual desire, sexual arousal, and orgasm. The most important sexual problems (or 'dysfunctions' as they are known technically) are shown in Table 1.

Nearly all illnesses are likely to be associated with reduced interest in sex, but this usually returns. However, certain conditions, especially those that are debilitating, are likely to be associated with persistent low sexual desire, perhaps reflecting depression or generally reduced energy levels. Many cases of erectile dysfunction, especially in older men, are due to organic factors. A history of a gradual onset to the problem, with a persistent pattern of erectile difficulties and absence of full erections in masturbation strongly suggests an organic cause. Female impaired sexual arousal may reflect hormonal disturbance. This may be associated with the menopause, especially after removal of the ovaries, or recent childbirth, particularly in breast-feeding mothers. Retarded or absent ejaculation and orgasmic dysfunction may be caused by certain types of medication (see Table 2).

Dyspareunia means that sexual intercourse is painful. While this can be due to anxiety and reduced arousal, it can be a symptom of a physical disorder such as endometriosis (fragments of tissue resembling the uterine mucous lining occurring at other sites in the pelvis). Vaginismus (sudden, painful contraction of muscles around the vagina) is usually a psychologically determined problem, the woman being unable to have sexual intercourse because of a phobia about vaginal penetration. However, it may also result from pain caused by, for example, an unsatisfactory episiotomy scar.

Table 1  Types of sexual dysfunction

| Aspect of sexuality affected | Men | Women |
| --- | --- | --- |
| Sexual desire | Low sexual desire | Low sexual desire |
| Sexual arousal | Erectile dysfunction | Impaired sexual arousal |
| Orgasm | Premature ejaculation | Orgasmic dysfunction |
|  | Retarded/absent ejaculation |  |
| Other |  | Vaginismus<br>Dyspareunia |

**Table 2** Medication that may cause sexual dysfunction

Antihypertensives (e.g. propranolol)
Diuretics (e.g. bendrofluazide)
Antidepressants, including tricyclics (e.g. imipramine),
  monoamine oxidase inhibitors (e.g. phenelzine), and
  serotonergic antidepressants (e.g. fluoxetine)
Major tranquilizers (e.g. chlorpromazine)
Hormones (e.g. steroids)
Anticonvulsants (e.g. phenytoin)

The dysfunctions most commonly caused by illnesses or their treatments are low sexual desire, erectile dysfunction and impaired sexual arousal, retarded (or absent) ejaculation, orgasmic dysfunction, and dyspareunia.

## Causes

Medical disorders that commonly cause sexual difficulties are listed in Table 3. Erectile dysfunction is particularly common in men with diabetes mellitus, 30–50% of such men eventually experiencing erectile difficulties. This occurs because diabetes can cause both circulatory problems and impaired nerve conduction. Hypogonadism in men may be caused by any condition that damages the testes or affects production of the hormones produced by the pituitary gland, which stimulate the testes. Its effects are due to reduced production of the male sex hormone, testosterone. This hormone is also important in female sexuality (being produced by both the ovary and the adrenal cortex in women) since it influences levels of sexual desire.

Arteriosclerosis is a common cause of sexual difficulties in older men, narrowing of the pelvic blood vessels reducing the blood supply to the penis and hence the ability to obtain and sustain an erection. Total section of the spinal cord will cause erectile and orgasmic dysfunction. Partial damage to the spinal cord, through injury or a disease such as multiple sclerosis, may result in difficulty, but not inability, to obtain erections and reach orgasm.

Surgery may affect sexuality because of direct interference with sexual anatomy. Examples include surgery to the rectum or bladder, which may disrupt nervous pathways to the genitals, major surgery involving the genitalia, and surgical procedures involving the spinal cord. Surgery may also affect sexuality because of the disfiguring effects of certain operations. Examples include mastectomy, amputation, and creation of an 'ostomy' (e.g. colostomy) because of bowel disease.

Many drugs used to treat physical or psychiatric conditions can affect sexuality. The more important drugs in this regard are listed in Table 2. Antihypertensives, diuretics, tricyclic antidepressants, and major tranquilizers often cause erectile dysfunction. Monoamineoxidase inhibitors and antidepressants may cause delayed or absent ejaculation or orgasm. Long-term use of steroids and anticonvulsants may cause diminished sexual interest, the latter because of induction of sex hormone-binding globulin, which binds with testosterone in the bloodstream and thereby inactivates it.

Excessive alcohol consumption is an important cause of sexual problems. In addition to its potential disruptive effects on relationships, it may cause peripheral neuropathy, hypogonadism, and liver damage (which may interfere with the metabolism of sex hormones). Sexual problems are common in drug addiction, probably because of the effects of consequent general debility on sexual desire. Sexual difficulties, particularly erectile dysfunction, may also be linked to smoking because of the increased risk of arteriosclerosis.

Sexual problems often occur because of the adverse psychological effects of physical illness or treatment on sexual adjustment. An individual may develop anxieties about sexual activity because of fears that it might cause a relapse of a physical condition, or because of concerns about the perceived effects of illness or surgery on sexual

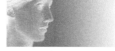
**Table 3** Examples of medical disorders that often cause sexual dysfunction

| System | Examples | Possible sexual dysfunctions |
|---|---|---|
| Endocrine | Diabetes mellitus | Erectile dysfunction<br>Impaired sexual arousal |
| | Hypogonadism (impaired function of testes or ovaries) | Low sexual desire<br>Retarded/absent ejaculation<br>Erectile dysfunction |
| Cardiovascular | Arteriosclerosis | Erectile dysfunction |
| | Myocardial infarction | Low sexual desire |
| Neurological | Spinal cord damage | Erectile and orgasmic dysfunction |
| | Multiple sclerosis | Absent ejaculation |

attractiveness. The partner may have similar concerns. Changes in roles because of illness in either partner may affect a couple's relationship. Depression after a severe illness is a common cause of reduced sexual desire. Lastly, the ways in which the implications of physical illness are managed by clinicians may be very important in determining subsequent sexual adjustment.

## Treatment

Management of sexual problems must be based on very careful assessment. It is usually appropriate and necessary to involve both partners in this. The clinician should endeavor to establish the extent to which physical and psychological factors have contributed to the problem. When treatment is provided for a member of a couple, both partners should be seen whenever possible.

Specific treatments that may help people with sexual problems caused by physical disorders or their treatments are listed in Table 4. For many people with medically related sexual problems, careful explanation and advice may be of considerable help. Explaining that a sexual problem is a recognized effect of a disorder (for example, diabetes) can reassure the patient. Advice may then be given about the benefits of spending more time on foreplay, and a couple may perhaps be encouraged to modify their sexual relationship if sexual intercourse is unlikely to be possible.

Sex therapy was developed at the beginning of the 1970s after the work of Masters and Johnson in the USA. In this approach, specific instructions are given to the couple about gradually rebuilding their sexual relationship, beginning with simple caressing. The aim is partly to remove the pressure the couple might be experiencing because of their not being able to have a full and satisfying sexual relationship, and also to help them to begin to enjoy their physical relationship in a non-demanding fashion. Improved communication is a major goal in this treatment. The therapist has to use skillful psychological intervention to help the couple when they encounter difficulties with the homework program. Education about sexuality is another important element of treatment. Sex therapy may

be particularly helpful for couples whose sexual difficulties are the result of a psychological response to an illness or surgery, or where psychological factors are amplifying the sexual consequences of a medical disorder.

Surgical procedures are reserved for people with special indications, such as young men with diabetic erectile dysfunction, or men with vascular abnormalities affecting the blood supply to the genitals. The vacuum constriction device is a relatively new and safe sexual aide for men with erectile dysfunction. Intracavernosal injections are used widely for men with organic erectile dysfunction but do have the risk of priapism (excessively prolonged erections) which can be harmful. Sex hormones are usually reserved for men with hypogonadism. Estrogen can be helpful for women with vaginal dryness associated with either a natural or a surgical menopause. The drug yohimbine may help some men with erectile dysfunction.

Where medication has caused a sexual problem, other types of medication might be tried. It is important that the minimal effective dose of medication is used. Doses of a drug might be timed so that it causes as little interference as possible with sexual activity.

Treatment for sexual problems may be obtained from several sources. Some general practitioners take a particular interest in providing such help. Some specialists in a variety of clinical disciplines, including psychiatry, clinical psychology, gynecology, family planning, and urology, will have special expertise in this type of work. In Britain the Relate organization has many trained sex therapists. There are also private therapists, although people seeking help should ensure that they only consult properly trained therapists providing bona fide treatments.      KH

*See also* ADVERSE DRUG REACTIONS; ENDO-CRINOLOGY; OBSTETRICS AND GYNECOLOGY

## SEXUALLY TRANSMITTED DISEASES — HISTORY

There are records of sexually transmitted diseases notably gonorrhea, from the earliest times. Only with the development of the city and the concept of travel — be it in the context of war, commerce, or expedition — was there some practice of venereology. Gonorrhea was mentioned by the ancient Egyptians, being described in the EBERS PAPYRUS. It was mentioned in the Old Testament in *Leviticus* 15: 2–33: 'the man who has a running of the reins is unclean, even though his defilement, at certain times, dries up and causes a stoppage' (Knox translation). The Greek and Roman writers — notably Herodotus, CELSUS (p 806), and GALEN (p 324) — described gonorrhea and its sequels. In the Middle Ages AVICENNA (p 60) of Baghdad wrote at length on

Table 4  Help for people with sexual problems caused by medical disorders or their treatments

| Psychological | Sexual aids |
|---|---|
| Advice | Vacuum constriction device |
| Sex therapy | |

| Surgical | Medication |
|---|---|
| Penile prosthesis | Intracavernosal injections |
| Vascular surgery | of vasoactive drugs (e.g. papaverine) |
| | Sex hormones |
| | Yohimbine |

urethral discharge, recommending irrigations. Moses MAIMONIDES (p 59) of Cordoba aptly described gonorrhea as fluid escaping without erection or feeling of pleasure, doughy, and the result of disease including amorousness and excesses.

Scabies and louse infestation were also recognized at an early date, although the concept of different causes for skin disease has developed only in the past 300 years. Genital warts (condylomata acuminata), venereally acquired, have been recognized for 2000 years. Anal warts as a result of sodomy were exemplified by Juvenal in his satires. Much later they were described by the Restoration surgeon Richard Wiseman (1676) and the French physician John Astruc (1736).

SYPHILIS is among the most interesting of diseases from a historical standpoint, not only because of arguments about its origin, but because of its influence on morality and measures towards PUBLIC HEALTH and hygiene. There are conflicting views as to its origin in Europe. The pre-Columbian (Europeanist) theory is that syphilis was somehow endemic in Europe through the Middle Ages, becoming pandemic at the end of the 15th century and venereally acquired. The Columbian (Americanist) theory is that in 1493, after the return of Christopher Columbus from the New World to Spain, his sailors brought back with them this new disease. Another idea is the Unitarian theory of Hudson (1946), who pointed out that the infection yaws is widespread in equatorial regions. It has many similarities in its manifestations to syphilis. Hudson emphasized the evolutionary relationship of yaws, pinta, endemic syphilis, and sporadic syphilis, regarding them all as varieties of one disease caused by one parasite, *Treponema pallidum*, and originating from sub-Saharan Africa.

### Transmission of syphilis

Whatever the origin of syphilis, its transmission was well described after the siege of Naples (1495) and the passage of soldiers and travelers throughout Europe. Public health edicts against the disease stemmed from that time. One such was in Nuremberg (1496), which inspired the celebrated drawing attributed to Dürer of a syphilitic man, *The Cavalier*.

Physicians very soon described the signs and symptoms of early syphilis and accepted the concept of congenital syphilis. From its first epidemic ravages, treatment for syphilis had been by inunction with mercury ointment (unguentum Saracenicum). Preparations of mercury had long been in favor for treating skin diseases, being used by Arabian physicians. Mercury was also given as pills, by inhalation, and fumigation, and, much later in the 19th century, by injection.

Among the many references to syphilis in Shakespeare is the one to fumigation, which was carried out in the sweating tub, the patients often being confined for this purpose to the 'spital', the equivalent of the subsequent lock-hospital, and successor to the old lazar house. In *Henry V*, II.i Pistol tells us that Doll Tearsheet is in the 'powd'ring tub of infamy', and that '… my Nell is dead, the spital of malady of France' (*Henry V*, v.i.). Guaiacum, derived from a South American tree, was later introduced as an alternative treatment. It was imported into Europe by the mercantile house of Fugger of Augsburg.

Early descriptions called syphilis the Great Pox or Morbus Gallicus, the French disease, or, in France, the Neapolitan disease or Spanish disease.

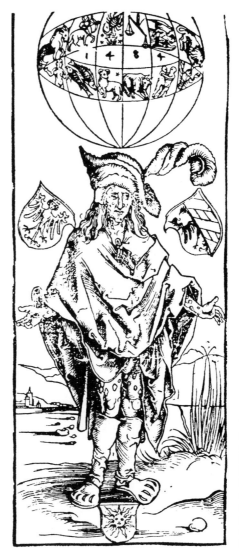

The earliest known portrayal of the eruption of secondary syphilis in a European cavalier, by Dürer. Prepared as an illustration for Theordoricus Ulsenius' Broadsheet of 1 August 1496. (Reproduced from *Graphische und typographische, Erstlinge der Syphilisliteratur aus den Jahren 1495 und 1496*, Munich, 1912.)

Jacques de Bethencourt of Rouen was the first to use the term venereal disease (lues venerea) in 1527. In 1530 Girolama Fracastoro of Verona wrote the celebrated poem *Syphilus sive morbus gallicus*. Syphilus, a swine-herd, was smitten when he refused to make sacrifices to Apollo. Syphilis must be the only disease to be named after an imaginary person in a poem. The term was not used in English literature until 1686, when the poet laureate Nahum Tate translated the work of Fracastoro. The first mention in English medical writing was the work of the surgeon-dermatologist Daniel Turner *On syphilis* (1717).

Although in modern times gonorrhea and syphilis have been regarded as different diseases, this has not always been so. The confusion between syphilis and gonorrhea seems to have been compounded during the first part of the 16th-century. For the next 300 years, until the final proof of their difference by the French physician Phillipe Ricord (1838), the medical world was divided on the pathology of venereal diseases. There were monists, such as the celebrated 17th-century English physician Thomas SYDENHAM (p 721), who believed that syphilis and gonorrhea were one and the same disease, and dualists, who stuck out for their being two distinct conditions. The frequent association of gonorrhea with syphilis, as well as the discharge due to a urethral syphilitic ulcer (chancre), doubtless explains the tendency of the old writers to regard 'clap' as the early stage and syphilis the late stage of 'the pox', a view idealized by Pope, 'Time that at last matures a clap to pox'.

During a long period in the history of syphilis in the 17th century nothing of special merit occurred. A posthumous publication of work by Lancisi (1728) correlated enlargement of the heart with syphilis — 'aneurysma gallicum'. In the same year the great innovative physician BOERHAAVE (p 121) of Leiden implicated syphilis as a cause of cardiovascular disease. In 1736 Jean Astruc, physician to Louis XV, summarized the whole corpus of knowledge on venereal disease in the most comprehensive and scholarly work on the subject yet written. He argued strongly for the American origin of the disease, but shared the then current belief that gonorrhea and syphilis were two stages of the same venereal disease. Among his descriptions of other sexually transmitted diseases is an accurate one of genital herpes.

John HUNTER'S (p 398) *A treatise on the venereal disease* (1786), although notable for scientific objectivity, was not one of his greatest works. But such was his eminence that perhaps more importance has been attached to it than would have been the case with a publication by a lesser man. Hunter's most important error was adhesion to the monist doctrine. Until recently it was thought that, in the celebrated experiment of 1767, Hunter, to prove the view of the single identity of gonorrhea and syphilis, inoculated himself with matter of gonorrhea on to his penis. Unfortunately, he chose the inoculum from a patient suffering from both syphilis and gonorrhea, after which he further strengthened his single-identity view. Some modern commentators state, on the other hand, that the experiment is described in the third person and argue that the experiment was carried out on a patient. Hunter thought that the only difference between the two diseases depended on the surface to which the inoculum was applied, that it caused ulceration when it acted on the skin, but only a purulent discharge without breach of surface, when applied to a mucous membrane. In Edinburgh, Benjamin Bell (1793) carried out inoculation experiments on medical students, showing that gonorrhea and syphilis were different diseases, but, at last, Philippe Ricord in Paris in 1838 showed conclusively, by experiments on 667 patients in a mental hospital, that gonorrhea and syphilis were different diseases. Ricord also classified syphilis into three stages: primary, secondary, and tertiary. He was the founder of a remarkable school of venereology in France in the 19th century.

Much progress in sexually transmitted diseases was made in the 19th century, often secondary to advances in scientific medicine using laboratory techniques such as microscopy and the disciplines of MICROBIOLOGY, serology, IMMUNOLOGY, and inorganic chemistry. Between 1857 and 1863 Jonathan Hutchinson of the London Hospital described the entities now known as Hutchinson's triad (interstitial keratitis in the cornea, nerve deafness, and Hutchinson's teeth (notching of the incisor both in the juvenile and adult dentitions)), important signs of established congenital syphilis. It was left to Alfred Fournier in Paris in 1875 to propose that syphilis was a cause of the symptoms of paralysis, incoordination of movement, and progressive unsteadiness of gait. Fournier formed the concept of parasyphilis — those diseases of which syphilis was essentially the cause, but which were not directly the result of the syphilitic organism, namely general paralysis, tabes dorsalis

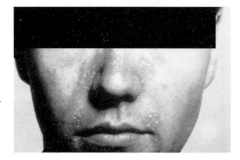

Seborrhoeic dermatitis, a manifestation of HIV infection.
(From Bradley, J. and McCluskey, J. (1997). *Clinical immunology*, OUP.)

(progressive destruction of sensory nerves), tabo-paresis, and primary optic atrophy.

## Advances in gonorrhea

Albert NEISSER (this page) in 1879 at Breslau, using KOCH's staining methods, conclusively described the causal agent of gonorrhea. Advances in the diagnosis and treatment of gonorrhea progressed quickly after Neisser's discovery. In 1881 Credé of Leipzig introduced instillation of silver nitrate drops into the eyes of newborns to prevent gonococcal inflammation (ophthalmia neonatorum), then a common cause of blindness in infants. Gram's stain (1884) provided a reliable staining technique for the microscopic diagnosis of gonorrhea. For about 100 years several commentators had noticed urethritis which did not seem like gonorrhea in its true sense. In 1907 Halberstaedter and Prowazek found inclusions in the eyes of infants with neonatal conjunctivitis, and then found genital discharge in their mothers. Lindner (1909) in Vienna advanced knowledge into the cause of non-gonococcal urethritis when he found the so-called elementary bodies, indistinguishable from those seen in inclusion conjunctivitis, in urethral discharge. However, it was not until the end of the Second World War that the concept of non-gonococcal urethritis was really established by the celebrated London venereologist, Harkness.

In 1903 METCHNIKOFF (p 412) and Roux showed that syphilis could be consistently transmitted to chimpanzees. Fritz Schaudinn, a protozoologist, collaborated with Erich Hoffman, a dermatologist, in examining specimens of preparations of primary and secondary syphilis stained with aniline dye. On 3 March 1905, in the CHARITÉ HOSPITAL (p 354) in Berlin, Schaudinn was able to demonstrate spirochetes (a microorganism resembling a spiral) in one of Hoffman's slides. Using dark-field microscopy, Landsteiner and Mucha recognized, in 1906, the spirochete responsible for syphilis, *Treponema pallidum*.

Their method is still in use today. In 1913 NOGUCHI (p 874) and Moore, using a silver staining method, were able to demonstrate *Treponema pallidum* in the brains of 12 patients with general paralysis of the insane, thus proving its causation by syphilis.

Immunology came into its own in the latter years of the 19th century. In 1901 Bordet and Gengou described the complement fixation test, with which an infection could be diagnosed by finding the antibody to the causative organism in the serum. Wassermann (1906) in Berlin showed the value of the complement fixation test in the diagnosis of syphilis. Over the next forty years many different serological tests for syphilis were devised. However, not until the early 1940s was it fully realized that many diseases could be responsible for a positive Wassermann reaction. The introduction of the test for specific antibody, the treponemal immobilization test by Nelson and Mayer in 1949, inaugurated an era of more accurate serological diagnosis.

In 1909 Paul EHRLICH (p 260) in Frankfurt found salvarsan (arsphenamine), his 'magic bullet', to be effective as a cure for syphilis. This was superseded in 1943, when Mahoney and co-workers from the USA showed that penicillin was effective and without serious side-effects in the treatment of syphilis.

A new era was ushered in; despite antibiotic resistance, the pharmaceutical industry has managed to maintain effective treatments for those sexually transmitted diseases caused by bacteria — namely, syphilis, gonorrhea, chancroid, granuloma inguinale, lympho-granuloma venereum, and chlamydial genital infection.                    MAW

*See also* AIDS-HIV; ANTIBIOTICS AND ANTI-INFECTIVE DRUGS

## SEXUALLY TRANSMITTED DISEASES

Sexually transmitted diseases are transmitted by sexual intercourse and by other direct contact between an infected and an uninfected mucous surface when two people come together intimately. Several may also be transmitted by contaminated blood or blood products. There are more than 25 such diseases, including SYPHILIS, gonorrhea, genital herpes, some varieties of viral hepatitis, and most lethal of all, HIV/AIDS. The WORLD HEALTH ORGANIZATION identifies sexually transmitted diseases as one of the most common classes of infection in young adults, resulting in serious illness, and in some conditions, such as acquired immune deficiency syndrome (AIDS), and genital cancer in women resulting from human papilloma virus infections, early death. The concurrent presence of some sexually transmitted diseases facilitates the transmission of HIV. Attention has also been drawn by the World Bank to the disastrous financial consequences in developing countries, not only of HIV/AIDS but other sexually transmitted diseases, especially those that cause pelvic inflammatory disease and infertility. If a sizeable group of the young adult wage-earning population is non-productive, economies, especially of poorer countries, suffer.

The management or study of sexually transmitted diseases used to be called venereology, but venereal diseases occasionally have legal implications that were established in developed countries at the turn of the 20th century. Venereal diseases are generally considered to include syphilis, gonorrhea, chancroid, and, in some countries, granuloma inguinale, and lymphogranuloma

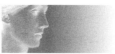

venereum. In the past 50 years a wide range of infections have been seen to be sexually transmissible, so 30 years ago the term genitourinary medicine was adopted to describe the study and management of sexually transmitted diseases, or venereology, in Britain. A new concept, sexual health, is emerging. This is a positive avocation of good sexual health, based on EVIDENCE-BASED MEDICINE and a partnership between health professionals and clients. It usually encompasses contraceptive advice, psychosexual practice, and health education. In Australia and New Zealand this concept has flourished: the Australasian College of Sexual Health Physicians is well established.

The situation is different in other countries. In some countries in Europe and Latin America, and many countries in Asia, venereology is a subspecialty of dermatology, dermatovenereology. Elsewhere the treatment of sexually transmitted diseases is even more fragmented. Urologists treat men who have a urethral discharge. Gynecologists treat female patients. Another trend in recent years has been specialization in HIV disease, prompted by the need to care for patients with AIDS.

### Gonorrhea

*Cause Neisseria gonorrhoeae* This may cause uncomplicated urogenital infection in both sexes. In addition, especially after homosexual activity or oropharyngeal contact, there may be rectal and pharyngeal infections, respectively. If left untreated in the male, inflammation of the testicles and prostatitis may result, and in the female, pelvic inflammatory disease may occur, with resultant sterility. Disseminated infection may occur infrequently with variable skin, joint, and blood-spread manifestations. Adult conjunctivitis is rare in developed countries. An untreated pregnant woman may give birth to a baby born with neonatal conjunctivitis. In recent years various strains of *N. gonorrhoeae* have developed which are completely resistant to penicillin and to some other antibiotics, especially ciprofloxacin (a quinolone); strains are found throughout the world.

*Non-specific genital infection* This is the name often used synonymously with non-gonococcal urethritis and non-specific urethritis. Though not completely accurate, 'chlamydial infection' is too frequently used to cover these infections, but it should be used only for proved chlamydial infection. Genital chlamydial infections are much more easily diagnosed now with new techniques based on DNA studies.

*Cause* In 70% of cases, the causative organism is *Chlamydia trachomatis*; *Ureaplasma urealyticum,* and *Mycoplasma hominis* are also implicated. These organisms may cause non-gonococcal ure-

thritis, post-gonococcal urethritis, epididymitis, proctitis, cervicitis, infection of Bartholin's ducts, salpingitis, and perihepatitis.

Infrequently in men, mostly after a urethritis, Reiter's syndrome may occur with associated arthritis, conjunctivitis, and other variable manifestations.

### Syphilis

*Cause Treponema pallidum*

1. Early infections: the primary stage gives rise to chancre (enlargement of the regional lymph nodes) at the site of inoculation — that is, the genitals, ano-rectum, mouth, or pharynx; the secondary stage gives rise to systemic manifestations, especially rashes.

2. Early latent: latent syphilis of not over 2 years' duration.

3. Latent: no manifestations but specific serological tests for syphilis are positive.

4. Late syphilis (tertiary or late syphilis): may lead on to cardiovascular, neurological, and systemic complications.

5. Congenital syphilis: acquired infection of the newborn from an untreated mother.

### Genital herpes simplex virus infections

*Cause Herpes simplex virus* (types 1 and 2). Genital herpes infection is a viral disease that may be chronic and recurring. It has become very common since the advent of the contraceptive pill encouraged unprotected casual sex; when the HIV/AIDS epidemic motivated wider use of condoms, genital herpes began to recede, but it remains a common sexually transmitted disease. Symptoms are variable, starting with a small blister (vesicle) leading on to recurrent, small, genital sores. There may be systemic complications. There is a potential danger to the child born to a pregnant woman who has had herpes genitalis.

### Venereal warts (condylomata acuminata, genital human papilloma virus infection)

*Cause Genital wart virus.* Soft infectious warts may occur in the anogenital region after sexual contact with a person also infected with human papilloma virus. Atypical warts should be biopsied. Cervical cytology should be performed in women with genital warts, which may be a factor in various genital cancers. New techniques based on genotyping may point out which human papilloma virus types are potentially likely to cause cancer of the cervix.

### Molluscum contagiosum

*Cause* A pox virus. This is not infrequently found in the genital region. Small, horny papules which may be mistaken for warts, are found in groups. It may occur on the trunk and the face in AIDS.

## Trichomoniasis

*Cause* *Trichomonas vaginalis*, a protozoan. This very common infection causes an unpleasant vaginal discharge. Men are symptomless carriers.

## Non-specific vaginitis: Gardnerella vaginalis

*Cause* *Gardnerella, Haemophilus vaginalis*, and various anaerobic organisms. This may cause a variable vaginal discharge.

## Genital candidiasis (thrush)

*Cause* This is a common disorder caused by a yeast, *Candida albicans*, which is often found on the skin and in the intestines, and symptomless carriage may occur in the vagina. It may be associated with other systemic disease, especially in recurrent cases. It may occur after antibiotic treatment for other conditions. It is not a venereal disease, but as it may present with genital symptoms is included in this list for completeness. It commonly occurs:

- in women, when it may present with a vaginitis
- in men, when it may present with inflammation of the glans and prepuce of the penis
- as a complication of AIDS. Oral thrush may occur in AIDS.

### Skin parasite infections, sexually transmissible

*Scabies* Caused by a mite, *Sarcoptes scabiei*. This causes an itchy rash. It is passed on by close body contact, which may include coitus. It may be treated with benzyl benzoate or 1% benzene hexachloride lotions to the body. Close contacts should be treated.

## Pediculosis pubis ('crabs') Caused by a louse, *Pediculosis pubis*, which makes the patient itch. It may be found in the anogenital area and also in pubic, abdominal, and axillary hair. The treatment for this is similar to that for scabies.

## Tropical sexually transmitted disease

The following diseases are more commonly found in the tropics (see TROPICAL MEDICINE). Travelers may occasionally bring them back to more temperate latitudes.

## Lymphogranuloma venereum

*Cause* Lymphogranuloma venereum serotype of *Chlamydia trachomatis*. After an initial transient genital lesion, the lymph nodes in the groin become inflamed, followed by various constitutional symptoms. There may be late complications resulting from fibrotic changes to the lymph vessels draining from the genitals.

## Chancroid

*Cause* Ducrey's bacillus (*Haemophilus ducreyi*). This may cause painful genital sores, which lead on to swellings with abscess formation in the groin.

## Donovanosis (Granuloma inguinale)

*Cause* *Calymmatobacterium granulomatis* (Donovan body) — a bacterium. This disease was first described by tropical medicine specialists in the INDIAN MEDICAL SERVICE at the turn of the 20th century. Ulcerating, enlarging, granulating sores leading to swellings with abscess formation in the groin occur.

## Other viral diseases

A sexually transmissible organism (and route) has been implicated in the following diseases.

*Epstein-Barr virus* This is the cause of glandular fever, which is common in young adults. It may be transmitted orally during coitus, or just by kissing, hence the common name 'kissing disease'.

*Cytomegalovirus* It causes mild glandular fever-like symptoms in young adults. It is a serious cause of neonatal congenital infection, and causes serious eye disease and blindness in patients with AIDS.

*Hepatitis A* The cause of fecally transmitted jaundice, especially in homosexuals. It may be prevented by an effective vaccine.

*Hepatitis B* The cause of jaundice and chronic ill-health, especially in homosexuals. There may be asymptomatic carriers. It may be prevented by an effective vaccine. Other types of hepatitis, that is C, may be transmitted sexually, the latter being more frequent in intravenous drug users.

In the late 1970s and early 1980s, hepatitis B was very common in the gay community in several large American cities: case-control studies demonstrated that it was transmitted by oral–genital contact and anal–genital intercourse. Understanding these modes of transmission became useful when it was realized that HIV/AIDS is also transmitted this way: effective health education campaigns in the gay communities of San Francisco, New York, and Los Angeles applied this 'knowledge'.

## Treatment

Treatments for sexually transmitted diseases mostly require specific antibiotics which vary according to the infecting organism and its known or presumed susceptibility or resistance to the principal anti-infective agents. A serious problem has arisen because of indiscriminate use of antibiotics such as penicillin, and default of patients before the treatment has been completed. Anti-infective agents alone are not enough: counseling about the dangers of casual unprotected sex is an essential part of the treatment regimen.

### The specialty in Britain

In 1917 the recommendations of the Royal Commission on Venereal Disease came into force. Its guiding principles were that free and confidential treatment under the supervision of qualified medical practitioners should be available to all who required treatment for what are now regarded as sexually transmitted diseases. This service is an essential part of the National Health Service and it is more than ever required, not only for the treatment of these conditions but also to aid in the prevention of sexually transmitted diseases and HIV/AIDS and their effects.

Apart from the treatment of bacterial infections, the control of sexually transmitted diseases in women and of sexually transmitted viral disease, such as genital herpes and genital warts, takes up more and more time. Partner notification and skilled contact tracing of these conditions are essential, coupled with informing the public about these conditions. Since 1982 most specialists in Britain have also taken on a major role in the care of patients with HIV/AIDS and play a major part in sexual health programs.

Postgraduate training is rigorous and follows that of any other medical specialty, with the added input of gynecological training. Clinics in genitourinary medicine are found throughout Britain, and the specialty has grown, with increasing numbers of consultants in the past twenty years, owing to the problems of HIV/AIDS and rising expectations of good sexual health in the population. Research has flourished, while professorial chairs have been instituted, and there is a postgraduate medical society in Britain, the Medical Society for the Study of Venereal Diseases, with similar societies throughout the world. There are two thriving British journals: *Sexually Transmitted Infections* and *The International Journal of STDs and AIDS*.

### Global situation

Where sexually transmitted diseases flourish, HIV infection is most prevalent. Sub-Saharan Africa, Southern Asia, and Latin America are all major areas where sexually transmitted diseases, and their interactions and consequences, are of major concern. Governmental action locally is required. There has been one outstanding success, that of Thailand, where an effective condom campaign has cut back the incidence of sexually transmitted diseases. This model has started to be taught to other neighboring countries.

The syphilis epidemic in a predominantly black population in some states of the USA has been contained. American research in both HIV/AIDS and sexually transmitted diseases, pharmacology and diagnostic methods is amongst the best in the world.

In the late 1990s the uncontained epidemic of syphilis in RUSSIA and former states of the Soviet Union caused much concern, as did the rapid spread of HIV-AIDS. There are many factors, not the least of which are the economic and social breakdown of society and poorly organized effective public health measures to contain the epidemic. The WORLD HEALTH ORGANIZATION has enlisted a task force to coordinate effective measures.

Sexually transmitted infections need effective measures for treatment and surveillance. 'The syndromic method' has evolved based on management of disease symptoms in sexually transmitted diseases. This method is most useful for poorer countries and its ideology is being taken up with alacrity by many health administrations. Efficient surveillance of sexually transmitted infections is needed and will be required for many years to come, as long as the human condition remains as it is.                                    MAW

*See also* AIDS

**SKEPTICS** Playwrights and film makers, philosophers and social scientists have all delighted in taking a skeptical view both of medicine, and of the doctors who practice it. From Molière (*Le médecin malgré lui*) to Alan Bennett (*The madness of George III*), they have poured scorn on the theories and practice of medicine. Satirists have always poked fun at those who have power over us in society, or at those we fear. Doctors amply fulfill both criteria.

Medicine's critics pose an array of challenging questions. Who determines the aims of modern medicine, and what are they? What is the evidence for the success of medical intervention? How does this compare with the improvements in health consequent not on medical discovery, but on social and economic advance? What harm is done by medical care, and by the medical profession? Is the cost of healthcare commensurate with the benefits? Has biotechnology damaged our perception of the human state, and redefined what we mean by life and death in mechanistic terms? Are we in danger of dehumanizing the very processes of care? As the power and effectiveness of medical interventions have increased, so medicine itself has come increasingly under skeptical scrutiny. Some have gone so far as to suggest that doctors have created a society of dependent patients, fearful of future disease, ill with the anxiety of it, and prepared to trade autonomous life choices for the slavery of medical prescriptions.

Such critique has been leveled at medicine by thinkers from both within and without the medical profession. In his Rock Carling lecture *The role of medicine* (1976), Professor Thomas McKeown advanced the argument that since Déscartes, medical science has been unhelpfully preoccupied by the image of the patient as a body-machine. Current medical theory postulates that this machine is inherently faulty and requires internal intervention. McKeown argued that this mechanistic approach neglects the powerful determinants of health and illness which are not amenable to medical interventions. He identified four determinants of health (genetic diseases; conditions associated with the genetically programmed wearing out of organs at the end of life; diseases in which the environmental influences are pre-natal; and those in which the environmental influences are post-natal).

The ability of modern medicine to intervene is limited largely to the last of the four categories, and McKeown suggested that even here it is easy to overestimate the effects of medical interventions. Although most of the major infections (pneumonia, scarlet fever, or measles) have declined dramatically during the century, the decline was already well established before the introduction of immunization and antibiotics. At the time that streptomycin was introduced in 1947 the major decline in the incidence of tuberculosis in Britain had already taken place.

Professor Archie COCHRANE (p 79) in his Rock Carling lecture (*Effectiveness and efficiency*, 1972) pleaded for greater scientific skepticism in the evaluation of healthcare. With hindsight, it is easy to look with horror on the excesses of unscientific medical care. The bleeding, cupping, and purging of earlier centuries were treatments based on imaginative theory, unsupported by evidence. The death of Charles II at the hands of his doctors is said to have been infinitely more cruel than his father's at the hands of an executioner.

### Faulty reasoning

In the 1930s TONSILLECTOMIES and CIRCUMCISIONS were carried out with the best of intentions, but on the basis of faulty clinical reasoning and with no evidence of benefit. From the 1970s onward there was a dramatic increase in interventional obstetrics, and in particular of cesarian sections, with little proved effect on infant or maternal health. McCormick and Skrabanek (*Follies and fallacies in medicine*) challenged the evidence that SCREENING for breast and cervical cancers, now public policy in Britain, does more

good than harm. They argued powerfully that mass screening programs (because of the unnecessary anxiety caused by false positive results, and the misleading reassurances of false negative findings) increase anxiety, not health. Cochrane's argument was that in the absence of rigorous evaluation, both doctors and public are easily seduced into enthusiasm for policies and interventions based only on hope and belief.

Zola and others criticized the medical profession for having 'medicalized society'. In the 19th century the relation between social conditions and disease was increasingly understood and acknowledged. Public health doctors became social reformers, and VIRCHOW (p 853), a pathologist and public health reformer, wrote 'Medicine is a social science, and politics nothing but medicine on a grand scale'. In the 20th century, new insights into the causes of chronic disease focused on the habits of human behavior — concerning diet, exercise, cigarette smoking, sexual intercourse, and so on. These human behaviors have been labeled 'risk factors' by doctors, who in the pursuit of disease prevention prescribe how we should live our lives. Summing up the evidence on so-called 'risk factors' in the development of coronary-artery disease, a physician has composed the following profile of a low risk individual:

> …an effeminate municipal worker or embalmer completely lacking in physical or mental alertness and without drive, ambition, or competitive spirit; who has never attempted to meet a deadline of any kind; a man with poor appetite, subsisting on fruits and vegetables laced with corn and whale oil, detesting tobacco, spurning ownership of radio, television, or motorcar, with full head of hair but scrawny and unathletic appearance, yet constantly straining his puny muscles by exercise. Low in income, blood pressure, blood sugar, uric acid and cholesterol, he has been taking nicotinic acid, pyridoxine, and long-term anticoagulant therapy ever since his prophylactic castration.

The critique of medicine in general has found a particular focus in mental health. Psychiatrists such as David Cooper (*Psychiatry and antipsychiatry*), Thomas Szasz (*The myth of mental illness*), and R. D. Laing (*The divided self*) challenged the very concepts and practices of contemporary PSYCHIATRY. They argued that the attempt to conceptualize a schizophrenic experience as a disease, using physical disease as the model, is not only misleading and fruitless, but also repressive. The control of feelings and behavior by drugs has been compared with the use of physical restraints in the past. FOUCAULT (p 313)(*Madness and civilization*) argued that the introduction of the madhouse into European society was part of a movement to shut away the social and political deviants in an age when social conformity was deemed an economic necessity. He described this as *The great containment* and traces a direct line of development from leper colony or lazar-house, to madhouse, workhouse, and hospital. During the bleakest years of the Soviet Union, political dissidents were treated as psychiatric patients, their protest hidden in psychiatric institutions, and muted by major tranquilizers.

Perhaps the most trenchant skepticism about the benefits of modern medicine was voiced by the moral philosopher Ivan Illich (*Medical nemesis*). He made much use of the term 'iatrogenic' — a word derived from Greek roots, and meaning 'caused by doctors'. He listed three levels of iatrogenic damage.

First, clinical iatrogenesis, the physical damage caused by the remedies that doctors employ. Illich referred to the many drugs that have unwanted effects which inevitably cause damage. In addition, drugs may be prescribed inappropriately, or the patient may mistakenly take an overdose, so that iatrogenic disease becomes a growing epidemic with the burgeoning of new healthcare institutions.

Second, Illich listed social iatrogenesis, what Zola and others had described as the medicalization of life, the creation of dependency on medical institutions, and so on.

Illich's third category is cultural iatrogenesis. This he describes as the expropriation of health:

> When dependence on the professional management of pain, sickness and death grows beyond a certain point, the healing power in sickness, patience in suffering and fortitude in the face of death must decline. These three regressions are symptoms of third-level iatrogenesis: their combined outcome is Medical Nemesis.

Despite the exaggerations of many of the attacks on medicine and the medical profession, despite the obscure language of of some of the philosophers and the barbed tongue of the playwrights, the medical skeptics are the allies of good medical care, not its enemies.

The keystone of modern research in medicine, as in all sciences, is mounting a challenging critique by the scientists themselves, on their own working methods, data, and conclusions. Indeed, the approach is the attempt by the researcher, in every possible way, to disprove the hypothesis which is to be tested. Skepticism is therefore at the center of modern medical scientific thought. It is essential to the biomedical advances of the 20th century, and in the future it will ensure the limitation of medicine's potential harm, and the maximizing of medicine's potential good.     MM

*See also* EVIDENCE-BASED MEDICINE

**SLEEP** We evolved upon a rotating Earth in which light and dark, warmth and cold, came and went about every 24 hours. In common with other animals we have within our genetic design an inherent rhythmicity that combines in a sensible manner with the alternation of light and dark. Some creatures have specialized and are nocturnal in habit, but humans are among the majority; during the light they are active and during the dark they rest. The nervous system imposes rest, sleep being a positive state of inertia and unresponsiveness to the environment.

Biological rhythms of about 24-hour periodicity (circadian rhythms) can be found in isolated tissues but are normally coordinated in the whole body by the brain. If we fly to the other side of the northern hemisphere, our biological rhythm continues to make us sleepy and inefficient at times when those around us are alert, and it makes us wakeful while they rest.

The mental life of sleep has always held a special fascination and in most cultures the soul has been thought to leave the body during sleep, to mingle with supernatural beings, so to receive guidance for the future. The interpretation of DREAMS for prophetic purposes is familiar, in the story of the boy Joseph, who grew to interpret Pharoah's dream, and in the dream-books of 19th century Europe. Sigmund FREUD (p 321) considered his greatest work to be his book *The interpretation of dreams* (1899), in which he saw the dream as a guardian against disturbance of sleep, and as revealing not the future, but the hidden personality traits of the individual.

Until the 1950s sleep was often seen as a negative state, of mere absence of arousal. It was a decade in which the regulatory role of the brainstem reticular formation came to be understood. Formerly, PAVLOV (p 729), the Russian physiologist, for example, had supposed that wakefulness was determined by the intensity of sensory information reaching the cerebral cortex. It emerged that this was not the case, and that there is a key part of the brain, situated in the central core of the brainstem, excitement of which would lead to ascending and descending impulses that would activate the forebrain and the spinal cord, raising their responsiveness to wakeful levels.

The most important determinant of falling asleep is to have arrived at that phase of the circadian cycle during which we have learned to fall asleep. Falling asleep is, however, also promoted by sheer lack of sleep, by immobility, monotony, warmth, or lack of immediate purpose. The heart slows, the blood pressure falls, the muscles relax, the electrical resistance of the skin rises as insensible sweating diminishes, the pupils become small, and the electrical brain waves (electroencephalogram or EEG) change in appearance.

We first flit to and fro between wakefulness and drowsiness, while imperceptibly the control of our thoughts escapes us. Environmental cues become missed and reactions delayed whenever, for a second or more, the EEG displays slower waves. The tired car driver may at such a point leave the road without any reason other than his inattention.

As sleep deepens, the EEG displays the characteristic sleep spindles or groups of waves at 12–14 cycles per second (Hz), while slower waves of 1–3 Hz become more and more prominent. The body's oxygen consumption falls and reaches its lowest while the EEG's slowest waves prevail. During this same slow-wave sleep of the early night the brain's blood flow and glucose consumption fall and growth hormone is secreted in greatest amounts. Circulating cortisol and adrenaline have by this time fallen to their lowest levels of the 24 hours. Soon afterwards body temperature falls to its lowest and near the end of the sleep period, cortisol begins to rise again in pursuit of its after-breakfast peak.

Within sleep there may readily also be seen an ultradian rhythm of about 100 minutes' periodicity with recurring periods of paradoxical (rapid eye movement, REM) sleep. In this form of sleep there are EEG waves in appearance near to those of drowsiness, jerky eyeball movements, extreme muscular relaxation, penile erection, enhanced brain blood flow, and irregularity of heart, blood pressure, and respiration. Although, in statistical terms, mental life most often deserves to be described as dreaming just after the very moment of one of the rapid eye movements during paradoxical sleep, mental life at any other time of sleep can be indistinguishable.

## The function of sleep

There is a widespread intuitive belief that sleep renews and restores. The apparent renewal is most evident for the brain. If total wakefulness is deliberately imposed on volunteers for several days and nights, they become unable to sustain attention or coherent thought because of brief 'microsleeps' that would lead them directly into full sleep were it not for relays of vigilant watchers. Judgement becomes impaired, visual and other misperceptions intrude, irritability and paranoid ideas erupt, volition diminishes, energy is conserved, body temperature and muscular strength fall, while nitrogen excretion rises and the immune system that fights infection functions less effectively. A couple of subsequent nights of unbroken sleep, during which long periods of slow-wave sleep have priority, restore normal function. We need to sleep.

Tissues such as skin or the epithelium of the gut are constantly worn away and renew themselves by cell division, whereas the brain renews its structural components, not by making new cells but by replacement of protein molecules ('turnover'). Most research into these renewal processes has been conducted in rodents, in which, in all tissues, there has been found to be a higher rate of renewal by cell division or by protein synthesis during that time of the 24 hours when rodents sleep, and this is true of brain protein synthesis.

## Poor sleep

The complaint of poor sleep is one of the most common any doctor encounters. Dissatisfaction with sleep is more frequent among women, among persons of anxious temperament, and among older age-groups.

A reduction of sleep duration below normal, with greater brokenness of sleep, is commonly a consequence of enhanced anxiety arising out of problems in daytime life. As worries recede, sleep improves again. Sometimes sleep is reduced for weeks or months as a result of mental illness, severely so in mania, characterized as it is by excess energy and confidence. The observed disorder, depressive illness, is more common and, especially in middle or later life, unaccustomed and persisting insomnia accompanied by a black cloud of gloomy worries unjustified by the circumstances of daily life should provide a proper reason for seeking medical advice.

Drugs taken to promote sleep were formerly provided by alcohol, the poppy, and extracts from plants containing hyoscine and related compounds, the mandrake root being the most famous. Conversely, caffeine and other xanthines in coffee and tea have been natural substances capable of delaying or disturbing sleep, especially for the middle-aged or older.

Chemical compounds of non-plant origin have come into use in the past two centuries as promoters of sleep: paraldehyde, chloral, bromides, barbiturates, and, most often used nowadays, benzodiazepine derivatives. They relieve anxiety and promote sleep.

The regular intake of any sleep-promoting, anxiety-relieving compound leads to compensatory adjustments in the brain. If intake of the drug ceases suddenly, then, as a consequence of the prior use of the drug, there is unnatural insomnia, with restlessness, anxiety, and an enhanced liability to fits. If large daily doses have been taken, the withdrawal picture may even be that of delirium tremens, although the less extreme syndrome is much commoner after benzodiazepines. Several weeks are then needed before the withdrawal phenomena fade and for return to a natural level of anxiety and a natural duration of sleep.

### Sleep disorders

Although complaints of insomnia are common among older adults, some 5% of adolescents regard themselves as sleeping badly, with associated feelings of unhappiness and low self-esteem. In even younger children, no fewer than 40% of parents of children under 4 years of age regard their child as having a sleep problem, with rapid improvement after that age.

Nightmares are common at any age and the true nightmare is a phenomenon of paradoxical sleep, made up of a relatively prolonged and fearful sequence within a dream, coupled with inability to move, and generally arising in the later night. Neither nightmares nor night terrors denote mental disorder, although they are commoner when daytime life is anxious, and nightmares are frequent after recent withdrawal of sleep-promoting drugs. Night terrors are features of the early night: they arise during EEG slow-wave sleep and are coupled with unelaborated mental life, such as a brief experience of being entrapped, and may be accompanied by shrieking and lashing out. Night terrors run strongly in families, together with a liability to sleep-walking and nocturnal shouting. They often begin around puberty and occasionally persist into adult life. The affected child remembers almost nothing of the nocturnal experience. The most important need is for reassurance of the family, together with simple precautions against injury while sleep-walking. It must be noted that any drug that acts upon the brain may provoke night terrors and sleep-walking in occasional individuals.

While many people complain of lack of sleep, there are a few who complain of falling asleep too readily. In some cases this must be attributed to a constitutional need for more than the average hours of sleep, or to getting up early for work and then trying to remain awake in the evening in company with other family members. Sometimes, however, the liability to fall asleep must be regarded as a disorder, usually of unknown origin. Often it is manageable only by attempts at losing weight, and by the judicious use of deliberate naps and of caffeine or amphetamine derivatives. Two syndromes that the average doctor may expect to encounter can, however, be defined.

One is known as idiopathic narcolepsy with cataplexy. It can begin at any age and is usually first manifested by spells of irresistible sleep, each lasting for about 10 minutes, a couple of times a day. The same person may during the day suddenly find himself or herself partly or totally paralyzed for a brief moment in response to an emotion characteristic for him or her, be it laughter, triumph, or anger. These brief paralyses are known as cataplectic attacks. About one person in a thousand suffers from idiopathic narcolepsy and the disorder should be more widely recognized as one that causes embarrassment and a liability to road accidents. Another reason for excessive sleepiness, particularly among males, is obstructed breathing that develops only during sleep. Children with large and infected tonsils and adenoids may be affected and also some obese adults. The obstruction means that every 20 seconds or so the sleeper almost awakens while engaging in violent snorting efforts to breathe, thereby greatly disturbing sleep.

### Hypnosis

The Greek god of sleep was Hypnos and because many people during hypnotic trances look like sleep-walkers, the term 'HYPNOTISM' came into use. However, despite the conventional instructions, 'You are falling asleep, you are falling asleep'; the trance that is induced by the suggestions of the hypnotist is not a state of sleep, but one of wakefulness and enhanced suggestibility.

It is advisable to keep regular hours for getting up and going to bed. We should minimize alcohol intake and smoking, avoid evening caffeine, take plenty of regular exercise, and avoid being underweight or severely overweight. We should take evening meals at regular times and let them be of easily digestible food. Above all, we should seek to be satisfied with ourselves as we are, accepting our failures and disabilities, and being forgiving of others. We should not worry about how many hours of sleep we get; the brain will look after its needs. 10

*See also* DREAMS

**SMOKING AND HEALTH** The second half of the 20th century saw the emergence of cigarette smoking as a major cause of illness and death. Given that many previously lethal conditions, such as infections (and particularly TUBERCULOSIS), could be cured, for example, with the newly discovered antibiotics, smoking thus came to the forefront as a cause of preventable premature death and serious illness, and has remained there.

Epidemiological research has shown that smoking causes about a third of cancer deaths — not only of the lung, but also of the mouth, larynx, esophagus, pancreas, kidney, bladder, and uterus. It has also a principal causative role in illness and death from serious lung diseases (chronic bronchitis and emphysema), coronary heart disease, and peptic ulcers. Smoking in pregnancy was found to increase the risk of small babies and the occurrence of sudden infant death syndrome, and passive smoking (involuntary inhalation of others' smoke) increased the risk of a child developing asthma.

# THE GREAT KILLERS: SMALLPOX

Smallpox occurs in a major form, *variola major*, and a less virulent form, *variola minor* or alastrim. These probably represented opposite ends of a spectrum of human smallpox, with differences in virulence and in some biological characteristics. (The fatality rates were about 25% for variola major and 1% or less for alastrim.) The smallpox virus is one of a species-specific animal DNA pox viruses, whose size (roughly 200 μm) and complexity place them at the top of the range of known viruses (for comparison, some of the smallest viruses, for example, YELLOW FEVER, measure *c*.17–25 μm). Smallpox infection was airborne and known through the centuries as an acute systemic disease characterized by pustular eruption, beginning as a rash on the face, forearms, and hands and spreading centrifugally to the legs and trunk. The lesions appeared as flat patches developing through raised spots to vesicles, pustules, and finally crusts, which became detached while still infective; thus contaminated bedclothes might still infect. During the incubation period, after infection via the upper respiratory tract, the virus would spread and multiply in the blood and internal organs until, after about 12 days, symptoms appeared with fever, headache, and prostration, and the patient became infectious.

The reason for the successful eradication of smallpox, when comparable scourges such as bubonic PLAGUE, MALARIA, and yellow fever still take their toll, is that, although animal pox viruses exist, smallpox is exclusively a human disease, transmitted by direct man-to-man infection; there is no vector and no intermediate host. There is also an effective vaccine, which, when it was applied by dedicated WORLD HEALTH ORGANIZATION teams trained to trace and vaccinate contacts of patients in outbreaks world-wide, however remote, gradually eliminated the disease. The impact of *variola major* on history in terms of human loss and misery in great epidemics of the past has been comparable with that of bubonic plague — BLACK DEATH — and of malaria and CHOLERA. With an average fatality rate of 25%, its role in intermittently drastically reducing populations in the Americas, Australasia, Africa, and Europe should not be underestimated in its shattering effects on small and large communities alike.

For those who survived, disfigurement by pock marks (such loss of her beauty left Lady Mary Wortley Montagu with a permanent dislike of the medical profession, turning her into a spirited campaigner for 18th-century variolation) and partial or total blindness were often lifelong reminders. Nor was the impact confined to more or less densely populated towns and cities: those who lived on estates and even in palaces were not spared, as shown by the effects of smallpox on world rulers in past centuries. Abraham Lincoln traveled to Pennsylvania to deliver the Gettysburg Address from a Washington in the grip of an extensive smallpox epidemic. By the time he returned to the White House in November 1863 he was unwell, suffering from what was eventually diagnosed as a mild attack of smallpox. He survived; but several European kings and queens were not so lucky. The Virgin Queen (Elizabeth I) was given up for lost by both herself and her medical attendants in October 1562, during her first month at Hampton Court Palace, but recovered against the odds to complete an illustrious reign, albeit forced to wear wigs in

*(continued overleaf)*

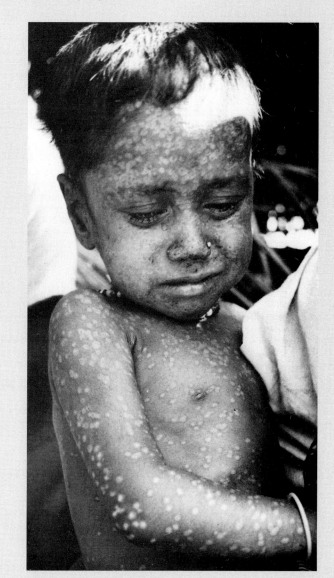

This 2-year-old Bangladeshi girl was the last case of smallpox to be seen on the Asian subcontinent, and the last case in the world of variola major, the most severe form of the disease. (Photograph courtesy of the World Health Organization.)

*(continued)*

public. Two centuries later the disease was instrumental in ending Stuart rule in England, when Queen Anne's son and heir, William Duke of Gloucester, died of smallpox after the deaths from the same cause of his aunt, William III's Queen Mary, in 1694, and of other relatives in the 1950s and 1960s. Thus smallpox paved the way for the accession on the English throne of the House of Hanover, when George I succeeded Queen Anne in 1714.

About this time, the practice of 'engrafting' (later known as 'variolation') was introduced into Britain. William Sherard brought the work on 'transference' by Giacomo Pylarino to the attention of the Royal Society, and Emanual Timone wrote on '…procuring the small pox by incision' in the Society's *Philosophical Transactions* in 1714. This practice of inoculating material from mild cases of smallpox was preceded by 'buying the smallpox' — children were sent to buy crusts from such cases in rural districts during outbreaks in several European countries. Lady Mary Wortley Montagu began her campaign promoting 'engrafting' in Constantinople in 1717; back in London during an outbreak in 1721, she joined forces with the then Princess of Wales. Until the announcement of JENNER's cowpox method (p 452), variolation was increasingly practiced in Britain, where Charles Maitland successfully inoculated Lady Mary's 3-year-old daughter, and Hans SLOANE (p 56) and James Jurin campaigned on behalf of the Royal Society. The Suttons, father and sons, developed their own successful system of inoculation from mid-18th century onwards.

Across the Atlantic, Cotton Mather and Zabdiel Boylston established variolation during severe epidemics in the 1720s. In France, on the other hand, acceptance was much slower, in spite of support from Voltaire, who, like Lady Mary, had himself suffered a severe attack early in the century. Only the death from smallpox of Louis XV in

May finally convinced the French court that a policy of variolation might be expedient, all the more so when a planned French–Spanish invasion of England via a poorly defended Channel coast was thwarted by an outbreak of smallpox in the Armada's ships. Yet the Italian, Angelo Gatti, working in Paris from 1761, was searching unceasingly for ways of attenuating the smallpox virus, or what he called 'weakening the variolous matter' without success. He died in 1798, the year JENNER (p 452) published his empirically conceived *Inquiry*.

Until after the end of the Second World War, efforts to control smallpox remained national rather than international, and vaccination programs focused on the personal protection of individuals. Where endemic smallpox was eliminated on a national scale, it was more as a byproduct of massive vaccination attempts involving whole populations: in Sweden as early as 1895 and Puerto Rico in 1899. The disease largely disappeared from Austria in the 1920s; from Britain, the Philippines, and the USSR in the 1930s; and from Canada and the United States in the 1940s. Other continents and more remote areas were less fortunate. Even after the new World Health Organization took over international health policy activities from the League of Nations in 1948, it was to be nearly another 20 years before concerted international action finally resulted in the adoption of a specific deadline for the eradication of smallpox. Then a resolution by the World Health Assembly in Geneva specified the goal of eradication within years from January 1967.

With smallpox cases still greatly under-reported (on average, globally only about 2% of cases were ever reported), the first step was to improve ratios of reporting, and then to provide advisers, equipment, and sufficient vaccine. Under the skilled leadership of Dr D. A. Henderson, a medical epidemiologist on secondment to the World Health

Organization from the United States Public Health Service, the smallpox eradication program scored an early victory in the face of considerable skepticism when smallpox was eradicated in less than three and a half years, in difficult circumstances, in no fewer than contiguous countries in West and Central Africa. From then on, the work gathered pace, helped by an efficient surveillance-containment strategy and the introduction of the bifurcated needle. Brazil, the last endemic country in the Americas, was declared smallpox free in May 1970. In spite of delays caused by political difficulties in Asia and Africa, Asia became smallpox free in October 1975, with the recovery of its last known case of *variola major* in a young girl in Bangladesh; in Africa, *variola minor* was eliminated from its final stronghold in Ethiopia and Somalia two years later.

In 1979 the WHO's Global Commission for the Certification of Smallpox Eradication was able to declare the world free from smallpox. When its Final Report was accepted the following year by the World Health Assembly it marked the first and so far the only time in history that a major infectious disease had been deliberately and successfully eradicated.

Smallpox eradication was possible because vaccination for a few days after exposure protects against the disease; this was the basis of the containment strategy. Fred Soper, of the USA, deserves the credit for first suggesting this in 1949, and the Soviet delegates to the World Health Assembly for insisting that Soper's strategy should be tried.

In 1806, Thomas Jefferson had written to Edward Jenner when congratulating him on his development of vaccination: 'You have erased from the calendar of human afflictions one of its greatest … future nations will know by history only that the loathsome small-pox has existed'. Jefferson's prophecy had traveled a long road to fulfillment by the time the World Health Organization's Final Report could be published in 1978–80.          LW

---

Such was the impact of the realization of the dangers of smoking that in 1967 Senator Robert F. Kennedy could state that every year tobacco was killing more Americans than had the First World War and later conflicts in Korea and Vietnam combined. The annual deaths were also almost equivalent to those due to battle in the Second World War, while another of the senator's comparisons was that every day the death rate was the same as three full jumbo jets crashing. Similar figures may be produced for other countries: for example, in Britain cigarette smoking kills 125 000 people prematurely every year, and it

is estimated that one in two smokers will die of the habit.

Self-evidently, unlike the earlier 'captains of the men of death', deaths from smoking are preventable. In most developed countries, moreover, there is good evidence that the general population recognizes the risks, if not their magnitude, Governments are faced with the major paradox that, if used as intended by the manufacturer, cigarettes are the only product advertised to the public that may well kill their users. Indeed, had cigarettes first come on to the market after 1960, they would never have got past the prevailing consumer product safety laws because tobacco contains several potent known cancer-producing chemicals.

After the scientific evidence was published in 1950, varying proportions of smokers gave up, depending on the country and the educational level. Even so, smoking has continued to stay at the same level or even to increase in particular groups: young women, blue collar workers, Afro-Americans, the former Soviet bloc countries, and the Third World. This is almost entirely due to aggressive and skillful marketing. Most governments have taken little action to contain such increase, and indeed in their subsidies to tobacco growers, and their initial failure to condemn the habit and subsequently to legislate against seductive advertising and sponsorship of prestigious sporting and artistic events have been held to have encouraged smoking. Globally, tobacco is the most widely grown non-food crop (China being the world's largest producer), with its return per hectare of cultivated land both absolutely and relatively high (twice that of coffee, the next most profitable crop). Governments like it for the tax revenues it engenders — which in Britain at one time were high enough to pay for the whole National Health Service.

Smoking was adopted by Europeans with the first encounter after their American Indians at the end of the 15th century. Not only was tobacco used as a medicine; it also alleviated hunger and thirst, while the growing cycle of the crop was short and it could flourish in various sites and climates. Early on, governments found that they could levy taxes on tobacco — one reason why it was never grown in Britain, given that it was easy to collect duties on imports initially from Virginia and North Carolina and later from other countries.

Until the latter part of the 19th century cigarettes were not smoked widely: most men preferred chewing tobacco or smoking cigars and pipes, while cigarette smoking by women was generally frowned on as 'fast'. The change came about, firstly, through the development of flue curing, which produced tobacco giving rise to smoke mild enough to inhale, and, secondly, by the invention of machinery to replace the laborious and expensive hand-rolling processes.

By the 1890s, mass production of cigarettes was world-wide, and smoking them gained momentum in the First World War, when they were handy for the fighting soldiers, and social attitudes relaxed towards smoking by women, who suddenly had money to spare through working in wartime factories. Hence consumption rose steadily — so that by 1963 the precise per capita consumption for an adult in the USA was 4345 cigarettes every year (compared with only 54 in 1900), and 80% of adults were smokers. As may be seen in movies of the time, cigarette smoking was almost universal and it was socially encouraged — with film stars and even doctors endorsing the mildness of particular brands throughout the media.

Concerns about possible health risks started just before the Second World War. At first these were largely conjectural or anecdotal, but shortly after the war the British Medical Research Council became concerned about the striking increase in the frequency of a once rare tumor — cancer of the lung — something also noted in other countries. Between the periods 1920–30 and 1940–44 cancer of the lung had increased sixfold in men and threefold in women. Asked to investigate (and suspecting that a rise might be due to atmospheric pollution, particularly from the tar on roads), two epidemiologists, Austin Bradford HILL (p 381) and Richard Doll, concluded in 1950 from a study of 709 patients with lung cancer and an equal number of control subjects that smoking was an important factor in producing the disease. Because their study had been carried out in London, they decided to extend it to other localities, and in the meantime, in the USA, Wynder and GRAHAM (p 762) had established a similar link — whereupon Doll and Hill published their original findings, going on to report the same association in a larger and wider study two years later. By the end of 1950, the link had been confirmed for several other countries, including Germany and the Netherlands.

Doll and Hill's next project was to begin a cohort study, seeing how over a period of years

The earliest picture showing the use of tobacco, from a work on Brazil published in Paris in 1558. In the center of the picture is a man suffering from syphilis; behind him, on the left, a man is smoking a large cigar over him as a curative measure, while to either side his arms are held by two figures who seek to suck the poison out of him. Above his head is a monkey, a parrot, and a bale of tobacco.

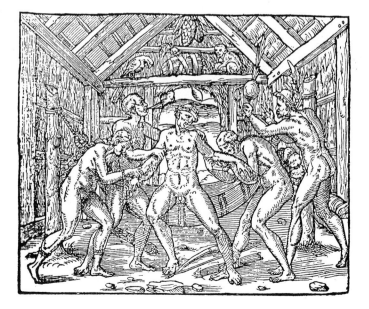

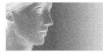

Evarts Ambrose **GRAHAM** (1883–1957). American surgeon. With Warren H. Cole he developed cholecystography. Later his interest shifted to thoracic surgery. He performed the first total pneumonectomy, and was among the first to call attention to the association of tobacco smoking with lung cancer.

While smoking among men is declining, it is tending to increase in women. (Reproduced courtesy of the National Cancer Institute, Bethesda, MD.)

the rates and causes of death compared in smokers with those in people who had given up the habit. They chose doctors, who had reacted to the publication of the original findings more sharply than the general population by giving up smoking. The epidemiologists found that stopping smoking reduced the risk of developing lung cancer within a few years, and that the risk became almost normal after ten years.

This and subsequent work in many countries showed conclusively that the risk of premature death and certain diseases was increased in pipe and cigar smokers (much more in inhalers), but rose 50-fold in heavy cigarette smokers. And Doll was to comment that there had been no greater a convincing epidemiological link since the 1850s, when John SNOW (p 48) had described the association between sewage-contaminated drinking water and CHOLERA outbreaks. Nevertheless, governments were slow to publicize the links or act against the promotion of cigarettes. They were a good source of tax revenue, smoking was popular, and the habit itself powerfully addictive (some said as addictive as heroin or cocaine). In 1961 and 1964 two path-breaking reports, one by the Royal College of Physicians and the other by the US Surgeon General (who had been asked by the President, John F. Kennedy, to produce a report along the British lines) gave good summaries of the scientific evidence.

### Official action

Nevertheless, all this had comparatively little effect on the general public, and, though some people stopped smoking, overall consumption rose. Further pressure, including in Britain a second report by the Royal College of Physicians, forced the authorities belatedly to take some action against the cigarette. Tobacco taxes were progressively raised, extensive publicity was given to the dangers of smoking, and restrictions on radio and television advertising were introduced. Ten years later semi-official organizations were started to keep the pressure up — GASP (Group Against Smoking Pollution) in the USA and ASH (Action on Smoking and Health) in Britain. In fact in 19th-century Britain there had been an anti-smoking movement concentrating on juvenile smoking and based on a strong religious element. Particularly after the revelations of the unfitness of many volunteers for service in the Boer War at the turn of the century, this movement gained momentum and its campaign resulted in a ban on smoking in children enshrined in the 1908 Children's Act.

In the last decade of the 20th century many airlines also introduced comprehensive bans on smoking, even on intercontinental flights. For latterly much attention has been concentrated on the hazards of passive smoking. The evidence for its harmful effects on non-smokers is less clearcut than for conventional cigarette smoking, but most experts agree that it does increase the risk of heart disease and lung cancer — hardly surprising given that cigarette smoke is known to contain 4000 chemicals, around 50 of them carcinogens (substances that cause cancer). The USA has taken the widest steps against passive smoking, with many states requiring the establishment of smoke-free environments — while Norway, followed by Sweden and Finland, has enacted some of the most stringent legislation against tobacco advertising in the world.

In other countries, conversely, restrictions have been much less draconian and in many countries they are almost non-existent. There is evidence that manufacturers are now shifting their campaigns to the former Soviet bloc and the developing world, where smoking among young people and women is still at low levels. Projections for the number of smoking-related deaths by the 2020s have suggested horrific figures for countries such as China, where male smoking is already at a high level. Future generations may be at a loss to discern why current societies failed to deal severely with a lethal addiction — what has become a preventable drain on the community's scarce health resources. Yet it remains true that, while very few things are as dangerous as the cigarette, very few things are as successful as products. Smokers are only part of a complex web of dependence on tobacco: growers, manufacturers, distributors, governments, advertisers, and sports and arts promoters have an equal, or possibly even more persuasive role, in ensuring that things go on as they always have.  SPL

*See also* EPIDEMIOLOGY; POLLUTION

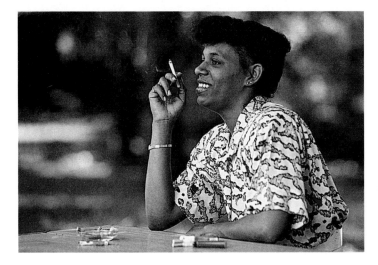

**SNAKE BITE** Less than a quarter of the 2500 species of snake are venomous. They have fangs which are either grooved or contain a venom channel to introduce the venom into their prey during a bite. Most snakes of medical importance belong to two families. The **Elapidae** include cobras, kraits, mambas, and coral snakes; Australasian snakes such as tiger snakes, taipans, and death adders; and the sea snakes. The **Viperidae** comprise the Old World vipers and adders; the pit vipers of Asia; and the lance-headed vipers, moccasins, and rattlesnakes of the New World, which possess a heat-sensitive pit organ, situated between the eye and the nostril, for detecting their prey. There are venomous snakes in most parts of the world except in icy regions, at altitudes above 4000 m, and on some islands. Sea snakes are found in the Indian and Pacific Oceans between latitudes 30°N and 30°S.

Bites by fewer than 200 species have proved life-threatening or caused permanent disability. In Europe a few thousand people are bitten each year and fewer than 100 die. In the United States some 7000 are bitten but only 12–15 die. In Australia bites amount to 1000–3000 but there are only two deaths each year. Snake bites are common in parts of the tropics, especially in Latin America, West Africa, the Indian subcontinent, and in South-East Asia. In Burma, snake bite has been the fifth most common cause of death. In parts of north-eastern Nigeria, there are 500 bites and 50 deaths per 100 000 population per year. The global death toll per year may exceed 50 000. Permanent physical handicap from gangrene of the digits or limbs is a not uncommon sequel to snake bite. Seasonal increases in the incidence of snake bite coincide with heavy rains, flooding, or agricultural activity such as rice harvesting in South-East Asia.

## Venomous snakes are not aggressive

They bite humans only when inadvertently trodden on, cornered, or intentionally handled. The people most frequently bitten are agricultural workers, herdsmen, hunter-gatherers, and children living in rural areas of the tropics. Bites are usually inflicted on the feet or ankles when the victim is walking in the dark or in undergrowth. Surprisingly, in only about half those bitten by venomous snakes is sufficient venom injected to cause symptoms of envenoming.

## Snake venoms

Snake venoms are the most complex of natural poisons, containing numerous components. Polypeptide neurotoxins act at where the nerves join the muscles (peripheral neuromuscular junctions) to prevent the binding of the physiological neurotransmitter acetylcholine. 'Cardiotoxins' damage cell membranes. Snake venoms are rich sources of enzymes such as phospholipases $A_2$ that can damage nerves, cell membranes, red blood cells, and muscle; 'procoagulant' enzymes that activate the blood clotting system; and hemorrhagins that can damage the endothelial lining of blood vessels. Other venom constituents include non-toxic proteins, such as nerve growth factor, carbohydrates, metals, lipids, free amino acids, nucleotides, and biogenic amines.

## Clinical effects of snake venoms

The potency and diversity of snake venom toxins have resulted from evolutionary selection, ensuring that the snake's natural prey, a small mammal, reptile, amphibian, or invertebrate, is rapidly immobilized, easily swallowed, and rapidly digested by the limbless predator. Human snake-bite victims receive a much smaller dose of venom in relation to their size than the prey, and some of the toxins may not be as effective.

*Local tissue damage (caused by vipers, African spitting cobras, and Asian cobras)* Cell-damaging and gangrene (necrosis)-inducing factors digest tissues, membranes, and muscles, causing blood and plasma to leak out of the blood vessels. The bitten limb swells, there is local bruising, red lines appear along the track of lymphatic vessels, and the skin may blister (Fig. 1). Lymph nodes draining the bitten area may become painfully enlarged. Gangrene and secondary bacterial infections lead to life-threatening septicemia, necessitating amputation, resulting in crippling deformity, or leaving a chronic ulcer that may eventually become cancerous.

*Neurotoxic (paralytic) effects (caused by many Elapidae and some Viperidae)* There is progressive paralysis of muscles supplied by the cranial nerves (Fig. 2): first drooping of the eyelids (ptosis) and paralysis of eye movements (external ophthalmoplegia), followed by inability to open the mouth, protrude the tongue, speak, swallow, and breathe. Finally, the whole body may become paralyzed.

*Generalized breakdown of skeletal muscle (rhabdomyolysis)(caused by sea snakes, some Australasian Elapidae, and some Viperidae)* Muscle pigment (myoglobin), muscle enzymes, and potassium leak from the damaged muscles into the circulation. Patients pass brown urine (myoglobinuria). The muscles are painful and tender and the jaws are clenched shut (trismus).

*Kidney damage (caused by sea snakes and some Viperidae, especially Russell's viper)* Venoms may damage the kidney in many ways, by lowering blood pressure by obstructing its small blood vessels with fibrin clots, through the effect of products of damaged muscles and red blood cells, and through the direct effects of venom toxins on the renal tubules.

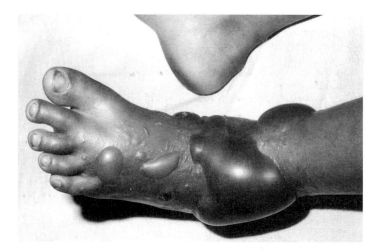

**Fig. 1** Local swelling and blistering developing 24 hours after a bite on the dorsum of the foot by a Brazilian lance-headed viper, the jararaca (*Bothrops jararaca*).

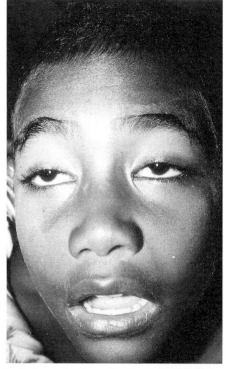

**Fig. 2** Drooping of the eyelids (ptosis), paralysis of eye movements (external ophthalmoplegia), and inability to open the mouth wide and protrude the tongue in a boy bitten by a taipan (*Oxyuranus scutellatus canni*) in Papua New Guinea.

***Bleeding and blood clotting abnormalities (caused by many Viperidae, Australasian Elapidae, and some Colubridae)*** Some snake venoms contain enzymes that activate specific steps in the mechanism of blood clotting. This results in formation of fibrin, which is simultaneously broken down by the body's fibrinolytic system. Eventually, when the liver's capacity to replenish clotting factors is exhausted, the blood becomes unclottable and the patient may bleed uncontrollably from sites of injury. This dangerous situation is made worse by other venom components that affect platelet function and 'hemorrhagins' that damage vascular endothelium, resulting in spontaneous bleeding from the gums (Fig. 3) and into the digestive system, brain, lungs, kidneys, or heart.

***Cardiovascular effects (caused by many Viperidae and Atractaspididae, some Elapidae)*** Blood pressure may fall and shock may develop because of blood loss into the bitten limb and elsewhere. Some venom toxins act directly on the heart, on the caliber of blood vessels, and on physiological mechanisms controlling the blood pressure. The usual result is a fall in blood pressure.

***Traditional first aid methods*** In general, methods such as the use of tight bands or tourniquets, cuts at the site of the bite, attempts to suck out the venom, application of 'snake stones', and electric shocks, have been abandoned as dangerous and ineffective. Patients should be reassured and transported to hospital as quickly as possible. Muscle contractions, especially in the bitten limb, increase absorption of venom into the bloodstream. The bitten limb should therefore be immobilized with a splint or sling. 'Pressure immobilization' of the bitten limb with a firmly applied long crepe bandage and splint may delay the spread of venom from the site of the bite.

***Antivenoms,*** introduced at the beginning of the 20th century, are the only specific antidotes for treating snake bite. They consist of serum from horses or sheep that have been immunized with increasing doses of a particular venom to stimulate production of neutralizing antibodies. Antivenoms are effective only against the venom or venoms used in their production or against a limited range of venoms from related species. Their use has reduced the case fatality of snake bite from up to 50% to less than 5% in the case of patients envenomed by the most deadly species. Antivenoms may produce serious reactions and so should be used only by medically-qualified people. Ancillary treatments for snake bite include mechanical ventilation (for patients with respiratory paralysis), surgical removal of dead tissue, and intensive care unit treatment of kidney failure, shock, and other complications.    DW

**SOUTH-EAST ASIA** Geographically, South-East Asia comprises the Indochina Penisula and the islands and peninsulas to the south-east of the Asian continent. The region extends over 2000 miles (3200 km) from north to south and 3500 miles (5600 km) from east to west, and encompasses the mainland nations of Thailand, Myanmar (Burma), Vietnam, Laos, Cambodia, (West) Malaysia, and the island nations of the Philippines, (East) Malaysia, Singapore, Indonesia, Brunei, Borneo (Indonesia), Timor, and a number of smaller islands.

### The development of medical education

In the early stages, medical education and health services in South-East Asian countries followed the trends of the former western colonial powers. Their influence may still be traced up to the present day. Western medicine came to South-East Asia along with the arrival of European merchants seeking to explore and dominate the region, particularly in the 16th century. Thus merchants of British, Spanish, and Dutch origin were the main groups traveling back and forth between Europe and the islands and peninsulas of the region. Conflicts of interest eventually brought to the region the naval fleets of those European powers, resulting in colonization of most South-East Asian nations.

It was not until the latter half of the 19th century that the first medical school was founded in South-East Asia. After several epidemics, a school of medicine was established in Batavia by the Dutch in 1851. However, lessons of modern western medicine may have been taught earlier in Bangkok by D. B. Bradley (1804–73), a well-known MD of New York University, who first arrived in Bangkok in 1835 and spent most of his life there. He was the owner of the first printing press in Thailand and published several treatises on medicine in the Thai language. The Dutch school in Batavia was attached to the military hospital and Dutch military physicians were the teachers. The purpose of the school was to train native practitioners, mainly to formalize widespread SMALLPOX vaccination. At first the course lasted for two years, leading to the title of Doktor Djawa or Javanese physician; these doctors were trained to diagnose common diseases, to perform minor surgery, and to treat some illnesses. By 1875 the course was extended to six years with Dutch as the main language of instruction. In 1902 the school, having been reorganized with more buildings added, was renamed School tot Opleiding van Inlandsche Artsen (School for the Training of Native Physicians) and the course was extended to nine years after elementary school; a three-year

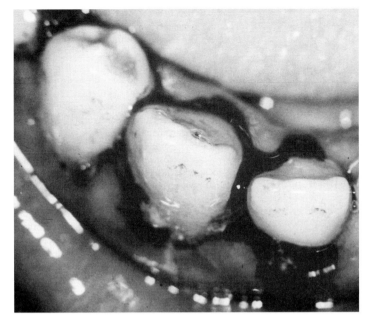

**Fig. 3** Bleeding from tooth sockets in the lower jaw in a boy bitten by a saw-scaled viper (*Echis ocellatus*) in Nigeria.

preparatory course equivalent to junior high school was compulsory before students were allowed to enter the six-year medical school course.

### Indonesian faculties

In 1913 the Dutch colonial government established a second medical school in Surabaya, East Java, named Nederlandsch-Indische Artsen School (Netherlands-Indies School of Physicians). Both schools later became faculties of medicine in the Universiteit van Indonesie, which was also established by the Dutch. The medical school in Surabaya later became a Faculty of Medicine of the University of Airlangga. In 1948 the Republic of Indonesia opened a new faculty of medicine in Jogjakarta in the newly established Universitas Gadjah Mada with Bahasa Indonesia (Indonesian language) as the language of instruction. All other medical schools came into being after Indonesia officially gained its independence in 1949; by the end of the 1990s there were 24 medical schools in Indonesia producing about 1100 doctors each year.

The oldest private medical school in the region was established in November 1871 at the University of Santo Tomas in Manila, the Philippines, under the auspices of the Roman Catholic Church. In June 1907, a second medical school sponsored and controlled by the government of the Philippines was opened. Since March 1923 it has been officially known as the College of Medicine of the University of the Philippines. These two medical schools were the main producers of doctors for the country for several decades. The past quarter of a century has seen some 25 privately owned medical schools opened to local as well as to a large number of foreign students who have sought to enter the medical profession and then to return to practice in their homelands.

The development of medical education in Thailand, the only country in South-East Asia which avoided western colonization, took a different course. The oldest medical school, originally known as Pattayakorn Medical School and shortly thereafter renamed the Royal Medical School, was established in the capital city of Bangkok by the royal decree of King Chulalongkorn the Great of Thailand in 1890 at Siriraj Hospital. The most prominent turning point in medicine in Thailand was due to the achievements of Prince Mahidol of Songkla, who initiated and, together with Prince Jainad, carried out successful negotiations with the Rockefeller Foundation. That foundation, for a 12-year period, from 1923 to 1935, helped the Royal Medical School at Siriraj Hospital in Bangkok to upgrade its standards to those of American medical education at that time. It became a Faculty of Medicine of Chulalongkorn University, which was founded in 1916 by King Rama VI in commemoration of his father. In 1943, by an Act of Parliament, the Faculty of Medicine and Siriraj Hospital were transferred to the newly established University of Medical Sciences, which eventually set up two more medical schools, one based at the Thai Red Cross Chulalongkorn Hospital in Bangkok and the other at the northern city of Chiang Mai.

The past few decades have seen six more medical schools established, two in the provincial cities of Songkhla in the south and Khon Kaen in the north-east, the others being in Bangkok, one of which belongs to the army. Recently a private medical school belonging to Rangsit University was opened. About 900 doctors graduated from the eight government medical schools in existence in 1992. All graduates of government medical schools are automatically given a license to practice by the Thai Medical Council.

## Malaysia and Singapore

Medical education in Malaysia and Singapore developed similarly as the two countries together formed a federation in the British Empire until independence in 1957. Western medicine was introduced to Singapore by Thomas Prendergast, a sub-assistant surgeon who accompanied Sir Stamford Raffles when he landed in Singapore in 1819. From 1870, suitably qualified young men were sent annually by the government to the Madras Medical College in India to train as assistant surgeons. In 1905, the Straits and Federated Malay States Government Medical School was founded in Singapore. After the school received a large donation in 1912 from the King Edward VII Memorial Fund, the name of the school was changed to King Edward VII Medical School in 1913, and to the King Edward VII College of Medicine in 1921.

In 1949, the College of Medicine amalgamated with the Raffles College to become the University of Malaya, and became its Faculty of Medicine. In 1959, the University of Malaya established two largely autonomous divisions, one in Kuala Lumpur, the other remaining in Singapore. Before Singapore became an independent republic in 1965, the school became in 1962, the Faculty of Medicine of the University of Singapore, which again, in August 1980, through the merger with Nanyang University became the National University of Singapore. The University of Malaya in Kuala Lumpur soon founded a new medical school in 1972. Recent decades have seen two more medical schools established in Malaysia under the National University of Malaysia, University Kabangsaan, in Kuala Lumpur, and the University Sains Malaysia, originally in Penang Island but later moved to Kota Baru in Kalantan State in the north-east of West Malaysia.

In Myanmar (Burma) the first medical school was established in the capital city of Rangoon (Yangon) at the turn of the century when the country was still a British colony. Like Singapore and Malaysia, early doctors who came to Myanmar were from Britain and were followed by those qualified from various medical schools in India; during the colonial period this reflected the policy of the British government. The development of medical education in Myanmar has been hampered considerably by several incidents when, because of political unrest, universities were closed, sometimes for prolonged periods. There are at present only three medical schools in Myanmar, two in Rangoon and one in Mandalay, qualifying about 550 doctors a year.

## Training programs

The curricula of medical schools in South-East Asia were influenced by the various stages of development and prevailing trends in each individual country. The systems of education in these schools varied considerably and still reflect the influence of the countries of colonial domination, which, in most cases, were British, American, or Dutch. The current medical curriculum leading to the Doctor of Medicine degree of all the medical schools in the Philippines is similar to that in the USA, namely, that a B.Sc. degree is a prerequisite for admission; there follows a four-year curriculum, consisting of a two-year preclinical period and two-year clinical period, followed by one year of internship. An examination is required for a license to practice in the Philippines. Many native MD graduates have emigrated to practice medicine outside the Philippines, mainly in the USA.

The medical curriculum in the Indonesian medical schools is, in general, based upon the European model, being divided into premedical, preclinical, and clinical phases. The minimum required period to complete the medical course is 6–7 years, which also includes internships in teaching hospitals. The responsibility of generating, implementing, and coordinating policy in relation to the training of doctors and dentists lies with the Consortium of Medical Sciences, a government agency under the aegis of the Ministry of Education and Culture.

In Thailand the medical curriculum of the Royal Medical School in Bangkok, when it first opened in 1890, began differently as the school had to induct students not familiar with modern western medicine into a three-year course combining components of western and traditional medicine. It was only after the subsequent developments funded by the Rockefeller FOUNDATION that the medical profession became attractive to students as the medical curriculum was then similar to American medical education, namely, a four-year course consisting of two years' preclinical and two years' clinical training.

The First National Conference on Medical Education, held in 1956, recommended several amendments in the medical curriculum and, through subsequent national conferences, substantial changes have been introduced into all medical schools. They have included the introduction of internship in 1961, compulsory government service for all graduates in 1968, and the realignment of the entire medical curriculum of all medical schools into a six-year course consisting of one year of premedical training, a two-year preclinical, and a three-year clinical course incorporating the internship period, as introduced in 1980. Recently, some medical schools in Thailand have opted for a problem-based curriculum. The reintroduction of The Thai Medical Council Act 1968 imposed several regulations and professional standards with which all medical schools must comply. The university administration system in Thailand is under the responsibility of a separate Ministry of University Affairs headed by a cabinet minister. A Consortium of Medical Schools was set up recently to coordinate educational and administrative matters relevant to medical schools.

Malaysia, Singapore, and Myanmar share a similar pattern of undergraduate medical education, reflecting the system of medical education in Britain. The entry requirements into the medical schools include the local Higher School Certificate or the British General Certificate of Education Advanced Level or equivalent examinations. The medical curriculum leading to an MB, BS (or MD) degree generally takes five years, consisting of a two-year preclinical and three-year clinical period. To obtain a license to practice, graduates must complete one year of internship (housemanship) in a recognized hospital. In Singapore, English is the language of instruction whereas in Malaysia the Malaysian language is used in medical schools. There as also been a trend to adopt the problem-based curriculum, particularly into the newer medical schools in Malaysia. The medical degree of the medical schools in Singapore is at present recognized by the General Medical Council of Great Britain as a primary qualification for full registration, enabling its medical graduates to be eligible for registration in Britain and some other Commonwealth countries.

## Postgraduate education

The systems of postgraduate medical education in South-East Asian countries differ greatly. The only common features are trends towards medical specialization and those 'academic' qualifications leading to higher degrees, namely the M.Sc. or Ph. D., or diplomas in subjects related to medical, clinical, preclinical, and allied disciplines.

In South-East Asia, 'professional' medical education, where a period of clinical training is obligatory, is generally under the responsibility of the respective medical councils or other similar professional bodies. In Indonesia, the Consortium of Medical Sciences is responsible for the residency training program in some 20 specialties. On the other hand, the Philippine Medical Association, through its affiliate societies, as well as the Board of Education, is responsible for the training of medical specialists. In Malaysia and Singapore, the university still remains the sole source of training with the granting of the Mastership diploma in various clinical specialties. The Thai Medical Council, an autonomous body, is responsible for the residency training program in some 30 specialties and subspecialties in the country. A formal specialist training program does not exist in Myanmar and the Indochinese countries.

One notable trend in medicine in South-East Asian countries during the past decade has been in regional co-operation; this has been achieved through the many regional professional bodies, such as the Medical Association of South-East Asian Nations, through which many academic and social activities are jointly carried out on a regular basis. Such activities have strengthened the development of various aspects of medicine in South-East Asia. AV

*See also* EDUCATION; HEALTHCARE SYSTEMS

**SPANISH-SPEAKING COUNTRIES** During the government of Emperor Octavius Augustus and following the defeat of the resisting Cantabrians and Asturians, its original inhabi-

## TWO SPANISH DOCTORS

**AVENZOAR** (Abu Merwan Abdúl-Malik Ibn Zuhr) (*fl.* 1162). Moorish physician. Born in Seville, where he practiced. AVERROES is said to have been his pupil. He was an empiricist who attached much importance to practice and did not hesitate to question GALEN's (p 324) views. He held strongly that surgery was an inferior craft with which physicians should not soil their hands. He first described the itch-mite (*Acarus scabiei*) of scabies.

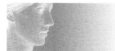

**AVERROES** (Ibn Ruyshd Abu'l Walid Muhammad ibn Ahmad Ibn Muhammad) (1126–98). Moorish physician. He studied in Seville and practiced in Cordoba where he became physician to the Caliph, lost favor in 1195, and fled to Marrakesh; his writings were burned.

tants, the Iberian peninsula finally became part of the political, cultural, and economical structure of the Roman Empire in 19 BC.

Subsequently, the humoral-based Hellenic medicine practiced by the Roman conquerors co-existed with the old, traditional, pre-Roman therapies related to the worship of water and mountains, which prevailed in the less civilized and romanized areas of the country. In the larger urban zones the colonizers built ambitious public works to improve hygiene and sanitary conditions; such were the aqueducts of Segovia and Mérida, and the dam of Proserpina that supplied water to Mérida. In addition, public baths were built in other towns and many hot-water sources were exploited for potential therapies, demonstrated by the abundant votive stars found around these sources of water. Additionally, many surgical instruments, similar to those found in distant provinces of the Roman Empire, have also been found. These findings demonstrate the extent of diffusion and acceptance of the Hellenistic–Roman type of medicine in the Iberian peninsula. Nevertheless, the distance of these provinces from Rome delayed the program of romanization and, consequently, the practice of medicine was not as contemporary as that practiced in other territories of the Empire, such as southern France.

After the fall of the Roman Empire, settlement of the Visigoths (originating in Germania) in Hispania (5th century AD) was followed by a period of cultural stagnation similar to that which occurred throughout the entire Christian world. During this period the most important Spanish contribution to medical knowledge was the concept that Saint Isidore of Seville (560–636) included in his *Etimologies*, a primitive medical encyclopedia which was soon widely referred to throughout Europe. While the book lacked originality, it was a useful synthesis, and Saint Isidore presented the ideas of some of the later Roman authors (for example, Cecilio Aureliano, Sorano) in a very comprehensive manner.

The geographical location of Spain allowed intellectual and cultural exchange with other European countries; this was very fruitful for the development of science and medicine. Arabic medicine, which resulted from the assimilation of Hellenic medicine by the oriental cities of Resaina, Nissibis, and Gondishâpur, was soon accepted. Several clinicians (AVERROES (this page), AVENZOAR (this page)) and surgeons (Abulcassis) wrote books which were widely read during the Middle Ages and the Renaissance. Hispano-Arabic physicians, especially Averroes, in accordance with the Islamic ideal of the *hakim* (a physician simultaneously interested in all aspects of knowledge and enquiry, including theology),

contributed greatly to the development of philosophical thought.

Military campaigns directed towards the expulsion of Muslims from the peninsula which, especially during the 11th century, constituted the *Reconquista*, provided a decisive impetus to the diffusion of classical medicine as reinterpreted by Arab physicians, throughout those countries remaining under Latin influence.

In different Spanish centers (Tarazona, Barcelona, Tarragona, Ripoll), but very specifically in the city of Toledo, work on translating Greek philosophy (ARISTOTLE (p 64) and Plato) and science into Latin from Arabic texts soon emerged, thereby prompting a wide diffusion of classical culture. Translation of the *Koran* was also regarded as fundamental in efforts to refute the Islamic faith and convert the Muslims to Christianity. Simultaneously, versions of medical texts (GALEN (p 324), Ionnitius, and AVICENNA (p 60), and a number of Hippocratic texts) decisively contributed to the incorporation of classical medicine into western European countries. For several centuries, translations written in Toledo, later corrected by commentators during the Renaissance, became the textbooks used to train successive generations of European physicians.

### Independent kingdoms

The subdivision of the Iberian peninsula into independent kingdoms allowed individual contacts between scholars from the eastern regions of Spain with those in the rest of Europe; such was the case with Arnau de Villanova (1235–1312), considered one of the most illustrious representatives of medieval scholastic medicine.

The many Jewish settlements in the Iberian peninsula determined the character of Spanish medicine from the Middle Ages onwards, because of the outstanding 'art of healing' of the Jewish physicians. The presence of Jewish physicians was habitual in Spanish society. Some openly expressed their traditional religious beliefs (MAIMONIDES (p 59)), yet others converted to Christianity, either sincerely or under pressure. Some of these physicians endured great conflicts under the Inquisition and its religious intolerance.

The first universities created in Spain (13th–14th century), emulating those already existing in Europe, contributed to the institutionalization of medicine as a discipline of academic standing. At the University of Salamanca, the Chair of Physic (medicine) was soon recognized, although it was never accorded the distinction of other disciplines such as law and theology. Despite these advances, it should be pointed out that the Islamic tradition (characterized by a more faithful adherence to the Arabic medical textbooks and Arabian Galenisms) prevailed for several centuries.

The 16th century undoubtedly represented the most brilliant period of Spanish medicine, paralleling the political hegemony and intervention in Europe which existed from the reigns of the Catholic kings (1476–1516) to that of Charles I (1517–55). The decisive factor leading to this scientific development was the movement of many Spanish physicians throughout Europe (P. Pintor, J. Almenar, G. Torella, L. Alderete, A. Laguna). Although Latin continued to be the scientific language *par excellence* until the 18th century, the peninsular languages (Castillian, Catalonian, and Portuguese), in differing degrees, although still lacking precision and maturity, gradually became the vehicle of scientific communication.

## Achievement of Servetus

The spectacular philosophical and scientific personality of Miguel SERVETUS (p 484) merits special attention. Born in 1511 in Villanueva de Sijena, a small town of Aragón, he soon showed a clear and non-conformist mind able to handle the problems that dominated Renaissance thinking. His writings covered topics as diverse as classical languages, biblical philology, astronomy, geography, mathematics, medicine, psychology, philosophy, history, and theology (the passion of his life). Although he was a self-made scholar he attended several European universities — Bologna, Toulouse, Strasbourg, Lyon, and Paris — eager to be in contact with the ideal humanism of the 16th century. His books, written in Latin, have been translated into Italian, English, Dutch, German and Spanish, and he maintained an extensive correspondence with his theological enemy Calvin, published as part of his famous *Christianism Restitutio* in Vienna in 1553 but written when he was 20 years old.

Inspired by the ideas of the Reformation, Servet denounced the corruption of official Christianity, the fall of the Church, and the errors of the Holy Trinity. His claim to scientific fame is his description of the pulmonary circulation, present in many manuscripts such as the *Restitutio* and written in Paris in 1546. When HARVEY (p 363) was writing in 1628 the technical description of the main circulation in his *De motu cordis* he traveled to PADUA (p 447) to study Servet's writings. In numerous notes Servet discussed concepts as complex as the 'tyranny of sex', 'the feeling of guilt', 'habit forming', and 'sociability'. Accused by Calvin as the author of controversial books, he was condemned to death after a long trial lasting two months, and burned alive in October 1553 in Geneva.

Until the 18th century, the *Protomedicato* served as the supreme political-administrative institution, exercising all medical and public health responsibilities. During this period the political establishment completely controlled the training of professionals (*protomedicos* examined all university graduates before authorizing their professional activity) as well as various aspects of sanitary activity (inspections carried out by the *protomedicos* and their delegates).

Dating from the reign of Phillip II (1556–98), a gradual process of isolationism contributed to the progressive marginalization of Spanish medicine and its exclusion from the innovative methodology which nourished medicine and science in the 17th century. Faithful to the so-called 'authorities', a highly systematized practice of medicine was imposed, impermeable to all innovation; capacity for dialectic argument was given precedence over observation and experimentation. This process was challenged by minority groups (*novatores*) in the later decades of the 17th century, but with little effect until more enlightened rulers came into power after 1750. The hiring of foreigners to fill offices and various occupations, including medicine, promoted this change. Moreover, the need for a more professional army motivated the state's interest in the training of surgeons; as a result, colleges of surgery were founded (Cadiz, 1748; Barcelona, 1760) and introduced new teaching methods. These new institutions were able to introduce learning techniques traditionally avoided in the universities.

## 19th century confrontations

Political confrontations in the 19th century between the partisans of an absolute monarchy and those who backed a mere liberal constitution had undesirable consequences upon medicine and public health. Successive purges and exiles generated such insecurity that any climate conducive to reflection and study was unthinkable; universities underwent a significant loss of independence and teaching facilities. Many properties belonging to the Catholic Church were also confiscated (desamortización), and the institutions established under its auspices were transferred to civil authorities. This instability meant that European science reached Spanish culture only after considerable delay. Only after the restoration of the Bourbon lineage in 1874 did progress become possible.

Until 1936, the year in which the Spanish Civil War began, there were uninterrupted attempts to further Spanish participation in, and knowledge of, European medicine and science. In basic science, the outstanding histologist, S. Ramón y Cajal, founded a brilliant school of research and was the main instigator, as President of the Board of Advanced Studies, of programs of research abroad for young scientists. The lack of a complex public health infrastructure allowed a much more restricted international reputation for the work of other able professionals: G.

Marañón, T. Ortega, G. Pittaluga, and A. Mírquez. The Spanish Civil War resulted in the nearly total dismantling of weak existing structures. Emigration of intellectuals was widespread from schools of medicine (especially among the basic disciplines) and also among professionals in many clinical specialties. The years immediately following the war were marked by international isolation and recurrent economic crises. Economic development only began in the 1960s. Various campaigns of preventive medicine were implemented (eradication of MALARIA in 1964, systematic VACCINATION of the infant population). A public assistance (national insurance) system was put into effect which covered the entire population, and new hospitals and centers for primary care were created. The incorporation of new generations of professionals, trained, for the most part, in other European or American centers, and the ever-increasing dedication of public funds to health (the Health Ministry was created in 1977), has characterized medicine in Spain during the past two decades.

## Medical care and training in present-day Spain

At the present time, there are 26 public medical schools in Spain and a private one in Pamplona, created by Opus Dei in 1954. In order to enter one of the medical schools, after finishing the baccalaureat, the students have to pass a national examination in science and the humanities, and are accepted or rejected according to their marks. Once accepted they have to complete a six-year academic program to obtain their license in medicine. The first two years are dedicated to basic disciplines (such as anatomy, physiology, biochemistry, genetics) and the following four years, in addition to theoretical lectures, involve the students in clinical activities within the hospitals associated with each medical school. There has been a reduction in theoretical lectures to enable a substantial increase in practical clinical training. This may take place in outpatient clinics, emergency rooms, or in hospital wards. Clinical cases may also be presented as seminars with active student participation.

On completion of medical studies, an official license to practice medicine and surgery is granted. However, most students receiving this license, in order to obtain specialty training, apply to a national postgraduate specialty program known as MIR (Médicos Internos y Residents). This postgraduate program, lasting 3–6 years, takes place in hospitals accredited by the national committee for each specialty. Every year some 20 000 young physicians apply to enter these programs, which have a training capacity for 4000 doctors. Once specialty training is completed,

physicians have the alternative of occupying hospital positions, starting their own private practice, working for private insurance companies, or joining local governmental medical facilities. The number of physicians trained since it was instituted 25 years ago has increased enormously; consequently, newly graduated specialists are encountering great difficulties in finding a job.

In recent years the organization of medical schools and the healthcare delivery by public institutions in Spain has undergone important changes. Since the establishment of a democratic parliamentary system after the long period of Franco's dictatorship, several provinces, now called *comunidades autónomas*, have obtained considerable administrative and political autonomy — as has been the case for Cataluña, Andalucía, Galicia, and Euskadi (Basque country). As a consequence, the central government has transferred to each province the responsibilities for the primary schools, baccalaureat, university, as well as the management of institutions providing public health. As expected, each *comunidad* has introduced its own changes, such as the compulsory use of written and spoken local languages in all teaching institutions and hospitals, an unthinkable prerogative during Franco's regime. Thus, at present, even at national scientific meetings held in Cataluña, Catalonian is the official language and a Spanish simultaneous translation has to be provided.

*Healthcare* Medical care in Spain is offered both in publicly and privately administered institutions. Public healthcare is delivered through the National Institute of Health, within the Ministry of Health. A network of publicly owned health facilities encompasses the entire territory of Spain and is administered both at a federal and regional level. All Spanish citizens are covered by this system and contributions are made through the workplace by the employer and by the employee as part of a national Social Security program. All medical specialties are covered, with the exception of dentistry and optical services. Patient care starts with primary care, but can also provide hospitalization. Most medication (80–90%) is also provided.

A private patient-care system exists in parallel with the National Health Care system. It takes the form of a fee for item of service system, provided by insurance companies or private physicians.

Several private patient-care systems have proliferated in the past ten years. Despite the fact that the National Institute of Health continues to deliver free healthcare to all Spanish citizens, roughly six million people now have additional private health insurance. These changes reflect the tendency towards privatization that the present conservative government is undertaking. The

Ministry of Health seems to have concluded that it is financially impossible to offer free global care and the high quality medical attention that patients present request. As in many other countries, high demand for healthcare is prolonging the already long medical and surgical waiting lists. It is also increasing the work and responsibilities of doctors without any proportionate compensation in their salaries.

## South America

Since the discovery of America in 1492, the development of the continent has been indivisibly linked to the history of Spain. Apart from the prolonged political dominance over much of the newly discovered continent, a lasting bond was created by the use of a common language. One of the more significant and lasting examples of this symbiosis was the creation of various universities (Santo Domingo, Mexico, and Lima). These basically reproduced the Hispanic model of the University of Salamanca, which, in turn, imitated the medieval model of BOLOGNA (p 447), wherein jurisprudence studies were given priority over those of medicine. For this reason, only some of the universities (Mexico, Lima, Guatemala, and Quito) offered studies in medicine, while others were quite late in offering these studies in their curricula (Havana, Caracás). European humoral medicine of Hippocratic–Galenic origin was first introduced by the doctors who arrived on the new continent (Álvarez Chaca arrived in Columbus's second trip, 1493) and subsequently by the universities created in the New World. European diseases reached the new continent and killed many of the local populations, isolated since their crossing of the Bering Straits (measles, LEPROSY, SMALLPOX, INFLUENZA), while others were brought back to Europe with increased virulence (SYPHILIS). The Africans shipped to America for slave labor carried their own diseases (YELLOW FEVER), as well as contributing to the ethnic mix. The great interest with which European doctors studied American therapeutic products was rapidly reported and widely distributed in various publications by the Sevillian doctor N. Monardes (1493–1588).

During the 18th century, the most ambitious campaign undertaken by the Spanish Crown in the colonies was the expedition of vaccination (1803) directed by Dr F. Balmis; lymph vaccine was transported first to America and then to Asia (the Philippine Islands, then under Spanish control) to try to combat smallpox, which had previously been introduced there by the colonists.

*Medical education in Mexico* Two stages may be identified: the colonial and the republican. In 1533 the first university in the American continent was founded in 'Nueva Espana' (now Mexico), entitled

the Royal and Pontifical University. In this university a medical school was inaugurated in 1519 and the opening lecture was given by Professor Juan de la Fuente, who received a salary of 150 gold pesos annually as chairman of the 'Catedra Prima'. In 1598 Dr Juan Plasencia established the second chair entitled 'Visperas'.

In June 1680 a chair of Anatomía y Cirurgia was created, Dr José García being elected as chairman at a salary of 50 gold pesos annually. To practice medicine in the 'Nueva España' three types of degree were necessary: bachelor, licensee, or doctor. To become a bachelor the completion of the programs of the three chairs Catedra Prima, Visperas, and Anatomía y Cirugía was compulsory. The degree of bachelor in medicine was not sufficient to practice medicine legally unless the degree of bachelor of arts had been obtained previously. To assess a candidate's competence, a committee composed of a teacher in arts, a teacher in medicine, the rector of the university, and a neutral referee was set up. To practice as physicians, the candidates had to work for two additional years in the school of medicine, followed by a promedicato final evaluation. To become licensee in medicine the following were necessary: a bachelor's degree, not to have debts with the Holy Office, not to be a descendant of a slave, and to own medical books.

In 1768, under the responsibility of two surgeons, Antonio Vezquez de Leon and Domingo Rusi, the Royal College of Surgery was founded, following the pattern of the same institutions in Barcelona and Cadiz. The 'Real Hospital de los Naturales' was used for patient care, and the first chair (Clinical Surgery, Operations, and Legal Medicine) was inaugurated in 1770.

The Medical School and the College of Surgery functioned independently. In the medical schools a six-year program of training was required but only four years in the College of Surgery. In 1833 the two institutions merged and a unified degree of Medical Doctor and Surgeon was granted. While this process evolved in Mexico City, in 1792 a medical school was established in Guadalajara under the auspices of the Royal Literary University.

The Republic of Mexico became an independent free and confederate state in 1824, 3 years after Mexico became independent from Spain. The first elected authorities created a new medical school in Oaxaca in 1827, followed by others in Nuevo León (1828), Morella (1829), Yucatan (1833), and San Luis de Potosi (1877).

In 1826 Don José María París, the first Governor of the state of Nuevo León, published the following decree: 'If a generous citizen would sponsor a chair of medicine in Monterrey the government would designate him as a benefactor and his portrait and name would be exhibited at the door of the 'institution'. Unfortunately no one considered himself capable of founding a medical school. Two years elapsed until the new governor, Don Joaquín García, ordered his first federal deputy, Dr Manuel De Llano, to travel to Mexico City and find a talented professor capable of creating the first school of medicine in Monterrey. Dr Pascual Costanza, a prestigious practitioner of Italian origin who graduated in Naples, was the chosen physician. He accepted the proposal after a six-year contract had been signed in the presence of a public notary and a salary of 1000 pesos was settled as a director of El Rosario Hospital. He arrived in Monterrey on 13 October 1828 and five days later was inaugurated as professor attended by five students who followed the adopted program of the School of Mexico. Unfortunately through financial problems the school closed six months later on March 1829.

An unexpected political event was to change the teaching of medicine in Mexico. In 1859 the President of the republic, Don Benito Juarez, promulgated the laws of the *Reforma* and as a consequence a civil college was founded in Monterrey with two faculties, one of law and the other of medicine. From then on the responsibilities of superior teaching were no longer under religious control.

The new school of medicine opened its doors on 30 October 1859 with fifteen students and six professors under the direction of Professor José Eleuterio González. The Civil Hospital was then nominated the University Hospital.

***Medical education in Venezuela*** Venezuela was discovered by Columbus during his third voyage in 1498. There are records indicating that until 1763 medical practice was carried out by individuals acting empirically and independently. The following merit mention: surgeon Alonso and the pharmacist Bernal were the first Europeans to practice medicine in Venezuela; Don Diego Montes 'The Venerable' (1531) treated poisoned arrow wounds by using cauterization; in 1696 surgeon Guerra Martinos performed the first AUTOPSY in Venezuela on a person who had died of yellow fever ('black vomiting'); Albertus Millier, a physician from Vienna, signed a death certificate on a patient believed to be the first documented case of tuberculosis in Venezuela; the first craniotomy was performed in Caracas by Pedro Roberto Diget on 5 April, 1736; in 1908 Dr Balmis began a program of smallpox vaccination.

In 1763 the first organized teaching of medicine at university level was developed by Dr Lorenzo Campins y Ballester, who established a 'license' in the so-called 'Protomedicato de Medicina' following Spanish and European models. In 1827, after Venezuela became an independent nation, Dr Vargas, Rector of the Central University of Venezuela, created a faculty of medicine, where modern teaching techniques were used. Many other medical schools and hospitals were also founded in other cities.

Several other important events also deserve mention. In 1904 the National Academy of Medicine was founded, and in 1930 the Ministry of Health was created, followed by a compulsory public health insurance program. In 1954 the Institute of Neurology and Cerebral Research was inaugurated.

More recently, the influence of the North American method of teaching and practicing medicine has been clearly apparent. Many private hospitals have been developed to compensate for the administrative difficulties of the public institutions.

**Conclusion**
The process of emancipation and independence of the colonies from Spain in 1821 promoted a nationalist tide which also sought to develop science and health. The political convulsions suffered by most of these countries, however, proved a decisive factor in the relegation of social as well as scientific development. The first medical schools in Spanish-speaking American countries imitated European, principally French, models. However, the influence of the USA in the 20th century has resulted in the current general acceptance of that model. Numerous medical doctors, researchers, and teaching professionals, exiled after the Spanish Civil War and the Second World War, relocated in various Latin American countries, which profited greatly from their expertise. In recent decades, political instability and economic crises have forced many young Latin American doctors to emigrate to the USA, where working conditions and research possibilities are more attractive.                 APor-S, AC, PPon, RR

*See also* EDUCATION; HEALTHCARE SYSTEMS

**SPECIALIZATION** as we know it today has a history of little over 150 years. Its progress, achieved against the determined opposition of the established profession, was at first slow but inexorable. By the end of the 19th century a handful of specialties were recognized but constituted a very small element in medical care. Their role was enlarged by technical advance or medical ambition, by rising public expectations, and by increased spending on healthcare. At present, hospital medicine and most of private medical practice in the developed countries of the western world is irreversibly specialized. The European Union currently lists some 70 specialties for which a postgraduate training period is prescribed; in practice, some of those listed are already extensively subspecialized. Paradoxically, general practice, with its specific training program and defined aspects of operation, must for many purposes now be considered a specialty.

Specialization is costly; it expands the range of treatment but increases hospital staffing and multiplies technical facilities. It denigrates the synoptic view of clinical problems and for effective care it demands, but does not always compel, a cooperative team approach. It undermines the capacity of teachers to convey to undergraduates a broad understanding of the whole of medicine. Nevertheless, its inevitability is disputed by few. The enormous range of medical knowledge, the profundity of the sciences which support it, and the extraordinary variety of investigative and therapeutic procedures have made it inconceivable that any single individual could comprehend the information available, let alone apply it. Historically, however, it was not the spectacular increase in knowledge that initiated specialization; often, it was the reverse. The concentration of attention upon a limited aspect of medicine, as in many aspects of reductionist science, hugely added to the knowledge base to such an extent that only by specializing could it be assimilated and brought to bear in practice.

## Specialist and specialties

In contemporary British medicine, specialists ordinarily see patients referred to them by general practitioners. This was not always so and is still not customary in many countries. Specialization evolved later in Britain than elsewhere, and for many years the term specialist carried derogatory overtones.

Originally physic and surgery were seen as the natural divisions of medicine in the broad sense, and specialization was a segmentation of either of these divisions. During the 19th century, as the élite physicians and the surgeons relinquished primary care to the growing band of general practitioners they became, collectively, consultants not specialists. The specialists, it was believed, might be expert in their narrow discipline but lacked the balanced vision of the consultants and could not aspire to the higher ranks of the profession. The fact that the patients and the public generally did not share this view only sharpened the aversion of the generalists towards them.

Today the great majority of specialists, now admitted to the consultant ranks, practice within a recognized specialty. Individual specialism necessarily preceded the emergence of these recognized groups and may now initiate subspecialization. For ambitious young doctors, some element of specialization is part of the enterprise culture by which they assert their individual abilities. For the older doctors, specialization may be a welcome retreat from the turmoil of generalist practice into a discipline where their experience and authority are fully recognized.

The specialties now listed by the regulatory bodies have arisen at various times and in various circumstances but they have certain features in common. A specialty is defined by both technical and social factors. It has an acknowledged territory, a corpus of relevant knowledge, and a range of skills not readily acquired by others. The territory is most often limited by the anatomic and physiologic systems of the body but may also relate to specific patients or diseases, to a method of investigation, or to a particular treatment. The knowledge may be derived from the appropriate science or from accumulated clinical experience. The skills are normally manual — hence the priority of surgical specialization — but may consist of expertise in pattern recognition, in a specific discipline.

The social structure of a specialty is first evident when the leaders pass on their expertise to their successors. In the next stage, specialists are appointed, or advertise themselves, to teach the subject. Later, designated hospital posts are created, a journal appears, and a society is founded. To begin with, the society is concerned with academic discussion and its membership is broad based, but it soon comes to represent the interests of the specialists as well as affording opportunities for exchanges of information and taking on a medicopolitical function. A specialty may be considered to be fully established when a training program for it has been accepted by a national authority and when the specialist group controls entry to its own ranks. In Britain the final accolade for the favored few comes with the foundation of Royal Colleges devoted to their interests.

A specialty needs a name. It may take that of the science which existed before, such as ophthalmology or neurology, terms that had long appeared in the literature. Conversely, however, some of the first specialists needed to free themselves from the opprobrious descriptions with which they were lumbered. Man-midwives became accoucheurs and then obstetricians. Mad doctors became alienists and then psychiatrists. Aurists became aural surgeons and then otologists. Older titles such as physician for the diseases of the skin and genitourinary surgeon gave way to dermatologist or urologist when specialists could be proud of their expertise, but higher status was also sought by venereology in becoming genitourinary medicine.

## Origin of specialties

A technical and social definition of a specialty as it exists today may give no clue to its origin. Specialization is a process common to many human endeavors, but its precise form depends greatly upon circumstances. Medical specializa-

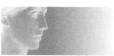

tion took place at a time of rapidly increasing knowledge but the major specialties did not arise from any planned division of labor of the type seen in industry.

A biological analogy might be closer to the medical model. Specialization is then visualized as the process by which in a competitive world a species diversifies to exploit the potential of a varied and changing environment. The medical specialties arising in the 19th century exploited aspects which were then little regarded by mainstream medicine yet having the potential for furnishing sufficient business to occupy the time of a group of practitioners and provide them with a livelihood. The continued popularity of such traditional fringe practitioners as oculists, aurists, and bonesetters in aspects avoided by the established profession because of the taint of quackery, suggested the territory for some new specialties. Often, however, it was opportunity to study a large number of cases with similar diseases that revealed the possibilities of new understanding and interventions.

### Roots of psychiatry

Lunacy had been the subject of speculation by physicians and philosophers, but psychiatry as a specialty had its roots in the mad houses and ASYLUMS; it was essentially custodial, which perhaps accounted for its intellectual stagnation through much of the 19th century. DERMATOLOGY as a specialty started in post-revolutionary France when Louis Alibert was put in charge of Hôpital St Louis, to which had been allocated huge numbers of Parisians with skin and venereal diseases. The very numerous small special hospitals in London, set up for a variety of reasons, noble or ignoble, were the breeding ground for several specialties.

During the world wars there was almost inevitably a grouping together of casualties with particular injuries, and once again this encouraged specialization. PLASTIC SURGERY soon achieved specialty status as a result of the work of Gillies in the First World War and of McIndoe and others in the second. NEUROSURGERY had been pioneered by Victor Horsley and Harvey CUSHING (p 537), but was not taken seriously until the huge numbers of head injury cases during the WAR required expert attention. ORTHOPEDICS was granted new respect after Sir Robert JONES (p 773) had persuaded the British Army to set up a series of military orthopedic hospitals in 1916. In each case, there was a father figure for the specialty, much revered by his pupils, but his success depended upon there being an entity ripe for exploitation.

An invention or discovery can trigger the emergence of a new specialty. Thus Stromeyer in 1830 introduced subcutaneous tenotomy for the correction of club foot, and thereby gave fresh impetus to the treatment of all deformities — the start of specialist orthopedics. Czermak's demonstration of the laryngeal mirror in 1857 created the specialty of laryngology. In recent years renal biopsy and dialysis have separated the nephrologists from the general physicians; cardiac catheterization and angioplasty have transformed CARDIOLOGY into a fully fledged specialty. Attempts to use the discoveries in microscopy, bacteriology, immunology, and radiology in the practice of general physicians and surgeons soon failed, and their complexities demanded new specialties which cut across older territories.

### International comparisons

The first specialists were everywhere met with hostility and accusations of quackery from the established medical profession. In Britain, the opposition was more effective and lasted considerably longer than elsewhere and designated posts, journals, and societies were later in their appearance. There are those who ascribe this resistance to the good sense and respect for a balanced clinical approach of the British profession, but more readily recognizable factors are to be found in the structure of the hospital service, the institutional dominance of the two Royal Colleges, and the strength of the general practice sector.

The hospital service in 19th century Britain was characterized by the multiplicity of small but prestigious voluntary hospitals and by the low status accorded to the larger Poor Law or local authority institutions. Sub-division of clinical facilities in the teaching hospitals, small by international standards, was difficult and likely to be resisted, staff appointments were inevitably few, and the general physicians and surgeons were understandably reluctant to share their privileged position with the specialists. By contrast, the huge state-funded hospitals in the continental capitals provided ample opportunities for the segregation of patients according to their diseases and therefore for their special study. Moreover, in the great hospitals of Vienna and Berlin specialization was encouraged not only by the designation of wards but by the well-funded university system. By contrast, in London the university influence was minimal before the inter-war period, and the consultant ranks were dominated by the Royal Colleges. The council members belonged to the teaching hospital staff but they were without any significant departments in which academic diversity could flourish and were themselves busy in private practice. In such conservative bodies there was no inclination to allow the radical change which a proliferation of specialties would involve. Moreover, the fee-paying classes in Britain had accepted the role of general practice, and direct self-referral for specialist consultation was unusual, thereby depriving the young specialists of the trivial 'bread and butter' cases, which in other countries — particularly in France and the USA — enabled them to get started. Evidently there was a range of cultural differences responsible for the relative tardiness of specialization in Britain.

## Late 20th century

By 1950, the major specialties were well established, but the following decades witnessed an accelerating process of subspecialization which has not yet been stemmed by the funding crisis or the holistic medicine movement. Increased spending on healthcare encouraged the development of new aspects of expertise, which in turn demanded even more financial support. In the USA, patient self-referral for specialist opinion has fueled this spiral leading to the demand by insurers for MANAGED CARE. In Britain, the National Health Service has allowed salaried consultants to expand those aspects like child care which under the private practice system were seriously underfunded. Pediatrics and its numerous subspecialties have, therefore, seen major growth aided by the charitable support for specialist research groups where there is a strong public appeal. Technological advance has opened up for exploration branches of both medicine and surgery which were previously inaccessible, and new treatments have created specialties such as oncology and intensive care.

It is statistically evident that specialist centers acting within their own limited range can deliver safer and more effective, if more expensive, care. The demand for monitoring performance thus drives the hospital service towards specialization and the increasing volume of medical negligence litigation makes doctors wary of operating outside their expertise.

As a reaction against this, there has been a growing movement in favor of 'whole person medicine' and a return to 'natural' cures. Within the profession some changes have been hailed as moves away from specialism. Thus general practice has in recent years enlarged its horizons and reclaimed from the clinic long-term management of some chronic disorders. However, this could hardly be considered a portent of more fundamental change. Specialized hospital services are the natural corollary of a well-organized general practice. Expert opinion will always be required for the difficult case and the current trend undermines the position of the general physician and the general surgeon rather than that of the specialist. The specialties are now so deeply entrenched within diagnostic complexities and

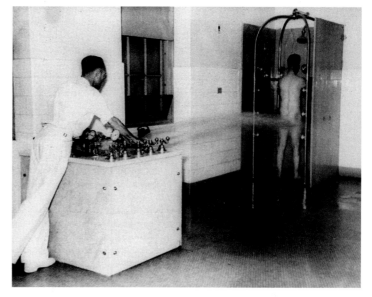

Hydrotherapy was well on the way to becoming a specialty in the early years of the last century, but its place has been overtaken by treatment from rheumatologists and physiotherapists. (Reproduced courtesy of the National Library of Medicine, Bethesda, MD.)

technical skills that it is inconceivable that their work could be returned to the generalists.

Further subspecialization may be halted by lack of funds but it is difficult to visualize the return of the internist and general surgeon.        DIWil

*See also* EUROPEAN UNION – IMPACT ON MEDICINE; HEALTHCARE SYSTEMS; JOURNALS

**SPORTS MEDICINE** The International Federation of Sports Medicine, founded in 1928, adopted the most satisfactory of many definitions of sports medicine:

> Sports Medicine embodies theoretical and practical medicine which examines the influence of exercise, training and sports, as well as lack of exercise, on healthy and unhealthy people of all ages to produce results that are conducive to prevention, therapy, and rehabilitation as well as beneficial for the athlete himself.

Thus the subject is far more comprehensive than suggested by single factions (typically, claims that sports medicine is about injuries, or a matter for orthopedists), and the complex and interrelated aspects of athletic preparation far exceed the skills of any one group of professionals. In other words, sports medicine implies a high degree of interdisciplinary cooperation — all centered on the athlete (and perhaps family and school) — not only between doctor, therapist, and scientist but with coach, official, manager, sponsors, and media.

Selection and training seek to define the ideal properties required for success in the various sporting events. Keen children soon reach anatomical or physiological limits when they find that enthusiasm can no longer triumph over body

## SPORTING DOCTORS

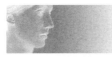

William Gilbert **GRACE**
(1848–1915). British physician
and cricketer. Trained at
Bristol, St Bartholomew's, and
Westminster Hospitals, Grace
practiced in Bristol from
1879–99. He was the most
celebrated of all cricketers and
a legend in his own time,
playing first-class cricket from
1865–1908, scored 54 869
runs, and took 2876 wickets;
he made 126 centuries and
his highest score was 400 not
out in 1876.

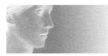

Robert Tait **McKENZIE**
(1867–1938). Canadian
physician and sculptor.
McKenzie taught anatomy
and physical education. In
1904 he was appointed
professor of physical
education at the University of
Pennsylvania. His sculptures
of athletes brought him a
decoration by the King of
Sweden at the Olympic
Games of 1912. In the First
World War he was a pioneer
in rehabilitation medicine. His
greatest work is the Scottish
War Memorial in Edinburgh.
Others include that at
Cambridge, General Wolfe at
Greenwich, the Young
Franklin at the University of
Pennsylvania, many athletes,
and memorial plaques and
medals including Osler, Weir
Mitchell, Robert Jones, and
Ronald Ross.

Forces acting on the human
body, an illustration from
Borelli's book *De motu
animalium*. (From Harries, M.
*et al* (eds.) (1998), *Oxford
textbook of sports medicine*,
2nd edn, OUP.)

size or shape. Ideally, early selection of children into or away from appropriate events should allow their better perserverance and enjoyment. For instance, short fat children will not excel at gymnastics or high jumping nor skinny youths at long-distance swimming, where the insulation of body fat is an important advantage. In casual and amateur sport, this does not matter. In the ever-increasing ranks of the serious competitors, small differences make for big discrepancies in outcomes.

The clinician's role is limited to routine examinations and health surveillance — a reason why few find this attractive work. The coach (teacher, parent, or sports coach) is the key influence in guiding the training schedules and progression. Technique skills bear meticulous instruction and endless repetition, routine stamina and flexibility maintenance are boring and take much judicious persuasion and inspiration. Equipment must be bought, tried, and mastered. Backing the coach might be the sports scientist, with a battery of physiological assessments, which should relate clearly to the event requirements rather than the investigator's curiosity. Such testing rarely has an immediate pay-off. Its sequential repetition over time reveals glimpses of meaning behind the athlete's constant fluctuations in form and occasionally may give important help.

The coach is chief motivator outside the athlete's own mind. Other managers may intervene here, and others including sports psychologists may be employed.

In the background, sports scientists study the biomechanics of the events and equipment. Track surface qualities, including traction (which must interrelate with shoe properties), jumping, and landing areas (especially the crucial safety factors of landing from high jump or pole vault); clothing properties in respect of the event and climate requirements and footwear design — all these are constant targets for scientific study. Event actions

themselves are now electronically dissected frame by frame from videos to search for improvements and corrections. Occasionally a whole new technique leaps from the scientific mind as did the Fosbury Flop technique, which rapidly became universal in the high jump.

In the athlete's body, chemical explanations are sought for movement, training, success, and failure by biochemists and the new breed of exercise physiologist. The sports nutritionist looks for a new advantage in fueling or refueling ever better exercise performance. For example, in the carbo-loading diet for marathons to increase his muscle glycogen store beforehand, the runner would learn to deplete his muscles by a long run; then take in an excess of carbohydrate to boost muscle levels beyond the normal physiological ones. Hence the custom of pre-race 'pasta parties', when the runner tops up his glycogen reserves. Hydration in sport has become an important topic of research and too many athletes ignore or even misunderstand the essentials of adequate hydration during exercise. Dehydration is disadvantageous because it impairs sweating and heat loss control, with a consequent danger of hyperthermia.

### Training at altitude

It is now a *sine qua non* at top level to train at altitude for endurance events. Originally, this was a self-defensive measure against the unreasonable and unphysiological burden of being forced to compete at medium altitude. (We now know that it is virtually impossible for a sea-level born athlete to win a long-distance race at altitude.) It has become a matter of using altitude to stimulate extra hemoglobin and myoglobin production for a subsequent limited span of supercharged sea-level competition. It works — numerous track records have been set in this way. However, the logical alternatives used by those disinclined to go to the mountains are declared illegal. First

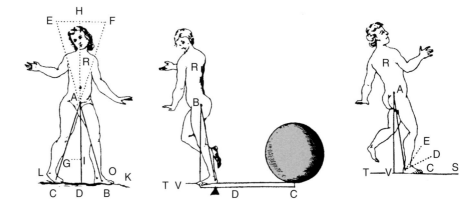

came blood transfusions, then autoretransfusion (whereby the athlete would donate himself a store of blood whose packed cells would be re-infused a few weeks later to boost the hemogloblin). Finally came erythropoietin, which stimulates the bone marrow to produce extra hemoglobin. As the last is now easily available through biosynthesis, it is difficult to educate athletes against its seductive advantages, in spite of unexplained sudden deaths and the dangers of mismanagement.

## Technical research

Sports science is engaged in technical research into all aspects of sporting equipment and clothing. These are important to safety as well as good performance at altitude and heat, so that designs and fabrics are carefully chosen — today's athlete is not just a fashion victim in the odd array of eccentric materials and uniforms used in top sport. The main shoe manufacturers are locked in permanent wars over every aspect of footwear style and function.

The ultimate goal of all this is competition. The art and science of training will bring the athlete gradually up over several years to a plateau at international level, from which a small élite will win medals. Many events feature the very young and immature — notably swimming and gymnastics. This leads to complex medical problems concerned with training, monitoring, and health. The glamor and adulation of a generation of little east Europeans caused a huge growth in pre- and adolescent sports participation. Now, after the collapse of the Iron Curtain, we have learnt that many or most were sustained by illegal hormonal

manipulation and in the west, without drugs, we have learned the full dangers of overtraining in the young, especially in girls. The 'female triad' is described — of amenorrhea, osteoporosis, and anorexia nervosa — with stress fractures a common complication. The causes are not fully understood.

So great is the training needed for success that overtraining has become a limiting factor in sport. Overuse injuries are self-induced (in contrast to impacts and sprains) and affect all the locomotor tissues ranging from bone (stress injury), joint (synovitis), and ligament strain through tenosynovitis and rarely rupture and peritendinitis to post-exercise muscle soreness and destruction, not forgetting the humble callus and blister. A common mistake is to train intensively without regularly interspersed adequate rest phases. Event needs, especially endurance and technical perfection, demand incessant hours of repetitive stereotyped movement patterns so that locomotor soft tissue injuries are both very localized and often very severe. As the injury is the direct result of the event, and the event cannot be safely resumed before remission, there is obvious scope for difficulty in clinical management and athletic rehabilitation. Add to this the depressingly usual pattern of top athletes breaking down with overuse injury in the countdown to championships because they rarely learn to abate the training stress in sharpening up into the big event and it becomes clear why the clinicians' impact in sport may be disproportionate to others.

Little has changed in our knowledge of orthopedic and soft-tissue medical treatments in recent

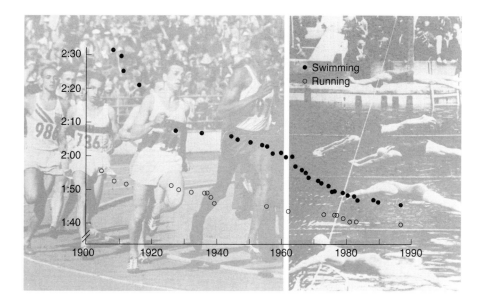

The development of world records in swimming and running is shown. Swimming speed for the 200 m freestyle has improved 27 per cent since the 1920s, whereas running 800 m has improved only 12 per cent. The left-hand photo shows Arthur Wint (of Jamaica) leading in the 800 m final at the 1952 Olympic Games in Helsinki (UPI photo; ressens Bild AB). One of the swimmers is Johnny Weissmuller, winner of five gold medals in the 1924 and 1928 Olympic Games, better known for his movie role as Tarzan. (From Harries, M. *et al* (eds.) (1998), *Oxford textbook of sports medicine* 2nd edn, OUP.)

years. The challenge remains one largely of applying the simple effective treatments and skills we have. Even so, there have been many transformations in the diagnostic and early management of overuse and soft tissue injuries. Imaging by ultrasonography has altered radically, but still depends greatly on the skill of the operator. Future developments might introduce computer assessments of findings, so that more clinicians can proceed with an initial expert assessment and accurate

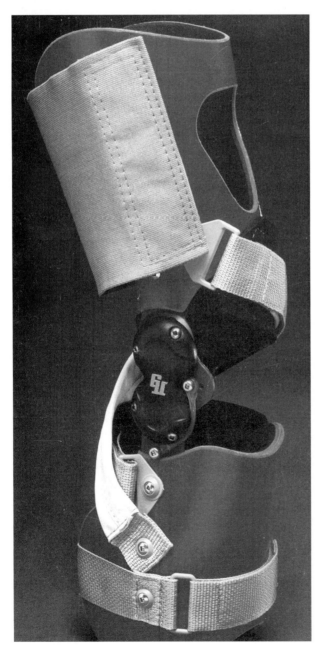

A custom-made derotation knee brace designed to control anterior cruciate instability. (From Harries, M. et al (eds.) (1998), *Oxford textbook of sports medicine* 2nd edn, OUP.)

diagnosis. Leading clinics now use active imaging techniques in the detailed diagnosis and interventional management of injury. For instance, direct vision aspiration or injection under ultrasound allows early precision techniques and quicker recovery. The place of soft tissue surgery — for instance, early exploration and treatment of tendon injuries — is well applied in leading units but remains alien elsewhere.

Physiotherapy continues to offer little except the enthusiasm of more intensive rehabilitation programs for those lucky enough to be treated.

The clinician continues to be the key to team medical care, and ideal preparation of teams will involve the close participation of doctors, physiotherapists, and psychologists well in advance of important championships. Among the routine duties is the medical screening of the team, and correction of any medical neglect.

One of the bizarre curiosities is ensuring that the team's females are indeed as advertised, an arcane ritual introduced by elderly male officials for female athletes, but not men. Doping is the bane of modern sport. Despite the millions of pounds and dollars thrown at the problem, clearly the issue has not been dealt with seriously and will not disappear. Indeed, the recent statement by the President of the International Olympic Committee that some loosening of controls might be reasonable, suggests that the problems may even get worse. This is of intimate importance to the sports doctor concerned with élite sport. Team doctors in Britain have been removed for refusal to cooperate in doping procedures and continued disclosures show that most sports are affected. All this symbolizes the ruthless pursuit of limitless achievement at any price. A well-quoted survey showed that young athletes would sacrifice lifespan and health for that moment of Olympic gold — and that survey predated the professionalization of amateur sport, when an athlete can acquire a lifetime's earnings in weeks, or even moments.

The sports doctor's role is complex at the top, but rather simpler at amateur levels. For most, the challenge remains of bringing a few well-worn clinical essentials to every practice.     PNS

*See also* ATHLETES; ORTHOPEDIC SURGERY

**STAMPS** In South America centuries ago the Incas sent messengers hundreds of miles aided only by knots on a length of string. Since ancient times the majority of the world has used writing. The messages and the container in which they were sometimes carried had marks put upon them showing their destination, occasionally the route by which they were to travel, and sometimes the distance. In 1840 a new system was developed in Britain, whereby the cost of transmission was covered by an adhesive stamp fixed to the message. The collection and study of adhesive postage stamps is known as philately.

The first adhesive postage stamp – the famous Penny Black of Great Britain – featured the head of Queen Victoria, as it was considered a design extremely difficult to forge. In the years since 1840 every country in the world has issued its own distinctive postage stamps. Because Great Britain pioneered the use of stamps the Universal Postal Union allows it to be the only country whose name does not have to appear on the stamp, only the monarch's head is necessary.

Last century it was common for collectors to try and obtain a copy of every stamp issued throughout the world. Nowadays, when tens of thousands of different stamps are issued each year, this is impossible. Collectors have, therefore, started limiting their field of interest. Postal issuing authorities have taken note of this change and deliberately issue stamps to cater for it. Stamps can provide, therefore, a secondary role for education, information, advice, and occasionally propaganda.

This diversity of design and subject means that collectors have been able to subdivide their fields of interest even further. An original theme of 'medicine on stamps', for example, can be broken down into RED CROSS issues, famous medical practitioners, anatomical drawings, plant medicine, and so on. These themes can be divided yet again at the whim of the collector into, for example, famous anesthetists, NOBEL PRIZE-winning doctors, human skulls on stamps, surgical operations, diseases, etc.

Collectors can have great fun tracking down an elusive point of interest on a stamp issue, for example, spotting medical 'howlers'; very few issues have spelt 'diphtheria' correctly, sometimes the wrong doctor is depicted, or occasionally some impossible anatomical condition is shown.

The American Topical Association, among others, has published a series of handbooks dealing with various aspects of medical philately. Several journals of special interest to medical philatelists are produced regularly, the American monthly *Scalpel and Tongs* and the British quarterly *Medi-Theme* are amongst the better known.

The Disinfected Mail Study Circle was founded in 1973 and publishes a quarterly journal, *Pratique*. Its foundation was due to the fact that until early this century, postal administrations considered that letters and postal packets could spread infection. To counteract any possible spread of disease the items were treated in various ways. These included slitting or punching holes in the surface, then fumigating them with superheated steam. Alternatively, they were toasted or

chemicals were sprinkled over them. They were usually handled with tongs.

The Medical Philately Study Group, founded in 1982 has a world-wide membership of doctors, dentists, pharmacists, and others. It is always happy to encourage anyone interested in both medicine and philately to contact them for the sharing of information.                JMDun

**STATISTICS** The term *statistics* initially referred to information summarized as numbers, specifically information about individuals which was relevant to the state. Thus the Romans and the Egyptians conducted regular censuses. Interest in collecting and interpreting statistics developed during the 19th century. Several learned societies were founded, including the Statistical Society of London (1834), later to become the Royal Statistical Society. Early work in statistics relating to medicine was directed towards issues of PUBLIC HEALTH. An early pioneer was Adolphe Quetelet, a Belgian astronomer who turned to social statistics, whose body mass index (weight/height$^2$) is still used as a measure of body fat. In Britain the physician William FARR (p 780) was appointed to the then newly established General Register Office, which was created to record all births and deaths in Britain. He stayed over forty years, during which time he made major contributions to vital statistics and helped to define classifications of diseases and occupations, which aided the collection and tabulation of statistics. Farr had studied medicine in Paris with LOUIS (p 780). Louis tried to introduce a more scientific approach to medicine based on the compilation and analysis of extensive patient records. By his 'numerical method' he showed (in 1835) that blood letting, then in common use, was ineffective.

A key figure in moving statistics to a higher level was Karl PEARSON (p 782). He was one of the most influential statisticians, not least because of his focus on using numerical information to try to answer specific scientific questions, such as the effect of heredity on personal characteristics. A famous study of his related the heights of parents to the heights of their offspring, using these measurements to illustrate his 'correlation coefficient' to quantify the degree of association. Pearson argued for the use of 'inferential' methods not just in medicine — a subject that became known as biometrics — but potentially into all aspects of science.

Between the two World Wars many developments in statistical methods took place in agriculture. A particularly influential figure was Sir Ronald Fisher, a British statistician. A key element of his work was the development of a systematic approach to designing scientific exper-

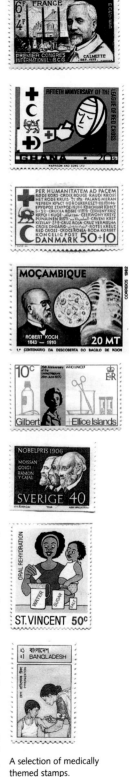

A selection of medically themed stamps.

## EARLY STATISTICIANS

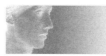

Pierre Charles Alexandre **LOUIS** (1787–1872). French physician. Working at first at La Charité, Louis was later on the staff of La Pitié and the Hôtel Dieu. A practical clinician, he attracted large numbers of students and introduced the 'numerical method' into clinical medicine, thus founding medical statistics. He analyzed large series of cases of pulmonary TUBERCULOSIS (1825) and of typhoid fever (1829), giving the second the name 'TYPHOID'.

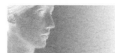

William **FARR** (1807–83). British physician and medical statistician. In 1839 he was appointed compiler of abstracts to the Registrar-General and was Commissioner of the Census in 1851 and 1871 and president of the Statistical Society in 1872 and 1873. Farr was the pioneer British medical statistician; he compiled life tables, tables of causes of death, and vital statistics.

(continued on p 782))

iments. Fisher developed the concept of randomization as a method for eliminating bias when comparing crop yields from areas of land treated in different ways.

Fisher's work was to have a profound influence on medicine, in particular through the work of Austin BRADFORD HILL (p 381). Bradford Hill is best known as the statistician who introduced the concept of randomization to medicine. In 1946 there was a new anti-tuberculosis drug called streptomycin but it was in short supply. Bradford Hill helped to design a controlled trial under the auspices of the Medical Research Council, in which random numbers were used to determine whether patients would receive streptomycin or not. This carefully designed first randomized trial (technically the first to be published rather than the first to be started) provided clear evidence of the effectiveness of streptomycin. It introduced many key features of controlled trials that are still practiced today.

The early post-war years were notable for developments in EPIDEMIOLOGY — studies of the causes of disease. Here too Bradford Hill was very influential. He developed criteria for considering whether an observed association may reasonably be thought to indicate a causal relationship. With Richard Doll he carried out a series of studies which helped to demonstrate, together with studies elsewhere, that smoking was a serious health hazard, especially in relation to the development of lung cancer. Their prospective study of British doctors was especially important, as most previous studies had been retrospective (and as a consequence less reliable). Hill and Doll were both subsequently knighted.

Over time, but especially in the 20th century, 'statistics' came to mean not just numerical information but also the collection of techniques developed for collecting, analyzing, and interpret-

ing information collected on individuals and groups, usually but not necessarily numerical. Although statistical methods include a lot of mathematical aspects, statistics, especially as applied in medicine, is as much about concepts as calculation.

### Types of medical research

Nowadays the primary focus of statistics in medicine is in medical research. The modern era may perhaps be dated to the publication in the *Lancet* in 1937 of a series of articles on statistical principles by Bradford Hill. Apart from treatment and causes of disease, statistical methods are also important to varying degrees in other aspects of medicine, including diagnosis and decision-making in general (for example, genetic counseling), interpretation of laboratory results, quality control, and audit. In essence, statistical methods are relevant to any medical activity that involves numerical information, from fetal ultrasound scans to forensic studies.

An essential idea that underlies all medical research is that we make observations on a sample of individuals and use them to make inferences about the population of interest. The term 'population' here does not mean the general population but a specific group of people. In medical research the population is often patients with a particular disease, such as epilepsy or diabetes. The validity of any inferences based on a sample of patients with a disease thus relies upon the sample being representative of all patients with the disease.

Systematic lack of representativeness is one form of *bias*, which is the main impediment to valid research. For example, a study of diabetic patients attending a hospital diabetes clinic may not be relevant to all patients with the same disease because they are a highly selected subgroup. Bias may also arise from a representative sample if observations are not obtained from some individuals; patients who do not agree to participate in a study or who do not complete their treatment are often rather different from those who do.

Medical research may be passive, in which patients are simply observed, or active, in which treatments or other interventions are evaluated. The choice of research design depends upon both circumstances and ethical considerations. The relative strengths of different types of study design may be assessed largely in relation to the potential for avoiding bias. The most reliable research results come from RANDOMIZED CONTROLLED TRIALS, studies which compare the effects of different ways of treating patients with some condition or disease. It is vital that the groups of patients receiving each treatment differ only in the nature of their treatment; otherwise the

## STATISTICS USED WELL: CHOLERA

Several others besides William Farr made good use of health statistics in England in the 19th century. John SNOW (p 48) investigated a CHOLERA epidemic in a localized area of Soho; he suspected that the cause was contaminated water from the Broad Street pump. When epidemic cholera returned to London in 1854, Snow was able to test his theory. He obtained the records of cholera deaths from the General Register Office, where William FARR (this page) was in charge; he ascertained the source of drinking water by visiting the homes where cases had occurred and worked out the death rates in relation to the source of the

water supply of affected houses (see EPIDEMIOLOGY — HISTORY). This was a convincing demonstration of the capacity of vital records to investigate and identify the cause of an epidemic. Florence NIGHTINGALE (p 548), like William Farr, was a Fellow of the Royal Statistical Society and the London Epidemiological Society. She designed a medical records system at St Thomas's Hospital, and showed how this could be used to compile statistics of hospital use and the outcome of medical care, both there and among wounded soldiers during the Crimean war.

comparison would not be fair. Bias is eliminated by letting each patient's treatment be chosen at random. ('Random' is a technical term meaning that all patients have the same chance of getting each of the treatments — it is equivalent to tossing a coin, although more complex procedures are used.) The ethical basis for this approach is that the trial is being carried out because doctors do not know which treatment is better. Many controlled trials compare a new treatment with the current best treatment. Controlled trials are also used to assess measures for preventing disease, such as health education or screening of apparently healthy people for early signs of life-threatening disease — for example, some cancers.

There have been hundreds of thousands of randomized trials comparing different health procedures or treatments. Most have been carried out in the last 20 years as, in the aftermath of the THALIDOMIDE disaster, governments introduced legislative requirements for the thorough testing of new drugs.

Whereas controlled trials are used to assess treatments, observational studies are needed to study the causes of disease. Such 'epidemiological' studies may be either retrospective, in which existing data are used, or prospective, when data are usually collected specifically for the study. Observational studies may involve relating different pieces of information obtained from a single group of individuals or comparing information from two pre-existing groups. These studies are prey to a wide number of potential problems that may lead to systematic differences between the groups and so to misleading findings.

Consider a study to see if there is an association between eating carrots and good eyesight. In a *cross-sectional* study people would be interviewed or complete a questionnaire to ascertain consumption of carrots and probably other foods, as well as demographic and clinical information, and they would have their eyes tested. It is then simple to see if there is a relation between the quantity of carrots consumed and their visual acuity. In a *case-control* study groups of individuals with poor eyesight (cases) and good eyesight (controls) would be identified and asked about their past consumption of carrots. Unfortunately, such recalled information is often unreliable. In a *cohort* study people with good eyesight would be classified according to their consumption of carrots and then followed up, perhaps for many years, to see which of them develop poor eyesight.

All of these designs have potential problems. If a clinical trial shows a clear difference in outcome between treatment groups we can reasonably conclude that the difference was the result of the treatments given. Findings from other types of study are open to many potential biases, and so their findings must be treated very cautiously. For example, an association found in a cross-sectional study would not necessarily indicate cause and effect, as it is possible that carrot consumption and eyesight are both affected by something else. The cohort study is the most reliable, but such studies take much longer to carry out.

### Basic principles

There are two basic approaches to statistical analysis. The more intuitive is known as *estimation*, in which we measure the aspect of interest in the sample and infer that the same applies in the population of similar subjects. For example, we may observe the average (mean) reduction in blood pressure in a sample of patients treated with a particular drug, or the difference between such means for groups of patients treated with

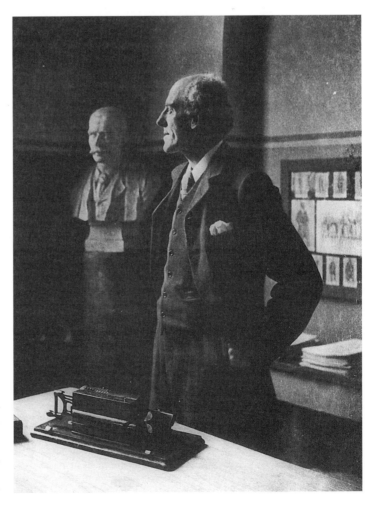

Karl Pearson (1857–1936), one of the most influential statisticians of his day. (Reproduced courtesy of the National Library of Medicine, Bethesda, MD.)

(continued)

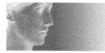

Karl **PEARSON**
(1857–1936). British biologist and mathematician. Pearson was appointed Goldsmith's professor of applied mathematics and mechanics in London in 1884, and in 1891 became Gresham professor of geometry. Thereafter he became increasingly interested in biometry and eugenics. In 1911 he was made the first Galton professor of eugenics. He founded the journal *Biometrika* in 1901 and was an influential teacher of statistics and biometry.

different drugs. A further, crucial aspect is that each estimate, such as a mean or a proportion, is accompanied by a measure of its uncertainty. A range of values is obtained extending either side of the observed value, which is highly likely (usually 95%) to include the true population value. This range of values is known as a *confidence interval*. Put simply, the estimation approach is one of measurement of the quantity of interest plus explicit assessment of uncertainty.

The alternative approach of *hypothesis testing* is much less intuitive. First, a 'null hypothesis' is set up, which is usually the opposite of the research hypothesis. It might be that two drugs are equally effective, or that smoking does not increase the risk of developing cancer of the colon. The second step is to collect relevant data and then calculate the probability of getting the observed data if the null hypothesis was in fact true. If this probability *P* is very small the null hypothesis is rejected in favor of the alternative — for example, that the two drugs do differ or that smoking does cause colon cancer. By convention a *P* value of 5% (1 in 20) is taken as the cut-off point for such an interpretation, so that if the *P* value is less than this level the difference or association is termed 'statistically significant'. This is the concept referred to when scientists refer to having significant results. Although standard practice, the value of 5% is arbitrary and has no clinical relevance.

The hypothesis testing approach dominated medical research for many years. Recently estimation has become more popular, although most papers still contain *P* values. The two approaches are in fact closely related mathematically, but their interpretations are different. There are several difficulties associated with hypothesis testing (often called significance testing). In particular, there is widespread practice of equating statistical significance with clinical importance. Thus an observed difference is taken as both real and clinically important only if it is statistically significant. Such inflexible use of *P* values may lead to important differences in interpretation when the data change slightly and so push the *P* value across the 5% boundary. By contrast, the estimation approach gives virtually the same results whether or not the extra patient is included, which accords with common sense. For the foreseeable future the most common presentation is likely to remain a mixture of both forms of analysis.

Statistical estimates based on small samples have considerable uncertainty, as shown by the wide confidence intervals. Sample sizes are frequently too small to allow a clear interpretation of research results. This is one of the motivations behind the recent development of methods to carry out a systematic overview of all the available research evidence on a topic, as discussed below.

## Methods of analysis

Many of the simpler forms of statistical analysis involve comparing two or more groups of patients. The data might be measurements, such as serum cholesterol concentrations or birth weight (known as continuous variables); they might be attributes, such as presence of a certain disease or symptom, or whether or not the individual was a smoker (known as categorical variables); or they might be the time elapsed since some event, such as diagnosis of a disease; and there are other types of data too. Different methods of analysis are used according to the type of data and the design of the study, but all fall within the estimation and hypothesis testing framework outlined above.

A large body of research takes a rather different line, looking at the relationship between the values of different variables measured in the same individuals. Pearson's correlation coefficient may be used to assess the strength of association between two variables — for example, between serum cholesterol concentration and blood pressure. A more useful, although closely related, approach is to use *regression* to try to predict one variable from another. Thus, for example, it is possible to obtain an equation to predict someone's blood pressure from his or her age. This type of analysis underlies the use of ultrasound measurements of a fetus to estimate the elapsed duration of the pregnancy and thus the expected date of delivery.

Regression is also used to make predictions based on values of several variables. Unfortunately, such predictions are usually imprecise for individuals. For example, there is major uncertainty in predicting a baby's birth weight, even though it is well known that birth weight is affected by the length of the pregnancy, the number of previous children the mother has had, the sex of the baby, whether the mother smokes, and some other factors. When the outcome of interest is not a measurement but an event which may or may not occur, the uncertainty is usually considerable.

It is common to compare an individual risk of an event in relation to the presence, absence, or amount of a risk factor. Thus we can say that a heavy smoker has a relative risk of about 10 for developing lung cancer. In other words, she is 10 times as likely to develop lung cancer as a nonsmoker. Even though one cannot make precise predictions for an individual it may still be valuable to make predictions based on data from large groups. An index of the relative risk of a particular event may be derived from a regression model. One such is the Dundee coronary risk score, used to estimate the risk of coronary heart disease within five years in relation to age, blood pressure, serum cholesterol concentration, and smoking behavior.

## Diagnosis

Considerable research effort is devoted to the development of improved ways of diagnosing a disease. The ideal *diagnostic test* is one which always gives a positive result for people who do have the disease in question, and always gives a negative result among those who do not. Such tests are exceptionally rare. The usual case is that the test will miss some patients with the disease (called false negatives) and wrongly identify some patients who do not have the disease (called false positives). The question then arises whether the test is reliable enough to be used in clinical practice. Various clinical considerations come into play here, as does the true prevalence of the condition among patients with the symptom in whom the test will be used. An example of a diagnostic test is the use of acute abdominal pain as a means of diagnosing appendicitis. Because such pain is not specific to appendicitis, some patients will have healthy appendices removed.

Similar considerations apply when SCREENING apparently healthy people for possible disease, such as cancer of the large bowel or heart disease. However, because disease is rare in the general population, even a small false positive rate can lead to the vast majority of patients with positive tests being free of disease. For example, suppose that 1% of the population has the disease of interest, that a test correctly identifies 95% of

## STATUES

For much of history societies have honored special persons or commemorated events by raising statues or building monuments. Statues of famous personages were erected in ancient Egypt, Greece, and Rome, but the practice lapsed until the 16th and 17th centuries. Then only sovereigns and their kin had the prerogative of an elevated public effigy. A notable exception was Fracastorius, who gave syphilis its name; his statue, the first to a doctor if we exclude Greek and Roman physicians, was placed in Verona in 1559.

In the 18th century other great men were acknowledged by public statues. One was Sir Hans SLOANE (p 56), the only person to combine the presidencies of the Royal Society (he succeeded Isaac NEWTON, p 544) ) and the Royal College of Physicians. His natural history collection was the nucleus of the British Museum. His statue was placed in Chelsea Physic garden in 1748, during his life.

The erection of statues was common in the 19th and early 20th centuries; not only were great men commemorated, but also many prominent only in their own community. Now the honor is given to few. The custom has been confined largely to Europe, and to countries ruled by those of European stock, such as the Americas and Australasia. It is proscribed on religious grounds by Jews and Muslims, but in Cordoba in Spain there are statues of the Arab doctors, AVERROES (p 768) and Al Ghafiqi, and also of MAIMONIDES (p 59), the great Jewish physician and Talmudist, who forbade making human likenesses in the round, though permitting it in painting and tapestries.

Many of the great names in medicine have statues in their honor. William HARVEY (p 363) at Folkestone, Ashford (Kent, outside the William Harvey Hospital), London, Oxford, and

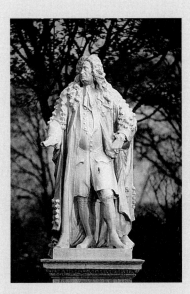

Sir Hans Sloane.

Cambridge; one which stood outside the Royal College of Physicians is now in the garden of a tavern in Willesborough, Kent. JENNER (p 452), of SMALLPOX vaccine fame, has statues in London's Kensington Gardens and St George's Hospital, Gloucester Cathedral, Boulogne, Tokyo, and Guatemala City; the second was unveiled in 1996, the bicentenary of vaccination. There is a large bust of LISTER (p 473) in London's Portland Place, and a handsome statue in Glasgow's Kelvingrove Park. There are many statues in Paris — including Claude BERNARD (p 102) outside the Còllege de France; PINEL (p 77) near the Salpêtière; and Bichat in the École de Médicin (also in Bourg-en-Bresse) — although many

were removed in World War II. Statues of LAENNEC (p 461) stand in Quimper in Brittany, Paul Bert in Auxerre, VESALIUS (p 846) in Brussels, SEMMELWEISS (p 479) in Budapest and Vienna, BOERHAAVE (p 121) in Leiden, Egas MONIZ (p 538) in Lisbon, FREUD (p 321) in London, and Ramon y Cajal in Madrid, where FLEMING (p 50) also has a handsome monument outside the main bullring.

Several military surgeons are commemorated by statues. Baron LARREY (p 796), Napoleon's chief surgeon, who introduced 'Ambulances volantes' to bring the injured back from the front line for surgery, stands outside the Val-de-Grâce, the French military hospital in Paris. Sir James McGrigor, first director general of the British Army's medical department, served with Wellington; he has a London statue near the Tate Gallery, and a 72 ft obelisk in Duthie Park in Aberdeen. That of another Scot, Sir James Wylie, is in the grounds of the Wylie hospital in St Petersburg; he was director of the medical department of the Russian war ministry.

Many doctors were famous because of their work outside medicine. There are statues to the authors Schiller (Vienna), RABELAIS (p 700) (Meudon and Chinon in France), NOSTRADAMUS (p 76) (Salon de Provence), and Oliver Goldsmith (Dublin). Clemenceau, the former French premier, has a statue in Paris, and SUN YAT-SEN (p 178) stands in Canton and Macao (and also has a bust at the Inns of Court in London).

Doctor-explorers are well represented. LIVINGSTONE (p 503) has five statues — in London (outside the Royal Geographic Society), Glasgow, Edinburgh (on Prince's Street near a statue of Sir James Young SIMPSON (p 43)), at Nassau in the Bahamas *(continued overleaf)*

(continued)

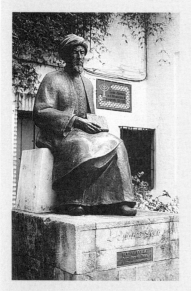

Maimonedes in Cordóba, Spain.

(in the gardens of the Ocean Club Hotel, the former home of the millionaire Huntington Hartford), and overlooking the Victoria Falls (which he named). His fellow Scot, Mungo Park, whose statue is in Selkirk, had died in Africa trying to find the source of the Niger river. Surgeon Major Thomas Heazle Parke has a statue in Merrion Square in Dublin. He went with Stanley in the famous rescue of Emin Pasha (also a doctor) and is commemorated

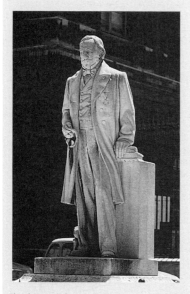

Claude Bernard.

by a stone cairn on the banks of the Nile. Edward Wilson was Scott's medical officer on his two Antarctic expeditions, and died with him on the return from the South Pole in 1912; Wilson's statue is in Cheltenham. George Bass, the British naval surgeon who discovered the Bass Straits between Tasmania and the Australian mainland, has a statue in Sydney. John Logan Campbell, an early settler in New Zealand and 'father' of Auckland, is commemorated there by a statue and a large obelisk. Paccard, a local doctor, and his guide Balmat were the first to climb Mont Blanc (in 1786); their statues are combined in a monument in Chamonix.

At some locations there are many statues. The senate of London University chose twenty-two worthies to grace the front of its building in London's Burlington Gardens, subsequently the British Museum's ethnography department and now part of the Royal Academy of Arts. Five were doctors — GALEN (p 321), Harvey, John HUNTER (p 398), John Locke, and Linnaeus, the botanist. In the Capitol Building in Washington, D.C. each state can place two statues of prominent citizens in the National Statuary Hall Collection. Six are of doctors: John Gorrie (Florida), the father of refrigeration and air-conditioning; Crawford Long (Georgia); Marcus Whitman (Washington); John McLoughlin (Oregon); Ephraim McDowell (Virginia); and Florence Sabin (Colorado), one of five women commemorated in the Capitol Building. There are also statues to Gorrie, Long, and McDowell in their respective states.

There are many other medical statues in the USA. Washington D.C. has statues to Benjamin RUSH (p 726), Samuel Gross, and HAHNEMANN (p 391), the father of homeopathy. Marion Sims is portrayed in New York, Columbia (S. Carolina), and in Montgomery (Alabama), where his son-in-law, John A. Wyeth, also has a statue. Statues of the MAYO brothers (Charles and William) and of their father, William Worrell MAYO (p 799), are in Rochester, Minnesota. Horace Wells's representation stands in Hartford, Connecticut, and that of Morton in Charlton, Massachusetts. Joseph Warren, who fought the British in the War of Independence, has two statues in Boston, Massachusetts. There is a statue of Hunter McGuire in Richmond, Virginia. Edward Livingston TRUDEAU (p 831) is commemorated at the Trudeau Sanitarium in Saranac Lake, New York, and William E. B. Davis in Birmingham, Alabama. In Canada, Sir William GRENFELL (p 299) has statues at St Anthony and St John's in Newfoundland; in Montreal there is a statue of Norman

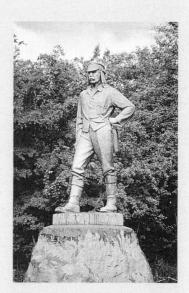

David Livingstone at Victoria Falls.

BETHUNE (p 180), who was a patient at the Trudeau Sanitarium; he also has a statue in Peking in China.

There are few public monuments to women doctors. Tavistock Square in London has a monument to the surgeon Louisa Brandreth Aldrich Blake, Dean of the London School of Medicine for Women (later the Royal Free Hospital School of Medicine). In the south island of New Zealand there is, in the small town of Waimate South, a statue to Margaret Cruickshank, the local general practitioner, who died herself of influenza after tending her patients during the pandemic of 1918.

There are statues to other local practitioners. Jenner, Park, Gorrie, McLoughlin, and Long, are mentioned above. In England, Sir James MACKENZIE (p 332), the cardiologist, has a monument in Burnley, where he practiced for twenty years. Bolton has statues to two local doctors, Chadwick and Dorrian, and Leamington Spa one of Jephson in Jephson Gardens. In Scotland, there are statues of John Grigor in Nairn, James Gorman in Rutherglen near Glasgow, and David Macbeth Moir in Musselburgh, near Edinburgh. In Wales, Evan Pierce stands on top of an enormous column in Denbigh, and in Llantrisant, there is a statue of William Price, the eccentric pioneer of cremation.

This account is necessarily brief, incomplete, and highly selective, but it gives a flavor of the high regard in which doctors have been held over the last few centuries.    NM

those with the disease, and only 2% of healthy people are wrongly diagnosed. This seems like a good test, but in fact only about 1 in 20 patients identified will have the disease, with serious implications of unnecessary worry and financial cost.

## Uncertainties of medical research

Research rarely provides clear answers to scientific problems. The usual pattern is a slow evolution of understanding until the truth emerges. Even the association between smoking and lung cancer, which is easily the strongest known effect of a common environmental influence, was not suspected before 1948, and was not widely accepted until twenty years or more after the first report suggesting the link. Most risks are very much smaller than those of smoking, so advances in the understanding of disease and the development of improved treatments are inevitably slow. Also, it is unavoidable that various false trails will be followed: the history of therapeutic medicine is full of abandoned 'wonder' treatments. Often the first optimistic reports are from small uncontrolled series of patients, and the new procedure is taken up enthusiastically. Subsequent controlled studies then show that the new treatment is ineffective, or at least no advance on existing treatments, and the wonder treatment is abandoned. An example was the use of gastric freezing as a treatment for ulcers, which was introduced, widely adopted, and then abandoned within eight years. Many treatments in current use have never been fully evaluated in controlled trials, such as epidural anesthesia in childbirth.

Also, because medical research studies often have small numbers of subjects, the inevitable consequence is that there will be much confusion, misunderstanding, and controversy. Some apparent controversies are simply due to the expected variation among several small studies, especially if using different methods. Others are, at least in part, due to inadequate statistical design or analysis.

Individual studies rarely provide a definitive answer to a research question. It is common for several similar studies to be carried out over several years, probably in several countries. A systematic review examines all the available reliable data to assess the evidence. Often it makes sense to combine the numerical information from them all, in a 'meta-analysis'. In recent years there has been a large increase in the number of systematic reviews, as part of the movement known as EVIDENCE-BASED MEDICINE. Usually such studies relate to controlled trials of treatment, but the same principles are now being applied more widely.                                                        DGA

**STIGMA** Any identifying mark or 'fingerprint' which is characteristic of a particular condition. The plural form stigmata when otherwise unqualified refers to marks, usually hemorrhagic or purpuric, located in the sites of the wounds of the crucified Christ; such marks are alleged or recorded as having appeared on the bodies of numerous saints, mystics, and others over the last 2000 years, as, for instance, those which were impressed on St Francis of Assisi on 15 September 1224 by a seraph with six wings. The full set of stigmata includes marks corresponding to the crown of thorns and to the spear wound as well as to the wounds on the hands and feet.

*See also* MARTYRS; SAINTS

**STROKE** See NEUROLOGY

**SUBSTANCE ABUSE** Since prehistory, almost every society has found a place in its practices, traditions, and values, for psychoactive drugs. These are substances used primarily for their effects on consciousness, mood, and the way we feel and react to the world around us and inside us. The appeal of such drugs may be a universal feature of mammalian biology. Rats, mice, dogs, monkeys, and other species may easily be trained to do work that is rewarded with small doses of alcohol, morphine, cocaine, amphetamine, sedatives, or tranquilizers. Human taste in drugs is similarly broad: the traditionally accepted drugs in pre-industrial societies were those found in the natural surroundings, regardless of their pharmacological actions, so long as they made the user feel differently from the sober state. Thus, alcohol, tobacco, coffee, tea, betel nut, coca, khat (qat), opium, cannabis, and kava all found acceptance in different societies long before heroin, cocaine, or barbiturates appeared.

In the brains of all mammals (and probably birds as well) there exist special nerve circuits that alert us to things we need for survival (such as food, water, sex), increase our attentiveness to them, and give us a sense of reward or pleasure when we use them. Conversely, things that threaten our survival activate other parts of this circuitry to produce negative feelings that make us avoid these things in the future. The psychoactive drugs appear to activate the same circuitry and produce effects ('reinforcement') that make us more likely to consume the drugs when we again become aware of their presence. This is how we come to 'like' them.

The intensity of the reinforcing effects varies from one drug to another (soft versus hard drugs), as well as with the dose given and how it is taken. Since drugs that are smoked or injected intravenously get into the brain much more rapidly than those that are taken by mouth or injected under the skin, the reinforcing effects are felt more rapidly and more intensely. For example, heroin injected intravenously or inhaled (by smoking or by 'chasing the dragon') carries a major risk of addiction, but may be taken by mouth as a cough remedy with relatively little risk.

Yet most users never encounter serious problems from these drugs, keeping their use within limits that avoid physical, mental, or social harm. This is because people have learned, from their own experience or from their elders, that the drugs may give rise to many problems.

Several different types of problems arise from using psychoactive drugs. If taken in excessive amounts, many produce distinctive patterns of acute intoxication, affecting alertness, judgement, speed and accuracy of reactions, muscular coordination, emotional self-control, and level of consciousness. Much individual and social harm may ensue such as automobile and other accidents, violence, impaired work performance, and foolish behavior that may harm interpersonal relations. At higher doses, vital physiological functions such as circulation and breathing may be affected. Many of the drugs (alcohol, barbiturates, heroin, and other opiates) may cause death by depressing breathing. Others (cocaine, amphetamines, ephedrine, and other psychostimulants) may cause death by excessive raising of the blood pressure causing brain hemorrhages, or by excessive increase in the heart rate and irregularity of the heart rhythm.

### Chronic health problems

Repeated and heavy use of these drugs can give rise to chronic health problems, such as alcoholic cirrhosis, septicemia from repeated unsterile intravenous injections of heroin or amphetamine; chronic bronchitis, and lung cancer from smoking tobacco or cannabis; and psychiatric disorders such as paranoid delusional states in heavy users of cocaine or amphetamines. Chronic exposure of the nervous system to these drugs may lead to adaptive changes. Such changes offset the drug actions and increase the user's tolerance, so that more drug than originally is needed to produce the same effect. Some of these changes are also maladaptive in that they constitute the basis of physical dependence, recognized by withdrawal reactions when the drug is suddenly stopped or prevented from acting.

The withdrawal reaction is generally opposite to the effects of the drug: if the drug (for example, alcohol or benzodiazepines) produces sedation and decreased excitability, the withdrawal reaction includes sleeplessness, hyperexcitability, and possibly convulsions. If the drug suppresses appetite and causes increased arousal, prolonged wakefulness, excitement, and euphoria (such as

cocaine or amphetamine), the withdrawal reaction includes profound depression, deep sleep, and voracious appetite. If the drug (for example, morphine) slows the movements of the intestines and thus causes constipation, the withdrawal reaction includes excessively rapid peristalsis, causing cramps and diarrhea.

Social problems may arise from chronically poor performance at school or work, loss of employment, family break-up, and social withdrawal because of criticism or ostracism by friends and family. If the drug is illegal, such as heroin, cocaine, or cannabis, the cost of continued heavy use may exceed the user's income and lead to theft, embezzlement, or fraud, or to prostitution or drug trafficking, in efforts to obtain the money needed to purchase the user's own supply. This in turn may lead to legal problems, if the user runs foul of the law.

### Drug abuse and addiction

This term is widely used in the lay press and the clinical and scientific literature. It is even part of the name of the National Institute on Drug Abuse in the United States. The term 'abuse' has been variously applied to any non-medical use, to use high enough to cause problems, or to any use of illicit drugs.

Probably the best definition of abuse is that given by the first 'drug czar' of the United States, Dr Jerome Jaffe, who wrote that drug abuse is 'any use that deviates from the approved medical or social patterns within a given culture'. It is essentially a term of disapproval rather than a specific description or explanation.

Like abuse, drug addiction has no universally accepted meaning. Under ancient Roman law, a person found guilty might be punished by being 'addicted' or given in bondage to a master. During many centuries, those who used too much alcohol or other drugs, and suffered some of the problems of acute intoxication or chronic excess, were regarded as being of bad character or weakness of will. The idea that such a person might be 'in bondage' to the drug, and not able to act with freedom of will, is a new one in human history. Although morphine had been isolated from opium in 1803, not until the invention of the hypodermic syringe, and the massive use of hypodermic injection of morphine to ease pain in wounded soldiers in the American Civil War, did physicians became aware of the powerful control that the drug could exert over the physiology and the behavior of some individuals.

### Adaptive changes

Most of those who receive a few injections of morphine or a related drug for postoperative pain do not experience intense euphoria or craving for the drug; instead, they usually have some nausea, dizziness, drowsiness, and loss of appetite, that are tolerable because of the welcome relief from pain. However, some of those in the American Civil War who received too many injections for too long developed adaptive changes, and if they tried to stop the drug they had a disturbing withdrawal reaction that might be promptly relieved by taking some more of the drug. This led to a self-perpetuating use of the drug, long after the original cause had gone, that came to be known as 'soldier's disease'.

Others found the immediate effects of the drug intensely pleasurable, and continued to inject themselves with morphine not for relief of pain, but for its rewarding effects now known to be produced by the action on the 'reward system' in the brain. The term addiction came to be applied to both these patterns of use, as well as to similar non-medical use of opium, cocaine, and various other drugs, whether injected, swallowed, sniffed, or smoked. For many years, the concept of addiction was dominated by the idea of physical dependence, as shown by the withdrawal reactions on sudden termination of drug use. Indeed, many people, including many physicians, still tend to equate addiction with physical dependence.

However, in the 1960s an expert committee of the WORLD HEALTH ORGANIZATION recognized that the two terms were not synonymous. Patients in hospital might experience physical dependence if treated with frequent doses of morphine for a long period because of severe chronic pain, yet once they recovered, they would probably not go searching for morphine or heroin in the illicit drug market. On the other hand, those who found the effects intensely pleasurable might become so engrossed in the search for the drug that their lives became disrupted even though they never experienced a withdrawal reaction. The committee concluded that the essential features of this form of drug bondage or addiction were the intense desire to use the drug, the preoccupation with getting it, and the inability to stop using it despite the serious problems attributable to the drug use. This is known as psychological dependence, and is always present in these cases, whereas physical dependence might or might not be.

The World Health Organization recommended that the term addiction should be dropped from use, with the problem being called drug dependence — which was primarily psychological and sometimes physical too. However, 'addiction' has continued to be used widely, and slightly different definitions or concepts of it continue to circulate.

## Causes

All humans have a 'reward system' in the brain, and indeed would not survive without it. Yet only a minority of those who try psychoactive drugs become addicted. In Canada, for example, 5–10% of adults who use alcohol are alcohol-dependent; the figure for marijuana is probably also in the range of a few per cent. Even with hard drugs such as heroin and cocaine, probably fewer than 20% of those who try them become addicted. Why are only some users affected in this way?

One factor is genetic vulnerability. Children of biological parents who are alcohol-dependent, even if they have been brought up by non-alcoholic adoptive parents since early infancy, have a three- to four-fold greater risk of becoming alcoholic than adopted children of non-alcoholic biological parents. A similar genetic risk may exist for addiction to other drugs. But many different genes appear to contribute to the overall risk: for example, some determine that the children of alcoholics are less sensitive to the unpleasant effects of alcohol when they first try it, and possibly more sensitive to the rewarding effects; other genes allow them to acquire tolerance more rapidly; yet others permit them to metabolize alcohol more rapidly, and therefore to eliminate it more rapidly from the body. There is similar evidence of genetic differences in the way the body handles other drugs. All of these separate genes contribute to the overall risk that a person may become dependent on a drug. Nevertheless, genetic predisposition does not cause dependence; most children of alcoholics do not become alcoholic. The genetic background merely increases the degree of risk.

Other environmental factors affect the probability of using enough drug to cause problems as a result. One is availability. The easier it is to obtain a drug, the more people tend to use it. Thus when the open hours of pubs in Britain were reduced during the First World War, the total consumption of alcohol dropped significantly, as did alcohol-related problems in the population. Another factor is price. The consumption of alcohol and of cigarettes has been found in many countries to be inversely related to their price, when corrected for changes in average income and cost of living. A similar relationship seems to exist for illicit drugs such as cocaine, marijuana, and heroin. Another important factor is social perceptions and beliefs that determine the approval or disapproval of a drug in a population at a given time. For example, throughout the 1980s the use of alcohol and marijuana by North American young people decreased steadily, because it was seen as not being compatible with the athletic outdoor life popular at that time, and the use of these drugs was regarded as not very clever or fashionable. Peer group pressure and social networking are important influences in the propagation of such attitudes for or against drug use. For reasons not entirely clear, that trend reversed in the early 1990s, and drug use has again become more widely accepted. Fad and fashion undoubtedly play a part in such changes of acceptance, and the example set by sports and entertainment figures, as well as the prominence of drug use in the media, probably contribute.

A third causal factor is individual emotional problems. Situational worry, anxiety, tension, frustration, depression, and schizophrenia all increase the likelihood of use of alcohol, cannabis, and other drugs. The ability of the drugs to relieve such problems even temporarily is another mechanism of reinforcement of their use, even though problems created by excessive use can eventually come to outweigh the relief. Much clinical interest is directed toward the problem of co-morbidity — that is, the concurrent existence of an alcohol or other drug problem and a psychiatric problem, that interact with and aggravate each other.

### Treatment of addiction

Given the many factors that cause addiction, not surprisingly various treatments have been used, with varying success. A few addicts recover spontaneously after some years. This is sometimes referred to as 'maturing out', and may reflect a spontaneous decrease in emotional or environmental factors that originally contributed to causing addiction.

Medical treatments are based on several principles. The first is reduction or complete cessation of use. If the person is willing to stop completely, the drug use may be discontinued abruptly (cold turkey) and benzodiazepines, clonidine, chlormethiazole, or other sedatives are given to minimize the withdrawal symptoms. Alternatively, the dosage of the addicting drug is decreased gradually until it may be stopped with no noticeable withdrawal reaction. The interruption of drug use is not by itself a full treatment of addiction because relapse is common unless the person is also helped to resist this with psychological and social measures.

Another principle, for patients unwilling to give up the drug entirely, is maintenance therapy to prevent withdrawal symptoms, but with a substitute drug that produces very little of the euphoria. For example, a heroin addict may be given methadone by mouth to replace intravenous heroin. During maintenance therapy, the primary goal is the patient's social rehabilitation after contact with the illicit drug environment has been broken.

A third principle is the treatment of psychiatric problems that may have contributed to the addiction. For example, the use of antidepressant, antipsychotic, or antianxiety drugs may make it easier to let the person stop using the drug of addiction.

A fourth principle is to use drugs to block the rewarding or reinforcing effects. In treating alcoholism, this first took the form of giving disulfiram (Antabuse), which blocked the metabolism of acetaldehyde (the first product formed from alcohol in the body), and thus caused the toxic acetaldehyde to accumulate. The hope was that the person who experienced the disagreeable effects of the acetaldehyde after drinking alcohol would stop drinking; unfortunately there is also the possibility that he or she will stop taking the disulfiram. More recently, drugs have been developed which may prevent activation of the reward system. Naltrexone, a blocker of the morphine receptor, prevents opiate drugs such as morphine and heroin from producing their reinforcing effects. Interestingly, it also prevents alcohol from producing these effects. Naltrexone has given very promising results for preventing relapse in opiate and alcohol addiction.

### Psychological treatments

Psychological treatments are similarly varied. Individual counseling or psychotherapy is usually directed toward solving situational or psychiatric problems. Group therapy enables the addicted person to share problems and derive support from others coping with the same difficulties. Self-help groups such as Alcoholics Anonymous and Narc-Anon provide such support on a non-professional and long-term basis. Various types of brief intervention, involving either the family physician or an addiction counselor, are designed for those who do not wish to take part in extended formal therapy, but seek simple guidance on how to cut down their drug intake to a harmless level. Such programs may also include coping skills training, to help the patient anticipate and avoid situations in which the risk of relapse is greatest.

Social therapies include measures by which addicted persons are forced to reshape their pattern of life by changing their environment, their friends, their beliefs, and their values, so as to build a drug-free life-style for themselves. These methods include long-term residential programs, some of which unfortunately have authoritarian and cultist overtones. A more benign form is constructive coercion by employee assistance programs to require employees whose job performance has been impaired by alcohol or other drug problems to accept treatment as a condition of continuing employment.

The results of treatment are better than is widely believed. If treatment is begun while the affected person is still employed, still has valued personal relationships, and has community support available, as many as 70% may recover from their drug-related problems.

### Prevention

Population studies have shown that there is no clear dividing line between normal use and dependent use of these drugs, with respect to the amounts used. Most users of any of these drugs (with the exception of tobacco or cigarettes) are occasional, light, or moderate users. Small numbers use larger amounts, the pattern being described by a smooth continuous curve with a low modal value and a skewed tail extending toward the high-use end. Anything that shifts the modal value of use by the general population also shifts the high end of the consumption curve in the same direction.

# SUDDEN INFANT DEATH SYNDROME

This term was first described by a group in Seattle in 1969 and was defined as: the sudden death of an infant or young child, which is unexpected by history, and in which a thorough post-mortem examination fails to demonstrate an adequate cause of death. Cot death is the same condition. There is a peak in prevalence between 8–17 weeks of age with a few cases occurring in the rest of the first year of life. More boys are affected than girls and the risk is increased in low socio-economic groups. There is an increased risk to the infants of young mothers, to infants with a large number of other siblings, and when there is only a short interval following the previous pregnancy. The risk is greater if the child is one of multiple births, is preterm, or is of low birthweight. There was a peak incidence in winter months but this has become considerably less marked during the past 7 years. Cot death is the most common cause of death in the age group one month to one year and despite extensive research the causes have not been found. For some cot deaths the cause, previously unsuspected, is found at the post-mortem examination, for example, a severe pneumonia or a severe abnormality of the formation of the heart; however, in most cot deaths no cause of death is found. At present it is considered that a combination of factors affect a baby at a particularly vulnerable stage of development.

The prevalence of cot death in England and Wales remained at about 2 per 1000 live births from 1971 to 1988 and then began to decline. Since 1993 the rate has remained at about 0.6 per 1000 live births. This trend has occurred in other western countries and has been attributed to the simple four-point advice in a campaign launched in Britain in November 1991. It should be noted that the incidence of sudden infant death syndrome had started to fall a few years before this campaign.

## Historical aspects

Cot death has been known since biblical times and was described in the famous Judgement of Solomon, when a baby was found dead in the mother's bed and it was considered that she had slept over the baby and suffocated him. (1 Kings 3: 21). Until recently, cot death was considered to be due to unintentional suffocation. Following the surge of research in the 1970s with more detailed investigation of the social background and post-mortem examinations by a pediatric pathologist, the theory of multifactorial causes was started and generally accepted.

Using the epidemiological risk factors research workers in Sheffield (Britain) delineated high-risk infants at birth who were then visited intensively by a health visitor (public health nurse). The incidence of cot deaths in the region was considerably reduced but similar results could not be obtained in other regions. The incidence of cot deaths in New Zealand was particularly high and a retrospective case-control study published in 1991 showed that 44% of cot death victims slept on their fronts compared with 3% of an unmatched control group. In the same year a Hong Kong study showed that 73% of cot death victims were found lying on the their fronts compared to 7% of controls. From 1956 there had been studies from different parts of the world of small groups of infants either with no or poorly defined controls which had come to a similar conclusion. Subsequent prospective studies identified three risk factors which were potentially amenable to change. They were prone (on their fronts) sleeping position of the infant, maternal smoking, and bottle feeding. These variables appeared to act independently. A practice of placing babies on their fronts was to reduce the risk of inhaling vomit. During the late 1960s and 1970s in special care baby units for preterm or sick infants, the practice was to nurse infants on their front. This was based on physiological studies which showed that oxygenation was more efficient in the prone position and regurgitation was reduced. Gradually the practice was used more generally without evidence that it was of benefit to the mature infants.

In 1991 an expert group on the sleeping position of infants and cot deaths convened by the Chief Medical Officer of England and Wales launched a national campaign to avoid the prone sleeping posture, to encourage reduction in maternal smoking, and to encourage breast feeding. Follow-up studies have shown that the majority of infants in England and Wales are now sleeping on their backs and the incidence of cot death has fallen although no scientific explanation of this fall has been found and several factors may have been responsible. In addition to the sleeping position, which has now been modified to ensure that the infants' feet are at the foot of the cot, the campaign emphasized the importance of preventing infants from becoming too warm by avoiding a duvet or baby nest. The importance of severe social adversity and poor parenting was addressed in the earliest intervention studies and it may be receiving better attention now.

A recent study from Italy showed an association between an abnormality of the newborn electrocardiograph (prolongation of the QT interval) and later risk of sudden infant death. This was a prospective study of 33 000 infants; half of the infants who died of sudden infant death had an abnormal electrocardiogram compared with none in the survivors. This suggests that if there is a family history of sudden infant death or other unexplained life-threatening events, selective electrocardiograms could be carried out in the newborn period. At present there is no evidence that treatment would be helpful for these infants at risk.

## Conclusion

The incidence of sudden infant death syndrome has fallen considerably during the last ten years although there has been little advance in knowledge of the causes. Although these infants usually have no or apparently minor symptoms before death, retrospective and prospective studies have produced checklists (Baby Check) which may be helpful to parents in deciding whether particular symptoms warrant medical attention and the speed with which this should be sought. Improved awareness of the significance of potentially lethal symptoms by parents and doctors and changes in local medical services as a result of the confidential inquiries may be important factors in the fall in the number of cot deaths. The Confidential Inquiries into Sudden Infant Deaths in Britain look into every infant death and ensure an assessment of the social background as well as the evaluation of the post-mortem findings. Discussion of these findings with the parents is an important therapeutic action in their grieving for the most dramatic event in their lives.          BV

Thus, increased price of the drug, decreased availability, and social disapproval of its use all tend to reduce use by the whole population and also by the heaviest users. All of these factors are used in efforts to reduce heavy use and dependence. For example, increases in taxes on alcohol and tobacco, efforts to increase street price of illicit drugs by intercepting the supply, and education campaigns to encourage non-use or low levels of use, all form part of the prevention strategy. For individuals, the most useful approaches are the early recognition of hazardous levels of use, and of warning signs of risk factors, followed by efforts to refer the affected person to physicians or agencies which offer help. The effectiveness of legal PROHIBITION for prevention is not entirely clear. On one hand, there is good evidence that the prohibition of alcohol in the 1920s did sharply decrease the death rate from alcoholic cirrhosis. On the other, it is not clear whether the legal prohibition of cannabis deters many adolescents from using marijuana. This topic requires careful scientific analysis, as a basis for wise policy decisions on legal restraints on drug use. HK

*See also* ALCOHOL; PATIENTS' ASSOCIATIONS; PROHIBITION; SMOKING AND HEALTH

**SUICIDE** is a major social, psychological, and medical problem. In most developed nations it is among the first 10 causes of death. Each year about 25 000 persons in the USA and about 5000 persons in Britain kill themselves. In men the suicide rate increases with age; in women the rate reaches a peak in the 50s and then gradually declines.

### History

In ancient Greece, suicide was in disfavor except under a few specific circumstances, such as incurable illness, old age, or grief. In the Roman Republic, with its emphasis on civic duty, moral virtue, and individual sacrifice, recorded suicide was predominantly of the heroic type; however, it was also permissible as an alternative to shame or chronic incurable disease. Early Christians, such as St Augustine, considered that suicide was a mortal sin and a crime because it precluded the possibility of repentance and because it violated the sixth commandment against killing ('Thou shalt not kill'). Social condemnation of suicidal behavior became embedded in legal and religious prohibitions.

After the social upheavals of the Renaissance and the Reformation was there some softening of the harsh medieval attitude toward suicide. Early studies linked insanity, alcoholism, physical illness, family conflicts, and love problems with suicide. As medical studies enhanced understanding of the deep-seated psychological reactions preceding suicidal acts, cultural attitudes began to change. Gradually the laws against suicide behavior were repealed; now few nations retain such legal restrictions.

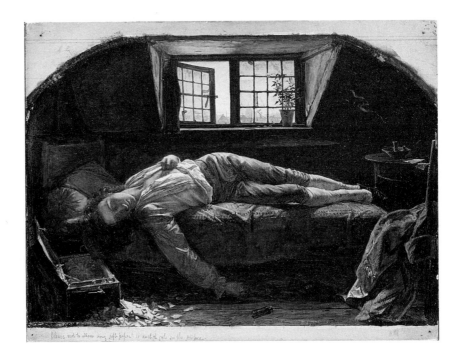

A tragic suicide. *The Death of Chatterton* by Henry Wallis, 1856. (The model for this painting was the novelist George Meredith.) (Reproduced courtesy of the National Gallery, London.)

The modern era of the study of suicide began at the turn of the 20th century with two main types of investigation, psychological and sociological, associated with the names of Sigmund FREUD (p 321) and Emile Durkheim, respectively.

In his classic sociological study *Le suicide* (1897), Durkheim used statistical comparative studies of suicide rates among different groups to support his argument that suicide is the result of a society's strength or weakness of control over the individual. He postulated three basic types of suicide, each associated with an individual's relationship to his society. One type, the 'altruistic' or institutionalized suicide, is required by the customs of the society. In India, since time immemorial, suttee has been practiced, influenced by the religious belief that death was followed by living again with the lost one. Most commonly wives, but also mothers, were burnt with the dead on the funeral pyre to avoid being separated from the lost loved one. Suttee is now forbidden by law in India, but it is still occasionally carried out. Although the altruistic type of suicide is rare today, it was more common in the past.

Most suicides in western countries are 'egoistic' — Durkheim's second category. Egoistic suicide is brought about by the individual's weak ties to or integration with the social group. The high rate among unmarried older men is accounted for in Durkheim's theory by their lack of ties to social groups.

The last category, 'anomic' suicides, occur when there is a traumatic disruption of the accustomed relationship between an individual and society. This results in weak social control and the resultant emergence of unrestrained self-destructive forces in the individual (for example, the divorced or those with loss of money or status).

Investigations in the USA and Europe show that suicide, as other forms of social deviance, occurs more frequently in the central business districts and contiguous areas of large cities. Suicidal behavior tends to be associated with urban districts that have high levels of social disorganization and social isolation.

Since World War II, suicidal behavior among the young has been recognized as a PUBLIC HEALTH problem of increasing importance. In most industrialized countries, the rates of attempted and completed suicide among young people have increased significantly. For example, suicide rates among young adults (aged 15–24) in the United States and Canada have trebled since 1950. Suicide rates among young people are particularly high in groups that have been marginalized, for example, by colonization of aboriginal societies in which cultural roots have been avulsed.

## Psychiatric and psychoanalytic contributions

Freud (1917) emphasized the importance of unconscious hostility and unresolved grief over lost loved ones (BEREAVEMENT) as causes of suicidal reactions. The loss or threatened loss of a loved person often causes the individual to turn his aggression unconsciously back upon the self in self-destructive ways.

The numerous psychiatric studies of depression and suicidal behavior have contributed to our understanding, but have not produced a broadly accepted theory explaining the complexities of suicidal behavior. The conscious and unconscious meaning of suicide varies with individuals, both in the same society and between different cultures. Some of the more important, predominantly unconscious, suicidal motivations include the following: a desire for escape, sleep, surcease, or death; a guilt wish for punishment, atonement, or sacrifice; a hostile wish for revenge, power, and control, or to punish and to commit murder; an erotic wish for masochistic surrender or for reunion with a dead loved one; and a hope for rescue, rebirth, rehabilitation, or a new life.

Systematic psychiatric studies in Britain and the USA show that at least 94% of those who commit suicide have a serious psychiatric illness. About half have a depressive illness, roughly one-

## FACTS AND FABLES ABOUT SUICIDE

Shneidman wrote about popular misconceptions of suicide: these are listed below, together with the authenticated facts demonstrated by those who have carried out research on suicide in the past sixty years.

• *People who talk about suicide do not commit suicide*. Fact: eight out of ten individuals communicate their intention to kill themselves before they commit suicide. Usually, they express their intention explicitly, although sometimes they may make indirect and non-verbal communications about their suicide wishes.

• *Suicide occurs precipitously and without warning*. Fact: studies reveal that nearly all suicidal persons give many clues, warnings, and threats concerning suicidal intentions.

• *Suicidal individuals are fully committed to dying*. Fact: most suicidal persons are ambivalent and undecided about living or dying, and they 'gamble with death,' leaving it to others to rescue them.

• *Suicide is a problem of lifelong duration*. Fact: individuals who wish to kill themselves most often are suicidal only for a limited period of time.

• *Improvement after a suicidal crisis means that the suicidal risk is over*. Fact: remobilization of suicidal morbidity can ensue after apparent improvement. The individual should be considered vulnerable for several months after suicidal crisis.

• *The poor or the rich are most likely to kill themselves*. Fact: all socio-economic strata are proportionately represented.

• *The propensity to commit suicide is inherited*. Fact: there is no scientific evidence that a self-destructive potential is inherited.

• *All suicidal persons are insane*. Fact: studies demonstrate that a minority of individuals who commit suicide are psychotic at the time of their death. Most suicidal persons are extremely unhappy and depressed.

quarter suffer from chronic alcoholism, and a smaller but significant number suffer from schizophrenia, borderline personality disorder, or drug addiction.

### Attempted and completed suicide compared

About ten times as many people make unsuccessful suicide attempts as commit suicide. More men than women commit suicide (about three to one) and more women than men attempt suicide (again about three to one). People completing suicide are considerably older (about 50) than the mean age of those who attempt suicide (about 34). Completed suicides tend to use more lethal methods, such as firearms and hanging, whereas attempters commonly employ drugs.

A basic difference between the attempted and completed suicide populations is the degree of suicidal intent. Persons attempting suicide show a continuum of suicidal intent ranging from a suicide gesture group, who show little or no suicidal intention; through a large group of ambivalent attempters; and finally to a serious suicide attempt group, who, like the completed suicides, have a high degree of intent to kill themselves. Many serious suicide attempters would die were it not for intensive medical efforts to save their lives.

### Treatment and prevention

Individuals posing a serious suicide risk are often referred to a psychiatrist and hospitalized in psychiatric hospitals. Treatment depends on the patient's needs and the clinical diagnosis. Individual, group, and family psychotherapy, electroconvulsive therapy, and the use of antidepressant drugs are the main therapeutic approaches.

The pioneer suicide prevention service, the Samaritans, was founded in 1953 in London and has over 150 centers in Britain. In the USA, the crisis intervention work and the suicide prevention services of the Los Angeles Suicide Prevention Service, established in 1955, have been widely emulated. Today there are over 320 suicide prevention centers in the USA. Typically they are 24-hour telephone answering centers that use both professional and lay volunteer staff to provide short-term crisis intervention services.

The study of suicide as an interdisciplinary subspecialty has developed since 1950. Most of those involved are also mental health professionals — that is, psychiatrists, psychoanalysts, psychologists, or social workers. Some are anthropologists, sociologists, clergy, or other professionals, and they, together with mental health professionals, are involved in suicide research, education, prevention, and intervention.                    TLD

*See also* PATIENTS' ASSOCIATIONS; PSYCHIATRY; SUBSTANCE ABUSE

**SURGERY, GENERAL — HISTORY** The origins of surgery in prehistory cannot be separated from speculation and fantasy. Trepanning or trephining is one of the early operations of which we have definite proof. There seems no reason to doubt the popular notion that it was to release some demon entrapped in the skull. Examples have been found dating back to 10 000 BC, in which the growth of new bone around the site of trepanning suggests that some people lived after the operation. The practice had evidently spread widely and trepanned skulls have been found not only in Europe but also in Mexico and Peru. However, none has been found in India, China, or Egypt.

The instruments used would clearly have been the implements available at the time and not specifically designed. Initially, flints are likely to have been used but eventually metal instruments would have become available. Flints would also have been suitable for scarification. Cautery at the site of an abscess or as a counter irritant over a dermatome related to a deeper internal pain (which is still common in the Middle East and the African continent) may also have been undertaken, but no proof remains.

### The primitive and ancient world

Speculation gives way to pictorial and written record about 2000 BC in Babylon, with the seal of the surgeon Urlugaledin and the stele (column) of the great law-giver Hammurabi defining a code of medical practice with some specific instructions serving to illustrate the development of the art of surgery by then:

> If a physician operates on a man for a severe wound (or makes a severe wound upon a man) with a bronze lancet and save a man's life, or if he opens an abscess (in the eye) of man with a bronze lancet and saves that man's eye, he shall receive 10 shekels of silver (as his fee).

From this time the rod and serpent Sachan, the signs of the god Ninazu and his son, Ningischzida, were used as symbols of healing. The existence of surgical implements from Nineveh fashioned in bronze with both smooth and serrated edges confirm the transition of medicine from something magical to a developing art determined by the experience of those engaged in its practice.

Accounts of Egyptian surgery are to be found in various papyri dating from about 2000 to 1500 BC. The EDWIN SMITH PAPYRUS (somewhat speculatively attributed to IMHOTEP (p 412), physician to King Zoser) gives a good but limited account of medicine in the 2nd millennium BC, and also suggests a link with Babylonian and Assyrian medicine. It shows that the art of examination and observation was already regarded as important in the clinical assessment which, in the developing science of surgery, had to precede treatment. In the papyrus there are records of detailed examinations of 48 patients and from these we know that the pulse was thought to be important in assessing patients with head injuries, and that wounds were probed to establish their depth before treatment. After such an examination it became possible for the surgeon to give some prediction of the probability of cure. Methods of wound closure and splinting are also given in some detail.

The EBERS PAPYRUS is a collection of medical texts. Some of the material belongs to an earlier period, but the rest records the extensive practice at the time. It is of surgical interest because of the account of CIRCUMCISION, which was apparently carried out at the age of 14 among Egyptians, Ethiopians, and Copts. Whether the reason was for hygiene or a supposed increase in fertility is obscure.

The Kahun medical papyrus from Faiyum, which is entirely devoted to gynecology, may mean that some specialization and instruction was organized in schools or through apprentices, as was the custom in surgical training in the Middle Ages. From the 3rd millennium BC, knives were probably used for evisceration before burial, as well as for circumcision and other simple operations. Formal anatomical records were not made until the Alexandrian School in the 3rd century BC.

Between the third and first millennium BC there were significant migrations into the Mediterranean Basin, bringing primitive civiliza-

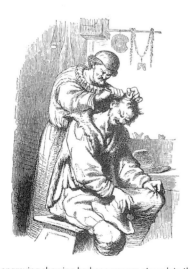

An engraving showing barber surgeons at work in the 17th century. (Reproduced courtesy of the Mary Evans Picture Library.)

tion and culture, which then spread to India. There was, therefore, a certain uniformity of medical practice spreading centrifugally from the eastern Mediterranean.

The development of INDIAN surgery, however, seems to have been in advance of that of classical Greece. An operation for fistula in ano and some plastic operations on ears, nose, and cheeks are described in sacred Indian texts such as the *Sushruta*. These included the most suitable incisions in different regions, indicating some knowledge of lines of stress and tension, which predate the formal description of Langer's lines. The use of metals in India and China preceded that in Europe and the Mediterranean Basin, and the availability of instruments must have indicated the development of surgery.

There is a tradition that acupuncture with metal needles was started in CHINA by the Emperor Shen Nung in the 3rd millennium BC. Castration was certainly practiced at this time and was accomplished by a combination of ligation and amputation.

## Classical times

More detailed documentation is available for the Greek world, about 500 BC. Initially, we learn from the Homeric writings such as the *Iliad* that wounds were accurately described and that there was considerable knowledge about extracting foreign bodies and stopping hemorrhage. Achilles binding Patroclus's wound is illustrated on the bowl of Sosia (5th century BC) and is, incidentally, an early example of the application of a spica (figure of eight) bandage.

However, the cult of ASCLEPIUS (p 710), which came to dominate medical thinking in Greece and Asia Minor, being introduced in Athens in 429 BC, was largely mystic, with little relevance to surgery. Such medicine as was practiced was by the priests rather than the laity, as in the Homeric period.

From the many cult centers in the Aegean a form of cleansing and treatment developed, which was to herald the start of medicine and surgery as both an art and a science. Traditionally, the school at COS with HIPPOCRATES (p 382) was the most important, although others, such as that of Alcmaeon of Croton, who practiced anatomical dissection, must surely have contributed.

The Hippocratic writings describe several surgical instruments — sounds knives, curettes, trephines, forceps, and specula — which indicate an increasing range of surgical skills. Some procedures, such as the reduction of dislocated joints, operations for fistula in ano, hemorrhoids, and cataracts, are also described in some detail. Pure, boiled water or wine was known to benefit wound healing, although there was no knowledge of asepis.

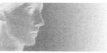

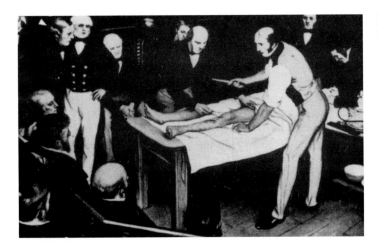

The first amputation under ether at University College Hospital, London, December 21, 1846, at which the young Joseph LISTER (p 473) was a spectator. (Reproduced courtesy of University College Hospital, London.)

The empirical school at Alexandria and particularly Herophilus of Chalcedon, who around 300 BC practiced both animal and human dissections, advanced anatomical knowledge. Its greatest development came when Heracleides of Tarentum in the 2nd century BC undertook operations for hernia, vesical calculi (bladder stones), and cataracts.

With the Roman Empire inevitably medicine reached a certain pre-eminence, and the documentation of this we owe largely to Aulus Cornelius CELSUS (p 806), who died about AD 50. In the sixth and seventh book of *De artibus* are detailed accounts of surgical procedures. The techniques he records and of which there was no good evidence previously are the resection of protruding fragments of bone in open fractures and of the omentum after penetrating injury of the abdomen. Operations for phimosis, abdominal paracentesis, gut anastomosis, and certain plastic operations, including one for exomphthalmos, are also described. Although he recommends excision for early breast cancer, he records that surgery aggravates the problem when the tumor is advanced.

A Greek physician who came to Rome was GALEN (p 324). Born in Pergamum, an ancient shrine of Asclepius, he was destined to dominate medical thought for some centuries. Of surgical interest, he records that an escape of air from the thorax indicates that a penetrating injury has perforated the lung, and describes the new technique of resection of the ribs and sternum for empyema and tracheotomy. Undoubtedly, procedures of this complexity were being attempted in various centers in the Roman Empire and perhaps even in the Orient. The lack of development of analgesia and ANESTHESIA were among the factors that clearly limited the possibility of undertaking more complicated operations. Probably Hua T'o, the father of Chinese surgery, had a greater

knowledge and access to opiates, allowing him to perform difficult procedures under the influence of narcotics. He had a powder that effervesced in wine and produced some anesthesia. ANTYLLUS (p 793), also from Pergamum, gave a good account of arterial aneurysms and details of exposure and ligation above and below. He discussed indications for PLASTIC SURGERY of the eyelid, nose, and cheek.

Actinus of Amida, a Byzantine writer of the 6th century, who studied medicine in Alexandria, described TONSILLECTOMY and ligation above an aneurysm of the brachial artery. The importance of Alexandria as a center of medical learning continued into the 7th century. The last great Byzantine physician, Paul of Aegina, who studied there in the mid 7th century, discussed in his *Epitome* cancer of the uterus and breast, recommending surgery. He gives detailed accounts of lithotomy (stone removal) with the patient positioned in what was to become the classic lithotomy position, and also repair of inguinal hernia by reducing the intestines with a sound and uniting the bulges on either side with sutures.

Important surgical writings gradually dwindled. Medicine, which had thrown off empirical priestly and mystic associations, to flower in the period of Hellenic philosophy and science and to be consolidated during the great period of the Roman Empire, declined. Many of the ideas and traditions of Greek medicine, however, were kept alive in the Arab world.

## Arab legacy

The schismatic dispute in AD 431 involving Nestorius and the Patriarch of Constantinople caused the former to flee with followers to Mesopotamia, where a medical school was eventually established. This had far-reaching implications for surgery in that the Greek writings and thought were preserved. Even when the Nestorians were subsequently expelled from Edessa, they took their libraries with them to Jundishapur, which was to become the nucleus of the Muhammadan tradition of surgery. Some of the Greek documents were translated by Hunain ibn Ishaq, and when he was eventually appointed court physician to Al-Mamun, Caliph of Baghdad, the center of learning was transferred there and became an important center with a large hospital. Here Al-Razi (RHAZES (p 59)) came from Teheran to study in the late 9th century, and it was from Baghdad that he published his encyclopedic medical work, *Hawi* or *Continens*. This records bleeding by cupping and the applications of leeches. It also suggests the use of animal gut for suturing wounds, which is therefore traditionally attributed to Rhazes.

Among the writings of this time is the *Canon* of AVICENNA (p 60). This Canon suggests that pig bristles should be used for sutures, and also has the first main reference to obstetric forceps for extracting a dead fetus. Despite the advances for which he was responsible, his acceptance that surgery was a separate branch of medicine to be practiced by inferiors, took centuries to eradicate and undoubtedly hindered surgical progress.

The Arab world embraced the Mediterranean Basin not only in the east but also in the west, with an important presence in SPAIN. Albucasis, born in Córdoba in AD 936, kept alive the ideas of Paul of Aegina, which he disseminated in the *Altasrif* within the western Arab world. It became a valuable surgical source book with good accounts of the techniques of cautery, lithotomy, and amputation.

## Medieval renaissance

The reawakening of surgical interest and practice in Europe was in a climate of thought created by religious dogma that was certainly restrictive, if not openly hostile. Although St Benedict of Nusia had founded a monastery at Monte Cassino in AD 529, whose work was largely directed towards healing, the belief in the evils and uncleanliness of the body was firmly held. It was considered wrong even to cut for stone — especially as the site of the operation required the exposure of parts of the body not fit to be observed. A further blow was dealt in 1215 by Pope Innocent III, who formulated the views of the Church in *Ecclesia abhorret a sanguine*. Shedding blood was thought to be so abhorrent that occupations which entailed bloodshed were relegated to the lowly strata of society.

It was against this background of opinion that surgical activities, even of monks committed to surgical work, had been restricted by the Council of Tours in 1163. However, the Church was unable to stop the Arab influence coming back into European culture. Constantine the Moor, born in Carthage in AD 1010, eventually arrived in Monte Cassino in AD 1072 and translated the *Pantegni* of Heli ibn al Abbas, an Arabic version of an original Greek text, into Latin. The section devoted to surgery discussed suturing methods, the ligating of blood vessels, fractures, and inflammation. None of this was new, but when reintroduced to Europe it was natural that it would be looked at objectively. One center where this happened was SALERNO (p 448). Constantine himself had been there before going to Monte Cassino and the city was already a center of healing and destined to have one of the first universities. *Regimen sanitatis Salernitanum*, by tradition compiled and edited by John of Milan, was published from Salerno. This and *Practica chirurgiae*, compiled in

1170 by Guido Aretino (a pupil of Roger Frugardi, who was one of the most distinguished surgeons of this period in Salerno), bear witness to the preeminence of this university in medicine and surgery. This remained so for some 150 years, with the *Practica*, or *Rogerina*, being developed through several editions (for example, *Glossulae quatuor magistorium super chirurgium Rogerii et Rolandi*) as the most important working surgical treatise of the time, with sections on wounds of the head, fractures of the skull, and diseases of the neck and limbs.

In addition to the preoccupation of surgeons with battle wounds, they now began to think about such matters as incision as opposed to cautery in healing (Guglielmo SALICETTI (p 446) in *Cyrurgia*, 1210) and the differential diagnosis of benign breast lumps and cancer (Lanfranck, *Chirurgia magna*).

## Foundation of European surgery

The French School was pre-eminent in the 14th century. Lanfranck, in addition to technical achievements, clearly understood that a knowledge of medicine was also essential for the surgeon. The belief that he should not merely be a technician but a physician who practices surgery — and able to appreciate and be able to meet the whole needs of the patient and his family — was suggested by Lanfranck's contemporary Henri de Mondeville. He wrote about the qualities of the ideal surgeon, including the need to counsel both the patient and relatives about prognosis.

Among the technical advances, Lanfranck's pupil Jehan Yperman described a metal shield for allowing cautery at small precise points. The great Guy de CHAULIAC (p 320), surgeon to three popes, wrote a comprehensive textbook of surgery (1363), in which he described radical cure for hernia, but he is perhaps popularly remembered now for the chain hoist still seen hanging over many surgical beds. His textbook of surgery was translated into English (the *Questyonary of surgeons*), French, Provençal, Dutch, and Hebrew. It maintained its importance until the writings of Ambroise PARÉ (p 320) 200 years later.

In England, the Guilds of Barbers and Surgeons (officially recognized in 1368) increased in importance and began to exercise jurisdiction over the practice and standards of the profession. A system of apprenticeship was established by the early guilds, but it was not until 1629 that this was eventually supplemented by a series of lectures.

Barber-surgeons performed venesections and many operations in France. Ambroise Paré was at first refused admission to the College of St Come because he could not write Latin and was, therefore, considered unworthy of the honor. The court, Church, and universities had a somewhat

(continued)

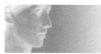

**Dominique-Jean LARREY** (1766–1842). French military surgeon. After training Larrey became a surgeon in the navy (1787) but later transferred to the army. He was *chirurgien aide-major* in 1787, director of medical services on the Egyptian expedition (1798), and became inspector-general of the health services of the army in 1805 and professor at the Val-de-Grâce. He introduced the 'ambulances volantes' in 1793 and traveled with the army through Germany, Austria, Spain, and Russia. Napoleon regarded him with affection and respect, leaving him 100 000 francs in his will.

(continued on p 798)

greater influence on the structure of the developing profession in the rest of Europe than the guilds and colleges in England.

Some important English surgeons emerged at this time. John of Gaddesden, physician to Edward II and probably the model of Chaucer's doctor of physic, and John of Mirfield spanned the 14th century. From their writings, *Rosa anglica* and *Breviarium Bartholomei*, respectively, we get a good idea of clinical practice at this time. They described injuries, hygiene, diet, and dressings. The development of surgical techniques clearly changed little during this time but John of Mirfield is credited with observing that an injury on the right side of the head may lead to paralysis on the left side of the body.

The greatest English contribution during the 14th century was that of John of Arderne. His experience was obtained largely on the battlefield, but the writings for which he is justly remembered were on fistula in ano. Until his detailed account of treating it with a grooved probe, ligature, and scalpel, his contemporaries considered it as largely incurable. His manuscript *De arte phisicale et de chirurgia* (1412) is a good record of his practices.

Despite the importance of surgeons to the armies of Europe, over many generations, they remained socially and academically inferior to physicians. The development of specialized techniques did nothing to remove this trend.

It was not unnatural that surgeons and barbers, being denied university education, should protect their interests by forming guilds. In France during the 13th century the Collège of St Come was founded (or refounded, for Malgaigne states that it was originally established in 1033) and to some extent protected the interests of surgeons. In Britain a Company of Barbers and the Guild of Surgeons fulfilled a similar function between 1300 and 1540, when the two merged and were incorporated in the City of London as the Company of BARBER-SURGEONS, with Thomas VICARY (p 91) as first Master. Not until 1745 was the definitive Company of Surgeons founded, and until 1840 that it was given a royal charter. Progress towards academic and social acceptance had been faster on the European continent, and, as early as 1672, Louis XIV of France had ordained that public demonstrations of surgery be given annually in the royal garden.

By the mid-16th century the barber-surgeons, phlebotomists, and the traveling lithotomists were fused into a recognizable profession in Europe, with leaders emerging in each country. One of the greatest of these was Ambroise PARÉ (p 320).

He started life as a military surgeon and arrived in Paris in 1532, ignorant of Latin and Greek but with an intelligence and originality which were to dignify surgery and leave us with the important and immortal concept that, although the surgeon dressed wounds, God healed them. Compared with his personality and independent mind, and the fact that he helped release surgery from dogma, his reintroduction of ligatures in amputation and belief that treating gunshot wounds with boiling oil harmed the tissues were modest advances. His contemporaries in Britain were William Clowes, who described ligating an omental mass and leaving long tails on the ligatures so that they could be extruded and William CHAMBERLEN (p 493), a Huguenot who designed the midwifery forceps. An ingenious technique was introduced about this time by Jean Tagout of Belgium, who in 1543 described the injection of alum and silver into a sinus tract to find where a bullet had lodged. These were minor advances and somewhat pedestrian compared with lithotomy or cutting for stones so skilfully practiced by Jermain Colot, Pierre Franco, and Frère Jacques, who developed an approach lateral to the midline to avoid damaging central structures.

**Anatomical and pathological understanding**

The rising status of surgeons and commitment to their profession inevitably led to an interest in anatomy. Andreas VESALIUS (p 846) and his contemporaries in the Italian school founded the modern science of anatomy in the 16th century. This had been stifled by religious scruples between the 2nd and 16th centuries, except for the remarkable textbook written in 1316 by Mondino de Luzzi (Mundinus) of Bologna. Vesalius performed dissections in BOLOGNA (p 447), Pisa, Basle, and PADUA (p 447), which formed the basis of his book *De humani corporis fabrica* published in Basle in 1543. Gabriel Fallopio, a pupil of Vesalius, succeeded him as professor in Padua in 1551. He is chiefly remembered for his description of the human oviducts.

Although a human body had been dissected publicly in Venice in 1308, resistance remained, largely from the Church, and in Britain it was not until 1540 that the barber-surgeons were given permission to have four bodies each year to dissect (although clandestine dissection had been carried out frequently in the past). The first proposal that the Company of Surgeons in England should build an anatomical theater, was by Michael Andrews in 1636; it was opened two years later.

Surgeons were understandably preoccupied with the organization of their profession, raising standards of surgical practice, and improving the education of barber-surgeons' apprentices. Society was still served by quacks and pseudosurgeons, including cutlers, cooks, tooth-drawers, sow gelders, and witches, who had little honesty and skill in surgery. However, out of the disorder important figures emerged. John Woodall is remembered surgically for abandoning the method of amputating gangrenous limbs by cutting through the dead tissue below the line of demarcation of viability; he recommended cutting through the healthy tissue above. His *The surgeon's mate* (1617) was a comprehensive surgical handbook for ships' surgeons, their mates, and probably ships' captains who found themselves without a surgeon on board and might need information about instruments and their use in accident surgery, bowel obstruction, and other topics. The range of operations was limited and the art of surgery still primitive as a result of sepsis and the lack of anesthesia.

Many leading surgeons, despite the knowledge in basic sciences developing in parallel, were both critical and scornful of attempts to investigate the causes of disease rather than concentrating on surgical technique. Operations without anesthesia on a delicate organ such as the eye demanded great manual dexterity. Understandably, therefore, many thought that surgery could not be refined or advanced further. In 1734 Percivall Pott, assistant surgeon to St Bartholomew's Hospital, took a contrary view:

> Many and great are the improvements which the chirurgical art has received in the last 50 years, and many thanks are due to those who contributed to them; but when we reflect how much still remains to be done it should rather excite our industry than inflame our vanity.

This reference to vanity reflected the mental attitude of many of his contemporaries, who were not only individualists but had fixed ideas preventing their accepting or seeking any innovations apart from minor modifications in technique.

Surgery then largely entailed removal of any affected part. The lack of knowledge about the cause and treatment of infection prevented surgery from being used for anything but minor conditions such as hernias. Operations on the body cavities were extremely dangerous. However, developments took place during the 18th century that mark an important advance in the approach to various serious clinical problems.

The true founder of scientific surgery in the 18th century was undoubtedly John HUNTER (p 398). His scientific argument, with a clarity of inductive and deductive reasoning, allowed him to approach and solve problems far ahead of others of his generation. This was seen not only in his ability to advance surgical technique but also in his enunciation of the general principles of inflammation and their application to various diseases. He always tried to link structure and function and to know not only the diseases but their causes. The founder of the science of experimental and surgical pathology, he could convince his generation, and subsequent generations, that processes of disease could be studied scientifically.

The scientific approach to PATHOLOGY and the understanding of function are most strikingly displayed in John Hunter's (Hunterian) Museum at the Royal College of Surgeons in London.

The time had now arrived for the European tradition to be carried to the New World. Philip Syng Physick was an American pupil of John Hunter, who having qualified in Edinburgh returned to Philadelphia in 1792. His inventive and unrestricted American mind brought modifications in techniques and instrumentation. With Alexander MONRO (p 41) of Edinburgh, he became the first to wash out the stomach, and undertook CESAREAN SECTION in 1824. He designed a wire snare for removing tonsils, and a flexible pewter cannula for insertion into the ventricle of the brain through a trephine hole. He was the first full professor of surgery at the University of Pennsylvania — a position he held for 13 years.

A great American tradition developed. Henry Jacob Bigelow of Boston was an inventive genito-urinary surgeon who favored crushing bladder stones and bladder irrigation, designing his own instruments. A similarly ingenious surgeon, John B. Murphy, developed a 'button' for end-to-end anastomosis of the intestine. Charles McBurney is remembered for his grid-iron abdominal incision for appendicectomy. The international pre-eminence of W. S. HALSTED (p 746) and of Harvey CUSHING (p 537), the leading neurological surgeon, both of JOHNS HOPKINS HOSPITAL (p 840) in Baltimore, consolidated the position of American surgery. Halsted introduced his radical mastectomy in 1882, and Cushing's classic monograph on pituitary diseases and surgery was published in 1912.

In 1881, a year after von MIKULICZ-Radecki (p 798) had operated on a patient with a perforated peptic ulcer, Theodore BILLROTH (p 518) successfully removed a carcinoma of the pylorus (distal aperture of the stomach). This was a momentous step in surgery, acclaimed the world over. It was, however, the third hazardous operation he had introduced, for in 1872 he had resected the esophagus and in 1873 performed a laryngectomy. Not until 1897 was total gastrectomy undertaken by Schlatter. Such developments attracted many visitors from around the world. Travel was not easy, but these visitors could then reproduce the complex operations in their own countries.

(continued)

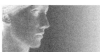

Johann Von **MIKULICZ-RADECKI** (1850–1905). Polish surgeon. After serving as Billroth's assistant, Mikulicz-Radecki became professor of surgery in Cracow (1882), Königsberg (1887), and Breslau (1890). One of the leaders in abdominal surgery he devised the esophagoscope and was the first to operate in a mask and cotton gloves. He described the enlargement of lacrimal and salivary glands known as Mikulicz's syndrome (1892).

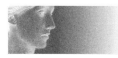

Robert **LISTON** (1794–1847). British surgeon. He was the first British surgeon to operate on a patient under ether anaesthesia. His splint (the 'long Liston') is still occasionally used today.

(continued opposite)

## Pain and anesthesia

Many potions and concoctions have been used through the ages to relieve the PAIN and suffering of injury and surgery. Opium prepared from poppy seeds and Indian hemp (*Cannabis indica*) were known to the ancients, as well as mandrake (*Atropa mandragora*) and henbane (*Hyoscyamus*). More recently alcohol was employed for its analgesic and paralytic qualities. Joseph Priestley discovered nitrous oxide in 1772, and Humphry Davy experienced its ethereal qualities in 1799, suggesting that it might be used for the relief of pain. The discovery of morphine and its soporific effects by Friedrick Wilhelm Sertürner in 1806 was another important milestone.

In January 1842 William Clarke, a medical student, used ether while a tooth was extracted from a friend, and Long, of Athens, Georgia, gave ether later in 1842. William Morton used it in a public demonstration in Boston in 1846. Chloroform was popularized by James SIMPSON (p 43) of Edinburgh, when on 15 November 1847, he anesthetized a 4-year-old patient. The benefits that followed the introduction of general and local anesthesia were inestimable. They were to release the patient from fear and pain, and surgeons from the need to exercise excessive speed. Anatomic dissections were to become possible and injury to tissue was to become less. The surgeon could seek a better anatomical and physiological solution to operative problems. Anesthesia was to prove the catalyst of surgical development between 1850 and 1950, when John Gillies introduced hypotensive anesthesia to reduce the loss of blood during surgery. Since then the supportive role of anesthetics has diversified even further, with resuscitation, CRITICAL CARE, and pain control.

## Infection

The tide of history has often been ruled by disease and plague. In surgery, infection remained, after anesthesia, as the factor preventing its advance. The key to a greater understanding of surgical infection had existed since Alexander Gordon of Aberdeen claimed in 1795 that infection and fever were carried from woman to woman by MIDWIVES. However, not until Ignaz Philipp SEMMELWEISS (p 479) in 1846 formulated his doctrine of puerperal fever was the message clearly received.

Joseph LISTER (p 473) started his medical studies at University College Hospital the year after Semmelweiss published his views on puerperal fever (though he did not hear of his discovery). As a child he had developed an interest in microscopy from his father, who had been made a fellow of the Royal Society for work on microscopical lenses. By 1860 Joseph Lister was appointed regius professor of surgery at Glasgow. His contributions to general surgery were important by any standards, devising an amputation of the thigh through the condyles (1860), a new operation for excision of the wrist joint (1865), radical mastectomy planned on anatomical principles (1867), and various operations and instruments for urethral surgery. However, as we read in the *Lancet* in 1855, the excision of the wrist joint led to six cases of gangrene and one of pyemia.

Fortunately, Lister was acquainted with the growing influence of the ideas of PASTEUR (p 620). This led him to speculate about how micro-organisms could be destroyed by some chemical agent. Lister himself had seen carbolic acid used to disinfect sewage at Carlisle, and hence he tried carbolic acid in a case of compound fracture in 1865. Initially it was applied undiluted with lint. This damaged the tissue, so that in 1866 he mixed the carbolic acid with linseed oil and common whitening. The cases of compound fracture on which he used this less-damaging mixture were recorded in the *Lancet* in 1867. Nine of the 11 patients were alive with intact limbs 6 months after surgery. With the confidence of this success he recommended that even silk ligatures should be carbolized to prevent secondary sepsis and hemorrhage at the site of ligated vessels.

In an attempt to kill the micro-organisms in the air which might settle on wounds and lead to infection Lister attempted to operate within a sterile environment, created and maintained by a small hand-spray filled with dilute carbolic acid. Even though this was developed into a more powerful steam projected spray, Lister abandoned it in 1887. However, his recommended simple gauze dressings impregnated with carbolic acid were used widely until 1889, thereafter being replaced by gauze impregnated with mercuric cyanide and zinc. His thinking was generally accepted and immediately led to developments such as that by Karl THIERSCH (p 653) of Munich, who, in 1874, introduced a method of skin grafting which would otherwise have been impossible.

Although this method did much to reduce sepsis, the latter still occurred, and Lister's shrewd surgical judgement led him to advocate the adoption of India-rubber drains, first used by Chassaignac in 1859, to allow any pus that might form to drain away freely. Lister's great contribution to surgery resulted from his ability to relate advances in other fields to those of his own, and to solve problems that had eluded surgeons for generations. Perhaps this can be described as genius; Lister's mind was, happily, not as inward-looking as those of his surgical contemporaries, and therein lay his greatness.

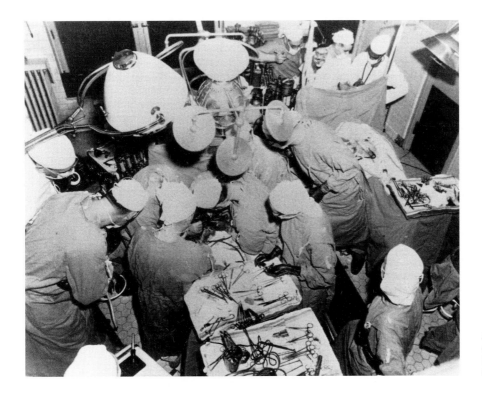

A view from above the operating room during Lillehei's 1954 first cross circulation operation.

## Modern times

The surgery of trauma and WAR has always been a sad and urgent necessity and has, through the ages, led to advances. One notable development, which became an important and life-saving advance, resulting from the impetus of war, was the science of BLOOD TRANSFUSION. This had been anticipated in the 16th century when Hieronymus Cardanus and Magnus Pegeius suggested cross-transfusion. Between 1814 and 1836 James Blundell at Guy's Hospital in London demonstrated the value of cross-transfusion in resuscitating exsanguinated dogs. George Crile of Cleveland in 1907 successfully performed transfusions in seven patients. Thereafter, work on blood groups, anticoagulation, and the preservation of blood enabled transfusion to become a realistic possibility, and the collection and preservation of blood was an important by-product of the First World War.

PLASTIC SURGERY was stimulated by the work of plastic surgeons, such as Sir Harold Gillies at this time and subsequently Sir Archibald McIndoe in rehabilitating badly burned air-crew during the Second World War in Britain.

The miracle of penicillin, discovered by Alexander FLEMING (p 50) and later developed during the Second World War with dedication and single-mindedness by Howard FLOREY (p 52) and E. B. Chain, would not have been possible in

a time of peace and security. Apart from the impetus of two world wars, progress in elective surgery was steady. Ingenious surgeons began to take liberties and make advances establishing them as pioneers in the new science. This was justified once the pain, mortality, and morbidity of infection, as well as shock, had been reduced to an acceptable level. Almost all organs now became amenable to elective surgery.

In 1885 Sir Victor Horsley carried out physiological experiments on the function of various parts of the brain. He developed an antiseptic modeling wax from beeswax and almond oil to reduce the bleeding from the edges of cranial bones. Although he did not fully appreciate the mechanism, he found that applying living muscle tissue to the bleeding surface of the brain reduced hemorrhage. In 1887 he successfully removed a tumor of the spinal cord — the first operation of its kind.

TUBERCULOUS disease was a widespread scourge. Various methods of draining tuberculous abscesses were devised, in conjunction with artificial pneumothorax, which temporarily rested the lungs. Occasionally tuberculosis appeared to demand removal of part of the lung. This reached a sufficiently advanced stage in 1931 for Rudolf Nissen to achieve complete removal of one lung.

After the initial success with intestinal surgery in the second half of the 19th century, Vincenz

(continued)

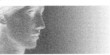

William Worrall **MAYO** (1819–1911). Mayo was the founder of the Mayo Clinic in Rochester, Minnesota: later joined by his two sons, William James (1861–1939), American surgeon; and Charles Horace (1865–1939), American surgeon. The sons established the Mayo Foundation for Medical Education and Research, affiliated with the University of Minnesota. Charles Horace Mayo was specially skilled in surgery of the thyroid gland, while William James Mayo had a special interest in surgery of the stomach.

Czerny resected the upper esophagus in 1877 for cancer, and Franz Torek removed the thoracic esophagus in 1913. Removal of the small and large bowels for tumors, diverticular disease, vascular lesions, and regional enteritis became common. Success depended on great skill and also on techniques learned from those thought of as the old masters, but who were merely the great men of the previous generation; the specialty was moving fast.

Pediatric surgery did not lag behind, despite the specialized anesthetic techniques required. Conrad Ramstedt in 1912 described two cases of severing the muscle fibers in the stomach (pyloromyotomy) for congenital hypertrophic pyloric stenosis. The abundance of vascular injuries produced an early interest in vascular surgery. Von Eck joined the portal vein, draining the liver, to the inferior vena cava (the first portacaval anastomosis) in 1877, and Berkeley Moynihan excised an aneurysm of the subclavian artery, in 1895. It was not, however, until 1944 that John Alexander and F. X. Byron successfully resected a congenital stricture (coarctation) of the aorta. The modern age of vascular surgery was ushered in when, in 1964, Michael De Bakey used synthetic Dacron grafts to repair blood vessels.

In the early days elective, or so-called 'cold' surgery (as distinct from emergency surgery), had understandably been preoccupied with solving mechanical problems. Stones had been removed from the bladder from early times, and by 1905 Howard Lilienthal had reported 31 suprapubic transvesical prostatectomies without death. This was refined by Terence MILLIN (p 838), who in 1945 described retropubic prostatectomy. Intestinal obstruction from various causes and perforated peptic ulcers posed little problem now for surgeons, and the mortality of cesarean section, even for placenta previa, first undertaken by A. C. Bernays in 1893, was now acceptably low. Delicacy of technique and perfection of sutures allowed the restoration of continuity of even small structures such as the bile duct, which was accomplished by W. J. MAYO (p 799) in 1905.

Classically, operations had primarily been directed towards solving mechanical problems, and clinical benefit resulted with restoration of function. Many interesting physiological observations were ultimately made on the alteration of function of organs before and after such surgery. Renal failure and diuresis, for example, were studied in patients after surgery for urinary obstruction. Astley Cooper undertook experimental thyroidectomies in animals to elucidate the changes seen after the technical problems of thyroidectomy (for goiter obstructing the larynx). These had been mastered by pioneers such as Theodor Kocher, who published a series of 13

thyroidectomies in 1872 with only two deaths. In studies of function after surgery, physiologists and physicians worked closely with surgeons. It soon became evident that surgery was a tool by which normal function could be altered and also through which physiological normality could be restored, after removal of an abnormally functioning organ.

**Endocrine operations**
An early example of normal function being altered by surgery was castration, which had been practiced from the earliest times — initially on those in charge of harems and subsequently to prevent the breaking of voices of ecclesiastical choristers. In 1881 tubal ligation for sterilization was introduced by W. P. Langren and, in recent times, both oophorectomy and adrenalectomy (respectively, removal of the ovaries and of the adrenals) have been used to alter the hormone environment of certain tumors, such as breast cancer, in an attempt to reduce their dissemination.

Given a greater understanding of thyroid function and its control of the basal metabolic rate, Sir Patrick Watson in 1872 undertook a partial thyroidectomy for exophthalmic goiter. The first subtotal thyroidectomy for this condition was done by Ludwig Rehn in 1884. The possibility of ablative endocrine surgery having far-reaching metabolic consequences led to a close association between physicians and surgeons, heralding a new cooperation between specialists with differing but complementary skills.

**Heart transplantation**
A similar cooperation was to exist in heart surgery. The optimal timing of surgery was clearly within the discretion of the physician as well as that of the surgeon. Such a cooperation enabled Henry Souttar in 1925 to attempt breaking open with a finger a narrowing of the mitral valves through the upper part of the heart. Subsequently, Dwight Harken of Boston used instruments to achieve the same result, in 1948. Two other successes in cardiac surgery took place, first when Robert Gross in 1939 successfully ligated a connection between the pulmonary artery and the aorta (patent ductus arteriosus) in children, and later when Alfred Blalock in 1949 joined the left subclavian and left pulmonary artery to reduce the effect of the congenital abnormality of Fallot's tetralogy.

After the development and insertion of artificial, mechanical, and denatured animal valves into failing hearts, with considerable clinical success, the ultimate goal in cardiovascular surgery appeared to be transplantation of a healthy heart from a donor who had suffered irreversible brain damage. Such a dramatic achievement was accomplished in man by Christiaan

Barnard in 1967. This followed considerable pioneering work in many laboratories throughout the world, possible only through enormous advances in understanding of IMMUNOLOGY. However, many scientific and ethical problems were posed by the achievement; techniques had, to some extent, advanced too rapidly.

Organ TRANSPLANTATION had been a dream for generations and had become a reality in the mid-1950s when Hume performed nine kidney homotransplants in patients and Goodrich undertook the first successful liver transplant in man. However, despite the initial enthusiasm for spare-part transplantation surgery, the problems of immunological rejection, availability of organs, finance, and ethics all dictated that the apparent ultimate goal might not be so. In 1982 the first artificial hydraulic heart was inserted into a patient.

The topic of ORTHOPEDICS illustrates what has, in many respects, been a happier revolution, raising less controversial ethical and financial problems. In addition, the surgical techniques have developed in parallel with related disciplines, such as those of immunology. After the days of external fixation of fractures, the inevitable progress to internal fixation took place with plates and intramedullary nails. By the mid-1960s, the development of biologically inert implantable material was such that satisfactory artificial hip joints of varying design were being widely inserted, after pioneering work in many centers. These demanded a high technical ability and a close liaison with mechanical engineers and chemists, who developed biological cements.

Clearly, such a stage of complexity and technical skill has been reached in various branches of surgery that the classic concept of general surgery has become somewhat outmoded. It will, however, always remain the training ground of all super-specialists, and within it there will always be aspects of special expertise demanding skills and experience equal to those that are now regarded as the specialized branches of surgery. These have previously been organ-specific, such as ophthalmology, or system-specific such as gynecology and gastroenterology, but may in future need to be disease-related.

All general surgeons treat cancer, for example; the multidisciplinary approach required now dictates that, at least in some specialized centers, there should be surgeons who have a greater commitment and knowledge in this aspect. At one time cancer surgery meant merely more radical surgery, as when Wertheim in 1900 developed his radical hysterectomy or when Ernest Miles of the Royal Marsden Hospital, London, undertook the first synchronous combined abdomino-perineal excision of the rectum. Now, however, cancer surgery is undertaken in close association with physicians who supervise chemotherapy and radiotherapy. A new aspect of specialization within general surgery has been born and is now called surgical ONCOLOGY.

The general surgeon is now being confined to history. With technical developments — lasers, endoscopes, invasive radiology, joint implants, and tissue banks, to name but a few — super-SPECIALIZATION is required. The range of operative skills developed by each surgeon (such as microvascular anastomoses) becomes limited and the training more targeted. This may now involve simulated virtual reality training, with complicated models leading to accepted standards of proficiency and specialist accreditation. The expectation of the public is greater, and surgical audit is now in the public domain, with complications and success rates being available not only for procedures but also for the operators themselves. This is demanded by the public and the profession after a certain inertia is now meeting this expectation.

Pressure of funding has led to a rapid development of MINIMALLY INVASIVE SURGERY with great benefit — particularly in reducing the time in hospital and the morbidity of surgery. This depends on the expertise of anesthetists and much of the work is now carried out as a day case. Scars are smaller and healing is rapid. The removal of the gall bladder and appendix lend themselves particularly to this technique. Fiberoptic technology and flexible instruments have brought with them amazing advances, not only in treatment but also in diagnosis (for example, stomach lesions) and even preventive medicine (such as the removal of pre-cancerous colonic polyps).

For some years laser beams have been used to destroy small lesions such as laryngeal polyps and cervical erosions. Now there is the possibility of photo-sensitization of some lesions with chemicals, so that they are selectively susceptible to laser beams of tuneable wavelengths.

A variety of implanted manufactured joints, pacemakers, pumps, and erectile devices are being developed by bio-engineers working in close collaboration with clinicians, but for some indications this will probably be superseded by tissue culture and gene engineering. Human ingenuity leads inevitably to new ways of solving age-old problems.

In the 16th century Ambroise Paré defined the duties of a general surgeon 'to remove what is superfluous, restore what has been distorted, separate what has grown together, recreate what has been divided, and redress the defects of nature'. Although the developments since then have been momentous, the contention of Percivall Pott that much still remains to be done and that this should 'excite our industry' is as true today in third millennium as it was in 1745.                    HWhi

# SYPHILIS

Syphilis, except when it is endemic or congenital, is a SEXUALLY TRANSMITTED DISEASE. It is caused by a bacterium, a spirochete, *Treponema pallidum*. Before the advent of penicillin, it was the most serious of the venereal diseases, the others being gonorrhea and chancroid. Historically, it has been called *lues venerea*, the pox, the Spanish, French, and Neapolitan disease, reflecting periods in its romance. OSLER (p 602) at the start of the 20th century stated that to know syphilis was to know medicine. In its time it has infected millions. Its control depends on effective PUBLIC HEALTH surveillance combined with good clinical services for sexually transmitted diseases. Where this does not occur, as today in Russia, India, parts of Africa, and in some black populations in the United States of America, it is still frequent.

There have been several often controversial classifications of syphilis, and it is easier to divide it into early (infectious) syphilis and late syphilis. After infection there is an incubation period of 10 to 90 days before the primary stage occurs. In the primary stage, there is an ulcer called a chancre, at the point of inoculum, be it penis, vagina, anus, or mouth, with enlarged lymph nodes locally. Blood tests for syphilis become positive during this stage. If untreated at some variability, but usually 6–8 weeks later, secondary syphilis occurs. A rash, which may often be atypical, appears affecting the skin and mucous membranes. There may also be constitutional symptoms such as fever and feeling off-color. These symptoms gradually subside leaving the patient in the early latent stage which may be up to two years. Syphilis is considered to be contagious in these stages.

Control depends on excellence in diagnosis, the organism being demonstrated by a microscopical technique, dark field examination, and verification of positive tests in the blood specific for syphilis. Usually a prolonged course of penicillin by injection is required. In certain clinical cases other antibiotics of the tetracycline, macrolide, or cefalosporin groups may be used. Partner notification and contact tracing are essential in well-controlled public health systems.

If the diagnosis is not made the disease enters the latent period. There are no symptoms or signs of disease but blood tests are positive.

After the period of latency, late manifestations of syphilis will appear in some of the untreated patients. These may occur from three years onwards, but often much later, 10 to 20 years after infection where serious forms of neurosyphilis, such as tabes dorsalis and general paralysis, may occur. The heart and aorta may be affected in cardiovascular syphilis. Though all these late manifestations are uncommon now in western societies, occasional cases are still seen. A rare late manifestation is a gumma, a mass of syphilitic diseased tissue which can affect the skin, the muscles, and the bones. Although prolonged courses of effective antibiotics help to some extent, damage to major structures is often irreversible.

Congenital syphilis is rare in societies where the level of syphilis is low, and where there are effective public health, obstetric, and pediatric services combined with antenatal screening for syphilis. The fetus is infected through the placenta of an untreated infected mother. It may abort. There may be a stillbirth, or a specific sign of congenital syphilis may occur after birth and on into adult life. Some more frequent signs are called stigmata of congenital syphilis.

Some treponemal diseases, although caused by treponemes, are probably the same as *Treponema pallidium*, but are not venereally acquired, and generally do not damage the nervous system or the heart or blood vessels but may cause unpleasant and disabling effects on the muscles and bones. They are often contracted through close body contact in moist, warm, unhygienic conditions in childhood. Endemic syphilis used to occur in Iceland, Scotland, the Baltic States, and Bosnia, and still occurs in Kurdistan and parts of southern Africa. It has to be differentiated from yaws, caused by *Treponema pertenue* occurring throughout the Tropics, and pinta, caused by *Treponema carateum*, occurring in South America, both of these presenting with skin manifestions in childhood.

In parts of the world where ulcerative sexually transmitted disease is common and where HIV infection is spreading, syphilis is thought to be a factor in the transmission of HIV infection. In Europe and North America it has been noted that in HIV immune suppressed individuals, the treatment response in syphilis may be depressed.

Like many of the chronic infectious diseases, syphilis, because of its rarity in western countries, is forgotten about by some physicians, but it is an old adversary which needs constant respect. MAW

*See also* EHRLICH; TUSKEGEE SYPHILIS STUDY

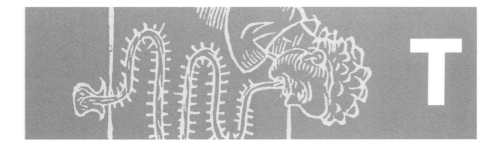

**TATTOOING** produces an indelible mark or design on the skin by introducing permanent dyes through a needle puncturing the epidermis into the dermis. Transmission of hepatitis B is an obvious hazard when the instruments are inadequately sterilized. The word 'tattoo' is derived from the Tahitian *tatu*, which means a puncturing. In Britain, except for Northern Ireland, the tattooing of persons under the age of 18 is forbidden by law.

**TELEMEDICINE**, medicine at a distance, is an umbrella term for many separate applications of electronic medical care. It depends on transmitting clinical information from one location to another electronically. For example, teleradiology involves capturing a digital X-RAY image and transmitting it to a different site for display. Telepathology requires a system that can capture an image from a microscope, transmit it, and display the image at a remote site. Teleconsulting involves videoconferencing equipment installed at both the local and remote site so that doctor and patient can see and talk to each other. Diagnostic equipment of this sort can also be used for education and the broad definition of telemedicine covers the whole range of medical activities including education and treatment.

Distance education in medicine is a well-tried technique, likely to be increasingly important in future as teaching hospitals become more and more specialized, and pressures on the participants' time grow ever greater. Distance treatment includes telesurgery, where a surgeon operates on a patient at a distance with the aid of remotely controlled instruments. In contrast to distance education, there has been little clinical experience of distance treatment and it is difficult to envisage a mainstream role for it in routine health service practice.

Most telemedicine activity around the world concerns the third aspect — that of diagnosis and clinical management at a distance. Great things are promised for this sort of telemedicine: the decentralization of healthcare delivery beloved of politicians, bringing improved access for rural communities, accelerated referrals, better communication between primary and secondary care,

and reduced costs. There is, however, little proof of cost-effectiveness. This is important, because few healthcare providers are likely to implement new techniques on an appreciable scale without solid evidence that they are at least as good as traditional methods. Regardless of the lack of formal proof, certain telemedicine applications, such as teleradiology, have become major commercial successes, especially in the USA. Other telemedicine applications, such as telepathology, remain the subject of intensive research effort. Teleconsulting applications lie somewhere between these two extremes. Although the main work occurred in the 20th century, particularly in its last 20–30 years, the history of telemedicine is much older than that.

### Pre-electronic telemedicine

Diagnosis and treatment at a distance have been practiced for hundreds of years. The scientific basis of Greek medicine is well known but the Greeks also practiced religious healing. Sufferers could stay overnight at a major TEMPLE, allowing the priest to act as an interpreter for Gods such as ASCLEPIUS (p 710). This kind of healing was probably cheaper and more accessible for the patient than using the services of a physician directly — something that is still being claimed for telemedicine 2500 years later.

Telemedicine was also practiced in the Middle Ages. There is at least one recorded instance of a physician examining a patient for PLAGUE in 1666, with the patient and doctor on opposite sides of a river to minimize the risks to the latter. It was also common for wealthy families to send urine samples to their doctor, who could use a urine chart to arrive at a diagnosis.

The development of national postal services in the mid-19th century facilitated prescribing by post: a sick person would write to an eminent physician enclosing his medical history. The physician's reply would include a diagnosis, directions for a regimen, and a prescription. Prescribing by post was also practiced well before national postal services were established, and there is a well-documented example from 1726.

### Electronic telemedicine

Telemedicine really developed with the expansion of electronic communication. Initially analog methods were employed, but these have been largely supplanted by modern digital communication techniques.

*Telegraphy* Telegraphy — signaling by wires — began in the mid-19th century and was used for distance medicine. For example, equipment was developed which permitted an X-ray film to be transmitted by telegraph, a forerunner of the fax machine in many ways. In the USA teleradiology for dental X-ray films was offered as a commercial service as early as 1929. In much of Europe and the USA the telegraph was rapidly superseded by the telephone as a general means of communication. However, because of the enormous distances in Australia telegraphy survived much longer. In a famous episode in telemedicine the telegraph was used to instruct a postal official how to perform first a perineal and subsequently a suprapubic cystostomy on a patient with severe pelvic injuries in an inaccessible region of north-west Australia.

*Telephony* The telephone has been used for medical work since its invention in the late 19th century and is still widely used for this purpose. However, the telephone may be used for other purposes than voice communication. As early as 1910 a tele-stethoscope was described, which amplified the sounds from a stethoscope and transmitted them through the telephone network. Similar devices are still in use today to permit a physician to carry out remote auscultation using low cost equipment. Other medical uses for the ordinary telephone network include the transmission of electrocardiograms using a computer modem and also the use of fax machines. An episode of brain surgery by fax has been recorded in the case of a rural emergency. The telephone network is now becoming widely used as a method of providing INTERNET access to medical information.

Although the newer methods of telemedicine are often criticized for lack of formal evidence of cost-effectiveness, almost no such evidence exists for techniques such as the fax and the telephone. One of the few scientific studies that has been carried out, a randomized control trial, showed that regular telephone calls to patients with hypertension were effective in improving compliance and controlling blood pressure.

*Radio* At the end of the 19th century, communication by radio became possible, initially by Morse code and later by voice. The potential of radio to provide medical advice for seafarers was recognized very quickly, and by the 1920s most of the maritime nations had established their own services. In Italy, for example, over 35 000 shipborne patients were treated by radio in the 60 years from 1935. The growth in long-distance air travel has brought a new medical problem: the provision of medical advice to passenger aircraft. In-flight medical incidents which require professional help occur at a rate of about 1 in 50 000 passengers carried. In cases where there is no doctor on board, airlines maintain an on-call service, by which the aircraft captain can obtain radio medical advice from the ground.

Television closed-circuit television was used in the 1950s by the Nebraska Psychiatric Institute for consultations between specialists and general practitioners. Another early example of television was its use for the provision of medical care to travelers at the Logan International Airport (Boston) from doctors at the Massachusetts General Hospital. Subsequently there has been growth in such techniques with the wide avail-

## TREATMENT BY TELEGRAPH

**(1917): excerpt from the obituary of John Joseph Holland (1876–1959)**

"In 1952 Holland received the CBE for the invaluable work he had done for the Ambulance Services in Western Australia. His interest in this work dated back to his Kanowna days. One of his pupils in first aid was a postal official named Tuckett. In 1917 Tuckett was the postal official at Hall's Creek. A man, James Darcey, fell from his horse, and was brought in a distance of 40 miles over extremely bad country by his brothers. Darcey's condition was critical. He had severe pelvic injuries and retention of urine. It would have taken a week to get him to the nearest doctor at Wyndham, and of course, he could not have survived. Then was enacted the epic case of treatment by telegraph.

Wires were sent back and forth between Tuckett and Holland several times a day, each wire (the first of 279 words) costing about $40 (perhaps $5000 in today's money). There were pages of them, at a total cost of about $600. Holland instructed Tuckett how to perform first of all a perineal and later a suprapubic cystostomy. There was immediate relief; but it was arranged that Dr Holland and a nurse should go up, as Darcey's condition was precarious. The 2000 mile journey in those days presented many difficulties. Because of regulations, Dr Holland had to sign on as a cattleman on the SS *Moira*. From Derby he set out for Hall's Creek with Jack Haly, and after a nightmare journey, partly by car, partly by horses, through terrible country and crocodile-infested creeks, they reached their goal. Twenty miles from Moolaboola natives brought word that Darcey's condition was deteriorating. They drove their 'T' model Ford all through the night at top speed in order to maintain the lights. (It was the first time a car had been driven at night in the Kimberleys.) They arrived at Hall's Creek to find that Darcey had died three hours previously. A post-mortem examination disclosed that the operations had been skilfully performed, there was no sepsis, no peritonitis, and the kidneys were normal. There was a very large spleen and it appeared that the patient had succumbed to a very severe malarial attack, starting two days previously.

When Dr Holland returned to Perth he was met on the railway station by Dr John Flynn. He recounted his adventures, and said: 'The next time I go to Hall's Creek, I'll fly'. 'Good idea', said Flynn. It was at that moment that the seed of the Royal Flying Doctor Service for our north-west was planted, and we all know how it has borne fruit. Dr Holland was one of the founders of this service, and always took an active interest in it."

(Holland JJ. Obituary. *Medical Journal of Australia* 1959; **1**: 549–50.
©Copyright 1959 *Medical Journal of Australia* — reproduced with permission.)

ability of videoconferencing. Indeed, the costs have now fallen to the stage where much of the equipment is based on personal computers.

***Wireless communication*** The development of mobile phones has allowed mobile telemedicine, and current research includes the transmission of slow-scan video pictures from ambulances, as well as emergency electrocardiogram transmission from the roadside. Wireless techniques also include the use of satellite communications. One of the first uses of telemedicine in the developing world was the use of a low-cost satellite system to enable internet access (for e-mail) for healthcare workers.

## Conclusion

There are two reasons why telemedicine is used: either because there is no alternative, or because telemedicine is better than traditional medicine. Thus telemedicine has been used very successfully in emergencies, when there is no alternative. More recently, telemedicine has been used to improve access to healthcare in rural areas where the alternative is the cost and inconvenience of patient or doctor travel. Much telemedicine has been driven by enthusiastic experimenters, and it is suspected of being financially unsustainable. However, evidence is beginning to emerge about the cost-effectiveness of certain applications. For example, telemedicine is cheaper than transporting prisoners to hospital in Texas; it is also cheaper than patients or doctors traveling for specialist consultations in rural areas such as Queensland. Even in urban areas, introducing telemedicine can speed up referral, reducing unnecessary referrals and improving the consistency and quality of healthcare.

Telemedicine is an exciting new technique for healthcare delivery. The technique is acceptable to doctors and patients are enthusiastic about it; although it certainly changes the doctor–patient relationship, it does not do it irreversible damage. Telemedicine is not simply about technology and new equipment. It is a *process*, whose successful exploitation requires organizational changes in the structure of the relevant health service. Given this, the experience suggests that in the right context telemedicine may be effective in improving access to healthcare, in raising the quality of service, and even reducing the costs.　　RWOO

*See also* EDUCATION; FLYING DOCTORS

**TEMPERAMENT** is a combination of the characteristic qualities of people's emotional nature, their constitutional tendency to react to their environment in a certain way, and the quality and lability of their mood. GALEN (p 324) recognized four types of temperament reflecting a preponderance of one or other of the supposed four body 'HUMORS', namely, sanguine, choleric, melancholic, and phlegmatic. There have been other more recent attempts to categorize differences in temperament. One such proposes a dimension based on proneness to a particular type of mental disorder: at one extreme of this is the 'cyclothymic personality', often jovial, friendly, and outgoing but with swings of mood and prone in the event of breakdown to develop manic-depressive psychosis: the associated bodily habitus is 'pyknic', that is, short, thick, and stocky. At the other end of this spectrum is the 'schizothyme', who is introverted, withdrawn, and shy, and liable to develop schizophrenia: here the habitus is tall, thin, and 'leptosomatic'.

**TEMPLE MEDICINE** The temple medicine of ancient Greece probably began some time in the 8th century BC, when temples were first erected to ASCLEPIUS (p 710), the god of medicine; they were called *asclepieia* (singular *asclepieion*). The medicine practiced took the strange form known as 'incubation'. The patient, after sacrifice and purification, lay down to sleep near the altar of the god, whereupon the remedy for his illness was revealed to him, either in a dream or by a priest dressed to represent Asclepius. On recovery, thank-offerings were presented to the temple, including models of the affected part in gold, silver, and wax, and a tablet was erected describing the illness and treatment. Other persons than the patient could incubate on his behalf, and in some temples there were professional dreamers who could be hired for the purpose. Over 300 such temples were mentioned by classical writers, the most famous being at Epidaurus, Cnidus, COS, and Pergamum. HIPPOCRATES (p 382) is said to have been indebted to the clinical material accumulated on the tablets at Cos, but the Hippocratic school, though partly contemporaneous with the temple movement, was independent of it.
*See also* GREECE

**TERATOLOGY** See ANATOMY; THALIDOMIDE

**TERMINAL CARE** See PALLIATIVE CARE

**TEXTBOOKS** serve to synthesize and summarize knowledge for students and others. Books have long been produced to provide this function. Several of the Hippocratic and Galenic treatises fall into this category, and a Latin version of AVICENNA'S (p 60) *Canon of medicine* enjoyed long currency as a comprehensive synthesis for students and young practitioners. It was translated into French and in use as late as the 17th century. A 10th century Leechbook prepared in Old English for a physician named Bald has been described as the oldest English medical textbook. General medical works by physicians such as Jean

## EARLY ENCYCLOPEDISTS

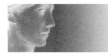

Aulus Cornelius **CELSUS** (*fl.* AD 25). Roman writer. Celsus, a contemporary of the emperor Tiberius and a member of a noble family, was not medically trained. He compiled an encyclopedia of which only the eight books dealing with medicine, *De re medicina,* survive. They were largely translations and drawn from many sources. Written in elegant Latin, they give details of operative methods, discuss pediatrics and dentistry, and provide graphic descriptions of disease. His were the first medical works to be printed, appearing in 1478.

Fernel and Lazarus Riverius were often used in medical faculties during the Renaissance and early modern period; although they were occasionally translated into the vernacular, Latin continued as the primary language of medical instruction.

Despite the existence of the object, the word textbook did not appear in English until the 18th century. The growth of more formal educational structures within medicine created greater demand for textbooks. During the first half of the 18th century, these were supplied above all by Hermann BOERHAAVE of Leiden (p 121), the *Communis Europae praeceptor.* His *Institutiones medicae* (1708) was frequently pirated and translated into many European languages. The original faculty of the medical school at the University of Edinburgh had all studied with Boerhaave. Despite the success of the Edinburgh school, a textbook tradition developed there only slowly, primarily because professors' incomes depended on student fees, and they feared that the students would stop attending their lectures if they were able simply to read their textbooks.

William CULLEN (p 129) of Edinburgh inherited Boerhaave's mantle as the most visible medical teacher in the second half of the century. His *First lines of the practice of physic* (1778–9) acquired wide usage and influence, in English and other languages. Yet this and other Cullen textbooks on nosology and materia medica were produced late in his career, and largely in response to unauthorized, pirated editions of his lectures, based on notes taken by students. Philippe PINEL (p 77)

### PRINCIPLES AND PRACTICE OF MEDICINE

This is the title of the famous textbook of medicine published in 1892 by Dr (later Sir) William OSLER (p 602), the Canadian-born physician, who became professor of medicine successively at the universities of MCGILL (p 139), PENNSYLVANIA (p 839), JOHNS HOPKINS (p 840), and Oxford, where he occupied the regius chair. The last edition to be published during Osler's lifetime was the eighth in 1912; the ninth appeared in 1920 shortly after his death. The book was subsequently revised by McRae and later by Christian until 1939. It was revived again after the Second World War by Harvey and colleagues from Johns Hopkins and continues.

translated Cullen into French, and then produced his own synthesis of medical practice, arranged, like Cullen's, nosologically.

By the early 19th century, most textbooks were being written in the vernacular, with translations being adapted to local diagnostic conventions and treatments. Cullen was also adapted to American practice, and British textbooks dominated the American scene until mid-19th century. Whatever

the original language, these textbooks were generally the product of a single author who was a successful teacher; they tended to be based on a combination of lectures and clinical teaching. As French lesion-based pathology came to dominate medical thinking, textbooks began to be organized around the diseases of systems and organs, and to be rooted in hospital practice. In the German-speaking lands, the textbooks of Carl Friedrich Canstatt and Felix von Niemeyer dominated the middle decades of the century; in France, Armand TROUSSEAU's (p 29) achieved classic status; in Britain, the published lectures of Sir Thomas Watson replaced Cullen as the student's bible; in the United States, Austin Flint produced a highly successful indigenous textbook.

### Centrality of examinations

Examinations became more central to medical education and licensing during the 19th century, and textbooks also began to take into account what the student would need to know to pass. For the ambitious, larger, multi-authored works began gradually to appear. In Britain, John Russell Reynolds and, at the end of the century, Thomas Clifford ALLBUTT (p 812) edited such synthetic compilations. They have become the standard format in more recent times, a reflection of the complexity of medical knowledge and the specialization within the discipline. Throughout the 19th century, however, single-author manuals and textbooks were the norm, including an increasing number of smaller, handy-sized guides aimed directly at the student. The most successful would go through many editions, sometimes becoming a millstone around the author's neck.

Reasons for success varied and might rely on an author's reputation or prose style, combined perhaps with special features of the approach. William Aitken's *Science and practice of medicine* was popular for three decades from the 1860s partly because it incorporated generous treatment of tropical diseases, before Patrick Manson's great specialized monograph on that branch of medicine. John S. Bristowe's *Treatise on the theory and practice of medicine* acquired a niche from the 1870s because of its up-to-date consideration of the relevance of laboratory science for clinical practice. That Bristowe was also a regular examiner for the University of London undoubtedly helped the sales of his book. Adolf Strümpell's phenomenally successful (18 editions in German plus several translations into English) *Lehrbuch der speziellen Pathologie und Therapie der inneren Krankheiten* represented an authoritative voice at a period of German dominance of international medicine and medical science.

The decades from the 1890s, however, belong to William OSLER (p 602), whose *Principles and practice of medicine* (1892) quickly established itself as the gold-standard of medical textbooks. By 1906, his textbook was recommended by most American medical schools, and, unusually, the first edition (and subsequent ones) were published in both America and Britain, as the publishers obviously anticipated a success. They were correct, of course, and Osler's later translation to the Regius chair of medicine in Oxford did nothing to harm his transatlantic reputation. Appropriate for the times, the *Principles* was therapeutically conservative, but it contained vivid, elegant descriptions of diseases and how to diagnose them, and assimilated the latest Continental thinking into the text. It was translated into French, German, Spanish, and Chinese.

Osler also lent his name and editorial skills to a multi-author encyclopedic tome which survived him. The edited format dominated 20th-century textbooks, the successful ones enjoying long life and changes of editors and authors. Students tend to refer to them in shorthand: *Cecil-Loeb*, *Harrison*, *Price*, or, more recently, *The Oxford textbook*. Shorter, single-authored textbooks also have had some success. All modern medical textbooks have the problem of assimilating rapid change in diagnostic criteria, therapeutic indications, and favored therapy. It has been suggested that textbooks should carry health warnings. Electronic publishing will eventually make updating easier, but will probably not render extinct the printed versions.

Textbooks have been extraordinarily adaptable, and students will continue to use them as well as their companions in the medical sciences and in the medical and surgical specialties. *Mutatis mutandis*, stories similar to the one summarized here could be told about the textbook tradition of each of these other disciplines within medicine.    WFB

*See also* BOOKS AND LIBRARIES; EDUCATION

**THALIDOMIDE** a sedative drug first synthesized in 1953, created one of the most dramatic tragedies in the history of medicine. A highly effective cure for morning sickness of pregnancy, it deformed thousands of unborn babies, mostly in their limbs, producing its characteristic *phocomelia*, or limbs like seal's flippers. These deformities were particularly common in Germany, where the drug had been available without prescription, but there were also hundreds in Britain and other countries where it had become a popular prescription drug. The result of this debâcle was to introduce mandatory testing in pregnant animals of all new drugs before marketing them and follow-up monitoring once they were licensed.

From 1958 thalidomide had been widely praised, advertised, and prescribed on the grounds that it was highly effective and almost impossible to use for suicide. There seemed to be no reason to doubt its safety. The tragedy was without precedent and unlike anything that had gone before. It was then widely believed that the human placenta was impervious to poisons except in such doses as killed the mother. Yet there was already widespread evidence that this was untrue and that fetuses could be deformed by external influences, including poisoning and therapeutic drugs, infection, X-rays, and malnutrition. Some of this evidence, particularly in relation to SYPHILIS and rubella, had been accepted and acted upon by the medical profession (for example, by Wassermann tests for pregnant women and rubella parties for prepubertal girls), but most of it had been ignored because this suited the contemporary mind-set or *Denkstil*.

Thalidomide was soon discovered to affect the peripheral nerves but little notice was taken of this. Antenatal care did not include advice about drugs. Routine testing of new drugs on pregnant animals was perfunctory or non-existent. Why did the medical profession ignore the extensive existing evidence that teratogenic substances (causing developmental abnormalities in the fetus) could cross the placenta? It is useful to look at the question as part of a mind-set or a shared view of reality that controls, organizes, and limits perception and understanding. We all tend to ignore what does not fit the theories and beliefs with which we live. The placenta was deemed to be impermeable to harmful substances and so evidence to the contrary was ignored until something occurred that was so startling, anomalous, and public, that it could be ignored no longer. Then the belief was challenged and changed.

To some extent this rearrangement involved a return to past theories and beliefs, which raises the question of why these had ever been abandoned. The idea that maternal impressions can affect an unborn child for better or worse is old. Interest in monsters goes back at least to ancient Egypt. For many centuries they were seen as warnings or divine omens and were often confused with mythological beings. It was an ancient Jewish custom to put a beautiful child at the door of public baths to help women to 'have children as fine as he'. In ancient Carthage it is said that alcohol was forbidden to a bridal couple in case a fetus was damaged by it. Later, monsters became objects of interest, to be collected and described. Most museums of pathology still possess a collection of them.

**Maternal impressions**

In the 18th century there was much interest in maternal impressions. In the mid-19th century it was believed in the English-speaking world that heredity could be altered by external circumstances at any point between conception and weaning. Physicians warned against sexual intercourse under the influence of drugs or alcohol as they believed that these could affect the constitution of a child.

In the late 19th century this kind of belief was falling into disrepute for being linked with magic and 'unscientific' thinking. As medicine became more 'scientific', magic came into contempt. The placenta was steeped in myth and mystery. Belief in the placenta as a perfect barrier against damaging influences in the environment was reinforced by the Victorian tendency to put 'woman' on a pedestal, which led to idealization of the womb as well as of the woman. Women's reproductive organs were regarded as different and special and also as the source of all women's symptoms and ills not visibly due to something else. Only a few practicing doctors disagreed. One of these was F. W. Ballantyne, a teratologist and lecturer in antenatal pathology in Edinburgh, who initiated many advances in antenatal care. In 1904 he listed 'varieties of fetal morbid states', including transmitted diseases and toxicological states such as lead poisoning, alcoholism, morphine poisoning, etc. Few took notice, and as late as 1937 a popular textbook discussed the diagnosis of fetal abnormalities but not their causes. In 1941, when the damaging effects of German measles (rubella) to the unborn baby were demonstrated, the peculiarity of the infection was emphasized but it was not taken as a general warning about the vulnerability of fetuses.

Another possible reason why little notice was taken of environmental dangers in pregnancy was that fetuses, stillbirths, and newborn babies had been regarded as expendable, or at least as not very important. They created danger for their mothers at a time when maternal mortality was high. Accounts of obstetric cases in the 19th century seldom mention whether or not the infant survived, clearly regarding it as trivial. A deformed fetus was likely to arouse even less interest unless it had rare abnormalities, in which case it might be described in a journal. By the 1930s the maternal mortality rate was falling, birth control was spreading, families were smaller, and there was greater interest in infants and their survival. Also, decline in mortality from infection and improved antenatal care meant that congenital defects became more prominent as a cause of illness and death, which at least provided a reason for studying them.

Thus an analysis of the historical context of the thalidomide disaster suggests that it occurred largely because human teratology was not regarded seriously by clinicians, who had no reason to take it seriously. An attitude of mind idealized the placenta and ignored most of the existing evidence of fetal damage through environmental influences.

Thalidomide changed the way in which the medical profession regarded drugs taken in pregnancy, and indeed at any time. It also played a part in breaking down the idealization/denigration of women that has been so prominent in western medical history. However, it was a useful and effective drug and recently it has been used again in some parts of the world in the treatment of myeloma (a tumor of the bone marrow) and leprosy — with the inevitable result that 'thalidomide babies' are once again being born.     AD

See also ADVERSE DRUG REACTIONS; MISADVENTURES; PHARMACOLOGY, CLINICAL PHARMACOLOGY, AND THERAPEUTICS

**THEORIES OF ILLNESS** Severe, unexpected illness poses extraordinary demands on the individual. The afflicted person is plunged into a new and frightening world, where familiar ways of feeling and acting have vanished. Questions immediately arise: What has caused this illness? Why has it happened to me? What can I do to get well? The answers will be shaped by the way individuals and their cultural group understand health and illness. Most immediately relevant are the proximate causes of the illness, its 'how?'. Perhaps the cause is thought to be a viral infection, a dietary imbalance or a problem of overheating, conditions arising from the natural world. Treatment to help the person heal at this level may include various pharmacological, herbal, dietary, and physical remedies. But there are many deeper levels of illness causation recognized by people around the world. These levels are seen as the 'ultimate' causes of illness, the 'why?' of the illness. Here, illness is seen as a disruption in the normal state of balance between an individual and the social or supernatural world, and is understood in a moral, spiritual, or religious context. Treatment of these causes of illness may include secular, magical, or sacred rituals, which serve to restore proper relationships between afflicted individuals and their environment. Often, an illness is seen to have both a proximate and an ultimate cause, and treatment must be directed towards restoring balance at both levels.

People make this journey towards the healing of illness in an extraordinary variety of ways. Theories about illness deal with the explanations people give for why they become ill. They may include such ideas as offending dead ancestors, breach of taboo, soul loss, upset in the hot–cold balance of the body, or a weakening of the body's immune system. Theories of illness causation derive from the underlying cognitive orientation of the cultural group. Therapeutic practice follows the same cultural logic. Theories and practices are seen as irrational only by people outside the group who cannot accept the fundamental cognitive assumptions underlying the theories.

Anthropologists divide theories of illness into two broad categories: personalistic and naturalistic. In a personalistic system, illness is believed to be caused by the intervention of a sensate agent, who may be a supernatural being (a deity, or a dead ancestor), or a human being with special powers (a witch, or a sorcerer). The sick person's illness is a direct result of these malign influences. In naturalistic causation, illness is explained in impersonal terms. When the body is in balance with the natural environment, a state of health prevails. When that balance is disturbed, illness results. These two theories of illness causation are not mutually exclusive. Often, people may invoke both types of causation in explaining an episode of illness, and both theories may be involved in treatment.

In many traditional cultures, the world is seen as alive, and all natural objects are filled with some form of animating essence. The life force ('anima') of the natural world is seen to interact with the life force of each individual in multiple ways. In this animistic view, the natural world is intimately linked with a supernatural world. Sickness is often seen to have underlying causes that are moral or spiritual, and healing practices in such societies generally have strong spiritual elements.

### Personalistic theories of illness

Illness may be linked to transgressions of a moral and spiritual nature. If someone has breached a religious taboo, or violated a behavioral norm, he or she may invoke the wrath of a deity. Sickness is often seen as a form of divine punishment. Evil spirits are thought to cause illness in many cultures, and the treatment of such illnesses often involves the performance of complex rituals by religious specialists. Possession by evil spirits is sometimes thought to be a result of inappropriate behavior on the part of the patient, or it may be purely bad luck. If the spirit belongs to a dead ancestor, the inappropriate behavior in question is often the failure to carry out the proper rituals of respect for the ancestor. Sometimes, other humans are thought to be the cause of illness through supernatural means. The evil eye is an example of this form of thinking. Here, one person's envy of another's good fortune is believed to exert a malign influence which can result in illness or other calamities.

In magical healing, a substance or process is used therapeutically that in some way symbolizes the symptoms of the illness. For example, if someone develops jaundice and his eyes and skin become yellow, then this doctrine suggests that help might be obtained from an animal of yellow color — perhaps the sacrifice of a yellow bird. In rural INDIA, traditional midwives treat prolonged labor by unlocking all doors and windows in the birthing room, and undoing all knots in the woman's sari. A magical connection between obstructions in the birth process and physical symbols of locking and knotting is established.

### Naturalistic theories of illness: the humoral system

Naturalistic theories of disease causation tend to be empirico-rational in their approach. Health is seen as a state of harmony between the human being and the environment; when this balance is upset, illness will result. The humoral system is a widespread naturalistic approach to illness whose roots are over 2000 years old. Humoral concepts of health and illness are widely found in India, SOUTH-EAST ASIA, and CHINA. Humoral medicine in a somewhat different form was practiced in ancient Greece, and spread from there to Arabia and the Middle East, and later to Spain. The system came to the New World with the Spanish conquerors, and humoral medicine is still widely practiced in Latin America.

In a humoral understanding of health and illness, the healthy body is seen in a dynamic equilibrium with its environment. An excess of hot or cold in the environment causes illness, and therapeutic measures are directed towards righting this imbalance. Foods are classified into heating and cooling foods. 'Hot' foods tend to be those that are brightly colored, spicy or pungent, high in protein (such as meat and eggs), and fried. 'Cool' foods are commonly green, yellow, or white, bland, and raw or lightly cooked. Maintaining humoral balance requires attention to diet — one should eat heating foods in the cool season and cooling foods in the hot season. Illnesses are similarly categorized into those due to excess heat and those due to excess cold. Treating an illness of overheat would involve measures such as giving cooling foods and applying cool compresses. Perhaps the humoral theory is still so prevalent today because it is a system which has some philosophical elegance and seems to be logical under many circumstances. It is a gentle form of treatment which is seldom harmful and often beneficial.

*Ayurveda* In India, the ancient system of Ayurveda encompasses many examples of naturalistic illness causation. Ayurvedic medicine encompassed a complex medical system that relied on empiricism and explanations of observ-

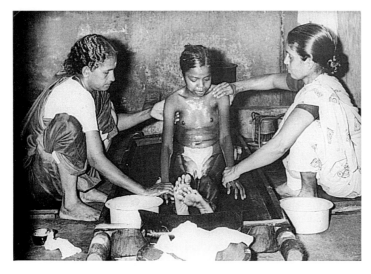

A young girl with rheumatoid arthritis is treated by trained Ayurvedic practitioners. (WHO photo by A. S. Kochar.)

gious way of thinking about the world, as well as a therapeutic approach to maintaining and restoring health.

***Biomedicine*** The concept of the self as an observing and reflexive 'I' that stands apart from the body may be traced through western philosophical tradition, deeply influencing the way modern biomedicine has evolved. Illness tends to be located within the physical body and is conceptualized as a breakdown in the mechanics of bodily functioning. The 'body-as-machine' metaphor has been a powerful way of conceptualizing the body and an enormous variety of effective treatments have developed within biomedicine. Biomedical theories of disease are generally naturalistic, with an empirico-rational basis to therapy. A core assumption of the value system of biomedicine is that diagnosis and treatment should be based on scientific data. However, many treatments in biomedicine have little or no scientific evidence to support them. Early in the 20th century, surgeons removed part of the colon for 'autointoxication', a procedure that had no demonstrable therapeutic value and left patients with chronic diarrhea. Brain surgery for psychiatric conditions, including severing the connections between the frontal lobe and its underlying structures (lobotomy), had the support of the medical community in the mid-20th century. Operations to remove prolapsed intervertebral discs (laminectomies) were commonly performed only a few years ago; these treatments have largely been supplanted by more conservative management.

Biomedicine is not purely empirico-rational in its approach. Ritual and symbolism have important roles in its healing process, as they do in other healing systems. For example, coronary artery bypass grafting is far more commonly performed in the United States than in Canada or Europe. There is little scientific evidence to show that it significantly extends lifespan, although it may relieve symptoms. Much of its therapeutic value may lie in its dramatic ritual and symbolic context.

Popular ideas about illness causation in the western world often locate the origin of ill health within the individual — perhaps the person has behaved inappropriately (such as wrong diet or lack of exercise); or perhaps the person is vulnerable to illness in some way (hereditary or psychological factors). Popular ideas about illness that locate the cause of illness external to the individual include ideas about infection; exposure to heat or cold; and, increasingly, exposure to environmental contaminants.

Conditions caused by disturbances in mental functioning or by strong emotions do not fit well into the biomedical model. People who are oppressed or in distress may feel their emotional

able phenomena. It was a philosophical system as well as a set of medical practices, incorporating detailed advice on how to lead a long and healthy life. Treatments in Ayurveda included a vast pharmacopeia of preparations made from herbs and minerals. Dietary advice also formed part of every prescription. Techniques of surgery and midwifery were described in ancient Ayurvedic texts, although these are no longer a part of the practice. Ayurveda is actively practiced in India today and has shaped the way Indians think about their bodies in health and in illness.

***Vital energy and healing*** An important cognitive orientation to health and illness, widespread in China, and South and South-east Asia, links health with energy states of the body. Some authors have called these 'vitalist' theories about the body. The body is perceived to be in dynamic harmony with the surrounding environment. Vital forces within the body flow in a harmonious pattern, providing energy for the proper functioning of body and mind. Illness results when this smooth flow of energy is disrupted, and therapeutic measures are aimed at restoring a normal flow of energy in the body. In China, this vital force is known as 'chi'; in India it is called 'prana'.

Therapeutic approaches to balance energy in the body are manifold. In China, the ancient art of acupuncture is based on this understanding of the body. Acupuncture needles are inserted at various points along the 'meridians', or energy orientations, in the body. The stimulation of the needles helps to restore a proper flow of energy within the body. In India, yoga (particularly hatha yoga, the physical postures) is used therapeutically to restore a balanced energy flow through body and mind. Yoga is a philosophical and relipain in their bodies, often experiencing appreciable psychosomatic illness. Perhaps because there is no recognizable organic defect in the body, this form of illness tends to be poorly understood and treated within a biomedical framework.

*Alternative medicine* The traditional split between mind and body in biomedicine is facing challenges from many sides. Proponents of 'mind–body medicine' pose a strong philosophical critique of biomedicine, suggesting that the time has come for a 'paradigm shift' in medicine towards a more integrated understanding of the interaction between mind and body. The links between mind and body are being explored in many different ways. In research, epidemiologists have long shown links between psychological stress levels and patterns of disease. Now, scientists are exploring topics such as psychoneuroimmunology, examining the links between the central nervous system and the immune system and proposing physiologic mechanisms for ways in which mind/body integration may occur. Clinical research is beginning to show evidence that mind–body approaches may be successful in treating a variety of disorders.

There has been a rapidly growing interest in various forms of alternative therapy (also called COMPLEMENTARY MEDICINE) in western countries. These therapies are diverse, ranging from traditional ones adapted from their lands of origin, such as acupuncture and Shiatsu, to newly developed forms such as therapeutic touch. Some have been well established for many years, such as chiropractic, while others are just beginning to gain some acceptance. Homeopathy is one form of alternative therapy that is generally not well accepted in North America, yet is quite well established in European countries such as Germany.

Many alternative therapies have underlying theories of illness causation that are different from that of biomedicine. In therapies such as acupuncture, Reiki and Shiatsu the concept of vital energy, or chi, is the basis for the practice. Successful treatment is that which regulates and harmonizes energy flows. In iridology, particular areas on the iris of the eye are thought to correspond to specific body organs. Diagnosis of malfunction of the organs can be made by an examination of the iris. A similar assumption is made in reflexology, using the foot as the reference area. Conceptually, these theories of illness link to an ancient philosophical system of 'homologies', prevalent in the East, that makes connections between the cosmic and the terrestrial; the outer environment and the inner; the external body and the internal body. Such theories have little congruence with scientific patterns of thought, and thus can be conceptually difficult to understand.

Alternative medicine may focus more on ultimate causes, or the 'why' of the disease than on the immediate, biological cause of the disease. Afflicted individuals need to examine their lives, searching for emotional conflicts of life-style issues which may have had an influence on the development of the disease. This approach may be appealing to people who are ill, because the questions of 'why me?' and 'why now in my life?' often become issues of central concern. Such an approach may help the patient assume responsibility for the illness and work actively towards healing; however, some people face the dangers of self-blame and guilt.

The controversy swirling around the alternative medicine movement has much to tell us about people's dissatisfaction with biomedicine. Clearly, many people are searching for a broader way of thinking about the body — the notion of the body as a machine seems too rigid and sterile a view. Practitioners and researchers in mind–body medicine attempt to go beyond the dualisms of biomedicine. While this is a subject of great complexity and confusion, promising directions are emerging. There is a second aspect to the public's dissatisfaction with biomedicine. Medical doctors are highly trained in the technical aspects of their disciplines, yet may not spend much time on the human, personal sides of the patient's illness. Therapists in many alternative medicine approaches tend to be less powerful and intimidating than doctors, and spend far more time talking with their patients. Patients feel attended to, and often feel more in control of their own healing process.

What is the difficulty at the interface between the systems? Biomedical practitioners feel that the alternative therapies have little scientific basis, and also feel that alternative practitioners sometimes make unsubstantiated claims about the efficacy of their treatments. Alternative practitioners feel that doctors too frequently 'medicalize' problems that are really emotional and social issues. On both sides, practitioners tend to take an 'either–or' approach that forces the patient to choose one system or the other.

Perhaps there is room for more flexibility. Increasingly, people are seeking alternative treatments as well as conventional biomedical treatments. This approach works in many parts of the world — in rural India, patients move pragmatically between one system and another, often employing several different modalities at once, even if the underlying philosophical basis of the treatment is very different. There may be circumstances when alternative therapies are much more appropriate than biomedicine, or vice versa, and other circumstances when both could be used together.

### Conclusion

Illness creates a crisis of meaning for afflicted people, in whatever cultural context they live. The primary task of the healer anywhere in the world is to create a meaningful context for the illness — a way for sick people to understand why they became ill and what they can do to get better. This context of meaning arises from underlying theories about illness causation, and usually reflects core cultural values. A meaningful context may be created by the use of ritual, in which signs and symbols express powerful cultural orientations. Rituals help to order the chaotic world of serious illness, and help the individual to regain some sense of control in a frightening situation. Sometimes, healing ceremonies are held which may help to mobilize support for patients and permit an acknowledgement of their suffering. When the underlying cause of the illness is disturbed relationships between the patient and his or her social group, a healing ceremony can help to heal these rifts.

In many parts of the world, the healer is one who has experienced serious illness. Such people are thought to have learned some of the secrets of suffering by direct experience, and are thus in a better position to help the one who has fallen ill. The personal attributes of the healer are often held to be paramount rather than the technical knowledge that the healer possesses. Perhaps this speaks to the deep human need to have one's suffering acknowledged at the time of serious illness. Sufferers need to tell the story of their suffering, and the healer must always remember that listening to that story is an essential part of the therapeutic process.      KK

*See also* CHIROPRACTIC; HOMEOPATHY

**TITLES AND DEGREES** Medical titles and degrees may mean different things in different countries and be confusing. In the United States, students enter medical school after completing a bachelor's arts or science course in college (BA or BS) and graduate after four years as doctors of medicine (MD). The terms doctor and physician are used interchangeably, and surgeons are at times included in these all-embracing labels. After completing residencies of varying length (three years of internal medicine or family practice, five years for surgery) doctors become board qualified; after passing the board examinations

---

## THERMOMETERS

A Jesuit priest Jean Leurechon coined the term thermometer in 1624; before that, thermometers were called thermoscopes. Galileo is accredited with the invention of the thermometer in 1592. His air-filled bulb was the size of a hen's egg and the glass column two spans long and the width of straw. The lower end of the column was placed in a beaker of water. The bulb was warmed in the hand, causing downward displacement of the water level in the glass column. SANCTORIUS (p 743) was the first physician to use such a device for measuring body temperature. His adapted thermometer was convoluted, with glass bead graduations. The bulb was placed in the mouth. The influence of barometric pressure on these devices was not foreseen, as the barometer was invented only in 1643.

In 1631 Rey initiated the search for the ideal thermometric liquid when he invented a water-filled thermometer. It looked like an inverted Galileo thermometer with the beaker removed. The upper end was left open so that readings were more affected by evaporation than barometric pressure. The first hermetically sealed alcohol thermometer was invented in 1641 by Grand Duke Ferdinand II. Various liquids were incorporated in thermometers, including linseed oil, which NEWTON (p 544) used. In 1714 Fahrenheit invented the mercury thermometer, after which mercury was mostly used.

With the invention of the thermometer there was a need for a standardized scale. The lower and upper extremes of the Sanctorius thermometer were the temperature of snow and a heated candle. In 1694 Renaldi first proposed the boiling and freezing points of water as the extremes, with 12 degrees between. Réaumur proposed boiling point (steam) and the temperature of a salt and ice mixture as his extreme reference points. His scale had 60 degrees to correspond with clocks and geometric instruments. Fahrenheit used Réaumur's reference points, but changed the scale. In his scale the coldest point was 0°, freezing 30°, and boiling 212°. The freezing point was subsequently changed to 32°. In 1742 Celsius designed a 100° (centigrade) scale, 0° being boiling point and 100° freezing. The following year Linnaeus and Christian independently reversed the scale to its present form.

The use of the thermometer was given impetus by Wunderlich, who showed for the first time that fever was a sign of disease and not a disease *per se*. Influenced by Wunderlich, Aitken arranged for thermometers to be made for him by Casella. Aitken's thermometers were straight or curved. The straight thermometer was removed from the axilla before reading; the curved was read *in situ*. Their size made them cumbersome and limited their use. In 1867 ALLBUTT (this page)

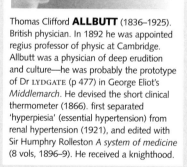

Thomas Clifford **ALLBUTT** (1836–1925). British physician. In 1892 he was appointed regius professor of physic at Cambridge. Allbutt was a physician of deep erudition and culture—he was probably the prototype of Dr LYDGATE (p 477) in George Eliot's *Middlemarch*. He devised the short clinical thermometer (1866). first separated 'hyperpiesia' (essential hypertension) from renal hypertension (1921), and edited with Sir Humphry Rolleston *A system of medicine* (8 vols, 1896–9). He received a knighthood.

announced that he was using a pocket version, which was made by Messrs Harvey Reynolds. It was 6 inches (15 cm) long, the diameter of a pencil and cost 7s 6d (38p). Thermometers were later shortened to 3 inches (7.5 cm). Early thermometers were round and rolled on flat surfaces; however, subsequently to prevent breakage a triangular shape was created. Fortuitously the new shape also magnified the bore. The 'lens front' thermometer was patented by Peroni and marketed in 1878.

(*continued opposite*)

*(continued)*

In the second half of the 20th century, ecological concern about mercury spawned an array of new thermometers. Electronic thermometers are of two types, thermocouples or thermistors. Seebeck discovered the thermocouple in 1821, noting that heat applied to one end of dissimilar fused wires produces a force at the other end. Siemens discovered the thermistor in 1871 when he noticed that resistance to a current was temperature dependent. Callandar produced a resistance thermometer, which in 1897 was first used in clinical practice by Atwater and Rosa. Electronic thermometers became generally available at an affordable cost in the 1960s.

Disposable chemical thermometers were first used in the 1970s, with the onset of AIDS in the 1980s popularizing their use. These are flexible plastic strips which contain liquid crystals or organic chemicals. Temperature-induced color change occurs when crystals change from solid to liquid or when organic chemicals cause dye release.

Ear thermometers are a 1990s innovation. In 1959 Benzinger showed that the ear and body core temperature are similar. The temperature regulation centre (hypothalamus) and the tympanic membrane have a common blood supply. Tympanic membrane heat is measured with an infra-red sensor. IB

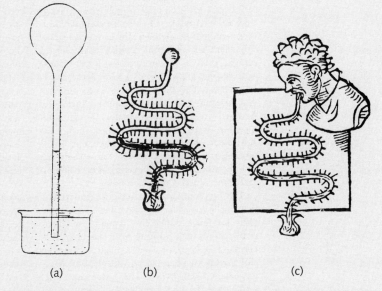

(a)                    (b)                         (c)

(a) Galileo's thermometer; (b) Sanctorius's thermometer; (c) Sanctorius's thermometer in use.

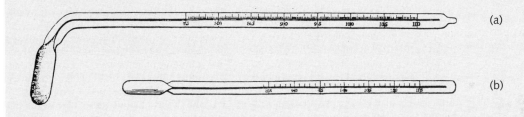

(a)

(b)

Aitken's thermometers: (a) the curved thermometer is for *in situ* reading, (b) the straight thermometer, which could be removed before reading.

they become board certified; subsequently they may take two or sometimes more further years of training and become board certified in sub-specialties such as gastroenterology or cardiology. Such training periods tend to be longer in Canada.

Doctors certified in internal medicine may apply to be inducted into the American College of Physicians and become fellows thereof. They may then use the letters FACP after their name but rarely do so, especially in recent years, since the American College of Physicians has concentrated on emphasizing primary care; it has recently merged with another internal medicine association, the American Society of Internal Medicine. Doctors who are board certified in internal medicine call themselves internists. They provide consultations to surgeons and other specialists, but tend to act as primary contact or primary care

doctors in internal medicine. They confine themselves to internal medicine, unlike family medicine doctors, who may also practice pediatrics and uncomplicated obstetrics, but from whom they are for practical purposes barely distinguishable.

Doctors may also undertake further postgraduate work and obtain master's degrees in public health or business administration, or carry out research and be awarded a doctor of philosophy (Ph.D.) degree from a university.

### Osteopathy degrees

Americans may also graduate from one of several osteopathic colleges with a doctor of osteopathy degree. Their training, though emphasizing the laying on of hands, is basically the same as that of allopathic doctors, from whom they are for practical purposes indistinguishable. MD or DO degrees are generally recognized as being equivalent, which is not the case for chiropractic practitioners.

In Britain there have been traditionally three paths to licensure. The most common is a bachelor's degree (MB, BS or MB, BChir), awarded by universities. Another is to take the conjoint licensure examination offered by the Royal Colleges of Physicians and Surgeons, leading to the degree of MRCS, LRCP (Member of the Royal College of Surgeons, Licenciate of the Royal College of Physicians). The third pathway is to obtain a qualification from the Worshipful Society of Apothecaries. All these graduates, though commonly referred to as doctors, have in fact the equivalent of a bachelors of medicine. To be officially recognized as MD (Doctor of Medicine) or to be awarded a Ph.D. qualification they must carry out research and write a thesis.

If they wish to follow a more pure clinical path they might undertake the prescribed years of specialist training and then pass higher postgraduate examinations (equivalent to American boards) to become fellows of the Royal College of Surgeons (FRCS) or members of the Royal College of Physicians (MRCPUK). The latter may after several years be elected to become fellows of one of the Royal Colleges, of London or Edinburgh, in which case they become FRCP (London) or FRCP (Ed). Additionally in Britain, a higher surgical degree is obtainable (the Mastership of Surgery — MChir or MS), usually by examination. There are similar higher examinations in both the surgical specialties such as orthopedics and ophthalmology, as well as the other specialties such as radiology and pediatrics. In Britain, but not in the United States, board certified surgeons are called Mr, a throwback to the days when the surgeons (and barbers) were sharply differentiated from physicians (and apothecaries).

Of the other English-speaking countries, Canada follows most closely the United States pattern, doctors graduating as MD. On passing their higher examinations they become fellows of the Canadian Royal College. Several other countries, however, follow the British system, their students graduating with bachelor degrees and the doctorate and specialty degrees being obtained after several more years of postgraduate study. In Australia physicians become FRACP and surgeons FRACS. In other European countries the pattern varies, but is usually more like the American than the British pattern, with the qualifying degree being MD.

In the United States the lowest university rank is that of instructor, a title sometimes given even to chief residents and research fellows. The most common level of entry, however, is at assistant professor level (corresponding to lecturer in Britain). After several years, commonly six, this may be followed by promotion to associate professor (in Britain, senior lecturer or reader) and after more years, perhaps six, to professor, though this may involve competing with outsiders for the post. Some universities make promotion to a certain rank a condition for awarding tenure. In any medical faculty department there may be several professors, one of whom would be the chairman of the department, and perhaps several others who might be associate chairmen. Department chairmen may elect to also be the program directors, responsible for training residents or students, and they may delegate such titles to other department members. Some chairmen of medical departments have separate vice-chairmen in charge of research, education, and clinical services. University departments are usually divided into sections (or divisions), each with its own chairman or director. These are largely devoted to subspecialties, such as cardiology or nephrology, orthopedics, or urology, but frequently there are also sections of general medicine and surgery.

In some universities, especially in the departments of medicine, all appointments at a certain level (for example, associate professor) are equivalent in status. Some schools, however, distinguish between research and clinical tracks, or between full-time and part-time university appointees. Accordingly the professor title may be unqualified, or qualified as professor of clinical medicine (usually full time but more clinical and not as prominent in research) and clinical professor (often private practitioners devoting a few hours each week to teaching or making patient rounds). Hospital appointments are commonly distinct from university ones and, depending on the institution, may range from senior attending to attending or to courtesy staff. They are generally referred to as attendings, whereas in Britain they are called consultants.

In Britain, university and hospital appointments also tend to be separate. Academic appointments start as lecturer, progressing through reader to professor. The latter, in general, are fewer than in the United States and are mainly the department chairman. Professors in Britain and Australia are generally called professor, whereas in the United States professors of medicine are usually called doctor.                          GD

*See also* INTERNAL MEDICINE – USA; PROFESSIONAL REGULATION

**TOBACCO** See CHEST MEDICINE; SMOKING AND HEALTH

**TORTURE** is defined by the British Medical Association as the deliberate, systematic or wanton infliction of physical and mental suffer-

# TONSILLECTOMY

The tonsils were once thought to be an aid to digestion. Then they came to be regarded as dangerous organs, often infected and better removed. The modern view is that they are part of the immune system, more protective than infective, especially in childhood. Like other lymphatic structures, they are large in small children and shrink as the child grows. At the same time, small children tend to get upper respiratory infections while they build up their immunity. This has confused the issue and a powerful myth persists to this day that tonsils actually cause infections.

Since antiquity, tonsils have occasionally been removed surgically (tonsillectomy), usually for an abscess (quinsy). During the 19th century it became customary to remove them because they were thought to be large or recurrently infected. This fashion peaked in the middle of the 20th century and lasted, with diminishing enthusiasm, until the present day.

As surgery became safer, there developed a tendency to remove organs whose function was not known, seemed unnecessary, or merely were thought to be 'enlarged'. The history of tonsillectomy demonstrates this clearly.

### Class bias

There was a class bias in tonsillectomy, which was more commonly carried out on middle-class patients, whose family doctors usually performed the operation themselves in the patient's home, often on several siblings at a time. Hospitals were also keen on the operation and provided a service for the working class. Infection, or the presence of inflammation or pus, was always the main indication for operation but size was an important source of argument. People believed passionately that large tonsils were abnormal and dangerous.

The tonsillectomy rate in one area could be as much as 30 times the rate in another similar one. These differences could be explained not by need but largely by the attitudes and practices of the local doctors. A local rate often changed dramatically with a change of a surgeon or medical officer of health.

Why did this operation become so popular with both doctors and parents? First, it occurred against a background of increasing confidence in doctors, growing enthusiasm for surgery, and improving techniques — with anesthesia, antisepsis, and improved instruments such as the 'guillotine' — which cut off tonsils near their roots. It is notable that operations which became fashionable were those performed chiefly on women and children and in parts of the body that were relatively easy to reach.

Second, there was increasing medical interest in children. Before the mid-19th century doctors took little interest in children and often regarded them as unimportant and expendable. A new climate developed, but there was widespread ignorance of many of the differences between adults and children. Where a child differed from a normal adult, it was apt to be regarded as abnormal and treated as such, often drastically. One such difference was the relative size of the tonsils. Once developed, the desire to label large tonsils as abnormal and to remove them was extraordinarily powerful. Some even thought that the very existence of a tonsil was a disease. Many different illnesses and disabilities were attributed to their existence. Arguments often concerned the best method of operating rather than whether or not the operation should be carried out. Those making the most extreme claims were not all 'fringe' doctors trying to be important or to make a living. They included many professional heavyweights, though others opposed the wholesale removal of tonsils.

Third, parents, especially in the middle classes, became keen for their children's tonsils to be removed. Tonsillectomy became almost part of childhood. During the late 20th century, as surgical enthusiasm for tonsillectomy waned, pressure from parents was often the strongest reason for the operation. There are still remnants of this pressure today and there are parents who believe that tonsillectomy is necessary to prevent recurrent colds or chest illnesses.

Fourth, by the second decade of the 20th century, the theory of focal infection was gaining ground, leading to the belief that tonsils were a breeding ground for bacteria. Even established surgeons believed that enlarged tonsils might cause epilepsy, bedwetting, laryngismus (spasm of the larynx), and night terrors. For many, the argument shifted from whether all enlarged tonsils should be removed to whether all tonsils should be removed.

Fifth, doctors needed to carve out practices for themselves. In private practice they were paid directly. Operating in public hospitals often led to power: prestige, and that great symbol of medical power: beds. Tonsillectomy became the most frequent operation and was a powerful political tool.

Meanwhile, the opponents of routine operations were gaining power. They showed that the benefits of the operation were marginal and that selection of patients was highly subjective. The evolution of the tonsil, which diminishes in size during childhood, became known. The psychological effects of operating on small children were also causing concern. There was new awareness of the suffering of children when they were in pain, in strange surroundings, and separated from their mothers. Pediatricians began to insist that they, rather than social workers, ear, nose, and throat surgeons, or parents should screen children referred for tonsillectomy. This may have been a bid for power in a growing specialty, but it produced some sanity in the race for maximum tonsillectomy.

Amid all this, no controlled trials of tonsillectomy were begun until 1962, but evidence was accumulating that the tonsil played a positive part in the defence against infection and should be retained whenever possible. Yet in 1948 there was a large increase in the number of tonsillectomies performed in England. That year the National Health Service began and many doctors were scrambling for beds and power and trying to demonstrate the needs of their particular specialty. Others were struggling to reduce the incidence of tonsillectomy. After that, the incidence declined gradually, until today the operation is performed comparatively rarely.

AD

*See also* ENT; EVIDENCE-BASED MEDICINE

ing by one or more persons acting alone or on the orders of an authority, to force another person to yield information, to make a confession, or for any other reason which is an outrage on personal dignity.

In 1982, the UN General Assembly adopted the document *Principles of medical ethics relevant to the protection of prisoners against torture*. This was published multilingually; in English, French, Spanish, Russian, Chinese, and Arabic.

In 1998 about one third of the world's governments routinely tortured their own citizens. The reasons usually lie in the repression of unwanted minorities or as an example to others rather than a desire to extract information which would otherwise be withheld. The target group for torturing regimes tends to expand over time, from 'enemies of the state' to eventually include such a wide variety as drug addicts, prostitutes, homosexuals, 'corrupt' lawyers, and street children.

In some countries where torture is legally forbidden, practices are condoned which seem to be indistinguishable from torture. In 1970s Britain sleep and food deprivation, hooding, enforced uncomfortable postures, and the use of continuous noise were employed in Northern Ireland 'depth interviews'. In 1990s Israel the Landau Report allowed interview techniques to include 'moderate physical pressure such as shaking'. At least one previously well adult male suspect died of widespread brain damaged after being so shaken. Most countries which torture their own citizens in defiance of the law minimize the frequency or severity of the problem or attempt to justify their actions.

Those who are about to be tortured are frequently held incommunicado in cells which are usually filthy and often very small. Lighting is customarily either nearly or wholly absent, or incandescent and unceasing. Sleep deprivation seems to be routine. Torture often occurs at night, when guards may come on duty drunk, or is applied randomly — the unpredictability amplifying the effect. The impression is given that no one is aware of the victims' whereabouts and that they might easily die undetected.

The methods of torture employed are too numerous to even attempt to list but include simple beatings with boots or fists, electrocution, near-drowning, suspension or fixation in unnatural positions, placing irritants on to mucous membranes, and rape and other sexual humiliations. Adjunctive techniques are isolation from all the usual indicators of place and time and some sensory deprivation. An additional factor sometimes used is that of beating, raping, or killing prisoners in front of or in earshot of members of their own family or forcing the other members of that family to do such things to them.

New technology would seem to have increased the torturer's armament. Sophisticated Chinese-built electroshock batons have recently been used and the chemical substance P is said to have been used. The Dubai Special Branch commissioned a British firm to build a torture chamber equipped with stroboscopic lights and a white noise generator, which was said to reduce victims to submission within 30 minutes.

Torturers seem to believe that those they torment are somehow less than human, or that their job is grim and unpleasant but vital in terms of national security. They are usually selected as potential torturers from a section of the population which to some extent already believes this of the tortured people's class. Their training usually features prolonged periods of isolation in selected camps away from routine society, in which time their pre-existing hatred of 'enemies of the state' is reinforced and they are forced to be humiliated and to beat each other in order to raise the threshold of violence they routinely tolerate. After this they are invited to swear special loyalty oaths which win admission to an 'élite corps', whose function is not at first known. Initial duties in the élite corps involve simply watching torture or minor, 'kindly' participation in torture such as carrying victims back to cells or attending their injuries. Full participation as a torturer is achieved gradually, no act seeming to be much more outrageous than those that preceded it.

### The role of doctors?

The role of doctors in torture varies greatly. The commonest are such things as the refusal to treat a torture victim because they are a 'police case' or to fully or accurately to describe or attribute such things as pathological findings. This may occur as the consequence of an unthinking compliance with authority, through a fear of official or unofficial retribution, or through active complicity with torture. Some doctors have had an active role as supervisors of torture, using their knowledge to advise how much or what sort of torture should be applied. Other doctors, such as Radovan Karadiç, promote torture by spearheading a political regime which makes such things possible rather than actually participating in themselves.

By its nature torture destroys feelings of security and self-worth. Victims are often filled with guilt, self-doubt, and shame. Doctors reflect this, as they did with childhood sexual abuse, by seeming never to ask those torture-related questions whose answers they might find too difficult to deal with. As a consequence of this effect, almost all doctors in clinical practice in the developed world have encountered patients (often refugees) who have been tortured, and have usually done so entirely unknowingly since torture is rarely spontaneously raised by either doctor or patient.

Tortured people frequently complain of pain and stiffness in limbs, which is often ascribed to previously endured cramped and cold prison conditions but which might equally well be due to the convulsive movements made when attempting to avoid being beaten. Scars over bony points are caused by beating but may have other causes. More easily defined nerve damage may follow long suspension in unnatural positions, and very characteristic foot pain follows beating on the soles of the feet (*falaka*). Chronic lung damage may follow near drowning in contaminated water, head blows may result in optic nerve, retinal, or middle ear damage.

Sometimes such long-standing pains as from peptic ulcers or headaches are attributed by victims to continuing physical damage of some sort when the psychological after-effects of torture are likely to be largely or wholly responsible. Whether these symptoms are linked to torture by the attending physician depends on whether the victim chooses to discuss what has happened to them, or the doctor chooses to ask.

In those patients who do talk about being tortured the problems commonly presented have some similarities to those seen in POST-TRAUMATIC STRESS DISORDER. There are, however, crucial differences. The trauma has often been repetitive and prolonged rather than a single event. Crucially, as with CHILD ABUSE, the trauma has been intentionally inflicted and not the product of accident.

Whether there is a commonly seen 'post-torture syndrome' is doubted, not least because some people seem less susceptible to the longer term psychological sequels and because it is not known how many people are tortured and never come to the attention of medical services.

### Psychological recovery

A fairly frequently seen pattern is for victims to initially show daytime hyperarousal, irritability, poor concentration, and failure to engage in previously meaningful activities. Daytime flashbacks triggered by evocative circumstances are usual. Very poor sleep is usually reported and substance misuse may occur and may need treating in its own right.

## TOURETTE SYNDROME

Tourette syndrome is a hereditary neuro-behavioral disorder that is characterized by a triad of motor tics, involuntary vocalizations, and compulsive behavior.

The tics may be simple repetitive motor movements such as blinking or facial grimaces, shoulder shrugging, finger or foot tapping, and sometimes self-hitting or finger biting. Other movements may be very complex motor acts such as hopping, twirling, squatting, body twisting, or bending. The vocalizations can be repetitive words or phrases (palilalia), repeating the words said by others (echolalia), or, in a few cases, profanities (coprolalia). Most often the sounds are throat clearing, coughing, squealing, barking, blowing, or whistling. The compulsive behavior is often doing things over and over in the same way, having to arrange objects, and to carry out actions in a repetitive manner. Patients often feel a building inner sensation that is relieved by the tic or vocalization, and, although they may be able to suppress these for a short time, most cannot do this for long. Over the years the pattern of tics and vocalizations may change, with some features disappearing, others taking their place, and old patterns returning. In adults the manifestations often wax and wane and may decrease, and in a few they may disappear.

The symptoms often appear around ages 8 to 12, just when the normal tics and behaviors of childhood are coming under control. The symptoms increase for a few years and then stabilize, waxing and waning to some extent, but remaining for the rest of the patient's lives. It is more common in boys and occurs in all ethnic groups, although more often in Ashkenazi Jews. It has a hereditary basis, and, although it appears to have a dominant genetic pattern in some studies, some have inheritance from both sides of the family, suggesting a polygenic basis. Others in the family may have aspects of the triad, such as tics, or obsessive compulsive traits.

Initially the child may be thought to be just a troublemaker in school or have a behavior problem. It is not surprising that the disorder was thought to be due to emotional or psychological disturbance, but it is now known to be an inherited central nervous system disorder, perhaps a neurochemical abnormality that affects inhibitory networks in the cortical–basal ganglia connections. Recent studies using magnetic resonance imaging have suggested that there are some differences in these regions in patients compared with normal brains.

One of the first cases described was a French noblewoman, the Marquise de Dampierre, who shocked her family by her strange behavior, not the least of which was the tendency to repeatedly blurt out, 'Shit and fucking pig'. She was described by J. M. G. Itard in Paris, and 60 years later by George Gilles de la Tourette, when he published details of other cases and recognized that it was a specific disorder. For the next century it was thought to be an interesting but rare condition, but when haloperidol was found to improve the symptoms, Arthur and Eileen Shapiro identified hundreds of patients and it is now known to be common, occurring in 30 cases in 100 000 people.

Recent research has focused on the genetic factors, the neurochemical changes, and pharmacological treatment. Several helpful drugs are available, including haloperidol, pimozide, clonidine, fluxetine, risperidone, deprenyl, and the transdermal nicotine patch. About half the patients take no medication and appreciate the reassurance and understanding that comes from realizing the nature of the disorder and that they are not alone in this. Greater knowledge of the disorder by teachers and the public has helped Tourette patients cope both in school and in society.

Many young people are interested in others that shared their disorder. Claudius, the Roman Emperor, had the features of Tourette syndrome, as did numerous members of five generations of his family. A Bohemian secular priest was thought to be possessed by the devil during the Inquisition, described in the *Malleus Maleficarum*. Samuel Johnson, the 18th century lexicographer, had all the features of Tourette syndrome, which surprised those who first met the great man, but later they regarded his bizarre behavior as the eccentricities of a great genius. Others with the features of Tourette syndrome include Prince de Condé in the Court of Louis XIV, the French author André Malraux, and a British Columbia surgeon described by Dr Oliver Sacks. Joseph Bliss described his own case and the experience of having these symptoms.

Although some patients have associated learning difficulties, most are otherwise normal and successful in life despite the symptoms, perhaps because aided by their compulsive personalities.　　　TJM

*See also* LANGUAGE

Later, sleep improves in length and daytime flashbacks become less frequent. Unconscious processing of the torture is demonstrated by frequent nightmares. As daily functioning improves, the nightmares become less frequent and less frightening and assume a dreamlike quality. The rate of improvement varies greatly between individuals, and may be increased with expert psychotherapeutic help and socially and culturally congruent support from a refugee association, church, or suchlike body.

Torture changes people forever, and given a strong enough reminder any tortured person will collapse under the weight of agonized memories. Most, however, build a new life with which they are satisfied, and it is perhaps the role of medicine to realize that those who have been tortured are simply normal people who have undergone abnormal experiences and thus to aid their return as close to their previous abilities and life as they can or want to be.　　　　　　　　　　JB

See also BIOETHICS; OATHS AND CODES OF CONDUCT

**TRANSPLANTATION** In 1800 the Italian surgeon Baronio reported the first clearly defined scientific experiment on tissue grafting. He showed that free 'autografts' of skin (taken from the same animal to be grafted) took permanently if the surgery was skilful, but skin 'allografts' (taken from another individual) were destroyed after a few days.

Over a century later, in the classic 1943 experiments of Gibson and MEDAWAR (p 819), this destruction process was shown to be an immune reaction. These researchers found that after skin grafts taken from a donor rabbit were rejected by the recipient, 'second-set' grafts from the same donor were destroyed more rapidly. As a result of exposure to the donor's skin, the recipient become specifically sensitized in a similar manner to the immunity to measles that follows infection with the measles virus.

Billingham and his colleagues then showed that the destruction immune response could be prevented if the donor antigens were presented to the recipient *in utero* or during the neonatal period before the reticuloendothelial cells, the lymphocytes, and macrophages of the immune system had developed. The recipient animals were unable to recognize these grafts as foreign and accepted subsequent grafts from the same donor origin. They had developed specific 'immunological tolerance'.

No progress was possible until a reliable method of joining blood vessels together was devised by Alexis Carrel at the turn of the century, which permitted surgeons to investigated grafted organs. In a series of experimental kidney grafts, Carrel

concluded that if the surgery was correctly performed, renal autografts were accepted permanently, whereas allografts were destroyed after a period of function of a few days. Thus, he duplicated Baronio's experiments but with a vascularized kidney instead of skin. Further studies of kidney grafting in a dog along similar lines led Joseph Murray and his colleagues to perform the first clinical renal transplant at the Peter Bent Brigham Hospital in Boston between identical twins.

Confidence in the surgical technique of kidney grafting had become established. Some of the early patients still have functioning transplants after 40 years, showing that, when rejection is avoided, the kidney graft can remain in excellent condition. These two unrelated early experiments were a signal to many surgeons that organ grafting might one day become a more general form of surgical treatment. Nevertheless, tentative trials of allografts from both unrelated and familial donors were extremely disappointing. Initially, large doses of total body X-irradiation were given to the recipient, which damaged the immune system but was extremely toxic and usually did not prevent rejection. However, there were two important exceptions; both of these grafts were between non-identical twins, one was performed in Paris, the other in Boston. The advantage of familial donors has been established subsequently. Moreover, the main transplantation tissue group, the major histocompatibility complex (determining the acceptance or rejection of cells), has been largely unraveled and we know that the complex resides on the sixth human chromosome.

### Graft rejection

It became clear that without immunosuppressive treatment, rejection was to be expected for all grafts, except those between identical twins, and that total body X-irradiation could not prevent rejection, except in recipients of particularly well-matched familial donors. Rejection in the kidney is manifested by two destructive processes. Lymphocytes from the blood penetrate the capilary walls of the graft and divide rapidly in the substance of the kidney, causing swelling of the organ and impaired function. This infiltration by white blood cells can often be dispersed with high doses of corticosteroid drugs, leaving little damage behind. The second immune response is due to circulating antibodies secreted by plasma cells (secretory B lymphocytes) in the lymph nodes and spleen. The antibodies are specifically active against the graft blood vessels, destroying their lining and eventually blocking them. This second response is not easily controlled and much of the damage is irreversible.

It was then found that rabbits given the antileukemia drug 6-mercaptopurine did not pro-

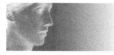

duce antibodies when challenged with a foreign protein. Hence a 'drug-induced immunological tolerance' had been produced. Next, it was found that the rejection of renal allografts in dogs was also impaired by 6-mercaptopurine. Subsequently, a newly synthesized drug, azathioprine (a derivative of 6-mercaptopurine), was found to be even more effective and this, combined with the corticosteroids, became the sheet anchor of clinical immunosuppressive treatment for recipients of organ grafts for 20 years.

## Transplantable organs

The kidney was the first organ to be transplanted successfully because the surgery is straight-forward. In addition, patients dying from kidney disease can be restored from a moribund state to reasonable health by hemodialysis, which can also be used to maintain the patient if the graft is slow to function or is rejected. With the same immunosuppression, grafts of heart and liver were performed, the results initially being poor as there were no adequate substitutes for function if the organ failed or was rejected. With the liver, rejection is less severe than with other organs, an intriguing observation that in some species can be remarkable. In man, immunosuppressive drugs are needed but the main danger is the operation itself, which is a major trauma in an already sick patient.

With the exception of kidney transplantation, organ grafting did not really enter into general treatment until a new immunosuppressive agent, cyclosporin, was introduced. This agent was discovered in 1976 by Borel at Sandoz Laboratories, Basle, to have powerful immunosuppressive properties. Studies in animals with organ grafts confirmed its efficacy, and when it was first used in human renal transplantation in Cambridge graft survival at a year increased from around 60 to 80%. Unfortunately, cyclosporin was found to damage the kidney and, therefore, the dose has to be watched very carefully. To reduce toxicity of all the agents used to prevent rejection, a strategy of multiple treatment has been adopted by most centers, giving small non-toxic doses of azathio-prine, corticosteroids, and cyclosporin together, so that the agents' immunosuppressive effects are additive but side-effects are minimized.

Organ preservation is an important requirement if the benefits of tissue typing are to be applied. Throughout the world there is a shortage of donor organs, and in many countries super-stitious taboos preclude cadaveric transplanta-tion. The ideal donor is a person, otherwise healthy, who has died as a result of head injury, intracranial hemorrhage, or primary cerebral tumor, who does not harbor sepsis or cancer outside the brain. Such cases managed on a venti-lator can be maintained so that the organs to be grafted are in perfect condition until they are removed and cooled. They may then be stored in ice for several hours. Cooling the organs is accomplished by immersion in cold fluid and perfusion through the blood vessels of special cooling solutions which slow down the inevitable damage which occurs with time. With modern perfusion fluids, the kidney can be kept in good condition for 36–48 hours, the liver and pancreas for 12–24 hours, and the heart and lungs for 4–6 hours. These time intervals are important to make use of the advantages of getting good tissue matches and also to move the organs to the appropriate recipients.

The world-wide shortage of donor organs means that many potential recipients never have the chance of a graft.

## Present situation

In the last few years several new agents have become available which are effective in inhibiting the immune system at different points in its activation. These include monoclonal antibodies produced by culture techniques that are effective and much less toxic. The new chemical immuno-suppressive agent, FK506, is very powerful and effective in remarkably low doses. It seems to act at the same point as cyclosporin and therefore has most of the same side-effects, but does not cause increase of hair growth. The new antiproliferative drug mycophenolate mofetil seems to be more effective than azathioprine and has replaced it in many centers in North America. Other new agents are in clinical trial and the clinician will soon have more than sufficient drugs with which to control rejection. Indeed, there is a danger of causing over-immunosuppression.

## Present — and future

With each new agent difficulties arise as to how or if it should be combined with other, better estab-lished treatments. With the current control of rejec-tion, liver and heart grafting have become routine, the lungs and pancreas are also frequently trans-

(continued)

Sir Peter **MEDAWAR** (1915–87). British zoologist and immunologist. His work on the rejection of skin grafts in animals laid the foundations of modern cellular immunology, and his subsequent studies of human leukocyte antigens, along with work on T lymphocytes, led to his being awarded the NOBEL PRIZE for physiology or medicine in 1960.

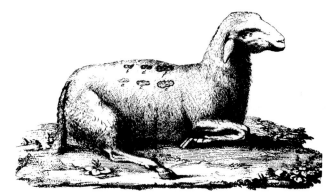

Baronio's skin-grafting experiment. Autografts, below, took satisfactorily; allografts, above, were rejected.

planted, and the small bowel has been grafted, alone or together with other organs. The pancreas is usually grafted together with the kidney in patients with diabetic renal failure, and the results are good. The functional survival of most organ transplants is around 70–80% at one year, although, with well-matched kidneys, over 90% functional survival is expected at five years. Really long-term survival has now been achieved in recipients of allografts as well as in identical twin transplants.

Throughout the world there are several patients with renal transplants still living between 30 and 35 years after transplantation from cadaver donors. The longest surviving recipient of a liver transplant is 26 years and of a heart 23 years; pancreas, 13 years; heart and lung, 10 years. Thus prolonged survival is possible and rehabilitation can be excellent. Recipients of organ transplants can lead normal lives and have children.

Interest is now returning to the possibility of achieving immunological tolerance in humans, using donor cells together with short courses of powerful immunosuppression. As results of organ transplantation improve, so will the demand for this form of treatment. Already there are many ethical worries concerning the payment of living donors who are not related to the patients, inducing them to give organs or parts of organs. The questions of coercion, the use of organs from executed criminals, and how to decide on priorities in organ allocation are all difficult problems.

As immunosuppression improves, so there will be an inevitable extension of the organ graft repertoire to transplantation of other tissues, such as limbs (an arm has been transplanted in France) and the sex organs. (Transplantation of testes and ovaries would certainly cause many new ethical and moral concerns.)

The world-wide donor shortage has inevitably led to attempts to use alternative sources — namely, organ xenografts (organs from animals). In the 1960s several kidneys were transplanted from chimpanzees to man, and one of these functioned in a human patient for nine months. Subsequently, a liver was transplanted from baboon to man; this functioned for 70 days, when the patient died from infection. Transplantation from non-human primates to man is between two closely related species, and overcoming rejection would seem to be a goal that might soon be achieved, the so-called 'concordant' xenograft.

Grafts from widely disparate species, for example, from pig to man, are destroyed almost instantaneously, and understanding and overcoming this 'discordant' reaction is the subject of intense research. Natural antibodies in man cause activation of the complement system and destroy pig organs usually immediately. A new approach has been to produce a strain of pigs that has the human complement-controlling protein. Studies show that transplants of organs from these transgenic pigs have not been subjected to immediate destruction and hence the first hurdle for discordant organ transplantation may have been overcome. Nevertheless, there are other factors to consider besides immunological rejection, for example, the physiology and metabolism of the organs from a foreign species might not be suitable for man.          RYC

*See also* BIOETHICS; IMMUNOLOGY

**TRAUMA — HISTORY** The history of trauma management is mainly the history of military surgery. Written evidence is scanty before the end of the 18th century, but Ambroise PARÉ (p 320) wrote in 1545 of the benefit of wound exploration and débridement. However, his advice was largely ignored for almost 400 years, because of the surgical obsession with closing wounds.

LARREY (p 796) created the first army medical team in 1792, by providing ambulances with trained attendants and equipment to collect the wounded on the battlefield. However, the mortality from wounds in battle was horrendous. An open fracture was regarded as a sentence of death, with the only question being would death occur before or after an amputation? The mortality rate for all kinds of open fractures in the Franco–Prussian war (1870–71) was 41%. Of 13 173 amputations performed on the French side, 10 006 patients died.

Up until 1915 it was policy in all armies that penetrating abdominal wounds should be treated non-operatively. In the American Civil War, there was an 82% mortality rate following penetrating abdominal wounds treated in this way. The concept of exploration for penetrating abdominal wounds was developed by the Russian army in the Russo–Japanese war (1903–5), but it was not until 1915 that operative care of abdominal wounds became the rule. However, there was no concept of the cause of shock and the reported mortality rate, even with surgical exploration, remained between 50 and 60%. As the First World War evolved, the role of wound excision became regulated and wounds were excised and left open. In 1917, the Allies issued an edict that all war wounds should be left open.

However, at this time the physiology of shock was not appreciated and the importance of blood volume replacement was not recognized until the late 1930s. During the Spanish Civil War and Second World War, the concept of early blood volume replacement became established and was a significant factor in reducing the mortality after penetrating wounds. The American army also paid particular attention to reducing the time between injury and treatment, and the mortality rate after penetrating abdominal wounds fell to 24%.

**TRAUMA SURGEONS**

Alexander **TIETZE** (1864–1927). German surgeon. Having studied medicine at Breslau, gaining his doctorate in 1887, he worked in the surgical clinic, becoming a lecturer in surgery in 1894 and later professor. In 1896 he joined the Allerheiligen Hospital. He wrote widely on surgical subjects and published a textbook on emergency surgery (1927). He gave his name to costochondritis (Tietze syndrome or disease), an inflammation of the rib cartilages where they join the breastbone.

*(continued opposite)*

In the Korean War, the American army introduced the widespread use of the helicopter, together with mobile army surgical hospitals to further reduce the therapy-free interval. The mortality rate following abdominal wounds fell to under 12%. During the Vietnam War, advances in understanding of the pathophysiology of shock and pulmonary failure led to vastly improved systemic care of the patient, with data showing that the mortality rate after abdominal wounds in the American army was under 9%.

Knowledge and interest in the management of the injured were much slower to develop in civilian practice. Gissane established the Birmingham Accident Hospital in 1941; this was an experiment designed to improve the care of the injured by providing continuous cover by trained consultant surgeons and anesthetists, supported by appropriate technical and transfusion services. In the USA, the stimulus to improve trauma care came with the end of the Vietnam War and the return into civilian practice of experienced surgeons, anesthetists, and paramedics, who translated their military experience into the care of the civilian injured.

In 1976 the Committee on Trauma of the American College of Surgeons called upon hospitals to commit themselves to provide facilities and personnel to deal with the seriously injured. This group has set standards for staffing and equipment for hospitals dealing with injuries in North America, and has also pioneered the concept of trauma centers, where the management of severely injured patients is concentrated in suitably staffed and equipped units.

The Federal Republic of Germany also set up an integrated trauma care system in the early 1970s. This was based on 35 designated trauma centers, each supported by a air/ground ambulance system. Skilled medical care was deployed to the scene of accidents, and patients were rapidly transported back to the designated trauma centers.

However, the lessons learnt from North America and central Europe have not been widely accepted within Britain, which continues to lag behind other western nations in provision of care for the injured.      PW

*See also* BLOOD TRANSFUSION; RED CROSS/ RED CRESCENT; WAR

**TRAUMA** (*trauma* Gr, wound) implies injury. It is the leading cause of death at all ages from 1–34, commonly outnumbering all other causes put together. When all ages are considered, it still ranks very high. For example, in the USA in 1995, deaths due to unintentional and intentional injury accounted for about 5.4% of all deaths; they were exceeded only by heart disease (32%), cancer (24%), and stroke (6.8%). But, unlike patients with heart disease, cancer, and stroke, the victims of trauma are predominantly young. Not only are most trauma victims young, they seldom have pre-existing diseases or disabilities and are usually male — indeed, in some categories such as gunshot wounds, they are overwhelmingly male in the USA and many other countries.

In the USA, about 150 000 people die annually from causes related to trauma (classified as injuries, poisoning, and violence, and including burns). There are about 7 million non-fatal injuries and about 340 000 people are permanently disabled every year. A high proportion of those disabled are people who suffer permanent neurological damage — impaired brain function, paralysis of limbs due to fractures of the spine and severing of the spinal cord — and whose long-term care is costly and often has to be provided in institutions. Other categories are permanent damage to eyesight, and to joints and bones. Altogether, trauma accounts for about 40% of total long-term disability; it is responsible for over 4 million years of potential life lost compared with 2 million years lost due to heart disease and 1.7 million years due to cancer.

Trauma occurs in several settings: at work, in the home, on the roads, and in sports and other recreations. In the industrial nations the proportions are very roughly 30%, 30%, 30%, and 10% respectively (it is hard to be more precise because reporting is inadequate for some categories). There are some well-defined and easily recognized features of each. The victims of work-related trauma are more often male than female; the most common varieties are back injuries associated with lifting heavy weights, foreign bodies in the eye, and lacerations. At home, the pattern is quite different. The most affected victims are the very young, toddlers, and preschool children, who drown in the bath, get burned, consume poisonous substances, or have serious falls; and the old, notably old women living alone, who fall and break a hip or other bones.

All ages and both sexes are affected by traffic-related trauma. With the rising popularity of bicycles in city traffic, an increasing proportion of serious injuries and deaths occur when a poorly protected cyclist is struck by a fast-moving car or truck. At the same time, better-engineered and safer cars, the use of airbags and seat-belts, and improved roads (especially controlled access highways) have all helped to reduce the toll of death and serious injury due to traffic crashes. Alcohol and other substances that impair judgement and skill contribute to a high proportion of traffic crashes, and some are associated with the syndrome called road rage. In some countries, including the USA, firearms are associated with much intentionally caused trauma and premature

(*continued*)

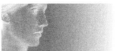

Josep Anthony **TRUETA** (1897–1977). Spanish surgeon. Trueta specialized in the surgery of trauma. In 1929 he was appointed chief surgeon to Caja de Provisión y Socorro, which dealt with thousands of accident cases a year and in 1935 became professor of surgery at Barcelona University. During the Spanish Civil War he treated air-raid and battle casualties, perfecting the 'closed plaster technique' rather than amputating limbs; he personally treated over 1000 casualties with only six deaths. As a liberal, after the Spanish Civil War he came to Britain and in 1949 was appointed Nuffield professor of orthopedic surgery. During the Second World War his experience made him one of the British government's foremost advisers on the treatment of casualties. He was a pioneer in the treatment of bone infections (osteomyelitis) with penicillin, and continued to do research not only into orthopedic problems but also into kidney function after injury.

## REDUCING THE IMPACT OF TRAUMA

Attempts to reduce the impact that trauma exerts upon our population have classically been approached in three ways: pre-crash, crash, and post-crash.

- Pre-crash — preventing an injury from occurring. Strategies to prevent blunt or unintentional trauma include safer driving habits, prohibitions against drunk driving, seat belts, air bags, safer vehicles, better roads and lighting, and restrictions on speeding. Strategies to prevent accidental falls include handrails for the elderly, for example, slip-proof mats in bathrooms, more secure floor rugs. The difficulties in preventing intentional injuries are enormous and reflect the problem of VIOLENCE in society.

- Crash — refers to the possibility of diminishing the actual amount of injury once preventive strategies have failed, and includes efforts to improve the safety of vehicles and, in intentional injuries, reducing the types of weaponry available to the population.

- Post-crash — the medical response is most evident; even the best prevention strategies may fail and result in seriously injured patients. The approach here is through a trauma system.

death. Recreation-related trauma effects mostly young men. There are some well-known serious and fatal varieties — for instance, fractured cervical spine ('broken neck'), with paralysis of arms as well as legs, caused by diving head-first into shallow water or by a rough tackle playing football. Sprains, fractures, and dislocated joints are other common recreational injuries.

### Underfunding in research

Trauma is poorly nourished with research funds. In the USA, despite its heavy cost in years of potential life lost, trauma research receives only about $112 million per annum, compared with $624 million for heart disease and $998 million for cancer. Part of the reason for this might be the association of trauma with the word 'accident', implying that nothing can be done to prevent it happening. This is far from the truth: many forms of trauma are predictable and preventable. Traffic crashes have been extensively studied by epidemiologists, using the frame of reference that has worked well for studying infectious disease epidemics: the environment, the agent, and the host. The environment (the road) is especially hazardous at dusk, when it is slippery, has many blind corners, and carries merging traffic. The agent (the car) has been made much safer in recent years by improved design and the use of safety belts and airbags. The host (the driver) is

safest when educated about proper driving behavior and free from alcohol, drugs, or medical conditions such as unstable diabetes that may impair consciousness and cloud judgement. More research is needed on prevention of trauma in the other settings described above.

Trauma has been classically divided into blunt trauma and penetrating trauma. Blunt trauma most commonly results from automotive crashes or falls; penetrating trauma is caused by gun shot wounds, stabbing, or shotgun blasts. From a prevention point of view, it may be more rational to classify trauma into unintentional (automotive crashes and falls) or intentional (deliberately inflicted, such as gunshot wounds, stabbing, shotgun blast, and personal assaults).

### Trauma system — experience in the USA

This comprises three components and aims at getting the appropriate patient to the appropriate hospital in an appropriate time.

- The appropriate patient. Not all injured patients have immediate life- or limb-threatening injuries. In fact, 95% of trauma patients have small or minor injuries that can be safely managed in any adequate hospital. A few patients, however, have immediate serious life- or limb-threatening injuries that need to be recognized at the scene and such patients need to be transported to appropriate hospitals. This process is referred to as 'field triage'.

- The appropriate facility. The appropriate facility is generally a designated trauma center. This differs from a normal hospital emergency department in having a separate trauma service, generally staffed by surgeons who are totally separate from the general surgery service. Such trauma centers must also provide needed subspecialty services such as neurosurgery, pediatric surgery, and vascular surgery. Operating rooms must be constantly available, adequately staffed by nurses and anesthesiologists; radiology departments with computerized tomography scanning and angiography capability, and blood banking are also necessary. A commitment by an institution to become a trauma center is accordingly more than just providing a trauma service; it is an institution-wide commitment which implies that the resources of the entire institution are mobilized and prioritized for the care of the seriously injured patient. The designation of a trauma center may be disruptive to the life of the hospital: elective surgical cases may have to be deferred or canceled to allow for urgent operative intervention in the more seriously injured trauma patients. In addition, the implied priority given to trauma patients from hospital resources such as computerized tomography scanning, angiography, or blood banking capabilities may well preclude elective patients from accessing these same facilities.

- A reasonable time scale. In the United States the accepted time taken to move a seriously injured patient from the site of the injury to an appropriate trauma center or trauma care facility is 20 minutes. In the city this is generally achieved by ambulance; in rural areas aeromedical evacuation may be needed.

Setting up trauma systems involves discussions between government agencies, hospitals wishing to become trauma centers, and those hospitals that do not but are worried about losing patients to such centers. The question may therefore be reasonably asked whether such systems are worth while developing. The first such system was established in Orange County, California. Before the establishment of an organized trauma system almost three-quarters of patients' deaths were from 'a preventable trauma death' — that is, an injury that would have responded to treatment. Examples of such injuries are ruptured spleens, causing the patient to bleed to death, and epidural hematomas not treated soon enough by neurosurgeons. Following the implementation of a designated trauma system in Orange County — where these seriously injured patients were taken to hospitals with trauma centers — the preventable deaths dropped significantly to about 4%. In 1983 Donald Trunkey reviewed the work of trauma systems, concluding that preventable deaths from inadequate trauma care vary between 30–40%, and that a decrease of 30–40% is consistently seen when trauma systems are implemented, showing that they work. It has been estimated that if trauma systems were implemented in the whole of the USA, some 25 000 lives would be saved every year.

### Creation of trauma systems

In the late 1960s David Boyd of Cook County Hospital persuaded Illinois Governor Richard Ogilvie to finance a system of trauma care consisting of pre-hospital triage, rapid transport, and designated trauma centers. This system was instituted originally in Illinois, and subsequently similar systems were introduced in other states in America. There are two types: the urban X model or the rural Y model.

The urban X model is most frequently used in the urban areas where there are dense populations with a high prevalence of trauma; there are often large numbers of hospitals that provide tertiary care; ground transportation is mostly used to transport the injured patients to the designated trauma center; and the journeys tend to be short.

The Y model is more commonly used in rural or suburban areas characterized by scattered populations, low prevalence of trauma, and long transport times by ground, frequently implying that aerial medical evacuation is more efficient. In the X model the solution is to designate among the tertiary care facilities in the city a small number of Level I trauma centers. All trauma patients are taken directly to a Level I trauma center, staffed with certified surgeons present in-house 24 hours a day, and equipped with constantly staffed and immediately available operating rooms.

Under the Y model the distance from the scene of the injury to a tertiary care facility may be so great that it exceeds the recommended limit of 20 minutes. Under these conditions community hospitals may be used as 'Level II trauma centers'. Such hospitals would be within 20 minutes of transportation of the injured patient, and though not possessing all the characteristics of the Level I trauma center would have made a commitment to the care of the injured patient. Typically they will have surgeons on call available to respond to the hospital within 30 minutes and able to provide rapidly needed operative intervention for injured patients, though perhaps not immediately. Some patients who cannot be managed in Level II trauma centers would be stabilized there and then transported to the more distant Level I trauma center. It is these inter-hospital transports that have used aero-medical evacuation facilities so successfully.

### Field triage

This is an attempt to separate the 5% of patients with an immediate life- or limb-threatening injury from the other 95%. Various triage schemes have been proposed. Essentially they recognize patients with clearly life-threatening injuries who require rapid transport to an appropriate facility (particularly hemorrhagic shock, depressed level of consciousness, or airway problems). Another group of patients are those who show no clear physiological consequence of their injury but are considered at risk because of the kinetics of the mechanism that caused their injury. Such mechanism would include penetrating injuries to the head, neck, or torso; evidence of spinal cord injury; amputations; falls from heights of over 30 feet; automotive crashes from speeds at over 30 miles per hour, death of another occupant in the same vehicle, ejection from the vehicle or major damage to it. Some schemes have also considered the extremes of age and pre-existing medical conditions as indications for triage to trauma centers. It is important to recognize that the pre-hospital care provider is probably the best judge of the condition of the patient at the scene and the necessity for bypass to a trauma center.

These requests from the pre-hospital care provider to bypass patients to trauma centers should in general be approved.

One of the dangers in creating a trauma system is to designate too many trauma centers. Many hospitals consider it advantageous to become a designated center and there may be competition among institutions. It has been argued that a certain level of volume is necessary in order to maintain the skills of a Level I trauma center. The American College of Surgeons has recommended that at least 1000 seriously injured patients should be seen every year in a designated trauma center, and studies have shown a direct correlation between the total number of trauma admissions to a trauma center and the mortality rate. Nevertheless, the setting up of trauma centers systems, though difficult to achieve and frequently dogged by political considerations and hospital politics, when successfully implemented has resulted in a significant decrease in preventable deaths among the young population at risk.                    JBarr

*See also* VIOLENCE

**TROPICAL MEDICINE** is a specialty defined by the part of the world where the illness was acquired. The ties of tropical medicine to PUBLIC HEALTH of developing countries (traditionally called tropical hygiene) are so close that they have to be considered together, and both are related to the natural history of the agents and vectors of warm climate diseases: the science known as PARASITOLOGY. For the first half of the 20th century tropical medicine and parasitology were closely intertwined and almost synonymous.

### History
Although medical practice in the tropics originally comprised the traditional medical systems of indigenous peoples, except for the use of quinine as an antimalarial originally among the Incas, indigenous medical systems had little impact on 'tropical medicine', as usually defined, until recently. Rather, the subject arose from the problems encountered by explorers and the military, and developed as a necessary aspect of the colonial system.

Mortality among Europeans visiting the tropics, from the time of the earliest Portuguese and Spanish explorers, was very high. In addition to the nutritional problems of long sea voyages, visits to tropical ports were accompanied, or shortly followed, by fevers with or without jaundice, diarrheal diseases, and many other illnesses. In both West Africa and the Caribbean the most lethal were MALARIA and YELLOW FEVER, with men of the garrisons in Jamaica dying at the rate of 13% per year in the early 19th century. Even in South and South-East Asia, where yellow fever

was absent, 45% of a military expedition to Burma in 1824 died of disease.

The initial discovery that linked medicine in the tropics to specific biological processes was, however, made by a civilian British physician working in Amoy (Xiamen) in China, on the spread of elephantiasis (swelling of the limbs), which had been shown by Lewis and by Bancroft to be caused by a filarial WORM. Patrick Manson (1878) demonstrated that the embryos of the worm were found in the peripheral blood only at night and that they underwent development in a night-biting mosquito which was responsible for transmission of the infection. This was the first demonstration of an INSECT vector of human disease, adding two further connotations to the idea of tropical disease: firstly, that many are transmitted by insect vectors, and, secondly, that the life cycle of many agents of tropical disease involves development outside the human body, and that this stage is temperature-dependent.

In the decades that followed, corresponding to the golden age of bacteriology, mosquitoes were shown to be responsible for the transmission of malaria and yellow fever, and many other diseases peculiar to the tropics were shown to be insect-borne, while the role of ticks and snails in the transmission of infections was discovered, together with the role of mammalian reservoirs of viral, bacterial, and parasitic diseases.

### Epidemic disease control
The 19th century scientific advances in understanding parasitic disease transmission were accompanied by, and sometimes due to, concern for practical problems of epidemic disease control in the tropics. Interest in tropical countries moved from exploration to colonization, and the period 1890–1910 was marked by disease outbreaks on a scale that could not be ignored by governments. In particular, sleeping sickness was responsible for the death of perhaps one-third of the population of southern Uganda. India was affected by epidemics of PLAGUE and of KALA-AZAR, while the great Punjab malaria epidemic of 1908 led to an intensified interest in malariology. In the New World the building of the Panama canal depended on adequate measures for control of yellow fever and malaria. The complex life cycles of the major parasitic and other vector-borne diseases were elucidated, usually by the military or by expeditions from industrial countries, but the life cycle of SCHISTOSOMIASIS was first determined by Japanese workers in their own country.

To control epidemics in the absence of adequate chemotherapy, emphasis had to be placed on the environmental control of vectors. It had been found that malaria is transmitted only by

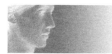

anopheline mosquitoes, and that in a given area only a few species are important vectors, with specific breeding habitats: some species live in swamps, others in small sunlit pools, and yet others in shaded streams. Environmental modifications directed to removing the specific habitats of the major vectors achieved good results at moderate cost, an approach known as species sanitation. Sleeping sickness was similarly controlled by selective removal of vegetation to make the area unattractive to tsetse flies.

## Tropical healthcare systems

As colonial governments became involved with the welfare of indigenous populations as well as colonists, there was a gradual expansion of healthcare systems. Schools of tropical medicine were set up at the beginning of the 20th century, gradually taking over the lead from the military. They reflected the shift from military to trading ventures and colonization, and were usually sited at major ports. They gradually became more associated with imperial power (for example, the Royal Tropical Institute in Amsterdam), and the corresponding national colonial territories. France and Britain, with a widespread distribution of their colonies around the globe, tended to have a world-wide interest.

Research laboratories were often established in the tropics in response to a particular problem, but some had a broader function, such as the Institute for Medical Research in Kuala Lumpur, founded at the beginning of the century. The Rockefeller Foundation founded laboratories specifically to study yellow fever in Belem, Trinidad, Poona, and several places in Africa. Other research institutes were of indigenous origin, such as the Oswaldo Cruz Institute in Brazil. In Britain, the early part of the 20th century saw the emergence of the London and Liverpool Schools with a focus on East and West Africa, respectively, as the intellectual centers. The Indian Medical Services provided bases for research on malaria under such workers as Christophers, Sinton, and Shortt, who extended the pioneer work of Ross; on cholera by ROGERS (this page); on kala-azar by Shortt; and on dysentery by Boyd. They were gradually replaced by a distinguished group of Indian national research workers.

The American tradition in tropical hygiene has a strong military component, exemplified by the outstanding work of Walter Reed on the transmission of yellow fever and of GORGAS (p 824) on its control, together with malaria, in Cuba and Panama. Civilian parasitological work, involving biologists rather than doctors, focused particularly on helminthology in the USA, and then in China and the Philippines. The Second World War was a notable stimulus to tropical medicine. It speeded up the introduction of residual insecticides, synthetic antimalarials, and antibacterial chemotherapy. Whereas before the Second World War the British focus in tropical medicine was in India, the post-war focus was on Africa, for the obvious reason of Indian political independence. The focus also shifted from sleeping sickness, epidemics of which had wrought such havoc in Uganda and the West African Sahel but were now under control, to the other parasitic diseases. Malaria and filariasis were studied, and especially the extreme degree of malarial endemicity seen only in sub-Saharan Africa and New Guinea.

## The recent past

*Malaria* Malaria dominated much of the world scene in tropical medicine until the 1960s and is returning to this position at present. After the Second World War, DDT became widely available and its use in the Mediterranean islands controlled malaria to a dramatic extent because its persistent insecticidal properties reduced mosquito numbers but also reduced the long-term mosquito survival which is needed for malaria transmission. It was found that when spraying was discontinued after several years, in some instances malaria did not recur, as the reservoir of infection in man had died out. This was developed into deliberate national campaigns aimed at malaria eradication within specific time limits, rather than control. These were capital projects of immense cost in relation to national health resources, and organized separately from the general health service of developing countries. They required international financing and specialized expertise, often provided through the WORLD HEALTH ORGANIZATION, which achieved international importance through malaria eradication which dominated its activities in the 1960s. The program was highly successful in Europe and North America and on many islands. An initially successful campaign in Asia was followed by a resurgence of infection in the 1970s, while in the highly endemic areas of stable malaria in sub-Saharan Africa little impact was made on the disease. The problems of malaria control increased with the emergence of insecticide resistance among vectors and drug resistance among the parasites, twin problems of so many control campaigns.

*Medicine in the tropics* As this intensive public health endeavor developed, medicine in Africa and the Caribbean moved in other directions. Medical colleges were founded in the postwar period. Heart disease and cancer in Africa were investigated and many important and fascinating new diseases and syndromes were studied, such as

(continued)

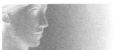

Leonard **ROGERS** (1868–1962). British physician and pathologist. Rogers was commissioned in the Indian Medical Service in 1893 and became professor of pathology in Calcutta in 1900. He returned to England in 1920 and was appointed physician to the Hospital for Tropical Diseases in London. One of the pioneers of TROPICAL MEDICINE, Rogers identified *Entamoeba histolytica* as the cause of amebiasis and introduced emetine in its treatment; he was the first to use antimony in treating KALA-AZAR and hypertonic intravenous saline in CHOLERA. He received a knighthood.

(continued overleaf)

(continued)

**Cicely WILLIAMS**
(1893–1992) was primarily
responsible for identifying in
the 1920s kwashiorkor, a
nutritional deficiency disease
which had ravaged children in
drought and war-torn areas of
maize-eating developing
world countries. As a
pediatrician and nutritionist,
she was a pioneer of women's
progress in the medical
profession. She was the first
adviser in maternal and child
health to the WORLD HEALTH
ORGANIZATION, from
1948–51. She was a forceful
proponent of breast-feeding
and in a blistering speech in
1939 entitled 'Milk and
murder' accused proprietary-
brand baby-food
manufacturers of causing
infant deaths.

Burkitt's lymphoma. There grew an interest in what has been called 'medicine in the tropics' to distinguish it from those parasitic infections which were the traditional content of 'tropical medicine'. The two approaches remained relatively separate in Africa, with the consequence that medical students were educated in the first tradition, and for too long the focus of the first generation of indigenous physicians educated in modern medicine was not primarily upon the tropical parasitic diseases. Nutritional research, after the early description of tropical vitamin deficiency syndromes, was given new impetus by the description of kwashiorkor by Cicely WILLIAMS (this page) in Ghana.

The late stages of the World Health Organization's efforts at malaria eradication prepared the way for changes in the perception of tropical medicine. It became clear that a prerequisite for the consolidation phase of eradication was effective health service coverage. This required better management and organization. The focus of attention moved away from building up excellence in medical schools and towards the periphery, with emphasis on health centers rather than large hospitals. Medical schools acquired teaching health centers and their adjacent small communities as pilot or demonstration areas, with emphasis on effective coverage, or access by people to the health services; recognition that disease control and health promotion may be the only feasible routes to follow; attention directed towards childhood, where mortality is greatest; and an implied use of lower-cost approaches if coverage was to be achieved.

***The medicine of poverty*** These issues emphasized coverage, and achieving it by healthcare largely delivered by paramedical workers. The community diagnosis concept meant that the key causes of death and disability emerged as cosmopolitan infections such as TUBERCULOSIS and acute gastrointestinal and respiratory infections, the ages most at risk were the very young and mothers during delivery, and the importance of malnutrition was apparent. These were not intrinsically tropical problems — similar disease predominated in the poverty-stricken parts of temperate countries, most dramatically during the industrial revolution — but they were the principal health problems of the tropics. Thus a third view of tropical medicine emerged, as the 'diseases of poverty', and this predominated during the 1970s. It clearly united health with development, although in the converse of the earlier way. Instead of health being viewed as a prerequisite for economic productivity, disease in the tropics was thought of as primarily being a consequence of poverty, with socio-economic development representing the

road to health. Thus, malnutrition might be reduced more effectively by land reform than by specifically nutritional supplementation.

This change of viewpoint had three significant implications for tropical health. If disease was due to poverty, the reduction of disease was, in the long run, not primarily a matter of medical professional intervention. Either the doctor accepted that his role was peripheral or else he became involved in developmental issues requiring more than clinical skills. To achieve the necessary population coverage the doctor could no longer practice on a traditional doctor–patient basis; his role became that of a teacher and manager of paramedical workers. Thirdly, if tropical medicine comprises the diseases of poverty, it follows that the resources available to provide care will be extremely limited, and only low-cost interventions will be feasible: the 'medicine of poverty' for the diseases of poverty. These problems attract a different sort of person from the clinically oriented physician. There is a strong component of humanitarian administration and a tendency to minimize professional skills of diagnosis and one-to-one patient care, while the elements of social engineering are often uncongenial to the independently minded physician. This approach grew out of the charities such as Oxfam and non-governmental organizations played an increasing part along with charismatic individuals, outside the government health services and in remote places. Religious groups often led the way. Meanwhile, the World Health Organization had progressed from the faltering attempts at malaria eradication to an emphasis on building up basic health services, then on self-help and 'community participation', leading to locally recruited and trained paramedical staff providing preventive as well as curative 'primary healthcare'. This global program, launched at a meeting at Alma Ata in 1978, marked the extreme of de-professionalizing tropical medicine in an effort to improve access to healthcare for the entire populations of tropical and other developing countries. This needed cheap, simple, and effective interventions.

***Treatment and control interventions*** An example of what is involved in a 'medicine of poverty' is oral rehydration therapy for the acute watery diarrheas. This was developed from work on the physiological mechanisms whereby a mixture of saline and glucose allowed fluid absorption. A series of investigations has determined how far other sugars or starches could be substituted for glucose; the possible replacement of bicarbonate by citrate for easier storage; whether packets of salts will be made up correctly in villages, and how far domestic ingredients can substitute; as well as how best to make the therapy both available and widely used in villages of the tropics. Such studies have something in common with the research needed for successful environmental control of malaria vectors: a detailed understanding of the ecological and cultural milieu, precise definition of a relatively simple and low-cost intervention, and through field study of its operational deployment. Other agents for the treatment and prevention of tropical infections have involved more complex laboratory work.

### The present day

The subject once known as tropical medicine is now full of activity. The different aspects and perceptions of the subject — as parasitic disease, as diseases of poverty, as tropical variants of disease, and as the medicine of poverty — are all jostling for position in a rapidly evolving scene. Whereas formerly it was possible for one person to have expert knowledge and do research while working at the cellular level, the level of the sick patient, and the level of the community. The rate of progress in all these topics is now such that this is no longer possible.

Thus the subject is settling into three main parts: molecular parasitology has become an accepted aspect of basic scientific research; international health has developed greatly, with links to development studies — the continuum of problems from the least developed countries through to affluent ones is now more apparent than the previous dichotomous approach; and clinical tropical medicine is becoming closely aligned with the specialty of INFECTIOUS DISEASES. Internationally, the dominance of the World Health Organization in health is being challenged by the activist approach of UNICEF, with its tendency towards vertical programs and emphasis on child mortality, and by the World Bank in policy analysis. The Bank reflects the economic approach to health interventions. The role of non-governmental organizations is now accepted. Tropical health continues to be a rapidly moving topic conceptually, while what is happening on the ground moves slowly. The public in richer countries are better informed. Many tropical health issues are easy to explain visually, and television has increased their visibility. The health consequences of FAMINE, environmental change, refugee situations, and poverty are now well known. The challenge is to develop new and cost-effective interventions to control the major diseases of developing countries, and to make them effectively available to the people of the tropics.

DJB

*See also* HEALTHCARE SYSTEMS; MISSIONARIES – MEDICAL AND MISSION HOSPITALS; POVERTY AND HEALTH; SNAKE BITE

**TRUANTS — DOCTORS IN OTHER WALKS OF LIFE** The idea seems to have emerged that doctors are a unique profession in deserting their calling for another. Some have even justified this in expansive terms: 'It has always been one of the salient characteristics of medical men in all countries, and at all times,' wrote Lord Moynihan in his *Truants*, 'that they have ardently followed other pursuits than that of their own profession … They have developed what the Greeks called *parergon* — work by the side of work.' The special relevance of medical experience to author echoes Somerset Maugham's conclusion of the importance of medical training for a lesson about life, as well as giving an elementary knowledge of science and scientific method.

Nevertheless, we have no data to show whether medicine really has had proportionately more truants than others — the law, for instance, where 90% of barristers are said never to make a satisfactory, permanent living, or Holy Orders, which can show some bizarre final occupations for some of its members. What follows, then, is an account, without any special claim, of the more distinguished or interesting truants from medicine, drawn largely from Dr Alec Cooke's contribution to the first edition of this book, Lord Moynihan's *Truants*, and 'Outside medicine', a series of articles published some years ago in the *British Medical Journal*.

### Scientists

Berzelius, Joseph (1779–1848). Swedish chemist; made important contributions to theory and nomenclature.

Black, Joseph (1728–99). Scottish chemist; discovered concepts of latent heat and specific heat.

BOYLE, Robert (1627–91). English chemist, a founder of the Royal Society; formulated Boyle's Law (p 125).

Brown, Robert (1773–1858). Scottish botanist; discovered Brownian motion.

Copernicus, Nicolaus (1473–1543). Polish mathematician and astronomer; showed that the Earth and other planets revolve round the sun.

Flett, Sir John Smith (1869–1947). Scottish director of the Geological Survey of Great Britain and of the Museum of Practical Geology.

Forel, Auguste (1848–1931). Swiss authority on ants.

Galvani, Luigi (1737–98). Italian expert on electricity.

Genser, Conrad (1515–65). Swiss professor of botany, natural history (and Greek).

Gerard, John (1545–1612). English botanist; wrote *The herball*.

Gilbert, William (1540–1603). English pioneer of magnetism.

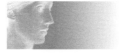

Sir Charles **WYNDHAM** (1841–1919). British physician and actor. Wyndham was born Charles Culverwell, changing his name when he went on to the stage in 1862. He served as a surgeon in the Federal Army during the American Civil War. He was manager of the Criterion Theatre in London from 1876–99, when he opened Wyndham's Theatre.

Grew, Nehemiah (1641–1712). English botanist; first to recognize the existence of male and female sexes in the plant kingdom.

Henry, Augustine (1857–1930). English botanist, having many genera and species named after him.

Hill, John (1716–75). English botanist; wrote *The vegetable system*.

Hooker, Sir Joseph Dalton (1817–1911). English botanist, Director of Kew Gardens, and president of the Royal Society.

Hutton, James (1726–97). Scottish geologist; emphasized the importance of volcanic action for the formation of rocks.

Huxley, Thomas Henry (1825–95). English naturalist, who contributed fundamentally to the study of evolution; president of the Royal Society.

JENNER, Edward (1749–1823). English naturalist; wrote in detail about the life and habits of the cuckoo (p 452).

Linnaeus, Carl (1707–78). Swedish botanist, who introduced the modern system of biological nomenclature.

Lister, Martin (1638–1712). Scottish naturalist; expert on spiders and shells.

Mantell, Gideon Algernon (1790–1852). English geologist; his extensive collection of fossils was sold to the British Museum.

Muffett, Thomas (1553–1604). English naturalist; wrote *Insects, or lesser living creatures*.

Owen, Sir Richard (1804–92). English zoologist and president of the Royal Society.

PETTY, Sir William (1623–87). English founder of the Royal Society, and polymath; creator of economic science (p 219).

Prout, William (1785–1850). English chemist; propounded the hypothesis that the atomic weights of all elements are exact multiples of either the atomic weight of hydrogen or half that of hydrogen (Prout's law).

Scarburgh, Sir Charles (1615–93). English mathematician; wrote a treatise on trigonometry.

SLOANE, Sir Hans (1660–1753). Irish botanist and collector, who refounded Chelsea Physic Garden; president of the Royal Society (p 56).

Stensen, Nicholas (1638–86). Danish geologist; distinguished between rocks containing fossils and those predating this period.

Thompson, Sir Henry (1820–1904). English astronomer, with his own observatory; he donated much apparatus to the Greenwich Observatory.

Thompson, John Vaughan (1779–1847). English marine biologist, who made important studies on barnacles, crabs, and other crustaceans.

Tyson, Edward (1650–1708). English zoologist, who published accounts of dissections of numerous different animals.

Ward, Nathaniel Bagshaw (1791–1868). English botanist; inventor of the Wardian case.

Wollaston, William Hyde (1766–1828). English chemist; invented the reflecting goniometer, enabling the exact measurement of crystals.

Woodward, John (1665–1728). British geologist; created the first geological museum, at the University of Cambridge.

## The Church and humanists

BARNARDO, Thomas John (1845–1905). English instigator of the Custody of Children Act and founder of refuges for homeless children (p 169).

Chance, Frank (1826–97). Englishman, on the committee that prepared the revised version of the *New Testament*.

Cogan, Thomas (1736–1818). English founder of the Royal Humane Society.

GRENFELL, Sir Wilfred Thomason (1865–1940). Scottish missionary who established local services in Labrador (p 299).

Hicks, John (1840–99). English Bishop of Bloemfontein.

Legg, John Wickham (1843–1921). English expert on the liturgy.

LETTSOM, John Coakley (1744–1815). English Quaker prison reformer; freed his slaves on his West Indian estates (p 242).

LIVINGSTONE, David (1813–73). Scottish missionary in Africa; prominent in antislavery movement (p 503).

Petrus, Julianus (1215–77). Italian priest, who became Pope John XXI in 1276.

Secker, Thomas (1693–1768). English divine: successively Bishop of Bristol, Bishop of Oxford, Dean of St Paul's, and Archbishop of Canterbury.

SCHWEITZER, Albert (1875–1965). Alsatian missionary (musician and philosopher) in the Congo (p 504).

## Bibliophiles

Askew, Anthony (1722–72). The sale of his books and manuscripts took 27 days, the principal purchasers being the British Museum and the kings of England and France.

Bernard, Francis (1627–98). English linguist and scholar; his library contained 50 000 volumes.

KEYNES, Sir Geoffrey (1896–1985). English book collector and bibliographer of Berkeley, Blake, Hazlitt, Harvey, etc. After his death part of his collection passed to the Cambridge University Library (p 119).

Maty, Matthew (1718–76). Dutch–Huguenot Principal Librarian of the British Museum.

Mead, Sir Richard (1673–1754). English collector of books, manuscripts, statuaries, coins, gems, and drawings — said to be the largest collection of its time.

Morton, Charles (1716–99). English Principal Librarian of the British Museum.

OSLER, Sir William (1849–1919). Canadian scholar whose library after his death passed to MCGILL University (p 139), where it forms an important part of the university library (p 602).

Williams, Sir John (1840–1926). Founder of the National Library of Wales.

## Linguists

Brown, Edward Granville (1862–1926). An expert in Islamic languages and professor of Persian at Cambridge University.

Good, John Mason (1764–1827). He knew 13 languages.

Latham, Robert Gordon (1812–88). Professor of English language and literature at University College, London, and an authority on the Scandinavian languages.

Leared, Arthur (1822–79). Wrote a book in Icelandic.

Macalister, Sir Donald (1854–1934). A Scotsman who spoke more than a dozen European and Eastern languages; while he was principal and vice-chancellor of Glasgow University it was said that the university had no foreign visitors with whom MacAlister could not converse in their native tongues.

Young, Thomas (1773–1829). An English polymath who helped to decipher the Rosetta Stone.

Zamenhof, Louis (1859–1917). The Russian who invented Esperanto.

## The law and politics

ADDISON, Sir Christopher (later Lord) (1869–1951). English Member of Parliament: successively Minister for Munitions, Minister for Reconstruction, and (first) Minister of Health (p 129).

Bickersteth, Henry (later Lord Langdale) (1783–1851). English Master of the Rolls.

Clemenceau, Georges Benjamin (1841–1929). French Prime Minister and Minister of War.

Crosby, Sir Thomas (1842–1929). English Lord Mayor of London.

Elliott, Walter (1888–1958). Scottish politician: successively Minister for Agriculture, Secretary of State for Scotland, and Minister of Health.

Fernando, Sir Hilariose Marcus (?–1936). Sri Lankan statesman; Director of the State Mortgage Bank.

Finch, Sir John (1626–82). English ambassador to Turkey.

Finlay, Robert (later Viscount Finlay) (1842–1929). Scotsman: the only doctor to be appointed Lord Chancellor.

Foster, Walter Balthasar (later Lord Likeston) (1840–1913). Irish Member of Parliament, and Parliamentary Secretary to the Local Government Board.

HUGGINS, Geoffrey (later Viscount Malvern) (1883–1971). English Prime Minister of the Federation of Rhodesia and Nyasaland (p 15).

JAMESON, Sir Leander Starr (1853–1917). English Prime Minister of Cape Colony: earlier led the Jameson Raid into the Transvaal (p 16).

Knighton, Sir William (1776–1836). English private secretary and keeper of the Privy Purse to the Prince Regent.

Marat, Jean Paul (1743–93). French revolutionary, stabbed to death in his bath by Charlotte Corday.

Summerskill, Edith (later Baroness) (1901–80). English Minister of National Insurance.

SUN YAT-SEN (1866–1925). Chinese revolutionary; first President of the Chinese Republic (p 178).

Tanner, Charles (1850–1901). Irish nationalist politician.

Tupper, Sir Charles (1821–1915). Canadian High Commissioner in London and subsequently Prime Minister of Canada.

Wood, Leonard (1860–1927). US general who became successively governor of Santiago, Cuba, Moro, and the Philippines.

## Philosophy

Bridges, John Henry (1832–1906). English authority on Comte and the editor of Roger Bacon's *Opus major*.

James, William (1842–1910). US professor of philosophy at Harvard.

Locke, John (1632–1704). English philosopher and founder of political economy.

MAIMONIDES (1135–1204). Noted Jewish theologian and philosopher (p 583).

## The arts

BORODIN, Alexander Porfiryevich (1833–87). Russian army officer and composer (p 188).

Cathcart, George Clark (1860–1951). English sponsor of the Promenade Concerts.

Haden, Sir Francis Seymour (1818–1910). English founder and President of the Royal Society of Painter Etchers.

Knowles, James Sheridan (1784–1862). Irish actor and playwright; colleague of Kean, Macready, and Kemble.

Neel, Louis Boyd (1905–81). English musicologist conductor, and founder of an orchestra.

TONKS, Henry (1862–1937). English Slade professor of fine art at London University: among his pupils were Augustus John and William Orpen (p 66).

Wall, John (1708–76). English founder of the Royal Worcester Porcelain Factory.

WYNDHAM, Sir Charles (1837–1919). English actor-manager (p 827).

## Miscellanea

Birkbeck, George (1776–1841). English founder of the London Mechanics Institute, subsequently Birkbeck College.

CAIUS, John (1510–73). English co-founder of Gonville and Caius College, Cambridge (p 135).

*(continued on p 831)*

# THE GREAT KILLERS: TUBERCULOSIS

Tuberculosis is an infectious and, in the absence of treatment, commonly fatal disease. Its bacterial cause (*Mycobacterium tuberculosis*) was isolated in 1882 by Robert KOCH (p 455), the great German bacteriologist. The bacillus is spread by droplet infection, mainly by coughing and sneezing, and inhaled droplets lodge in and infect the lungs. Drinking milk from a tuberculous cow may produce infection. Before the introduction of pasteurized milk (generally around the time of the Second World War) this was a common form of tuberculosis among children, usually starting in the lymph nodes.

Tuberculosis may affect any part of the body, but the dominant site of infection is the lungs. This form, causing over 80% of all deaths from the disease, was commonly known before the 20th century as consumption or phthisis. Other sites of infection include the bones and joints, the lymphatic nodes (a form known as scrofula), the abdomen, the meninges and central nervous system, and the skin (lupus vulgaris). Tubercle bacilli may also become widely distributed throughout the body through the bloodstream, causing a generalized infection called 'miliary tuberculosis'.

All age groups are susceptible, but respiratory tuberculosis has always struck hardest among young men and women. As the poet John KEATS (p 659) wrote two years before his death from tuberculosis in 1821 aged 26, 'Youth grows pale, and spectre thin, and dies'. Sometimes the course of the disease was so rapid in this age group that it became known as 'galloping consumption'.

While by all accounts tuberculosis is as old as mankind, there is little evidence to indicate how widespread it was before the 19th century. Diagnosis was problematic and tuberculosis might easily be mistaken for other diseases. Impressionistic accounts suggest that it was increasing in prevalence in the 17th century (when the author John Bunyan described it as 'The captain of all these men of death'). The major peak in prevalence and mortality came in the early to mid-19th century, when it reached epidemic proportions in Europe and America, generally being associated with the conditions arising from the industrial revolution. A decline set in during the latter half of that century, which historical epidemiologist Thomas McKeown has related to nutritional improvements but which other historians have attributed to improved sanitary infrastructures. Most modern historians agree that medical intervention in the form of treatments had little if any affect on the course of the disease before the 1950s.

The 19th century romantic 'consumptive' poets, Keats and Shelley, formed part of a great pilgrimage from the northern fog to the southern Mediterranean sun. From the mid-19th century other British sufferers (such as Robert Louis Stevenson, or D. H. Lawrence) set out for the South Seas or the warmer British colonies of South Africa, Australia, and New Zealand, where the customs and manners were thought to be less alien to them than were those of continental Europe. In America the West became the destination of many tuberculosis sufferers, who in the process shaped the communities of Colorado, Arizona, and California. Others set out on sea voyages, regardless of destination, in search of a cure.

From the late 19th century high altitudes were thought to have a curative effect, and mountain resorts in Germany and Switzerland became popular for tuberculosis victims. When the SANITARIUM movement was under way in Britain and elsewhere by the turn of the century the institutions were usually located well above sea-level. A new generation of tuberculosis specialists emerged from these institutions. They practiced rest and work therapy (also known as 'graduated labor') and from the 1920s introduced surgical interventions, such as collapse therapy or artificial pneumothorax, and later thoracoplasty. There is no evidence to suggest that any of these regimens had any appreciable influence on the course of the disease.

(continued opposite)

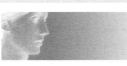

Charles **MANTOUX** (1877–1947). French physician. Mantoux practiced in Cannes with a special interest in the care of tuberculous patients. He devised the intradermal tuberculin test (1908).

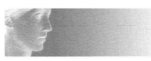

Jean Antoine **VILLEMIN** (1827–92). French physician. Villemin joined the army medical service and eventually became professor at Val-de-Grâce. In 1868 he firmly established the infectivity of tuberculosis by transferring it from man to rabbit. This was before KOCH (p 655) had isolated the mycobacterium and Villemin's work was discounted.

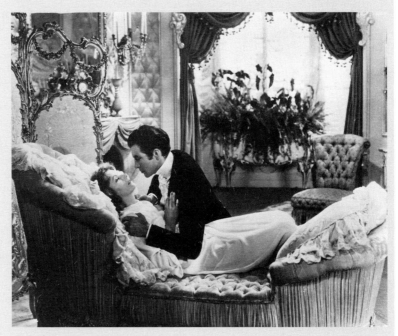

Greta Garbo as Camille, dying of consumption, with Robert Taylor in the 1937 film *Camille*. (Reproduced courtesy of Popperfoto.)

*(continued)*

In the 19th century a romantic iconography grew up around tuberculosis, because of its tendency to attack youth and because of the way in which the disease progressed, 'consuming' its victims. Alexandre Dumas's novel, *La dame aux camelias* (1848), Verdi's opera, *La traviata* (1853), and Puccini's *La Bohème* (1896) came to epitomize the frail consumptive heroine often of the demimondaine, or dubious virtue sanctified through illness and death. By the 20th century, however, the image of the 'lunger' had changed. No longer romantic, they were ostracized and shunned as suffering from an hereditary taint, or as part of the 'unclean poor'. Many were suspected of being guilty of miscreant behavior causing the disease. Sufferers from tuberculosis became stigmatized and often became social outcasts.

After the Second World War the image changed once again. With the promise that tuberculosis was curable if caught at an early stage, thousands of people were persuaded to be X-rayed using the new mass miniature radiography techniques which had been developed during the decade before the war. This campaign, which successfully lessened the stigma attached to the disease, predated but was greatly assisted by the availability of effective anti-tuberculosis drugs. In 1944 Selman Waksman discovered the antibiotic streptomycin, the first effective biomedical treatment for tuberculosis, and inaugurated the drug era in the treatment of the disease. With a cocktail of drugs including

streptomycin, paraaminosalicylic acid (1943), isoniazid (developed in 1912 and rediscovered in the 1950s), and rifampicin (1966), side-effects were effectively eliminated and it was believed that the 'white plague' was finally conquered. In some places this process was thought to have been aided by preventive immunization with BCG (Bacillus Calmette–Guérin), which had been discovered in 1921.

Recently there has been the fear of drug-resistant strains of tuberculosis evolving and in particular a recrudescence of tuberculosis among AIDS sufferers, whose immune systems are impaired. Moreover, while the western world was talking of the conquest of the disease in the early 1980s, the incidence in developing countries remained high. On a world-wide basis an estimated one billion people, or a third of the global population, were believed to be infected in 1981 and the disease was thought to be killing about a million people per annum. In the 1990s tuberculosis remained a disease of poverty and of the socially disadvantaged. René DUBOS (p 247), a leading microbiologist and philosopher of medicine, insisted that tuberculosis is not caused by the tubercle bacillus: a healthy individual can generally withstand the primary infection. But *M. tuberculosis* allied with poverty, poor housing, poor nutrition, overcrowding and ignorance of elementary personal hygiene (such as not covering the nose and mouth when coughing, and spitting out infected phlegm

on the ground where children play) is a lethal combination. LBry

*See also* ANTIBIOTICS AND ANTI-INFECTIVE DRUGS; CARDIOTHORACIC SURGERY – HISTORY; CHEST MEDICINE; DANCE; OPERA

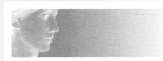

Edward Livingston **TRUDEAU** (1848–1915). American physician. Trudeau began practice in New York City, but soon developed symptoms of pulmonary tuberculosis. He went to the Adirondack Mountains to rest, expecting to die of the disease, but his health gradually improved and he attributed that to rest and mountain air. He remained in the Adirondacks, founding and directing the Saranac Lake Sanatorium. Trudeau carried out some laboratory and animal experiments with tuberculosis, following discovery of the organism by KOCH (p 655). He became a leading US authority on pulmonary tuberculosis, and played a prominent part in national medical societies. He is sometimes credited with the well-known maxim, thought now to be a 15th century folk-saying, of a physician's goal: 'to cure sometimes, to help often, to comfort always'.

---

*(continued)*

Gann, Thomas (1867–1938). English expert on Mayan archaeology.

Gibbons, William (1649–1728). English introducer of mahogany into the UK.

GRACE, William Gilbert (1848–1915). The most celebrated of all English cricketers (p 776).

Longstaff, Tom George (1875–1964). English Himalayan climber and member of the second Everest expedition in 1922: president of the Alpine Club.

Moore, Francis (1657–1715). English originator of *Old Moore's almanac* (p 587).

Park, Mungo (1771–1806). Scottish explorer of the Niger River.

Pim, Joshua (1870–1945). Irish tennis singles champion at Wimbledon 1893 and 1894, and doubles champion in 1890 and 1893.

Stallard, Hyla Bristow (1901–73). English international and Olympic athlete.

Stokes, Lennard (1856–1933). English rugby player; secured Rectory field for the Blackheath Club.

In conclusion, some medical students who for various reasons did not qualify in medicine, but attained distinction in other walks of life, may be mentioned:

Berlioz, Hector (1803–69). Composer.

Brecht, Bertolt (1898–1956). Dramatist.

DARWIN, Charles Robert (1809–82). Zoologist, botanist, and geologist (p 214).

Davy, Sir Humphry (1778–1829). Chemist.

Foucault, Jean Bernard (1819–68). Physicist who determined the speed of light.

Galileo, Galilei (1564–1642). Physicist and astronomer.

GALTON, Sir Francis (1822–1911). Writer on anthropology, heredity, and EUGENICS (p 285).

Goethe, Johann Wolfgang (1749–1832). Poet, dramatist, and philosopher.

Leech, John (1817–64). Caricaturist and cartoonist.

Smith, Sydney (1771–1845). Dean of St Paul's and a noted wit.

Thompson, Francis (1859–1907). Poet. SPL

**TUSKEGEE SYPHILIS STUDY** The Tuskegee Syphilis Study was initiated by the US Public Health Service in Macon County, Alabama, in 1932 to examine the natural history of untreated, latent SYPHILIS in black men. (A study of untreated syphilis among whites had been undertaken in Oslo, Norway, between 1891 and 1910, and arsenic compounds had become standard therapy for syphilis by 1932.) In the early 1930s, Macon County had one of the highest syphilis rates in the United States but there were insufficient resources to treat all cases. The men in the study (400 men with syphilis and 200 uninfected men) were predominantly poor and medically underserved. The participants were not offered treatment with penicillin, the more effective therapy that became available in the 1940s. In fact, on more than one occasion over the course of the study, Public Health Service investigators sought to ensure that participants did not receive antibiotic treatment from other sources so that the ability to examine the natural course of untreated syphilis would not be impaired.

Other ethical problems surrounding the study included the lack of informed consent and the use of incentives for participation that were manipulative or deceptive (for example, free burial after autopsy and spinal taps described as special treatment rather than diagnostic examination for neurosyphilis). Although the study has become known in recent decades as one of the most notorious episodes of abuse in the history of human subjects research, scientific reports of the study appeared in the literature every few years, from 1936 to the 1960s without any significant protest from the medical or scientific community.

In 1972, after critical accounts of the study first appeared in the popular media, the Public Health Service was forced to halt the study. At that time, 74 of the participants were still alive, while at least 28 participants (and possibly as many as 100) had died from advanced syphilis. The disturbing accounts of poor black men in the southern USA who were denied potentially life-saving treatment prompted widespread public criticism. Questions were raised about how a study that today seems so clearly to have violated medical research ethics could have continued for so long.

After the public disclosure of the Tuskegee Syphilis Study, an *ad hoc* advisory panel was formed to investigate the study and make recommendations to the Assistant Secretary for Health, Department of Health, Education, and Welfare. The panel, which included representatives from medicine, law, religion, labor, education, health administration, and public affairs, deliberated until early 1973. The panel's report strongly criticized the study for the lack of informed consent, the presence of methodologic weaknesses, and the failure to offer penicillin when it became available. The panel's report also examined US policies for protecting research subjects and made several recommendations, including the creation of a national board on human experimentation.

After these developments and revelations about other controversial studies involving people, Congress passed the National Research Act of 1974, which promulgated regulations for the protection of human research subjects and mandated institutional review board (research ethics committee) approval of all federally funded research involving human subjects. The Act also established the National Commission for the Protection of Human Subjects of Biomedical and Behavioral Research, which by 1978 had made several important recommendations.

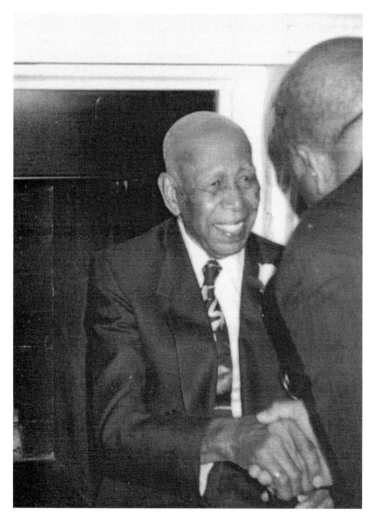

Herman Shaw, a Tuskegee Study participant, after the White House ceremony during which President Clinton apologized on behalf of the United States Government. (Reproduced courtesy of Joan Echtenkamp Klein.)

As a result of these regulatory changes, all institutions in the United States that receive federal funds for research involving people must have an institutional review board approval before it can proceed. Federal agencies within the Department of Health and Human Services have established such review boards that approve research protocols proposed by departmental investigators. Institutional safeguards and policies for protecting human subjects are overseen by the Office for Protection from Research Risks.

## Consequences for Public Health Agencies

Social scientists have suggested that the Tuskegee Study has contributed to the discontent many African–Americans feel about the public health system and has helped lay the foundation of a pervasive sense of distrust among African–Americans of public health authorities and biomedical research today. Some researchers have argued that the unfortunate legacy of the Tuskegee Study now hampers efforts to control AIDS and other public health problems in African–American communities.

Although some social scientists have emphasized racism in their analysis of the ethical problems that surrounded the Tuskegee study, other social scientists have argued instead that the mindset of the research scientists and their large stake in the project contributed to their unethical behavior. David Rothman has argued that 'social deprivation ought not to become the occasion for conducting a seemingly natural experiment, for researchers place themselves in an ethically untenable position'. In Rothman's view, researchers become accomplices to the problem in such situations, and not simply observers of it.

On May 16, 1997, President Bill Clinton apologized for the Tuskegee Syphilis Study on behalf of the US government.

In a follow-up to the presidential apology, Donna Shalala, Secretary of the Department of Health and Human Services, took several steps to build trust by ensuring and demonstrating commitment to the highest ethical principles in all of the department's activities, especially in the conduct of research involving people. The Department awarded a planning grant to Tuskegee University to pursue establishing a center for bioethics in research and healthcare, took steps to offer fellowships and short-term training programs in research ethics, and began develop training materials for bioethics courses in collaboration with public and private partners. The department also began developing and disseminating strategies to assist researchers in their outreach to communities — especially minority communities — to foster partnerships and enhance the involvement of minorities in research studies.

Thus, the legacy of the Tuskegee Syphilis Study, which stands as a powerful metaphor of misconduct in research in human subjects and racism in medicine and public health, is being transformed as federal agencies and individual researchers give greater attention to high ethical standards and attempt to build public trust. SSC, DES

*See also* BIOETHICS; HELSINKI, DECLARATION OF; INFORMED CONSENT; NUREMBERG CODE; SYPHILIS

## THE GREAT KILLERS — TYPHOID

Typhoid is an acute, infectious disease characterized by fever and headache, accompanied by a transient abdominal rash, often identified as 'rose spots'. Although individual responses to infection are dose related, and may be very mild, possible complications include intestinal hemorrhage, perforation, and pneumonia. Fatality is about 10%. Another 2%, often women, become permanent carriers of the typhoid organism and continue intermittently to excrete it in their stools. The organism concerned is *Salmonella typhi*, transmitted by the fecal–oral route, usually in contaminated food

and water. Typhoid's historical record is largely derived from the experience of western communities, but the disease is found throughout the world and remains endemic in many tropical countries.

Although typhoid has a long history, it may be clinically difficult to distinguish from TYPHUS. Only in the 19th century did doctors begin to separate the two, especially after William Wood GERHARD of Philadelphia (1837) (p 834) and William Jenner of London (1849) had published descriptions of their different clinical features. The disease had, however, probably become much more

common in the early 19th century. Certainly, doctors at the London Fever Hospital noted the presence of a new type of fever, requiring different management from the indigenous fever (typhus) of the city, during the 1830s.

The enormous growth of cities and lack of sanitary planning in western Europe and America in the 19th century resulted in the emergence of typhoid as a serious endemic killer. At that time the introduction of the flushing toilet and urban sewage networks also resulted in the pollution of river waters used for drinking with raw and often infected fecal matters. In addition, rising premiums on
(continued overleaf)

*(continued)*

urban land meant that wells and cesspools began to be sunk in close proximity, resulting in leakage, soakage, and further contamination of drinking waters. In London the critical transition from a relatively fecally uncontaminated environment to a highly fecally contaminated one took place in the late 1820s and early 1830s — the time when citizens first began to complain of serious deterioration in the quality of Thames water.

Like typhus, with which it was then confused, typhoid was quickly associated with insanitary conditions, especially with unwholesome air. In the 1840s, however, an English country doctor, William BUDD (p 274), noted the connection between typhoid outbreaks and fecally contaminated food and water. The gradual acceptance of Budd's idea, together with continuing sanitary emphasis on the dangers of 'sewer gas', contributed to appreciable improvements in urban water supplies across the developed world in the later decades of the century. It was by no means a uniform or uninterrupted progression: until at least 1900, for example, the Parisian authorities regularly topped up filtered water supplies with raw Seine water during the summer months, provoking repeated typhoid outbreaks in the city.

In England (where 19th-century cause of death data are the most reliable), sanitary improvements produced a reduction in typhoid deaths before the new techniques of bacteriology began to extend scientific understanding of the disease in the 1880s. Between 1870 and 1885, typhoid death rates in England and Wales fell from 32 per 100 000 people to 17, but then stabilized, falling again only after 1900 with more extensive hospital isolation of cases and recognition of the role of the healthy carrier in transmitting the disease. The latter was, perhaps, the landmark contribution of bacteriology to the control of typhoid, although of less importance than Budd's initial identification of the route of transmission.

In 1880 the typhoid bacillus was first identified by Carl Eberth and Edwin Klebs; in 1884 Georg Gaffky succeeded in culturing it; by 1900, vaccines against typhoid had been developed by several European bacteriologists, including Almroth Wright in England and Richard Pfeiffer and Wilhelm Kolle in Germany. In 1902 Robert KOCH

(p 455) suggested that endemic typhoid might be sustained by healthy carriers, and this suggestion was confirmed during an intensive anti-typhoid campaign conducted in south-western Germany between 1903 and 1905.

The discovery of the healthy carrier had a variable impact on public health programs in the West. In American cities, for example, efforts were made to identify, monitor, and regulate individual carriers, following the publicity surrounding Typhoid Mary Mallon, the immigrant Irish cook identified in 1906 as the first typhoid carrier in America. In Britain no such efforts were made, because they were widely regarded as an infringement of individual liberty. By 1914, however, in the context of the First World War, the problem of the typhoid carrier assumed new proportions. In both the Spanish American War (1898) and the Boer War (1899–1902), typhoid had outstripped wounds as a cause of casualties among the troops. As a result, sanitary training and immunization programs were implemented, resulting in negligible typhoid casualties among troops on the western front.

For many years after 1918, typhoid remained a present danger in European countries with defective water regulation systems. The novelist Arnold Bennett, for example, who died of typhoid in 1931, was reputed to have contracted his illness by drinking tapwater in Paris. (He was the last person for whom straw was laid in the London streets to deaden the traffic noise while he was dying.) The enduring public health problem presented by the healthy carrier was well recognized by western health authorities in the years to 1940.

While the potential for accidental outbreaks remains, the discovery from 1948 of antibiotics such as chloramphenicol has reduced the danger for individual patients. Yet the global prevalence of the disease means that it continues to be an active threat to public health. The internationalization of trade in foodstuffs, greatly accelerated since 1945, poses a threat where sanitary regulations are inadequate. The last major outbreak of typhoid in Britain occurred in Aberdeen in 1964, after the distribution of a consignment of contaminated tinned Argentinean corned beef. Newly arrived

immigrants and travelers returning from developing countries continually re-introduce the disease into non-endemic areas, and both as active cases and as unidentified carriers offer the potential for epidemic outbreaks and for re-establishing endemic foci.          AHar

*See also* EPIDEMIOLOGY; INFECTIOUS DISEASES; MICROBIOLOGY; WAR; WATER

---

**TYPHOID VERSUS TYPHUS**

Pierre Fidele **BRETONNEAU** (1771–1862). French physician. He studied at the École de Santé in Paris under Corvisart, but discouraged by failing an examination returned to his native Tours as an *officier de santé*. After graduation he was appointed chief physician to Tours hospital. He noted the intestinal lesions of typhoid fever (1820) and foretold that it would prove different from typhus (1828). He distinguished diphtheria from scarlet fever (1826) and was the first to carry out tracheostomy in croup (1825).

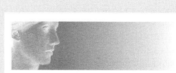

William Wood **GERHARD** (1809–72). American physician. Gerhard went abroad for further study and learned the clinical and pathological features of typhoid fever from Pierre LOUIS (p 780) in France. He returned to practice in Philadelphia. During an epidemic of typhus fever in that city he was able to call attention to clinical features which clearly differentiated it from typhoid fever: suffusion of the conjunctivae, petechial eruption, mildness of abdominal symptoms, and, in fatal cases, lack of swelling of Peyer's patches in the intestine. Typhoid and typhus were recognized as different diseases thereafter.

# THE GREAT KILLERS — TYPHUS

Typhus is an infectious disease transmitted by the human body louse: the infecting organism, *Rickettsia prowazekii*, is ingested by the lice in infected human blood and excreted in their feces. The infected feces in turn transmit the disease to man when they make contact with broken human skin, usually when louse bites are scratched. However, the rickettsiae may survive for months in the dust of dried louse feces, and in this state infect through the eye or nose.

The disease causes fever, prostration, head and body aches, and an extensive rash. It is usually more severe in adults than in children. Case fatality varies from 5–40% or more, and, although one attack generally confers life-long immunity, Brill–Zinsser disease, a relapse of mild type, may be triggered by later stress. Typhus has often been confused with TYPHOID, from which it was clinically distinguished only in the 1830s and 1840s. The human body louse is happiest in the warm environment of unwashed worn garments, so that typhus has a definite seasonal curve, occurring chiefly in the winter. It is above all a disease of social dislocation — of war, famine, and mass migrations — and of unwashed populations in confined, dirty spaces. Its many popular names reflect these associations: famine fever, ship fever, camp fever, gaol fever. The characteristic rash has also given it the name 'spotted fever' or the equivalent in many different languages.

Typhus may be a fairly new disease. Accounts of typhus-like disease occur from the 15th century, but the first clear description comes from Fracastorius, who observed an epidemic among French troops besieging Naples in 1528. By the late 18th century it had become endemic in many European cities; in London a special hospital was established in 1801 to treat its victims. Typically, endemic urban typhus was found in the poor quarters, where cleanliness was a problem for both humans and houses, but the disease repeatedly showed its epidemic potential in the 19th century. It harassed Napoleon's troops on their disastrous expedition to Moscow; ravaged Ireland between 1816 and 1819, and again during the Irish Great Famine of the 1840s; and flared up in eastern Europe, notably in Upper Silesia, during the 1848 Year of Revolutions.

In Britain, London experienced a serious epidemic in the 1860s, when a combination of major railway construction and building trade strikes led to extensive dislocation and deprivation in the city. The disease also appeared briefly in Lancashire during the Cotton Famine, but was dispelled by intensive philanthropic efforts among the cotton workers. By the 1870s, endemic typhus was retreating from cities throughout Europe, and by the 1880s it had become a disease of Europe's margins, surviving in Ireland, Russia, Austria, and Turkey; in the Eastern Mediterranean; and in North Africa.

While several observers, in Russia and elsewhere, made a connection between typhus and lice during the 19th century, the role of the louse in transmission was first elucidated by Charles Nicolle, of the Pasteur Institute in Tunis, between 1906 and 1909. Following as it did several similar discoveries (including that of the role of the rat in transmitting PLAGUE), Nicolle's work was quickly accepted by the scientific and public health communities. The causal organism was isolated in 1910, by Howard Taylor RICKETTS (p 433), who was investigating an epidemic of typhus in Mexico City, and who died of the disease shortly afterwards. It was subsequently named for Ricketts and a Bohemian scientist, Stanislaus von PROWAZEK (this page), who died of typhus while investigating an outbreak in a Russian prisoner-of-war camp in 1915. However, the bacterium could not be cultured on sterile media, and it was not until the American researcher H. R. Cox discovered, in 1937, that it grew in the yolks of fertilized hens' eggs, that attempts to produce a vaccine met with success.

With the outbreak of war in 1914, typhus showed its ability to evolve rapidly into a major epidemic threat. Although absent from the western front, it was rampant in Serbia by early 1915, causing some 150 000 deaths before measures taken by a British sanitary mission brought the epidemic to a halt in May. Railway communications, and association between troops and civilians, were central in generating this epidemic and continued to play a part in typhus activity throughout the war. In particular, the disease smoldered among Russian troops and civilians, and with the severe winter of 1917–18 was fanned to flame.

Between 1918 and 1922, an epidemic of unprecedented scale engulfed Russia and her provinces. An estimated 25–30% of the population were infected, and some 2.5 million people died. Against a background of war and revolution, of food and fuel shortages, and of economic collapse, the country's railways helped to spread typhus among people fleeing fighting, hunger, and destitution in countryside and town alike. It was in this context that Lenin uttered his famous remark: 'All attention to this problem, comrades. Either the louse will defeat socialism, or socialism will defeat the louse'. The return of political stability, more than rising levels of immunity or intensive delousing and disinfection campaigns, ended the epidemic in the closing months of 1922.

Typhus again caused international anxiety during World War II, but the availability of vaccines, and of the delousing agent DDT (dichlorodiphenyl-trichloroethane) in powder form meant that control of the disease among troops was easy. Major outbreaks did, however, occur among civilians in German concentration camps, and in Yugoslavia, North Africa, Japan, and Korea. In 1948 the broad-spectrum antibiotics (tetracyclines and chloramphenicol) were found to be effective against typhus. Prevention has since centered on these antibiotics. Nonetheless, typhus continue to be active in areas that are socially and politically marginal: the Andes, the Himalayas, and the Horn of Africa, notably in famine-torn Ethiopia, and Russia. Whatever safety is conferred by modern standards of hygiene, there is the potential for the return of epidemic typhus, given the right social circumstances, remains.                     AHar

*See also* HOLOCAUST, INFECTIOUS DISEASES, WAR

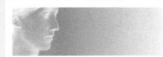

Stanislaus Josef Mathias **PROWAZEK** (1875–1915). Bohemian protozoologist. Prowazek discovered the cause of trachoma and fowl pest while working as an assistant to Schaudinns whom he followed at the Institut für Schiffs- und Tropenkrankheiten, Hamburg, in 1906. He died of typhus investigating an outbreak in a Russian prisoner-of-war camp in 1915. Henrique da Rocha-Lima, who also acquired the disease but recovered, elucidated the cause and named it *Rickettsia prowazeki* in his honour and in that of H. T. RICKETTS (p 433), who also died investigating it.

# U

**UNITED KINGDOM** See BRITAIN

**UROLOGY** or urological surgery encompasses the care of the urinary tract and the male genitourinary system, including infertility and impotence. It overlaps nephrology in the care of renal disease; endocrinology in male infertility, adrenal diseases, and metabolic stone disease; and gynecology in the care of female incontinence.

The symptoms of urological disease are most commonly disturbances in the voiding pattern. Frequent voidings (frequency), pain or burning with voiding (dysuria), and the urgent need to void (urgency) are the most common, usually indicating inflammation or irritation of the lower urinary tract. A slow stream or the need to strain to urinate is indicative of lower tract obstruction, while back or flank pain, nausea, and vomiting may accompany upper tract obstruction. Chills and fever are usually indicative of kidney or prostate infections. Blood in the urine may be a sign of early cancer. All of these symptoms should be investigated.

The development of urology was inseparable from the technological explosion of the late 19th and 20th centuries. Its practitioners are the intellectual descendants of the lithotomists (stone-cutters), the venereologists, and the general surgeons. They became expert in the diagnosis of urinary tract disease through their mastery of urethral instrumentation, which included the use of the cystoscope. This gave them the opportunity to compete with general surgeons in certain cases, and eventually urology became a subspecialty of surgery.

## Stone disease

Some of the most colorful urological history concerns the treatment of urinary calculus, or stone disease. Cutting for stone (which until 100 years ago included only bladder calculi) was separated from the main body of medicine and surgery long ago by HIPPOCRATES (p 382), who stated in his oath 'I will not cut persons laboring under the stone but will leave this to be done by practitioners in this work'. Hippocrates regarded wounds of the bladder as fatal ('Death commonly follows wounds of the brain, spinal cord, liver, diaphragm, bladder, and the great vessels'), and apparently preferred his disciples not to be involved.

The earliest descriptions of the operations for stone were those in the Sushruta Samhita from India and of CELSUS (p 806), both written before AD 600, describing essentially the same operation, with a perineal exposure, going up through the bladder floor. The operation had changed little by the time of Frére Jacques. He was an itinerant French lithotomist, setting up operating clinics in villages. He is said to have operated on 5000 people by the end of his career.

For a while the leadership in lithotomy went to Britain, where Cheselden, a trained anatomist who was also a lithotomist, tried the suprapubic approach (through the lower abdomen), only to abandon it because of problems with patients straining. Straining was a help in the perineal approach since it helped to push the stone out of the incision, but with a suprapubic approach straining tended to push the bowel into the incision and made it difficult to avoid opening the peritoneum. With adequate relaxation the suprapubic approach is by far the safest and easiest, but it did not come into popular use until anesthesia was available, and at that point the treatment of stones came into the mainstream of surgery.

A completely non-invasive treatment of renal calculi, the electro-hydraulic lithotriptor, was developed in the late 1970s. In this technique the patient is placed in a tub of water and an underwater spark-gap is used to produce a shock wave, which is then focused by an ellipsoidal reflector on the stone. The stone is strong to compression, but as the shock wave passes through, a negative pressure pulls off small fragments, which are then carried away by the urine. This treatment is suitable for stones in the kidney which are not bigger than 2 cm. Stones in the ureter and even some stones in the bladder may also be treated by this method. Larger stones in the kidney have to be treated by a form of 'keyhole surgery', in which a track is made from the skin surface into the kidney. By using a special endoscope together with some disintegrating device the stone fragments are then removed.

The prevention of stones by medical treatment has not advanced significantly since the 1950s. Although in many patients a metabolic cause for the stone formation can be identified, attempts to prevent new stones by modifying the diet or by giving medical treatment are not very successful. One of the most common causes of stone formation is an excess of calcium in the urine (hypercalciuria), which may be classified into absorptive (too much calcium from the gut), resorptive (excess mobilization of calcium from the bone), or renal (tubular wasting and loss of calcium from the kidney). The advice that often used to be given, to reduce the dietary intake of dairy products, which contain calcium, has now been shown to be wrong. If the dietary calcium is lowered more oxalate is absorbed from the gut and since oxalate is less soluble in urine than calcium there is an increased risk of stone formation. The most effective prophylaxis is to have a balanced diet which is not too high in meat products. Oxalate is found in tea, coffee, and colas and these fluids should be taken in moderation. In addition patients must maintain a high fluid input so that they have a urine output of at least $1^1/_2$–2 liters each day.

Another common cause of stone formation is urinary infection. After a stone has been removed it is then essential to eradicate infection if stone recurrence is to be prevented.

**Instruments**

The age-old problem of an obstructed, over-filled bladder has been relieved by catheters made of reeds, straws, palm leaves, or the leaves of the onion family. The double-lumened retention catheter, with a balloon on the end to keep it in place, was invented in the 1820s by Reybard in France, although Foley designed the modern version in 1933.

The first cystoscope (a telescope for visualizing the bladder) was invented by Bozzini in 1804 and Nitze developed the first adequate lens system in 1879; however, the first really useful cystoscope had to await invention of the Edison electric-light bulb in 1880. In 1887 Harwig of Berlin and Leiter of Vienna both placed Edison's light in Nitze's scope and the interior of the bladder could be routinely and safely visualized. Modification of these instruments by Brown of Baltimore allowed insertion of catheters into the ureters, and when x-rays were available contrast medium could be injected into the ureter to obtain an image of it for the first time. In the 1960s the Hopkins solid-rod lens system increased clarity considerably. Fiberoptic light bundles increased the amount of light available and were much more reliable. The use of coherent fiberoptics allowed the image-carrying portion of the 'scope' to be flexible and led to the development of flexible nephroscopes and ureteroscopes, permitting direct visualization of the entire urinary tract.

**Tumors**

The era of modern open urological surgery, as with all surgery, began with the development of anesthesia and asepsis. Simon carried out the first planned nephrectomy (removal of the kidney) in 1869 and the development of X-ray techniques made possible the preoperative diagnosis of most larger lesions. Smaller tumors may now be identified much earlier with the use of computerized tomography, magnetic resonance imaging, and ultrasonography. Since the incidence of metastatic spread is proportional to the size of the primary renal tumor, this early diagnosis should carry with it a better prognosis.

In childhood renal tumors (Wilms's tumor, or nephroblastoma), even though the diagnosis is still made late after the discovery of an abdominal mass, the prognosis has changed from less than 40% survival to better than 90%, largely through a combination of surgery, anticancer chemotherapy, and radiation.

*Bladder* The first recognized cause of bladder tumor was the so-called aniline dye workers' tumor described by Rehn in a German chemical plant in 1895. Actually, the tumor was probably produced by exposure to beta-naphthylamine, a by-product in the manufacture of alpha-naphthylamine, but that was not shown until the 1930s, when Heuper produced tumors in dogs by feeding beta-naphthylamine. Rats and mice metabolize naphthylamines by a different pathway than humans and dogs, and the same carcinogenic effects cannot be demonstrated in rodent experiments. Since then many chemicals, and even bracken fern, have been reported to be carcinogenic to the bladder. However, the most important clinical factor is cigarette smoking, which increases the incidence of bladder cancers fourfold.

Such tumors can now be produced reliably in animal models by several agents. The carcinogen is thought to be metabolized in the liver, and excreted in an inactive form in the urine, where the conjugate is broken up by urinary enzymes to release the active carcinogen.

This hypothesis fits with clinical experience in two important respects: firstly, bladder tumors are 10 times as common as tumors of the renal pelvis, where the urine rests for only a short time, and the carcinogen has not been released from its conjugated form; secondly, the clinical behavior of the tumor, with multiple recurrences over time in different parts of the bladder, and even in the

## PROSTATECTOMIST

Terence John **MILLIN**
(1903–80). Irish surgeon.
Millin was a big-hearted
Irishman who trained in
Dublin but whose extensive
urological practice was mainly
in London. He introduced the
then revolutionary retropubic
approach to removal of the
prostate gland. This allows
access to the organ, which is
frequently enlarged in older
men causing obstruction to
urinary outflow, by getting
into the space behind the
pubic bone and in front of
the bladder. The Millin
operation was tidier and
attended with fewer
complications and greater
comfort for the patient
postoperatively. It became
standard international surgical
practice for many years. He
made several other urological
advances, including total
bladder resection for cancer.
In his youth he played rugby
football for Ireland.

lining of the kidney and ureter, can best be explained by exposure of the lining of the urinary tract to the same carcinogenic stimulus. Because of their tendency to recur, bladder tumors require close follow-up with cystoscopy. This is often supplemented by urine cytology, which can detect malignant cells in the urine, much as is done with early detection of cervical carcinoma.

Tumors limited to the mucosal lining of the bladder may be treated locally with cautery or intravesical agents, but invasive tumors require radiation or surgical removal of the bladder. Removal of the bladder creates the problem of how to manage (divert) the urine. One solution was to bring the ureters to the skin, as performed by LeDentu in 1889, but this frequently resulted in stenosis (narrowing of the ureters) or infection. Over the next 100 years almost all segments of the intestinal tract, from the stomach to the rectum, were used; it is now possible to build a continent pouch which is emptied by catheterization, avoiding the need for a collection bag.

### Prostate gland

The prostate gland is that part of the sexual apparatus responsible for ejaculatory contractions. It might be considered as the weak link of the male urinary tract as it suffers from three common diseases: benign prostatic hyperplasia, which affects one-third of men over 60; carcinoma of the prostate, which is the second most common male cancer and is present at least in some form in 80% of men over 80; and prostatitis, which is one of the more common male complaints between the ages of 25 and 50.

The first reported prostatectomy was performed by Amussat, who in 1827 incidentally removed an obstructing intravesical prostate while removing a bladder calculus. The patient recovered completely. Eugene Fuller of New York, in 1894, was the first to describe a technique for the complete suprapubic removal of a prostatic adenoma. Fryer popularized the operation in Britain. In 1904 Young described his perineal approach to prostatectomy, and then Terence MILLIN (this page), in 1947 described the retropubic approach, coming down in front of the bladder directly on to the anterior prostatic capsule. However, the most common type of prostatectomy in the developed world at present is the transurethral resection (that is, using an instrument passed down the urethra). The first resectoscope was developed by Maximilian Stern in 1926, using a squarewave (spark gap) current for cutting and a sine-wave current for coagulation. Some operators were able to remove several hundred grams of prostatic tissue at a single procedure, but usually the large glands were dealt with by open surgery. The advantage of the transurethral approach is that

there is little discomfort and the patient may be out of the hospital in a few days. Many new methods of control of prostatic enlargement have been proposed, ranging from medical treatments to laser surgery. None has been tested over a prolonged period of time.

Cancer of the prostate is now a leading cause of cancer deaths in men, second only to that of the lung. Until the 1940s very little could be done for these patients, except for the fortunate few (usually less than 5%) in whom the disease was diagnosed while still localized. The treatment for localized cancer was then surgical removal by a radical prostatectomy. This differs from simple prostatectomy in that the entire gland is removed and the bladder is then re-attached to the urethra; while in a simple prostatectomy only the central obstructing portion is removed, leaving the outer capsule intact.

In 1941 Huggins (an American urologist) published his work describing the hormonal control of the prostate in dogs and the use of stilbestrol or orchidectomy (removal of the testes) as a clinical treatment for widespread carcinoma of the prostate. The results of orchidectomy were immediate, with dramatic relief of severe bone pain within a few hours. Huggins later received a NOBEL PRIZE for his work, the first surgeon to do so since Alexis Carrel. Bagshaw reported on the use of megavoltage treatment in localized prostatic cancer. It seemed to be as good as radical surgery for up to 10 years, but was followed by an increased number of recurrences after this period. Another approach has been implantation of radioactive material into the prostate, but the long-term results are still not available.

Significant side-effects occur after all forms of treatment for carcinoma of the prostate. Impotence is expected after hormonal therapy or surgery, and occurs in up to 60% of patients after external beam therapy. Careful preservation of the nerves on either side of the prostate may make it possible to maintain potency after a radical prostatectomy. Incontinence may follow radical surgery in 1–5% of cases. Rectal and bladder irritability may occur after radiation therapy.

Recently, screening for prostate cancer with prostate-specific antigen in the blood and digital rectal examination, supplemented by ultrasonically guided needle biopsies, has multiplied the percentage of operable lesions found by a factor of at least four. The use of complete androgen ablation by luteinizing hormone-releasing hormone antagonists and anti-androgens offers to those men reluctant to undergo an orchidectomy, an alternative therapy, albeit an expensive one.

### Pediatric urology

About 40% of the more serious congenital malformations occur in the genitourinary tract, and most of the urological surgery in the young is concerned with their correction. In the past the management of these problems was in the hands of general surgeons and until Meredith Campbell published his textbook on pediatric urology in 1937 there was little concerted effort to pay special attention to pediatric urology. Sir David Innes Williams held a similar position in Britain, as did Gregoire in France.

Obstruction, with dilated urinary tracts above the obstruction, is the most common problem. These obstructions are being recognized earlier, partly because of the availability of ultrasound scans, which are non-invasive. It is now possible to diagnose obstruction in utero. However, such babies are usually those who have most severe obstruction and attempts to drain such obstructions in utero have proved very disappointing, since the damage has often occurred by the time the dilatation is identified.

### Neurogenic bladder and urodynamics

It is important that urine is delivered to the outside at a low pressure and without infection. The recognition that urine flow is not simply a matter of static pressure but of dynamic flow has led to the development of a discipline of urology called urodynamics.

In spite of the incompleteness of our theoretical knowledge, much has been done in the practical treatment of incontinence. Female stress incontinence due to weakness of the muscles of the pelvic floor is a common problem, often related to the after-effects of childbearing. For years it was treated with pessaries inserted into the vagina to hold the bladder in place. Then anterior vaginal repairs advocated by Kelly gave considerable relief. In the 1950s the Marshall-Marchetti-Krantz procedure was devised. This involved securing the periurethral and bladder neck tissue to the underside of the pubis to give a solid support to the bladder neck. Later, Perrera developed a simpler technique, inserting a long needle down either side of the bladder neck and placing a stitch to lift the bladder neck up towards the abdominal wall. This procedure has gained wide popularity because of reliability and lack of upset.

In rare cases an artificial sphincter may be used. This consists of an inflatable silastic cuff which is placed around the urethra, a reservoir, and a pump or control valve which controls the flow between the reservoir and the cuff. Fluid is pumped into the inflatable cuff to hold the urine and is released into the reservoir to empty the bladder.

The importance of these problems and the results of increased understanding are most obvious in the improved prognosis, both early and late, in patients with spinal cord injury. Before the 1960s if the patient survived the acute injury or the first few years of life, the major cause of death was renal failure, usually from a combination of obstruction, infection, and stone. Expectant treatment is now begun immediately and the disastrously damaged urinary tracts that were once so common in paraplegics are now seen infrequently.

In patients with acute spinal cord injury, a program of intermittent catheterization is begun almost immediately. Without the initial insult of an overdistended, often infected bladder, they are managed with either an intermittent catheterization program, a sphincterotomy (cutting the sphincter to allow continual flow of urine), or a timed voiding program. The situation is much the same in patients with spina bifida and meningomyelocele (neural tube defects). Previously, almost all of the latter patients had some urinary tract abnormality noted by the age of 4 years. Now many patients can be kept free of difficulty, either with medication or with intermittent catheterization.                    WHC, HNwhi

*See also* MINIMALLY INVASIVE SURGERY; NEPHROLOGY; SCREENING; SPECIALIZATION

**USA** The central fact of medical practice in the USA is that it is organized and largely paid for by private insurance: no universal government program guarantees medical care for all, or constrains its cost. In the absence of government control too many doctors have been trained and too many of those trained become specialists; too many hospitals have been built, with too many beds and too much expensive technology; and there is overtreatment of the insured and undertreatment of the uninsured. Many factors contribute to the resultant overinvestment in medical care, most notably overconfidence in the capacity of medical care to cure and prolong life, combined with incomplete information on the basis of which to judge the benefits of many treatments. Many doctors overestimate the benefits and underestimate the risks of the procedures they perform. As a result, the public has grown to expect results beyond what medicine can provide. If these excesses are the direct consequence of privatization and a free-market organization of medical care, and in the absence of government regulation, as they surely are, how was it allowed to happen?

The need for a national health service with universal health insurance has not gone unrecognized. President Theodore Roosevelt first suggested a universal plan at the turn of the 19th century. President Franklin D. Roosevelt considered one at the beginning of his second administration in 1937, but it was forgotten as America

### USA PIONEERS

John **WARREN** (1753–1815). American surgeon. Warren was born in Roxbury, Massachusetts, USA, and took an active part in the Boston Tea Party of 1773. At various times he was prominent in helping control of SMALLPOX and YELLOW FEVER epidemics. He gave anatomical lectures at the military hospital in Boston, helped to found the Boston Medical Society, and established the first school of medicine associated with Harvard in 1782, becoming the first professor of anatomy and surgery there.

(continued on p 841)

## JOHNS HOPKINS HOSPITAL,

in Baltimore, Maryland, USA, with its University School of Medicine and University School of Hygiene and Public Health. It began under the will of Johns Hopkins, a wealthy businessman, who, when he died in 1873, left $7 million to establish a university and a hospital. The will required careful consideration and expert advice for the site and the building, the provision of physicians and surgeons of the highest character and greatest skill, and a school for nurses. Most far-sighted was his wish that ultimately the hospital would form a part of the medical school of the university.

The hospital, opened in 1889, attracted a galaxy of talent, including William Welch, William OSLER (p 602), William S. HALSTED (p 746), and Howard A. Kelly. At first they taught graduate students, and an undergraduate school began in 1893, four years after the nursing school. These famous men and their distinguished pupils inaugurated and carried into practice what has become commonplace in the idea of the university hospital and medical school with full-time staffs and integration of service to patients, with research and education. When Abraham FLEXNER (p 258) produced his report of 1910 Johns Hopkins was the model of what was best for the future of medical education.

Discoveries and advances have included the first use of rubber gloves in surgery, fundamental work on rickets, the discovery of epinephrine (adrenaline) and heparin as well as many other important developments, but especially well-known is the 'blue-baby' operation developed by Helen TAUSSIG (p 150) and Alfred Blalock.

## MASSACHUSETTS GENERAL HOSPITAL

is the third oldest teaching hospital in the USA. Founded in Boston in 1811, building was delayed by the war, so that it was opened to patients in 1821, and became the first teaching hospital of the Harvard Medical School. The first building was named after its architect Charles Bullfinch. It was there that in 1846 William T. G. Morton, a dentist, first administered ether to a patient operated on by John Collins Warren, an achievement commemorated in the Ether Dome. Other important developments included the identification of appendicitis as an entity by Fitz in 1886; the introduction of CLINICOPATHOLOGICAL CONFERENCES; the first replantation of a severed arm (1962); the first practical method of freezing blood (1964); the introduction of photochemotherapy (1974); and the development of artificial skin for grafting (1981). The hospital has 820 beds, admits 35 000 inpatients each year, and handles over a million outpatients at its main campus and its health centers. Its staff perform nearly 30 000 operations and deliver over 2100 babies each year; and conduct research with an annual budget of $200 million. The hospital has over 10 000 employees, 3700 doctors, and 2300 nurses. In 1994 the hospital merged with the Brigham and Women's Hospital to form an integrated healthcare system.

## PENNSYLVANIA, THE MEDICAL COLLEGE OF,

was founded in 1850 as the Female Medical College of Pennsylvania. Among the QUAKERS of Philadelphia, women were accepted more as the equals of men than in most other societies. Many male Quaker doctors were more willing to take women as apprentices — the pattern of medical education of the time — than other contemporaries. However, as in Europe, women still found difficulty in obtaining degrees from medical institutions. An Act of incorporation was granted in 1850 by the Legislature with very little opposition. Forty women began medical studies in the first year.

The Civil War temporarily closed the College, but then, under a succession of able deans, it flourished. One was Ann Preston, who founded The Women's Hospital in 1861, to provide clinical facilities for education because of male opposition to women attending the practice of other hospitals in Philadelphia. By 1867 the name was changed to that of The Women's Medical College of Pennsylvania. In 1969 the name was changed again to that of The Medical College of Pennsylvania. Men were then admitted to its courses, to its staff, and to the offices of dean and president.

focused on the Second World War. President Harry Truman made a brief, unsuccessful, effort in 1949. President Richard Nixon proposed the first employer mandate plan in 1971, suggested by his Health, Education, and Welfare Undersecretary, John Veneman, a former Californian Assemblyman who was the author of his state's Medicaid law six years earlier. Senator Edward Kennedy introduced a plan that almost succeeded in 1974. And, most recently, President Bill Clinton's proposed Health Security Plan would have mandated employer-based insurance that would have reduced but not eliminated the numbers of uninsured, 41.4 million individuals in 1998.

Only once did the effort to provide universal coverage succeed, and then only in part. This was the enactment by Congress in 1965 of Medicare (for the elderly) and Medicaid (for the poor) at the height of President Lyndon Johnson's 'Great Society'. Over the years the legislation of government-funded universal insurance received wavering support, and ultimately the opposition, of doctors. The American Medical Association, their political arm, vigorously opposed government control and probable loss of income. Looking over their shoulders at the National Health Service in Britain, where income for general practitioners is sharply limited under capitation based on the number of patients for whom the doctor provides care, and consultant specialists are reimbursed by salaries that are tightly constrained under limits imposed by the government, their fears of loss of income and government control can be readily appreciated.

American doctors feared government and instead got investor-owned, for-profit medical corporations. Instead of the government as single payer, payment now comes from multiple, mostly for-profit corporations, each attempting to minimize costs in order to maximize fiscal returns to its investors (only the Kaiser Health Plan and a diminishing number of Blue Cross-Blue Shield plans were still non-profit in 1998). Instead of a global budget, as in the British National Health Service, under which the medical profession has retained relative autonomy and clinical freedom, budgetary control has been imposed by micro-management of clinical practice and veto power over clinical decisions.

### Why costs of medical care have risen rapidly

Early in the 20th century, when medicine's therapeutic potential was limited, the need for medical insurance may have seemed small. Charges for care that was provided by physicians and hospitals were modest, and care was provided without charge to those too poor to pay. Costs and charges have risen rapidly in the decades that followed, and at the beginning of the 21st century approach $4000 on average for every individual. Yet there is still no universal national health insurance.

Medical care, practiced with a full armamentarium at its disposal, is expensive. It is expensive anywhere in the world and it is particularly so in the USA, where procedure and hospitalization rates are high; where research funding, estimated at $33 399 million in 1994, promotes the rapid introduction of new medical technology into practice; and where the overhead costs of its fragmented system are the highest in the world, as high as 35 cents on the dollar, about 20% of which represents insurance carrier administrative costs and profit and 15% provider administrative costs (informal US government estimates).

It is generally appreciated that newly developed 'high-tech' medicine is inherently costly. Less well understood are why the costs of medical care, even after adjusting for its increased potential, have risen more rapidly than in many other aspects of the economy. The American economist William Baumol, in his 1995 Office of Health Economics Annual Lecture in London, explained why the costs of medical care, a labor intensive enterprise, can be expected to rise more rapidly than elsewhere in the economy. Automation and computerization in manufacture, agriculture, transport, and communication have resulted in enormous increases in productivity, requiring a much smaller workforce. Computers and automation have made important contributions to medical care, but the workforce needed has risen, not fallen. Salaries for that workforce may be expected to rise as well, in keeping with those of workers in jobs with increased productivity. In a country in which the fiscal budget depends on taxes and is tightly controlled, as in Britain, salaries for health workers and for other state employed workers in labor intensive occupations, most notably teachers, incomes have not kept pace with the rapidly changing economy. In the USA, where there have been few fiscal limits, the cost of medical care has risen in parallel with an expanding economy, but there has been little appreciation of the simple economic principle expounded by Baumol.

### Bias to treat; the technological imperative

The ostensibly unlimited budget available for medical care in the USA in the past must be acknowledged as a major determinant of how much medical care has been given. But it is not simply, or even primarily, the result of an effort by doctors to earn large incomes. The American economist Victor Fuchs, in his seminal book *Who shall live?*, wrote that: 'a common mistake is to think that the behavior of physicians can be understood only in terms of their desire to maximize income ... during their medical school and

**MAYO CLINIC**, in Rochester, Minnesota, USA, began with William Worrall MAYO (p 799), who migrated to the USA from Manchester, England. His surgeon sons worked in St Mary's Hospital and in practice, and such was their fame that patients were sent to them from far afield; the use of the term 'Mayo Clinic' crept into general use about 1900. In 1914 the brothers and their associates moved into a purpose-built five-storey building to continue their form of group practice. This was revolutionary because all fees were pooled and the doctors were paid a salary, since they believed that they should not vastly enrich themselves but receive only just and fair compensation for their work. To this end the Mayo Foundation was ultimately started with a large gift from the brothers. This still receives all the income, and administers the Clinic, paying the doctors a salary. The philanthropy does not stop there since the Mayo Graduate School of Medicine was founded in 1915 and the Mayo Medical School (for undergraduates) in 1972, and there is also a Mayo School of Health-Related Sciences. The Clinic is associated with two private hospitals — St Mary's and the Rochester Methodist — which are staffed entirely by Mayo Clinic doctors. There is now a vast range of buildings and services, donated and supported by many benefactors, devoted to the enterprise. The Mayo brothers were legendary in their contributions to surgery, and Edward C. Kendall and Philip S. Hench of the Clinic received the NOBEL PRIZE for medicine for their work in isolating cortisone and using it in the treatment of arthritis, so opening a new era in endocrinology.

residency training physicians are "imprinted" with what they understand to be "best medical practice", to which they try to conform throughout their careers', a process for which he coined the phrase 'technological imperative' — namely, the desire of physicians to do everything they have been trained to do, regardless of the benefit–cost ratio. But firm data needed to estimate such a ratio are available for no more than 15 or 20% of medical procedures, and when the benefits of treatment are uncertain, doctors tend to overestimate benefits.

How medical care is paid for has a widely publicized effect on how much is provided. When re-

(continued)

John Collins **WARREN** (1778–1856). American surgeon. John Collins Warren was born in Boston, USA, one of John Warren's 17 children. He studied medicine with his father at Harvard, and followed his father in the chair of anatomy and surgery. He was Dean of the medical school at Harvard from 1816–19, and surgeon at Massachusetts General Hospital. Warren performed the first operation for strangulated hernia in the USA, and in 1846 invited the dentist Morton to administer ether anesthesia to a patient from whom he removed a tumor of the neck. The Warren Museum of Harvard Medical School was founded on the geological, paleontological, and other specimens he left. He was also a founder of the *New England Journal of Medicine and Surgery*.

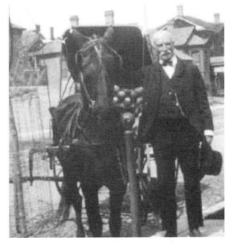

Dr William Worrall Mayo, 1904. Dr Mayo emigrated from England to the United States in 1846, and became a doctor in 1850.

imbursement is by fee-for-service the yearly costs for individuals may be as much as 50% greater than costs for individuals enrolled in prepayment, capitation plans. The importance of fee-for-service indemnity plans is diminishing, however, as the proportion of their subscribers has fallen from 59% in 1991 to 29% in 1998.

## Choice of specialty

Income may play a greater part in its effect on choice of specialty. Primary care, at least in part because of the smaller incomes it offers, attracts many fewer doctors in America than the medical and surgical specialties. The resultant weakness of primary care has direct effect on treatment rates. The primary care doctor is in a unique position to exercise what the sociologist Eliot Freidson has called 'the flexible discretionary judgement that is necessary to adapt services to individual patients' needs', and to balance the individual patient's values against the gains or losses of therapy at the margin, where risks and benefits are small and evenly matched. The primary care doctor, sometimes called the 'gate-keeper', has the advantage of being able to observe the patient over time and to assess the progress of illness, possibly opting to 'wait and see'. The specialist, on the other hand, may have one opportunity to diagnose an episode of illness, and but a single opportunity to intervene. This may explain the well-documented observation that in countries where primary care is strong, there are many fewer hospital admissions for medical and surgical care.

## Privatization of care

The privatization of medical care and its control by investor-owned corporations in America represent the culmination of a stream of events that began early in the 20th century. As Professor Paul Starr recounts in his Pulitzer Prize winning book, *The social transformation of American medicine*, the trajectory from solo practice fee-for-service medicine to employer insured, corporate medical care was very gradual. 'The dislike of physicians for "socialized medicine"', he wrote, 'is well known, but their distaste for corporate capitalism was especially strong. They had no more desire to be dominated by private corporations than by agencies of government, and consequently resisted the two forms in which business corporations threatened to move into medical services — the provision of treatment for their own employees through "company doctors" and the marketing of services to the public'.

Beginning with the hiring of company doctors late in the 19th century to treat industrial injuries, and against the concerted opposition of the medical profession, employers in larger corporations gradually accepted responsibility for most medical costs of their employees, and ultimately for their families. As the costs of care have mounted, to the extent that they now represent a significant fiscal handicap in a competitive business world, industry has become an important participant in the effort to restrain further increases.

The need to contain costs for the care of the poor and medically indigent became equally acute, and California was one of the earliest to attempt corrective action. By 1982 California's annual appropriations for Medicaid (or MediCal as the state calls it) were approaching $5 billion, despite the fact that the program was paying hospitals and doctors progressively less than were private payers. The Federal government's Medicare costs were similarly out of control. In the same decade private sector healthcare expenditures nationwide had increased from 7.5% to 10% of gross domestic product. Employer groups were forming health cost study coalitions, searching for ways to slow the runaway costs of health insurance.

In 1982, for the first time in California's history, marketplace competition was injected into healthcare. The state legislature mandated that MediCal would do business only with hospitals that offered favorable rates, competitively negotiated in advance. The system established came to be called selective provider contracting. When the state's actions came to be known to private health insurance leaders, they knew that an equally radical effort would have to be made to control rates in the private sector. The legislature agreed to give private insurers the same selective provider contracting authority, and marketplace competition had come to California healthcare, private as well as public.

Selective provider competition worked. In the first two years MediCal saved $1.5 billion. Selector provider contracting quickly spread from California across to USA and became known as 'the managed care industry'. It has come to dominate the reform movement in California and in the process has almost eliminated the free choice of doctor on which patients place high value, and the fee-for-service provision of care so important to doctors.

## Cost savings

The results of the implementation of selective provider contracting were startling and unexpected. Policy makers believed that, if costs were brought under control, more people would have health insurance because it would become affordable for employers purchasing it for their workers and families, and for individuals and families buying their own insurance. Remarkable cost savings were in fact achieved, but selective contracting led to more aggressive medical insurance underwriting and the elimination of cost shifting, the cross-subsidy of those unable to pay by charging higher rates to those insured. Individuals and defined groups, rather than communities, became the targets of 'experience rating', thus diminishing the sharing of risk that underlies a fundamental principle of all insurance.

Another unexpected result was a burst of entre-preneural speculation in medical care. Medical insurance 'carriers', as they are called, had started as non-profit corporations. They made small sur-pluses ('underwriting gains' in insurance par-lance), but they had no stockholders, and profit was not an objective. Selective contracting, and the harsh underwriting practices that it fostered, together with the restriction of cost-shifting, enabled medical insurers to operate with profit. The new ability to generate large sums of money stimulated the conversion of prepaid group prac-tices to stockholder-owned for-profit commercial enterprises, and the MANAGED CARE industry became big business.

## Consequences of managed care and for-profit medicine

Managed care, together with the privatization and 'corporatization' of medical practice, has pro-foundly altered the practice of medicine, as well as how it is financed. Clinical freedom in decision making and the autonomy prized and jealously guarded by doctors have been severely eroded. The new investor-owned medical corporations, reimbursing doctors and their practices by fee-for-service, micromanage medical decision making, require preadmission certification before hospital admission, and enforce rigid adherence to clinical management guidelines. To the extent that this may help constrain some of the poor practices of the past this can represent an improvement. But to the extent that it impairs the discretionary flexibility to tailor treatment in response to patients' values, interference with medical decisions, often by administrators unfa-miliar with the uncertainty or reliability of medical evidence, can only do harm. The greatest of the potential harms is that administrative over-sight, together with emphasis on cost-contain-ment, will compromise the quality of care and access to quality care. Fearing this, purchasers of health services, when negotiating contracted rates, are demanding assurance that quality will not suffer, but documentation of the protection of quality is not easily achieved.

Patients, on their part, worry that choice of doctor, access to specialists, assurance that medical decisions will be limited to qualified practitioners, the right to appeal such decisions, and the right to sue for alleged malpractice may be jeopardized. Their concerns are heightened by the current existence of laws in many states that shield managed care systems from liability for the actions of employed and contracted professional providers. Some relief may be provided by legisla-tion of a so-called 'patient bill of rights', a package of reforms pending in the Congress and in many state legislatures.

## The future

Managed care as a dominant force in the delivery of medical services in the USA is 'a work in progress', according to Paul Ellwood, an import-ant figure in the development of market-based health plans. He writes that 'it is unrealistic to expect to return to unmanaged, autonomous, fee-for-service medicine where those who paid the bill often exerted little influence over medical practice'. But the doctors themselves, most of whom have remained passive observers of what they have seen as a growing nightmare, can now take advantage of the potential of managed care to improve the organization and delivery of medical services. Writing from the Board of Governors of the New York Academy of Sciences, Henry Greenberg predicts that 'as managed care organizations lead the profession in the ways of efficiency and cost reduction, a reasonable and predictable reaction will occur from within the profession … Physician groups will replace the insurance entities with their own organizations. With no shareholders to enrich, such groups can undercut the for-profit companies by 15%–20% and carry the field.'

As fee-for-service is replaced by capitation and a fixed budget, professional incomes can be expected to diminish. On the other hand, and given the demise of for-profit enterprise, the need for micromanagement of clinical decisions should also be sharply reduced, and, as a result, pro-fessional autonomy largely regained. David Blumenthal at Harvard writes that some doctors 'undoubtedly will find themselves with unprece-dented opportunities to put their training to work for their patients. Freed by capitation to innovate in healthcare delivery, supported by professional management and state of the art information systems, newly sensitive to consumer wishes, and spurred by the example of competing organiza-tions, these physicians will deliver care of unprecedented quality and efficiency…This result seems most likely to occur when savvy, enlight-ened purchasers with highly educated workforces are able to identify and form partnerships with well-managed provider organizations that employ competent, conscientious physicians.'

The politics of medicine in the USA, its organ-ization and financing, are in transition at the present time. The Clinton Health Security Act, though not enacted by the Congress, would have been no more than a step along the way. The Clinton Plan would have built usefully on the current system of medical insurance voluntarily provided by employers. Employers would have been required to provide insurance, and small employers would have been allowed to join forces in alliances for the purpose. But a great deal would have remained to be accomplished. Many of the 17–18% of the non-elderly population currently uninsured would have remained so. The employers, who together with the insurance industry successfully lobbied against the Clinton reforms, believed that they would have been further handicapped by the employer mandate in competing for international business. The need for a single source of payment, 'the single payer' provision that was proposed but dropped in the final legislative draft, would have remained unresolved, with the enormous overhead costs of the current system of multiple 'third party payers' still in place.

The practice of medicine itself is in transition. Doctors still rely primarily on what the late Lewis Thomas called 'half way technologies', designed to ameliorate symptoms and improve function but that do not cure the underlying pathology. As better treatments are developed, and as better information on their effectiveness becomes available, medicine will move on beyond the current and unpopular guidelines or rules of thumb to a scientific practice that is based, at last, on evidence. JPBun, EBD, RWS

*See also* HEALTHCARE SYSTEMS; INTERNAL MEDICINE — USA; SPECIALIZATION

### Editor's comment

An alternative perspective might suggest that it was private enterprise, its occasional excesses notwithstanding, that made the United States the world's undisputed leader in medicine. Nor does the experience of the last century inspire much confidence in the efficacy of universally centralized government run systems. In America most patients not covered by private or government third party payers go to municipal, university, or Veterans Administration hospitals and clinics, where they receive a level of care at least comparable to the "socialized" medicine of many other developed countries. GD

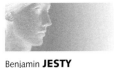

**VACCINATION** The term 'vaccination' owes its origin to a pamphlet published in 1798 by Edward JENNER (p 452): *An inquiry into the causes and effects of the variolae vaccinae.* It described for the first time in print, and on an experimental basis, the use of inoculation of cowpox as a protective measure, less dangerous than variolation (inoculation with smallpox matter practiced in the 18th century to produce a milder form of the natural disease), against SMALLPOX. Variolation had been introduced to western Europe by Lady Mary Wortley Montagu. She had encountered it in Constantinople, which it had reached via the Silk Route from China, where it was practiced from around 1000 AD.

The protective effect of cowpox against later infection with smallpox, often observed in milkers in contact with infected udders of the cows, was known among country people in Gloucestershire; as well as elsewhere in Britain and Europe, in the second half of the 18th century. Jenner was not the first to make the observation; but he was the first to carry out vaccination professionally, and as a scientific experiment.

Jenner's experiment was not entirely flawless, and would certainly not have passed today's barrier of medical ethics. After earlier observations involving 'swinepox' and his own 10-month-old son and the latter's nurse, Jenner in the 1790s went on to observe cowpox in milk maids as recorded in the *Inquiry*, with the one new experimental observation which has earned a lasting place in medical history: the inoculation on the arm of James Phipps, 8 years old, from a pock on the hand of milkmaid Sarah Nelmes, naturally infected with cowpox while milking cows. James had no serious reaction; and less than seven weeks later he was inoculated with true variolous matter, with only a local effect observable on the arm. That was the only real experiment at first included in the *Inquiry*, supplemented by secondary information on resistance to variolation, and on the role of cowpox and horse 'grease'. In fact, the origin of *vaccinia* virus, the active component of the 'cowpox' vaccine used throughout the 19th and 20th centuries, remains a matter for speculation.

Controversy has surrounded Jenner's 'discovery' from its very beginnings. In the annals of PUBLIC HEALTH he deserves every credit for firmly establishing vaccination as a valuable tool, which eventually led to the eradication of a dreaded disease. On the other hand, he maintained to the end of his life that the original cowpox vaccination would protect the recipient for a lifetime, although observers elsewhere soon recognized the necessity for regular revaccination. In 1802 the government awarded him £10 000 in recognition of his achievement — a gesture which added fuel to the fire of attacks from his critics.

**Homage to Jenner**

Arguments between those who admired Jenner and his contribution unreservedly, and others who, like Crookshank, claimed that he had 'discovered nothing', or worse, like Creighton, that he was a mere 'charlatan' and his work a 'tissue of inconsistencies and absurdities', continued until the end of the 19th century. PASTEUR (p 620) thought otherwise. For the better part of the 19th century, 'vaccine' and 'vaccination' had referred exclusively to inoculation with 'cowpox' to prevent smallpox. But when, in the 1880s, Pasteur began using attenuated bacteria and viruses to protect animals and man against chicken cholera, anthrax, and rabies, he adopted the terms. At the international medical congress in London in 1881, he announced the results of successful vaccination against anthrax in livestock; and in flowery French he duly paid homage to Jenner, whose introduction of vaccination over 80 years before had preceded his own deliberate attenuation procedures.

From then on, 'vaccination' and 'vaccine' were established terms for immunization against an infectious disease, usually by inoculation with an appropriate vaccine, which in turn now means a preparation of killed or attenuated micro-organisms (bacteria or viruses) able to stimulate production of antibodies to combat the disease in question. Despite many advances and the use of many different vaccines, several new ones, especially against parasitic diseases such as MALARIA, are still at an experimental stage.  LW

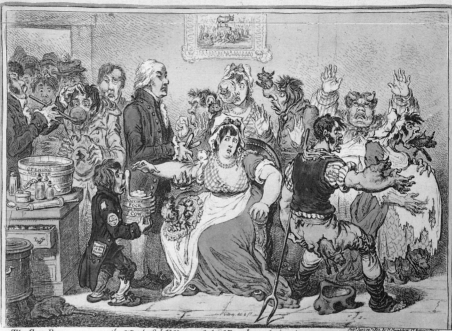

Edward Jenner and inoculation: a Gilray cartoon (1802). (Reproduced courtesy of the Wellcome Institute Library.)

*The Cow-Pock — or — the Wonderful Effects of the New Inoculation!* Vide. the Publications of ÿ Anti-Vaccine Society.

Andreas **VESALIUS** (1514–64). Born in Brussels, Vesalius carried out his medical studies at the University of Louvain and in Paris. After a period as a military surgeon, he entered the University of PADUA (p 447) in 1537 and within a year was offered the chair of surgery and anatomy. He gave lectures and carried out public dissections and in 1543 published his most famous work, the anatomical text, *De humani corporis fabrica*, showing the bones, muscles, ligaments, blood vessels, and organs of the human body. The book met with much opposition as it disagreed with the long-held views of GALEN (p 324) whose works on human anatomy were based on research into barbary apes. The controversy led Vesalius to resign his chair in Padua, and become court physician to the Emperor Charles V in Madrid and later to Philip II of Spain. Vesalius left Europe on a pilgrimage to Jerusalem and died in a storm on his return.

### VETERANS AFFAIRS, US DEPARTMENT OF

The Department of Veterans Affairs (VA) provides medical care annually to some 3.5 million persons. It has an annual medical budget of about US$18.5 billion and operates 172 hospitals; over 130 nursing home-care units; 70 comprehensive home-care programs; and over 600 outpatient, community, and outreach clinics. The Veterans

Affairs healthcare system is organized into 22 integrated service networks that provide comprehensive healthcare with emphasis on primary care and outpatient services. US programs for the care and pensioning of veterans of military service began after the American Revolutionary War. By the early part of the 19th century there were 'homes' in many parts of the USA for elderly and disabled veterans, many of whom required medical care. After the American Civil War, several veterans' hospitals were created and maintained by the federal government. By the early part of the 20th century, the number of veterans' hospitals had increased to about fifty. Additional hospitals were established to accommodate the increased veteran population that resulted from the two world wars.

Each of today's 25.5 million US veterans is potentially eligible for VA medical care. Care is provided based on seven congressionally mandated priorities. The highest priority is for veterans whose illness or disability was incurred during military service. At the end of World War II, VA initiated a process to establish affiliations between VA hospitals and US medical and associated health schools. Today, the VA healthcare system is the largest provider of graduate medical education and other health professional training in the USA. Each year, about 91 000 medical and other students receive some or all of their clinical training in VA facilities through affiliation with over 1200 educational institutions. VA funds about 9000 residency positions at some 130 medical school-affiliated hospitals, through which over 34 000 residents rotate each year. Over half of all US-trained physicians receive some of their training at a VA medical center and 70% of all VA physicians have medical school faculty appointments. VA is also one of the largest health research organizations in the USA. VA researchers pioneered the treatment of tuberculosis and high blood pressure, kidney and home dialysis techniques, development of the computerized tomography and magnetic resonance imaging, and cardiac pacemaker implantation.

Three VA scientists have received the NOBEL PRIZE for medicine. Dr Rosalyn S. Yalow received the Nobel prize for her work in the development of radioimmunoassay, and Dr Andrew V. Schally for his research on brain hormones. Dr Ferid Murad received the 1998 Nobel prize in medicine in part for research he conducted while working at the VA Medical Center in Palo Alto, California. VA continues to perform pioneering research across a broad medical spectrum, including post traumatic stress disorder, AIDS, diabetes, epilepsy, pain, and geriatric and women's health issues. The Department of Veterans Affairs is exceeded only by the Defense Department in number of federal employees. About 185 000 of VA's 205 000 total employees work in the department's healthcare system. The motto of the Department of Veterans Affairs is a phrase from the second inaugural address of Abraham Lincoln: 'To care for him who shall have borne the battle and for his widow and his orphan'.                    GD

**VETERINARY MEDICINE** In this post-Darwinian age, when scientists have placed humanity firmly as one species among many comprising the biosphere, it seems odd that one would even suggest that veterinary medicine and human medicine might *not* be related. Indeed, some of us have proposed, only partly in jest, that human medicine is a subspecialty of veterinary medicine, being dealt with by primate veterinarians with a particular interest in naked apes. That said, the practice of medicine is as much related to culture as to science, and culture dictates that people and other animals be treated in different ways. This split between the scientific and cultural lenses in observing disease has resulted in a schizophrenic history of relationships between human and veterinary medicine. Nevertheless, this relationship has a positive side.

### Comparative medicine
This draws on the understanding that humans are part of a larger, complex biological evolutionary

history, and applies this to solving both human and animal health and disease problems.

Rudolf VIRCHOW (p 853), one of several great 19th-century 'veterinary-physicians', exemplified these ideas of 'one medicine' when he said that 'between animal and human medicine there is no dividing line — nor should there be. The object is different but the experience obtained constitutes the basis of all medicine'. These ideas formed the foundation for all the basic biomedical sciences, as well as epidemiology, in which the principles of diseases and their prevention are the same. Such disciplines have become the cornerstones of our understanding of disease, therapeutic interventions, and toxicological assessments in the 20th century. From heart transplants and ear drum grafts to treatments for leprosy and AIDS, human medicine defines its problems, then works with non-human animals for solutions, and only much later returns to testing on humans. All of this assumes that animal models are trustworthy guides and that veterinary medicine is a sound basis for human medicine. Furthermore, it assumes that such scientific testing is more humane toward all species than *ad hoc* extrapolations from natural 'experiments'.

Calvin Schwabe documented much of the history of medical and veterinary practices and their common roots. The prehistoric religious and healing practices in ancient Egypt, which formed the basis for rational medicine in the western world, drew on a common pool of comparative disease knowledge, often derived from animal sacrifices, and translated it into both human and animal medical practices. ARISTOTLE (p 64) showed that Greek biology and medicine were rich in comparative biology. Greek thought was rooted in pre-historical legends. Chiron, for instance, the Centaur and legendary teacher of veterinary medicine, also fostered ASCLEPIUS (p 710), bringer of health to both animals and people, who in turn fathered Hygeia, the goddess of health.

Not until the 18th and 19th centuries would Europe and North America see again such a flourishing of veterinary and medical collaboration. This sprang from the foundation of the first two veterinary schools (Lyon, 1762; Alfort, 1765) in France, where the infectiousness of several animal diseases was firmly established, and whose graduates founded the National Academy of Sciences and the Health Council of France. H. M. O. Delafond, director at Alfort, cultured the anthrax bacillus *in vitro* in 1860, 15 years before KOCH (p 455), and the physician Jean VILLEMIN (p 830) and veterinarian Jean-Baptiste Auguste Chauveau demonstrated the infectiousness of TUBERCULOSIS in 1868. Henri Bouley, a French veterinarian, and president of the National Academy of Sciences and Academy of Medicine, was a lifelong

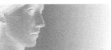

**LEADING VETERINARIAN**

Bernard Laurits Frederik **BANG** (1848–1932). Danish veterinary surgeon. After veterinary training he graduated in medicine and became director of the Royal Veterinary School in Copenhagen. In 1897 he discovered the bacterial cause of infectious abortion in cattle, abortus fever, now known as *Brucella abortus*. He was the leading veterinary surgeon of his time and made useful studies of smallpox vaccination, actinomycosis, and tuberculosis.

friend of Louis PASTEUR (p 620). Indeed, much of Pasteur's work on vaccines was carried out in collaboration with, or built upon, the work of veterinarians such as Henri J. Toussaint (on anthrax) and Victor Galtier (on rabies).

In North America, Duncan McEachran, a veterinarian, collaborated with William OSLER (p 602), at McGill University (p 139), where Osler was a member both of the medical faculty and of the Montreal Veterinary College. Osler took his comparative medical ideals with him to JOHNS HOPKINS UNIVERSITY MEDICAL SCHOOL (p 840), where veterinarians are still members in the Division of Comparative Pathology. Publication of *The Journal of Comparative Medicine and Surgery* started in the late 19th century in the USA, and organizations such as the Academy of Comparative Medicine and Surgery were founded in New York City. At the University of Pennsylvania, medical and veterinary students shared many of the same courses in the first two of their three years. Indeed, Christopher Graham, co-founder of the MAYO CLINIC (p 841), spent his first two years in a veterinary curriculum before finishing his training in human medicine.

The great visions and collaborations, however, were lost for much of the 20th century, when the illusion that veterinary medicine and human medicine are distinct enterprises was emphasized and much of the excitement of open collaboration was lost. A sign of the times was the demise of the McGill faculty of comparative medicine after only 13 years.

While open professional collaboration slipped from public view, basic biomedical research continued apace, and in one aspect in particular, veterinarians continued to play an acknowledged part in human medicine. Until the 1960s veterinarians were active in public health units in North America and Europe, particularly in subjects related to food safety and zoonoses (animal diseases which can be transmitted to humans) and this interest has been revived at the end of the 20th century.

## Food and nutrition

The great animal plagues have had devastating effects on human health and welfare because of the loss of work potential, food, and accumulated wealth. In some cases, such as the rinderpest epidemics in late 19th century Africa, these animal disease epidemics resulted in tens of thousands of human deaths and the collapse of societies, changing the course of history. Human nutritionists then focused on fortification and supplementation to redress nutrient deficiencies created through economic and agricultural policies. In recent years, however, more eco-systemic approaches have been proposed by such organizations as the International Food Policy Research Institute in Washington and the micronutrient initiative of the Federation of American Scientists. These systemic approaches look for solutions to simultaneous crises in micronutrient malnutrition, environmental degradation, and economic underdevelopment, and veterinarians and physicians have begun to make common cause. Clinical trials among Kenyan schoolchildren, for instance, have shown the beneficial effects of animal protein supplements on learning, and the judicious use of livestock in agricultural systems has been shown to benefit both the human population and the ecosystem of which they are a part.

Issues related to residues of agricultural and veterinary chemicals in foods, and the development of antibiotic-resistant bacterial populations from both veterinary and human medical use, have also led to a wide range of collaborative research and regulatory initiatives between human and veterinary medical practitioners.

## Infectious diseases

Several studies have suggested that 40 to 50% of serious human infections are either transmitted from vertebrate animal reservoirs to people (true zoonoses, according to the WORLD HEALTH ORGANIZATION definition), or are shared with other animals. The latter include diseases caused by infectious agents, such as blastomycosis and histoplasmosis, which thrive in environments altered by animal products. In the case of those diseases naturally transmitted from other vertebrates to people — rabies, TUBERCULOSIS, brucellosis, and some foodborne infections — the interests and practice of veterinary and medical research converged with general biology in the 19th century under the polymathic guidance pioneers such as Daniel Elder Salmon (a veterinarian), Sir William OSLER (p 602) (a physician), and Louis PASTEUR (p 620) (neither physician nor veterinarian).

This broad collaboration was largely lost in the mid-20th century, when practitioners on both sides tended to focus on more species-specific diseases (for instance, MALARIA in people, or foot and mouth disease in livestock which ravaged Britain and Europe in 1967 and 2001) or on chronic diseases in humans, where comparative biological research (animals in the service of humans), rather than a common practical agenda (animal and human health as rooted in common contexts) was deemed important. The practice of 'two medicines' has been found wanting, as old zoonotic diseases re-emerge, and new ones are described, in response to changing social and ecological conditions. Two classes of disease — the spongiform encephalopathies, and vero-toxin-producing *Escherichia coli* (and foodborne illnesses in general) — have been particularly important in re-establishing open veterinary–human medical collaborations.

*E. coli* 0157:H7 and related organisms first emerged as important human pathogens in the 1980s, associated, on the one hand, with such serious diseases as hemolytic uremic syndrome in children and hemorrhagic colitis in nursing home populations and, on the other, with foods of animal origin, especially ground meats (hence the popular name 'hamburger disease'). While more recent outbreaks have been traced to contamination of a wide variety of foods, the early associations with meat led to a flurry of research initiatives, initially as parallel veterinary–human medical activities, and then as full-scale collaborations. Researchers in Canada have created one of the most formidable, interdisciplinary collaborative teams anywhere, drawing on universities, hospitals, and government researchers.

In the mid-1980s, bovine spongiform encephalopathy emerged as a serious epidemic disease in cattle in Britain. Such diseases — CREUTZFELDT–JAKOB DISEASE and KURU in people, scrapie in sheep, and similar diseases in mink and several other species — were once thought to represent *only* cases of parallel evolution. When scrapie crossed the species boundary from sheep into cattle, however, public health officials and researchers were given cause for reconsideration. Initial work on the epidemic was carried out almost entirely by veterinary researchers, with a few parallel investigations in people. Subsequent investigations have shown that the new bovine form of this disease probably has crossed over into people, resulting in a few cases of 'new variant' Creutzfeldt-Jakob disease, and underlining the importance of ongoing veterinary and human medical collaboration and communication. Many publications are now appearing showing both comparative pathologies of these 'prion' diseases and cross-species transmission.

## Companionship and health
Keeping animals as human co-workers and companions is neither new nor restricted to affluent western societies. Dogs have been associated with human cultures for over 14 000 years, and cats were venerated in ancient Egypt. Fruit bats, lizards, and parrots were once kept as pets by Fijians; Samoans kept pigeons and eels; Australian Aborigines associated with dingoes. The reasons for these associations are manifold; a study of dog populations in Kathmandu, Nepal, showed that they were valued not only as companions, but as community police, guarding temples from thieves and keeping the streets clear of strangers at night.

Human relationships with animals may, and sometimes do, become pathological, just as

A disease chart for a dog, from an 18th century French textbook on veterinary medicine, *Cours complet d'agriculture*, Rozier, Paris. (Reproduced courtesy of the National Library of Medicine, Bethesda, MD.)

human interrelationships may degenerate into strange dependencies. On the positive side, companion animals improve various health measures in different settings. Dogs, for instance, have been used as 'co-therapists' to provide non-threatening, unconditional affection in several institutional programs to help psychologically and mentally disturbed people develop better social skills. Other research studies have focused on the lowered blood pressure and better survival after heart surgery provided by exposure to pets. Clearly there are also risks in such programs, since companion animals themselves may exhibit a range of psychological disorders, as well as being able to transmit some zoonoses. The success of any such programs depends largely on selection of people and animals, which in turn depends on excellent veterinarian–physician cooperation. Recent studies have shown that for elderly people living at home, in times of crisis, dogs and cats can substitute for human social support networks in preventing ill health.

## Sustainable development
In the 1980s, the World Commission on Environment and Development, chaired by a physician, Gro Harlem Brundtland, defined the term 'sustainable development'. Faced with the prospects of economic development being pitted against both human health and environmental integrity, it became clear that new ways of thinking about health, the environment, and the economy would need to be developed. Under the auspices of such organizations as the International Society for Ecosystem Health and the International Geosphere-Biosphere Program,

human and animal health workers have begun to seek each other out to find creative solutions.

In the 1980s and 1990s, veterinarians, physicians, ecologists, economists, geographers, and others began to define a new discipline which might be referred to as 'ecosystem health', or 'ecosystem approaches to health, agriculture, the environment, and socio-economic development'.

Good health, according to the World Health Organization, is 'a state of complete physical, mental and social well-being and not merely the absence of disease or infirmity'. The Ottawa Charter for Health and the WHO declaration at Alma Ata both focused on what was needed to promote healthy communities; these pronouncements suggested that health is not an 'objective for living', but a 'resource for everyday life'. Similarly, veterinarians have tended to develop definitions of health in relation to the particular expectations, or goals, which animal owners have for their charges.

Although these ideas were developed in relation to individuals, groups, and interacting communities in both human and animal populations, some researchers have begun to argue that they can provide a basis for assessing sustainability at a much greater scale. Indeed, veterinary and human medical researchers, searching for the root causes of diseases in different species, are increasingly looking at systemic interactions: economic activities, for instance, create environmental conditions which facilitate, or retard, the spread of different diseases. Climate and land use changes, both local and global, have become driving forces for changing disease patterns in many species in different parts of the world. In applying notions of health and disease to entire ecosystems, and devising ecosystemic solutions to problems in health, agriculture, and the environment, veterinarians and physicians are increasingly finding common cause with concerned citizens from a wide variety of other scientific and professional backgrounds.

In the 1990s, 'ecosystem health' courses have been implemented in several veterinary and medical schools; in professional training, these courses still tend to operate in parallel, although they may share case studies and other basic materials. This 'dual track' development is largely driven by the different cultural expectations placed on veterinarians and physicians.

In 1998, Gro Harlem Brundtland was appointed Director General of the World Health Organization. These, and other shifts in several global organizations, signal that such systemic approaches to human and planetary health, incorporating the work of both the medical and veterinary establishments as partners in a grander enterprise, can be expected. For the sake of future generations, this re-awakening of a common vision for veterinary and medical practitioners cannot come too soon.    DW-T

*See also* GLOBAL ENVIRONMENTAL CHANGE; HEALTH, DEFINITIONS; WORLD HEALTH ORGANIZATION

**VIOLENCE** Aggression is dispelled harmlessly in a peaceful society in many forms of sport but is manifest in several health problems. The most prominent are assaultative violence including homicide; domestic violence, which includes woman battering, CHILD ABUSE, ABUSE OF OLD PEOPLE; rape and sexual assault; road rage; and violence directed against the self.

In 1996, the WORLD HEALTH ORGANIZATION defined violence as 'the intentional use of physical force or power, threatened or actual, against oneself, another person, or a group or community, that results in, or has a high likelihood of resulting in injury, death, psychological harm, maldevelopment or deprivation'. Three types of violence are identified in the WHO document:

- Self-inflicted violence, where SUICIDE is the most severe manifestation.

- Interpersonal violence between individuals. This includes domestic violence, violence among acquaintances, and violence between strangers, as in robbery with violence.

- Organized violence, which is planned to achieve political, social, or economic ends. This includes riots, civil disturbances, and in its most extreme form, armed conflict, that is WAR.

Over 560 000 deaths annually world-wide, about 1.1% of all deaths, are due to interpersonal violence. Homicide rates of over 40 per 100 000 per annum occur in sub-Saharan Africa and in Latin America. Among the Organization for Economic Cooperation and Development (OECD) nations, the USA is an outlier with 10.1 deaths per 100 000; rates in others range from 0.6 in England to 2.1 in Canada. Homicide caused by firearms is 12 times more common in the USA than in other OECD nations. In the USA in 1994, firearm-related homicide and suicide together caused 38 805 deaths, compared with 42 524 motor vehicle-related deaths; the latter are declining while firearm-related deaths are increasing. If present trends continue, firearm-related homicide will soon cause more deaths annually than automobile accidents.

Homicide rates everywhere are highest among young men. In the USA firearm-related deaths are the leading cause of death in men aged 15–34, and are especially common among young black men in deprived inner-city regions.

Assaultative violence causes about 10–15 hospital admissions for every death, a huge number of lesser injuries, as well as incalculable psychological harm and social disruption. This is why WHO has designated violence as a PUBLIC HEALTH problem.

The causal factors associated with violence are biological, psychological, and sociological. The biological factors include psychiatric conditions and aggression related to male sex hormones. Psychological factors include neuroanatomical and biochemical aberrations and are relatively rare causes. The sociological factors are related to the process by which children learn the rules of social behavior; to cognition (violent and non-violent people may perceive social situations in different ways); and to social settings (such as stressful events, social environments in which violent behavior is the norm, presence of weapons, prevalence of alcohol, mood-altering drugs). Thus violence is a learned behavior and therefore it is preventable. Alcohol is consistently associated with violence. At the time of an assault or homicide the victim and the perpetrator have commonly been found to have been drinking. Illegal drugs have also been incriminated, but the relationship is complex. In controlled studies they have not consistently been found to cause aggression, but rather it is the context in which they are used that may be important. Alcohol may be used in dangerous situations and may remove inhibitions and embolden victims to take risks. Much of the violence surrounding the introduction of crack cocaine use was actually due to rivalry between street gangs attempting to expand their drug distribution markets.

## Cultural conditioning

The high homicide rates in the USA compared with other OECD nations are associated not only with the availability of guns but also with cultural conditioning: the portrayal of violent behavior on television fosters positive attitudes towards violence, the notion that disputes can be settled by using guns rather than by discussion and negotiation. The availability of guns in the USA makes them a preferred suicidal implement too; in 1994, firearms were used in 18 765 suicides and 17 866 homicides. Firearms also caused at least 1356 unintentional deaths. The availability of handguns in the United States associates them with serious injury and is arguably the greatest factor in the country's excess homicide rate. Ten thousand Americans died in 1990 of gunshot wounds compared with 22 in Britain and 13 in Sweden. A comparison of two similar cities close to each other, Seattle in the USA and Vancouver in Canada, showed a much lower rate of homicide in Vancouver, attributed to the lack of availability of handguns. A firearm obtained for protection is rarely put to that use but it is much more likely to kill an occupant of the household in which it is kept. Even a handgun carried by the victim of a robbery increases the risk of that person being shot in the course of the crime. Contrary to the common perception that an assault or a homicide is usually committed by a stranger, it has been shown that the victim and the perpetrator usually are acquainted, the situation being most often an argument, and the victim and perpetrator most often similar to each other, of the same race and age group. Men, however, are more likely to be the perpetrator when women are victims.

## The victims

Victims of violence are high users of medical care. Often they do not present with complaints related to their victimization but instead have multiple vague and somatic complaints. Such victims need to be identified in the course of the medical interview, and screening for violence has been recommended for high-risk patients and in clinical situations where such high-risk patients are seen most often. This will identify ongoing or recurrent victimization, avoid serious harm, and treat the effects of the victimization appropriately. It is particularly important to screen women because victims of domestic violence, though frequently seeking medical attention, may not reveal ongoing abuse unless specifically questioned. The American College of Obstetrics and Gynecology recommends that every woman be asked whether she has been struck or threatened in the last year. Pregnant women should also be questioned, because there is an increased incidence of abuse during pregnancy. The cost in years of potential life lost, the cost of emergency and long-term medical care of the victims, are huge. The social and psychological harm produced by violence cannot be measured in financial terms but they are huge too.

It follows from recognizing violence as a public health problem, and from the above account of causes, that prevention of violence requires concerted actions: reducing the cultural acceptance of violence, improving social conditions, restricting access to firearms, and reducing consumption of alcohol and drugs that are associated with a great many assaults and street crime. It is a challenge that no nation has yet confronted, let alone attempted to solve.

An aggressive nature probably enabled our hominid ancestors to survive in a hostile world. In civilized societies, however, aggression expressed as violent behavior may harm others. Perhaps organized communities invented competitive sports and stage plays to blunt or dispel aggressive impulses against others. Violence thus becomes a spectator sport, as in BOXING, ice hockey, and football, or in the tragedies and even comedies of classical and modern theater. A well-conceived play can arouse strong emotions, but is an improbable and infrequent cause of violent aggressive acts by an individual against another. In the 20th century, for the first time in history, entertainment could be mass produced. Performers and spectators no longer had to encounter each other face to face: radio and moving pictures, silent at first, then with sound and color and an illusion of being three dimensional, replaced actors on stage. Spectators may sit in darkened rooms, at the cinema or watching television in their homes, and emerge into the world of reality with their minds affected and their emotions roused by the behavior of the characters they have seen on the screen. Vicariously they can share in their hopes and fears, their loves and hates, their aggressive and often violent conduct.

What is the impact of observed violence on the aggressive impulses and violent tendencies of the observer? Does the age and suggestibility of the viewer make a difference? What, in particular, is the impact of exposing young children to excessive and repeated violence? Such concerns date back at least to the beginning of the 20th century. Indeed, as early as 1910 parents were urged to look into what children saw at theaters and stage performances. Then as now, editors, doctors, churches, and citizens' organizations complained with 'cries of protest' about this 'mental problem' and 'environmental issue'. Then came television, in the 1930s to Britain and Germany, and to the USA at the World's Fair in 1939, beginning its penetration into American households in the late 1940s so that within 20 years 95% of American households had a television set. In the USA, unlike in other countries, television began not as a public service but as an entertainment designed to sell goods and services. Over the years it has evolved into the prime medium on which millions of families rely for information, education, entertainment, and convenient baby-sitting. Most American children begin to watch television at the age of 3, spending an average of 28 hours per week sitting in front of a set, so that at any one time millions of children are watching television. It has been estimated that a child may see as many as 20 000 commercials during one year; may have been exposed to some 15 000 hours of television by the time of graduation from high school (compared with 11 000 hours of instruction); and in the process have witnessed 18 000 murders and many more episodes of robbery, arson, beatings, and torture. It has truly been said that 'never before has so much violence been shown so graphically to so many'. Children's programs contain six times more violence than adults', ranging from an average of five hourly violent acts to as many as 30 during prime time. An estimated 25% of the television industry's profits come from the 7% of its programs directed at children.

Professional concerns about the quality of its programs, and especially about the effects of the violence offered, began in the USA with the 1952 Surgeon's General Study, followed later by many other studies and commissions, such as the 1969 Kefauver senate hearings, the 1969 Milton Eisenhower report, the 1972 Surgeon's General Advisory Committee, the 1982 study by the National Institutes of Health, and the 1992 study by the American Psychological Association, and there were similar studies in Britain, New Zealand, and several European countries. Most of the hearings, field studies, reports, and analyses have concluded that children who watch a lot of television become more aggressive in their behavior, 'are more likely to view aggression and violence as the preferred means to resolve conflict', become less caring, compassionate, and cooperative, 'are less sensitive to the pain and suffering of others', and are prone to develop The Mean World Syndrome, believing that the real world is as mean and dangerous as it appears on television.

There is also abundant anecdotal evidence on this issue. When a character in a popular television series commits SUICIDE, there is a small epidemic of suicide among people who have identified with that character. When a schoolboy uses an automatic rifle and kills his teacher and several classmates, he later says that he did not really believe they would die: like the television characters with whom he was familiar, they would get up and reappear in another setting. When a gang of teenage kids set upon and beat up someone they don't like, they not only ape the behavior of the characters they watched on television or at the movies, using the same methods of assault; they also expect their victim to be as resilient as the fictional victim they had seen on the screen. Rigorous scientific evidence of a cause–effect relationship, however, is more elusive. It comes mainly from observational epidemiological studies. Violent young offenders exposed to television and movie violence express stronger preference for violent programs than similar young persons who have committed non-violent offenses or not committed offenses of any kind. But the associations are weak, perhaps not convincing enough to persuade legislators and makers of television and movie entertainment that it is not in the public's interest to purvey graphic scenes of violence in programs that are widely watched by young people.

Some common sense on this issue may have been injected by a 1995 position paper of the British Columbia Civil Liberties Association. It points out that science alone cannot provide all the answers and that absolute proof would require a prolonged controlled study carried out over a lifetime, or at least twenty years, clearly an impossibility. Instead it reminds us that societies, beginning with warrior societies and later with Plato, have had an interest in inculcating societal values in their young; that this responsibility is not entirely the parents' but also the state's, 'that young children are not full members of the polity', and that they do not vote. It concludes that some degree of censorship and regulation of what children can see is permissible in a democratic society, does not contravene the libertarian opposition to censorship in general, and that society has the responsibility to exercise some control over children's experience and be vigilant about what values they grow up with.

## Discontent with commercial television

Over the years the American public has expressed increasing dissatisfaction with the content of commercial television. A poll in 1995 found that 82% of Americans thought that it did not carry enough educational material and that there were good reasons to regulate children's programs more strictly than adults. At least in part in response to these concerns, Congress passed in 1990 a Children's Television Act, limiting violent programs and requiring more educational and informative programs. The initial rules implementing the law, however, were vague, ineffectual, and largely ignored. Then in 1996 the government reached a much hailed new agreement with the broadcasting industry, the latter promising to 'begin work tomorrow morning' on the 'urgent need' to improve programs and develop a ratings system. It was also settled that stations wishing to renew their television licenses automatically must air a minimum of three hours' educational programs a week, could provide shorter features as an alternative, and would institute a rating system of all programs. Such a rating system could be used in conjunction with a 'V-chip', allowing parents to deny access to programs with a high content of violence by impressionable children. So far, the impact of these efforts has been minimal, the new rating system having been criticized as useless and most likely representing merely another step in the process of how society chooses to deal with media violence and to go about exposing children in their most receptive and formative years to programs of a high educational value.

## Road rage

The combination of congested roads, poor driving, bad manners, frustration, and impatience to reach their destination as rapidly as possible, makes many automobile drivers angry. Within the apparent security of a metal and glass shell that is the late 20th century equivalent of a medieval suit of armor, drivers seem to feel invincible, taking risks with their own and other people's lives that they would never consider under any other circumstances. The bad temper that is so prevalent in peak-hour city driving conditions — when people shake their fists, make rude gestures, and can be seen, if not heard through closed windows, to utter curse words — occasionally boil over in an explosive bout of aggression and violence. Drivers weave dangerously from one traffic lane to another, flash their headlights to dazzle oncoming traffic, and deliberately ram other cars that are blocking their way. When all the cars grind to a halt in a serious traffic jam, drivers have been seen physically attacking each other, even in the otherwise polite and orderly city of Geneva. Worse still, gunshots have been exchanged on Los Angeles freeways, in Paris, and many other places. Every year increasing numbers of people, including innocent bystanders, have been injured or killed in this way.

These are manifestations of road rage. This new form of violent aggressive conduct was identified and named as a distinct syndrome in the late 1980s. An internet search in December 1998 yielded several thousand references to the problem. It has been studied systematically in the USA and in Australia, where nearly half of all fatal road traffic crashes are said to be associated with it. In the USA, about 90% of drivers have experienced aggressive and dangerous conduct on the roads by other drivers; about 20% have experienced aggression directed at them or their car by other drivers; about 1% have been physically assaulted by another driver.

Road rage therefore merits mention among the varieties of violence that afflict humans in modern society. Drivers who have committed sufficiently blatant acts of road rage to attract the attention of law enforcement officials can be suitably punished, and compelled to take remedial anger-management treatment. A better solution would be early driver education that includes sensitivity training to enhance awareness and emphasize how essential it is to live and let live.            JML, GD, TCon

*See also* ALCOHOL; SUICIDE; TRAUMA; WAR; WORLD HEALTH ORGANIZATION

Rudolf Karl **VIRCHOW** (1821–1902). German pathologist. Virchow enrolled at the Friedrich-Wilhelms Institut in 1839 undertaking to serve in the army after graduation. In 1847 he became prosector at the CHARITÉ (p 354). When he was sent to report on an epidemic of typhus in Upper Silesia his experiences turned him into a politically active radical and his consequent part in the uprising of 1848 led to his expulsion from the Charité. He was made professor of pathological anatomy in Würzburg in 1849 and in the following seven years built such a reputation that in 1856 he was invited to the chair in Berlin and to be the director of the pathological institute. Elected to the City Council three years later, he initiated great improvements in Berlin's hygiene and public health. Later as a member of the Prussian Lower House his radical views and his taste for polemics led him to oppose Bismarck on more than one occasion. During the Franco-Prussian war he organized the ambulance corps for the Prussian army.

Virchow, an outstanding figure in 19th century medicine, has been accounted the greatest pathologist of all time. Although not of great originality he avoided metaphysical speculation and his opinions were founded on his own observations and experience. His most famous work *Die Cellularpathologie* (1858) applied the cell theory to pathology and allowed him to proclaim his doctrine of '*omnis cellula e cellula*'. He regarded all disease as disease of cells. He described leukemia (1845), invented the term 'amyloid', studied thrombosis and introduced the idea of embolism (1846–56), and observed and defined leukocytosis. He first described the neuroglia (1846) and the cerebral perivascular spaces (Virchow-Robin spaces, 1851). In his later years he became interested in anthropology and wrote widely on the subject. In 1847 he founded the still extant *Archiv für pathologische Anatomie* (*Virchows Archiv*). Virchow was a man of powerful personality, unbounded energy, and strongly held opinions.

**VIROLOGY** See MICROBIOLOGY

**VITAMINS**, or accessory food factors, comprise a group of unrelated organic compounds which

**VITAMIN PIONEER**

Sir James **LIND** (1716–94). British naval surgeon. After apprenticeship, Lind became a surgeon in the Royal Navy in 1739. Although he showed that lemon juice prevented scurvy in *A treatise on the scurvy* published in 1754, its use was not enforced in the navy until 1795.

Vitamins and their roles

| Vitamin | Principal metabolic functions | Deficiency disease |
|---|---|---|
| A (retinol, B-carotene) | Vision — forms the visual pigments in the retina; cell differentiation; B-carotene is an antioxidant. | Night blindness, xerophthalmia, keratinization of skin |
| D (calciferol) | Maintenance of calcium balance — enhances intestinal absorption of calcium and mobilizes bone mineral | Rickets in children = poor mineralization of bone; osteomalacia in adults = bone demineralization |
| E (tocopherols, tocotrienols) | Antioxidant, especially in membranes | Extremely rare, serious neurological dysfunction |
| K (phylloquinone, menaquinones) | Coenzyme in formation of proteins required for blood clotting and some bone proteins | Impaired blood clotting, hemorrhagic disease |
| B1 (thiamin) | Coenzyme carbohydrate metabolism, also a role in nerve conduction | Peripheral nerve damage (beriberi) or central nervous system damage (Wernicke-Korsakoff syndrome) |
| B2 (riboflavin) | Coenzyme in many energy yielding reactions | Lesions of corner of mouth, lips, and tongue, dermatitis |
| Niacin (nicotinic acid, nicotinamide) | Coenzyme in many energy yielding reactions | Pellagra, photosensitive dermatitis, depressive psychosis, fatal |
| B6 (pyridoxine, pyridoxal, pyridoxamine) | Coenzyme in amino acid and glycogen metabolism; role in steroid hormone action | Disorders of amino acid metabolism, convulsions |
| Folic acid | Coenzyme in transfer of one-carbon fragments | Megaloblastic anemia |
| B12 (cobalamin) | Coenzyme in transfer of one-carbon fragments and metabolism of folic acid | Pernicious anemia = megaloblastic anemia with degeneration of spinal cord |
| Pantothenic acid | Coenzyme in fat metabolism | Peripheral nerve damage (burning foot syndrome) |
| H (biotin) | Coenzyme in carbohydrate and fat metabolism | Impaired fat and carbohydrate metabolism dermatitis |
| C (ascorbic acid) | Coenzyme in collagen synthesis antioxidant, enhances absorption of iron | Scurvy, impaired wound healing, loss of dental cement, subcutaneous hemorrhage |

have in common the twin attributes of being necessary in trace amounts to the normal metabolic functioning of an organism and yet cannot be synthesized by it; to remain healthy, the organism must therefore obtain them from the environment, in man normally from the diet (See Table). Vitamins are peculiar to species; what is a vitamin for one organism may be synthesized by another and is not therefore a vitamin for that species. For example, vitamin C (ascorbic acid) is an essential part of man's diet but of few other animals. The defining qualifications 'organic' and 'in trace amounts' should be noted. Essential amino acids and essential trace elements are not vitamins.

Adequate amounts of the various vitamins are necessary to the human diet to prevent corresponding deficiency disorders. For recommended daily dietary allowances, see NUTRITION. There is no good evidence that excessive amounts are ever beneficial, and, as in the case of vitamins A and D, they may be harmful. Sir Frederick Gowland HOPKINS (this page) first proposed the existence of accessory food factors in 1906, although deficiency diseases such as SCURVY, beriberi, and rickets had been treated empirically with appropriate foodstuffs for many years before that.

*See also* NUTRITION; DIET AND DISEASE

**VIVISECTION** See ANTIVIVISECTION; ANIMAL RIGHTS MOVEMENT

**VITAMIN DISCOVERER**

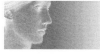

Sir Gilbert **BLANE** (1749–1834). British physician. Blane sailed to the West Indies as physician to Admiral Rodney in 1779 and acquitted himself so well that he was made physician to the fleet. Returning to London he was appointed to the staff of St Thomas's Hospital in 1783 and later physician-in-ordinary successively to the Prince of Wales, George IV, and William IV. Blane did much to improve the hygiene and discipline in the navy and introduced lemon juice as a preventive against scurvy. He wrote *Observations on diseases of seamen* (1785).

**'VITAMINE' DESCRIBER**

Casimir **FUNCK** (1884–1967). Polish nutritionist. Having trained at Bern, and the PASTEUR INSTITUTE (p 620) in Paris, Funk moved to Berlin. He became interested in nutrition and from 1911 he worked successively in London, the United States, Warsaw, Paris, and New York, where he settled permanently in 1939. While in London, Funk worked on vitamin research and deficiency diseases, isolating the thiamine present in rice husks that would prevent beri-beri. He was the first to suggest that similar substances, ascorbic acid, niacin, and calciferol would respectively prevent scurvy, pellagra, and rickets. Funk coined the term 'vitamine' (later vitamin) for these substances, believing initially that such substances were amines, chemical compounds derived from ammonia.

**VITAMIN ELUCIDATOR**

Sir Frederick Gowland **HOPKINS** (1861–1947). British biochemist. Hopkins's researches were wide-ranging and of fundamental importance. He identified tryptophan (1901), showed that lactic acid was formed by muscular contraction (1906), established the role of VITAMINS (1912), and identified glutathione (1921).

# W

INVOLVED IN WAR

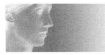

Johannes Friedrich August von **ESMARCH** (1823–1908). German surgeon. Although Esmarch was professor of surgery in Kiel in 1857, he is best known as a military surgeon, having served in the two Schleswig-Holstein wars of 1848 and 1864, and in the Franco-Prussian war of 1870 when he was surgeon-general. He devised the 'first field dressing' (1869) and the rubber bandage for rendering a limb bloodless before amputation (Esmarch's bandage, 1873).

(continued opposite)

**WAR** One of the ironies of medical history is the alleged benefit of medicine from war. For all the horrors of war, it has nevertheless brought benefit to medicine; out of bloodshed has come progress. Rarely savored is the implicit militarism of this attribution, and avoided entirely are the awkward political questions it raises about the allocation of resources for medicine in peacetime. Instead, historical legitimacy is lent the irony, typically by wheeling out in its support the view of the ancients. HIPPOCRATES (p 382), we are told, maintained that 'war is the only school for the surgeon'.

In fact, the notion of war as good for medicine is recent. Few medical 'lessons' of war were asserted before the mid-19th century, however much some of the medical and surgical heroes of the past may have been involved with armies and navies. Generally, the notion rests retrospectively on impressions from the Second World War, founded on the apparent transformation of medicine by the wartime introduction and mass production of penicillin. Thereafter, as biomedicine entered its golden age, it became 'commonplace … to speak of the stimulation of medical progress by the demands of modern warfare, the good that cometh out of evil'.

The criterion for assessing war's value to medicine thus tends to be based on medical–technical achievements, as in the essay 'The medical balance sheet of war' by the surgeon Zachary Cope (one of the editors of the official British medical history of the Second World War). Cope located on the positive side of his balance sheet every war since the Franco–Prussian of 1870–1, as antiseptics were first used on a large scale in that conflict (though only by the Germans). Cope also included the Crimean War, not, as he might have done for its increased use of chloroform, but on the basis of the reforms in army hygiene and nursing popularly ascribed to Florence NIGHTINGALE (p 548). He might have gone further back to encompass the innovation of the 'flying ambulance' by Napoleon's surgeon, Baron LARREY (p 796), though presumably not (given his 'progressive' standards) to the British trial of indiscriminate venesection on the wounded during the Peninsular Wars. He also might have entertained the American Civil War, which further developed the rapid rescue of the wounded as well as techniques for the systematic gathering of medical records, and the routine anthropometric measuring of conscripts. Often regarded as the first 'modern' war because of its introduction of mechanized technologies, the American Civil War is now reckoned 'modern' for its organizational innovations, including those in medicine: for the first time in warfare, combatant officers began to value medicine as a managerial and technical resource crucial to waging war.

The First World War easily meets Cope's criterion. Besides witnessing the launch of aviation medicine and the quickening of developments in reconstructive surgery and the design of artificial limbs, the 1914–18 conflict promoted research into a wide variety of conditions and techniques. Advances in BLOOD TRANSFUSION, and understanding wound shock and gas asphyxia were some of the gains. In Britain, the Medical Research Committee (later Council) was itself a major beneficiary; founded shortly before the war, its institutional prestige was consolidated through orchestrating much of the wartime research. The wartime gains might also include the tests devised to outsmart malingerers, or even the Weil–Felix test for TYPHUS, devised in 1917. The research on shell-shock is familiar. Despite its questionable therapeutic outcomes this did much to promote interest in psychotherapy. Psychology gained further ground professionally through the application in the USA of intelligence tests to recruits, which after the war were extended to schoolchildren.

The First World War also did much for emergent medical specialisms such as orthopedics and cardiology, which were effectively molded by the war into their modern forms. Other specialties benefited through the war-time supply of large groups of patients, special facilities, state-funding, and military vetting of would-be specialists. While the last also served generally to keep out quacks and to strengthen professional boundaries, the military's desperate need for medical personnel temporarily leveled some of the existing prejudices against women doctors. As during the Second World War, the shortage of medical personnel occasioned trimming medical education requirements, thus permitting many to qualify faster and more cheaply.

There were practical professional gains beyond those for specialist élites. Many general practitioners were introduced to new or unfamiliar technologies, such as X-rays, bacteriology laboratories, and chemotherapy (via the antisyphilitic drug, Salvarsan). They were introduced to the disciplines of the record card. Other managerial techniques and practices became familiar, such as triage, teamwork (first spoken of as such at the battle of Arras in April 1917), continuity of care, and, more broadly, the principles and procedures of primary and secondary care.

## Other advances

The health and nutrition of troops were other advances of war. For many recruited to the two world wars, medical and dental inspections, vaccinations, treatments, and health education may have been their first real encounter with medicine. Thus those whose lives and limbs were spared by the skills of military surgeons may not have been the only ones to return home with greater awareness, as well as higher demands for and expectations of orthodox medicine than when they left.

The civilian population also benefited. In one of the few monographs specifically to address the question of the effects of war on public health, the historical demographer Jay Winter has argued from life expectancy figures that the health of the poorest section of British society was much improved during the Great War. In concluding that the so-called residuum of British society had never had it so good, Winter's thesis stands alongside that of the social policy analyst, Richard Titmuss, who viewed both world wars as having had a positive effect. Superficially, at least, this argument is given backing in British history by the formation of the Ministry of Health immediately after the First World War, and the National Health Service immediately after the Second World War. Food shortages resulting from the German submarine campaigns made rationing necessary and led to the establishment of a national food policy based on scientific understanding of human nutrition. This had visible consequences in the improved growth of children, particularly after the Second World War.

In general, the outlook of Winter and Titmuss accords with the familiar story of how recruitment for the Boer War encouraged programs in maternal and child health and welfare, school medical services, health visitors, and so on in the 'quest for national efficiency'. Arguments for these causes (as well as for the EUGENICS movement) were bolstered by the lurid light cast on 'the people's health' whilst recruiting for the First World War. The medical inspection of recruits for the Second, however, directed more attention to mental health (partly from the 'medicalization of mind' stemming from the 1914–18 experience with shell-shock). In the USA the rejection of hundreds of thousands of draftees for psychiatric reasons is said to have been a major impetus to mental health policy and to the evolution of PSYCHIATRY during the postwar years. In Britain during the Second World War the case for the systematic reform of health services was strengthened not only by revelations of the physical and mental state of the military recruits, but also by the poor health of many of the schoolchildren evacuated from London. Once again, war brought to light inadequacies and inequalities in healthcare.

## Negative implications

For all this, however, the medical audit of war has its darker side. The negative implications of war and medicine are less frequently pointed out, though it would be wrong to suggest that they have been wholly ignored. Medical authors themselves have sometimes expressed doubt and dissent, even in relation to supposed medico-technical advances. The military medical practitioner turned historian, Fielding Garrison, reflected in 1929 that in contrast to the remarkable administrative achievements of the Great War 'the medical innovations and inventions … seem clever, respectable, but not particularly brilliant'. And in 1946, in the flush of media enthusiasm for 'the miracles of modern military medicine', the welfare columnist Albert Deutsch opined in an article in the first volume of the *Journal of the History of Medicine and Allied Sciences*: 'The melancholy truth seems to be that wars generally have contributed but little to the progress of medical science. War undoubtedly does spread skills in medical practice as a result of the opportunities it gives doctors for operating on men in masses… . Yet, in spite of the ballyhoo, I fail to recall a single medical discovery of primary importance that has come out of this or any war….'

Furthermore, one might question the extent to which even the alleged wartime advances in therapeutics have actually been incorporated into peacetime medicine. Few innovations have in fact been war born. Even the study of shell-shock — perhaps the nearest example of a war-born development — fails to 'pass muster' because it evolved

*(continued)*

Edith **CAVELL**
(1865–1915). British nurse. Edith Cavell was born in Norfolk, England. She was matron of a Red Cross hospital in Brussels during the First World War when Belgium was conquered by the Germans. With others, and using the hospital as a base, she helped about 200 Allied military to escape capture by the invaders. When caught she confessed, and was tried and shot. Since she was not a spy this caused an outcry throughout the neutral and combatant countries opposed to Germany. She has remained a heroine and a statue of her is placed near Trafalgar Square in London. On its plinth are inscribed her last words before execution: 'Patriotism is not enough. I must have no hatred or bitterness towards anyone'.

from work in the 1860s on 'railway spine' and 'traumatic neurasthenia'. For the most part, war has accelerated research into old medical problems of military importance. The treatment of gunshot and shrapnel wounds, gas asphyxia, gas gangrene, and trench foot, for instance, are rarely called for in peacetime.

Wartime research priorities with obvious civilian applications, such as treating fractures, flat foot, and venereal disease, have normally reverted to low status in peacetime because they are not very remunerative in private medical practice. Thus, while war has sometimes shed new light on neglected patient populations (such as the physically disabled) and on neglected problems (for example, the treatment of fractures), sustaining this post-war has often been another matter. So, too, in relation to acute injuries, wartime conditions have often been so different as to render the experience virtually irrelevant to peacetime and vice-versa. The need for urgency in wound treatment and amputations, for example — well appreciated since the Napoleonic wars, and a major impetus to the development of front line dressing stations — was less essential in the controlled and eventually aseptic hospital environment with its anesthetized patients. As noted during the Franco-Prussian War, 'errors may be committed by being too exclusively guided by the experience gained in civil hospitals'. Neurologists during the Great War found that their rule of thumb in civilian practice for assessing the gravity of a head injury — loss of consciousness — was often misleading when it came to gunshot wounds of the head.

### 'Lessons' of war

Because every new war since the mid-19th century has been substantially different medically and militarily from its predecessor, and because civilian medicine changed rapidly in the intervals between, the lessons of one war have often been of little value to the next. The 'lessons' of previous wars, when remembered, might in fact seriously deceive. A well-known example is that of the misplaced confidence that surgeons gained of the power of antiseptics to disinfect wounds during the Boer War. In the bacteria-infested battlefields of Europe and Mesopotamia, unlike the Transvaal, nearly all wounds resulting from explosions were septic, and conventional treatment was impotent to check the progress of infection. Since the Franco-Prussian War, when the amputation rate on the wounded was brought down from its usual 30–40% to 16.7%, the rate had continued to fall — to as little as 0.5% among the Japanese during the war with Russia in 1905. But during the Great War the rate soared to 80% of cases until new methods of wound treatment could be found.

Previous war experience in fact rendered the whole issue of wound treatment problematic from the start of the 1914–18 conflict; since greater mortality among troops had always resulted from non-combat causes, military medicine was preoccupied with disease prevention — the more so, as the amputation rate was reduced. Although the Franco-Prussian and Russo-Japanese wars (from the victors' sides) signaled the possibly greater medical importance in future wars of attending to wound treatment, the turn-of-the-century wars in South Africa and Spanish America reinforced an abiding faith in, and focus on, the importance of disease prevention.

Medico-technical considerations are not the only reasons for modifying callow impressions of war's benefit to medicine. Medicine suffers enormously in war. The priority given to military medicine usually cuts deeply into existing medical provisions for the weak and vulnerable in society — the elderly and the mentally and physically handicapped, in particular. In Britain during both world wars many civilian hospital wards and outpatient facilities were closed down. Mental asylums in London during the First World War saw death rates soar from 11% in 1914 to 27% in 1918. And the Great War was anything but 'great' for sufferers from TUBERCULOSIS — indeed, this was among the largest single causes of civilian casualties in all the belligerent nations. In Germany gout is said to have disappeared, but there was an eightfold increase in rickets, hunger edema, and other problems. In Russia, obesity, alcoholism, gout, gastritis, appendicitis, biliary disorders, and constipation all but disappeared, but enteritis, peptic ulcer, pyorrhea, and arteriosclerosis markedly increased. The consequences of the privations caused by the Second World War are better known. Some are still coming to light through the long-term follow-up study of the child-bearing descendants of the women who were born during the famine in Holland in the winter of 1944–5.

Far less is known about the immediate effects on public health and civilian medical services during other wars in other societies. That the effects could have been beneficial is doubtful, if only because fighting forces have always been major carriers of disease, spreading infection in their wake. In 1876 in the Turco–Serbian war, the misery and suffering imposed on the native population were out of all proportion to the extent of the war. In words that have since become only too familiar in relation to wars in Africa and again in Serbo-Croatia, the suffering was described as 'something perfectly frightful'.

### Balance sheet

Aspects of professionalization also need review, for not all medical personnel experienced war in career-enhancing ways. Many rank and file doctors *and* nurses during the world wars (when they were not totally frustrated by War Office mismanagement, red tape, and the incompetence of the military's own medical corps) experienced only boredom. Nurses witnessed dilutions of professional standards as a result of the involvement of volunteers and government hiring policy. While less well-off practitioners may have welcomed the security of military service, most resented the loss of their civilian incomes as much as they resented their lost autonomy. For some, experiencing bureaucratic salaried service cemented a distaste for 'socialized medicine'. Aware, too, that the worth of medical procedures during war was assessed differently than in peacetime, doctors often bore only grudgingly the deviations from their ethical norms, deeply resenting, for example, their enforced detection and exposure of malingerers.

For others, war simply brutalized. Though pale by comparison with the atrocities committed by Nazi and Japanese doctors on prisoners of war during the Second World War, the activities of many other practitioners in war have clearly not been over-governed by deep humanitarian impulses. Examples of butchery and barbarity abound — the garb of uniform and officer status, it seems, has affected authoritarian transformations in some doctors above and beyond what was encouraged by the military's imperative to care for the line not the man. And, as journalist Michael Herr discovered during the war in Vietnam, doctors were as much given to nationalist and racist propaganda as anyone else: overhearing a doctor bragging that he refused to allow wounded Vietnamese into his wards, Herr asked him '"Didn't you take the Hippocratic oath?" But he was ready for me, "Yeah", he said "[but] I took it in America"'.

Of course, since at least the 16th century practitioners plying their trade in the military have been warned by their peers to 'worke according to arte, not practisinge newe experiments upon a poore souldier'. But the advice has usually fallen on deaf ears; few enterprising physicians and surgeons have been able to resist the opportunities afforded by the mobilization of vast numbers of 'subjects' under ideal authoritarian conditions. For Cope, two positive factors of medicine in modern war were that the discipline of the forces renders it 'more easy to test any method or drug on a sufficiently large scale to endure a definite result'; and, '[that] it is possible to introduce compulsion and in this way confirm by large-scale experiment that which had been previously proved on a smaller scale'. Such candor in itself reflects how professional values with regard to human experimentation were strengthened by the Second World War and its memory.

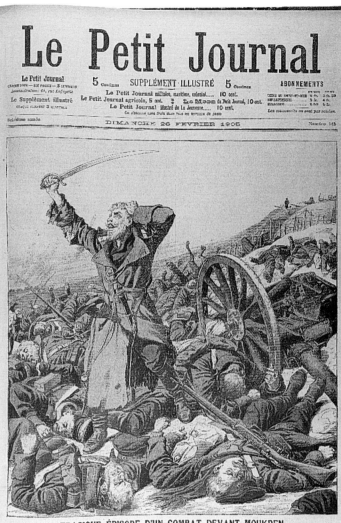

TRAGIQUE ÉPISODE D'UN COMBAT DEVANT MOUKDEN
Officier russe atteint de folie

A picture in *Le Petit Journal* (1905) showing a Russian soldier driven mad by fighting at Moukden in the Russia–Japan War. (Reproduced courtesy of the Mary Evans Picture Library.)

## Conclusion

Although some aspects of medical knowledge and practice have obviously been accelerated and expanded by war — or altered, elaborated, and transformed — others have remained unaffected, while still others have been temporarily interrupted, demoted in political importance, marginalized, or halted altogether. Generalization is thus impossible. Quite apart from whether the perspective is that of patients or professionals, or whether the reckoning is made in the short or the long term, the worth of war for any aspect of medicine varies according to the type of the war as well as its time, place, duration, and not least, its political and economic outcome. In selected cases, perhaps for selected periods, it might be possible to claim that medicine reaps in peace

## MILITARY HYGIENE

Military leaders from Julius Caesar to Napoleon to modern times have understood the importance of keeping their fighting forces fit. 2000 years ago, Romans had latrines to discourage casual defecation in their camp sites. The first systematic treatise on military hygiene, Sir John Pringle's *Diseases of the army* (1752), outlined the principles of military sanitation, including ventilation of hospital wards where wounded soldiers were treated. Pringle knew that antisepsis was important, and that TYPHUS was a disease of campaigning armies. Pringle's commanding officer and his French counterpart at the Battle of Dettingen (1743) reached an understanding that military hospitals should be regarded as neutral territory. This understanding persisted for almost 200 years and enabled Henri DUNANT (p 706) to develop the concept of the RED CROSS that led to the Geneva Convention of 1864.

Until World War I, many wars were decided not so much on the battlefield as by the ability of the combatants to withstand infectious and other diseases. Diseases took a heavy toll in some campaigns, but vaccines and sera and new epidemiological insights into methods of spread and control protected many of the troops against diseases that had sapped the vitality of fighting forces in earlier wars. By World War II, a wider range of prophylactic measures had become available. In tropical conflict zones, the use of yellow fever vaccine and effective antimalarials ensured that servicemen who would otherwise have succumbed to YELLOW FEVER or MALARIA were fit for combat. Venereal diseases incapacitated far fewer troops than in the previous generation's armies. Preventive medical services have advanced rapidly in the half century since the end of World War II. They are highly developed in the US armed services and in those of many other nations, and now embrace health promotion (smoking cessation, physical fitness programs, etc.) as well as specific preventive measures such as immunizations.

what it sows in war; but equally it might be argued that medicine reaps in war only what it sows in peace, or that wars are but testing grounds (primarily for the benefit of the military). The claim that war is good for medicine might well be regarded as a species of apology for medicine's collaboration with war. At the very least, it has to be conceded that the irony of medicine's profit through war may be far more apparent than real.          RCOO

See also BATTLE NEUROSIS; NUREMBERG CODE; SURGERY, GENERAL – HISTORY; RED CROSS/RED CRESCENT; TRAUMA

### Public health

In the barbarous times that have become customary in this era of total war, such niceties as neutrality of the Red Cross and hospitals have vanished. Civilian as well as military hospitals are deliberately shelled and bombed, and hospital and clinic staff murdered, for instance, by the Nicaraguan Contras and the Bosnian Serbs. Noncombatants are by far the largest proportion of those killed and maimed, often over 75%, mainly women and children. Sidel and Levy's book, *War and public health* (1997), describes many ways in which armed conflict is a massive public health problem. Almost all of the 20 million refugees and a similar or greater number of displaced persons in the world are homeless as a result of armed conflicts. Often their homes, farms, and other sources of sustenance are destroyed as part of military strategy. Caring for refugee populations presents challenging public health problems, especially as refugees often retreat to harsh and unsanitary environments lacking access to safe water supplies, food, and shelter. Humanitarian disasters abound in the late 20th century, a terrible demonstration of human destructiveness and an almost insuperable problem for the United Nations High Commission for Refugees and the non-governmental organizations and voluntary agencies that attempt to deal with such situations.

Nevertheless, war and epidemic disease go together: refugee communities can easily become a site for dangerous outbreaks, as illustrated by the CHOLERA and other diarrheal disease epidemics in refugee camps after the genocidal conflict in Rwanda in 1996.          JML

**WATER** All living things need water to survive. The unique physical property of water, its maximum density at a temperature just above freezing point, means that ice floats. This prevents lakes, rivers, and the sea from freezing solid in cold winters; makes it possible for marine animals to survive severe prolonged cold such as Ice Ages; and probably played a part in the evolution of life on earth. The amount of water needed in relation to an organism's weight varies greatly: some insects need almost none, and succulent plants may turn over several times their own weight of water every 24 hours. The human body is made up of over 70% water by weight, and the daily requirement for an adult man weighing 70 kg is about 2.5 liters, varying greatly with ambient temperature and humidity, physical activity, state of health, and other factors. Water is needed for all vital bodily functions — for example, the chemical processes of digestion, metabolism, and excretion, moistening of respiratory passages. Water enters the body in everything we drink, and as an ingredient in most of the foods we eat. It leaves the body in urine, feces, sweat, and as water vapor in expired air.

Water is needed to cultivate the crops that provide our food, so water has considerable strategic importance. The tension among nation states in some parts of the world is related to scarcity of water, which is said to be an underlying cause of a high proportion of the violent armed conflicts in the Middle East and in Africa. Water for drinking and irrigation is in short supply in regions supporting about a fifth of the world's population. By 2025 this shortage might become the most important limiting factor on the growth of population and the development of the affected regions, which include the Middle East, all of southern Africa, much of northern China,

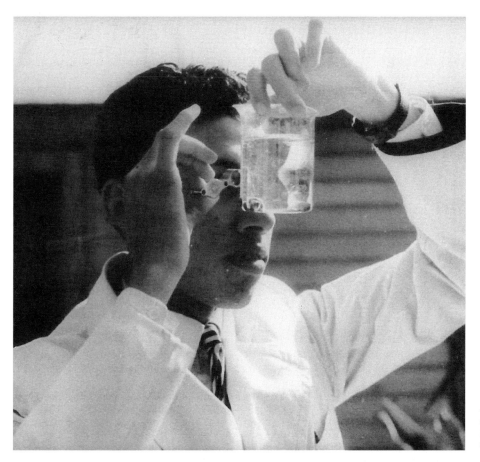

A doctor examines a beaker of water through a magnifying glass. (Reproduced courtesy of the WHO.)

the south-west of the USA, and northern Brazil, all of them heavily populated regions.

## Water and disease

Life on earth began in water, and water is the habitat of a vast variety of living creatures. These include many agents of disease — viruses, bacteria, protozoa, and parasitic worms that sometimes have complex life cycles involving fish or snails, and mammals, including humans. Water is the habitat too for part of the life cycle of mosquitoes, black flies, and other dangerous disease vectors.

Often water has to be treated before we can drink it safely. Some deadly diseases and many dangerous or debilitating ones are transmitted by drinking water: diarrheal diseases from CHOLERA to mild gastro-enteritis, several kinds of viral hepatitis, POLIOMYELITIS, and giardiasis. Huge numbers of people may be affected by a water-borne epidemic. In Milwaukee, Wisconsin, in 1994, over 400 000 people had diarrhea caused by a protozoan infection, cryptosporidiosis.

When there is any doubt about the safety of drinking water, it is always wise to boil it. This kills virtually all dangerous pathogenic organisms.

The custom of drinking infusions of herbs such as tea leaves in boiling water may have been reinforced by the observation that those who indulged were less likely to get diarrhea than those who did not. In a village in rural India hot tea is certainly a safer drink than water from a polluted stream.

The provision of safe drinking water was probably the most important step ever taken towards the advancement of good health for everyone. Now we regard safe water as a basic requirement of all human settlements. Rendering water safe to drink requires the segregation of human and animal waste from sources of supply and storage of drinking water. This was the great achievement of the 'Sanitary revolution' in the industrial world in the late 19th and early 20th centuries. Until then, over a third of all babies born alive had died before their 5th birthday, many of them from diarrheal diseases, which continued to exact a toll of premature deaths throughout later childhood — and, indeed, at all ages. The discoveries of John SNOW (p 48), Robert KOCH(p 655), and others, of the causes of cholera and other dangerous diarrheal diseases, transformed this state of affairs through the collaboration of PUBLIC HEALTH scientists and sanitary engineers.

Human feces and other dangerous pollutants can be segregated from drinking water in several ways. In rural areas and other places without sewage systems, a septic tank, or even a pit privy strategically located far enough away from springs, dams, or wells so that seepage from it cannot contaminate the source of drinking water, usually suffices. In urban regions it is necessary to use more elaborate methods of ensuring that human and animal excreta and other pollutants do not contaminate the water supply. The usual method is a water-carried sewage disposal system that begins at flush toilets and carries domestic wastes of all kinds to sewage treatment plants, where a series of processes render sewage harmless.

### Water supply systems

In urban areas, water supply and storage facilities are needed. The supply may come from a convenient river or lake, which may provide enough water for a metropolitan area, with purification as described below to remove bacterial and chemical contaminants. Dams or reservoirs often provide secure water supplies and also kinetic energy that is used to generate hydroelectric power.

In reservoirs, water is purified in several ways. Many pathogenic organisms die for lack of suitable hosts in which they can breed. Reservoirs nearly always have further safeguards. Alum may be added to promote flocculation and sedimentation of suspended particulate matter, to which many pathogens adhere. A filtration system, usually gravel beds, clears the water of suspended particulate matter. Algae growing in these filtration beds act as biological filters, consuming many of the bacteria. A further safeguard is disinfection of the water, using a chlorine-based chemical or ozone that kills almost all of the remaining pathogens. Filtration and chlorination or ozonation are the main defenses when rivers or lakes are the source of supply. Sometimes special methods must be used to remove toxic chemicals from the water supply. People who live downstream on rivers such as the Rhine and the Mississippi may have to drink water that has already passed through the bodies of many other people further upstream; is contaminated by agricultural runoff that includes pathogens and pesticides; and has been used in numerous industrial processes. It takes considerable technical capability to ensure that drinking water in Baton Rouge or New Orleans, or Cologne or Rotterdam, is as fit to drink as water in Minneapolis or Basle.

Drinking water usually contains trace amounts of chemicals, some required for normal growth and development. Among these is fluoride, which is essential to form dental enamel. Excessive fluoride produces unsightly blemishes on the tooth enamel, but fluoride deficiency, which is not uncommon in large water storage systems, makes the teeth vulnerable to decay. Therefore, public health officials in many communities advocate addition of trace amounts of fluoride to drinking water; the optimum concentration is one part per million. Unfortunately adding fluoride to drinking water has become a highly charged emotional and political issue: for obscure and mainly illogical reasons, fluoridation of drinking water is strongly opposed in many communities, leading to defeat of local polls and of political candidates who advocate fluoridation. The ethical argument, that fluoridation is paternalist and deprives people of the right to choose to drink 'pure' water, is hard to refute, but infants and children whose teeth benefit from the trace amount of the essential fluoride, are the victims, not the adults who demand the right to choose for themselves not to drink 'poisonous' additives.

This debate was renewed when chlorination of drinking water was found to have possible adverse effects. Organic matter in water reacts with chlorine to form hundreds of chlorinated compounds, including substances known to produce cancer in animals. Epidemiological evidence suggests that lifelong consumption of chlorinated drinking water slightly increases the risk of bladder cancer. The risk is small, and has to be considered in the context of the far greater risk of serious or fatal disease transmitted in untreated water. Moreover, if we abandon chlorination of drinking water, we will have to use other, perhaps more costly, ways to protect the water supply from bacterial contamination. Clearing the water of organic contaminants before chlorination improves the efficiency of the process and greatly reduces the cancer risk.                    JML

*See also* DENTISTRY; INSECTS; WORMS

**WELLCOME FOUNDATION, THE** See FOUNDATIONS

**WISTAR INSTITUTE, THE**, See FOUNDATIONS

**WOLFSON FOUNDATION, THE**, See FOUNDATIONS

**WOMEN IN MEDICINE** Although in medieval and other distant times women were healers, in many modern societies, women physicians are still a minority. As Samuel Johnson said of a woman minister: 'A woman preaching is like a dog's walking on his hind legs. It is not done well; but you are surprised to find it done at all'. One may, therefore, be naturally curious about women practicing medicine, and interested in finding whether they do so well. In many countries the frequency of women in medicine is high or increasing tremendously, and they are therefore a cohort that should be better understood. Since it has been unusual for women to be physicians, or members of any other profession of the highest socio-economic status (high education, income, and occupational prestige), several interesting issues and myths have emerged, and these should be addressed. Women physicians have been well studied in several western countries, and I present some of their findings here.

## US women physicians

Elizabeth BLACKWELL (p 117) graduated from medical school in 1848, the first woman to do so in the USA, and there were over a dozen women's medical schools in the second half of the 19th century. In the late 19th and early 20th century, most of these schools were closed, and women were discouraged from becoming doctors or formally excluded. In 1910, over half of US medical schools barred women, and others had quotas limiting admissions, while the American Medical Association was closed to women until 1915. When women regained more access to training, they were typically encouraged to consider disciplines such as pediatrics or obstetrics and gynecology, specialties where their 'womanly skills' would be most useful, and they would not confront male anatomy.

Even now few women are in leadership roles: women medical school deans currently number between zero (as recently as 1991) and the low single digits, and about half of state delegations to the American Medical Association have no women delegates. Such phenomena may be explained in part by fewer women having accumulated sufficient experience or years to become eligible for senior positions; but many other reasons also contribute to their exclusion, ranging from cumulative inadvertent obstacles to overt sexism.

The picture is far brighter when examining entry levels. Women now make up slightly more then 40% of US medical school applicants, and a slightly smaller percentage of enrollees. Similarly, although women still represent a very small percentage of residents in such disciplines as surgery subspecialties (typically in the single digits), those percentages are slowly increasing. As the US medicine becomes more 'pink collar', the profession will change in several ways, probably including the continued increased prevalence of women in non-traditional specialties and in leadership positions. Encouragingly, in 1998–9, the American Medical Association had its first woman president.

There are some interesting ways in which women and men practice medicine differently in

## WOMEN IN MEDICINE

Harriot Kezia **HUNT** (1805–75). With her sister, Sarah, she practiced in Boston. Having trained solely by apprenticeship, Harriot continued well into the 1870s, amassing a sizeable fortune. In 1847, wishing to legitimize her practice, she applied to Harvard Medical School for permission to attend the public medical lectures. Oliver Wendell Holmes, MD, as dean, was favorably inclined, but he was overruled. In 1859, Harriot was accepted for attendance at the lectures only. Meanwhile, Harvard had also accepted three black men to the MD program, and the medical students protested publicly against all four. Hunt and the three men withdrew. Although Hunt's practice was 'irregular' and she had no degree (save for an honorary MD she was awarded by the Female MEDICAL COLLEGE of PENNSYLVANIA (p 840) in 1853), she is accredited as the first woman 'to practice medicine successfully' in the USA.

Sophia Louisa **JEX-BLAKE** (1840–1912). British physician and pioneer of the right of women to practice medicine. She studied medicine under Elizabeth BLACKWELL (p 117) in New York and in 1869 was accepted for training by Edinburgh University at her second request, but later the Appeal Court decided that the university had acted *ultra vires* in so doing. In 1874 she founded the London School of Medicine

for Women and in 1877 clinical studies were permitted at the London (later Royal) Free Hospital. In 1877 she was permitted to practice. In 1878 she settled in Edinburgh and founded the Women's Hospital and School of Medicine, which survived until the university admitted women in 1894.

Susan **LA FLESCHE** (1865–1915), a member of the Omaha Indian Tribe, received her MD degree from the FEMALE MEDICAL COLLEGE of PENNSYLVANIA (p 840) in 1889. She carried on her practice among the 1300 widely scattered members of her tribe, acquiring an influence that made her *de facto* leader of the tribe.

Augusta **DEJERINE** (née Klumpke) (1859–1927). Franco-American neurologist. She determined to train in medicine and, against strong opposition, was admitted as an extern in 1882 and an intern in 1885. In 1888 she graduated MD and married Joseph Dejerine, thereafter devoting herself to working with her husband in neurology. She described with her husband the paralysis resulting from damage to the lower part of the brachial plexus (Dejerine–Klumpke paralysis, 1885).

Rebecca **LEE** (*c.* 1840–?) received her MD degree in 1864 from the New England Female Medical College. She is generally acknowledged to be the first black woman to receive the degree.

the USA. Women are less likely to practice in a rural area or be self-employed, and are more likely to be primary care practitioners and to see fewer patients. They also spend somewhat more time with their patients, and are more likely to emphasize prevention. However, many of these gender-based differences are small, especially when compared with the enormous differences within gender. The Women Physicians' Health Study queried 4501 US women physicians in 1993–4. About fifty articles will eventually come from this survey; several have already been published regarding demographics, and personal and clinical behaviors, and experiences that may be of interest. In the the first published report of physician ethnicity of either gender, we found that women physicians were more likely to be Asian, and somewhat less to be Black or Hispanic than Whites. Women physicians had healthier habits than did other women, even when compared with other high socio-economic status women, and they exceeded national goals in all examined health behaviors: only 3.7% smoked, and those who had previously smoked had stopped younger than had non-doctor women.

Women physicians spend less time on domestic activities such as cooking and other housework (three hours for each of these activities per week) than other US women, and somewhat less on childrearing. Regarding women physicians' clinical practices, the most important predictors of counseling patients about prevention were being a primary care practitioner and practicing healthy personal practices oneself. Importantly, 48% of women said they had been harassed in a medical setting on the basis of gender, and 37% said they had been sexually harassed; it was more common to be harassed during training than in practice.

### Canadian women physicians

The first woman to practice medicine in Canada was a British Army medical officer. Dr 'James' BARRY (p 158). Dr Barry posed as a man to gain entry to Edinburgh University in 1809, where she trained in surgery. She kept her secret throughout a long military career, during two years of which (1857–9) she served as the chief military doctor in Canada. Dr Barry's gender was discovered on her death. The first Canadian woman to become a doctor was Dr Emily Stowe, who studied medicine in the United States, and began practice in Toronto in 1867. Following Dr Stowe, several other Canadian women attended US medical schools, as no Canadian university admitted women until the Women's Medical Colleges were founded in Toronto and Kingston in 1883.

In 1993, women outnumbered men entering Canadian medical schools for the first time: 51% of entering students were women. The large proportion of women entering medical schools is a recent phenomenon (reaching 40% for the first time in 1980), and, as in the USA, there are still relatively few women in senior positions in Canadian medical schools and professional organizations. This situation might be expected to change as younger women move up through the ranks, and recent research suggests that increasing numbers of women in Canadian medicine might also bring about other qualitative changes in medical practice. As in other countries, Canadian female physicians are more likely to enter family practice, pediatrics, and obstetrics/gynecology, rather than technical specialties such as surgery. They typically practice fewer hours than do men physicians, are less likely to participate in professional medical organizations and committees, and are less likely to carry out academic research. On the other hand, women physicians spend more time on each patient visit, and are more likely to question patients about the social context of the presenting problem.

Female and male physicians also have differing views on healthcare policy and funding. Little research has been conducted on the health of Canadian women physicians, but a survey in 1993 found that women find medical practice more stressful than do men. A recent survey of Québec female physicians found that, while women have better health behaviors, they report a higher level of stress and distress than their male colleagues. They are less likely to smoke tobacco and to drink alcohol 'frequently' (20 days/month or more) than men, but are more likely to use codeine. As women become the majority of Canadian medical practitioners, preferences in life-style, career choice, practice patterns, and attitudes will affect the delivery of medical services in Canada.

### British women physicians

As in the USA and Canada, the proportion of women training to be doctors in Britain has grown enormously, from less than 10% of medical students being female in the early 1970s to more than 50% in the mid-1990s. As in North America, a greater percentage opt for general practice and, since 1993, over half of all GP registrars (the final training grade for the specialty of family practice) have been women. Some 32% of general practitioner partners in a practice were female in 1997, compared with 23% in 1987. More women than men work part time; a follow-up of doctors qualifying in 1986 found that two thirds of women doctors were working full time in clinical medicine compared with 90% of men. But 'full-time' hours of work are very long, with an average of 65 hours per week for all those in work (including both full- and part-time workers).

Two-thirds of general practitioners who are employed by other family doctors rather than being partners in the general practices, are women. Many prefer to work for a few sessions per week for disproportionately less pay, but a corresponding reduction in responsibilities.

Women doctors are more likely than men to be single, and if they do have children, they are more likely than men to be the parent with responsibility for caring for a child when the child is sick. Women physicians' disproportionate family responsibilities may also cause more stress at work; and more conflicts between domestic and work commitments, and career and personal lives. Many British women physicians believe that medicine in Britain is a male dominated profession, in which they have to work harder to compete, have less status, get passed over for promotion, and find it more difficult to get a general practice partnership. There are few senior women consultants in traditionally masculine hospital specialties such as general surgery and orthopedics; many fewer senior

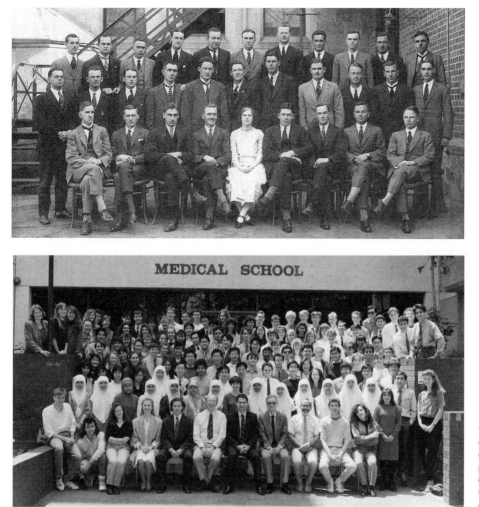

The increasing proportion of women in medicine is strikingly illustrated by these photographs of graduating classes in (a) 1924 and (b) 1992, University of Adelaide.

women physicians receive financial merit awards compared with men; and several studies record women's self-reports of discrimination occurring throughout their career paths.

## Norwegian women physicians

Over a century has passed since the first woman graduated in medicine from the University of Oslo in 1893, and only 18 women had graduated by the end of 1900. Despite these small numbers, until the 1930s, medicine was the academic field which attracted most women. From the interwar period until the end of the 1970s, about 12–14% of all Norwegian doctors were women. As in most western countries, enrollment and graduation data have increased greatly since the end of the 1970s; during the last ten years, women have made up about half of the enrollees to medical schools. In 1998 female physicians were 30% of all working

doctors in Norway. As in other western countries, female physicians have historically specialized to a lesser degree than their male colleagues; have tended to choose primary care, psychiatry, gynecology, and pediatrics; and have been under-represented in higher administrative and academic positions. Younger female physicians now specialize to the same extent as their male colleagues and are choosing among a broader array of specialties than before, yet women doctors are still very seldom found as residents in subspecialties of surgery and internal medicine.

Both men and women doctors work more hours per week than other working Norwegians. Women work fewer hours per week as a physician than do men (47 compared with 55), but do much more housework, so that they work more hours per week than their male colleagues. Among Norwegian women physicians, 16% work part time, a smaller proportion than that of other working women.

For working conditions, Norwegian physicians experience less control over their work than do other professionals and employees in Norwegian society, but female physicians report less autonomy than their male colleagues. About one-third of women physicians say that the doctor–nurse relationship is influenced by the doctor's gender, that is, women doctors often report that they are treated with less respect and confidence and are given less help than their male colleagues. However, women doctors seldom report experiencing other forms of discrimination or sexual harassment, and do not report having been passed over for promotion significantly more often than do men.

### Women physicians in other countries

The first record of a woman physician was an Egyptian named Peseshet, 'Overseer of Women Physicians', around 2500 BC (the first known male physician was Hesy Re, who lived about 200 years earlier). Unfortunately, subsequent records in many countries have been sparse. Unsurprisingly, the percentage of women is increasing most in the countries where they have been least represented. In some countries this has occurred because medicine became a less prestigious, powerful, and well-paying profession, in others because of increased access for women. The proportion and growth of women in medicine are not correlated with a country's per capita income. They are, however, correlated with political systems: socialist countries have had more women physicians, as well as more women dentists and pharmacists. In countries such as Russia, where most physicians are women, the physicians' salaries and prestige are low, and women are still severely underrepresented in the upper strata of teaching, research, and administration.

### Common characteristics of women physicians

Despite a paucity of supporting data, myths still exist about women physicians. Many assume, for example, that women will practice more compassionate medicine, though this has been poorly studied, and it is likely that the differences between women and men in this and other aspects are less than the differences between individuals of the same gender. Some gender-based differences do seem to be clear, however. Women physicians, despite an increasing presence, have not achieved parity with men in several dimensions. They tend to remain underrepresented in medicine, and are underrepresented in leadership and higher medical positions. They practice somewhat differently than men, and this may contribute to inequities even before consideration for leadership. For example, US women physicians typically earn two thirds of men's salaries, even to look at only physicians practicing the same specialty, or those of the same age, or in the same type of employment. However, when one combines all those factors, differences between men and women do diminish, especially for younger physicians.

Although it might be reasonable to have the profession not perfectly gender-balanced, it seems unlikely that medicine profits from gender inequities and a dearth of women leaders. There is much more to learn about physicians of both genders. Are there unique or especially valuable things that women may bring to medicine? Just as some men may prefer to have same-gender physicians, especially for discussions or management of intimate problems, so too may some women prefer to have women physicians. Women physicians may also improve medical practice by being particularly interested in issues such as female genital mutilation, breast cancer research, effects of hormone replacement therapy, or inclusion of women in cardiovascular disease trials.

Why might things be different for women than for men physicians? There are clearly still institutional and other professional barriers to women physicians' advancement that may create 'glass ceilings' or provide repeated micro-inequities that may be difficult to overcome. Moreover, many contemporary societies, and individuals within those societies, still believe that it is primarily a woman's responsibility to provide or coordinate childcare, cooking, cleaning, and other such domestic activities. Women physicians' lesser professional accomplishments may partly result, then, from conscious or unconscious barriers that they or others erect. While these 'others' may be colleagues, a critical problem to address, they may also be family members or physicians themselves. I believe that one of the greatest barriers western women physicians now face in their professional advancement is having a woman and her partner who do not both act on the premise that the woman's career is critically important, at least as important as her partner's.                        EF

*See also* SPECIALIZATION

**WORLD HEALTH ORGANIZATION** International conferences aimed at standardizing quarantine regulations, and other contagious disease control measures, were held periodically from 1851, and led to the formation of l'Office International d'Hygien Publique in 1907. This and the Pan-American Sanitary Bureau were the precursors for the health office of the League of Nations, which was established after the Great War of 1914–18. After World War II the functions

# WORKHOUSES

The Victorian workhouse was the creation of the 1834 New Poor Law in Britain, designed to curtail public spending on poverty. Workhouses were erected by unions of parishes, funded by local taxation. They were managed locally by Guardians of the Poor and centrally overseen by the Poor Law Board. By the mid-19th century, the workhouse system had become the largest civil organization in the country, comprising some 700 institutions.

To deter applicants the regime governing most of these institutions was deliberately harsh, as typified in Dickens's *Oliver Twist*, and workhouse masters were universally feared and reviled. Where ratepayers appreciated the effects upon the poor of epidemics and trade cycles, attitudes could be more benign, and the directives of the Poor Law Board and its officious secretary Edwin Chadwick to some extent resisted. To receive any assistance in time of need, poor people were required to live inside the workhouse, which entailed loss of citizenship, sale of personal belongings, break-up of homes, and separation of families. Called 'bastiles' by the poor, workhouses effectively imprisoned the sick, the unemployed, disabled, insane, and the old alongside the fit they were intended to deter.

Hundreds of people might be accommodated in a single workhouse. Because illness and old age were the primary causes of poverty, only a small proportion (less than 10%) was likely to be classified as 'able bodied', and required to work at such tasks as stone-breaking or carpet-beating.

It was well known that conditions within workhouse walls predisposed to disease, and were worse than those in prisons. Workhouse food was poor, monotonous, and inadequate. At Andover, for example, inmates fought each other for shreds of meat adhering to bones they had been directed to crush. Hygiene was also deficient. In some places, unscreened public latrines were situated inside workhouse wards, badly plumbed, and with no toilet paper provided. Epidemics of diarrhea and fevers were commonplace.

Workhouses had no casualty or surgical facilities, and many lacked separate infirmary buildings. The possibility of segregating sick patients suffering from acute, chronic, infectious, or terminal illnesses was limited by poor accommodation. The numbers of ill and infirm meant that even where such designated wards existed, sick and dying patients were to be found throughout the workhouse. Inevitably, mortality was high. Thomas WAKLEY (p 453), medical coroner, MP, and founding editor of the *Lancet*, described workhouses as 'Ante-chambers of the grave'.

Medical expenditure in these places was necessarily low. Nursing was provided by inmates at no cost. Doctors were awarded Poor Law work by competitive tender, to include all medicines, with contracts awarded to the lowest offer. The medical care of these large communities of the sick was expected to be only part time, and was sometimes in the hands of the worst type of doctor. One is recorded as having pocketed his entire salary by administering — even to those in severe or terminal pain — *colored peppermint water*. Others were of an altogether different stamp and, to give proper care, suffered both overwork and financial loss. However well qualified, workhouse doctors were nominally inferior in rank to workhouse masters, which could cause friction and difficulties in the medical management of cases. Doctors voicing criticism were induced to leave.

The mid-1860s was a key period of reform. A decade after the need for improvements in military hospitals had been revealed in the Crimea, the *Lancet* appointed a commission to investigate the state of British workhouse infirmaries. The three doctor-commissioners looked first at the workhouses of London. the *Lancet* Sanitary Commission's reports appeared in the journal at intervals during 1865–6. Although some recent improvements (such as the introduction of paid nurses in a few districts) could be reported, the Commission's conclusions were damning:

Patch up the present systems as we may ... it will still continue to be a scandal and a reproach ... The State Hospitals are in workhouse wards. They are closed against observation, they pay no heed to public opinion; they pay no toll to science. They contravene the rules of hygiene; they are under the government of men [Guardians and workhouse masters] profoundly ignorant of hospital rules ... The doctor and patient alike are the object of a pinching parsimony. There is neither uniformity, nor liberality, nor intelligence in the management.

Publication caused a furore. The government swiftly announced its own investigation, which subsequently largely confirmed the commission's findings, paving the way for change.

At the same period, Dr Joseph Rogers founded the Association for the Improvement of London Workhouse Infirmaries. It immediately attracted support from numerous public figures, such as Charles Dickens, who despised 'Poor Law mindedness'. The Association's aims were to establish six Poor Law hospitals for London, each with 1000 beds, to reclassify and rehouse the workhouse population, and to group the Metropolitan workhouse districts into one hospital region, so that the costs of healthcare for the poor were fairly spread. As medical officer of the Strand Union Workhouse since 1856, Rogers had been the victim of penny-pinching petty officialdom, but stayed to fight for his patients. Rogers was the NIGHTINGALE (p 548) of workhouse medicine. He had been a key influence on the *Lancet* Sanitary Commission, and went on to establish the Poor Law Medical Officers' Association to lobby for reform, proposing the provision of preventive medicine with dispensaries, improved dietaries for the institutionalized sick and infirm, payment by capitation, and work security for public sector doctors. (Rogers was also key to the passage in 1870 of the Medical Officers' Superannuation Bill, before which no pension provision had existed for doctors in the public sector.) Despite victimization designed to silence him, Rogers eventually won the day, and lived to see implemented much of what he had fought for.

Rogers's organizational lobbying and the *Lancet* investigation prompted the great hospital building boom of the 1870s. Hospital care for the sick poor was henceforth separated from the punitive treatment meted out to the unemployed and workshy. Slowly, as public hospital medicine developed a distinct institutional identity, workhouse medicine became a thing of the past.

RR1C, BH

of the Health Office were taken over in 1948 by the World Health Organization (WHO). Next to the UN General Assembly and the Security Council, WHO has been called the most important agency of the United Nations. However, as so much of the debate in the General Assembly and the Security Council seems to have little or no impact on the human condition, WHO may be the most important UN agency. It has a very impressive record.

In its first ten years WHO faced enormous challenges. In the aftermath of the Second World War,

George Brock **CHISHOLM** (1896–1970). Canadian psychiatrist. In 1945 he was chairman of the drafting committee whose work led to the creation of the World Health Organization. He served as its director-general for its first five years. His army years as a major-general and his practical experience as a psychiatrist enabled him to found and develop a strong organization.

massive public health problems oppressed populations in many parts of the world, especially in the tropics and many of the countries that had been ravaged by the war. MALARIA was out of control in Africa, South and South-East Asia, and Central and South America. Other vector-borne diseases and parasitic infections debilitated huge numbers of people in these regions. TYPHUS was among the ancient epidemics that had broken out towards the end of the war; as at Naples, it was rapidly controlled for the first time ever, by de-lousing those at risk with the newly developed insecticide, DDT. SMALLPOX, one of the world's worst scourges, smouldered in many war-torn nations, and a pandemic was always possible; in 1947 smallpox occurred in New York. Nutritional deficiency diseases and even famine as another aftermath of war or a consequence of coincident droughts snapped the vitality of populations in some regions. The infrastructure of PUBLIC HEALTH services had to be completely rebuilt in many nations and established for the first time in others.

The priority in the first ten years of WHO was the control of communicable and parasitic diseases. Another priority was to restore, or establish from a zero base in nations that had never had such things before, the infrastructure of essential public health services, including epidemiological surveillance and health information systems.

WHO's early actions included setting up disease control programs to deal with malaria and other vector-borne diseases, TUBERCULOSIS, SEXUALLY TRANSMITTED DISEASES, yaws (a tropical infectious disease), epidemic virus diseases, and zoonoses. Until DDT-resistant mosquitoes evolved, malaria control programs were very successful, enabling healthy workforces to flourish for the first time ever in some parts of the world. International quarantine procedures were revitalized, sharply reducing the risk of pandemics of dangerous contagious diseases. Epidemiological and health statistical services were established, and WHO became the clearing-house for worldwide reporting and notification of communicable and other diseases of public health importance.

## Dissemination of information

Another useful clearing-house function has been collection, collation, and dissemination of information about public health laws and regulations that often are relevant beyond the borders of the nations that enacted them. Other WHO initiatives deal with environmental sanitation, nutrition, maternal and child health services, mental health services, nursing services, veterinary public health, standard-setting in pharmaceutical and biological preparations such as vaccines and sera. WHO sponsors and arranges training programs for public health workers from developing coun-

tries that lack specialists in essential public health disciplines (for example, epidemiologists, microbiologists, and sanitary engineers).

Technical reports by expert working groups and authoritative monographs on the most important aspects of public health have been published frequently throughout the first fifty years of WHO's existence. Health education, especially in countries with poor sanitation and inadequate understanding of personal hygiene, has been another important function since the early days of WHO. Indeed, there is no aspect of public health science and practice that WHO has overlooked as it pursues its aim — the attainment by all people of the highest possible level of health.

To conduct its work, WHO established world headquarters in Geneva and regional offices for the Americas, Europe, the Middle East and Eastern Mediterranean, Africa, South-East Asia, and the Western Pacific. Political tensions produced irrational allocations of nations to certain regions, ignoring that epidemic diseases may easily penetrate national frontiers. But decentralization is useful for strategic approaches to health problems that are regionally rather than globally distributed. Over the first fifty years of WHO, regional collaboration among nations has generally become more effective, even when nations within a region have been at war against one another.

At the headquarters in Geneva and in the regional offices, a nucleus of permanent staff, constantly reinforced by temporary advisers, short-term consultants, and skilled experts seconded by the governments of member nations, manage all these activities, striving to enhance health and the human condition everywhere.

## Eradication of smallpox

In 1958, the Soviet Union proposed a smallpox eradication program to the annual World Health Assembly. At first the program was inadequately funded and poorly planned and coordinated; but in January 1967 a determined effort began to achieve the goal of total smallpox eradication by December 31 1976. Eradication was technically feasible because vaccination after exposure to a case but before the disease takes hold, can prevent smallpox from occurring among contacts. Smallpox was successfully eradicated from Asia by October 1975. The last remaining focus of infection in the world was in Somalia, and the last known case occurred in October 1977 — missing the target date for eradication by ten months, but none the less a remarkably successful effort. A laboratory infection occurred subsequently in Birmingham, Britain, but the World Health Assembly declared eradication successfully accomplished in 1980. Many people regard this as

WHO's greatest achievement, but the less spectacular and never-ending drive to improve the health of all the world's people deserves at least as much admiration.

## Health for all

Before the eradication of smallpox had been accomplished, WHO was already looking for new challenges. At an international conference held in Alma Ata, Kazakhstan, in 1978, the rallying cry of 'Health for all' was sounded. This is, of course, a slogan, not a realistic target. However, it was reasoned that if primary healthcare could be provided for all the world's people and if the people had the means and the understanding needed to take control of their own health, considerable improvements in levels of population health would be accomplished.

The delegates at the Alma Ata conference, and at subsequent conferences on health promotion in Ottawa and Adelaide, believe 'Health for all' had important consequences. One is a definition of 'health' that is action-oriented: 'Health is the extent to which an individual or a group is able to realize aspirations and satisfy needs, and to change or cope with the environment. Health is a resource for everyday life, not the objective of living; it is a positive concept, emphasizing social and personal resources as well as physical capabilities'. This embodies the concept of active participation by all people in actions aimed at promoting good health, rather than passive acceptance of sanitary services, vaccines, and whatever other routine services the public health authorities offer.

Another consequence is the 'healthy communities' movement. This focused first on industrial cities such as Liverpool and Düsseldorf, later on rural and isolated communities. The healthy communities concept recognizes that to solve health problems there has to be a coalition of public health workers with local government, town planners, teachers and other educational specialists, industry, labor, management, community groups — indeed, every sector of society — because health is everyone's business. Though skeptical critics find fault with it, the concept of healthy communities, led initially by staff in the European regional office of WHO then extending to other regions, showed measurable improvement in health indicators, such as sickness absences from work, reduced smoking rates, improved school performance. One feature of this initiative has been an emphasis on defined targets: the aim is to achieve a measured degree of improvement by predetermined dates — for example, to reduce cigarette smoking rates among teenage children by specific amounts each year. Road traffic fatalities, neonatal mortality rates, unwanted pregnancies among adolescent

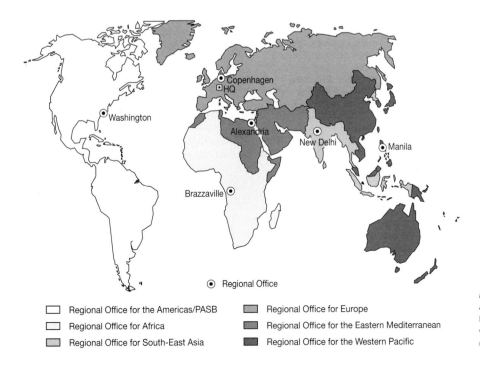

Regional Office

☐ Regional Office for the Americas/PASB
☐ Regional Office for Africa
▨ Regional Office for South-East Asia

▨ Regional Office for Europe
■ Regional Office for the Eastern Mediterranean
■ Regional Office for the Western Pacific

Map showing WHO regions and the areas they serve as of December 1994. (Reproduced with permission from the WHO report 1995.)

girls and associated terminations, the incidence of sexually transmitted diseases, and many other indicators of levels of community health can be assessed to evaluate progress towards the highest possible level of health. These actions and measures, of course, are carried out by the public health services of individual member states of WHO, not by WHO itself: WHO's role is to provide leadership and, where necessary, advice and technical assistance.

## Shortcomings and limitations

Inevitably, as with any large and complex organization, WHO has had problems. It has been accused of cumbersome bureaucracy, and during the tenure of a recent director-general, of lack of leadership and fragmented, ineffective action against pressing health problems. Other UN agencies have a role in human health. The Food and Agriculture Organization (FAO) is directly concerned with nutrition. The over-riding concern of the United Nations Children's Fund (UNICEF) is child health, including control of diarrheal diseases, vaccine-preventable diseases, acute respiratory disease, nutritional deficiencies. The United Nations Fund for Population Activities (UNFPA) promotes family planning as well as demographic data-gathering. The World Bank recognizes that health and economic well-being are related, and established a health division. From time to time there have been rivalries and poor cooperation among these and other UN agencies that have a stake in health. For example, collaboration between WHO and UNICEF has not always been close. The health division of the World Bank picked up financial support for tropical diseases research, one of many essential activities which had been starved of funds because of the budget cuts. These budget cuts were made necessary by the failure of the USA to pay its share of dues to United Nations agencies; under a series of Republican administrations, the United States accumulated debts of over $1.4 billion. The Clinton administration reduced but did not entirely eliminate these debts, which had led to staff cuts and sapped the morale of remaining staff.

The HIV/AIDS pandemic presented a daunting challenge to WHO. WHO established a Global Programme on AIDS in the early 1980s, soon after the pandemic began. Jurisdictional and financial problems impeded effective functioning of this program in WHO and it was made a direct United Nations program in 1991.

As with other UN agencies, WHO is reactive to the needs of member nations. The criticism that WHO should not be advocating health policies that run counter to political and cultural realities of member nations, is ill-founded: it is not WHO or its permanent staff, but the delegates from member nations who advocate health policies, exercise a leadership role, and indeed take most of the initiatives. WHO permanent staff implement the policies agreed upon at the meetings of the world health assembly, and try to remain aloof from national politics. This can be a difficult balancing act, for instance, when widely acclaimed health policies run counter to the internal policies of nations that do not recognize the rights of women to education, or access to maternal and infant care, family planning facilities, etc. The resolutions of the world health assembly sometimes conflict with the politics and culture of certain nations in this respect. Delegates of such nations may abstain, or vote against resolutions that are unacceptable to them. When the health of women and their infants, and women's reproductive rights are concerned, WHO staff and its temporary advisors and short-term consultants face severe ethical dilemmas in such nations.

## Recent developments

The recent annual reports of WHO address the prominent remaining challenges to world health: the growing gap between the nations that have health — and wealth — and those that have neither; recently emerged and often dangerous pathogens (and the re-emerging old ones like tuberculosis); and the need to begin serious planning to meet the new challenges. The annual report for 1998 reviewed the progress made in the first fifty years of WHO and addressed the present and future challenges, such as the increasing toll of premature death and chronic disability due to tobacco smoking.

In 1998, Dr Gro Harlem Brundtland, a physician, public health specialist, and a former Prime Minister of Norway who had previously chaired the United Nations Commission on Environment and Development, was appointed as the Director General of WHO. She immediately began a reorganization, reducing the layers of bureaucracy, setting up a small senior management team and an internationally representative advisory cabinet. Accountability has been enhanced, and determined efforts made to improve working relationships at all levels, including those between headquarters and the regional offices. Three programs with short time horizons are aimed at yielding rapid measurable results in prevention of tobacco addiction, control of malaria, and partnerships for the development of the health sector. The outcome of this strategy will become apparent early in the this new century. JML

*See also* HEALTHCARE SYSTEMS; HEALTH, DEFINITIONS; MALARIA; SMOKING AND HEALTH; VACCINATION

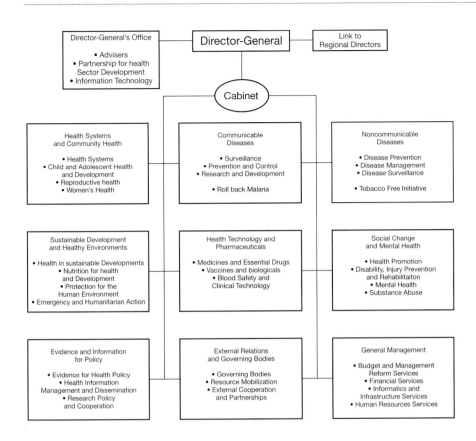

Diagram showing the organizational structure of the WHO's headquarters in Geneva (September 2000.).

**WORMS** Well over half the human race plays host to roundworms, flatworms, tapeworms, hook-worms, whipworms, pinworms, or combinations of these. All are parasites that feed on their human hosts, consuming food that the host has eaten, fastening on the intestinal wall or lurking in blood vessels and drinking the host's blood or body fluids. A few, such as pinworms, are harmless, but most impair or endanger the health of their host. They may sap vitality, cause wasting, anemia, or chronic debility, or predispose to cancer, and in one or more of these ways lead to premature death. Most of the worms live their adult lives and sexually reproduce in the human host, but humans are the intermediate host for two important varieties which cause trichinosis and hydatid cysts. The adult stage and sexual reproduction of these two worms occur in pigs with trichinosis, usually dogs with hydatids. But trichinosis cysts in the brain and elsewhere, and large hydatid cysts in the liver or brain of the human intermediate host may be dangerous, even lethal.

Some common parasitic intestinal worms — for example, the pinworm and the roundworm — rely only on one mammalian species for their livelihood, reproducing and laying eggs in the gut; the eggs are excreted in the feces and infect another host of the same or a similar species when ingested. But a striking feature of many parasitic worms is their dependence on two, or even three, disparate and seemingly unrelated species, in which they pass different stages of their complex life cycles. The life cycles of worms that involve several species raise provocative questions about evolutionary biology: how did these parasitic relationships ever evolve in the first place?

For example, the fish tapeworm lives as an adult in the intestine of humans or carnivorous (fish-eating) mammals such as bears, seals, mink, cats, or dogs. The eggs, discharged in feces into fresh water lakes, are consumed by tiny shrimp-like insects called cyclops, in which they undergo the first stage of their development life cycle. When the cyclops are eaten by fish such as pike or salmon, a further developmental stage takes place in the fish; when the fish are eaten by a mammal, the life cycle is completed with development of adult tapeworms that lay eggs which are excreted in feces, and another generation begins.

SCHISTOSOMIASIS (bilharziasis) is probably the most widespread serious worm infestation at the start of the 21st century.

### Hookworm disease

Hookworm disease was formerly common in parts of the southern USA when poor people in unsanitated regions defecated indiscriminately, spreading hookworm eggs widely. These hatch, and the larvae penetrate the skin to begin their complex migration through the body before arriving at their destination in the small intestine. Here they fasten on the lining and drink the host's blood and body fluids, causing anemia and debility.

Roundworms are very common in many rural regions of Africa. These are a little larger than common earthworms. Infestation may be very heavy: emaciated children with swollen bellies sometimes have this appearance because their intestines are stuffed with a mass of these worms, so many that they can be felt wriggling around below the skin, and give the abdomen a characteristic doughy feel when a doctor palpates it. The combined weight of all the worms sometimes equals or exceeds the weight of the child.

Several effective treatments are available for hookworm and for roundworms, but reinfection must be prevented by improved sanitation, or treatment is a waste of time.

Beef and pork tapeworm infection occurs when people eat poorly cooked meat containing the larval cysts; fish tapeworms are acquired in the same way from poorly cooked or raw fish. These three varieties of tapeworm may grow to a prodigious length, sometimes many meters, and consist of as many as several hundred segments, each containing male and female genital organs. The eggs, and mature segments, are shed in the feces. Heavily infected people suffer malnutrition, anemia, and wasting. Treatment is effective only if the head of the worm is killed, or paralyzed by drugs for long enough to release its grasp of the intestinal wall and be excreted; if the head of the worm remains attached it soon grows new segments and the infected person is no better off.

Pinworms are common among children in institutions such as orphanages and boarding schools. The worms emerge from the anus and may be seen, tiny wriggling white objects a few millimeters in length; they lay their eggs around the anus and the child re-infects himself or herself by scratching to relieve the itch, carrying the eggs to the mouth, where they are ingested. They are annoying, even disgusting, but usually they do not harm health appreciably. JML

*See also* PARASITOLOGY

Some important parasitic worms

| Worm (Disease) | Definite host of the adult worm | Intermediate host(s) | Distribution (habitat) |
|---|---|---|---|
| *Dracunculus medinensis* (guinea worm) (Dracunculiasis) | Humans | Water-fleas | Tropical Africa, Yemen, India |
| *Onchocerca volvulus* (Onchocerciasis, river blindness) | Humans | Blackfly | West Africa |
| *Wuchereria vancrofti, Brucia malayi* (Filariasis, elephantiasis) | Humans | Mosquito | Humid tropics |
| *Trichinella spiralis* (Trichinosis) | Pig, dog, rat, etc. | Humans, mammals | World-wide |
| *Taenia solium* (pig tapeworm (Taeniasis) | Humans | Pigs | World-wide |
| *Taenia saginata* (beef tapeworm (Taeniasis) | Humans | Cattle | World-wide |
| *Clonorchis sinensis* (fish tapeworm (Taeniasis) | Humans | Fish, crustacea | Northern Europe, Midwest USA |
| *Echinococcus granulosus* (canine tapeworm) (Hydatid disease) | Dog | Sheep, humans | Arctic tundra, S. America; eliminated in Australia, New Zealand |
| *Ancylostoma duodenale, A. americanus* (*Necator americanus*) (Hookworm) (Ancylostomasis, hookworm disease) | Humans | None needed | Tropics, subtropics |
| *Schistosoma haematobium, S. japonicum S. mansoni* (Schistosomiasis, bilharziasis) | Humans | Freshwater snails | Africa, East Asia |
| *Enterobius (Oxyuris) vermicularis* (pinworms, threadworm) | Human | None needed | Worldwide |

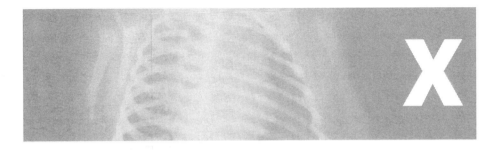

# X

**XENOPSYLLA** is a genus of rat fleas, many species of which are vectors of human disease, particularly PLAGUE (notably the Asiatic rat flea, *Xenopsylla cheopis*).

**XENOTRANSPLANTATION** See TRANSPLAN-TATION

**X-LINKED DISEASE** describes sex linkage in which the abnormal gene responsible for the disease is carried on the X chromosome. In the case of a dominant gene, an affected father will transmit the condition to all his daughters but none of his sons, an affected heterozygous mother to half her children of whatever sex.

Recessive X-linked conditions are much more common; they occur virtually only in males, who are hemizygous, and are transmitted only through heterozygous females (the classic example being hemophilia); females are affected only in the unusual case of a homozygote resulting from the union of a male sufferer with a female carrier.
*See* GENETICS.

**X-RAYS** are electromagnetic radiation (that is radiation of the same non-particulate type as light, gamma rays, and radio waves) whose wave-length is shorter than that of ultraviolet light but longer than that of gamma rays, ranging from 5 nanometres to 6 picometres.
*See also* IMAGING; RADIATION

### DISCOVERER OF X-RAYS

Wilhelm Conrad **ROENTGEN** (1845–1923). German physicist. Roentgen occupied the chair of physics successively at Strasbourg (1876), Giessen (1879), Würzburg (1888), and Berlin (1899). It was at Würzburg that he discovered X-RAYS. On 8 November 1895 while experimenting with a highly evacuated vacuum tube on the conduction of electricity through gases, he noted fluorescence of a barium platinocyanide screen lying nearby. Further investigation of this radiation showed that it could pass through some substances impervious to light. In view of its unusual features he suggested the name X-rays. For this discovery he was awarded the Nobel Prize in physics in 1901.

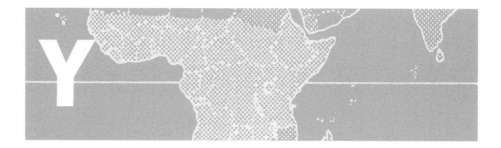

# THE GREAT KILLERS: YELLOW FEVER

The yellow fever virus is a mosquito-borne so-called flavivirus, belonging to the large group colloquially known as arboviruses (arthropod-borne viruses). It is also known as *fiebre amarilla*; colloquially 'Yellow Jack'. It is among the smaller RNA viruses. The most common vector, and the first to be identified as such in the man–mosquito–man transmission of yellow fever, is *Aedes aegypti* in urban epidemics. The later discovered sylvan cycle involves monkeys and forest-dwelling mosquitoes of the *Haemagogus* and *Sabethes* species in South America, and *Aedes africanus* and *A. simpsoni* in East Africa, where the last provides a link between monkey and man. In West Africa a number of *Aedes* species act as vectors.

The historical diagnoses of some early outbreaks of infectious diseases have to be taken with some caution. It is said to have almost wiped out the population of Hispaniola in 1493, leaving few survivors from early settlements of sailors from Columbus's wrecked ship, the *Santa Maria*. In the 17th century there were outbreaks in the Americas — at New York and Boston; Charleston, South Carolina; and Barbados — and a century later Mathew Carey and Benjamin RUSH (p 726) both famously described the devastating 1793 Philadelphia epidemic, a classic example of an outbreak in a '…low level town, hottest and dampest of all the American seacoast', with its swamps, marshes, stagnant water, no water system, and only one sewer. The term 'yellow fever', referring to the jaundice usually apparent only in convalescing patients, had first been used by Griffith Hughes in 1750 in his *Natural history of Barbados*. On the other side of the Atlantic there were short, soon controlled, outbreaks in and around European ports of yellow fever imported on ships carrying cargo from across the Atlantic — in southern Spain in Andalusia (1820) and Gibraltar (1828), but also further north, at Nantes (1861), and even in cool Swansea (1865).

The question of whether yellow fever originated in Africa or in the Americas has long been debated. Arguments on both sides involve dates of early recognition of the disease (the frailty of retrospective diagnosis should be kept in mind); the relative immunity of West African populations of both monkeys and humans; and the prevalence in Africa of the *Aedes aegypti* vector and many related species. These are, of course, arguments which could come to the fore only with the knowledge of much 20th century research.

The gradual realization of the rôle of mosquitoes as vectors in yellow fever began in the 19th century, before Carlos Finlay published his observations in 1881, 1886, and 1891, when he even experimented with what he claimed were preventive inoculations with 'contaminated mosquitoes'. His human guinea pigs were acknowledged as members of communities of Jesuit and Carmelite fathers in Havana 'under my medical charge', who had given their consent to the inoculations. Definitive proof of mosquito involvement came — not without loss of life — when at the turn of the century Walter Reed headed the US Army Commission on Yellow Fever in Havana. The American army officers suffered greater losses than enlisted men, despite their much better living conditions and it was suspected that poor sanitation was not the primary cause of the disease. While Cuban physicians suspected an unknown toxin injected by mosquitoes, an Italian graduate of the Pasteur Institute, bacteriologist Guiseppe Sanarelli, was sure that a bacterium was at work, even naming it *Bacillus icteroides*. Two of the commission group, Dr James Carroll and Dr Jesse Lazear, allowed themselves to be bitten by the same infected mosquito. Both men contracted the disease: Carroll survived, but Lazear died from yellow fever 12 days later. Reed and his co-workers confirmed Finlay's mosquito transmission theory, and at the same time established the agent of yellow fever as the first discovered 'filterable virus' to

cause human disease (after tobacco mosaic virus in plants and foot-and-mouth disease virus in cattle). Putting the Reed Commission's results to good use, and consulting Ronald ROSS (p 481) on mosquito control, William GORGAS (p 824) was shortly afterwards able to control the disease in Havana and most of the rest of Cuba; and eventually also in Panama, to finally allow building of the Panama Canal, after earlier severe difficulties.

In spite of the Reed Commission's evidence, the virus theory was disputed by Hideyo NOGUCHI (this page), who defended his own theory of a visible germ '*Leptospira icteroides*' as the agent of yellow fever — in fact, defended it against mounting evidence to the contrary, until he himself died of the disease at Lagos, West Africa, during the

*(continued opposite)*

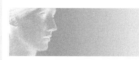

Hideyo **NOGUCHI** (1876–1928). American bacteriologist and immunologist. Born in Japan, Noguchi joined Simon FLEXNER (p 257) in the department of pathology at the University of Pennsylvania, then moved with Flexner in 1904 to the newly opened Rockefeller Institute in New York. He continued to be affiliated with that institution until his death in 1928, from yellow fever in West Africa while he was carrying out experiments regarding its etiology. He and Flexner confirmed that *Treponema pallidum* causes syphilis. In Peru he discovered that a species of *Bartonella* is the cause of Oroya fever. He also recovered *Leptospira icterohaemorrhagica* from cases clinically diagnosed as yellow fever, and thought this to be the cause of the disease.

(continued)

Rockfeller Foundation's Second Yellow Fever Commission's work there. Although the commission's work had by then established the susceptibility of rhesus monkeys to yellow fever, thus obviating the need to use human volunteers, the risks remained. Not only Noguchi, but also Adrian Stokes and colleagues Young and Hayne died at Lagos in the late 1920s, sadly before the development of the 17D vaccine by Max Theiler and co-workers.

Work on a vaccine began in earnest in the late 1920s, when in London Edward Hindle realized the importance of the discovery by Stokes and his colleagues of the susceptibility of rhesus monkeys to yellow fever. Working in relative isolation, he was soon overtaken by events. Work by Soper in Brazil confirmed the existence of jungle yellow fever, with a monkey–mosquito–monkey cycle, depending on mosquito vectors other than *Aedes aegypti*. It was the end of hopes for eradication of yellow fever, and at the Rockefeller Institute Max Theiler and colleagues intensified their efforts to attenuate the yellow fever virus in strains of white mice. During the 1930s they developed the 17D live virus vaccine, which is now a necessary precaution for travelers in Africa and South America.                              LW

*See also* INSECTS; TROPICAL MEDICINE

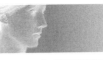

George Miller **STERNBERG** (1838–1915). American military surgeon and bacteriologist. Sternberg served in the US Army during the Civil War, the Indian campaigns in the American West, and the Spanish-American War, having by then become surgeon-general. One of several workers who independently discovered the pneumococcus, he also developed the technique of photomicrography. As surgeon-general he organized and supported Walter Reed's yellow fever commission in Cuba, which established the role of the mosquito in transmitting the causative agent.

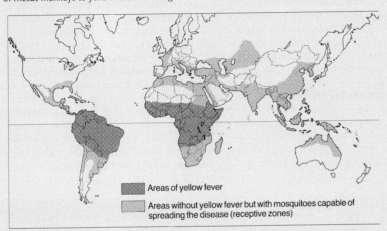

Areas of yellow fever

Areas without yellow fever but with mosquitoes capable of spreading the disease (receptive zones)

Map showing geographical distribution of yellow fever and of mosquitoes capable of spreading yellow fever. (From Dawood, R. (ed.), (1994). *Travellers' health*, OUP.)

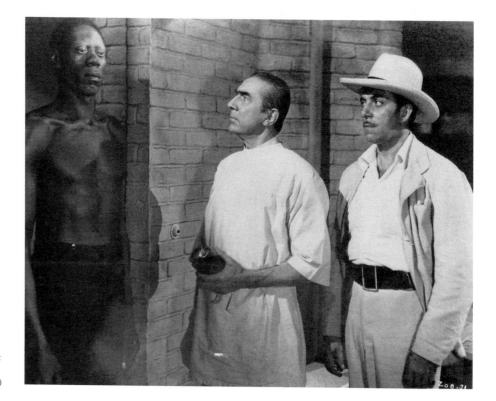

**ZOMBIFICATION** The zombie is a familiar figure from horror films, a stumbling but dangerous creature of the 'living dead'. Is there any real basis for its occurrence? Zombification became a subject of popular interest during the occupation of Haiti by the United States between 1915 and 1934. The United Nations intervention a few years ago has again focused international attention on a phenomenon regarded as exotic and improbable by most people, yet one which is taken by most Haitians as a distinct and verifiable state. Along with the related religious practice of *vodu*, Haitian medical practitioners regard zombification as a very real state — the consequence of poisoning — while the local clergy accept it as the product of sorcery. Zombis are frequently recognized by the

local population, and clinical estimates of their number are of about 1000 new cases per year.

Zombification is a crime under the Haitian Penal Code (Article 246), where it is considered as murder although the zombified individual is still 'alive'. Local interpretation is that either by poisoning or sorcery (and the two are not easily distinguished, for *poison* can act at a distance), a young person suddenly and inexplicably becomes ill, is subsequently recognized by the family as dead, placed in a tomb, only to be stolen by a *boko* (sorcerer) in the next few days, and secretly returned to life and activity but not to full awareness and agency. Haitians are seldom buried but interred in painted concrete family tombs above ground, which in country areas are on family land next to

A still from the film *Zombies on Broadway*. (Reproduced courtesy of the Kobal Collection.)

the houses; generally secured with a metal plate or door; they are vulnerable to being broken open.

Several different local schemata of body, mind, and spirit all recognize something like a separation of the *corps cadavre* (physical body) with its *gwo-bon anj* (loosely glossed as animating principle) from the *ti-bon anj* (agency, awareness, and memory). The last is retained by the sorcerer, usually in a fastened bottle or earthenware jar, where it is known as the *zombi astral*; the boko either extracts it through sorcery, which leaves the victim apparently dead, or else captures it after a natural death before it has gone too far from the body. The animated body remains without will or agency as the *zombi cadavre*, which becomes the slave of the sorcerer and works secretly on his land or is sold to another for the same purpose; it is induced to remain a slave only through chaining and beating, or through further poisoning and sorcery. This *zombi cadavre* is the 'zombie' popularized by western cinema, and indeed is locally referred to simply as the *zombi*.

Different explanations as to how a zombi cadavre may escape back to its original family suggest that: either the bottle containing the zombi astral breaks, or the boko inadvertently feeds his zombis salt, or he dies and they are liberated by his family, or rarely they may be released through divine intervention. On release, their mental and physical status remains the same, and they are vulnerable to recapture and continued enslavement: few Haitian bokos or doctors claim to be able to return a zombi cadavre to its original state of health and agency, and the matter is reserved for the mercy of *Le Grand Maitre* (the rather remote God recognized by vodu practitioners, who is only invoked briefly through Latin prayers before they begin their ceremonies). Zombies are recognized by their fixed staring expression; by their nasal intonation; by repeated, purposeless, and clumsy actions; and by limited and repetitive speech. They are generally regarded with commiseration; fear is reserved only for the possibility of being zombified oneself. Concern that a deceased relative may be vulnerable to zombification justifies prevention through the not infrequent decapitation of the corpse before burial, or poisons and charms are placed in the coffin to deter resurrection.

There has been recent medical interest in the possibility that zombification may be an empirical state — catalepsy or motor paralysis — which is induced by neurotoxins followed by retrieval and revival of the 'dead' person extracted from the tomb. Among the poisons which have been implicated, is tetrodotoxin (from the puffer fish *Sphoeroides testudineus* and *Diodon hystrix*), with *Datura stramonium* used to revive and then control the zombi. Tetrodotoxin has been studied biomedically in Japan, where the puffer fish is a

dangerous delicacy whose consumption may result in apparent but temporary death. Other ingredients mentioned by Haitian bokos as zombifacients include human remains, a polychaete worm ('sea snake'), toads, lizards, and tarantulas. No research on live people has been carried out with the suggested toxins, and, while local medical practitioners are familiar with the phenomenon of zombification, they have not published on its clinical characteristics. Studies of the one well-documented instance of a returned zombi concentrated on his symptoms at the time of presumed death, little on his mental and physical state at the time of the post-return interview; another well-known case who was hospitalized has been argued as an instance of mistaken identity.

Occasional success in the second and third (see box), if they do occur, would reinforce the more plausible first option — mistaken identity. That bokos actually enslave *zombis jardins* on secret agricultural grounds is implausible given the high population density of Haiti, with the close proximity of most tombs to houses, and thus to observation. Zombies have never been identified in these slave compounds but only on their 'return'. RLit

*See also* THEORIES OF ILLNESS

---

It is unlikely that there is a single explanation for all cases of recognition of zombies. The likely possibilities include:
• Mistaken identification of a wandering mentally ill stranger by bereaved relatives is the most likely explanation. People with a chronic schizophrenic illness, brain damage, or learning disability are not uncommon in rural Haiti, and they would be particularly likely to be identified as lacking volition and memory, whose absence are characteristic of a zombi; interpretations of mental illness as an alienation of some vital faculty of agency (and thus recalling death) are common in Central America and in the Caribbean. The ready local recognition of zombies and their generally considerate treatment on 'return' might even argue that this might be seen as an almost institutionalized restitution of the destitute mentally ill: recognition and incorporation of a zombi into a family provide public recognition and sometimes material advantage.
• The local understanding that the unexpected death of a young adult is

never a properly 'natural' death, together with the frequency of sorcery suspicions, may suggest the breaking open of tombs by an optimistic sorcerer in the belief that this has been achieved. Given that death is locally recognized without access to medical certification, and that burial usually occurs within a day of death, it is not implausible, if presumably rare, for a retrieved person to be alive; in some cases they might be well enough to recover with minimal care. The use of datura to 'revive' them, and its possible repeated administration during the period of zombi slavery might produce a schizophreniform state of extreme passivity.
• Discounting physical consequences of sorcery, one cannot exclude a specific neuromuscular toxin, topically administered together with a local irritant by a boko, to induce catalepsy followed by secret retrieval of the individual. Japanese evidence of tetrodotoxin poisoning indicates that a full and rapid recovery can occur spontaneously.

---

**ZOONOSES** See ANIMALS AS CARRIERS OF DISEASE; VETERINARY MEDICINE

# Topic Index

## The arts

Architecture 63, Art 40, 65, Authors, doctors as 83, Creativity 202, Dance 212, Detective stories 232, Emblems 261, Illustration and photography 406, Literature 473, Media 484, Music 514, Numismatics (Coins and medals) 190, Opera 593, Poetry 657, Statues 783, Truants 83, 827

## Basic sciences

Anatomy 41, 91, 388, 793, Autopsy 88, Cell and cell biology 153, Immunology 412, Microbiology 488, Molecular biology 505, Nutrition 569, Pathology 621, Pharmacology 633, Physiology 457, 645, 743, Statistics 779,

## Bioethics

Abortion 1, 107, 218, 582, 730, Abuse of old people 4, Advertising 11, Antivivisection movements/Animal rights 53, Aristotle 64, Beecher 94, Bioethics 105, Brain [stem] death 125, Chemical and biological warfare 109, Child abuse and neglect 168, Chinese 712, Christian Science 713, Circumcision 182, Code of Hammurabi 14, 363, Communication 191, Confidentiality 669, Declaration of Geneva 71, Declaration of Helsinki 71, 373, Ebers Papyrus 14, 253, Errors 283, Eugenics, 285, Euthanasia [in the Netherlands] 292, Executions 296, Experimentation 389, Experiments on children 176, Fraud and misconduct in research 719, Genetics 336, Hansen 431, Hippocrates 382, Hippocratic Oath 573, Holocaust 385, India 420, Informed consent 430, Islam 712, Jehovah's Witnesses 714, Justice 108, Life insurance 437, Nazis 385, 559, 573, 678, Non-maleficence 108, Nuremberg code 177, 431, 559, Nuremberg trial 389, 431, Oaths and codes of conduct 573, Old Order Amish 714, Palliative care 613, Pappworth 616, Patients' associations 625, Percival 629, Principles 107, Professional regulation 669, Quakers 695, Respect for persons 107, Red Cross, Red Crescent 706, Religion, philosophy, and medicine 709, Religious sects 713, Scientology 714, Self-experimentation 743, Seventh Day Adventists 713, Shinto 712, Torture 814, Transplantation 107, 818, Tuskegee Syphilis Study 832

## Communication

Advertising 11, Bible 103, Books and libraries 121, Communication 191, Computers 198, Diagnosis 234, Education 254, 257, Emblems 261, Encyclopedias of medicine 263, Historiography 382, History of medicine 383, Illustration and photography 406, Internet 122, 444, Journals 22, 122, 142, 173, 189, 349, 422, 452, Language 465, Media 484, Obituaries 574, Pamphleteering 616, Poetry 657, Quotations 698, Telemedicine 195, 803, Television 852, Textbooks 805, Wireless radio 308, 804,

## Countries

Africa 14, 18, 219, Arab countries 59, Australia 80, 230, Austria 352, Belgium 690, Britain 129, 330, 365, 394, 563, Canada 135, China 177, 366, 503, 809, Cuba 365, Denmark 690, 736, Egypt 509, European Union 286, Finland 736, France 319, 321, 690, Germany 352, 364, 385, 477, 690, Greece, 359, 365, 690, India 420, 503, 651, 809, Ireland 690, Italy 392, 446, 690, Japan 449, Mexico 771, Netherlands 292, 690, New Zealand 544, 552, Norway 737, Pakistan 606, Poland 387, Portugal 690, Russia 728, Scandinavia 734, South-east Asia 765, Spanish-speaking 690, 767, Sweden 553, Switzerland 352, USA 366, 394, 567, 691, 839, Venezuela 772

## Disciplines and specializations

Academic medicine 5, Allied health professions 34, Anesthesia 42, 603, Blood transfusion 117, Cardiology 146, Cardiothoracic surgery 150, Chest medicine 162, Child health 173, 174, Clinical chemistry 182, Clinical pharmacology 633, Community pediatrics 176, Complementary and alternative medicine 197, Craniomaxillary facial surgery 650, Critical care 204, Cytopathology 624, Dentistry 222, 224, Dermatology 227, Ear, nose, and throat (ENT) 248, 249, Endocrinology 267, Forensic medicine 309, Gastroenterology 324, 325, General practice 132, 330, Genetics 335, 336, 337, Geriatrics 347, 349, Gynecological oncology 581, Gynecology, 575, 579, Hematology 374, Homeopathy 390, Imaging 408, Infectious diseases 423, 425, Internal medicine [in USA] 441, Interventional radiology 411, Laboratory medicine 457, Microsurgery 655, Midwifery 34, 493, Minimally invasive surgery 498, 580, 801, Molecular biology 505, Nephrology 522, Neurology 526, 529, Neurosurgery 536, 538

## Economics

## Education and research

## History

## Institutions

## Other systems of medicine

## Therapeutic drugs

# List of Individual Conditions and Diseases

# People Index

**Note:** Inclusion in this list of non-living people implies a separate biography (page number in **bold** face) or a substantial mention in the text.

Abbott, MES (1869–1940) **145**
Addison, C, Lord (1869–1951) **129**
Addison, T (1795–1860) **263**
Adler, A (1870–1937) **675**
Albright, F (1900–69) **265**, 502
Albers-Schonberg, HE (1865–1921) **409**
Albertus Magnus, Saint (1206–80) **732**
Allbutt, Sir TC (1836–1925) **812**
Almeida Lima, PM de (1903–83) **536**, 538
Alzheimer, A (1864–1915) **39**
Andral, G (1797–1876) **375**
Antyllus (*fl.* 3rd century BC) **793**
Apollo **359**
Arbuthnot, J (1667–1735) **474**
Aristotle (384–322 BC) 36, **64**, 526
Armstrong, G (1720–89) **174**
Asclepius **710**
Auenbrugger, JL (1722–1809) **165**
Avenzoar (*fl.* 1162) **768**
Averroes (1126–1198) **768**
Avicenna (980–1037) **60**, 720

Babes, V (1854–1926) **49**
Babkin, BP (1877–1950) **515**
Baillie, M (1761–1823) **622**
Bancroft, J (1836–94) **473**
Bang, BLF (1848–1932) **847**
Banting, Sir FG (1891–1941) **236**
Barnardo, TJ (1845–1905) **169**
Barry, JMS (1795–1865) 158, **864**
Becquerel, AH (1852–1908) 409, **700**
Beecher, HK (1904–76) **94**
Bell, J (1897–1987) 232
Bernard, C (1813–78) **102**, 103, 458, 784
Best, CH (1899–1978) **236**
Bethune, N (1890–1939) **180**
Bevan, A (1897–1960) **130**
Beveridge, W, Lord (1879–1963) **131**
Billroth, CAT (1829–94) **518**
Black, GV (1836–1915) **224**
Blackwell, E (1821–1910) 117, **863**
Blane, Sir G (1749–1834) **855**
Bleuler, E (1857–1939) **675**
Boerhaave, H (1668–1738) **121**, 643, 806
Borodin, AP (1833–87) **186**
Bostock, J (1773–1846) **522**
Boyd Orr, J, Lord (1880–1971) **570**
Boyd, Sir JSK (1891–1981) **421**
Boyle, R (1627–91) **125**

Bretonneau, PF (1771–1862) **834**
Bright, R (1789–1858) **522**
Brown-Séquard, CE (1817–94) **708**
Browne, Sir DJW (1892–1967) **174**
Bruce, Sir D (1855–1931) **857**
Brunton, Sir TL Bt (1844–1916) **633**
Budd, W (1811–80) **274**
Bulgakov, M (1891–1940) 87

Cabot, RC (1868–1939) **190**
Caius, J (1510–73) **135**
Calmette, LCA (1863–1933) **621**
Cannon, WB (1871–1945) **189**
Cardano, G (1501–76) **139**
Castle, WB (1897–1990) **375**
Cavell, E (1865–1915) **858**
Celsus, AC (*fl.* AD 25) 794, **806**
Chamberlen, H the Elder (?1632–?) **493**
Chamberlen, H the Younger
  (1664–1728) **494**
Chamberlen, P (1601–83) **493**
Chamberlen, P (1635–1717) **494**
Chamberlen, P the Elder (d. 1631) **493**
Chamberlen, P the Younger (1572–1626)
  **493**
Charcot, JM (1825–93) **400**, 404
Charnley, Sir J (1911–82) **601**
Chauliac, G de (c. 1300–68) **320**, 795
Chekhov, A (1860–1904) 84, 87
Chisholm, GB (1896–1970) **868**
Cochrane, AL, (1909–1988) 79, **704**
Cole, R (1876–1966) **714**
Collip, JB (1892–1965) **265**
Cook, Sir A (1870–1951) **503**
Copernicus, N (1473–1543) **201**
Crichton-Brown, J (1840–1938) 77
Crippen, HH (1862–1910) **310**
Cullen, W (1710–90) **129**
Cumpston, JHL (1880–1954) **82**
Curie, MS (1867–1934) 409, **556**, 589
Curie, P (1859–1906) 409, **556**, 589
Cushing, HW (1869–1939) 267, **537**

Da Costa JM (1833–1900) 146
Dale, Sir HH (1875–1968) **212**, 716
Dandy, WE (1886–1946) **537**
Darrier, JF (1856–1938) **228**
Darwin, CR (1809–82) 214, 215, **599**
Darwin, E (1731–1802) **214**

Dawson, BE, Lord (1864–1945) **130**
Dee, J (1527–1608) **76**
Dejerine-Klumpke, A (1859–1927) **863**
Denys, JB (?1640–1704) **121**
Dick, G (1881–1963) **423**
Domagk, G (1895–1964) **50**
Doyle, Sir AC (1859–1930) **233**, 474
Drinker, CK (1887–1956) **664**
Dubos, RJ (1901–81) **247**
Dunant, JH (1828–1910) **706**

Eddy, MB (1821–1910) **713**
Ehrlich, P (1854–1915) **260**, 459
Eijkman, C (1858–1930) **569**
Ellis, HH (1859–1939) **747**
Enders, JF (1897–1985) **490**
Esmarch, JFA von (1823–1908) **856**

Fairley, Sir NH (1891–1966) **482**
Farr, W (1807–83) **780**
Fauchard, P (1678–1761) **222**
Fleming, Sir A (1881–1964) **50**
Flemming, W (1843–1905) 336
Flexner, A (1866–1959) **257**, 258, 306
Flexner, S (1863–1964) **257**
Florey, HW, Lord (1898–1968) **52**
Folin, O (1867–1934) **186**
Forssman, W (1904–79) **147**, 743
Fothergill J (1712–80) **695**
Foucault, M (1926–84) **313**
Frederick, Crown Prince of Germany
  (1840–88) **249**
Freud, A (1895–1982) **676**
Freud, S (1856–1939) **321**, 403, 686, 791
Funck, C (1884–1967) **855**

Galen (AD 129–199) **324**, 446, 522, 569,
  794
Galileo **446**
Gall, FJ (1758–1828) 526, **641**
Galton, F (1822–1911) **285**, 347
'Gamp, Mrs Sairey' **495**, 562
Gerhard, WW (1809–72) **834**
Gorgas, WC (1854–1920) **824**
Grace, WG (1848–1915) **776**
Graham, EA (1883–1957) **762**
Greenwood, M (1880–1949) **274**
Grenfell, Sir WT (1865–1940) **299**
Guillotin, JI (1738–1814) 296, **297**

# General Index

**Note:** See also entries under individual indexes for anything not included in this index